Avery's Neonatology Board Review

Certification and Clinical Refresher

Avery's Neonatology Board Review

Certification and Clinical Refresher

SECOND EDITION

Patricia R. Chess, MD, MS Health Professions Education

Professor, Vice Chair of Education
Pediatrics (unlimited tenure), Division of Neonatology, and Biomedical Engineering
University of Rochester School of Medicine and Dentistry
Rochester, New York

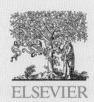

ELSEVIER

Elsevier
1600 John F. Kennedy Blvd.
Ste 1800
Philadelphia, PA 19103-2899

AVERY'S NEONATOLOGY BOARD REVIEW, SECOND EDITION   ISBN: 978-0-443-10638-5

Notice

Previous edition copyrighted 2019.

Executive Content Strategist: Sarah Barth
Senior Content Development Specialist: Rishabh Gupta
Publishing Services Manager: Deepthi Unni
Senior Project Manager: Manchu Mohan
Design Direction: Brian Salisbury

Printed in India

Last digit is the print number: 9 8 7 6 5 4 3 2 1

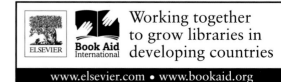

Preface

When preparing for the neonatal-perinatal board exam, it is helpful to utilize a variety of tools. This second edition of *Avery's Neonatology Board Review*, partner to *Avery's Diseases of the Newborn*, has been created as an aid to neonatologists preparing for their subspecialty boards, as well as for neonatologists interested in brushing up on their neonatal knowledge. Additional educational tools are available through the American Academy of Pediatrics, including *Neoreviews*, *Neoreviews-Plus*, and *NeoPREP*. The outline and content are based on the 2022 American Board of Pediatrics Content Outline for Neonatal-Perinatal Medicine. I would like to thank all of the authors and section editors for their contributions to this book.

Acknowledgments

I would like to thank my mentors, patients, and their families, as well as to the Neonatology fellows past, present, and future, who have been the inspiration behind the creation of this book. Additionally, I extend my thanks to the authors and section editors, particularly Dr Burris for providing a critical review of the entire book. I would like to thank my family, especially my husband Mitch, who has been my rock and my wings, I am also thankful to our children Rachel, Laura, Daniel, and Stephen, and our grandchildren Jaimie, Evan, Cora, Eliana, and Jason—our greatest joy.

In fond memory of our Neonatology colleague, book coauthor, and friend, Laura Price, MD.

Notice

While this book has been thoughtfully written by experts in the field and edited carefully, the authors, editors, and publisher cannot ensure there are no errors or omissions and assume no liability from any injury or damage that may occur from content contained in this material.

Understanding of this field is constantly changing. It is important for physicians to review any material for current relevance in light of updated research and understanding.

Any drug indication or dosage needs to be reviewed by appropriate references including manufacturer's information before prescribing.

Contributors

Rebecca Abell, DO
Associate Professor
Department of Pediatrics, Division of Gastroenterology
University of Rochester School of Medicine and Dentistry
Rochester, New York

Jeffrey R. Andolina, MD, MS
Associate Professor
Department of Pediatrics, Division of Hematology and
    Oncology
University of Rochester School of Medicine and Dentistry
Rochester, New York

Georgianne Lee Arnold, MD, MS
Professor
Department of Pediatrics, Division of Genetics
University of Pittsburgh Medical Center
Pittsburgh, Pennsylvania

Andrea Avila, MD
Assistant Professor
Department of Ophthalmology
University of Rochester School of Medicine and Dentistry
Rochester, New York

Gal Barbut, MD
Assistant Professor
Department of Pediatrics, Division of Neonatology
University of Rochester School of Medicine and Dentistry
Rochester, New York

Sonia Lomeli Bonifacio, MD
Clinical Professor
Department of Pediatrics
Stanford University School of Medicine
Palo Alto, California

Jennifer Burnsed, MD
Associate Professor
Departments of Neurology and Pediatrics; Division of
    Neonatology
University of Virginia
Charlottesville, Virginia

Jonathan Ryan Burris, MD
Assistant Professor
Department of Pediatrics, Division of Neonatology
University of Rochester School of Medicine and Dentistry
Rochester, New York

Melissa Carmen, MD
Associate Professor
Department of Pediatrics, Division of Neonatology
University of Rochester School of Medicine and Dentistry
Rochester, New York

Mitchell Chess, MD
Professor
Departments of Diagnostic Imaging and Pediatrics
University of Rochester School of Medicine and Dentistry
Rochester, New York

Patricia R. Chess, MD, MS HPE
Professor, Vice Chair of Education
Departments of Pediatrics and Biomedical Engineering,
    Division of Neonatology
University of Rochester School of Medicine and Dentistry
Rochester, New York

Bernard A. Cohen, MD
Professor
Departments of Pediatrics and Dermatology, Division of
    Dermatology
Johns Hopkins Children's Center
Baltimore, Maryland

Nina D'Amiano, MPH
Medical Student
Department of Dermatology
Johns Hopkins University School of Medicine
Baltimore, Maryland

Carl T. D'Angio, MD
Professor
Departments of Pediatrics and Health Humanities &
    Bioethics, Division of Neonatology
University of Rochester School of Medicine and Dentistry
Rochester, New York

Rita Dadiz, DO
Professor
Department of Pediatrics, Division of Neonatology
University of Rochester School of Medicine and Dentistry
Rochester, New York

Colby L. Day, MD
Assistant Professor
Department of Pediatrics, Division of Neonatology
University of Rochester School of Medicine and Dentistry
Rochester, New York

Andrew M. Dylag, MD
Associate Professor
Department of Pediatrics, Division of Neonatology
University of Rochester School of Medicine and Dentistry
Rochester, New York

Alison Falck, MD
Clinical Professor
Department of Pediatrics, Division of Neonatology
University of California
San Francisco, California

Emer Finan, MB, MEd, MRCPI, FRCPC
Staff Neonatologist
Department of Paediatrics
Sinai Health
Toronto, Ontario, Canada

Megan E. Gabel, MD
Associate Professor
Department of Pediatrics, Division of Neonatology
University of Rochester School of Medicine and Dentistry
Rochester, New York

J. Christopher Glantz, MD, MPH
Professor
Departments of Obstetrics & Gynecology and Public Health
　Sciences
University of Rochester School of Medicine and Dentistry
Rochester, New York

Lisa M. Gray, MD
Associate Medical Director of Maternal Fetal Medicine
Department of Obstetrics and Gynecology
Carle Health
Urbana, Illinois

Catherine K. Hart, MD, MS
Associate Professor
Department of Pediatric Otolaryngology Head and Neck
　Surgery
Cincinnati Children's Hospital Medical Center
University of Cincinnati College of Medicine
Cincinnati, Ohio

Marlyse F. Haward, MD
Clinical Associate Professor
Department of Pediatrics
Albert Einstein College of Medicine; Children's Hospital at
　Montefiore
Bronx, New York

William W. Hay, Jr., MD
Retired Professor
Department of Pediatrics
University of Colorado
Denver, Colorado

Matthew Lloyd Haynie, MD
Assistant Professor
Department of Ophthalmology
University of Rochester School of Medicine and Dentistry
Rochester, New York

Kendra Hendrickson, MS, RD, CNSC
Clinical Dietitian III
Department of Neonatal Intensive Care
University of Colorado Hospital
Aurora, Colorado

Narayan Prabhu Iyer, MBBS, MD
Clinical Assistant Professor
Department of Pediatrics
USC Keck School of Medicine
Los Angeles, California

Annie Janvier, MD, PhD
Professor
Department of Pediatrics, Clinical Ethics
University of Montreal, CHU Sainte-Justine
Montreal, Quebec, Canada

Angelina S. June, MD
Neonatologist
Department of Pediatrics
Fairfax Neonatal Associates
Fairfax, Virginia

Igor Khodak, MD
Assistant Professor
Department of Pediatrics, Division of Neonatology
University of Rochester School of Medicine and Dentistry
Rochester, New York

Deepak Kumar, MD
Professor
Department of Pediatrics, Division of Neonatology
Case Western Reserve University, MetroHealth Medical Center
Cleveland, Ohio

Jonathan Lai, BA
Medical Student
School of Medicine, Johns Hopkins University
Baltimore, Maryland

Echezona T. Maduekwe, MD, DCH
Associate Professor
Department of Pediatrics, Division of Neonatology
Stony Brook Children's Hospital
Stony Brook, New York

Tracey L. McCollum, PharmD
Pediatric Clinical Pharmacist
Department of Pharmacy
University of Rochester Medical Center, Golisano
　Children's Hospital
Rochester, New York

Niranjana Natarajan, MD
Associate Professor
Department of Neurology, Division of Child Neurology
University of Washington
Seattle, Washington

Allison H. Payne, MD
Associate Professor
Department of Pediatrics, Division of Neonatology
Rainbow Babies and Children's Hospitals/Case Western
    Reserve University
Cleveland, Ohio

Laura Price, MD
Assistant Professor
Department of Pediatrics, Division of Neonatology
University of Rochester School of Medicine and Dentistry
Rochester, New York

Erin Rademacher, MD
Associate Professor
Department of Pediatrics, Division of Nephrology
University of Rochester School of Medicine and Dentistry
Rochester, New York

Aarti Raghavan, MD, FAAP, MS
Associate Professor Clinical Pediatrics, Medical Director
    NICU, Director for Quality and Safety, Program Director
    Graduate Programs in Quality and Safety
Department of Pediatrics
University of Illinois at Chicago
Chicago, Illinois

Julie Riccio, MD
Associate Professor
Department of Pediatrics, Division of Neonatology
University of Rochester School of Medicine and Dentistry
Rochester, New York

Justin Rosati, MD
Fellow
Department of Neurology
University of Rochester School of Medicine and Dentistry
Rochester, New York

Vicki Roth, MS
Assistant Dean & Executive Director, Retired
Center for Excellence in Teaching & Learning
University of Rochester School of Medicine and Dentistry
Rochester, New York

Kristin Scheible, MD
Associate Professor
Departments of Pediatrics and Microbiology and
    Immunology
University of Rochester School of Medicine and Dentistry
Rochester, New York

Jotishna Sharma, MD, MEd
Professor
Department of Pediatrics, Division of Neonatology
University of Missouri Kansas City School of Medicine
Kansas City, Missouri

Ashley L. Soaper, MD
Fellow Physician
Department of Pediatric Otolaryngology Head and Neck
    Surgery
Cincinnati Children's Hospital Medical Center
Cincinnati, Ohio

Laurie Steiner, MD
Professor
Department of Pediatrics, Division of Neonatology
University of Rochester School of Medicine and Dentistry
Rochester, New York

Angela K. Tyson, DO
Assistant Professor
Department of Pediatrics, Division of Neonatology
University of Rochester School of Medicine and Dentistry
Rochester, New York

Kimberly Vera, MD, MSCI
Associate Professor
Department of Pediatric Cardiology
Vanderbilt University
Nashville, Tennessee

David R. Weber, MD, MSCE
Assistant Professor
Department of Pediatrics
The Children's Hospital of Philadelphia and the Perelman
    School of Medicine at the University of Pennsylvania
Philadelphia, Pennsylvania

Geoffrey A. Weinberg, MD
Professor
Department of Pediatrics, Division of Pediatric Infectious
    Diseases
University of Rochester School of Medicine and Dentistry
Rochester, New York

The authors, publishers, and editor would like to thank the following section editors for carefully reviewing their associated section chapters, and to Dr Burris for reviewing the entire book:

Section	Editors
1. Respiratory	Gal Barbut
2. Cardiovascular	Irina Prelipcean
3. Neurology and Neurodevelopment	Gal Barbut
4. Immunology and Infectious Diseases	Thornton Mu
5. Nutrition	Jotishna Sharma
6. Gastroenterology and Bilirubin	Alison Falck
7. Maternal-Fetal Medicine	Lynnette Johnson
8. Resuscitation and Stabilization	Thornton Mu
9. Genetics and Dysmorphism	Thornton Mu
10. Water, Salt, Renal	Alison Falck
11. Endocrine, Metabolic, Thermal	Alison Falck
12. Hematology and Oncology	Deepak Kumar
13. Head (Ears, Eyes, Nose, Throat), Neck, and Skin	Jotishna Sharma
14. Surgical and Complex NICU Patient Management	Burris, Khodak
15. Basic Pharmacology Principles	Deepak Kumar
16. Management of Neonatal Care Systems	Lynnette Johnson
17. Scholarly Activities and Quality Improvement	Alison Falck
18. Diagnostic Imaging	Jonathan Ryan Burris

Thornton S. Mu, MD
Associate Professor, Associate Dean for Graduate Medical
    Education
Department of Pediatrics, Division of Neonatology
Uniformed Services University of the Health Sciences
Brooke Army Medical Center
Joint Base San Antonio
Fort Sam Houston, Texas

Irina Prelipcean, MD
Assistant Professor
Department of Pediatrics, Division of Neonatology
University of Rochester School of Medicine and Dentistry
Rochester, New York

Lynnette M. Johnson, DO
Assistant Professor
Department of Pediatrics, Division of Neonatology
University of Rochester School of Medicine and Dentistry
Rochester, New York

Contents

1 *Maximizing Test Performance*

VICKI ROTH and PATRICIA R. CHESS

Before Beginning Your Review

- Completing a self-assessment
  - Prior to the date you intend to begin your studies, take stock of your initial preparedness. Using the content outline for this exam, create a quick chart rating your fund of knowledge and experience with each topic.
  - As you know, the topics on this exam tap into a range of learning approaches (e.g., visual and quantitative learning, simultaneous vs. sequential reasoning, memorization vs. conceptual thinking). So, in addition to rating your readiness by topic, a good self-assessment also includes a brief evaluation of your preferences, strengths, and weaknesses as a learner (more on this issue later).

TIP: If you will not be attending an in-person review course that includes a self-assessment, use a portion of the items in your question bank to create your own pretest.

- Building a study map
  - A study map ensures that all topics are addressed well and that appropriate review strategies are employed for each one. A study map also makes life easier, as the decisions about what to study in a given week are front loaded.
  - A well-constructed study map begins with time finding. Short bursts of study time can appear spontaneously during the day; when they do, be prepared to use them (see "Deciding where to study" below). But, more extensive periods of review time are needed too, and finding them usually requires some detective work.
  - In addition to the start date for your study and your anticipated exam date, an effective map also includes the following elements:
    - Specific dates for the review of each topic
    - Dates for catch-up study sessions
      - Catch-up hours are earmarked for study but have no assigned topic until close to the study-session dates.
        - Catch-up hours make room for study when other work or life commitments have interfered with your map. They also provide opportunities for additional study of topics that prove to be more challenging than expected.
        - Candidates often significantly underestimate the number of catch-up study hours needed, so it is advisable to include many such sessions in the study map right from the beginning.
    - Dates for loop-back sessions
      - Loop-backs are brief and lightweight study periods designed to reconnect with material that you examined in more detail 1 to 2 weeks earlier. The goal of these study periods is to improve the student's ability to retrieve information across time and to reduce anxiety about retaining information that has already been studied.
    - Creating a map with the features described here requires about 1.5 to 2 hours.

TIP: Given the density and volume of material to review, it is easy to build ambitious study maps that are impossible to maintain. A good plan is one that takes into account the practical requirements of your other responsibilities (i.e., make a map that is livable). Organize your study map to include target dates and to-do boxes to check off work on a weekly basis to help break your studying down into manageable pieces.

TIP: If you have a disability that qualifies for testing accommodations under the Americans with Disabilities Amendments Act and you intend to seek an accommodation, your map should include the time needed to complete the request process.

- Assembling your study kit
  - Just as we are more likely to go to the fitness center for a workout if we pack a gym bag the night before, we make better use of our study time if we collect and organize a set of review materials in advance.
  - To prevent a scattered approach to study, it often works best to think of your study materials in three layers:
    - The first is your set of central resources, such as this text, that can provide the overall foundation for your review.
    - The second layer might include several resources, perhaps ones you already own, that you turn to for short, detailed study of specific subtopics that require more attention. These first two layers should provide most of the resources needed for your study.
    - The third layer of materials is only for limited occasions when you encounter a persistently difficult subtopic that must be looked at from another angle. It is likely you already possess much of what is needed for this third layer as well.
  - For your study kit, also collect other materials such as a notebook or portfolio, electronic and paper folders for copies of high-impact figures and tables, hard-copy flashcards and/or a flashcard application, markers, etc. In addition, if you will not have easy access to a white board during your study sessions, consider purchasing a large sketchpad.

- Deciding where to study
  - When you find yourself with a few moments prior to a meeting or while waiting in a queue, make use of this time by having quick-review materials close at hand (e.g., review notes on your phone or a deck of flashcards in your pocket). In these cases, deciding where to study is not a priority; rather, the goal is to benefit from these slivers of time when and wherever they appear. A fair bit of learning is additive, meaning that we take on about a flashcard's worth of information at a time. So, use these short study interludes during your day, even if your location is not ideal.
  - However, planning for longer sessions should include decisions about study locations. It may be simpler to study in a single accessible location, but this can be a suboptimal approach for board review. As we study, elements of our environment, such as the type of lighting or the color of the walls, can become embedded with the target information. Later on, when those environmental cues are no longer present, retrieval can then be more difficult than anticipated. Changing study locations from time to time helps build the geographic independence that allows you to remember concepts and details, regardless of where you are.

TIP: Sometimes the only plausible place to work on your board review is in your own home. When this is the case, set up a place to study that is dedicated solely for this purpose.

TIP: As you will not have control over the environmental conditions of your actual test location, consider working at times in a location that includes a slightly uncomfortable feature. For example, study for a few sessions in a chilly room if air conditioning annoys you; in a room with fluorescent bulbs if that type of lighting is irksome; and so on. This practice will help you plan ahead (e.g., by dressing in layers) or at least will build your capacity to cope with any irritating conditions in the testing room.

The Review Itself

- For each group of concepts and facts, make sure that your study approaches include all three stages of the learning cycle: input, quizzing, and testing steps.
  - The *input step* employs reading, listening, and watching study materials, such as texts and review guides, podcasts, lectures, and videos.
    - While you are engaged with these input activities, you are likely to be jotting something down. It may feel as if writing and drawing should cement your learning, but the making of study tools such as flashcards, charts, diagrams, and concept maps—although all good options—largely still fits within this first step of the learning cycle. It is true that creating a study tool requires selectivity about what you write down and the use of your own words or images, but merely creating study tools is typically not enough. It is likely that your retention of the materials written in these study tools will be less than expected.

- So, within each session, stop periodically to examine your retention of the material you have taken in during the input step. The essential feature of this *quizzing step* is asking yourself questions and then immediately checking the accuracy of your responses. Easy ways to complete this step include reviewing any flashcards you have just created and generating questions from the rows and columns of the charts you have made.
  - During this stage of the learning cycle, special attention should be paid to the power of drawing. A great deal of the material you need to review is visual and sequential in nature, so quickly made illustrations, flowcharts, and concept maps are effective ways to rehearse this material.
  - Do not spend time making artistically sophisticated illustrations and charts, however. The goal is to sketch out your ideas quickly from memory and then check your work.
- During the *testing step*, set up conditions that simulate some elements of the actual exam. While completing practice questions, add time limits and refrain from stopping in-between questions to check your answers. More information about this step can be found in the "Reviewing Practice Questions" section, later.

TIP: Given the amount of material you have to review, it can seem more productive to complete extensive swaths of input activities before turning to the quizzing or testing steps of the learning cycle. Resist the impulse to just remain in the input stage by remembering how productivity is calculated. Getting the optimal amount of output for the amount of input you invest is your goal; this typically requires frequent toggling between the three stages of the learning cycle.

TIP: At intervals, add a self-check about the learning cycle to your study map. As time goes on, it is easy for the balance among these steps to become skewed. A common issue, for instance, is to lapse into an approach dominated by one of the stages of the learning cycle (e.g., just reading or just doing practice questions). Although it is not necessary to allocate exactly one-third of study time to each of the stages, it works best if some attention is paid to all three for each set of concepts and facts.

- Pacing yourself
  - As mentioned, brief units of study time can be valuable, but some longer study sessions are also essential for adequate preparation. However, at times it can be difficult to maintain full engagement with your review materials during these more extensive sessions. Appropriate pacing helps to offset exhaustion and distraction.
  - A recommended rhythm for longer sessions includes studying in about 50-minute periods followed by 10-minute breaks. To help you stay on track, use a timer on your phone for both the learning and the break portions of your study.
  - The nature of the mini-breaks has more influence than you might initially think. "Negative" breaks can lead to reduced concentration in the next cycle, whereas "positive" ones work in your favor.
  - Negative breaks are those that introduce other agendas, even those that are entertaining. So, avoid using the 10-minute breaks to check messages, make calls,

watch videos, surf the Internet, watch television, and the like. Nobody concludes such breaks feeling energized and ready to take on the next learning challenge. (It may be that your work and family obligations require you to take messages, but the time devoted to these duties should not be counted as mini-breaks.)

- Positive mini-breaks are those that allow you to recenter for a few minutes. A light snack, a few minutes of stretching, a quick walk around the block, listening to a favorite song—all of these can help you get ready for the next 50 minutes of study, and they neatly fit within the recommended 10-minute time frame.

TIP: Because you are so pressed for time in general, you may have developed an approach to work that propels you through long sessions without stopping. If so, keep in mind that this work habit leads to diminishing returns during board review sessions. Let yourself take those short breaks so your learning can become consolidated.

TIP: The 50:10-minute study cycle dovetails well with the steps of the learning cycle described earlier. For instance, you might designate the first 50 minutes for input practice by reading a text, taking a short break next, and then going on to a 50-minute period of quizzing yourself about the material you just read. Another helpful pattern is to devote your first session of the day to timed questions about the material studied earlier that week. Subsequent 50-minute sessions can include the input, quizzing, and testing pattern with new material.

Reviewing Practice Questions

This section details how to make the best use of the testing stage of the learning cycle. To efficiently process a group of timed questions that you have already completed, try labeling each of your answers as follows:

- *A correct answer that was easy for you to get right.* Some review of the explanatory material provided for the wrong answers can be helpful, but keep this part of your review light so you can devote sufficient time to the following answer categories.
- *A correct answer that required more effort for you to achieve.* To clarify, this category is for questions that made you hesitate because you had difficulty recalling the required information. You may have been able to narrow down the answers to two choices, and, in this case, you selected the correct one. The most efficient way to make use of such items for further review is to answer this question: *What would I have known if I had been able to answer this question easily?* This question helps you zero in on the precise information or steps in reasoning that you need to practice.
- *A correct answer that you selected for the wrong reason or through a lucky guess.* Treat these like wrong answers as per D, E, and F below.
- *An item you got wrong because you never knew the needed information.* For these questions, sometimes the explanations provided in the answer key are enough to master the subject at hand. However, some of the time, you need to read additional material. In these cases, it is smart to assign a value to the concept to be reviewed,

and then set a timer accordingly. For instance, you may have missed a question that reveals a gap in your knowledge base that would take about 10 minutes to remediate, whereas another topic might require 20 minutes of work. Timing these extra reviews helps you return to your original task promptly. (If you uncover the need for extensive review of a topic, it is often a good idea to move this larger unit of study to one of the upcoming catch-up periods that you have scheduled on your study map.)

- *An item that you got wrong because you partially knew the needed information.* This category is the flipside of B; that is, you may have been able to make some headway toward the answer, but you were unable to pinpoint the correct choice. Again, the strategy here is to look for those small elements of information that would allow you to answer a question on this topic correctly in the future.
- *An item that you got wrong because of a misconception about the topic.* This category differs from D and E, above, in that the learner believes something to be true when in fact it is not. For instance, many young students believe that plants increase in mass by taking it up from the soil, and others think that seasonal changes in temperature result from an increase or decrease in the Earth's proximity to the sun. Although you undoubtedly understand carbon fixation and the tilt of the Earth's axis, we all have errors in our overall base of knowledge. However diligent we may be, our own misconceptions can be difficult to spot. A clue that a misconception might be in play can be found when we answer items incorrectly but the correct answers do not make sense, even after careful review. An efficient way to remedy misconceptions is to work collaboratively with a study partner. More on this next.

More Advice

- Studying with a colleague
  - Although finding time to review board material with a colleague can be an issue, the payoff can be significant. In addition to rooting out misconceptions, these sessions can provide the chance for needed repetition and a motivational boost.
  - It is optimal during these sessions for the person who knows the least about a given subtopic to explain what he or she can and then to allow the other to make additions and corrections.
  - Use Zoom or other videoconferencing applications when in-person sessions are not practical.
  - Studying with colleagues can be stressful, but recognize that if they know more content than you, they can help you learn more.
- Visiting the testing center or location of exam at institution
  - If this will be your first time taking an exam at the testing center where you are registered, plan a visit to this location. This will allow you to gauge more accurately the time needed to get there, to check out parking options, and to evaluate the location where the test will be taking place. There is movement to allow medical boards to be taken at one's home institution. In this case, it is recommended to visit the room in which the exam will be proctored.

- Attending to diet, sleep, and exercise
  - Also essential is finding time for a reasonable level of self-care. Because reviewing for this exam adds to your workday, it is easy to let nutrition, rest, and exercise fall by the wayside. However, both the review process and the exam itself require stamina, so looking after your well-being is part of good preparation.
  - Self-care does not need to be perfect to be good. If you are not able to fit in an entire workout routine, for example, then a brisk walk can still be beneficial. Similarly, although long sessions of home cooking might not fit into your day, making better choices at the hospital cafeteria is probably doable.
  - The goal of the day before the test date is to set up conditions that optimize knowledge retrieval during the exam. So, do not spend this day trying to force in one last set of facts or asking yourself to answer another set of practice questions. Instead, to the extent your work and family duties allow, make this a day for light activity, fun distractions, and rest.
- Thinking positively
  - As sports psychologists know, the way we visualize our future performance has an impact on how we ultimately do. So, as the exam gets closer, try these positive images:
    - Recalling a prior time when you did well on a challenging exam
    - Imagining a question on your upcoming board exam that you do not answer with full confidence, shaking it off, and continuing onto the next item
    - Picturing success with a complicated question
    - Visualizing yourself dispelling nervousness by using short relaxation strategies
    - Imagining yourself answering the last question on the exam knowing that you have acquitted yourself well overall
    - Picturing yourself walking out of the testing center knowing that this was a successful day

Respiratory

ECHEZONA T. MADUEKWE, ANDREW M. DYLAG, NARAYAN PRABHU IYER, DEEPAK KUMAR and PATRICIA R. CHESS

2 Respiratory Embryology and Physiology

ECHEZONA T. MADUEKWE and ANDREW M. DYLAG

Anatomy and Development of the Respiratory System

ANATOMY OF THE RESPIRATORY SYSTEM

- The respiratory system is comprised of the structures responsible for air conduction and gas exchange.
- It is made up of the upper respiratory tract (nose, nasal cavity, sinuses, larynx, and trachea) and the lower respiratory tract (bronchi, bronchioles, and lungs, which contain the alveoli).
- Bronchi and bronchioles are responsible for gas transportation and humidification.
- Lungs are divided into lobes; the right lung has three lobes, and the left lung has two lobes.
- Lobes contain tiny air sacs (alveoli) on the end of the bronchioles that are the sites for gas exchange (O_2 and CO_2) at the pulmonary capillary beds.
- Congenital alveolar capillary dysplasia (ACD) is a disorder affecting the development of lung alveolae and blood vessels (misaligned capillaries and alveolae).

STRUCTURAL AND MORPHOLOGICAL DEVELOPMENT

- Lung development can be divided into five stages: **E**mbryonic, **P**seudoglandular, **C**analicular, **S**accular, and **A**lveolar. These can be remembered with the mnemonic **E**very **P**erson **C**an **S**tudy **A**lone (see Fig. 2.1 and Table 2.1.).
  - The gestational age weeks can also be remembered by "the rule of 6's":
    - 3–**6**: Embryonic
    - 6–1**6**: Pseudoglandular
    - 16–2**6**: Canalicular
    - 26–3**6**: Saccular
    - 3**6** and after: Alveolar
  - Development encompasses two major phases: growth (structure) and maturation (function).
  - Growth starts with the formation of conducting airways and continues after birth with an increase in alveolar number.
  - Respiratory insufficiency of the newborn results from delivery before the completion of both the structural and functional development.

EMBRYONIC STAGE: 3 TO 6 WEEKS' GESTATION

- The respiratory diverticulum (lung bud) originates as an outgrowth from the ventral wall of the foregut at 4 weeks.
- The bud pinches off the foregut at the tracheoesophageal ridges and forms the primitive trachea separating itself from the esophagus.
- Failure to separate can lead to tracheoesophageal fistula and/or atresia.
- The bud septates to form left/right bronchial buds; main stem bronchi form at around 5 weeks.
- Further formation of major bronchopulmonary segments includes secondary bronchi followed by eight tertiary bronchi (left lung) and ten tertiary bronchi (right lung).
- Respiratory endothelium originates from the endoderm, and the surrounding cartilage, muscle, and connective tissue originates from the mesoderm.
- Trachea and bronchi are lined with columnar epithelium.
- Airway development and differentiation are facilitated by retinoic acid signaling that induces TBX4 expression in endoderm, HOX, and FGF genes.
- Vitamin A deficiency is implicated in pulmonary agenesis and stenosis of the trachea.
- Vascular development of primitive arteries and veins mediated by vascular endothelial growth factor (VEGF) and extracellular matrix (fibronectin, laminin, type IV collagen) interactions
- Sixth aortic arch gives rise to pulmonary arteries.
- Pulmonary veins originate from an outgrowth of the left atrium.
- At the end of the embryonic stage, organization of the lobar and segmental sections is established.
- Aberrant development results in tracheal agenesis, tracheal stenosis, tracheoesophageal fistula, and possibly pulmonary sequestration (Table 2.1).

PSEUDOGLANDULAR STAGE: 6 TO 16 WEEKS' GESTATION

- Tubular branching (15–20 generations) occurs caudally to the level of the terminal bronchioles and completes by 12 to 14 weeks.
- Early branching is regulated by the insulin-like growth factor.
- Cellular differentiation (types: ciliated, goblet, and basal) occurs in a proximal-to-distal fashion under the control of fibroblast growth factor 10 (FGF-10) and FGF-7.
  - Disruption of FGF results in blockage of dichotomous branching of the conducting airways.
  - Excess FGF-7 leads to poor differentiation. This histologically resembles congenital pulmonary airway malformation (CPAM).

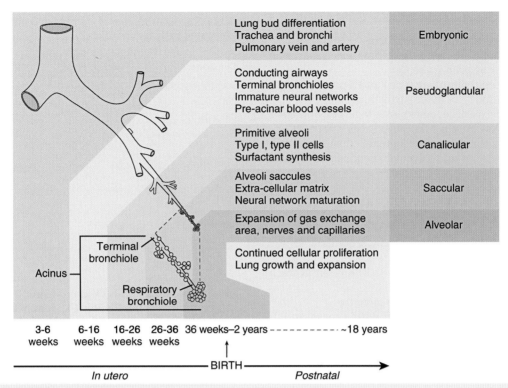

Fig. 2.1 Principal stages of lung development in humans. (Modified from Kajeckar R. Environmental factors and developmental outcomes in the lung. *Pharmacol Ther.* 2007; 114:129–145.)

Table 2.1   Clinical Implications of Abnormal Morphologic Development

Embryonic Stage (3–6 weeks)	Pseudoglandular Stage (6–16 weeks)	Canalicular Stage (16–26 weeks)	Saccular Stage (26–36 weeks)	Alveolar Stage 36+ weeks
▪ Atresia or fistula (esophageal, laryngeal, tracheal)	▪ Pulmonary sequestration	▪ Alveolar capillary dysplasia	▪ Alveolar capillary dysplasia	▪ Surfactant deficiency
▪ Bronchogenic cysts	▪ Pulmonary hypoplasia	▪ Surfactant deficiency	▪ Surfactant deficiency	▪ Pulmonary hypertension
▪ Pulmonary sequestration	▪ Pulmonary lymphangiectasia	▪ Pulmonary hypoplasia[a]	▪ Pulmonary hypoplasia	▪ Lobar emphysema
▪ Pulmonary aplasia	▪ Congenital pulmonary airway malformation	▪ Renal dysplasia	▪ Acinar dysplasia	
▪ Pulmonary agenesis	▪ Congenital diaphragmatic hernia			
	▪ Lung cysts			

[a]Second-degree oligohydramnios or premature rupture of the membranes (PROM).

▪ Columnar epithelial cell transition to cuboidal epithelium occurs in the bronchioles.
▪ Vasculogenesis (formation of new blood vessels) starts in the mesenchyme surrounding terminal lung buds.
  ▪ Removal of mesenchyme impairs branching morphogenesis.
▪ Aberrant development of the pseudoglandular stage results in bronchogenic cysts, congenital lobar emphysema, and congenital diaphragmatic hernia (Table 2.1).

CANALICULAR STAGE: 16 TO 26 WEEKS' GESTATION

▪ Gas exchange units are forming that include respiratory bronchioles, alveolar ducts, and a few terminal sacs toward the end of this stage.
▪ Angiogenesis (formation of new vessels from preexisting vessels) creates the prominent capillary meshwork within the mesenchyme from endothelial progenitor cells and promotes the ability to exchange gas, and a blood–air barrier forms.
▪ Canalization of lung capillaries and surfactant synthesis begins.
▪ Thyroid transcription factor-1 (TTF-1) increases the expression of surfactant proteins.
  ▪ Absence of TTF-1 leads to impaired lung morphogenesis.
▪ Simple cuboidal epithelial cells predominate with later formation of lamellar bodies.
▪ Primitive cuboidal cells differentiate into type I and II epithelial cells under the control of TTF-1, FOXa1, FOXa2, and GATA6.
▪ Canicular stage aberrant development results in pulmonary hypoplasia and alveolar capillary dysplasia (Table 2.1).

SACCULAR STAGE: 26 TO 36 WEEKS' GESTATION

- Terminal sacs or primitive alveoli form.
- Alveolarization begins with terminal sacs separating from each other by primary septa.
- Cells lining the epithelium are type I and II pneumocytes.
  - Type II pneumocytes make surfactant.
- The capillary network becomes closer together, and walls between the sacs contain a double-capillary network.
- Saccular stage aberrant development results in pulmonary hypoplasia and alveolar capillary dysplasia (Table 2.1).

ALVEOLAR STAGE: 36 WEEKS' GESTATION TO CHILDHOOD

- The terminal sacs are partitioned by secondary septae (adult alveoli).
- The number of alveoli increases (~100 million at birth up to 500 million in adult).
- Lung volume and surface area also increase.
- Alveolar epithelial cells are lined with type I and II pneumocytes.
- New double-capillary layers are formed, followed by remodeling to form a mature single layer (blood–air barrier).
- Alveolar stage aberrant development results in pulmonary hypertension and lobar emphysema (Table 2.1).

Physical Influences on Lung Growth

FETAL BREATHING AND RESPIRATION

- Fetal breathing movements (FBMs) are important for lung growth, development of respiratory muscles, and neural regulation.
- FBMs are episodic in nature and exhibit apnea in response to hypoxia.
- Net fluid flow is usually out of the lungs while maintaining a stable chemical environment, preventing entry of amniotic fluid or meconium.
- The principal breathing muscles are the diaphragm and glottis.
- The larynx is the major site of fetal lung fluid regulation by regulation of efflux.

FETAL LUNG FLUID DYNAMICS AND COMPOSITION (TABLE 2.2)

- Fetal lung fluid (FLF) and amniotic fluid are required for proper development of the lung.
- FLF maintains air spaces in a distended state, limiting amniotic fluid entry.
- FLF volume in air spaces is ~20 to 30 mL/kg (close to functional residual capacity) with flow rate averaging 4 to 6 mL/kg/hr.
- FLF production is a product of active chloride (Cl^-) secretion and bicarbonate resorption in the respiratory epithelium, generating an electrical potential difference of ~−4 mV across the pulmonary epithelium.

Table 2.2 Composition of Human Fetal Lung Fluid Compared to Other Body Fluids

Component	Lung Fluid	Interstitial Fluid	Plasma	Amniotic Fluid
Sodium (mEq/L)	150	147	150	113
Potassium (mEq/L)	6.3	4.8	4.8	7.6
Chloride (mEq/L)	157[a]	107	107	87
Bicarbonate (mEq/L)	3[a]	25	24	19
pH	6.27[a]	7.31	7.34	7.02
Protein (g/dL)	0.03[a]	3.27	4.09	0.10

[a]Bicarbonate, protein, and pH are less in lung fluid, but chloride level is higher in lung fluid.
Adapted from Gleason CS, Devaskar SU. *Avery's Diseases of the Newborn.* 9th ed. Philadelphia: Elsevier; 2012:577.

- FLF composition is different from that of fetal plasma or amniotic fluid: high Cl^-, low bicarbonate (HCO_3), and minimal protein.
- Late in gestation, K^+ concentration increases.
- This electrochemical gradient results in the flow of fluid from pulmonary microcirculation → interstitium → terminal sacs.
- Pulmonary epithelium restricts movement of protein (tiny openings); the endothelial membrane permits passage of proteins.
- As a result, lung lymph liquid protein content is 100 × greater than FLF.

FETAL LUNG FLUID CLEARANCE

- FLF absorption is mediated by the epithelial sodium channel (ENaC) and Na-K-ATPase.
- Fetal lung fluid changes during labor:
  - 35% is cleared antepartum
    - Decreased Cl^- secretion → decreased FLF production.
    - Na^+ transport from the alveolar space into interstitium is increased.
    - Increased lymphatic oncotic pressure leads to increased absorption into lymphatics.
  - 30% is cleared intrapartum
    - Active Na^+ absorption is mediated by ENaCs under the control of epinephrine (high during labor).
    - Cortisol upregulates ENaCs.
    - Mechanical forces ((chest is compressed during labor).
  - 35% is cleared postpartum
    - Transpulmonary pressure (lung distention) increases.
    - Lymphatic oncotic pressure (low fetal alveolar protein) increases.
- Mediators affecting fetal lung fluid clearance are shown in Table 2.3.

TRANSITION TO AIR EXCHANGE

- The first breath (and cry) results in air filling the lungs, increasing transpulmonary pressures and driving fluid absorption from the alveoli.

Table 2.3 Mediators of Fetal Lung Fluid Clearance

Hormones Involved in Na$^+$ Uptake and FLF Clearance	Channel Inhibitors	Channels	Inhibitor Function
Epinephrine	Amiloride	ENaC	Blocks fluid clearance
Glucocorticoids	Glucocorticoids	ENaC	ENaC upregulation
Vasopressin	Bumetanide	Na-K-2Cl	Impairs lung fluid clearance/liquid absorption
Aldosterone	Ouabain	Na-K-ATPase	Reduction in fluid clearance

ENaC, Epithelial sodium channel; *FLF*, fetal lung fluid.

- Lung inflation reduces pulmonary vascular resistance through several mechanisms:
  - Activation of stretch receptors
  - Increases in PaO_2, nitric oxide, and endothelin-1, resulting in pulmonary vasodilation
- The presence of blood in the alveoli completes the transition to air breathing with the absorption of oxygen and removal of CO_2.

PHYSICAL INFLUENCES DRIVING ABNORMAL LUNG DEVELOPMENT

- Abnormalities of chest wall, congenital diaphragmatic hernia (CDH), and oligohydramnios → lung hypoplasia
- Ablation of phrenic nerve → abolition of FBMs → lung hypoplasia (laryngeal, tracheal)
- Fetal pleural effusions → lung hypoplasia
- Laryngeal atresia → increased FLF → increased lung volume, surface area, and alveolar numbers
- Inadequate lung epithelial Na$^+$ transport (ENaC function) in term newborn → transient tachypnea of newborn
- Cesarean section → decreased clearance of lung fluid at time of birth → transient tachypnea of newborn
- There is increased risk of respiratory distress syndrome in preterm infants with deficient respiratory epithelial ENaC expression.

Functional Development of the Lung

OVERVIEW

- Lung maturation and achievement of functionality are mainly biochemical processes controlled by hormones.
- Production of surfactant (biochemical maturation) is independent of lung growth.

SURFACTANT

- Surfactant is crucial for maintaining the functional integrity of alveoli.
- It is produced by type II pneumocytes and is stored in the lamellar bodies.
- It is composed of 80% phospholipids, 10% neutral lipids (cholesterol), and 10% proteins.

HORMONES INVOLVED IN SURFACTANT PRODUCTION

- Glucocorticoids stimulate lung maturation → cortisol.
- Cortisol induces fetal lung fibroblast → fibroblast pneumocyte factor.
- Fibroblast pneumocyte factor stimulates surfactant production.
- Thyroid hormones are required for development of the surfactant system.

SURFACTANT LIPIDS

- Phosphatidylcholine (lecithin) is the most abundant phospholipid → 70% of total lipids.
  - ~25% unsaturated and ~45% saturated
- Phosphatidylglycerol accounts for 5%.
  - It is important for even spreading of the surfactant monolayer on alveolar surfaces.

SURFACTANT PROTEINS

- The protein part of surfactant has four types, SP-A, SP-B, SP-C, and SP-D.
- SP-B and SP-C are the hydrophobic principal proteins, and they reduce surface tension.
  - Both are induced by steroids.
- SP-A and SP-D are hydrophilic.
  - Their mRNA is detected earlier than 20 to 24 weeks.
- SP-A is required for tubular myelin formation and plays a role in host defense.
  - SP-A has little or no surface-active properties.
- SP-D is not located in lamellar bodies in type II cells and is involved in surface lipid homeostasis, host defense, and antioxidation.
- ABCA3 protein transports phospholipids into lamellar bodies for surfactant formation.
  - ABCA3 protein is involved in the formation of lamellar bodies.

FACTORS AFFECTING SURFACTANT PRODUCTION

- Gestational age—lecithin/sphingomyelin ratio increases in later gestation and has been used to predict respiratory distress syndrome (RDS) incidence (cutoff > 2).
- Accelerated production—maternal hypertensive disorders, intrauterine growth restriction, pregnancy-induced hypertension
- Delayed production—infants of diabetic mothers, Rh isoimmunization, male sex, cesarean delivery

ABNORMAL SURFACTANT DEVELOPMENT

- SP-B deficiency
  - Most common surfactant protein deficiency
  - Autosomal recessive
  - Histology shows pulmonary alveolar proteinosis, no lamellar bodies, and no tubular myelin.
  - Clinically shows non-sustained response to exogenous surfactant administration

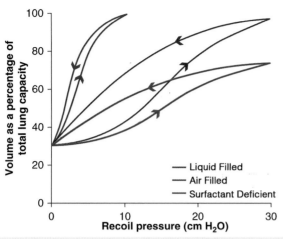

Fig. 2.2 **Effect of surface tension on recoil force.** Pressure–volume curves obtained on inflation and deflation of a fluid-filled lung (*blue*), normal air-filled lung (*red*), and surfactant-deficient lung (*green*). The horizontal difference between the curves reflects the effect of surface tension, which is greater on inspiration than expiration and abolished when the lung is liquid filled. (Modified from Culver BH, ed. *The Respiratory System.* Seattle, WA: University of Washington Publication Services, 2006. Data from Bachofen H, Hildebrandt J, Bachofen M. Pressure-volume curves of air- and liquid-filled excised lungs–surface tension in situ. *J Appl Physiol.* 1970;29:422–431.)

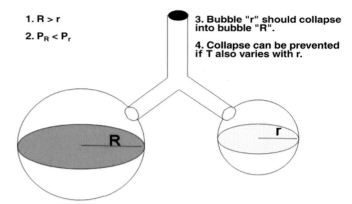

Fig. 2.3 **Law of Laplace as it applies to bubbles of equal radius.** *Pr,* Distending pressure of small alveolus; *PR,* distending pressure of big alveolus; *r,* radius of the small alveolus; *R,* radius of the big alveolus; *T,* surface tension. (From Prange HD. Laplace's law and the alveolus: a misconception of anatomy and a misconception of physics. *Adv Physiol Educ.* 2003;27:34–40.)

- Fatal without lung transplantation
- SP-B polymorphism is associated with RDS and bronchopulmonary dysplasia (BPD).
- SP-C deficiency
  - Autosomal dominant
  - Presents as chronic lung disease in infancy (rarely at birth) or interstitial (fibrotic) lung disease
- ABCA3 deficiency
  - Autosomal recessive
  - Mutation results in reduction or absence of protein function.
  - Decreased transport of surfactant phospholipids and impaired lamellar formation
  - Histology and electron microscopy show dense lamellar bodies or eccentrically placed electron-dense inclusions.
  - Clinically presents in neonatal period like RDS due to abnormal processing of SP-B and SP-C

SURFACE TENSION, SURFACTANT, AND LAPLACE'S LAW (FIGS. 2.2 AND 2.3)

- Surface tension is defined as a cohesive force of attraction experienced by molecules present at a gas–liquid interface.
- Surfactant forms a film between the two media, stabilizing their interactions with a resultant reduction in surface tension, preventing alveolar collapse and increasing pulmonary compliance.
- The relationship among surface tension (*T*), distending pressure (*P*), and radius of the alveoli (*r*) obeys Laplace's law: $P = 2T/r$.
- The pressure required to stabilize the system increases with increasing surface tension and decreasing radius.

- Insufficient surfactant at the alveolar air–liquid interface increases surface tension, increases the pressure requirement, and decreases compliance.
- Smaller surfactant-deficient alveoli also require more pressure because of their tendency to empty into the larger alveoli.
  - In RDS, lungs lacking surfactant exhibit decreased compliance, decreased lung volume, and increased intrapulmonary shunting and hypoxemia.
- Surfactant improves the pressure (P) requirement by decreasing *T* and increasing *r*.

MECHANICS OF RESPIRATION (FIG. 2.4)

- Lung volumes
  - There are differences in lung volumes between neonates and adults (Table 2.4).
    - Infants have higher respiratory rates and minute ventilation (despite lower tidal volumes).
    - Infants have smaller lungs as measured by lower total lung capacity (TLC), inspiratory capacity (IC), and vital capacity (VC).
    - Infants have higher lung resistance and lower lung compliance.
    - Infants have higher chest wall compliance.
  - The lung has no innate resting volume (collapses completely if separated from the chest wall).
  - Movement of air in and out of the lungs during respiration results in lung volume changes and can be measured with a spirometer.
  - Functional residual capacity (FRC) is the volume of gas that remains in the lung at the end of a passive expiration: Expiratory reserve volume (ERV) + residual volume (RV) = 20–30 mL/kg.
    - FRC can be maintained with noninvasive continuous positive airway pressure (CPAP) and invasive endotracheal intubation to deliver positive end-expiratory pressure and overcome alveolar collapse.
  - Residual volume is the volume of gas that remains in the lung after maximal expiration.

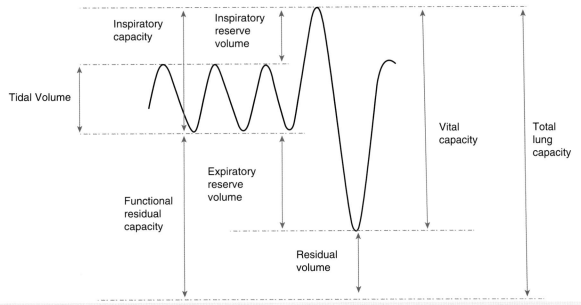

Fig. 2.4 Lung volumes. (From Davis RP. Neonatal pulmonary physiology. *Semin Pediatr Surg*. 2013;22:179–184.)

Table 2.4 Comparison of Lung Mechanics Between Neonates and Adults

Parameter	Neonates	Adults
Respiratory rate (RR)	Increased (40–60)	15
Tidal volume (TV)	4–6	Increased (5–8)
Minute ventilation (TV × RR)	Increased	—
Dead space	Similar (1.5–3)	Similar (1–2)
Lung compliance (mL/cm H_2O/kg)	1–2	Increased (3)
Chest compliance (mL/cm H_2O/kg)	Increased (5–10)	3
Alveolar ventilation ([TV – dead space] × RR)	Increased	—
Oxygen consumption	Increased	—
Resistance (cm H_2O/L/sec)	Increased (50–150)	2–3
Time constant	Very short (0.12–0.5 sec)	Long
Residual volume (RV)	Increased	—
Functional residual capacity (FRC)	Similar	Similar
Total lung capacity (TLC)	—	Increased
Inspiratory capacity (IC)	—	Increased
Vital capacity (VC)	—	Increased

- Pulmonary function testing
  - Pulmonary function testing is utilized in the evaluation of lung volumes, airway function, and gas exchange, and it includes spirometry, lung volume measurements, and diffusing capacity for carbon monoxide and arterial blood gases.
  - Pulmonary function test values are derived from current neonatal ventilators with capabilities for measuring lung mechanics and ventilator parameters. Some ventilator measurements are limited because of under-read tidal volumes and difficulty calculating compliance and resistance in small patients.

- Spirometry encompasses forced vital capacity (FVC), forced expiratory volume in 1 second (FEV_1), ratio of the two volumes (FEV_1/FVC), maximal voluntary ventilation, maximal inspiratory–expiratory pressures, and airway resistance.
  - Measure of volume against time
  - Flow volumes produced when air movement in and out of the lungs occurs during maximal inspiratory effort followed by maximal expiratory effort
    - Infant pulmonary function tests commonly require sedation and forced expiration maneuvers in a plethysmography chamber.
- Lung volumes can also be measured by spirometry: FRC, TLC, RV, minute ventilation, alveolar ventilation, and dead space.
  - Note that FRC and RV can only be measured through helium spirometry or plethysmography, not ordinary spirometry.
- Limitations to spirometry
  - Spirometry can detect obstructive abnormalities but is not sensitive to restrictive abnormalities.
  - Test results can show lung function abnormalities, but they are not disease specific.
  - A reduction of vital capacity indicates respiratory disease but cannot differentiate between restrictive and obstructive causes.
- Mechanics of breathing
  - Air flows from a region of higher pressure to a region of lower pressure (Boyle's law).
  - Normal breathing starts with active contraction of inspiratory muscles, resulting in:
    - Enlargement of the thoracic cavity
    - Lowering of intrathoracic and intrapleural pressures below atmospheric pressure
    - Enlargement of the bronchi, bronchioles, and alveoli
    - Air flowing into the lungs

- Inspiratory muscles, including the diaphragm (most important), external intercostal muscles, and accessory muscles, provide the forces required to overcome elastic recoil and frictional resistance.
- Expiratory muscles are the abdominal muscles (most important) and internal intercostal muscles. Expiration occurs due to elastic recoil of the pulmonary and thoracic tissues stretched during inspiration.
- Respiratory system resistance and gas flow
  - Airway resistance is affected by (1) radius, (2) velocity of airflow, and (3) physical properties of the inspired gas.
  - Formula for resistance: R = Change in pressure/Change in flow = $\Delta P/\Delta Q$
  - Flow (Q) mechanics depend on Poiseuille's law: $Q = \Pi P r^4/(8\eta l)$.
    - Flow is directly related to radius (r) to the power of 4 and pressure gradient (P) and inversely related to viscosity (η).
    - Example: Reducing r by one-half results in a 16-fold decrease in flow and 16-fold increase in resistance.
  - Gas flow pattern is dependent on airway size.
    - Laminar flow occurs in small airways.
      - Gas molecules travel in a straight line, with faster-moving molecules near the center.
    - Turbulent flow occurs in branching airways and large airways.
      - It occurs at high rates of gas flow with chaotic movements.
  - Lung tissue resistance is the resistance within the lung tissues generated during inflation and deflation.
    - It is high in neonates due to a low ratio of lung volume to lung weight and higher pulmonary interstitial fluid.
  - Chest wall resistance contributes to total resistance but is unlikely to increase with lung disease.
    - It is decreased in premature infants (less muscular rib cage).
  - Total resistance is the sum of airway resistance and tissue (lung + chest) resistance: R = chest wall ($\sim25\%$) + airway ($\sim55\%$) + lung tissue ($\sim20\%$).
    - Nasal resistance makes up the majority of airway resistance.
- Lung compliance (Figs 2.5 and 2.6)
  - Lung compliance is the relationship between the pressure and the volume of the lung.
    - Reflects the elastic properties of the lung
    - Calculated as change in volume/change in pressure = $\Delta V/\Delta P$
    - Elastance (tissue stiffness) is the inverse of compliance.
  - Static lung compliance is defined as the relationship between the change in lung volume and change in transpulmonary pressure (airway to intrapleural pressure change) *measured with no air flow.*
    - It is lowest at extremes of lung volume and highest in the middle (Fig. 2.5).
  - Dynamic lung compliance is *measured during spontaneous breathing*, but airflow is zero at the point of flow reversal during the normal respiratory cycle (Fig. 2.6).
    - Rate dependent

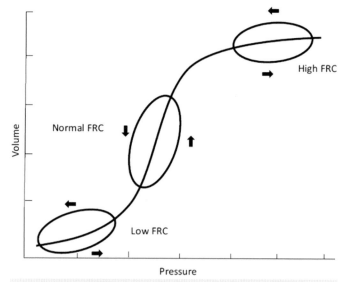

Fig. 2.5 Static compliance curve showing the relationship between changes in volume over pressure with superimposed dynamic flow volume loops. The bottom of the loop is consistent with positive end-expiratory pressure (*PEEP*) level, the top with peak airway pressure (*PIP*). *FRC*, Functional residual capacity. (From Davis RP. Neonatal pulmonary physiology. *Semin Pediatr Surg.* 2013;22:179–184.)

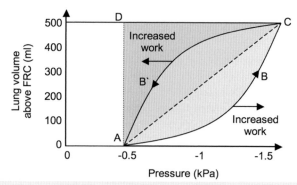

Fig. 2.6 The effect of airway and tissue resistance on the pressure–volume relationship within the chest. *ABC*, Traced line on inspiration; area *ABCA*, work done to overcome viscous resistance and friction on inspiration; area *ACDA*, work done to overcome elastic tissue resistance area; *CB'A*, traced line on expiration; area *CB'AC*, work done on expiration against airway resistance; *FRC*, functional residual capacity. (From Cross M. Respiratory physiology. In: Cross ME, Plunkett EVE, eds. *Physics, Pharmacology and Physiology for Anesthetists: Key Concepts for the FRCA.* 2nd ed. New York: Cambridge University Press, 2014:153.)

  - Reflects both elastic and resistive components and is measured from the end of expiration to the end of inspiration for a given volume
  - Decreased dynamic compliance is seen in conditions with prolonged time constant (e.g., emphysema) and increased respiratory frequency (failure of filling slower alveoli).
- Compliance decreases as lung volume approaches TLC.
  - Limitation of nonelastic components of the chest wall and lung
- After correction for volume, premature infants have more lung compliance compared to term infants.

- Chest wall compliance
  - Neonates have greater chest wall compliance than adults.
    - Infants have more cartilaginous material of the chest wall compared to an adult's rigid or calcified chest wall.
    - The rib cage is not well stabilized by the intercostal muscles in infants when the diaphragm contracts.
- Pressure–volume relationships (Figs. 2.2, 2.5, and 2.6)
  - Static pressure–volume curves represent the relationship between pressure and volume during passive inspiration and expiration.
  - Dynamic pressure–volume curves estimate the *work of breathing* (area contained in the loop) and can be measured during spontaneous breathing.
    - Work of breathing (Fig. 2.6)
      - Calculated from dynamic pressure–volume curve as the work required by the respiratory muscles to overcome the mechanical impedance to respiration
        - Work of breathing (kg cm) = Pressure × Volume
      - Directly proportional to the airway resistance and inversely related to lung-chest compliance
  - The slope of the line between the start of inspiration and expiration = compliance (Fig. 2.6, line AC)
  - A curved shift down and to the right (decreased compliance) occurs in interstitial lung disease, pulmonary fibrosis, post-abdominal surgery, and RDS (Fig. 2.2).
  - A curved shift up and to the left (increased compliance) is seen in BPD, emphysema, and chronic obstructive pulmonary disorders.
  - The pressure–volume curve does not reach zero volume due to trapping of gas in the small airways.
- Time constant (TC) (Fig. 2.7)
  - The time it takes the lung to fill or empty
  - Time constant = Resistance (R) × Compliance (C) = R × C
    - It takes three to five TCs for a relative complete inspiratory or expiratory phase (95–99% emptying).
    - Short TC = fast filling/emptying
      - Conditions: Infants versus adults, low C; RDS versus term infant, even lower C
      - Short TC allows for infants to breathe or be ventilated with relatively high respiratory rates.

- Long TC = slow filling/emptying
  - Conditions: BPD, high R; large-for-gestational-age baby with normal lungs, high C
  - Long TC is part of the reason why ventilation strategies in BPD favor high tidal volume and low rate.
- Hysteresis
  - The volume differences in the deflation and inflation arms of the pressure–volume curve
  - Hysteresis is caused by higher tension present in the lungs before inflation. As a result, higher pressure is required to inflate the lungs compared to expiration.

Ventilation–Perfusion Relationships and Gas Exchange

GAS EXCHANGE (THREE PROCESSES)

- *Ventilation*—exchange of air between lungs and the atmosphere (oxygen for carbon dioxide)
- *Diffusion*—spontaneous movement of gases (between the gas in the alveoli and the blood in the lung capillaries)
- *Perfusion*—passage of fluid through the circulatory system (process of pumping blood through the lungs by the cardiovascular system)

VENTILATION/PERFUSION RATIO (FIG. 2.8)

- V/Q = Alveolar ventilation/Cardiac output
  - The ventilation/perfusion ratio is the ratio between the amount of air getting to the alveoli (alveolar ventilation = V [mL/min]) and the amount of blood going to the lungs (cardiac output = Q [mL/min]).
  - Should be 1 for optimal gas exchange; anything else indicates V/Q mismatch and may lead to hypoxemia.
- The V/Q ratio can change *physiologically.*
  - Blood flow to different parts of the lung is dependent on gravity.

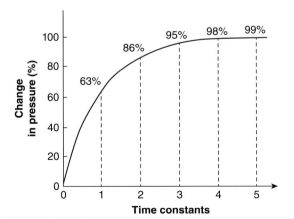

Fig. 2.7 **Percentage change in pressure in relation to time constants allowed for equilibration.** (From Waldemar A. Conventional mechanical ventilation: traditional and new strategies. *Pediatr Rev.* 1999;20:e117–e126.)

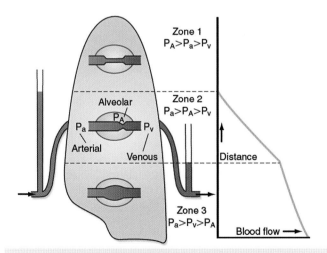

Fig. 2.8 **Distribution of ventilation and perfusion in an upright lung.** (Used with permission from West JB, Dollery CT, Naimark A. Distribution of blood flow in isolated lung; relation to vascular and alveolar pressures. *The American Physiological Society*; 1964.)

- Upper zone (zone 1):
  - Alveolar pressure (PA) is greater than both arterial (Pa) and venous (Pv) capillary pressures (PA > Pa > Pv).
  - It has the lowest pulmonary artery pressure → lowest perfusion.
  - The highest V/Q ratio occurs at rest.
- Middle zone (zone II):
  - Perfusion and gas exchange are influenced by pressure differences between arterial and alveolar pressures (Pa > PA > Pv), with a normal V/Q ratio.
- Lower zone (zone III):
  - Alveolar pressure is lower than both arterial and venous pressures (Pa > Pv > PA), and ventilation is reduced → intrapulmonary shunting.
  - It has the highest pulmonary arterial pressure → highest perfusion, but lowest V/Q ratio at rest.
  - Most of the neonatal lung is in zone III.
- V/Q ratio can change *pathologically*.
  - V/Q < 1 in cases of intrapulmonary or anatomic shunting
  - V/Q > 1 with increased dead space
  - Compensatory mechanisms include hypoxic vasoconstriction and bronchoconstriction.

DEAD SPACE

- Dead space (DS) is defined as the lung volume occupied by gas that does not participate in gas exchange.
- Anatomic dead space is gas that never reaches the alveoli.
  - V/Q > 1
  - Anatomic dead space is increased with smaller diameter endotracheal tube, greater endotracheal tube length, flow sensors, and acquired tracheomegaly.
- Alveolar dead space is gas that reaches alveoli with inadequate or no capillary flow.
  - Alveolar dead space increases with hyperinflation, heterogeneous inflation, and decreased pulmonary blood flow.
- Physiologic dead space = Anatomic DS + Alveolar DS = Total lung volume not participating in gas exchange
- Dead space is calculated by the Bohr equation.
  - $Vd/Vt = PaCO_2 - PeCO_2/PaCO_2$
  - Vd = dead space volume, Vt = tidal volume, $PaCO_2$ = carbon dioxide in the arterial blood, and $PeCO_2$ = partial pressure of carbon dioxide in the expired air

PULMONARY EDEMA

- Pulmonary edema is an increase in extravascular pulmonary water content.
- It occurs when transudation or exudation is greater than lymphatic drainage.
- Causes include:
  - Increased capillary pressure (edema protein < normal pulmonary lymph) due to over-transfusion, vasopressors, left ventricular (LV) failure, left-to-right shunt, or anemia
  - Increased alveolar–capillary permeability (edema protein content is very close to that of plasma) due to direct or indirect injury (sepsis)
  - Decreased lymphatic obstruction due to infection or tumor

- Decreased plasma oncotic pressure (seldom the primary cause of edema but common in very ill patients)
  - Miscellaneous causes include neurogenic (cerebral lesions), re-expansion (secondary to increased permeability), and high altitude.
- Effects on lung function
  - A venous admixture or shunt → increased PAO_2 – PaO_2 gradient and arterial hypoxemia
  - $PaCO_2$ may be normal or subnormal in mild to moderate edema due to hypoxia-induced increased respiratory drive.
  - Hypercapnia secondary to interference with gas exchange can occur when a high fraction of inspired oxygen (FiO_2) is used to treat severe edema.

INTRAPLEURAL PRESSURES AND CARDIOVASCULAR FUNCTION

- Changes in the intrapleural pressure caused by spontaneous mechanical ventilation can independently affect atrial filling (preload), impedance to ventricular emptying (afterload), heart rate, and myocardial contractility.
- Spontaneous inspiration → negative pleural pressure; reduced intrathoracic pressure is transmitted to the right atrium.
  - Systemic venous return depends on the pressure gradient between the extrathoracic veins and the right atrial pressure; spontaneous inspiration increases this gradient → accelerated venous return → increased right ventricular preload and stroke volume.
  - Right ventricular preload and cardiac output decrease with more positive intrathoracic pressure.
  - Changes in the intrathoracic pressure also have effects on the left ventricle; the thoracic aorta is within the thorax, so it is subject to changes in the pleural pressure.
  - The transmural pressure of the aorta is the difference between the pressure in the vessel and the pleural pressure.
  - During spontaneous (negative pressure) inspiration, there is a decrease pleural pressure greater than a decrease intravascular aortic pressure → increased transmural pressure → increased LV afterload and reduction in LV stroke volume.
  - In acute airway obstruction, inspiratory pleural pressure is already negative, and LV afterload is greatly elevated; a minimal further negative in intrathoracic pressure → acute increase in afterload → pulmonary edema.

CONTROL OF BREATHING

- The control of breathing ensures that the arterial PO_2 and PCO_2 are kept within a close range.
- The brainstem, chemoreceptors, and the respiratory muscles are the basic elements for breathing control.
- Brainstem includes the following:
  - Respiratory centers in the medulla and pons are responsible for generating the rhythmic pattern of inspiration and expiration.
  - Respiratory centers receive input from the chemoreceptors, the lungs, and the cortex, and they send output to the phrenic nerve.
- There are three main group of neurons in the brainstem: medullary respiratory center (floor of the fourth

ventricle), apneustic center (in the lower pons), and pneumotaxic center (in the upper pons).

- The medullary respiratory center serves as the primary respiratory control center responsible for sending signals to the muscles that control respiration.
  - The pre-Bötzinger complex in the ventrolateral region is essential for generation of the respiratory rhythm.
  - The dorsal respiratory group stimulates inspiratory movements.
  - The ventral respiratory group stimulates expiratory movements.
- The apneustic center increases the tidal volume by controlling the intensity of breathing.
  - It sends signals for long/deep breaths during inspiration.
  - At the maximum depth of inspiration, it is inhibited by the stretch receptors of the pulmonary muscles or by signals from the pnuemotaxic center.
- The pneumotaxic center decreases the tidal volume by sending signals to inhibit inspiration.
  - Its signals limit the activity of the phrenic nerve and inhibit the signals of the apneustic center.
- Apneustic and pnuemotaxic centers control the respiratory rate by working against each other.

CHEMORECEPTORS

- Chemoreceptors are located centrally (central chemoreceptors) or in the periphery (peripheral chemoreceptors).
- The central chemoreceptors located on the ventrolateral surface of the medulla oblongata are sensitive to changes in the brain PCO_2 or pH and contribute to the stimulation of breathing elicited by hypercapnia or metabolic acidosis.
- Peripheral chemoreceptors are located in the carotid and aortic bodies responsible for stimulating breathing in response to hypoxia ($\downarrow PO_2$, $\uparrow PCO_2$, and H^+).
- Ventilatory response to CO_2 and O_2:
  - The most important stimulus to ventilation is arterial PCO_2.
  - Most stimuli come from the central chemoreceptors, but the response to the stimulus from the peripheral receptors is faster.
- Peripheral chemoreceptors are the only chemoreceptors involved in hypoxia.
  - The control is negligible in conditions of normal oxygen levels but very important in long-term hypoxemia or at high altitudes.

ABNORMAL CONTROL OF BREATHING

- Neonatal apnea is the cessation of breathing for >20 seconds or shorter if accompanied by hypoxia or bradycardia.
  - Apnea is classified as central, obstructive, or mixed.
- The inability of the central chemoreceptors to timely sense the alteration in the PCO_2 secondary to a change in ventilation can lead to a condition called Cheyne-Stokes respiration.
  - Cheyne-Stokes respiration, which can be seen in patients with severe hypoxemia, is characterized by periods of apnea separated by equal periods of hyperventilation.

Principles of Diffusion and Oxygen Delivery

DEFINITIONS

- PaO_2
  - PaO_2 is the partial pressure of oxygen (O_2) in arterial blood plasma determined by:
    - Inspired oxygen concentration and barometric pressure
    - Alveolar ventilation
    - Diffusion of oxygen from alveoli to pulmonary capillaries
    - Distribution and V/Q matching.
- O_2 saturation
  - O_2 saturation is the percentage of hemoglobin binding sites occupied/saturated with O_2.
  - This does *not* describe how much O_2 is in the blood.
  - This may be *normal* in cases of anemia, carbon monoxide, and peripheral shunting; it is *not* dependent on hemoglobin (Hgb).
- O_2 content
  - O_2 content is a measure of how much oxygen is in the blood.
  - Formula: O_2 content = O_2 bound to Hgb + Dissolved O_2 = $1.34 \times$ Hgb $\times$ O_2 saturation + $0.003 \times PaO_2$
    - Hgb is the hemoglobin concentration (g/dL), and O_2 saturation is a decimal value (maximum 1).
  - O_2 content will *decrease* with lower Hgb.
- Oxygen delivery
  - Formula: O_2 delivery = O_2 content $\times$ Cardiac output
    - Cardiac output is measured in dL/min.
  - O_2 is essential for aerobic metabolism, but there is no oxygen storage system in the tissues.
  - A continuous tissue oxygen supply is dependent on metabolic requirements.
  - Tissue O_2 delivery depends on:
    - O_2 tension in the arterial blood
    - Adequate pulmonary blood flow
    - Adequate lung function
    - Appropriate V/Q matching (V/Q is relatively well matched in the middle zone)
    - Sufficient oxygen-carrying capacity
    - Adequate circulation and tissue perfusion.
- Oxygen consumption
  - Formula: Venous O_2 (VO_2) = Cardiac output $\times$ (Arterial O_2 content – Venous O_2 content)
  - Oxygen consumption is a measure of how much oxygen is extracted from the tissues.
    - VO_2 is increased in increased caloric intake, hypothermia, neonates, and term versus premature infants.
  - VO_2 increases in seizures, hyperthermia, and body size and decreases in peripheral shunting, cyanide poisoning, and hypothermia.
  - VO_2 is governed by the Fick principle.
  - Fick's equation of diffusion: $dQ/dt = (k \times A \times dC)/dL$
    - k = diffusion coefficient, A = area available for diffusion, dC = molecule concentration difference across membrane, and dL = length of the diffusion pathway
    - Expressed as diffusion per unit time (mL/min)

ALVEOLAR GAS EQUATION

- $PAO_2 = FiO_2 \times (PB - PH_2O) - (PaCO_2/R)$
- FiO_2 = fraction of inspired oxygen (decimal form); PB = atmospheric pressure (usually 760 mm Hg); PH_2O = water vapor pressure at 37°C; $PaCO_2$ = arterial carbon dioxide pressure; R = respiratory quotient (ratio of carbon dioxide eliminated divided by the oxygen consumed, typically 0.8)

ALVEOLAR-ARTERIAL OXYGEN TENSION DIFFERENCE (A-A GRADIENT)

- The A-a gradient is calculated by rearranging the alveolar gas equation:
  - $PAO_2 - PaO_2 = [FiO_2 \times (PB - PH_2O)] - (PaCO_2/R) - PaO_2$
- The A-a gradient will increase with V/Q mismatch, O_2 diffusion disorders or right-to-left shunting.
- Prolonged (8–12 hour) increase in the A-a gradient >600 is an indication for extracorporeal membrane oxygenation (ECMO) therapy.

HYPOXEMIC RESPIRATORY FAILURE

- Predicted using the oxygenation index (OI), where $OI = (FiO_2 \times MAP \times 100)/PaO_2$
  - FiO_2 = fraction of inspired oxygen (as a decimal), MAP = mean airway pressure, and PaO_2 = postductal arterial oxygen pressure
- Hypoxemic respiratory failure results from failure of oxygen uptake in the lungs:
  - Alveolar hypoventilation, respiratory depression, obstructive airway disease, respiratory muscle weakness
  - Impaired oxygen diffusion from the alveoli to the pulmonary capillaries, such as pulmonary edema
  - V/Q mismatch, such as pneumothorax, alveolar collapse, pulmonary vasodilators, and obstructive airway disease.

OXYGEN AFFINITY AND THE HEMOGLOBIN DISSOCIATION CURVE (FIG. 2.9)

- Factors affecting O_2 delivery to the tissues:
  - pH
    - Bohr effect: CO_2 and H^+ affect the affinity of the hemoglobin for oxygen.
    - High CO_2 and H^+ concentrations reduce the affinity of the hemoglobin for O_2, and vice versa.
    - **B O**xygen **H**ydrogen **R**eleased in tissue
    - Acidity shifts the dissociation curve to the right, and alkalinity shifts the dissociation curve to the left.
  - Temperature
  - 2,3-Diphosphoglycerate (2,3-DPG)
  - PCO_2
  - Fetal hemoglobin
  - Carboxyhemoglobin/methemoglobin → shifts dissociation curve to the left
    - Methemoglobinemia must be monitored during inhaled nitric oxide therapy.
  - Sulfhemoglobin → shifts dissociation curve to the right
- Haldane effect is a phenomenon where an increase in PaO_2 reduces the affinity of the hemoglobin to CO_2, and vice versa.
  - High O_2 concentrations enhance the unloading of CO_2 in the lung.

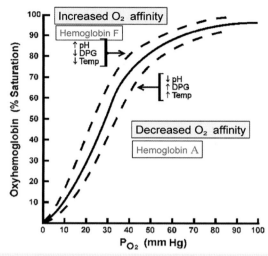

Fig. 2.9 Oxygen dissociation curve. (From Weindling MA. The definition of hypotension in very low birth weight infants during immediate neonatal period. *NeoReviews.* 2007;8:e32–e43.)

- Low O_2 concentrations promote loading of CO_2 onto hemoglobin in the tissues.
- Effects of altitude
  - At moderate altitude → right shift of the oxygen dissociation curve due to increased 2,3-DPG
  - At extreme altitude with hypoxia → stimulation of peripheral chemoreceptors → hyperventilation → respiratory alkalosis → left shift of the oxygen dissociation curve

CO_2 ELIMINATION

- $PaCO_2$ determined by $PACO_2 = CO_2$ production/(Alveolar ventilation)
  - a = arterial; A = alveolar
- Alveolar minute ventilation (MValv) = Tidal volume (TValv [in mL]) × respiratory rate (RR [per min])
- CO_2 elimination depends on alveolar minute ventilation, adequate pulmonary blood flow (V/Q matching), and effective diffusion across the alveolar–capillary membrane.
- Minute ventilation is affected by resistance, compliance, and time constants.
- Implications of increasing $PaCO_2$:
  - TValv falling leads to increased airway resistance, decreased lung compliance, air trapping, and instrumental dead space (endotracheal tube).
  - CO_2 production rising—sepsis, fever, and cold stress
  - Physiologic dead space rising—chronic lung disease and overinflation
  - Benefits of increased CO_2 (hypercapnia)—ensures maximal spontaneous respiratory drive, decreased complications of hypocarbia, protective effect on the lung, and decreased lung injury from decreased RR and tidal volume, in addition to ensuring the use of decreased minute ventilation

MEASUREMENT OF BLOOD GASES AND GAS EXCHANGE TESTS

- Methodologists of evaluation and monitoring:
  - Blood gas analysis
  - Capnography is a measurement of CO_2 concentration in an exhaled breath to determine the end-tidal

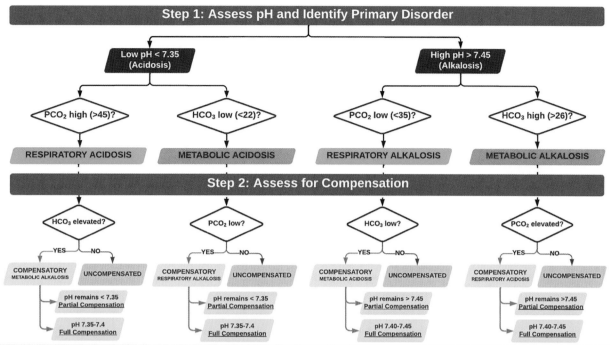

Fig. 2.10 Flowchart to interpret acid base balance and compensation. First, the primary disorder should be identified by the pH with the PCO_2 and HCO_3 values, then the degree (if any) to which there is compensation should be determined.

CO_2, which is displayed graphically or as a numeric read out.
- Pulse oximetry provides continuous information on peripheral oxygen saturation and heart rate; it is limited by a lack of data accuracy during hypoxemia, hyperoxemia, peripheral hypoperfusion, and body movements, as well as the need for regular calibrations.
- Blood gas interpretation (Fig. 2.10)
  - Overall assessment:
    - Step 1. Analyze the primary disorder.
    - Step 2. Assess degree of compensation (if any).
      □ Assess pH—Normal pH + Abnormal $PaCO_2$ + Abnormal HCO_3 = Complete compensation
      □ pH < 7.35 = acidosis with partial compensation; pH = 7.35 to 7.40, consider acidosis as primary cause prior to full compensation
      □ pH > 7.45 = alkalosis with partial compensation; pH = 7.41 to 7.45, consider alkalosis as primary cause prior to full compensation
    - Examples:
      □ pH 7.36, pCO$_2$ 62, PaO$_2$ 80, HCO$_3$ 29
        ○ Primary respiratory acidosis with *full* compensation
        ○ Compensatory mechanism is metabolic alkalosis
      □ pH 7.47, pCO$_2$ 26, PaO$_2$ 80, HCO$_3$ 21
        ○ Primary respiratory alkalosis with *partial* compensation
        ○ Compensatory mechanism is metabolic acidosis.
      □ See Fig. 2.10 flowchart for additional examples.
  - Check oxygenation (PaO$_2$)–it is reliable only if arterial.
    - PaO$_2$ ≅ 40–50 mm Hg = mild hypoxemia

- PaO$_2$ ≅ 30–40 mm Hg = moderate hypoxemia
- PaO$_2$ ≅ <30 mm Hg = severe hypoxemia
- Limitations of blood gas sampling:
  - Sampling errors cause alteration in blood gas values.
  - Arterial blood samplings are most reliable for pH, PaCO$_2$, and PaO$_2$.
  - Capillary blood samples are not accurate for PaO$_2$.
  - The most common sampling errors are dilutions with heparin → lower PaCO$_2$ and lower pH and alter PaO$_2$.
  - Therapeutic cooling leads to falsely high PaO$_2$ and falsely low pH and PaCO$_2$, unless corrected for temperature.
  - Air bubbles → increased PaO$_2$, lower PaCO$_2$, and increased pH
- Diffusing capacity tests
  - Measured using carbon monoxide gas (diffusing capacity of the lungs for carbon monoxide [DLCO]), corrected for the patient's hemoglobin (DLCOc).
  - The diffusing capacity test gives information about the size and integrity of the alveolar blood membrane.
  - It measures the diffusing capacity of gas across the alveolar membrane determined by surface area, integrity of the alveolar membrane, and pulmonary vascular bed.
  - Abnormal diffusing capacity:
    - Low total lung capacity (TLC)—intrapulmonary restrictive defect, interstitial lung disease, pulmonary edema, and pulmonary vascular disease (e.g., persistent pulmonary hypertension of the newborn [PPHN])
    - High TLC—emphysema

- Pulmonary emboli should be considered in patients with isolated reductions in DLCOc in the absence of any other respiratory cause.
- Limitations of diffusing capacity test:
  - Surface area in which the diffusion occurs
  - Capillary blood volume
  - Hemoglobin concentration
  - Properties of the lung parenchyma (e.g., alveolar–capillary membrane thickness)

Suggested Readings

West JB, Luks AM. *West's Respiratory Physiology: The Essentials*. 11th ed. Philadelphia: Wolters Kluwer Health; 2015.

Sivieri EM, Abbasi S. Evaluation of pulmonary function in the neonates. In: Polin RA, Fox WW, Abman SH, eds. *Fetal and Neonatal Physiology*. 4th ed. Philadelphia: Saunders; 2011:1011–1025.

Elias N, O'Brodovich H. Clearance of fluid from air spaces of newborns and infants. *NeoReviews*. 2006;7:e88.

3 Respiratory Distress Syndrome, Transient Tachypnea of the Newborn, and Bronchopulmonary Dysplasia

ANDREW M. DYLAG

Respiratory Distress Syndrome

OVERVIEW

- Respiratory distress syndrome (RDS) is the most common cause of respiratory disease in premature newborns.
  - Over 50% of babies born at less than 29 weeks' gestation will have RDS.
  - Maternal prenatal corticosteroids mitigate RDS risk if the pregnancy is between 22 and 34 weeks' gestation and delivery occurs 24 hours to 7 days after steroid therapy.
  - Maternal diabetes, male sex, and perinatal depression increase the risk of RDS.
    - Maternal diabetes impairs the production and affects the composition of surfactant.

PATHOPHYSIOLOGY

- RDS results from a developmental deficiency of pulmonary surfactant (see Chapter 2).
  - By the law of Laplace ($P = 2T/r$), as the radius of an alveolus decreases and surface tension rises during expiration, increased pressure is required to maintain patency.
  - During expiration, alveoli that lack surfactant collapse, resulting in decreased functional residual capacity, atelectasis, and ventilation–perfusion (V/Q) mismatching.
    - Positive end expiratory pressure (PEEP) mitigates some of these effects.
- During inspiration, surfactant-deficient lungs have decreased compliance and need increased negative intrathoracic pressure or increased positive pressure to open collapsed alveoli (Fig. 3.1) (see Gleason and Juulevaskar, 2018, Fig. 46.5).
- Shear stress from high inspiratory pressure in immature or surfactant-deficient lungs results in alveolar damage, inflammation, and protein leakage.

CLINICAL PRESENTATION

- Prematurity is the essential setting to develop RDS; respiratory symptoms in term patients are unlikely to be RDS, but late preterm infants are still at some risk.
- Typical symptoms include tachypnea, retractions, grunting, and hypoxia.
- Timing of symptoms is dependent on the degree of prematurity.
- Extremely premature infants may be symptomatic at birth, whereas more mature infants may develop symptoms over several hours as endogenous surfactant stores are depleted.
- Retractions reflect increased negative intrathoracic pressure during inspiration; grunting may prevent alveolar collapse by maintaining positive intrathoracic pressure during expiration.
  - Auscultation shows faint breath sounds and fine rales.
  - Persistent increased work of breathing may lead to apnea, hypotension, and respiratory failure.
  - Endogenous surfactant is generally produced in the first 3 to 4 postnatal days regardless of gestational age, mitigating RDS symptoms in some patients.

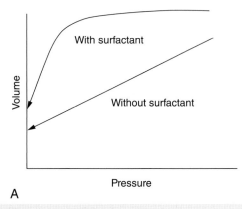

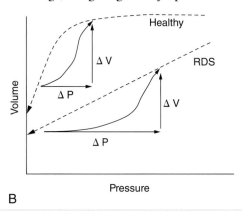

Fig. 3.1 Effects of surfactant on lung pressure–volume curves. Expiratory (A) and inspiratory (B) pressure volume curves for surfactant sufficient and deficient lungs. In both cases, the pressure required to achieve any lung volume is greater in the surfactant deficient lung. *ΔP*, Change in pressure; *ΔV*, change in volume; *RDS*, respiratory distress syndrome. (From Gleason CA, Juul SE. *Avery's Diseases of the Newborn.* 11th ed. Philadelphia: Elsevier; 2018.)

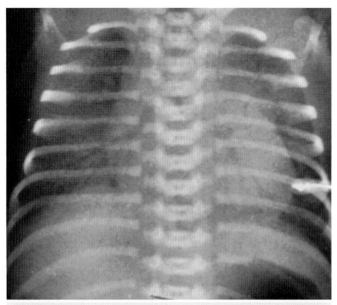

Fig. 3.2 Chest x-ray of respiratory distress syndrome (RDS). The chest radiograph of a patient with RDS shows decreased lung volume, air bronchograms, and a diffuse reticulogranular appearance. (From Gleason CA, Juul SE. *Avery's Diseases of the Newborn*. 11th ed. Philadelphia: Elsevier; 2018.)

DIAGNOSIS AND EVALUATION

- A diagnosis of RDS is supported by the clinical setting (prematurity), early onset (first few hours of life), and radiographic findings.
- RDS chest x-ray is characterized by poor lung volumes (diaphragm < 8 ribs), diffuse, homogeneous "ground-glass" appearance, and air bronchograms (Fig. 3.2).
- Hypoxemia that is responsive to supplemental oxygen supports the diagnosis of RDS rather than cyanotic congenital heart disease.
- Alternative diagnoses include sepsis, transient tachypnea of the newborn, cyanotic congenital heart disease, pneumothorax, and pulmonary hypoplasia.
- Early-onset sepsis, particularly group B streptococcal sepsis, may closely mimic the timing, symptoms, and chest x-ray of RDS.
- Distinguishing RDS from cyanotic heart disease may require an echocardiogram.
- Initial evaluation should include an anteroposterior chest x-ray (consider a decubitus view if a pneumothorax is suspected). Other components of the initial evaluation may include arterial blood gases, complete blood count (including a differential), blood cultures, and blood glucose.

TREATMENT

- Treatment of RDS rests on three major pillars: *maintenance of lung volumes*, *surfactant replacement*, and *supportive therapy*.
  - Maintenance of lung volumes
    - As summarized by the American Academy of Pediatrics (2014), use of *nasal continuous positive airway pressure* (nCPAP) shortly after birth is associated with improved survival, reduced need for mechanical ventilation, and decreased bronchopulmonary dysplasia compared to intubation and surfactant administration.
      - Despite this, failure of early nCPAP is common and may reach approximately 50% in patients between 25 and 28 weeks' gestation.
      - nCPAP failure is associated with a substantial increase in mortality and morbidity, including bronchopulmonary dysplasia (BPD).
      - A widely accepted definition of nCPAP failure requiring intubation is lacking, but a rising fraction of inspired oxygen (FiO_2) that crosses a threshold of 0.3 to 0.4 may be considered.
    - Additional considerations for early respiratory support:
      - Patients requiring resuscitation or with poor initial respiratory drive may *not* be candidates for early nCPAP and may require initial intubation and surfactant.
      - If intubation is required, administration of surfactant followed by rapid extubation (INSURE) is preferable to prolonged ventilation.
      - More recently, delivering surfactant by thin catheter while maintaining CPAP has showed favorable outcomes.
        - This strategy has two commonly used names: less invasive surfactant administration (LISA) or minimally invasive surfactant therapy (MIST).
    - Mechanical ventilation for RDS is addressed in Chapter 7.
  - Surfactant therapy
    - See Chapter 2 for additional information on surfactant.
    - *Surfactant* is synthesized, packaged into lamellar bodies, and secreted as tubular myelin by alveolar type II cells.
    - Hydrophobic surfactant-associated proteins (SP-B and SP-C) are essential for tubular myelin to spread and form a monolayer on the alveolar surface.
    - This monolayer reduces surface tension and thus keeps alveoli from collapsing.
    - Natural surfactants derived from animal sources (bovine or porcine) appear superior to synthetic surfactants.
    - Natural surfactants retain surfactant proteins B and C but not A and D.
    - Currently available natural surfactants seem equally efficacious.
    - For patients who are not eligible for early nCPAP or who fail early nCPAP, early surfactant administration within 30 minutes of birth (giving time for resuscitation and stabilization) has shown benefit.
      - Surfactant administration at >72 hours of life may not be efficacious.
    - Most patients require only one dose of surfactant, but indications for subsequent doses include rising FiO_2 above 0.3 to 0.4.
    - Complications associated with surfactant administration include those due to intubation and positive pressure, occlusion of the endotracheal tube,

and delivery of surfactant to the right main stem bronchus.

- Supportive therapy
  - Supportive care for patients with RDS includes maintaining a neutral thermal environment, judicious fluid management, careful monitoring of arterial blood gases and continuous oxygen saturation, and attention to nutritional requirements, likely through providing early parenteral nutrition.
  - Fluid management (addressed in Section 10) is important to prevent fluid overload, which may contribute to patent ductus arteriosus (PDA) and need for mechanical ventilation while avoiding hypovolemia due to increased insensible water loss.
  - Careful monitoring of blood gases will avoid hyperoxia, hypoxia, and overventilation, which are associated with lung injury, brain injury, and increased mortality.
  - Data are lacking on the management of hypotension in patients with RDS, particularly those with good peripheral perfusion.
  - Because of difficulty distinguishing between RDS and early-onset sepsis, antibiotics are routinely prescribed for premature patients with respiratory symptoms.
  - Complications of RDS include air leaks, such as interstitial emphysema, and chronic lung injury or BPD.
  - Despite improvements in RDS prevention and management, the incidence of BPD remains high in very premature infants, possibly due to increased survival at the lower gestational age limits.

Transient Tachypnea of the Newborn

OVERVIEW

- Transient tachypnea of the newborn (TTN) results from delayed clearance of fetal lung fluid.
- Risk is increased with following factors: cesarean section or precipitous delivery without labor, infant of diabetic mother, or delayed resuscitation with ineffective respirations.
- It can be difficult to differentiate TTN from more serious pathophysiologies, such as RDS or pneumonia.

CLINICAL PRESENTATION

- Tachypnea present at birth slowly improves over 2 to 3 days.
- There is a risk for aspiration with feeds due to tachypnea.

DIAGNOSIS AND EVALUATION

- Typically this is a clinical diagnosis unless significant tachypnea is present.
- O_2 saturation is normal or slightly decreased.
- The chest radiograph is hyperinflated with interstitial edema and perihilar streaking. Classically, "fluid in the fissure" can be observed on the right side of the chest.

TREATMENT

- Supportive care is the mainstay of treatment.

- Supplemental oxygen or CPAP is occasionally needed to avoid hypoxia.
- Consider nasogastric feeds if the respiratory rate is >70 breaths per minute or intravenous fluids if respiration is >80 breaths per minute to avoid aspiration until tachypnea resolves.
- If symptoms persist or worsen, assess for infectious, cardiac, or other serious pulmonary etiology.

Bronchopulmonary Dysplasia

OVERVIEW

- Bronchopulmonary dysplasia (BPD) is a chronic lung disease of premature infants that results from the confluence of lung immaturity with the injurious side effects of respiratory interventions necessary to support premature infants.
- The incidence of BPD is *inversely* related to gestational age and has not changed appreciably since the advent of surfactant therapy, perhaps due to increased survival of more immature infants.
- The incidence varies among institutions, as well as with various definitions classifying BPD.
- A genetic predisposition is suspected, but candidate genes have not been identified.
- There are two types of BPD: "old" vs. "new."
  - *Old BPD* is mainly a fibrotic lung as first described by Northway et al. driven by barotrauma and oxygen toxicity.
  - *New BPD* is mainly the arrest of alveolar and vascular development with a focus on the extrauterine environment.

PATHOPHYSIOLOGY

- Patients who develop BPD are generally in the late canalicular to early saccular stage of lung development (22–32 weeks), and contributing causes are multifactorial.
- The interplay of factors driving BPD pathogenesis are characterized by:
  - Expansion of distal respiratory surface area, extensive microvascularization of respiratory units, reduced interstitial space, and apposition of the distal capillaries to the respiratory epithelium
  - Surfactant deficiency, which results in increased surface tension, postnatal alveolar collapse, poor compliance, and need for mechanical ventilation
  - Deficiency of antioxidant enzymes (e.g., superoxide dismutase, catalase) and nonenzymatic antioxidant defenses
  - Immature mechanisms to remove alveolar fluid
  - Immature immunologic responses to prenatal and postnatal infections
  - Poor respiratory drive and a compliant chest wall, resulting in the need for positive pressure, including mechanical ventilation, even with minimal RDS
- The pathophysiology of BPD is complex (see Gleason and Juul, 2018, Fig. 48.1), involving the intrinsic immaturity of the premature lung and several extrinsic factors,

including relative hyperoxia, barotrauma/volutrauma, infection, inflammation, and pulmonary edema.

- Reactive oxygen species (ROS) produced by cellular metabolism of oxygen may overwhelm detoxifying mechanisms, resulting in damage to cell proteins, lipids, and nucleic acids.
- Increased oxidized lipids and proteins are found in the blood of patients who are treated with oxygen in the delivery room or who develop BPD.
- Elevated oxygen use in resuscitation and longer term cumulative oxygen exposure predict BPD. Interpretation of these studies is complicated by varying definitions of BPD, combined outcomes of BPD and death, and varying methods to measure oxygen exposure.
- Studies of oxygen administration suggest that higher saturation targets are associated with increased lung disease. However, appropriate oxygen saturations for premature infants are not known. The increased mortality at low saturations must be balanced with increased oxidant injury at higher saturations.
- *Mechanical ventilation*, particularly resulting in hyperinflation, is associated with BPD.
  - Premature infants with hypocarbia have a higher incidence of BPD.
  - Mechanical ventilation is associated with air leaks (e.g., pneumothorax, pulmonary interstitial emphysema), which may contribute to BPD.
  - BPD can consist of highly variable chest x-rays, ranging from diffuse haziness to areas of hyperinflation, atelectasis, and increased interstitial markings in more severe cases.
  - Mechanical ventilation resulting in hyperinflation, particularly in the presence of atelectasis, damages the pulmonary epithelium and endothelium, increases capillary leakage, and augments inflammation in experimental animals.
    - Institutions with less invasive approaches to respiratory support have a lower incidence of BPD.
- Infection, especially postnatal sepsis/pneumonia, increases the risk for BPD.
  - Respiratory colonization with *Ureaplasma* species is associated with BPD, but the role of specific antimicrobial therapy is not known.
  - Postnatal sepsis/pneumonia is strongly associated with an increased risk for BPD.
  - A prenatal inflammatory response to maternal chorioamnionitis may be mechanistically linked to BPD, but meta-analyses have failed to show a strong correlation.
- BPD must be distinguished from a PDA or sepsis/pneumonia, which may present as worsening respiratory status in the first several weeks of life.

LUNG FUNCTION IN BPD

- The chronic phase of BPD is characterized by heterogeneous lung disease with high resistance (R) and low compliance (C).
- Because of this, the lung time constant for BPD lungs is *high*.
  - The lung is slow to fill and empty.
  - Recall that time constant = $R \times C$.

- For BPD, the rise in R is greater than the drop in C, so overall the time constant lengthens.
- Therefore a ventilation strategy that utilizes a strategy of low rate, high tidal volume is efficacious in established BPD.
- Further information about respiratory support to treat BPD is covered in Chapter 7.

DIAGNOSIS AND EVALUATION

- There are many definitions of BPD in the literature. All definitions include a history of prematurity (typically <32 weeks' gestational age) and need for respiratory support (typically >28 days) *combined with* clinical outcomes:
  - A combination of respiratory support and supplemental oxygen requirement, based on the National Institute of Child Health and Human Development 2018 workshop definition (Table 3.1)
  - Respiratory support without consideration of supplemental oxygen requirement (Jensen et al., 2019)
  - Need for supplemental oxygen alone (either yes/no or FiO_2 range)
  - Physiologic challenge—for infants on nasal cannula at 36 weeks postmenstrual age, the FiO_2 is gradually decreased to 0.21; infants who can maintain a saturation of >88% for 60 minutes in room air are considered "no BPD"
    - Sometimes termed "room air challenge"

PREVENTION AND TREATMENT

- Treatment and prevention modalities include pharmacologic, respiratory, and supportive measures. Many current therapies lack a strong evidence-based rationale.
- Treatments with well-established evidence include the following:
  - Early CPAP compared to mechanical ventilation (with or without surfactant replacement therapy)
  - Caffeine initiated within the first 48 to 72 hours of life, which is associated with a reduced risk for BPD, possibly through effects on minute ventilation and CO_2 sensitivity
  - Vitamin A supplementation, which reduces the risk of BPD when administered during the first month of life
  - Volume-targeted ventilation (compared to pressure-targeted ventilation), which reduces death, BPD, pneumothorax, mechanical ventilation days, and intraventricular hemorrhage
  - Avoidance of infection
    - Infants with sepsis are at higher risk for BPD.
- Treatments that lack evidence despite common use include:
  - Systemic high-dose dexamethasone reduces the risk of BPD in mechanically ventilated infants; however, dexamethasone-exposed infants at less than 1 week of life have increased risk of cerebral palsy and gastrointestinal perforations. Dexamethasone treatment after 1 week of life is associated with smaller brain volumes in adolescence.

Table 3.1   NICHD BPD Definition for Bronchopulmonary Dysplasia

Must be <32 weeks' gestational age at birth

Respiratory Support	FIO_2 REQUIREMENT AT 36 WEEKS' CORRECTED GESTATIONAL AGE		
	Grade 1	Grade 2	Grade 3
Invasive mechanical ventilation	—	0.21	>0.21
Non-invasive high flow respiratory support (NIPPV, nCPAP, NC > 3 LPM)	0.21	0.22–0.29	>0.29
Non-invasive respiratory support (between 1 and 3 LPM)	0.22–0.29	>0.29	—
Non-invasive respiratory support (<1 LPM)	0.22–0.70	>0.70	—

BPD, bronchopulmonary dysplasia; FiO_2, fraction of inspired oxygen; NC, nasal cannula; nCPAP, nasal continuous positive airway pressure; NICHD, National Institute of Child Health and Human Development; NIPPV, Nasal intermittent positive pressure ventilation; LPM, liters per minute.
Adapted from Higgins RD, Jobe AH, Koso-Thomas M, et al. Bronchopulmonary dysplasia: executive summary of a workshop. J Pediatr. 2018;197:300–308.

- Because of these findings, the American Academy of Pediatrics recommends that high-dose dexamethasone not be used routinely to prevent BPD.
- Investigations into various dexamethasone treatment regimens (lower doses and shorter courses), different glucocorticoids, and improved patient selection may clarify the balance between the risks and benefits of glucocorticoid therapy.
- Inhaled glucocorticoids may have a role in preventing BPD, but data on long-term risks or benefits are lacking.
- Diuretics, particularly furosemide and thiazides, are frequently used in established BPD. Evidence suggests short-term improvements in pulmonary mechanics or oxygenation, but salutary long-term effects on BPD have not been proven.
- Beta-2 agonist bronchodilators may provide short-term benefits to ventilated infants with BPD, but evidence for a long-term benefit is lacking.
- Antenatal steroids may reduce mortality and RDS, but they do not reduce BPD.
- Inhaled nitric oxide, prophylactic indomethacin, and antioxidants have not been proven to be effective in the prevention of BPD.
- Surfactant treatment for RDS has also not been shown to reduce BPD.
- With regard to lower oxygen saturation targeting, meta-analyses of several randomized controlled trials of high (90–95%) versus low (85–89%) O_2 saturations have not shown differences in BPD rates.
- Supportive care for BPD disease modifiers:
  - BPD with pulmonary hypertension (BPD-PH) is common (5–29% of patients with BPD).
    - The etiology of BPD-PH is complex, involving hyperoxia, hypoxia, and other prenatal and postnatal factors that disrupt normal vascular development.
    - BPD-PH is a relatively late finding in BPD, occurring after ~6 weeks, and is a predictor of mortality.
      - No controlled trials of PH prevention or treatment modalities are definitive, but careful attention to preventing hypoxia, hypercarbia, and use of vasodilators in selected patients may be useful.
  - Symptomatic patent ductus arteriosus:
    - Pulmonary edema may increase the risk of BPD, but the data regarding optimal fluid management are still emerging.

- Fluid restriction that diminishes nutritional intake may be counterproductive.
- Patients with PDA are at increased risk for BPD, possibly due to pulmonary edema and decreased lung compliance.
- Growth failure
  - Poor postnatal growth is common in patients with BPD.
  - Energy requirements in BPD may be 20% to 25% greater than normal, requiring high caloric-density feeding to achieve acceptable growth.
  - Infants with more respiratory dysfunction are at risk for delayed enteral feedings and calorie restriction.
- Patients with BPD are at risk for the following postdischarge outcomes:
  - Increased mortality, particularly in the presence of pulmonary hypertension or respiratory infections such as respiratory syncytial virus (RSV)
  - Higher hospital readmission rates
  - Persistent respiratory function abnormalities, including:
    - Airway hypersensitivity
    - Increased use of bronchodilators and inhaled corticosteroids
    - Flow restriction in the mid- to later forced expiratory flows (FEF_{25-75}, FEF_{75}).
  - Poor postdischarge growth, although confounding variables may contribute
  - Impaired cognitive and motor function, cerebral palsy, deafness, and blindness that correlate with the severity of BPD
  - Learning deficits in language and visuospatial perception
  - Sleep disordered breathing and obstructive sleep apnea
  - Lower peak lung function with early obstructive lung disease
  - Diminished exercise capacity

Suggested Readings

American Academy of Pediatrics Committee on Fetus and Newborn. Policy statement—postnatal corticosteroids to prevent or treat bronchopulmonary dysplasia. Pediatrics. 2010;126:800.

American Academy of Pediatrics Committee on Fetus and Newborn. Respiratory support in preterm infants at birth. Pediatrics. 2014; 133(1):171–174.

Barkhuff WD, Soll RF. Novel surfactant administration techniques: will they change outcome? Neonatology. 2019;115:411–422.

Dargaville P, Gerber AR, Johansson S, et al. Incidence and outcome of CPAP failure in preterm infants. *Pediatrics*. 2016;138(1): e20153985.

Dylag AM, Kopin HG, O'Reilly MA, et al. Early neonatal oxygen exposure predicts pulmonary morbidity and functional deficits at 1 year. *J Pediatr*. 2020;223:20–28.e2.

Gleason CA, Juul SE. *Avery's Diseases of the Newborn*. 11th ed. Philadelphia: Elsevier; 2018.

Higgins RD, Jobe AH, Koso-Thomas M, et al. Bronchopulmonary dysplasia: executive summary of a workshop. *J Pediatr*. 2018;197:300–308.

Isayama T, Iwami H, McDonald S, Beyene J. Association of noninvasive ventilation strategies with mortality and bronchopulmonary dysplasia among preterm infants: a systematic review and meta-analysis. *JAMA*. 2016;316:611–624.

Jensen EA, Dysart K, Gantz MG, et al. The diagnosis of bronchopulmonary dysplasia in very preterm infants. An evidence-based approach. *Am J Respir Crit Care Med*. 2019;200(6):751–759. PMID: 30995069.

Kallapur SG. *Bronchopulmonary Dysplasia: An Update*. Amsterdam: Elsevier; 2015.

Northway WH, Jr., Rosan RC, Porter DY. Pulmonary disease following respirator therapy of hyaline-membrane disease. Bronchopulmonary dysplasia. *N Engl J Med*. 1967;276(7):357–368.

4 Aspiration, Pneumonia, and Persistent Pulmonary Hypertension

NARAYAN PRABHU IYER and DEEPAK KUMAR

Meconium Aspiration

OVERVIEW

- Meconium aspiration syndrome (MAS) is the occurrence of respiratory disease, otherwise unexplained, following aspiration of meconium-stained amniotic fluid (MSAF).
- MSAF occurs with 8% to 25% live births, of which 2% to 10% (around 0.4–1.8% of all live births >37 weeks) develop MAS.
- Meconium first appears in fetal intestines between 10 and 16 weeks' gestation and consists of water, gastrointestinal secretions, cellular debris, bile, mucus, blood, lanugo, and vernix.
- Meconium passage is rare between 20 and 34 weeks' gestation; the incidence of MSAF increases after 38 weeks and reaches a peak (30%) at 42 weeks' gestation.
- Increased amounts of motilin and parasympathetic innervation are thought to be the reasons behind the increased incidence of MSAF in postterm infants compared to the rare passage of meconium in preterm infants.
- Fetal hypoxia, with the resultant intestinal ischemia, can induce intestinal hyperperistalsis and relaxation of anal sphincter leading to in utero passage of meconium.
- Most cases of MSAF are not associated with fetal hypoxia, are not depressed at birth, and do not develop MAS. In the presence of fetal hypoxia (i.e., reduced/abnormal fetal heart tones) there is greater risk of developing MAS and a poor perinatal outcome. The risk of poor neonatal outcome in the presence of abnormal fetal heart tones is, however, similar in infants born with MSAF compared with infants born with clear AF. Therefore, the presence of abnormal fetal heart tones is a better predictor of poor outcomes than the presence of MSAF.

PATHOPHYSIOLOGY

- Lung abnormalities of MAS are related to airway obstruction, reduced lung compliance (due to surfactant inactivation), and parenchymal lung damage (due to inflammation induced by meconium).
- Airway obstruction is often partial, causing a ball–valve mechanism, which in turn leads to increased expiratory resistance and increased functional residual capacity (air trapping).

- Chronic in utero hypoxemia, which is typically associated with MSAF and MAS, is also associated with pulmonary vascular remodeling and persistent pulmonary hypertension of the newborn (PPHN).

CLINICAL PRESENTATION

- MAS covers a wide spectrum, ranging from mild respiratory disease to severe respiratory failure requiring extracorporeal membranous oxygenation (ECMO).
- Infants with MAS have respiratory distress and, in severe cases, show signs of air trapping such as barrel chest and prolonged expiratory phase. Thick meconium and extensive staining of meconium are associated with more severe MAS.
- PPHN is also associated with severe MAS.
- Symptoms of pneumonitis peak over 1 to 3 days after birth and resolve over the next 1 to 2 weeks.

DIAGNOSIS AND EVALUATION

- Chest x-ray
  - Coarse, heterogeneous patchy infiltrates, areas of hyperaeration
  - Increased incidence of pneumothorax, pneumomediastinum, and pleural effusion
  - Severity of chest x-ray findings may not correlate with clinical severity.
- Assess for PPHN using upper/lower saturations and cardiac echocardiogram.

TREATMENT

- Prevention
  - Early intervention when fetal hypoxia is noted.
  - Reducing post-term (≥41 weeks) deliveries
  - Intrapartum amnioinfusion is not associated with improved outcomes.
  - Oral and nasopharyngeal suction at the time of delivery, prior to the first breath, does not reduce MAS incidence or severity.
  - Routine tracheal intubation and suction after delivery are not recommended. Infants who are vigorous at birth may stay with the mother for initial steps of newborn care. Infants with poor respiratory

efforts should be resuscitated like those born without MSAF, and, as in all infants, airway suction and clearance should remain part of basic resuscitation when respiration is not established following stimulation.

- Supportive treatment
  - Management of temperature, electrolyte imbalance, acidosis, hypotension, reduced cardiac function, coagulopathy, and renal dysfunction
  - Hypothermia for moderate to severe hypoxic ischemic encephalopathy
  - Correction of hypoxia—if using mechanical ventilation, prolonged expiratory time and sedation are often required. High-frequency ventilation plus inhaled nitric oxide may have greater efficacy together than when used alone in MAS.
  - Exogenous surfactant decreases the need for ECMO if given early.
  - Treatment of MAS-associated PPHN
  - ECMO—in severe, refractory respiratory failure, ECMO is the final rescue treatment. The survival rate in infants with MAS who require ECMO is >95%.

Aspiration Pneumonia (Excluding Meconium Aspiration)

OVERVIEW

- Perinatal aspiration is due to aspiration of amniotic fluid (including infected amniotic fluid), maternal blood, and vernix.
- Postnatal aspiration occurs in preterm infants with swallowing difficulties or a displaced nasogastric tube, severe gastroesophageal reflux disease (GERD), laryngeal clefts, or esophageal atresia with tracheoesophageal fistula.

CLINICAL PRESENTATION

- Perinatal aspiration presents with respiratory distress soon after birth and can be indistinguishable from meconium aspiration syndrome.
  - Aspiration of maternal blood can be confused with pulmonary hemorrhage. The latter often has significant hemodynamic instability and coagulopathy.
- Postnatal aspiration presents with desaturation, apnea, bradycardia, and respiratory distress.

DIAGNOSIS AND EVALUATION

- History of antepartum hemorrhage and presence of meconium
- Infants with postnatal aspiration, especially if recurrent, often require extensive work-ups for gastroesophageal reflux disease (GERD), airway anomalies, dysphagia evaluation, and neurologic evaluation.

TREATMENT

- Respiratory support as indicated
- Antibiotics

Neonatal Pneumonia

OVERVIEW

- Pneumonia remains a major cause of morbidity and mortality.
- Incidence: 1% in term infants, 10% in preterm infants. Autopsy reports suggest pneumonia as a cause in 20% to 60% of stillbirths and liveborn neonatal deaths.
- Pneumonia is classified as early if presenting within 3 days after birth or late if presenting after 3 days.
- Congenital pneumonia is a subset of early pneumonia and can be acquired transplacentally (hematogenous spread) or through infected amniotic fluid (ascending infection from the birth canal).
- Ventilator-associated pneumonia (VAP) is a common cause of postnatal pneumonia.
- Microbial agents:
  - Transplacental—most commonly viral agents, including cytomegalovirus (CMV), rubella, varicella-zoster, herpes simplex virus (HSV), human immunodeficiency virus (HIV), enterovirus, and influenza. Bacterial agents include *Listeria monocytogenes*, *Mycobacterium tuberculosis*, and *Treponema pallidum*.
  - Perinatal (congenital, nontransplacental)—group B *Streptococcus* (GBS). Gram-negative organisms account for the majority (*Escherichia coli*, *Klebsiella*, *Haemophilus*, *Pseudomonas*, *Bacteroides*, *Proteus*, *Citrobacter*, and *Serratia*), as well as *Chlamydia trachomatis*.
  - Postnatal—*Staphylococcus aureus*, GBS, and gram-negative bacteria (e.g., *Klebsiella*, *Pseudomonas*, *Serratia*, *Acinetobacter*). Viral agents include RSV, influenza, parainfluenza, adenovirus, enteroviruses, and CMV, which can be acquired postnatally through breast milk or contaminated blood.

CLINICAL PRESENTATION

- There is often a history of maternal fever, skin rash (especially mothers with secondary syphilis), and joint swelling in infants with transplacentally acquired infection.
- Infants with listeriosis are often born with preterm labor and greenish-brown discoloration of the amniotic fluid. Their mothers may have a history of ingesting food contaminated with *Listeria*, including unpasteurized milk, raw sprouts, cold and uncooked hot dogs, soft cheeses, and smoked seafood.
- Perinatally acquired disease presents with respiratory distress and/or signs of sepsis at birth or within the first 2 days after birth.
  - *Ureaplasma urealyticum* in preterm infants is associated with chronic lung disease.
  - *Chlamydia trachomatis* pneumonia usually presents with staccato cough, apnea, and upper respiratory symptoms, often with antecedent conjunctivitis, between 2 and 8 weeks after birth.
  - Postnatally acquired pneumonia is most often seen in infants on invasive mechanical ventilation (IMV).
    - HSV pneumonia is most often due to HSV type II.
    - Viral agents such as RSV and influenza are associated with fever, respiratory distress, and sometimes apnea.

■ Fungal disease is usually seen in the context of disseminated disease and is more often seen in very low-birth-weight (VLBW) infants with prolonged antibiotic use, prolonged use of IMV, presence of a central line, intravenous nutrition, and postnatal use of corticosteroids.

■ Suppurative pneumonia—*S. aureus*, *Klebsiella*, *Pseudomonas*, *E. coli*, and fungi can cause suppurative pneumonia characterized by necrosis of lung parenchyma, microabscess formation, and formation of multiple air-filled pneumatoceles.

DIAGNOSIS AND EVALUATION

■ History of maternal illness helps guide workup.
■ Chest x-ray is usually nonspecific.
  ■ Interstitial pneumonitis is seen with viral infections, *Listeria*, mycoplasma, and *Chlamydia*. Pneumonia due to *Chlamydia* is also associated with radiologic signs of hyperinflation.
  ■ Congenital syphilis leads to pneumonia alba, a pathologic description for pale, firm, and enlarged lungs seen in autopsy. Chest x-ray often shows nodular and band-like opacities bilaterally.
  ■ Most bacterial pneumonias have a nonspecific lobar appearance.
  ■ Suppurative pneumonia is associated with pneumatoceles, usually thin-walled, and rarely with signs of empyema and lung abscess.
■ Tracheal aspirates are usually diagnostic, although it is often difficult to distinguish active infection from colonization. The presence of white blood cells (WBCs) can aid in distinguishing between the two.
■ Viral panels on nasopharyngeal swabs should be evaluated in infants with signs of upper respiratory symptoms or history of contacts.
■ A high index of suspicion is often required for the diagnosis of postnatal CMV and HSV. These require culture or polymerase chain reaction (PCR) analysis.

TREATMENT

■ Initially, broad-spectrum antibiotics
■ Influenza pneumonia requires early initiation of oseltamivir, often with antibiotics against secondary bacterial infections.
■ Management of specific agents (HSV, CMV, *Mycoplasma*, *Ureaplasma*, *Listeria*, *Chlamydia*, and fungi) is available.
■ It is important to treat early chlamydia conjunctivitis systemically to avoid later pneumonia.

Persistent Pulmonary Hypertension of the Newborn

OVERVIEW

■ PPHN is persistent elevation of the pulmonary arterial pressures (pulmonary vascular resistance [PVR]) during transition from in utero circulation to postnatal circulation.

■ Normally, there are four phases in the transition of decreased PVR:
  ■ *In utero phase*—in the in utero phase, PVR is higher than systemic vascular resistance. Oxygenated blood from placenta preferentially flows from inferior vena cava to the right atrium, left atrium, left ventricle, aorta, and head and neck vessels. Venous return from the head and neck flows through the superior vena cava and preferentially goes to the right atrium, right ventricle, pulmonary artery, ductus arteriosus (DA), and descending aorta, supplying the left upper extremity and lower half of the body.
  ■ *Immediate phase*—the immediate phase occurs in the first minutes after birth when the lungs are distended with fresh air, which is accompanied by a rapid reduction in PVR. Shear stress to the pulmonary arteries and oxygenation induce endothelial cell nitric oxide synthase (eNOS), which in turn leads to release of nitric oxide (NO). Oxygen and NO lead to further reduction in PVR. NO acts by inducing cyclic guanosine monophosphate (cGMP), which in turn activates protein kinase, which decreases intracellular calcium and leads to smooth muscle relaxation.
  ■ *Fast phase*—the fast phase lasts 12 to 24 hours after birth. NO and prostaglandin I2 (PGI2) cause progressive reductions in PVR, which falls rapidly.
  ■ *Final phase*—the final phase lasts for, on average, 6 to 8 weeks up to several months and is characterized by pulmonary vascular remodeling.
■ Causes of PPHN
  ■ Pulmonary vasoconstriction postnatally but normal pulmonary vascular development—acute perinatal hypoxia, MAS, sepsis, respiratory distress syndrome (RDS), and hypothermia. Increased PVR is transitory and reversible, and the prognosis is generally good.
  ■ Fixed decreased pulmonary arteriolar diameter—chronic hypoxia, in utero closure of the DA, chronic pulmonary venous hypertension (as in total anomalous pulmonary venous return [TAPVR]), and sometimes idiopathic disease processes can stimulate thickening of smooth muscle layer in the intraacinar and alveolar arteries. The prognosis is poor.
  ■ Decreased cross-sectional area of pulmonary vascular bed—hypoplasia of alveoli and associated vasculature as in congenital diaphragmatic hernia (CDH), lung hypoplasia (idiopathic or associated with renal problems), thoracic dystrophies, or oligohydramnios due to prolonged rupture of membranes). The prognosis is poor.
  ■ Functional obstruction of pulmonary blood flow—polycythemia and hyperfibrinogenemia. The prognosis is usually good.

CLINICAL PRESENTATION

■ Respiratory distress and labile hypoxemia, often disproportionate to pulmonary parenchymal disease
■ Right ventricular heave, single or closely split and loud S2, and low-pitched systolic murmur

DIAGNOSIS AND EVALUATION

- Preductal oxygen saturations are higher than the post-ductal when right-to-left shunting happens at the ductal level. This is also reflected in the arterial partial pressure of oxygen (PaO_2) difference between pre- and postductal blood samples.
- The hyperoxia test utilizes exposure to 100% oxygen for 5 to 10 minutes and typically results in an increase in PaO_2 to >100 in PPHN but not so in cyanotic heart lesions.
- Echocardiography rules out cyanotic heart lesions and demonstrates increased right ventricular pressures, deviation of interventricular septum to the left, right-to-left shunting across the patent ductus arteriosus, and intracardiac shunt across the foramen ovale.
- Chest x-ray may reveal opacities and hyperinflation in MAS or lobar opacities in pneumonia.

TREATMENT

- Supportive treatment includes correct shock, polycythemia, hypoglycemia, hypothermia, metabolic acidosis, and hypotension.
- High ambient oxygen while avoiding hyperoxemia and providing optimal mechanical ventilation—high mean airway pressures can increase the resistance inside pulmonary vasculature and worsen pulmonary arterial hypertension. Although respiratory alkalosis can counter the effects of metabolic acidosis, it is associated with later hearing issues, and the resultant low carbon dioxide can cause reduced cerebral blood flow. The strategy of hyperventilation is to be avoided.
- Specific pulmonary vasodilators:
  - Inhaled nitric oxide (iNO)—at doses of <20 parts per million (ppm), iNO dilates pulmonary vasculature. It preferentially vasodilates ventilated alveolar vessels, thus reducing ventilation perfusion mismatch. The combination of high-frequency ventilation and iNO has an additive effects. iNO reduces the need for ECMO.
  - Phosphodiesterase inhibitors inhibit the degradation of cGMP or cyclic adenosine monophosphate (cAMP) and reduce intracellular calcium and PVR. Sildenafil inhibits phosphodiesterase type 5 (PDE5), and milrinone inhibits PDE3.
  - Endothelin receptor antagonists (bosentan) block the action of endothelin 1, a potent vasoconstrictor.
- ECMO
  - ECMO can be considered for infants who have failed medical management. The success of ECMO depends on the underlying cause of the PPHN and has an overall survival rate of >80%.

OUTCOME

- Prematurity, acidosis, and hypoxia prior to ECMO and the need for ECMO for >7 days are independently associated with a poor prognosis and higher mortality.
- Long-term sequelae include chronic lung disease (25%), major neurologic abnormalities (13%), and poor growth. Infants with CDH have a worse prognosis than those with more reversible causes of PPHN such as MAS.

Suggested Readings

El Shahed AI, Dargaville PA, Ohlsson A, Soll R. Surfactant for meconium aspiration syndrome in term and late preterm infants. *Cochrane Database Syst Rev.* 2014;12:CD002054.

Lakshminrusimha S, Konduri GG, Steinhorn RH. Considerations in the management of hypoxemic respiratory failure and persistent pulmonary hypertension in term and late preterm neonates. *J Perinatol.* 2016;36(suppl 2):S12–S19.

Wyckoff MH, Aziz K, Escobedo MB, et al. Part 13: Neonatal resuscitation: 2015 American Heart Association guidelines update for cardiopulmonary resuscitation and emergency cardiovascular care. *Circulation.* 2015;132(18, suppl 2):S543–S560.

5 Pleural Disorders and Additional Causes of Respiratory Distress

NARAYAN PRABHU IYER and DEEPAK KUMAR

Extrapulmonary Lesions Causing Respiratory Distress

CONGENITAL DIAPHRAGMATIC HERNIA (CDH)

Overview

- Due to failure of development of posterolateral portion of the diaphragm, CDH results in persistence of the pleuroperitoneal canal or foramen of Bochdalek.
- Among these hernias, 80% to 85% are left sided and 90% to 95% are Bochdalek defects. The rest are retrosternal (Morgagni defect), anterior, and central in location.
- Abdominal viscera can slide through the pleuroperitoneal canal and occupy the chest cavity, compress developing lung tissue, and lead to ipsilateral pulmonary hypoplasia.
- The hypoplastic lung lacks all three components: alveoli, normal bronchiolar branching pattern, and pulmonary vascular structures. The remaining pulmonary arteries show muscular hypertrophy and postnatal pulmonary hypertension.

Clinical Presentation

- Scaphoid abdomen, typically decreased breath sounds on side of hernia
- Varying degrees of respiratory distress/failure and pulmonary hypertension
- Smaller lesions could be asymptomatic at birth and are often diagnosed incidentally.

Diagnosis and Evaluation

- Prenatal diagnosis is usually possible with demonstration of herniated abdominal viscera and mediastinal shift.
- Prenatal prognostic imaging measures done before 32 weeks have been shown to correlate with prognosis in fetuses with CDH. These include the lung-to-head ratio (LHR) assessed by ultrasonography (USG) and the observed-to-expected total fetal lung volume (O/E TFLV) assessed by magnetic resonance imaging (MRI). An LHR of <0.6 has been associated with close to 100% mortality and >1.6 with a favorable prognosis. O/E TFLV <20% carries a very poor prognosis, but >50% has a favorable prognosis

- Postnatal evaluation for other congenital and genetic abnormalities is also performed, given that 30% to 40% infants with CDH have additional anomalies.

Treatment

- Immediate intubation and nasogastric tube decompression of stomach and bowels
- Initial aim is to mitigate pulmonary hypertensive crisis and support gas exchange.
- "Gentle ventilation" in the form of permissive hypercarbia is practiced in order to minimize lung injury. Avoid peak inspiratory pressures >25 unless used as a bridge to extracorporeal membrane oxygenation (ECMO).
- Pre-repair use of iNO is controversial. If used, ready access to ECMO is important.
- ECMO is required in some infants with CDH, if standard therapy fails.
- Surgical repair is delayed until pulmonary hypertension improves. Some may benefit from repair on ECMO.
- Survival for isolated CDH varies from 70% to 90% and is lower (50%) for infants who require ECMO.

EVENTRATION OF THE DIAPHRAGM

Overview

- Musculature of the diaphragm is replaced by fibroelastic tissue, leading to thinning and abnormal movement.
- CDH may be congenital or acquired.
- Acquired causes include operative trauma and birth trauma.

Clinical Presentation

- Respiratory distress, occasionally requiring mechanical ventilation
- May be asymptomatic

Diagnosis

- Chest x-ray
- Fluoroscopy showing paradoxical movement of the diaphragm
- Ultrasound of chest showing lack of movement of hemidiaphragm (preferred initial diagnostic test)

Treatment

- Plication of diaphragm with nonabsorbable sutures to create a taut diaphragm

SPINAL CORD INJURY INCLUDING CORD TRANSECTION

Overview

- Spinal cord injury in the form of phrenic nerve injury and partial or complete spinal cord transection are rare causes of respiratory distress.

Clinical Presentation

- Respiratory distress, which is usually unilaterally, usually on the right side, and often associated with brachial plexus palsy
- Bilateral phrenic nerve injury and complete spinal cord transection are usually associated with respiratory failure and poor respiratory effort requiring mechanical ventilation.

Diagnosis

- Fluoroscopic examination of the chest shows paradoxical movement of the diaphragm in unilateral phrenic nerve palsy.
- Ultrasound of the diaphragm can be diagnostic, but sometimes phrenic nerve conduction studies are required.

Treatment

- Noninvasive and occasionally invasive mechanical ventilation is required to support affected infants.
- Phrenic nerve injury can improve over time, but many infants require diaphragm plication. Early demonstration of improvement and early plication are associated with better outcomes.

Airway Obstruction Causing Respiratory Distress

CERVICAL VASCULAR ANOMALIES

Overview

- Lymphatic malformations are the most common cervical vascular malformations noticed in the newborn period.
- They generally represent sequestered lymphatic channels that failed to communicate with larger lymphatics or draining veins.

Clinical Presentation

- Nearly half present prenatally or at birth, and the rest become evident during the first decade of life.
- The cysts can be macrocystic, microcystic, or mixed in morphology.
- Lymphatic malformations may shrink over time, but most do not, and some increase in size with intracystic hemorrhage or infection.

Diagnosis

- Prenatal or postnatal ultrasound
- MRI of neck to describe the extent of the malformation and its effect on surrounding tissues

Treatment

- Massive malformations require tracheotomy.

- Macrocystic lesions are amenable to sclerotherapy with OK-432, doxycycline, sirolimus, and ethanol. Microcystic lesions may respond to bleomycin.
- Surgical excision could be necessary, as often there is recurrence, and multiple surgeries are required.

PYRIFORM APERTURE STENOSIS

Overview

- Pyriform aperture stenosis is rare and is due to overgrowth of the medial nasal process of maxilla.
- The pyriform aperture is the narrowest region of nasal passage, and even small decreases in cross-sectional areas can cause significant respiratory distress.

Clinical Presentation

- Mild nasal congestion to apnea and severe respiratory distress
- Can be associated with midline maxillary incisor and other midline abnormalities

Diagnosis

- Nasal endoscopy
- Computed tomography (CT) scan

Treatment

- Nasal decongestion
- Surgical excision

CHOANAL ATRESIA

Overview

- Choanal atresia is the congenital absence of communication between the posterior nasal cavity and the nasopharynx.
- It is most commonly caused by a bony plate at the posterior nasal choana.

Clinical Presentation

- Females are affected more, and unilateral disease is more common than bilateral disease.
- Respiratory distress occurs, especially during feeding.
- Unilateral disease can present as persistent rhinorrhea.
- More than half, especially with bilateral disease, have associated abnormalities such as the CHARGE syndrome (coloboma, heart defect, choanal atresia, retarded growth, genitourinary and ear anomalies).

Diagnosis

- CT scan

Treatment

- Surgery to open posterior choanae

GLOSSOPTOSIS (RELATIVE MACROGLOSSIA)

Overview

- Glossoptosis is seen most commonly with the Pierre Robin sequence (PRS).

- PRS represents a sequence of events beginning with the arrest of mandibular development and micrognathia. The tongue rests higher in the oral cavity and prevents fusion of the palatal shelves.

Clinical Presentation

- Micrognathia, glossoptosis, and U-shaped cleft palate
- Presents with respiratory distress that is more severe in supine position and worsens during sleep
- Often associated with syndromes, most common being Stickler syndrome

Diagnosis

- Clinical exam
- Three-dimensional reconstruction of the face may be required to better assess the micrognathia.

Treatment

- Wait and watch, as the airway obstruction generally improves by the time the baby has doubled his or her weight
- Tracheotomy
- Mandibular distraction osteogenesis in selected patients

MACROGLOSSIA

Overview

- Macroglossia can have a focally or uniformly enlarged tongue.
- It can be isolated or associated with Beckwith-Wiedemann syndrome and trisomy 21.

Clinical Presentation

- Respiratory distress and feeding difficulty
- When associated with Beckwith-Wiedemann syndrome, findings include increased fetal and infantile growth, abdominal wall defects, visceromegaly, hypoglycemia, and embryonal malignancies.

Treatment

- Tongue reduction
- Tracheotomy

LARYNGOMALACIA

Overview

- Laryngomalacia is the most common cause of stridor in infants.
- There is inspiratory collapse of supraglottic structures, especially mucosa overlying the arytenoid cartilage and aryepiglottic folds.

Clinical Presentation

- Inspiratory stridor in the first few days after birth
- Feeding difficulties, aspiration
- Symptoms worsen with agitation and prone positioning and improve with supine positioning.

Diagnosis

- Flexible fiberoptic laryngoscopy

Treatment

- Most cases can be managed conservatively, as the symptoms resolve by 12 to 24 months.
- Supraglottoplasty to remove redundant supraglottic mucosa
- Tracheotomy

VOCAL CORD PARALYSIS

Overview

- Vocal cord paralysis is the second most common cause of stridor in infants.
- It can be unilateral or bilateral, acquired or congenital.
- Unilateral paralysis is usually iatrogenic, due to cardio-thoracic surgery and incidental trauma during endo-tracheal intubation. It can also be due to intrathoracic lesions causing compression of recurrent laryngeal nerve and birth trauma.
- Bilateral paralysis could be caused by Chiari malformation or other causes of brainstem compression.

Clinical Presentation

- Unilateral paralysis presents with stridor, weak cry, and feeding difficulties.
- Bilateral paralysis presents with prominent stridor, although it can be asymptomatic due to paramedian position of both cords.

Diagnosis

- Flexible laryngoscopy
- MRI brain/spine to exclude Chiari malformation in bilateral paralysis

Treatment

- Unilateral paralysis—spontaneous recovery; rarely medialization procedures
- Bilateral paralysis—treatment of underlying cause; 50% require tracheotomy

LARYNGEAL CLEFT

Overview

- Laryngeal cleft is due to inadequate development of tracheoesophageal septum.
- Laryngotracheal apparatus communicates with esophagus to varying degrees (types 1–4).

Clinical Presentation

- Aspiration, cough, respiratory distress, and stridor
- More than half are associated with other abnormalities.

Diagnosis

- Flexible laryngoscopy

Treatment

- Types 2 to 4 require surgical correction.

SUBGLOTTIC STENOSIS

Overview

- Subglottic stenosis is the third most common cause of stridor in infants.
- It can be acquired or congenital.
- Congenital subglottic stenosis results from fibrous bands or is due to cartilaginous deformities.
- Acquired subglottic stenosis results from trauma, especially traumatic and prolonged intubation.

Clinical Presentation

- Stridor and respiratory distress
- Congenital stenosis is prone to present as recurrent stridor and is often less severe than acquired ones.

Diagnosis

- Flexible laryngoscopy and tracheobronchoscopy

Treatment

- Treatment is conservative for congenital and less severe forms.
- Higher-grade stenosis can be managed by balloon dilatation, airway reconstruction, or tracheotomy.

SUBGLOTTIC HEMANGIOMA

Overview

- Hemangioma is a common tumor of infancy; subglottic site is unusual.

Clinical Presentation

- Asymptomatic during the first few weeks
- Tumor enters a proliferative phase after a few weeks, and tumor growth leads to stridor and respiratory distress.
- Symptoms are worse in the supine position.
- Cutaneous hemangioma is present in 50% of cases and has a "beard-like" distribution.

Diagnosis

- Direct laryngoscopy
- MRI/CT scan of neck

Treatment

- Watchful waiting is not acceptable.
- Propranolol
- Intravenous corticosteroids for symptomatic infants, given along with propranolol
- Surgical excision
- Tracheotomy

TRACHEAL STENOSIS

Overview

- Most cases of tracheal stenosis are congenital in origin. It can be acquired secondary to endotracheal intubation.

- Complete tracheal rings are important congenital causes.
- About 50% are associated with pulmonary sling.

Clinical Presentation

- Respiratory distress, and expiratory stridor
- Cough and wheezing while feeding
- Recurrent respiratory infections

Diagnosis

- Endoscopy
- MRI and CT of chest

Treatment

- Steroids and bronchodilators
- Physiotherapy
- Surgical intervention—resection with end-to-end anastomosis; slide tracheoplasty
- Balloon dilatation

TRACHEOMALACIA

Overview

- In cartilaginous tracheomalacia, the membranous ratio is normally horseshoe shaped (4.5:1), and there is less cartilage and resultant collapse of the trachea.

Clinical Presentation

- Respiratory distress, chronic cough, and wheezing
- Recurrent pneumonia
- Apnea

Diagnosis

- Bronchoscopy under spontaneous ventilation

Treatment

- Continuous positive airway pressure (CPAP)
- Tracheotomy or aortopexy

VASCULAR COMPRESSION (VASCULAR RING)

Overview

- The most common symptomatic anomaly is due to an anomalous innominate artery.

Clinical Presentation

- Chronic cough, dyspnea, stridor, and wheezing
- Reflex apnea
- Occasionally, dysphagia

Diagnosis

- Bronchoscopy
- For symptomatic cases requiring surgery, magnetic resonance angiography (MRA) and CT angiography

Treatment

- Aortopexy

Miscellaneous Lesions Causing Respiratory Distress

CONGENITAL LOBAR EMPHYSEMA (CLE)

Overview

- Emphysematous enlargement, usually of one lobe, is caused by air entry into the affected lobe with blockage of expiration and air trapping.
- Causes include bronchial stenosis, bronchomalacia, intraluminal obstruction, or extraluminal compression by a mass such as a bronchogenic cyst.

Clinical Presentation

- CLE usually affects the left upper lobe followed by the right middle lobe.
- Air trapping results in emphysematous lobar expansion, which can cause compression of adjacent lung and mediastinal displacement.
- Lobar hyperexpansion and adjacent lung collapse can be life threatening.

Diagnosis and Evaluation

- Chest x-ray shows characteristic finding of unilateral lobar hyperinflation with compression, atelectasis of adjacent lung, and mediastinal shift.
- CT of chest or MRI of chest may reveal any underlying cause for CLE.
- Echocardiography may reveal any vascular structures compressing the bronchi.

Treatment

- Observation is suggested if asymptomatic or mildly symptomatic.
- Thoracotomy and lobectomy are indicated for progressive respiratory distress and/or persistent/recurrent pneumonia.

CONGENITAL PULMONARY AIRWAY MALFORMATION (CPAM)

Overview

- CPAM is a group of lesions characterized by abnormal airway branching morphogenesis of the lower respiratory tract.
- It is the most common congenital lung lesion.
- Hamartomatous lesions that are cystic or adenomatous in nature (thus the previous terminology of congenital cystic adenomatous malformation [CCAM]) and contain epithelial elements from trachea, bronchial, and alveolar tissues.

Clinical Presentation

- Large lesions can present as hydrops in utero.
- Postnatally, CPAM could be asymptomatic or cause respiratory distress.
- It usually affects a single lobe, most commonly the left lower lobe.
- There is a 1% to 3% risk of malignant transformation.
- Five types of CPAMs:

- Type 0 is the rarest type, originating from tracheobronchial epithelium and small cysts.
- Type 1 represents 60% to 70% of CPAMs. Type 1 originates from distal bronchi and bronchioles and presents as 2- to 10-cm large cysts, thin-walled and affecting one lobe.
- Type 2 represents 15% to 20% of CPAMs. Type 2 consists of terminal bronchiolar epithelium and presents as 0.5- to 2-cm cysts that blend with normal tissue. Up to 60% of patients have other abnormalities, such as esophageal atresia, intestinal atresia, or renal agenesis.
- Type 3 represents 5% to 10% of CPAMs, which are often large and can involve multiple lobes. Acinar in origin, they can be cystic and solid or entirely solid. They are not associated with malignancy.
- Type 4 represents 5% to 10% of CPAMs, which consist of large cysts derived from alveolar lining cells. Type 4 carries the highest premalignant/malignant potential.

Diagnosis

- Can be diagnosed on prenatal ultrasound
- Cyst volume ratio (CVR) is the cyst volume divided by head circumference. Measured on prenatal ultrasounds, it can be used to predict outcome. CVRs > 1.6 are associated with a higher risk of hydrops.
- Chest x-ray and CT chest with contrast are used for diagnosis. Contrast is used to identify any systemic feeder vessels. Lesions with systemic feeding vessels are referred to as bronchopulmonary sequestration.

Treatment

- Fetuses with high-risk lesions (defined by size and CVR) can be managed with maternal steroids and, if needed, fetal resection of the lesion. Large cystic lesions can be managed with in utero thoracoamniotic shunts.
- Postnatally, surgical resection is recommended due to risk of infection and malignancy.
- The best time for surgery is between 2 and 6 months of age, although, symptomatic lesions may require more emergent resection.

Pleural Disorders Causing Respiratory Distress

PLEURAL EFFUSION

Overview

- Pleural fluid:
  - Produced by visceral pleura
  - Absorbed by lymphatics of parietal pleura
- Types of pleural effusion:
  - Congenital
  - Acquired
- Congenital pleural effusion:
  - Hydrops fetalis—abnormal fetal fluid collection in a minimum of two anatomic locations; usually bilateral pleural effusions. Causes include chromosomal abnormalities, congenital heart disease, immune and

nonimmune anemia, metabolic problems, and infections (herpes simplex, parvovirus).
- Congenital chylothorax—accumulation of chyle in the pleural space. Congenital chylothorax is due to abnormal development of the lymphatic system. Causes include chromosomal anomalies such as trisomy 21, Turner syndrome, and other genetic abnormalities.
- Acquired pleural effusion:
  - Iatrogenic effusions as complications of thoracic surgery (most common cause of acquired pleural effusion) or central venous catheter leak
  - Pneumonia
  - Hypoalbuminemia (nephrotic syndrome)
  - Superior vena cava syndrome

Clinical Presentation

- Congenital pleural effusions:
  - Usually seen antenatally
  - Large fetal bilateral pleural effusions may cause immediate respiratory distress at birth.
  - Associated pulmonary hypoplasia results in the need for prolonged assisted ventilation.
- In acquired effusions, symptoms depend on the size of the pleural effusions, with moderate to severe effusions causing respiratory failure.

Diagnosis

- Antenatal—fetal ultrasound. The cause for fetal hydrops is often ascertained during the same ultrasound exam.
- Postnatal—chest x-ray and fluid analysis for lactate dehydrogenase (LDH), protein content, lipid level and profile, and cell count with differential

- Fluid analysis leads to effusion classification as:
  - Transudate, which is low in protein and cellular elements and is due to increased hydrostatic pressure
  - Exudate, which has higher concentrations of protein and lactate dehydrogenase and is due to infection, extravasation of parenteral fluids, or lymphatic blockage
  - Chyle, which has a high protein and lipid content, especially after milk feed. Differential count reveals the lymphocyte predominance.

Treatment

- Needle aspiration is reserved for infants with respiratory failure. For persistent effusion, tube thoracostomy is done.
- Replacement of ongoing losses of fluid, albumin, immunoglobulin, and coagulation factors is necessary for prolonged chylous drainage.
- Chylous effusion treatment: medium-chain triglyceride (MCT) oil, nothing by mouth, octreotide (adverse effects include PPHN and NEC)

Suggested Readings

Chandrasekharan PK, Rawat M, Madappa R, Rothstein DH, Lakshminrusimha S. Congenital Diaphragmatic hernia – a review. *Matern Health Neonatol Perinatol.* 2017;3:6. doi:10.1186/s40748-017-0045-1.

David M, Lamas-Pinheiro R, Henriques-Coelho T. Prenatal and postnatal management of congenital pulmonary airway malformation. *Neonatology.* 2016;110(2):101–115.

Oluyomi-Obi T, Kuret V, Puligandla P, et al. Antenatal predictors of outcome in prenatally diagnosed congenital diaphragmatic hernia (CDH). *J Pediatr Surg.* 2017;52(5):881–888.

Wassef M, Blei F, Adams D, et al. Vascular anomalies classification: recommendations from the International Society for the Study of Vascular Anomalies. *Pediatrics.* 2015;136(1):e203–e214.

6 Apnea of Prematurity and Neonatal Respiratory Depression

NARAYAN PRABHU IYER and DEEPAK KUMAR

Overview

FETAL BREATHING

- Fetal breathing movements in utero are important for lung development and maturation of breathing control.
- Fetal breathing is not a continuous process; instead, it is characterized by periods of prolonged apnea lasting as long as 2 hours.
- Apneas in the fetus are more frequent and longer lasting at younger gestational ages.
- Fetal breathing increases with maternal CO_2 inhalation, suggesting intact central chemoreception.
- Fetal response to hypoxia is also centrally mediated and results in diminished or absent breathing movements.
- Diminished fetal breathing is associated with poor fetal health.
- During the fetal to neonatal transition, the discontinuous fetal breathing changes to a continuous neonatal breathing pattern. The sudden increase in arterial partial pressure of oxygen (PaO_2) at birth (compared to fetal PaO_2) silences the peripheral chemoreceptors. This silencing is not complete, as evidenced by the fact that supplemental O_2 compared to room air at birth may delay the onset of the first cry.

NEONATAL BREATHING

- Control of normal breathing resides within multiple centers in the bulbopontine region of the brainstem.
- Afferent inputs into the respiratory control centers include signals from central and peripheral chemoreceptors, pulmonary stretch receptors, upper airway mechanochemical receptors, reticular activating system neurons, and cortical inputs.
- Central chemoreceptors:
  - Are located in the ventrolateral surface of the medulla
  - Respond to hypercarbia and H^+ ions in the extracellular fluid (ECF)
  - Activation results in increased respiratory rate and depth.
  - Central chemosensitivity to hypercarbia is diminished in preterm infants, and this relative "insensitivity" is directly proportional to the level of prematurity.
  - Among preterm infants, those with apnea of prematurity (AOP) have greater insensitivity to hypercarbia than preterm infants of similar gestational age but without AOP.
- Peripheral chemoreceptors:
  - Are located near carotid artery bifurcation
  - Respond to changes in pH and PaO_2
  - Like central chemoreceptors, peripheral chemoreceptors also mature during the first few weeks of life in both term and preterm infants.
  - Peripheral chemoreceptors cause ventilation depression during acute hyperoxia. This response is blunted in preterm infants.
  - Peripheral chemoreceptors are activated during apnea and play a role in apnea termination.
- Biphasic response to acute hypoxia:
  - Adults show a sustained period of hyperventilation in response to acute hypoxia. In contrast, preterm infants and term infants up to 3 weeks' postnatal age show a biphasic response to acute hypoxia.
  - In response to acute hypoxia, preterm infants have a transient increase in rate and depth of respiration, and this is mediated through the peripheral chemoreceptors. This hyperventilatory response may be completely blunted in infants born extremely premature.
  - After about 30 seconds of hyperventilation, there is progressive depression of ventilation, and this response appears to be mediated by inhibitory signals from the bulbopontine region to peripheral chemoreceptors.
- Upper airway reflexes and breathing pattern:
  - Laryngeal mucosal receptors can elicit a strong protective airway reflex and can result in apnea, bradycardia, hypotension, and upper airway closure.
  - Negative pressure in the upper airways can also lead to decreased ventilation. During upper airway obstruction (obstructive apnea), respiratory efforts result in the development of negative upper airway pressure, which in turn can lead to central apnea.
  - Hypoxic ventilation depression and the blunted response to hypercarbia result in prolonged instability of respiratory pattern and apnea.
- Other reflexes:
  - In the Hering-Breuer (HB) inflation reflex, lung inflation stimulates stretch receptors, which send afferent impulses to the medulla. Efferent vagal nerve inhibition of further inspiration results in termination of inspiration.

- The HB reflex includes slowing of ventilatory frequency or apnea and bronchodilation.
- The HB reflex is strong in the first few months of life but weak in adults.
- The strength of the HB reflex is greater at 36°C than at 24°C in newborn rats, suggesting that newborns exposed to a warm environment are more susceptible to inhibitory inputs.
- Hyperthermia may predispose newborns to respiratory depression.
- Manifestations of immature breathing pattern:
  - Periodic breathing
    - Periodic breathing is a pattern of regular breathing alternating with pauses in respiration of at least 3 seconds, persisting through at least three cycles of breathing.
    - The prevalence of periodic breathing is up to 80% in full-term infants and almost 100% in extremely low-birth-weight infants.
    - The prevalence reduces to reach a nadir by about 44 weeks of postmenstrual age (PMA).
    - Low lung volumes, low pulmonary compliance, low baseline oxygenation, and immature central chemoreceptors make preterm infants prone to having more severe and prolonged episodes of periodic breathing.
    - Periodic breathing is associated with intermittent hypoxia and possibly bradycardia and may be associated with adverse neurodevelopmental outcomes.
    - The pattern of periodic breathing changes with the phase of sleep. During REM sleep, periodic breathing is irregular with inconsistent cycle durations. During quiet sleep, periodic breathing is regular with consistent duration and intervals of breathing pauses.
  - Apnea
    - Apnea is the cessation of ventilation of longer than 20 seconds; shorter breathing pauses (15 seconds) can be considered apneas if associated with bradycardia and desaturation.
    - The mechanism of bradycardia is unclear and usually follows apnea and oxygen desaturation but may be coincidental with apnea and may occur without oxygen desaturation.
    - Apneic episodes are classified as:
      - Central, with a lack of respiratory effort due to immaturity of the central nervous system and immature chemoreceptor functions/response causing an absence of chest wall movement.
      - Obstructive, with obstructed breaths in the presence of respiratory efforts; airflow cessation occurs due to absent coordination of respiratory musculature, pharyngeal instability, nasal obstruction, and neck flexion. Central regulation of the pharyngeal tone is important for airway patency maintenance.
      - Mixed, with an initial loss of central respiratory drive along with delayed activation of upper airway muscles superimposed on a closed airway; these combinations of events result in prolonged mixed apnea.

- Causes of apnea
  - Preterm infants—idiopathic (apnea of prematurity), involving central nervous system manifestations of immature breathing pattern causes (seizures, intracranial hemorrhage, hypothermia, depressant drugs), pulmonary causes (pneumonia, especially due to respiratory syncytial virus [RSV]; laryngeal reflex; vocal cord paralysis; pneumothorax; tracheal occlusion caused by neck flexion), sepsis, metabolic causes (hypoglycemia, hypocalcemia, hyponatremia, hypernatremia), and anemia
  - Term infants—intrapartum asphyxia, brainstem depression due to drugs (narcotics, magnesium sulfate, general anesthetics), airway obstruction (choanal atresia, mandibular hypoplasia), neuromuscular lesions (muscle weakness), trauma (phrenic nerve palsy, spinal cord transection), and central nervous system conditions (seizures, Dandy-Walker malformation, central hypoventilation syndrome)

Disorders of Control of Breathing

APNEA OF PREMATURITY

Overview

- Pathophysiology—AOP is the consequence of immaturity of central respiratory control centers and the altered ventilatory responses to hypercapnia and hypoxia. There is a genetic component to causation, as there is greater concordance of AOP in monozygotic twins compared to same-sex dizygotic twins.
- Incidence—the incidence varies: <10% of infants born >34 weeks' gestation, 60% of infants born with birth weight <1500 g, and >85% of infants born with birth weight <1000 g.

Clinical Presentation

- Clinical symptoms may manifest during the first day of life, but usually appear later. Peak incidence of symptoms is between 4 and 6 weeks after birth, corresponding with increased sensitivity of peripheral chemoreceptors and, therefore, greater respiratory instability. Mixed apnea is the most common type of apnea during AOP.

Diagnosis

- The diagnosis is made clinically using bedside observation of prolonged apnea (>20 seconds) on standard impedance monitoring, especially when such apnea is associated with bradycardia and oxygen desaturation. Although there is no consensus, at least one visually confirmed apnea associated with bradycardia and desaturation is required to diagnose AOP. Impedance-based monitors cannot be used to diagnose obstructive apnea, and prolonged episodes of obstructive episodes are diagnosed when resultant central apnea or bradycardia and oxygen desaturation trigger an alarm.

Treatment

- When other causes of apnea have been excluded (such as infection), treatment for AOP is considered.
  - *Methylxanthines*—caffeine, theophylline, and aminophylline are used but caffeine is preferred due to its high therapeutic index and long half-life, and monitoring its plasma concentrations is not routinely required.
    - Methylxanthines act both peripherally and centrally.
    - They activate central respiratory centers, increase sensitivity to hypercarbia, induce bronchodilation, and enhance diaphragm function.
    - Beneficial effects include increased minute ventilation, more stable respiratory pattern, and reduced hypoxic respiratory depression.
    - Side effects include increased metabolic rate, which may lead to transient slowing of physical growth, tachycardia, and irritability.
    - Although routine drug level monitoring is not recommended, if performed, the therapeutic level of caffeine is 5 to 25 µg/mL, and toxicities are generally not seen until the levels exceed 40 µg/mL.
    - Other benefits of methylxanthines include that its use facilitates extubation. Caffeine treatment started within 3 days after birth is associated with reduced bronchopulmonary dysplasia, less patent ductus arteriosus treatment, reduced severity of retinopathy of prematurity, and a reduction in some long-term neurologic deficits.
    - Methylxanthines are stopped when AOP symptoms resolve, usually around 33 to 36 weeks' PMA. Extended courses may be used to reduce frequent intermittent hypoxia. After caffeine is discontinued, infants are generally monitored for 5 to 7 days for the reemergence of clinically signifiacnt AOP, but a longer duration of observation may be considered for infants born at 25 weeks' gestation or less. It may be necessary to individualize specific duration of observation without events based on the gestational age at birth and or the severity of events noted during NICU stay. Caffeine levels may not become subtherapeutic for 11 to 12 days after discontinuation in extremely low-birth-weight infants.
  - *Respiratory support*—nasal continuous positive airway pressure (NCPAP), nasal intermittent positive pressure ventilation (NIPPV), high-flow nasal cannula (HFNC), and invasive mechanical ventilation (IMV) have been used to treat the symptoms of AOP.
    - NCPAP helps improve functional residual capacity and prevents pharyngeal collapse, leading to significant reductions in AOP symptoms.
    - HFNC reduces the amount of dead space and can also provide continuous distending pressure like CPAP. Safety concerns have been raised, as the pressure produced is unpredictable and can be very high.
    - If, despite methylxanthines and NCPAP, AOP symptoms persist, then NIPPV or IMV is required. When IMV is required, infants should be evaluated for infections, sepsis, and seizures.
  - *Doxapram*—doxapram is a nonspecific central nervous system stimulant sometimes used in the treatment of AOP. Doxapram requires continuous intravenous infusion, and side effects include hypertension, tachycardia, jitteriness, vomiting, and low seizure threshold.
    - With regard to treatment of gastroesophageal reflux (GER), most evidence suggests that there is no causal link between GER and AOP. Physiologic observations have shown that apnea is more likely to lead to, rather than be caused by, GER. Antireflux medications have not been shown to reduce the number of AOP-related episodes.
    - Other treatments include CO_2 inhalation, sensory stimulation, and low-flow nasal cannula delivering room air.
  - Resolution with time
    - AOP progressively improves over time and in most infants resolves by 34 to 36 weeks' PMA. In more immature infants, AOP symptoms may persist until 43 to 44 weeks' PMA.
    - Episodes of clinically intermittent hypoxia and bradycardia often continue beyond the resolution of clinically apparent apnea but are generally too brief to trigger an alarm or cause visible cyanosis.
    - Infants who had AOP-related symptoms within the last 5 days prior to neonatal intensive care unit (NICU) discharge have a greater likelihood of having a significant cardiovascular episode postdischarge. However, no consensus exists on the required number of AOP symptom-free days prior to discharging the infant.
    - Premature infants with a history of AOP are at higher risk of RSV-related apnea and apnea associated with exposure to general anesthesia (GA). The risk for apnea associated with GA does not reduce to <1% until after 54 to 56 weeks' PMA.
- Neurodevelopmental outcome in infants with AOP
  - Precisely defined predischarge apnea has been associated with lower developmental indices at 2 years of age.
  - Similarly, infants with greater cardiorespiratory events on home monitors after discharge are also associated with impaired neurodevelopmental outcomes.
  - The impact of treatment of AOP in the hospital or the prevention of cardiovascular events postdischarge on neurodevelopmental outcomes is unknown.

SUDDEN INFANT DEATH SYNDROME

- Sudden infant death syndrome (SIDS) is the sudden death of an infant that is unexplained by a thorough postmortem exam, which includes a complete autopsy, investigation of the scene of death, and review of the medical history.
- SIDS is the third leading cause of infant mortality in the United States, representing 8% of all infant deaths.
- A triple-risk model has been proposed to explain causation: critical developmental period (first 6 months), vulnerable infant (preterm infant, growth restricted infant, exposure to smoking or drugs in utero), and extrinsic factors (prone/side sleep position, soft bedding, overbundling, overheating, bed sharing, and parental smoking or alcohol use).
- The rate of SIDS peaks between 1 and 4 months of age, and 95% of cases occur by 6 to 8 months of age.
- Back to Sleep campaign—the annual rate of SIDS dropped from 1.3 to 1.4/1000 live births in 1992, before the Back to Sleep campaign, to 0.55/1000 live births in 2001 after the widespread use of supine sleep position began.

- Preterm infants have 2.5 to 2.7 times the risk of SIDS compared to term infants. Reasons for higher rates of SIDS in preterm infants include brainstem dysfunction and increased vulnerability to SIDS from prone positioning.
- The current American Academy of Pediatrics policy statement on SIDS does not recommend the use of home monitors for the prevention of SIDS.

BRIEF RESOLVED UNEXPLAINED EVENTS

- Brief resolved unexplained events (BRUEs) were previously known as apparent life-threatening events (ALTEs).
- A BRUE is defined as a sudden, unexpected change in an infant (color, tone, breathing, and/or level of responsiveness) that is frightening and perceived as life-threatening to the caregiver.
- Infants born preterm are at an increased risk for a BRUE. The incidence of BRUE varies from 0.5 to 10/1000 live births (the high variability is due to the different definitions), but the incidence in preterm infants is reported to be 8% to 10%.
- About half of BRUEs are idiopathic and are thought to be sleep related.
- There is no evidence that BRUEs are precursors of SIDS. Idiopathic BRUEs and SIDS may share some common mechanisms. The risk of SIDS may be as much as three to five times greater in infants who have experienced BRUE compared with healthy controls.

SLEEP DISORDERED BREATHING

- About 4% of children have sleep disordered breathing (SDB).
- Infants born preterm are at higher risk of SDB, with some studies showing a two- to threefold increased risk compared to infants born at term.
- SDB is associated with neurodevelopmental impairment in preterm infants and is likely mediated by intermittent hypoxia.
- Infants born preterm are also at higher risk for later obesity, which is an independent risk factor for SDB.

Suggested Readings

Doyle J, Davidson D, Katz S, et al. Apnea of prematurity and caffeine pharmacokinetics: potential impact on hospital discharge. *J Perinatol.* 2016;36:141–144.

Eichenwald EC. AAP Committee on Fetus and Newborn. Apnea of prematurity. *Pediatrics.* 2016;137(1):e20153757.

Moon RY. Task Force on Sudden Infant Death Syndrome. SIDS and other sleep-related infant deaths: evidence base for 2016 updated recommendations for a safe infant sleeping environment. *Pediatrics.* 2016;138(5):peds.2016–peds.2940.

Tieder JS, Bonkowsky JL, Etzel RA, et al. Brief resolved unexplained events (formerly apparent life-threatening events) and evaluation of lower-risk infants. *Pediatrics.* 2016;137(5):e20160590.

7 Assisted Ventilation, ECMO, and Pharmacologic Agents

PATRICIA R. CHESS

Assisted Ventilation

RESPIRATORY SUPPORT (TABLE 7.1)

- Respiratory support is utilized when oxygenation and/or ventilation are inadequate.
- Care is taken to optimize positive end expiratory pressure (PEEP) to avoid atelectasis (suggesting that PEEP is too low) and to avoid overdistention (suggesting air trapping or that PEEP is too high), which can lead to impeded venous return to the thorax/heart and subsequent hypotension pneumothorax.
- Regardless of method of respiratory support, in general, target lungs 9 to 9-1/2 ribs expanded assessed by chest x-ray (CXR) for most pathophysiologies, 8 to 8-1/2 ribs expanded if air leak occurs (pneumothorax [PTX], pulmonary interstitial emphysema [PIE]), pulmonary hypoplasia, or congenital diaphragmatic hernia (CDH). PEEP has the greatest impact on lung expansion.
- Targeted tidal volume in preterm is 4 to 6 cc/kg; term, 5 to 8 cc/kg.
- Any mode of ventilation that uses an endotracheal tube can lead to airway damage (acute or chronic) or subglottic stenosis (chronic), as well as present a risk of ventilator-associated pneumonia.
- Positive pressure ventilation, including noninvasive ventilation, can lead to overdistention and increase the risk of a pneumothorax.
- CO_2 is mostly affected by tidal volume, rate, and expiratory time.
- Oxygenation is mostly affected by the mean airway pressure and fraction of inspired oxygen (FiO_2).

TYPES OF VENTILATION

- Continuous positive airway pressure (CPAP) PEEP provides distending pressure to alveoli via CPAP prongs in nares to maintain alveolar distention and improve oxygenation in infants with adequate spontaneous respirations. There is a risk of pneumothorax and nasal septum breakdown.
- Synchronized intermittent mandatory ventilation (SIMV)
- Volume-targeted ventilation
  - Set rate, PEEP, inspiratory time (iTime), target volume; delivers pressure needed to establish the set volume; pressure limit set; risk of high pressure to maintain target volume; able to set pressure limit to minimize risk
  - Used for bronchopulmonary dysplasia (BPD) and homogeneous lung disease in full-term infants when compliance does not change significantly

- Pressure-targeted ventilation
  - Set rate, PEEP, iTime, peak pressure to be achieved; does not guarantee a set volume; risk of underventilation/atelectasis
  - Used for rapidly changing compliance to minimize risk of pneumothorax such as respiratory distress syndrome (RDS); with improved technology, volume-targeted ventilation with pressure limits can be used safely.
- Control mode (e.g., assist control)
  - Each breath is fully supported; there is a risk of gas trapping.
  - Used to fully support each breath in critically ill infants
- Pressure support mode
  - Delivers both mandatory and assisted (support) breaths; support breath peak inspiratory pressure is slowly decreased to wean from mechanical ventilation.
  - Used to facilitate gentle weaning
- High-frequency oscillator ventilator (HFOV)
  - Diaphragm in the oscillator moves to and fro, providing active inspiration and expiration (only mode where expiration is active).
    - Mean airway pressure (MAP) primarily affects oxygenation. To transition from conventional ventilation (CV) to HFO, typically set 1 to 2 cm H_2O above MAP on CV or consider MAP on CV if air leak; adjust MAP based on saturations and CXR to targeted desired lung expansion.
    - Frequency—rate reflects the number of to and fro movements of the diaphragm. In general,
      - Premature infants, 15 Hz
      - Term infants, 10 Hz
    - Power (amplitude, delta p) primarily affects CO_2 removal; it reflects the delta of the diaphragm from midline; target shaking to the groin.
  - There is a risk of over-/underdistention if PEEP is not optimized, an air leak if infant is not weaned when compliance improves, and impeded cardiac return if MAP too high.
  - Use in air leak and homogeneous lung disease.
  - Pressures are significantly attenuated before reaching the alveolae.
- High-frequency jet ventilator (HFJV)
  - Interrupted gas flow leads to a "jet" spike of air down central air spaces for inspiration and swirling of air up the periphery of air spaces of expired air.
  - Active inspiration, passive expiration
  - Peak inspiratory pressure (PIP) and PEEP are significantly attenuated.

Table 7.1   Modes of Respiratory Support

Name	Effects	Uses	Contraindication	Risks
Oxyhood	Provides supplemental O_2	Mild hypoxia without significant increased work of breathing or CO_2 retention	Inadequate ventilation	Hyperoxic end organ damage, primarily to lungs and in case of premature infants, ROP
Low-flow nasal cannula (LFNC, <2 LPM)	Dead space washout improves gas exchange	Weaning from mechanical ventilation	Apnea, NEC	Pneumothorax, gastric distention
High-flow nasal cannula (HFNC, >2 LPM)				
Nasal continuous positive airway pressure (NCPAP)	Avoids atelectasis, stabilizes FRC, improves apnea and intermittent hypoxia events	RDS, weaning from mechanical ventilation	Prolonged apnea, NEC	Pneumothorax, gastric distention, nasal bridge erosion
Noninvasive (asynchronous or synchronous) positive pressure ventilation (NIPPV or sNIPPV, respectively)	Avoids atelectasis, stabilizes FRC	Mild–moderate respiratory distress, weaning from mechanical ventilation	Early RDS, NEC	Pneumothorax, gastric distention, nasal bridge erosion
Synchronized intermittent mandatory ventilation (SIMV)	Maintains lung expansion	Respiratory failure	—	Pneumothorax, volutrauma, atelectotrauma
Pressure support ventilation	Helps overcome elastic and resistive forces	Typically used in SIMV mode during weaning	—	Pneumothorax, volutrauma, atelectotrauma
Pressure–volume control ventilation	Fully supports each breath	Severe respiratory failure	—	Pneumothorax, volutrauma, atelectotrauma, stacking breaths
High-frequency jet ventilation (HFJV)	Active inspiration, passive expiration	PIE, air leak, nonhomogeneous lung disease	—	Air trapping, hyperventilation
High-frequency oscillatory ventilation (HFOV)	Active inspiration and expiration	Homogeneous lung disease	Use with caution with cardiac dysfunction	Impeded blood return to heart

FRC, Functional residual capacity; *LPM*, liters per minute; *NEC*, necrotizing enterocolitis; *PIE*, pulmonary interstitial emphysema; *RDS*, respiratory distress syndrome; *ROP*, retinopathy of prematurity; *SIMV*, synchronized intermittent mandatory ventilation.

- Transitioning from CV to jet:
  - Set PIP and PEEP similar to CV and adjust based on exam, CXR, and blood gases.
  - Jet rate is based on gestational age and disease process but is typically 240 to 420 breaths per minute (typically lower in term, higher in preterm).
  - Initially set CV (provides "background rate," PIP) in tandem with jet until PEEP is optimized; wean rate on CV when possible with target CV rate zero.
- Used for nonhomogeneous lung disease, air leak, PIE, pulmonary hypoplasia, cardiac compromise when high-frequency ventilation is indicated, and aspiration syndromes

VENTILATION STRATEGIES BASED ON PATHOPHYSIOLOGY

- RDS—avoid atelectasis with optimal PEEP, adequate surfactant replacement, high rates, low tidal volume (lung has low compliance and short time constant so it empties quickly). Noninvasive ventilatory support, when tolerated, is optimal.
- BPD—provide low rates with higher tidal volumes to allow adequate time for expiration and minimize air trapping and overdistention (lung has high compliance and long time constant, so it empties slowly).
- Meconium aspiration syndrome (MAS)—provide optimized PEEP and MAP and ensure adequate expiratory time; there is a high risk of ball–valve air trapping/pneumothorax due to meconium plugs.

- Pneumonia is often homogeneous in neonates, as hematogenous spread is common. Ensure adequate PEEP to achieve 9 to 9-1/2 rib expansion.
- Air leak (PIE, pneumothorax)/pulmonary hypoplasia/CDH—target 8 to 8-1/2 ribs, avoid overdistention, and avoid PIP > 25 in full-term infants.

MONITORING BABIES ON MECHANICAL VENTILATION

- Standard intensive care unit monitoring can help give clues to issues. Prolonged periods of no spontaneous respirations can suggest oversedation, significant neurologic compromise, or overventilation/hypocapnea with loss of respiratory drive. Tachycardia with hypotension can result if MAP is impeding venous return to the heart.
- Change in saturation can suggest need for suction, pneumothorax, or change in compliance. Improved oxygenation suggests improved pulmonary function and need to wean. Weaning MAP should be considered, given the risk of a pneumothorax if compliance improves and MAP is not weaned. The use of a transcutaneous CO_2 monitor or frequent blood gas monitoring is suggested to follow CO_2 in infants on high-frequency ventilation, as large swings can occur. End-tidal CO_2 monitors can be used in term infants but will increase the dead space.
- Following pressure–flow and pressure–volume loops on CV can help guide management strategies, identifying changes in compliance, gas trapping, airway obstruction, etc. (Figs. 7.1 to 7.3).

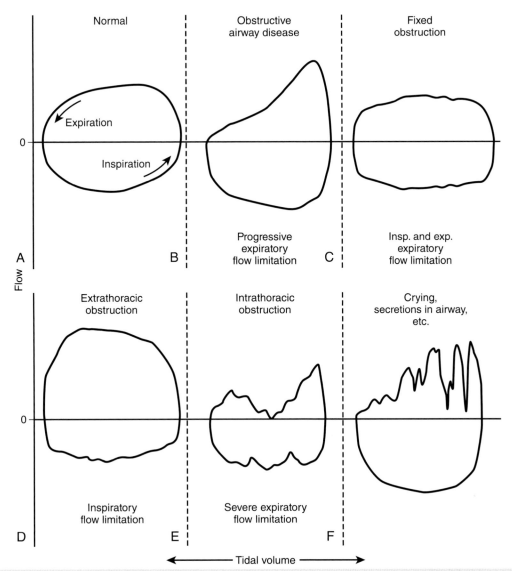

Fig. 7.1 Flow–volume loops in normal, abnormal conditions. Tidal flow–volume loops illustrating various manifestations of flow limitation that result from heterogeneity in airway resistance. (A) Normal loop. (B) "Ski-slope" loop observed with expiratory airflow limitation as seen in babies with bronchopulmonary dysplasia. (C) Extrathoracic airway obstruction with inspiratory and expiratory airflow limitation as seen in babies with subglottic stenosis or narrow endotracheal tube. (D) Intrathoracic inspiratory airflow limitation as seen in babies with intraluminal obstruction (close to the carina) or an aberrant vessel compressing the trachea. (E) Unstable airways or tracheomalacia. (F) This type of loop usually is suggestive of an erratic airflow limitation, as seen with airway secretions. (See Fig. 12.6 in Goldsmith et al., 2017.)

- Although there are limited data to support specific blood gas targets, Table 7.2 has been created based on relevant literature and expert opinion and can be used as a general guide to target blood gases. If one needs to utilize extreme settings on the ventilator to achieve these gases, consideration of modifying the type of ventilation or target blood gas range should be discussed.

Respiratory Pharmacologic Agents

- Surfactant is given intratracheally to improve compliance in surfactant deficiency (RDS) or reverse surfactant inactivation (aspiration syndromes). Risks include transient hypoxia/bradycardia due to airway obstruction and nonhomogeneous distribution with subsequent unequal aeration and pneumothorax if compliance rapidly improves and ventilator pressures are not weaned.

- Aminophylline and caffeine have been shown to increase respiratory center activity, decrease severe apneas in preterm infants, help facilitate extubation, and decrease BPD rates. Caffeine is preferred (see Chapter 6)
- Diuretics have been shown to facilitate extubation for premature infants but have not been demonstrated to change long-term outcomes.
- Dexamethasone, a synthetic glucocorticoid, improves compliance and decreases inflammation. It has been shown to increase the risk of cerebral palsy (CP) and gastrointestinal perforation when used early (<14 days). It can affect growth and alveolarization, in addition to increasing the risk of infection, leading to hypertension and hyperglycemia. Late glucocorticoids (>14 days) have been associated with decreased mortality and risk of BPD. The use and timing of glucocorticoids must

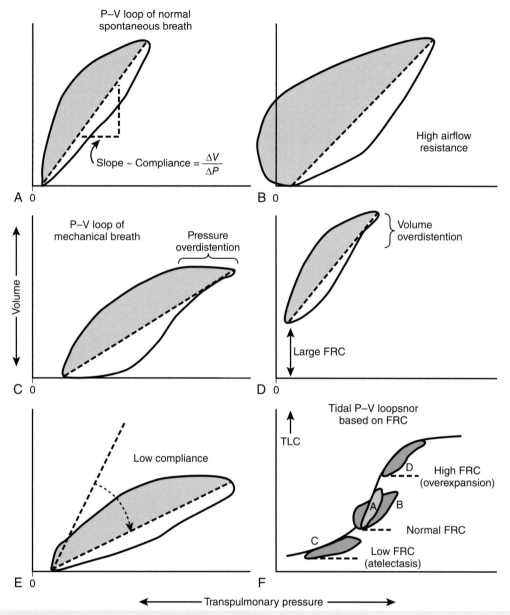

Fig. 7.2 Pressure–volume loops in normal, ventilated, and abnormal lungs. Pressure–volume (P-V) relationship illustrations show components of inspiratory elastic work and inspiratory elastic and resistive work. (A) A normal P-V relationship. (B) Increased expiratory resistive work (such as obstructive airway disease, meconium aspiration syndrome, or bronchopulmonary dysplasia). (C) Increased expiratory resistive work with excessive inspiratory pressure (such as overdistention due to high positive inspiratory pressure or high tidal volume). (D) Increased expiratory resistive work due to excessive functional residual capacity (such as overdistention due to air trapping, shortened expiratory time, etc.). (E) Decreased inspiratory elastic work (such as respiratory distress syndrome, pneumonia, atelectasis, etc.). (F) Comparison of P-V relationships affected by the functional residual capacity. *FRC,* Functional residual capacity; *TLC,* total lung capacity. (From Goldsmith P, et al. *Assisted Ventilation of the Neonate: Evidence-Based Approach to Newborn Respiratory Care.* 6th ed. Philadelphia: Elsevier; 2017:114.)

take into consideration the risk/benefit ratio, which is still under investigation.

- Hydrocortisone, a naturally occurring glucocorticoid, improves compliance, decreases inflammation, and increases the risk of infection, hyperglycemia, and hypertension.
- Inhaled glucocorticoids provide targeted delivery and reduce pulmonary inflammation, but there are only limited studies on long-term benefits.
- Inhaled nitric oxide (iNO)
    - iNO is US Food and Drug Administration (FDA) approved to treat respiratory failure from pulmonary hypertension in infants > 34 weeks' gestation.

- NO is naturally occurring in vascular endothelial cells, formed from L-arginine by nitric oxide synthase, which then diffuses into neighboring vascular smooth muscle cells activating guanylyl cyclase (GC). GC converts guanosine-5′-triphosphate (GTP) to cyclic guanosine monophosphate (cGMP), leading to vascular relaxation via calcium efflux and decreased intracellular calcium.
- Figure 7.4 shows the signaling pathway of NO.
- NO is used as continuous inhaled gas (due to a half-life of 15–30 seconds) to promote relaxation of pulmonary vascular bed in infants with hypoxic respiratory failure. Center-specific protocols should be developed,

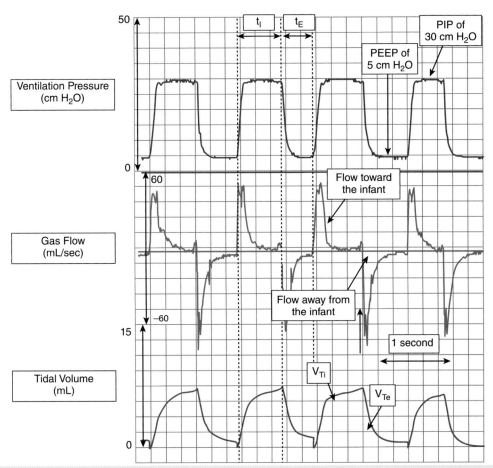

Fig. 7.3 Flow mechanics during positive pressure ventilation in neonate. Using this display on the conventional ventilator can give key information related to air leak, gas trapping, etc. *PEEP,* Positive end expiratory pressure; *PIP,* peak inspiratory pressure. (From Goldsmith P, et al. *Assisted Ventilation of the Neonate: Evidence-Based Approach to Newborn Respiratory Care.* 6th ed. Philadelphia: Elsevier; 2017:284.)

Table 7.2   Target Arterial Blood Gases for Various Disease Processes

Diagnosis	RDS	PPHN/PNA (Term)	PIE/PTX	CDH	BPD
pH	7.25–7.35	7.35–7.45	7.25–7.30	7.30–7.35	7.25–7.30
pCO_2	45–50	35–45	55–60	45–60	50–65
pO_2	50–70	60–100	50–60	60–80	50–60

BPD, Bronchopulmonary dysplasia; *CDH,* congenital diaphragmatic hernia; *pCO₂,* partial pressure of carbon dioxide; *pO₂,* partial pressure of oxygen; *PIE,* pulmonary interstitial emphysema; *PNA,* pneumonia; *PPHN,* persistent pulmonary hypertension of the newborn; *PTX,* pneumothorax; *RDS,* respiratory distress syndrome.

but in general an oxygenation index (OI) > 15 to 25 is used as starting parameter for iNO initiation after other factors such as pulmonary expansion and cardiac function are optimized.

■ iNO can lead to pulmonary edema if used in patients with left ventricular dysfunction or left-sided cardiac obstructive lesions, so it is important to obtain echocardiograms before starting.

■ Maximum dose typically used is 20 ppm. Wean infant quickly if no response, and stop within 1 hour of starting; otherwise, it is necessary to wean more slowly, especially when weaning from 5 to 0 ppm, due to downregulation of endogenous NO.

■ High oxygen and iNO can lead to direct damage from toxic reactive oxidants (peroxynitrites and nitrogen dioxide).

■ There is a risk of methemoglobinemia and elevated NO_2 at high doses. It is dose dependent, with lower risk at the current doses used.

■ Ensure extracorporeal membrane oxygenation (ECMO) availability or, at minimum if an ECMO center is not immediately available, the ability to transfer to an ECMO center on iNO before initiating iNO in case escalation of care is needed.

Extracorporeal Membrane Oxygenation

■ ECMO is used in cases of severe *reversible* cardiac or respiratory compromise not responsive to other therapies.

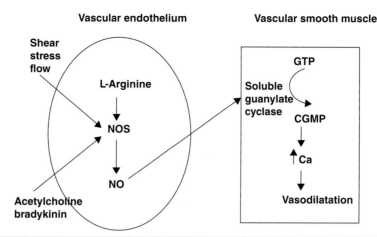

Fig. 7.4 Signaling pathway of NO. *CGMP,* Cyclic guanosine monophosphate; *GTP,* guanosine-5′-triphosphate; *NO,* nitrous oxide; *NOS,* nitric oxide synthase.

- Indications—original indications are based on the OI and alveolar–arterial (A-a) gradient that predicted an 80% mortality when ECMO first became available (OI > 40; A-aDO$_2$, 600–620). Subsequent medical advances (e.g., surfactant, iNO, high-frequency ventilation) have improved survival in those situations, so additional indications such as echocardiogram assessment of cardiac dysfunction, refractory lactic acidosis, hypotension, or hypoxia are also considered before starting ECMO.
- ECMO provides pulmonary (venovenous) or cardiopulmonary (venoarterial) support in infants with reversible cardiac and/or respiratory failure.
- ECMO requires anticoagulation to avoid circuit clotting with subsequent risk of hemorrhage.
- If an infant with CDH needs a PIP > 25 to maintain target blood gases (allowing permissive hypercapnia) or with iNO presurgical repair, ECMO should be strongly considered.
- When discussing ECMO as a treatment option, goals of care and expectations should be discussed with family before initiating, especially because infants sometimes are unable to wean from the circuit after an extended period of time.
- Venous cannula in right atrium via internal jugular vein (IJV), arterial cannula in internal carotid artery terminates as it joins aorta

- Risks include hemorrhage, infection, clots, long-term hearing loss, and neurodevelopmental impairment.
- Contraindications:
  - Irreversible fatal disease
  - Irreversible severe neurologic dysfunction
  - Uncontrolled bleeding
  - More than 7 to 10 days of injurious mechanical ventilation
  - Prematurity < 34 weeks due to risk of intraventricular hemorrhage (IVH) and technical limitations of placing an adequately sized cannula

Suggested Readings

Brodie D, Peek G, MacLaren, G et al., eds. *Extracorporeal Life Support: The ELSO Red Book.* 6th ed. Ann Arbor: Extracorporeal Life Support Organization; 2022.

Durand D, Courtney S. Neonatal respiratory therapy. In: Gleason CA, Sawyer T, eds. *Avery's Diseases of the Newborn.* 11th ed. Philadelphia: Elsevier; 2023:559–579.

Goldsmith JP, Karotkin E, Suresh G, Keszler M. *Assisted Ventilation of the Neonate: Evidence-Based Approach to Newborn Respiratory Care.* 6th ed. Philadelphia: Elsevier; 2017.

West JB, Luks A. *West's Respiratory Physiology: The Essentials.* 11th ed. Baltimore: Lippincott Williams & Wilkins; 2020.

Cardiovascular

KIMBERLY VERA

8 *Cardiac Development*

KIMBERLY VERA

Normal Cardiac Morphogenesis

- Cardiac progenitor cells migrate from the mesoderm to form a crescent shape in the lateral plate mesoderm (Fig. 8.1).
- The first heart field cells fuse in the midline to form the primitive heart tube, which begins to beat around day 17, becoming the first organ to function (Fig. 8.2).
- The cephalad portion of the primitive heart tube will become the future outflow region, and the caudal portion will become future atria.
- The primitive heart tube folds to the right as the second heart field cells migrate into the tube.
- First heart field cells give rise to the left ventricle and some of the atria; second heart field cells give rise to the remaining atria, right ventricle, and outflow tracts (Fig. 8.3).
- Folding of the heart tube places the outflow portion, or conotruncal portion, of the tube adjacent to the inflow portions and creates an outer curve, which develops into ventricles, and an inner curve, which develops into the atrioventricular canal and atrioventricular septum (Fig. 8.4).

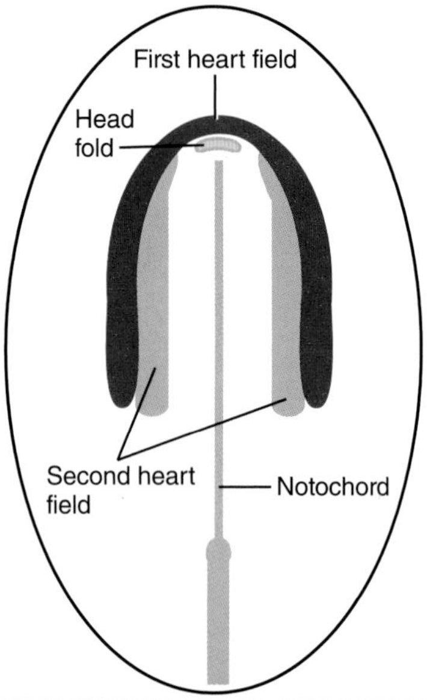

- The atrioventricular septum develops from the endocardial cushions to divide the primitive common atrioventricular valve into a tricuspid and mitral valve and must shift to the right. It aligns with the developing ventricular septum and positions the future tricuspid valve over the right ventricle and the future mitral valve over the left ventricle (Fig. 8.5).
- Conotruncal development:
    - The early common outflow tract, the conotruncus, is septated into an aorta and pulmonary artery, which rotates and then shifts to the left to align the conotruncal septum over the developing ventricular septum. This allows the aorta to arise from the left ventricle and the pulmonary artery to arise from the right ventricle (Fig. 8.6).
    - Conotruncal development requires extensive interaction between second heart field cells, neural crest cells, and pharyngeal tissues.
- Development of the great arteries:
    - The aortic sac contains six bilateral arches, which undergo complex remodeling.
    - The third, fourth, and sixth arches become mature arches and proximal pulmonary arteries.
    - Most of the right arches undergo programmed cell death to leave a left-sided mature arch.

Regulators of Cardiac Embryology

See Box 8.1.

- NKX2.5, GATA4, HAND1, and many Tbox transcription factors are major transcription regulators that drive the expression of myocardial-specific genes and lead cells to myocardial commitment.
- TBX20 is expressed throughout the heart tube to ensure specific chamber myocyte differentiation.
- Left–right asymmetry is mediated by the expression of Sonic hedgehog (Shh) in the left lateral mesoderm, which induces the expression of nodal and lefty proteins (members of the transforming growth factor beta [TGF-β] family). This drives the rightward folding of the primitive heart tube. Nodal pathways induce the transcription factor Pitx2c in the left limb of the cardiac crescent and also contribute to left–right differentiation.
- Left ventricular development is driven by NKX2.5, HAND1, and TBX5.
- Islet 1 is important in right ventricular development
- TBX5 and COUP-TFII are important in atrial development.
- TBX1 plays an important role in outflow tract development.

Fig. 8.1 Development of first and second heart field. Crescent-like shape is caused by progenitor migration pattern and cardiogenic induction signals. (From Schoenwolf GC. *Larsen's Human Embryology.* 5th ed. Philadelphia: Elsevier; 2015.)

Box 8.1   Major Transcription Factors in Cardiac Development

ISL1—Right ventricle
NKX2.5—Left ventricle
HAND1—Left ventricle
TBX5—Left ventricle, atria
COUP-TGII—Atria
TBX1—Outflow tract
Shh—Left–right differentiation
Pitx2c—Left–right differentiation

Abnormal Cardiac Morphogenesis

- Failure of the atrioventricular (AV) septum to shift to the right will lead to a double-inlet left ventricle.
- Incomplete shifting leads to an unbalanced AV septal defect, with the right AV valve only partially over the right ventricle.
- If the conotruncus does not shift to the left, a double-outlet right ventricle forms.
- If the conotruncus does not septate, a truncus arteriosus forms.

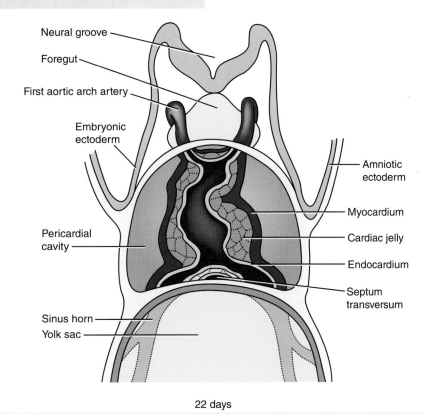

22 days

Fig. 8.2 Primitive heart tube. (From Schoenwolf GC. *Larsen's Human Embryology*. 5th ed. Philadelphia: Elsevier; 2015.)

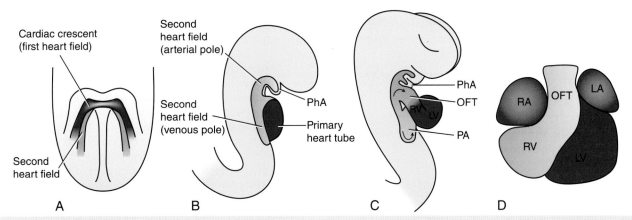

Fig. 8.3 Structures derived from the first and second heart fields. (A) Location of the second heart field relative to the first heart field before body folding. The second heart field is located within the splanchnic mesoderm just medial and slightly caudal to the first heart field (first heart field shown in *red*). (B) After formation of the primary heart tube, the second heart field becomes located dorsal to the dorsal mesocardium and runs along the cranio-caudal axis. (C) With rupture of the dorsal mesocardium, the second heart field is divided into a caudal segment, responsible for adding to the venous pole of the heart, and a cranial segment, responsible for lengthening the heart tube at the arterial pole. (D) Ventral view of the looped heart shows the contributions of the first and second heart fields (contributions of the second heart field to the atria are not visible in this view). *LA*, Left atrium; *LV*, left ventricle; *OFT*, outflow tract; *PA*, primitive atria; *PhA*, pharyngeal arch tube; *RA*, right atrium; *RV*, right ventricle. (From Schoenwolf GC. *Larsen's Human Embryology*. 5th ed. Philadelphia: Elsevier; 2015.)

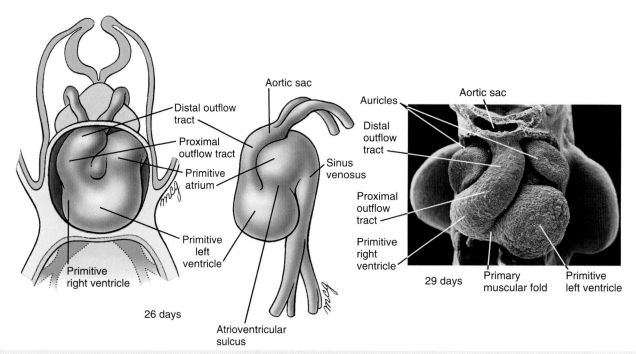

Fig. 8.4 Primitive heart tube folds to the right, creating an inner and outer curvature. (From Schoenwolf GC. *Larsen's Human Embryology.* 5th ed. Philadelphia: Elsevier; 2015.)

- If the conotruncus does not rotate, transposition of the great arteries develops.
- Incomplete rotation of the conotruncus can lead to tetralogy of Fallot because the conal septum is no longer aligned with the ventricular septum, leading to a ventricular septal defect, with the conal septum causing obstruction to pulmonary outflow.
- Arch anomalies arise from abnormal persistence and/or cell death of the six embryonic arches.
    - An interrupted arch develops from abnormalities of the fourth arch.
    - Abnormalities of the pulmonary arteries develop from abnormalities of the sixth arch.
    - Persistence of the right-sided dorsal and aortic arches, with abnormal regression on the left, leads to a right-sided aortic arch.
- Abnormal development of any proximal cardiac structures leading to decreased flow can cause secondary hypoplasia of downstream structures.

Developmental Changes of the Myocyte and Contraction

- The contractile unit of the myocyte is the sarcomere, which is made up of myofibrils.
- Contraction of the sarcomere is triggered by calcium binding to troponin.
- In the mature myocyte, membrane depolarization triggers calcium influx at L-type calcium channels found in the T tubules of the cell membrane. This small influx of calcium binds to the ryanodine receptor of the sarcoplasmic reticulum due to the close physical relationship of the T tubules and sarcoplasmic reticulum in the mature myocyte. The sarcoplasmic reticulum then releases a large amount of calcium into the cytosol allowing

calcium binding to troponin. This is termed *calcium-induced calcium release.*
- Immature myocytes have more physical separation of the sarcoplasmic reticulum and the cell membrane, as well as the absence of T tubules, leaving the cell dependent on calcium influx at the cell membrane alone. Calcium-induced calcium release does not occur in the immature myocyte; the sodium-calcium exchanger is primarily responsible for calcium influx into the cytosol.
- Several structural differences of the immature myocyte lead to less force generated with sarcomeric contraction:
    - Myofibrils are disorganized in fetal and early newborn hearts; organization of myofibrils along the long axis of the cell occurs with development.
    - Sarcomeric protein isoform expression changes with development; the troponin I isoform (TnI-s) is predominant in fetal life and changes to TnI-c by 9 months of age, allowing for increased force of contraction.
    - Mitochondria aggregate in the center of the immature myocyte and then become regularly distributed along the myofibrils with maturation.
- In immature hearts, lactate and carbohydrates are the primary energy sources, with transition to long-chain fatty acid in mature hearts.
- Cardiac growth in fetal life is mainly due to cell division, with resultant increase in cell number. After birth, cardiac growth is driven by hypertrophy in existing myocytes.

Maternal Diseases With Fetal Cardiac Manifestations

- Diabetes mellitus
    - There is a fivefold increase of cardiac anomalies in infants of diabetic mothers.

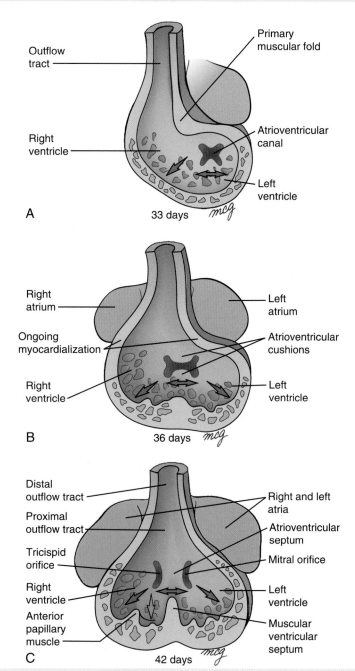

Fig. 8.5 Developing atrioventricular valve shifting to the right. (A–C) Realignment of the heart. As the atrioventricular septum forms during the fifth and sixth weeks, the heart is remodeled to align the developing left atrioventricular canal with the left atrium and ventricle, and the right atrioventricular canal with the right atrium and ventricle. *Red arrows* indicate the direction of realignment of the atrioventricular canal and outflow tract and formation of the muscular interventricular septum. The *blue arrow* in C indicates formation of an enlarging slit carved out of the muscular ventricular septum; this is responsible in part for repositioning of the tricuspid orifice to the right, as well as for formation of the moderator band.
(From Schoenwolf GC. *Larsen's Human Embryology.* 5th ed. Philadelphia: Elsevier; 2015.)

- Ventricular septal defects are the most common cardiac defect.
- Transposition of the great arteries is markedly increased.
- Other defects seen include hypoplastic left heart syndrome, coarctation of the aorta, and atrial septal defects.
- The frequency of anomalies increases with increasing first-trimester maternal hemoglobin A1c.
- Hypertrophic cardiomyopathy can develop in response to maternal hyperglycemia in the third trimester in response to increased insulin growth factor 1 (IGF-1) and increased deposition in the intraventricular septum. Hypertrophy gradually resolves within 6 months.
- Systemic lupus erythematosus
  - Maternal antibodies to Ro (SS-A) cross the placenta and can cause cardiac inflammation. Antibodies to La (SS-B) are no longer seen as high risk.
  - Neonatal lupus occurs in less than 5% of pregnancies with antibodies.
  - It can occur in asymptomatic mothers.

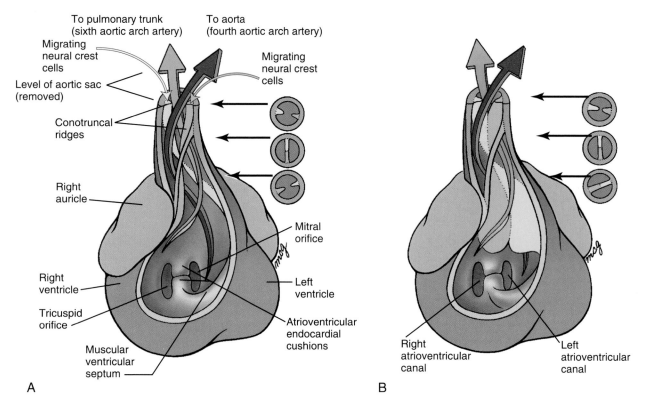

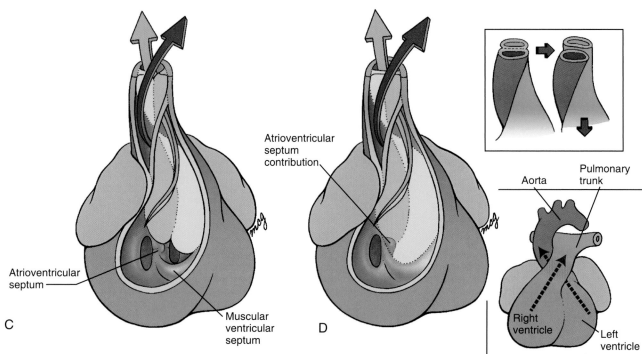

Fig. 8.6 Septation and rotation of primitive outflow tract and alignment with the developing ventricular septum. Septation of the cardiac outflow tract and completion of ventricular separation; right oblique view. The cranial–lateral wall of the right ventricle has been removed to show the interior of the right ventricular chamber and the presumptive outflow tracts of both ventricles. (A, B) Starting in the fifth week, the right and left conotruncal ridges grow out from the walls of the common outflow tract. These swellings are populated by endocardial and neural crest cell–derived cushion cells and develop in a spiraling configuration. They fuse with one another in a cranial-to-caudal direction, forming the conotruncal septum, which separates the aortic and pulmonary outflow tracts. The circular structures to the right of the developing outflow tract illustrate drawings of cross-sections at three proximodistal levels. (C, D). By the ninth week, the caudal end of the conotruncal septum has reached the level of the muscular portion of the ventricular septum and the atrioventricular septum. Here, it fuses with these others to complete the ventricular septum. (From Schoenwolf GC. *Larsen's Human Embryology.* 5th ed. Philadelphia: Elsevier; 2015.)

- Isolated complete heart block is the most common fetal cardiac effect, and risk increases with higher Ro titers.
- It usually presents with fetal bradycardia at 20 to 24 weeks of gestation.
- Poor cardiac function and valvular regurgitation secondary to bradycardia can result in fetal hydrops.
- Maternal treatment with dexamethasone and intravenous immunoglobulin (IVIG) can be used to treat the fetus with complete heart block and evidence of endocardial fibroelastosis, congestive heart failure, or hydrops.
- Maternal B-mimetics such as terbutaline can be used to treat a fetus with a critically low heart rate.
- Neonates with persistent complete heart block following birth require postnatal pacing and potential permanent cardiac pacemakers.
- Maternal hydroxycholoquine reduces the risk of recurrence in subsequent pregnancies.
- Maternal phenylketonuria
  - A strict diet followed during the mother's childhood no longer needs to be followed during adult childbearing years; however, elevated levels of maternal phenylalanine can cause a wide array of abnormalities in a developing fetus.
  - Cardiac malformations include tetralogy of Fallot, ventricular septal defect, aortic coarctation, and hypoplastic left heart syndrome.
  - Maternal serum phenylalanine levels correlate with the risk of cardiac anomalies.
- Maternal infections during pregnancy
  - Parvovirus can cause fetal myocarditis with poor ventricular contractility, as well as high output cardiac failure secondary to aplastic anemia.
  - Congenital rubella is associated with patent ductus arteriosus and pulmonary artery stenosis.

Suggested Readings

Bruneau BG. The developmental genetics of congenital heart disease. *Nature.* 2008;451(7181):943–948.

Hutson MR, Kirby ML. Model systems for the study of heart development and disease: cardiac neural crest and conotruncal malformations. *Semin Cell Dev Biol.* 2007;18(1):101–110.

Mahony L. Development of myocardial structures and function. In: Allen HD, Driscoll DJ, Shaddy RE, Feltes TF, eds. *Moss and Adams' Heart Disease in Infants and Children and Adolescents.* 7th ed. Philadelphia: Lippincott Williams & Wilkins; 2008:573–591.

Ruppel K. Molecular and morphogenetic cardiac embryology: implications for congenital heart disease. In: Artman M, Mahony L, Teitel DF, eds. *Neonatal Cardiology.* 2nd ed. New York: McGraw Hill; 2011:1–19.

Ziman AP, Gomez-Viquez NL, Bloch RJ, Lederer WJ. Excitation-contraction coupling changes during postnatal cardiac development. *J Mol Cell Cardiol.* 2010;24:949–965.

9 *Cardiovascular Physiology*

KIMBERLY VERA

Fetal Circulation

Fetal circulation is optimized to send oxygenated blood from the placenta to the left ventricle for distribution to the most metabolically active fetal organs, and deoxygenated blood is directed to the right ventricle to be pumped to the placenta (Fig. 9.1).

- Venous return to the fetal heart:
  - Deoxygenated blood from the upper body returns to the heart via the superior vena cava and is directed across the tricuspid valve and into the right ventricle.
  - Deoxygenated blood from the coronary sinus streams across the tricuspid valve to the right ventricle due to its location adjacent to the tricuspid valve.
  - Deoxygenated blood from the lower body returns via the inferior vena cava and streams across the tricuspid valve.

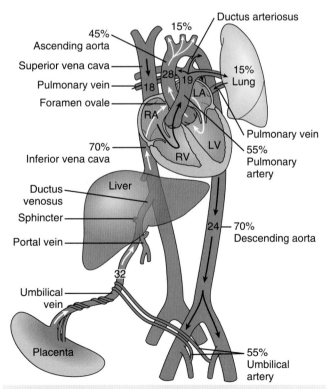

Fig. 9.1 Fetal circulation. Numbers within the vessels denote PaO₂; numbers outside the vessels denote the percentage of cardiac output. *LA,* Left atrium; *LV,* left ventricle; *RA,* right atrium; *RV,* right ventricle. (From Park MK. *Park's Pediatric Cardiology for Practitioners.* 6th ed. Philadelphia: Saunders; 2014.)

- Oxygenated blood from the placenta goes from the umbilical vein primarily into the ductus venosus, with a smaller amount directed to the left portal vein.
- The ductus venosus joins the inferior vena cava (IVC) near the entrance of the left hepatic vein into the IVC.
- These oxygenated streams within the IVC are baffled by the foramen ovale into the left atrium, resulting in more oxygenated blood entering the left ventricle.
- Ventricular output of the fetal heart:
  - The right ventricle is dominant in fetal life, pumping 55% to 65% of the cardiac output. The right ventricle has greater mass and thus directly affects the filling and ejection of the left ventricle in the fetus.
  - Most of the right ventricular output is directed away from the lungs due to the very high pulmonary vascular resistance in fetal life. Blood is directed across the ductus arteriosus, with one-third delivered to the lower body and two-thirds delivered to the placenta via the umbilical artery for oxygen uptake.
  - Left ventricular output supplies the oxygenated blood from the ascending aorta to the coronary arteries (7% of left ventricular output) and to the brain (55% of the left ventricular output).

Postnatal Transition of Circulation

- Pulmonary blood flow greatly increases due to rapid decrease in pulmonary vascular resistance:
  - Ventilation alone with lung distension and decreased carbon dioxide tension induces a two-thirds decrease in pulmonary vascular resistance.
  - Increased oxygen tension further decreases pulmonary vascular resistance.
  - Prostacyclin is produced by lung distention and is a potent pulmonary vasodilator.
  - Remodeling of the pulmonary vascular bed decreases the muscularity of the proximal arterioles and leads to mature levels of pulmonary vascular resistance by 2 months of age.
- Fetal central shunts (e.g., ductus arteriosus, ductus venosus, foramen ovale) close, creating a circulation in series:
  - Ductus venosus flow dramatically decreases with cord clamping. Anatomic closure is completed within hours to days after birth.
  - The flap of the foramen ovale is functionally closed at birth, with the dramatic increase in pulmonary venous return causing left atrial pressure to exceed right atrial pressure. Anatomic closure may not occur for months after birth and remains open in 25% of people.

- The ductus arteriosus typically closes at 12 to 48 hours of life in term infants. Variability exists for prematurity due to the cellular and muscular differences of the ductus.
  - Flow across the ductus arteriosus typically changes from right to left to left to right due to the decrease in pulmonary vascular resistance and increase in systemic vascular resistance after birth.
  - Ductus arteriosus constriction and closure are initiated by increased oxygen content and decreased levels of prostaglandins after birth.
- Ventricular output dramatically increases to meet new increased energy demands due to the work of breathing and thermoregulation:
  - Oxygen consumption triples at birth.
  - Left ventricular output increases by increases in heart rate and stroke volume due to catecholamine surge at delivery.
  - The left ventricle becomes the dominant ventricle in the transitional circulation as it pumps at higher pressure and ejects more blood due to the continued patency of the ductus arteriosus.
  - Cardiac output (CO) = Heart rate × Stroke volume
    - Or, CO = Systemic blood pressure/Total peripheral vascular resistance
  - Neonatal myocardium is more dependent on heart rate to increase CO due to stiffness of newborn myocardium. In premature neonates, functional cellular and mitochondrial immaturity of the ventricular myocardium results in poor stroke volume and accommodation of rapid changes in volume, as well.
- Systemic vascular resistance increases after birth due to removal of the low-resistance placenta and the constriction of systemic vascular beds, especially the cerebral and coronary beds, in response to the higher oxygen content of blood.

Monitoring Cardiovascular Function in the Fetus

- The fetal echocardiogram can assess for wall motion and valvular dysfunction.
- In response to stress, fetal arterial output is redistributed, with increased resistance in the placental and lower body vascular beds to maintain cerebral and cardiac oxygen delivery.
  - End-diastolic velocities decrease in the umbilical artery (Figs. 9.2 and 9.3).
  - End-diastolic velocities increase in the cerebral arteries (Fig. 9.4).
- When the arterial compensatory mechanisms are exceeded and fetal heart failure develops, abnormalities are seen in the venous system.
  - The first sign of decompensation is a larger A-wave in the inferior vena cava Doppler signal.
  - Development of a reverse A-wave in the ductus venosus Doppler trace develops as heart failure progresses.
  - Atrial pulsations in the umbilical venous Doppler trace occur in end-stage fetal heart failure.

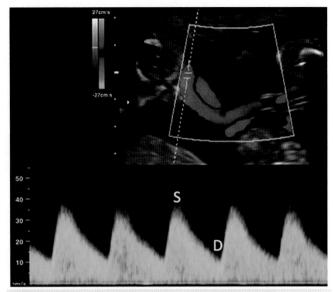

Fig. 9.2 Normal umbilical artery Doppler trace. *D*, Diastolic; *S*, Systolic. (From Norton ME. *Callen's Ultrasonography in Obstetrics and Gynecology.* 6th ed. Philadelphia: Elsevier; 2017.)

Hemodynamic Consequences of Perinatal Events

- Perinatal asphyxia
  - Perinatal asphyxia impairs the transition of fetal to postnatal circulation.
  - Hypoxia keeps the ductus arteriosus open and promotes pulmonary vasoconstriction.
  - Metabolic acidosis worsens pulmonary vasoconstriction.
  - Increased pulmonary vascular resistance promotes tricuspid insufficiency, which increases right atrial pressure and promotes continued right to left shunting at the patent foramen ovale.
  - Cardiac output is maintained in early asphyxia due to systemic vasoconstriction shunting flow away from less vital organs, such as the gut, muscle, and skin, and toward the heart and brain.
    - This redistribution maintains oxygen delivery to critical organs and leaves the less vital organs to rely on increased oxygen extraction.
  - Skin pallor is the clinical finding that occurs secondary to this redistribution of flow.
  - Bradycardia and hypertension result from the reflexes that drive the flow redistribution.
  - Central venous pressure rises in early asphyxia secondary to the vasoconstriction of capacitance vessels.
  - As hypoxia and acidosis worsen, cardiac function declines, causing hypotension and worsening bradycardia and leading to further increases in the central venous pressure. Right ventricle dysfunction is most commonly found.
  - Correction of asphyxia sequelae in the early stages can be done by establishing adequate ventilation and oxygenation.
  - If cardiac failure has developed, treatment must include rapid correction of the acidosis to improve the poor cardiac wall motion.

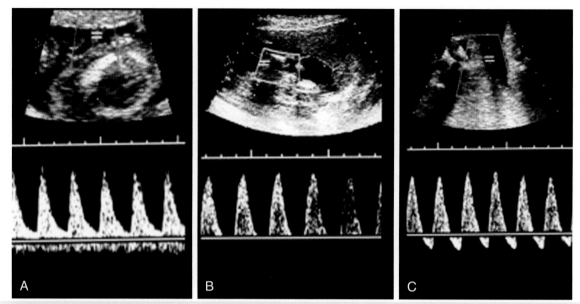

Fig. 9.3 Umbilical artery traces in fetal distress. (A) End-diastolic velocity decreases in response to fetal distress. It proceeds to absent end-diastolic flow (B) and ultimately reverse end-diastolic flow (C) as fetal distress progresses. (From Norton ME. *Callen's Ultrasonography in Obstetrics and Gynecology.* 6th ed. Philadelphia: Elsevier; 2017.)

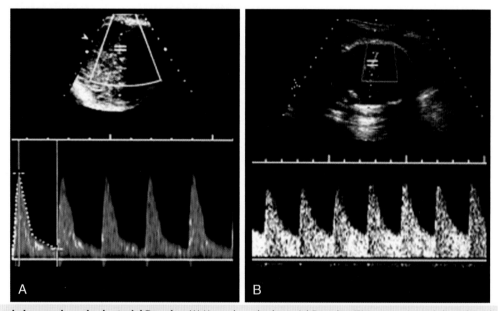

Fig. 9.4 Normal and abnormal cerebral arterial Doppler. (A) Normal cerebral arterial Doppler. (B) Increase in end-diastolic velocity in response to fetal stress. (From Norton ME. *Callen's Ultrasonography in Obstetrics and Gynecology.* 6th ed. Philadelphia: Elsevier; 2017.)

- Perinatal hypovolemia
  - Perinatal hypovolemia results in hemodynamic responses similar to those for asphyxia, including redistribution of the cardiac output to vital organs.
  - Acidosis and bradycardia can also be seen in hypovolemia.
  - Central venous pressure, however, is typically low in infants in the early stages of hypovolemia.

Suggested Readings

Hecher K, Campbell S, Doyle P, Harrington K, Nicholaides K. Assessment of fetal compromise by Doppler ultrasound investigation of the fetal circulation. Arterial, intracardiac, and venous blood velocity studies. *Circulation.* 1995;91(1):129–138.

Huhta JC. Fetal congestive heart failure. *Semin Fetal Neonatal Med.* 2005;10(6):542–552.

Polin RA, Fox WW, eds. *Fetal and Neonatal Physiology.* Philadelphia: Saunders; 1992.

Rudolph AM, Iwamoto HS, Teitel DF. Circulatory changes at birth. *J Perinat Med.* 1988;1(9):9–21.

Rychik J. Fetal cardiovascular physiology. *Pediatr Cardiol.* 2004;25(3):201–209.

10 Presentation of Congenital Heart Disease

KIMBERLY VERA

Congenital heart disease occurs in 1% of live births and can be associated with genetic syndromes or maternal medications (Table 10.1). Symptoms associated with congenital heart disease in a newborn include cyanosis, poor perfusion, tachypnea, poor feeding, or some combination of these symptoms.

- Cyanosis
  - Cyanosis due to heart disease develops secondary to inadequate pulmonary blood flow (PBF) or intracardiac mixing.
  - Cyanosis is clinically appreciated when 5 g/dL of hemoglobin is deoxygenated.
  - Babies who are severely anemic may appear pale, not cyanotic, when hypoxic, given the low hemoglobin level.
  - Cyanosis is not clinically apparent until oxygen saturation is <85%.
  - Differential diagnoses include congenital heart disease, persistent primary pulmonary hypertension of the newborn, and primary parenchymal lung disease.
  - Congenital heart disease is likely in a cyanotic infant with mild tachypnea without significant respiratory distress.
- Poor perfusion
  - Poor perfusion due to congenital heart disease occurs secondary to left-sided obstruction.
  - It presents with ductus arteriosus closure in the first days of life; however, ductal closure can occur as late as 3 to 4 weeks of age.
  - Poor perfusion can be caused by poor left ventricular function.
- Tachypnea
  - Tachypnea due to congestive heart failure develops slowly over the first weeks to months of life as the pulmonary vascular resistance drops and allows significant left-to-right shunting.

Evaluation of an Infant With Suspected Congenital Heart Disease

Cardiac auscultation includes identifying normal and abnormal sounds and can give indications to underlying pathology.

- S1 indicates the closure of the mitral and tricuspid valves and is best heard at the apex or left lower sternal border (LLSB).
- S2 indicates closure of the aortic and pulmonary valves. It is normally split into A2 (aortic closure) and P2 (pulmonary closure). The time between A2 and P2 normally increases with inspiration and decreases with expiration, causing the normal splitting of S2.
  - A narrowly split S2 occurs with pulmonary hypertension.
  - A widely split S2 occurs with volume overload that is seen in conditions such as an atrial septal defect or anomalous pulmonary veins.
  - A single S2 is found in anomalies with only one semilunar valve.
- S3 is a low-frequency, early diastolic sound best heard at the apex or LLSB. It is the sound of rapid filling of the ventricle.
  - It can be a normal finding; however, a loud S3 is abnormal and is seen in conditions with poor ventricular compliance, such as a cardiomyopathy.
- S4 is a low-frequency late diastolic sound that is always pathologic. An S4, also called a *gallop*, indicates poor ventricular compliance in conditions such as cardiomyopathy.
- An ejection click follows S1 closely and indicates pathology of one of the semilunar valves.
  - A pulmonary click is best heard at the second or third left intercostal space and is louder with expiration.
  - An aortic click is best heard at the second right intercostal space, apex, or mid–left sternal border.
- Murmurs should be graded by intensity (1–6), timing (systolic vs. diastolic), location, transmission, and quality.
- Systolic murmurs occur between S1 and S2.
  - Systolic ejection murmurs have intensity that grows from S1 and peaks at a midpoint before decreasing at S2.
    - These murmurs result from pathology of the semilunar valves and physiologic murmurs.
  - Regurgitant systolic murmurs begin from S1 with peak intensity and continue with variable duration throughout systole.
    - These murmurs result from ventricular septal defects, mitral regurgitation, and tricuspid regurgitation.
  - Location of the murmur is associated with the underlying lesion:
    - Upper left sternal border (pulmonary area)—pulmonary stenosis, atrial septal defect, and anomalous pulmonary veins
    - Upper right sternal border (aortic area)—aortic stenosis

Table 10.1 Syndromes and Medications Associated With Congenital Heart Disease

Disorder	Cardiovascular (CV) Abnormalities: Frequency and Types	Major Features	Etiology
Alagille syndrome (arteriohepatic dysplasia)	Frequent (85%), peripheral PA stenosis, with or without complex CV abnormalities	Peculiar facies (95%) consisting of deep-set eyes, broad forehead, long, straight nose with flattened tip, prominent chin, and small, low-set, malformed ears; paucity of intrahepatic interlobular bile duct with chronic cholestasis (91%), hypercholesterolemia, butterfly-like vertebral arch defects (87%); growth retardation (50%) and mild mental retardation (16%)	AD chromosome 22q11.2
CHARGE association	Common (65%); TOF, truncus arteriosus, aortic arch anomalies (e.g., vascular ring, interrupted aortic arch)	*C*oloboma, *h*eart defects, choanal *a*tresia, growth or mental *r*etardation, *g*enitourinary anomalies, *e*ar anomalies, genital hypoplasia	8q12 deletion
Carpenter syndrome	Frequent (50%); PDA, VSD, PS, TGA	Brachycephaly with variable craniosynostosis, mild facial hypoplasia, polydactyly and severe syndactyly ("mitten hands")	AR
Cockayne syndrome	Accelerated atherosclerosis	Senile-like changes beginning in infancy, dwarfing, microcephaly, prominent nose and sunken eyes, visual loss (retinal degeneration) and hearing loss	AR
Cornelia de Lange (de Lange) syndrome	Occasional (30%); VSD	Synophrys and hirsutism, prenatal growth retardation, microcephaly, anteverted nares, downturned mouth, mental retardation	Unknown; AD?
Cri du chat syndrome (deletion 5p syndrome)	Occasional (25%); variable CHD (VSD, PDA, ASD)	Cat-like cry in infancy, microcephaly, downward slant of palpebral fissures	Partial deletion, short arm of chromosome 5
Crouzon disease (craniofacial dysostosis)	Occasional; PDA, COA	Ptosis with shallow orbits, premature craniosynostosis, maxillary hypoplasia	AD
DiGeorge syndrome (overlap with velocardiofacial syndrome)	Frequent; interrupted aortic arch, truncus arteriosus, VSD, PDA, TOF	Hypertelorism, short philtrum, downslanting eyes, hypoplasia or absence of thymus and parathyroid, hypocalcemia, deficient cell-mediated immunity	Microdeletion of 22q11.2
Down syndrome (trisomy 21)	Frequent (40%–50%); ECD, VSD	Hypotonic, flat facies, slanted palpebral fissure, small eyes, mental deficiency, simian crease	Trisomy 21
Ehlers-Danlos syndrome	Frequent; ASD, aneurysm of aorta and carotids, intracranial aneurysm, MVP	Hyperextensive joints, hyperelasticity, fragility and bruisability of skin, poor wound healing with thin scar	AD
Ellis-van Creveld syndrome (chondroectodermal dysplasia)	Frequent (50%); ASD, single atrium	Short stature of prenatal onset, short distal extremities, narrow thorax with short ribs, polydactyly, nail hypoplasia, neonatal teeth	AR
Fetal alcohol syndrome	Occasional (25%–30%); VSD, PDA, ASD, TOF	Prenatal growth retardation, microcephaly, short palpebral fissure, mental deficiency, irritable infant or hyperactive child	Ethanol or its byproducts
Fetal trimethadione syndrome	Occasional (15%–30%); TGA, VSD, TOF	Ear malformation, hypoplastic midface, unusual eyebrow configuration, mental deficiency, speech disorder	Exposure to trimethadione
Fetal warfarin syndrome	Occasional (15%–45%); TOF, VSD	Facial asymmetry and hypoplasia, hypoplasia, or aplasia of the pinna with blind or absent external ear canal (microtia); ear tags; cleft lip or palate; epitubular dermoid; hypoplastic vertebrae	Exposure to warfarin
Friedreich ataxia	Frequent; hypertrophic cardiomyopathy progressing to heart failure	Late-onset ataxia, skeletal deformities	AR
Goldenhar syndrome (oculoauriculovertebral spectrum)	Frequent (35%); VSD, TOF	Facial asymmetry and hypoplasia, microtia, ear tag, cleft lip or palate, hypoplastic vertebrae	Unknown; usually sporadic
Glycogen storage disease II (Pompe disease)	Very common; cardiomyopathy	Large tongue and flabby muscles, cardiomegaly; LVH and short PR on ECG, severe ventricular hypertrophy on echocardiography; normal FBS and GTT	AR
Holt-Oram syndrome (cardio-limb syndrome)	Frequent; ASD, VSD	Defects or absence of thumb or radius	AD
Homocystinuria	Frequent; medial degeneration of aorta and carotids, atrial or venous thrombosis	Subluxation of lens (usually by 10 yr), malar flush, osteoporosis, arachnodactyly, pectus excavatum or carinatum, mental defect	AR
Infant of mother with diabetes	CHDs (3%–5%); TGA, VSD, COA; cardiomyopathy (10%–20%); PPHN	Macrosomia, hypoglycemia and hypocalcemia, polycythemia, hyperbilirubinemia, other congenital anomalies	Fetal exposure to high glucose levels

Table 10.1   Syndromes and Medications Associated With Congenital Heart Disease—cont'd

Disorder	Cardiovascular (CV) Abnormalities: Frequency and Types	Major Features	Etiology
Kartagener syndrome	Dextrocardia	Situs inversus, chronic sinusitis and otitis media, bronchiectasis, abnormal respiratory cilia, immotile sperm	AR
LEOPARD syndrome (multiple lentigenes syndrome)	Very common; PS, HOCM, long PR interval	*L*entiginous skin lesion, *E*CG abnormalities, *o*cular hypertelorism, *p*ulmonary stenosis, *a*bnormal genitalia, *r*etarded growth, *d*eafness	AD
Long QT syndrome; Jervell and Lange-Nielsen syndrome; Romano-Ward syndrome	Very common; long QT interval on ECG, ventricular tachyarrhythmia	Congenital deafness (not in Romano-Ward syndrome), syncope resulting from ventricular arrhythmias, family history of sudden death (±)	AR, AD
Marfan syndrome	Frequent; aortic aneurysm, aortic or mitral regurgitation	Arachnodactyly with hyperextensibility, subluxation of lens	AD
Mucopolysaccharidosis; Hurler syndrome (type I); Hunter syndrome (type II); Morquio syndrome (type IV)	Frequent; aortic or mitral regurgitation, coronary artery disease	Coarse features, large tongue, depressed nasal bridge, kyphosis, retarded growth, hepatomegaly, corneal opacity (not in Hunter syndrome), mental retardation; most patients die by 10–20 yr of age	AR, XR
Muscular dystrophy (Duchenne type)	Frequent; cardiomyopathy	Waddling gait, "pseudohypertrophy" of calf muscle	XR
Neurofibromatosis (von Recklinghausen disease)	Occasional; PS, COA, pheochromocytoma	Café au lait spots, multiple neurofibroma, acoustic neuroma, variety of bone lesions	AD
Noonan syndrome (Turner-like syndrome)	Frequent; PS (dystrophic pulmonary valve), LVH (or anterior septal hypertrophy)	Similar to Turner syndrome but may occur in both males and females, without chromosomal abnormality	Usually sporadic; apparent AD?
Pierre Robin syndrome	Occasional, VSD, PDA; less commonly, ASD, COA, TOF	Micrognathia, glossoptosis, cleft soft palate	In utero mechanical constraint?
Osler-Weber-Rendu syndrome (hereditary hemorrhagic telangiectasia)	Occasional; pulmonary arteriovenous fistula	Hepatic involvement, telangiectases, hemangioma or fibrosis	AD
Osteogenesis imperfecta	Occasional; aortic dilation, aortic regurgitation, MVP	Excessive bone fragility with deformities of skeleton, blue sclera, hyperlaxity of joints	AD or AR
Progeria (Hutchinson-Gilford syndrome)	Accelerated atherosclerosis	Alopecia, atrophy of subcutaneous fat, skeletal hypoplasia and dysplasia	Unknown; occasional AD or AR
Rubella syndrome	Frequent (>95%); PDA and PA stenosis	Triad of the syndrome: deafness, cataract, and CHDs; others include intrauterine growth retardation, microcephaly, microphthalmia, hepatitis, neonatal thrombocytopenic purpura	Maternal rubella infection during the first trimester
Rubinstein-Taybi syndrome	Occasional (25%); PDA, VSD, ASD	Broad thumbs or toes, hypoplastic maxilla with narrow palate, beaked nose, short stature, mental retardation	Sporadic; 16p13.3 deletion
Smith-Lemli-Opitz syndrome	Occasional; VSD, PDA, others	Broad nasal tip with anteverted nostrils, ptosis of eyelids, syndactyly of second and third toes, short stature, mental retardation	AR
Thrombocytopenia–absent radius (TAR) syndrome	Occasional (30%); TOF, ASD, dextrocardia	Thrombocytopenia, absent or hypoplastic radius, normal thumb; "leukemoid" granulocytosis and eosinophilia	AR
Treacher Collins syndrome	Occasional; VSD, PDA, ASD	Defects of lower eyelids, malar hypoplasia with downslanting palpebral fissure, malformation of auricle or ear canal defect, cleft palate	Fresh mutation; AD
Trisomy 13 syndrome (Patau syndrome)	Very common (80%); VSD, PDA, dextrocardia	Low birth weight, central facial anomalies, polydactyly, chronic hemangiomas, low-set ears, visceral and genital anomalies	Trisomy 13
Trisomy 18 syndrome (Edwards syndrome)	Very common (90%); VSD, PDA, PS	Low birth weight, microcephaly, micrognathia, rockerbottom feet, closed fist with overlapping fingers	Trisomy 18
Tuberous sclerosis	Frequent; rhabdomyoma	Triad of adenoma sebaceum (2–5 yr of age), seizures, and mental defect; cyst-like lesions in phalanges and elsewhere; fibrous-angiomatosis lesions (83%) with varying colors in nasolabial fold, cheeks, and elsewhere	AD
Turner syndrome (XO syndrome)	Frequent (35%); COA, bicuspid aortic valve, AS; hypertension, aortic dissection later in life	Short female, broad chest with widely spaced nipples, congenital lymphedema with residual puffiness over the dorsum of fingers and toes (80%)	XO with 45 chromosomes

Continued

Table 10.1 Syndromes and Medications Associated With Congenital Heart Disease—cont'd

Disorder	Cardiovascular (CV) Abnormalities: Frequency and Types	Major Features	Etiology
VATER association (VATER or VACTERL syndrome)	Common (>50%); VSD, other defects	*V*ertebral anomalies, *a*nal atresia, congenital heart defects, *t*racheoesophageal (TE) fistula, *r*enal dysplasia, *l*imb anomalies (e.g., radial dysplasia)	Sporadic
Velocardiofacial syndrome (Shprintzen syndrome)	Very common (85%); truncus arteriosus, TOF, pulmonary atresia with VSD, interrupted aortic arch type B, VSD, and D-TGA	Structural or functional palatal abnormalities, unique facial characteristics ("elfin facies" with auricular abnormalities, prominent nose with squared nasal root and narrow alar base, vertical maxillary excess with long face), hypernatal speech, conductive hearing loss, hypotonia, developmental delay and learning disability	Unknown; chromosome 22q11 (probably the same disease as DiGeorge syndrome)
Williams syndrome	Frequent; supravalvar AS, PA stenosis	Varying degree of mental retardation, so-called elfin facies (consisting of some of the following: upturned nose, flat nasal bridge, long philtrum, flat malar area, wide mouth, full lips, widely spaced teeth, periorbital fullness), hypercalcemia of infancy?	Sporadic, 7q23 deletion, AD?
Zellweger syndrome (cerebrohepatorenal syndrome)	Frequent; PDA, VSD, or ASD	Hypotonia, high forehead with flat facies, hepatomegaly, albuminemia	AR

AD, Autosomal dominant; *AR*, autosomal recessive; *AS*, aortic stenosis; *ASD*, atrial septal defect; *CHD*, congenital heart defect; *COA*, coarctation of the aorta; *D-TGA*, dextro-transposition of the great arteries; *ECD*, endocardial cushion defect; *ECG*, electrocardiogram; *FBS*, fasting blood sugar; *GTT*, gamma-glutamyl transferase; *HOCM*, hypertrophic obstructive cardiomyopathy; *LVH*, left ventricular hypertrophy; *MVP*, mitral valve prolapse; *PA*, pulmonary artery; *PDA*, patent ductus arteriosus; *PPHN*, persistent pulmonary hypertension of the newborn; *PS*, pulmonary stenosis; *TGA*, transposition of the great arteries; *TOF*, tetralogy of Fallot; *VSD*, ventricular septal defect; *XR*, x-linked recessive.
(From Park MK. *Park's Pediatric Cardiology for Practitioners.* 6th ed. Philadelphia: Elsevier, 2014.)

- Lower left sternal border—ventricular septal defects, tricuspid regurgitation
- Apex—mitral regurgitation, aortic stenosis
- Diastolic murmurs occur between S2 and S1 and signify aortic or pulmonary insufficiency.
- Continuous murmurs begin in systole and continue past S2 into part or all of diastole.
  - Patent ductus arteriosus and coarctation of the aorta can present with a continuous murmur.
- Pulse oximetry
  - Pulse oximetry is useful for measuring oxygen saturation (<95% abnormal).
  - Simultaneous measurements in right hand (preductal) and lower extremity (postductal) are useful to assess whether the ascending and descending aorta are being perfused by different ventricles via the ductus arteriosus (Table 10.2).
- Arterial blood gas
  - Obtain if the pulse oximetry is abnormal to evaluate for low partial pressure of oxygen (pO_2)
  - Demonstrates metabolic acidosis in infants with left-sided obstructive lesions
- Oxygen challenge test (*hyperoxia test*)
  - This clinical tool is useful in differentiating between primary lung disease and congenital heart disease in cyanotic infants.
  - Infant is placed on 100% fraction of inspired oxygen (FiO_2) for 5 to 10 minutes, and right radial arterial blood gas is measured.
  - Failure to increase pO_2 dramatically (absolute pO_2 < 100 mm Hg on 100% Fio_2 or increase of pO_2 by <30 mm Hg on 100% Fio_2) is suggestive of hypoxia secondary to cardiac disease.

Table 10.2 Differential Diagnosis of Differences in Preductal and Postductal Saturations

Preductal Saturation > Postductal Saturation	Postductal Saturation > Preductal Saturation
Pulmonary hypertension	Transposition of the great arteries with a coarctation
Coarctation of the aorta	
Interrupted aortic arch	
Critical aortic stenosis	

- Abrupt increase in oxygen tension may result in constriction of the ductus arteriosus, which is often detrimental in ductal dependent lesions.
- Four-extremity blood pressures
  - Upper extremity systolic blood pressure should be a lower value than in the lower extremities.
  - If the lower extremities have lower systolic blood pressures, coarctation of the aorta should be suspected.
  - Narrowing of the aorta results in elevated upper extremity blood pressure.
- Electrocardiogram (ECG)
  - Nonspecific diagnostic tool for most congenital heart disease
  - Normal neonate ECG will demonstrate right ventricular hypertrophy, with upright T waves in the right precordial leads.
- Chest radiograph
  - May show increased or decreased pulmonary vascular markings, heart size, and shape
  - Can suggest thymic absence and right-sided arch, which would support the diagnosis of 22q11 syndrome (associated with conotruncal cardiac defects)

- Echocardiogram
  - Gold standard to define anatomy and diagnose specific lesions

Medical Interventions in Infants With Cyanotic Heart Disease

- Severely hypoxic infants (saturation <75%) due to inadequate PBF should be treated with prostaglandins to open or maintain patency of the ductus arteriosus.
- Oxygen should be used sparingly to maintain saturation of 75% to 85% because the pulmonary vasodilatory response to oxygen can lead to excessive PBF and inadequate systemic blood flow in single-ventricle infants.

Common Surgical Interventions in Cyanotic and Single-Ventricle Infants

- Atrial balloon septostomy (*Rashkind procedure*)
  - Atrial septum is enlarged via cardiac catheterization to allow for atrial-level shunting, often performed emergently due to persistent hypoxia and inadequate mixing.
  - This procedure is performed in infants with hypoplastic left heart syndrome or transposition of the great arteries with a restrictive atrial septum.
- Systemic to pulmonary artery shunts
  - Typically performed in the first week of life in a prostaglandin-dependent infant to ensure stable PBF
  - Utility for stenting of the ductus arteriosus done via cardiac catheterization
  - The goal is to balance flow to the lungs (Qp) and flow to the body (Qs) to provide adequate oxygenation.
  - Careful attention should be paid to avoiding excessive PBF, which results in inadequate systemic perfusion and ventricular volume overload.
  - Balance is typically achieved with oxygen saturations of 75% to 85%.
- Blalock-Taussig shunt (Fig. 10.1)
  - Gore-Tex tube is placed to connect the subclavian artery to a branch of the pulmonary artery PBF.
- Bidirectional Glenn (Fig. 10.2A)
  - Anastomosis of the superior vena cava to the right pulmonary artery in an end-to-side fashion
  - Performed at 4 to 6 months of age
- Fontan (see Fig. 10.2B)
  - Direction of inferior vena cava flow to the pulmonary artery via an extracardiac conduit or via a baffle through the right atrium
  - Performed at 2 to 4 years of age

Left-to-Right Shunting Lesions

- Infant is asymptomatic at birth followed by signs of congestive heart failure as the pulmonary vascular resistance falls in the first weeks to months of life.
  - Premature infants may develop symptoms earlier because they are born with lower pulmonary vascular resistance.
- Lesions can be divided into those with pure left-to-right shunting with normal oxygen saturations versus lesions

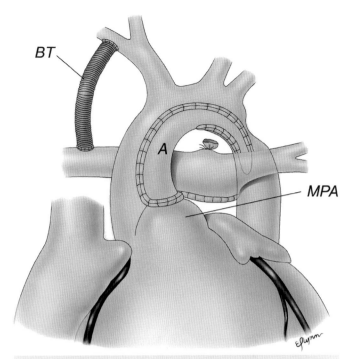

Fig. 10.1 Blalock-Taussig shunt (BT). *A*, NeoAorta; *MPA*, middle pulmonary artery. (From Keane JF. *Nadas' Pediatric Cardiology.* 2nd ed. Philadelphia: Saunders; 2006.)

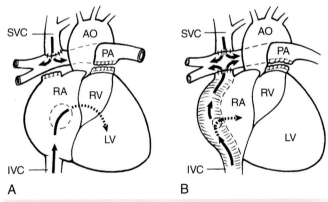

Fig. 10.2 Single-ventricle palliation. (A) The Glenn operation. (B) The Fontan operation. *AO*, Aorta; *IVC*, inferior vena cava; *LV*, left ventricle; *PA*, pulmonary artery; *RA*, right atrium; *RV*, right ventricle; *SVC*, superior vena cava. (From Park MK. *Park's Pediatric Cardiology for Practitioners.* 6th ed. Philadelphia: Elsevier; 2014.)

with bidirectional shunting and excessive PBF leading to mild desaturation (Table 10.3).

- Symptoms of congestive heart failure include tachypnea, diaphoresis, and failure to thrive.
- Chest x-ray demonstrates cardiomegaly with increased pulmonary vascular markings.
- Ventricular septal defect (VSD)
  - Anatomically, VSDs can occur at different locations: perimembranous, outlet, inlet, and muscular (Fig. 10.3).
  - Small defects are clinically asymptomatic and have a loud, high-pitched quality murmur.
  - Small perimembranous and muscular defects can spontaneously close.
  - Medium to large defects develop into symptoms of congestive heart failure develop at several weeks to months of age.

Table 10.3 Left-to-Right Shunting Lesions

Exclusive Left-to-Right Shunting	Bidirectional Shunting Present But Not Left-to-Right Shunt
Ventricular septal defect (VSD)	Double-inlet left ventricle with unobstructed outflow tracts
Atrioventricular septal defect	
Anteroposterior window	Truncus arteriosus
Patent ductus arteriosus	Total anomalous venous pulmonary return without obstruction
Atrial septal defect	

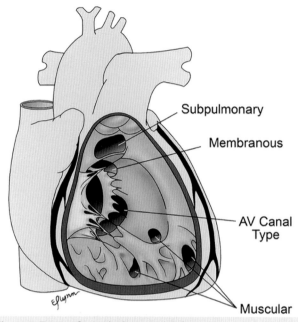

Fig. 10.3 Types of ventricular septal defects. (From Keane JF. *Nadas' Pediatric Cardiology.* 2nd ed. Philadelphia: Saunders; 2006.)

- Large defects have a lower frequency holosystolic murmur and can have a diastolic rumble.
- Medical management of congestive heart failure includes diuretics, digoxin, angiotensin-converting enzyme inhibitors, and maximization of nutrition.
- Surgical repair is preferably delayed until 4 to 6 months of age but is indicated earlier if congestive heart failure symptoms are refractory to medical management.

- Atrial septal defects
  - Secundum atrial septal defects occur in the fossa ovalis and are the most common defects.
  - Primum atrial septal defects are found in the inferior portion of the atrial septum and are part of the atrioventricular septal defect spectrum.
  - Sinus venosus atrial septal defects are found adjacent to the inferior or superior vena cava and are often found in association with partial anomalous pulmonary venous return.
  - Atrial septal defects rarely cause symptoms in infancy because the right ventricular compliance does not typically allow for significant left-to-right shunting.
  - Auscultatory findings can include a pulmonary outflow murmur at the left upper sternal border and a fixed split S2.
  - Surgical repair is indicated for those symptomatic from infancy to adolescence.

- Atrioventricular septal defects (AVSDs)
  - AVSDs are a class of cardiac lesions with endocardial cushion defects resulting in a common atrioventricular valve.
  - Atrioventricular valves are always abnormal and can have significant regurgitation.
  - Incomplete AVSDs
    - Primum atrial septal defects with a cleft mitral valve
    - Physiologically act as an atrial septal defect in the absence of severe valve dysfunction
  - Complete AVSDs (Fig. 10.4)

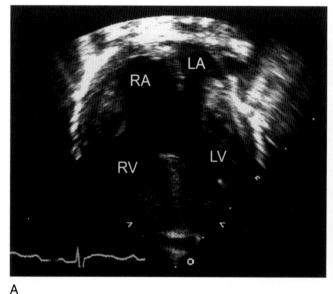

A

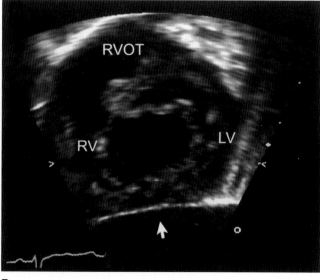

B

Fig. 10.4 Echo images of a complete atrioventricular septal defect. (A) Demonstrates the large inlet ventricular septal defect and large primum atrial septal defect. (B) Demonstrates the common atrioventricular valve. *LA,* Left atrium; *LV,* left ventricle; *RA,* right atrium; *RV,* right ventricle; *RVOT,* right ventricular outflow tract. (From Keane JF. *Nadas' Pediatric Cardiology.* 2nd ed. Philadelphia: Saunders; 2006.)

- Primum atrial septal defect, common atrioventricular valve, inlet ventricular septal defect
- About half of the infants with a complete AVSD will have Down syndrome.
- Electrocardiogram (ECG) shows a left superior QRS axis.
- Congestive heart failure symptoms develop at a few weeks to months of age.
- Infants with complete AVSDs often have mild cyanosis.
- Auscultatory findings vary widely, depending on the degree of atrioventricular valve insufficiency and the degree of left-to-right shunting at the ventricular level. Murmur may not be present.
- First-line medical management is with diuretics along with afterload reduction and nutritional support.
- Surgical repair is optimally done at 3 to 6 months of age.
- Patent ductus arteriosus (PDA)
  - Ductus arteriosus arises from the sixth dorsal arch and connects the pulmonary artery to the dorsal aorta at the isthmus (Fig. 10.5). The formation is complete by 8 weeks of fetal life.
  - The fetal structure normally closes spontaneously after birth depending on gestational age.
  - PDA in preterm infants is due to developmental immaturity. Persistent PDA in term infants may have a structural abnormality.
  - Persistence of ductal patency leads to symptomatology.
  - Moderate to large PDAs result in significant left-to-right shunting as the pulmonary vascular resistance falls after birth.
  - Pulmonary vascular resistance decreases in the first weeks of life, leading to increased shunting across PDA. Pulmonary edema and congestive heart failure symptoms develop due to increased PBF, increased pulmonary artery pressure, and increased left ventricular and atrial volume and pressure.
  - Premature infants can develop heart failure symptoms earlier than term infants due to the incomplete development of the medial musculature of small pulmonary arteries causing decreased pulmonary vascular resistance. The immature contractile function of the ventricles makes volume load more difficult to handle.

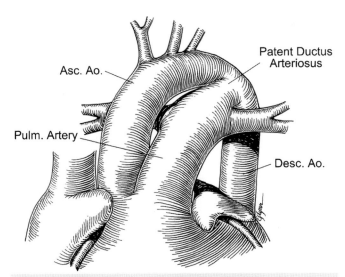

Fig. 10.5 Patent ductus arteriosus. *Ao,* Aorta. (From Keane JF. *Nadas' Pediatric Cardiology.* 2nd ed. Philadelphia: Saunders; 2006.)

- A crescendo systolic murmur or continuous murmur is present, but some premature infants have no murmur.
- Runoff from the aorta into the pulmonary artery lowers the diastolic blood pressure and leads to wide pulse pressure.
- Necrotizing enterocolitis and renal dysfunction may result from the aortic runoff, causing ischemia.
- Treatment
  - Symptomatic term infants can be managed medically with diuretics and afterload reduction.
  - Ultimately, symptomatic PDAs should be closed surgically or via percutaneously cardiac catheterization.
  - Asymptomatic term infants can be monitored without treatment, but PDA closure often is still done via catheterization during childhood to remove the risk of endocarditis.
  - Preterm infants with PDAs are medically treated with ibuprofen, acetaminophen, or indomethacin.
  - Ibuprofen is comparable to indomethacin with regard to closing PDA with less risk of acute kidney injury and necrotizing enterocolitis (NEC). There are no differences in the efficacy of ibuprofen or acetaminophen.
  - Indomethacin inhibits prostaglandin synthesis leading to ductal constriction; it also inhibits platelet function as a side effect.
  - Indomethacin produces PDA closure in 70% to 85% of preterm infants (medical treatment in first 7–10 days of life has higher chance of PDA closure) but is not effective in term infants.
  - Surgical or percutaneous closure is indicated in premature infants with symptomatic PDAs (worsening bronchopulmonary dysplasia (BPD), unable to wean off ventilator, high oxygenation requirement, renal insufficiency), despite medical treatment.
  - The risk of NEC is higher with reverse end diastolic flow in the aorta from PDA.

Left-Sided Obstructive Lesions

- Critical aortic stenosis
  - Critical aortic stenosis occurs when systemic output is dependent on a PDA. When the PDA closes, symptoms include congestive heart failure with pulmonary edema and cardiogenic shock.
  - The aortic valve is often bicuspid with thickened and doming leaflets.
  - Auscultation reveals a systolic murmur at the upper sternal borders, with a possible click.
  - A murmur may not be present if only a minimal amount of blood is passing through the aortic valve.
  - Chest x-ray demonstrates cardiomegaly and pulmonary edema.
  - Decreased left ventricular wall motion is common on echo.
  - Medical management includes prostaglandin E1 infusion and inotropic support.
  - Critical aortic stenosis should be treated urgently with balloon valvuloplasty via cardiac catheterization to improve aortic valve gradient and left ventricular outflow obstruction.
  - Mild to moderate aortic stenosis that is not critical is often asymptomatic and does not require intervention in the neonatal period.

- Coarctation of the aorta
  - Discrete coarctation occurs at the isthmus at the insertion of the ductus arteriosus.
  - Contractile tissue from the ductus can extend around the isthmus, resulting in further narrowing of the isthmus with ductal constriction.
  - Long-segment coarctation involves a long tubular narrowing of both the transverse arch and isthmus.
  - In severe discrete coarctation and long-segment coarctation, adequate perfusion of the lower body is dependent on maintaining patency of the ductus arteriosus. Presentation occurs with ductal restriction and closure.
  - A continuous murmur may be auscultated in the back.
  - Differential cyanosis can occur with lower postductal saturations.
  - Symptomatic infants have congestive heart failure, decreased lower extremity pulses, and leg blood pressures 10 to 15 mm Hg lower than arm blood pressures. Cardiogenic shock can develop.
  - Medical management includes prostaglandin E1 infusion and inotropic support before surgical repair.
  - Surgical treatment is required to augment the aortic arch.
    - Discrete coarctation can be treated with an end-to-end anastomosis from a thoracotomy without cardiopulmonary bypass.
    - Long-segment coarctations require arch augmentation from a sternotomy with cardiopulmonary bypass.
  - Balloon angioplasty of discrete coarctations can be used in infants who have a contraindication to operative repair; however, redevelopment of coarctation over time is common after angioplasty of a native coarctation.
- Interrupted aortic arch
  - Complete interruption of the arch
  - Type A—interrupted after the left subclavian artery (Fig. 10.6)
  - Type B—interrupted after the left carotid artery (see Fig. 10.6)
    - Most common type of interruption

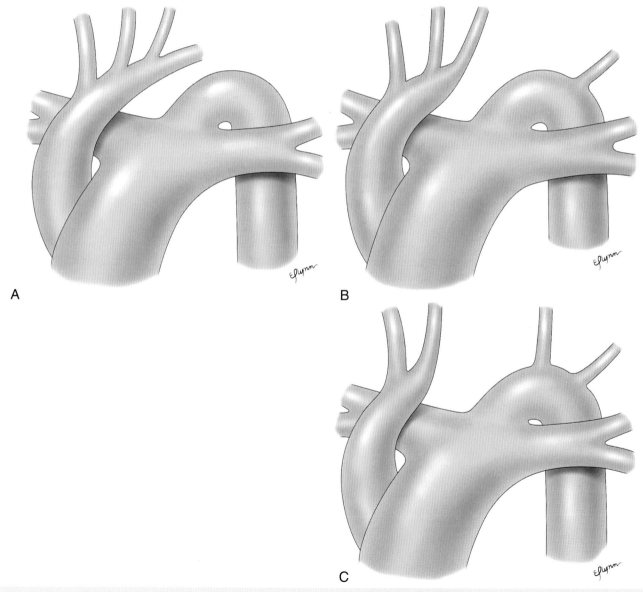

A

B

C

Fig. 10.6 Types of interrupted aortic arches. (A) Type A. **(B)** Type B. **(C)** Type C. (From Keane JF. *Nadas' Pediatric Cardiology*. 2nd ed. Philadelphia: Saunders; 2006.)

- Chromosome 22q11 deletion is found in 60% of infants with type B interruption.
- Type C—interrupted after the innominate artery (see Fig. 10.6)
- Interrupted aortic arch almost always occurs with a ventricular septal defect.
- It presents with congestive heart failure leading to cardiogenic shock when the ductus closes.
- It is treated with prostaglandin E1 infusion until surgical arch repair can be performed.
- Hypoplastic left heart syndrome
  - Hypoplasia of the mitral valve, left ventricle, aortic valve, and aortic arch with left-sided structures unable to meet the systemic output demands (Fig. 10.7)

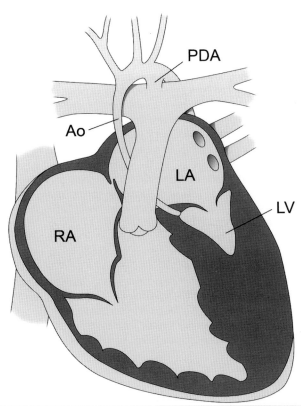

Fig. 10.7 Hypoplastic left heart syndrome. *Ao,* Aorta; *LA,* left atrium; *LV,* left ventricle; *PDA,* patent ductus arteriosus; *RA,* right atrium. (From Keane JF. *Nadas' Pediatric Cardiology.* 2nd ed. Philadelphia: Saunders; 2006.)

- To maintain hemodynamic stability, a PDA and patent foramen ovale must be present to maintain systemic output and to decompress the left atrium.
  - Infants with a restrictive or closed patent foramen ovale at birth will quickly develop profound cyanosis, pulmonary edema, and shock.
  - Emergent balloon atrial septostomy (Rashkind procedure) can be performed.
- Infants with an unrestrictive atrial septum are generally hemodynamically stable after birth.
- Medical management with prostaglandin E1 infusion is required to maintain ductal patency.
- Auscultation can be normal with a widely patent ductus arteriosus and a single S2 heard as the only indication of disease.
- Hemodynamic stability is dependent on the Qp/Qs (ratio of pulmonary to systemic blood flow) being roughly equal to 1, correlating with oxygen saturations between 75% and 85%.
- Following birth, as pulmonary vascular resistance falls, pulmonary flow increases and systemic flow decreases, leading to poor end-organ perfusion, with resultant lactic acidosis. Untreated, this leads to cardiovascular collapse.
- Supplemental oxygen should be used cautiously if saturations are greater than 75% to avoid stimuli for the pulmonary vascular bed to relax, resulting in overcirculation.
- Infants with high saturations and evidence of decreasing systemic perfusion whose ductus arteriosus is confirmed to be patent should be treated with measures to increase the pulmonary vascular resistance.
  - Supplemental carbon dioxide
  - Induced hypoventilation via the ventilator, with sedation and paralysis
  - Consider subambient oxygen with inspired nitrogen
- Enteral feeding of the infants must be done with caution, given the potential for decreased gut perfusion and NEC.
- Management options are palliative care, heart transplantation, or a three-stage, single-ventricle palliation. Most centers' first-line treatment is single-ventricle palliation.
- The Norwood operation is the first operation typically performed in the first week of life (Fig. 10.8).
  - The Norwood includes arch reconstruction, Damus-Kaye-Stansel anastomosis, atrial septectomy, and a Blalock-Taussig or Sano shunt (right ventricle to pulmonary artery).

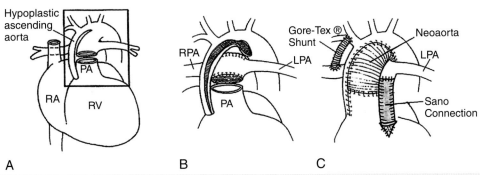

Fig. 10.8 Norwood operation. (A) MPA is transected. (B) Native aorta is opened. (C) Aortic arch is augmented and MPA is anastomosed to the arch; Sano connects the RV to the PA. *LPA,* Left pulmonary artery; *MPA,* middle pulmonary artery; *RA,* right atrium; *RPA,* right pulmonary artery; *PA,* main pulmonary artery. (From Park MK. *Park's Pediatric Cardiology for Practitioners.* 6th ed. Philadelphia: Elsevier; 2014.)

- Second-stage palliation is the Glenn procedure, which is performed at 4 to 6 months of age.
- Third-stage palliation is the Fontan procedure, which is performed at 3 to 4 years of age.

Right-Sided Obstructive Lesions

- Pulmonary stenosis
  - Narrowing can be subvalvar or supravalvar, but the most common level of obstruction is at the pulmonary valve, with thickened and doming leaflets.
  - Supravalvar pulmonary stenosis is associated with Williams syndrome and congenital rubella.
  - The degree of obstruction can vary from mild to severe.
  - Critical pulmonary stenosis requires a PDA to maintain adequate PBF.
  - Severe forms of pulmonary stenosis result in a degree of right ventricular hypertrophy.
  - Auscultation reveals a systolic ejection murmur with radiation to the suprasternal notch, and a click may be present, as well.
  - Severe obstruction along with ductal restriction and/or closure result in cyanosis.
  - Mild valvar stenosis only requires monitoring and rarely progresses.
  - Moderate stenosis requires close monitoring as progression can occur.
  - Severe forms of stenosis require prostaglandin E infusion until balloon valvuloplasty can be performed.
    - Dynamic subvalvar obstruction from right ventricular hypertrophy may limit PBF after a successful pulmonary valvuloplasty.
    - Prostaglandins may be needed for a time to ensure adequate PBF as the right ventricular hypertrophy regresses after the fixed obstruction is relieved.
  - Subvalvar and supravalvar forms of pulmonary stenosis are not amenable to catheter-based intervention, and severe forms require operative intervention.
- Tetralogy of Fallot
  - Most common cyanotic congenital heart lesion
  - The defect includes pulmonary stenosis, anteriorly malaligned ventricular septal defect, aortic override, and right ventricular hypertrophy.
    - Aortic arch is rightward in 25% of patients.
  - Chromosome 22q11 deletion is present in 15% of patients and is more common in those with right-sided aortic arches.
  - Auscultation reveals a systolic ejection murmur of pulmonary stenosis along the left sternal border.
  - A wide spectrum of presentations is possible, depending on the degree of right ventricular outflow tract (RVOT) obstruction.
  - Significant RVOT obstruction presents with cyanosis and hypoxia.
  - Initial management with prostaglandins is needed to maintain adequate saturation (<75%).
    - Infants with minimal RVOT obstruction will be normally saturated and may develop some signs of congestive heart failure.
  - Progressive development of increased RVOT obstruction is common.

Table 10.4 Treatment Options for Hypercyanotic Spells

Treatment	Effect
Knee–chest position	Increased systemic vascular resistance
Oxygen	Decreased pulmonary vascular resistance
Morphine	Decreased agitation
Propranolol	Decreased heart rate and infundibular spasm
Sodium bicarbonate	Decreased acidosis
Phenylephrine	Increased systemic vascular resistance
Ketamine	Increased systemic vascular resistance and decrease agitation
Extracorporeal membrane oxygenation	Rescue in refractory patients

- The chest x-ray demonstrates a boot-shaped heart with decreased pulmonary vascular markings.
- Hypercyanotic (Tet) spells often develop later in infancy. They are an acute dramatic decrease in PBF that leads to progressive cyanosis and acidosis.
  - Triggered by agitation and/or medical procedures
  - Theorized to be caused by infundibular spasm, tachycardia, and an imbalance between the systemic and pulmonary vascular resistances
  - Loss of murmur is a hallmark of a true hypercyanotic spell.
  - Treatment includes measures to increase systemic vascular resistance, decrease pulmonary vascular resistance, and decrease agitation (Table 10.4).
- Surgical repair in acyanotic infants occurs at 4 to 6 months of age.
- Development of hypercyanotic spells is an indication for surgical repair.
- Cyanotic neonates can undergo complete repair but may be palliated with a Blalock-Taussig shunt or ductal stenting via cardiac catheterization.
- Complete surgical repair includes ventricular septal defect closure and relief of the RVOT obstruction (Fig. 10.9).
- Tetralogy of Fallot with absent pulmonary valve
  - Rudimentary pulmonary valve is present, creating pulmonary stenosis and significant pulmonary insufficiency.
    - Marked dilation of the right ventricle and pulmonary arteries
    - Associated with significant airway anomalies secondary to compression from the pulmonary arteries
  - It is associated with 22q11 deletion syndrome.
  - A to-and-fro murmur is present due to pulmonary stenosis and insufficiency.
  - Varying degrees of cyanosis can be present, depending on the degree of RVOT obstruction.
  - Significant airway compression and obstruction can require mechanical ventilation and prone positioning.
  - Prostaglandins may be needed if PBF is inadequate.
  - Urgent surgical repair is needed in severe cases, which include VSD closure, pulmonary artery plication, and RVOT augmentation with a right ventricle to pulmonary artery homograft.
  - Outcomes are related to the degree of airway obstruction.

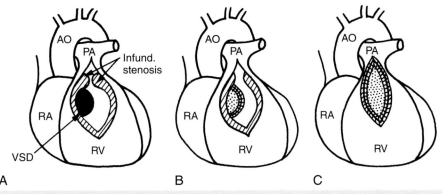

Fig. 10.9 Transannular patch repair of tetralogy of Fallot (TOF). (A) Anatomy of TOF showing a large ventricular septal defect (*VSD*) and infundibular stenosis seen through a right ventriculotomy. Note that the size of the ventriculotomy has been expanded to show the VSD. (B) Patch closure of the VSD and resection of the infundibular stenosis. (C) Placement of a fabric patch on the outflow tract of the right ventricle (*RV*). *AO*, Aorta; *PA*, pulmonary artery; *RA*, right atrium; *RV*, right ventricle; *VSD*, ventricular septal defect. (From Park MK. *Park's Pediatric Cardiology for Practitioners*. 6th ed. Philadelphia: Elsevier; 2014.)

- Tricuspid atresia (Fig. 10.10)
  - The tricuspid valve remains unformed as a plate so that all systemic venous return must pass through the patent foramen ovale into the left atrium.
  - Nearly all patients have a VSD.
  - If the VSD is large, the pulmonary valve is often normal in size, so there is adequate PBF without a PDA.
  - If the VSD is small, the pulmonary valve is often hypoplastic, so a PDA is needed for adequate blood flow.
  - The VSD can become smaller, causing the saturations to decrease later in infancy.
  - Transposition of the great arteries can occur, which results in a small aorta and inadequate systemic blood flow in the absence of a PDA.
  - Presentation depends on the degree of obstruction to pulmonary or systemic blood flow, but cyanosis and hypoxia are the most common symptoms.
  - The ECG demonstrates left axis deviation and left ventricular hypertrophy.
  - If the pulmonary or systemic blood flow is inadequate, initial medical treatment uses prostaglandins.
  - For tricuspid atresia with normally related great arteries and inadequate PBF, initial surgical palliation involves a Blalock-Taussig shunt, followed by a Glenn and Fontan procedure later in infancy. Infants with adequate initial PBF undergo a Glenn procedure as their first operative intervention.
  - For tricuspid atresia with transposed great arteries and a hypoplastic aorta, the initial operative intervention is a Norwood procedure followed by a Glenn and Fontan procedure later in infancy.
- Ebstein anomaly
  - Apical displacement of the septal and posterior leaflets of the tricuspid valve, with a large anterior leaflet (Fig. 10.11)
  - Severity widely varies with the most severe presentation causing fetal demise.
  - Severe cases include marked dilation of the right atrium with "atrialization" of the right ventricle, right ventricular hypoplasia, functional or anatomic pulmonary atresia, and severe tricuspid valve insufficiency.
  - Associated with Wolff-Parkinson-White syndrome with delta waves on the ECG

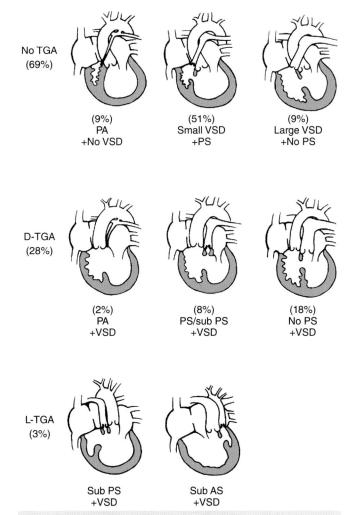

No TGA (69%)

(9%) PA +No VSD

(51%) Small VSD +PS

(9%) Large VSD +No PS

D-TGA (28%)

(2%) PA +VSD

(8%) PS/sub PS +VSD

(18%) No PS +VSD

L-TGA (3%)

Sub PS +VSD

Sub AS +VSD

Fig. 10.10 Anatomic variations of tricuspid atresia. *PA*, Pulmonic atresia; *PS*, pulmonic stenosis; *TGA*, transposition of the great arteries; *VSD*, ventriculoseptal defect. (From Park MK. *Park's Pediatric Cardiology for Practitioners*. 6th ed. Philadelphia: Elsevier; 2014.)

- Associated with maternal lithium use
- Infants with severe tricuspid valve insufficiency have a holosystolic murmur at the lower left sternal border and often a click and/or gallop.

- Significant cardiomegaly is seen on chest x-ray.
- Symptoms manifest as both cyanosis and congestive heart failure.
- Initial medical management in severe cases includes:
  - Prostaglandins to supplement PBF

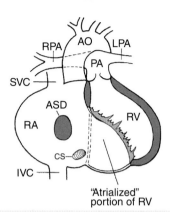

Fig. 10.11 Ebstein anomaly. *AO,* Aorta; *ASD,* atrial septal defect; *CS,* coronary sinus; *IVC,* inferior vena cava; *LPA,* left pulmonary artery; *PA,* main pulmonary artery; *RA,* right atrium; *RPA,* right pulmonary artery; *RV,* right ventricle; *SVC,* superior vena cava. (From Park MK. *Park's Pediatric Cardiology for Practitioners.* 6th ed. Philadelphia: Elsevier; 2014.)

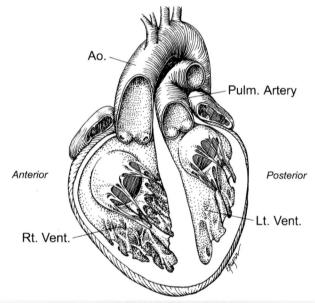

Fig. 10.12 d-Transposition of the great arteries. *Ao,* Aorta. (From Keane JF. *Nadas' Pediatric Cardiology.* 2nd ed. Philadelphia: Saunders; 2006.

- Measures to decrease the pulmonary vascular resistance, such as oxygen, nitric oxide, and inducing a respiratory alkalosis with ventilation
- A drop in pulmonary vascular resistance may allow sufficient PBF through the infant's right heart.
- If the infant continues to be ductal dependent, a Blalock-Taussig shunt can be placed.
- Long-term surgical treatment varies based on the degree of right-sided hypoplasia.
- Options include tricuspid valve repair later in life and single-ventricle palliation.

Mixing Lesions

- d-Transposition of the great arteries
  - The aorta arises from the right ventricle, and the pulmonary artery arises from the left ventricle (Fig. 10.12).
  - Circulation is in parallel, with deoxygenated systemic venous blood flow being pumped back to the body and oxygenated PBF being pumped back to the lungs.
  - Survival depends on shunting taking place at the level of the patent foramen ovale and PDA.
  - Infants present with cyanosis and hypoxia with expected saturations around 80% following birth.
  - Infants with an intact ventricular septum and/or intact or restrictive atrial septum present with profound cyanosis, hypoxia, poor perfusion, and lactic acidosis after birth.
    - Emergent balloon atrial septostomy is required for survival.
  - Auscultation reveals a single S2, as the anterior aortic valve obscures the sound of the pulmonary valve closing.
  - Chest x-ray demonstrates a narrow mediastinum or "egg on a string" appearance.
  - Medical therapy includes prostaglandin infusion to augment shunting and oxygen mixing between the two circulations.
  - Arterial switch surgical repair is performed in the first weeks of life (Fig. 10.13).
    - The aorta and coronary arteries are removed from their native root, as is the pulmonary artery.
    - The two great vessels are then switched, so that the aorta and coronary arteries arise from the left

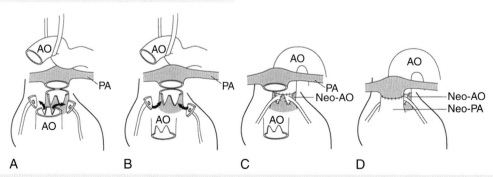

Fig. 10.13 Arterial switch operation. (A) Ao and PA are transected and coronary buttons are removed. (B) Coronary buttons are moved to the native PA. (C) Coronary buttons and arch are attached to the native pulmonary arteries. (D) PAs are attached to the native aorta. *AO,* Aorta; *PA,* pulmonary artery. (From Park MK. *Park's Pediatric Cardiology for Practitioners.* 6th ed. Philadelphia: Elsevier; 2014.)

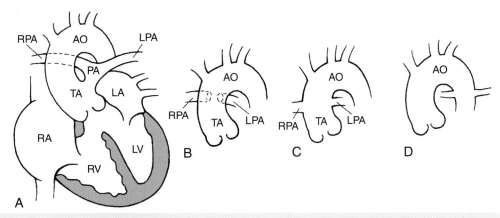

Fig. 10.14 Types of truncus arteriosus. The anatomic type of persistent truncus arteriosus (*TA*) is determined by the branching patterns of the pulmonary arteries. (A) In type I, the main pulmonary artery (*PA*) arises from the truncus and then divides into the right (*RPA*) and left pulmonary artery (*LPA*) branches. (B) In type II, the RPA and LPA arise separately from the posterior aspect of the truncus. (C) In type III, the PAs arise separately from the lateral aspects of the truncus. (D) In type IV, or pseudotruncus arteriosus, arteries arising from the descending aorta (*AO*) supply the lungs. *AO*, Aorta; *LA*, left atrium; *LPA*, left pulmonary artery; *LV*, left ventricle; *PA*, pulmonary artery; *RA*, right atrium; *RPA*, right pulmonary artery; *RV*, right ventricle; *TA*, truncus arteriosus. (From Park MK. *Park's Pediatric Cardiology for Practitioners.* 6th ed. Philadelphia: Elsevier; 2014.)

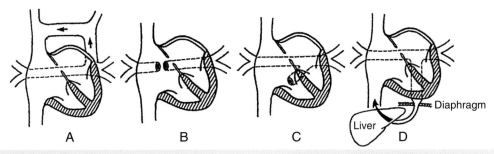

Fig. 10.15 Types of total anomalous pulmonary venous return (TAPVR). (A) Supracardiac TAPVR. (B) Cardiac TAPVR with the veins returning directly to the right atrium. (C) Cardiac TAPVR with the veins returning to the coronary sinus. (D) Infracardiac TAPVR. (From Park MK. *Park's Pediatric Cardiology for Practitioners.* 6th ed. Philadelphia: Elsevier; 2014.)

ventricle and the pulmonary artery arises from the right ventricle.

- Truncus arteriosus
  - A common arterial trunk gives rise to the aorta and pulmonary arteries. A VSD is always present (Fig. 10.14).
  - Truncus type is defined by the manner in which the pulmonary arteries arise:
    - Type 1—A main pulmonary artery arises from the truncus and bifurcates into right and left pulmonary arteries.
    - Type 2—The right and left pulmonary arteries arise from separate origins from the truncus but in close proximity to each other.
    - Type 3—The right and left pulmonary arteries arise from separate origins from the truncus at a distance from each other.
  - The truncal valve is often dysfunctional, with varying degrees of stenosis and insufficiency.
  - Murmur is dependent on the type and degree of dysfunction of the truncal valve.
  - Auscultation reveals a systolic ejection murmur with stenosis or a regurgitant diastolic murmur with truncal insufficiency.

- Both murmurs are present with a valve that is both stenotic and regurgitant.
- Murmur is associated with 22q11 deletion syndrome and a right-sided aortic arch.
- Infants are typically minimally cyanotic, with few symptoms initially.
- As the pulmonary vascular resistance falls, the infants develop significant congestive heart failure, which can be difficult to control medically.
- Surgical repair in the first weeks of life is typically performed with VSD closure and moving the pulmonary arteries from the truncus to a right ventricular to pulmonary artery conduit.
- Truncal valve repair is sometimes required in the neonatal period after birth.
- Truncal valve dysfunction is often the primary determinant of the long-term prognosis.

- Total anomalous pulmonary venous return (TAPVR)
  - All pulmonary veins return to a systemic vein or the right atrium, resulting in complete mixing, with all systemic output passing from right to left across the patent foramen ovale (Fig. 10.15).
  - TAPVR is classified as supracardiac, cardiac, or infracardiac.

- Supracardiac results from the pulmonary veins returning via an ascending vertical vein to the innominate vein.
    - All pulmonary venous flow returns to the heart via the superior vena cava to the right atrium.
  - Cardiac results from the pulmonary venous return entering the coronary sinus, which then empties into systemic veins or directly into the right atrium.
  - Infracardiac results from the pulmonary venous return descending through the diaphragm and joining the hepatic veins and/or inferior vena cava (IVC) before returning to the right atrium.
    - Infracardiac is frequently obstructed.
- The presentation depends on the degree of obstruction to pulmonary venous return:
  - Unobstructive TAPVR infants are minimally cyanotic initially and present with progressive congestive heart failure due to right ventricular volume overload and pulmonary overcirculation.
  - Obstructed TAPVR infants present with a marked degree of cyanosis and pulmonary edema.
  - Profound cyanosis with a white-out on the chest x-ray can result.
- Treatment is surgical anastomosis of the pulmonary veins to the left atrium in the first weeks of life. Obstructed TAPVR may require emergent repair or extracorporeal membrane oxygenation (ECMO) as a bridge to surgical repair.

Double-Outlet Right Ventricle

- This complex and highly variable group of lesions is characterized by a ventricular septal defect with both the aorta and pulmonary artery arising from the right ventricle.
- Outflow tract obstruction on the right or left is commonly seen.

L-Transposition of the Great Arteries

- This is also referred to as congenitally corrected transposition.
- A morphologic left ventricle is on the right, and a morphologic right ventricle is on the left.

- The aorta arises from the morphologic right ventricle, and the pulmonary artery arises from the morphologic left ventricle.
- This allows deoxygenated blood from the right atrium to go through the morphologic left ventricle to the pulmonary artery to the lungs appropriately. Also, oxygenated blood from the left atrium goes through the morphologic right ventricle to the aorta appropriately.
- Levo-transposition of the great arteries (L-TGA) is associated with VSDs and outflow tract obstruction.
- Complete heart block has an association with L-TGA but not D-TGA.
- Patients without VSD or outflow tract obstruction may never need surgery.
- Obstructive symptoms and congestive heart failure due to right ventricular dysfunction may warrant the use of diuretics, closure of VSD, and/or the potential for double-switch operation.

Arterial Vascular Lesions

- An anomalous left coronary artery is off the pulmonary artery.
- The left main coronary artery arises from some aspect of the pulmonary artery instead of the aortic root.
- These are typically asymptomatic at birth due to the elevated pulmonary artery pressures in the first weeks of life. As the pulmonary artery pressure drops, the coronary perfusion pressure decreases, leading to ischemia.
- Presenting symptoms are irritability, pallor, diaphoresis, and poor feeding, followed by tachypnea.
- Auscultations reveals a gallop and the holosystolic murmur of mitral insufficiency.
- The ECG shows deep Q waves in leads I and aVL.
- Q waves are common in V5 and V6.
- T wave inversion is also commonly seen in I, aVL, V5, and V6, as well as ST depression (Fig. 10.16).
- Chest x-ray demonstrates cardiomegaly.
- Diagnosis is often made by echocardiography, but cardiac catheterization may be needed to confirm the diagnosis.
- Inotropic support is used to support the infant, but urgent surgical reimplantation of the left main into the aortic root is the mainstay of treatment.

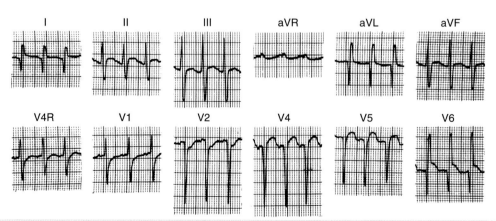

Fig. 10.16 **Electrocardiogram in an infant with anomalous left coronary artery from the pulmonary artery.** (From Park MK. *Park's Pediatric Cardiology for Practitioners.* 6th ed. Philadelphia: Elsevier; 2014.)

Suggested Readings

Alsoufi B, Bennetts J, Verma S, Calderone CA. New developments in the treatment of hypoplastic left heart syndrome. *Pediatrics*. 2007;119:109–117.

Khairy P, Poirier N, Mercier LA. Univentricular heart. *Circulation*. 2007;13:800–812.

Marshall AC, van der Velde ME, Tworetzky W, et al. Creation of an atrial septal defect in utero for fetuses with hypoplastic left heart syndrome and intact or highly restrictive atrial septum. *Circulation*. 2004;110:253–258.

Shinkawa T, Polimenakos AC, Gomez-Fifer CA, et al. Management and long-term outcome of neonatal Ebstein anomaly. *J Thorac Cardiovasc Surg*. 2010;139:354–358.

VanOvermeire B, Smets K, Lecoutere D, et al. A comparison of ibuprofen and indomethacin for closure of patent ductus arteriosus. *N Engl J Med*. 2000;343:674–681.

11 *Cardiopulmonary Dysfunction*

KIMBERLY VERA

Neonatal Cardiomyopathies

OVERVIEW

- Cardiomyopathies are a wide spectrum of disorders characterized by myocardial dysfunction in the absence of structural heart disease.
- Cardiac dysfunction often involves both systolic and diastolic components.
- The Frank-Starling curve graphically represents how increasing preload increases cardiac output in normal hearts. In hearts with decreased contractility, this curve is shifted downward and to the right. Pharmacologic treatments of cardiomyopathies attempt to shift the curve back upward and to the left (Fig. 11.1).

CLINICAL PRESENTATION

- Clinical manifestations include poor feeding, hepatomegaly, tachypnea, gallop rhythm, and murmur from valvar dysfunction.
- Signs of inadequate cardiac output include tachycardia, narrowed pulse pressure, diminished pulses, and oliguria.
- Chest x-ray reveals cardiomegaly and pulmonary edema.

DIAGNOSIS

- Cardiomyopathies can be divided into dilated cardiomyopathies and hypertrophic cardiomyopathies based on their echocardiographic findings.
- Some causative factors result in both dilation and hypertrophy.

TYPES OF CARDIOMYOPATHY AND RESPECTIVE MANAGEMENT

- Dilated cardiomyopathies are characterized by decreased ventricular wall motion and ventricular enlargement.
  - Dilated cardiomyopathies can have numerous causes, including hypoxia (birth asphyxia), infection (myocarditis), incessant tachyarrhythmias, and primary disorders of energy production (Box 11.1).
  - Neonatal myocarditis is a form of dilated cardiomyopathy that can be acquired perinatally or postnatally.
    - The most common causes are echovirus and type B coxsackievirus.
    - Beyond supportive measures discussed above, treatment can include immunoglobulin, interferon, and steroids.

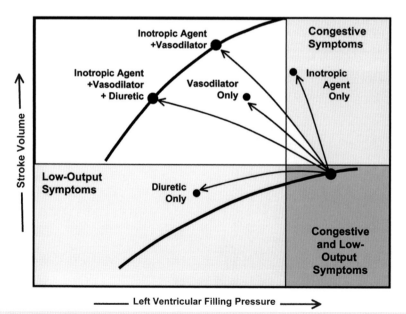

Fig. 11.1 Frank-Starling curve. The *upper line* is the curve in a heart with normal contractility. Decreased contractility shifts the line downward and to the right. Various treatment modalities shown can shift the curve back upward and leftward. (From Park MK. *Park's Pediatric Cardiology for Practitioners.* 6th ed. Philadelphia: Elsevier; 2014.)

Box 11.1 Causes of Dilated Cardiomyopathies

Infectious

Viral
Bacterial sepsis
Myocardial ischemia, birth asphyxia
Reversible electrolyte abnormalities
Hypoglycemia
Hypocalcemia
Hypophosphatemia
Incessant tachyarrhythmias
Genetic isolated cardiomyopathies
Familial dilated cardiomyopathy
Arrhythmogenic right ventricular dysplasia
Noncompaction of the left ventricle
Neuromuscular diseases
Duchenne muscular dystrophy
Becker muscular dystrophy
Friedreich ataxia

Metabolic Disorders

Carnitine deficiency syndromes
Disorders of pyruvate metabolism
Disorders of oxidative phosphorylation
Kearns-Sayre syndrome
Barth syndrome
Infiltrative storage disease
Glycogen storage diseases
Mucopolysaccharidosis
Hurler syndrome
Amino acid and organic acid disorders
Propionic acidemia

Box 11.2 Causes of Hypertrophic Cardiomyopathies

Endocrine Disorders

Maternal diabetes mellitus
Pheochromocytoma
Hyperthyroidism
In utero sympathomimetic exposure
Genetic isolated cardiomyopathies
Contractile protein mutation
Genetic syndromes
Noonan syndrome
Cardiofacial cutaneous syndrome
LEOPARD syndrome
Neurofibromatosis
Beckwith-Wiedemann syndrome
Neuromuscular diseases
Friedreich ataxia

Metabolic Disorders

Carnitine deficiency disorders
Disorders of pyruvate metabolism
Disorders of oxidative phosphorylation
Kearns-Sayre syndrome
Barth syndrome
Infiltrative storage disorders
Glycogen storage disorders
Pompe disease
Mucopolysaccharidosis
Hurler syndrome
Hunter syndrome
Sanfilippo syndrome
Fabry disease
Gaucher disease
Tyrosinemia

- Treatment is often driven by the exact cause, but supportive measures are common to most forms of dilated cardiomyopathies.
    - Correction of electrolyte abnormalities and acid–base status
    - Careful management of fluid status with fluid and diuretics to allow for enough volume to optimize cardiac output while minimizing pulmonary edema
    - Intravenous inotropic agents to augment cardiac output
    - Extracorporeal membrane oxygenation can be used in patients refractory to management in cases where the cause is thought to be reversible or as a bridge to cardiac transplantation.
    - Oral agents can be used in patients who do not need intravenous support.
        - Spironolactone, angiotensin-converting enzyme (ACE) inhibitors, and beta-adrenergic receptor blockers such as carvedilol and digoxin.
    - Cardiac transplantation can be considered for infants and children who appear to have an otherwise fatal course and no significant extracardiac pathology.
- Hypertrophic cardiomyopathy is characterized by inappropriate thickening of the ventricular walls with diastolic dysfunction.
    - Systolic function can be normal, hyperdynamic, or depressed.
    - Thickened ventricular walls can produce ventricular outflow stenosis and result in an outflow tract murmur.

- The electrocardiogram (ECG) can show diffusely increased QRS voltages as well as repolarization abnormalities.
    - Short PR interval is found in Pompe disease.
- Hypertrophic cardiomyopathies also have a wide range of causes, including genetic diseases such as infiltrative storage diseases and primary metabolic disorders of energy production (Box 11.2).
- Treatment of most is supportive and targeted at the primary cause.
    - Inotropes are often not helpful because they can worsen the outflow tract obstruction.
- Infants of diabetic mothers can develop a transient hypertrophic cardiomyopathy, primarily of the ventricular septum.
    - Left ventricular outflow tract obstruction can occur and can range from mild to severe.
    - It results from hyperinsulinemia produced by transplacental passage of a high maternal glucose load.
    - Hypertrophy slowly regresses over time postnatally.
- The most common hypertrophic cardiomyopathies are genetic disorders of one of the cardiac contractile proteins, most commonly of the myosin heavy chain.
    - Neonatal echocardiogram can be normal, but hypertrophy can develop later in childhood or adulthood.
    - Those presenting at birth have a poor prognosis.

Cardiac Tumors

OVERVIEW

- The most common type of cardiac tumor is a rhabdomyoma, which is strongly associated with tuberous sclerosis.

CLINICAL PRESENTATION

- Often occurs with multiple tumors throughout heart
- Natural history is to regress over months to years.
- May create hemodynamic compromise if the tumors block inflow or outflow of the heart
- Possible development of serious arrhythmias

DIAGNOSIS AND TREATMENT

- Depending on size, signs of obstruction based on echo will dictate continued observation with follow-up imaging to monitor if regressing versus symptoms developing.
- Removal requires an expert cardiothoracic surgical team.

Pericardial Effusion and Cardiac Tamponade

OVERVIEW

- Pericardial effusion is an accumulation of fluid, either blood or intravenous fluid, in the pericardial space.

CLINICAL PRESENTATION

- Complication of central venous catheters—perforation or local irritation by hyperosmolar parenteral nutrition fluids
- Present in neonates who had fetal congestive heart failure due to anemia, myocarditis
- Can happen post open-heart surgery
- Can be associated with neonatal pneumonia
- Accumulation of air in the pericardial space (pneumopericardium) can also happen as a complication of mechanical ventilation with similar hemodynamic effects as fluid.
  - Intrapericardial air can be easily differentiated from pneumomediastinum on a chest radiograph as it circumscribes the heart.
- The hemodynamic magnitude of a pericardial effusion and the development of tamponade physiology are dependent on the speed of fluid accumulation.
  - If the pericardial fluid accumulates gradually, intrapericardial pressure remains relatively low and symptoms do not develop until the effusion is large. Yet, much smaller volumes can lead to tamponade in rapid accumulations.

DIAGNOSIS

- Cardiac tamponade is a medical emergency that requires immediate recognition and treatment.

- A high index of suspicion is needed in any infant with early signs of poor cardiac output, tachycardia, and poor perfusion, given that the initial clinical signs are subtle.
- The typical sign of pulsus paradoxus (an exaggerated drop in systemic blood pressure during inspiration) is most easily observed with continuous blood pressure monitoring.
- A large cardiac silhouette can be seen on chest radiograph, but echocardiography offers diagnostic and hemodynamic impact value and should be performed when there is suspicion for tamponade based on the history and physical exam.
- Echo findings include systolic right atrial collapse (earliest sign), diastolic right ventricular collapse (high specificity), plethoric inferior vena cava with minimal respiratory variation (high sensitivity), and exaggerated respiratory cycle changes in mitral and tricuspid valve in-flow velocities (surrogate for pulsus paradoxus).

TREATMENT

- Pericardiocentesis can drain enough fluid or air to eliminate tamponade physiology and relieve symptoms.
- If there is a need for continuous drainage, a surgically or percutaneously catheter can be placed.

Systemic Blood Pressure Regulation

OVERVIEW

- Blood pressure is the product of systemic blood flow and systemic vascular resistance.
- In neonates, systemic vascular resistance is a larger determinant of blood pressure than blood flow.
- The measurement of the blood pressure in severely ill or preterm neonates is preferentially done with an intraarterial catheter.
- Complications include thrombosis and infections.

Hypotension

OVERVIEW

- Hypotension is a decrease in blood pressure so that tissue oxygen delivery does not meet tissue oxygen demand.
  - Hypotension is defined as mean blood pressure of <30 mm Hg, mean blood pressure below the patient's gestational age in weeks, or blood pressure where there is evidence of circulatory compromise.
- Autoregulation occurs with hypotension so that vital organ vascular beds, especially the brain, dilate, and less vital arterial beds constrict to maintain oxygen delivery to vital organs.
  - Autoregulation is impaired in preterm neonates so that blood pressure more clearly mirrors cerebral blood flow.
  - Factors that impair autoregulation include birth asphyxia, acidosis, infection, hypoglycemia, tissue hypoxia or ischemia, and sudden alterations in arterial carbon dioxide tension.

CLINICAL PRESENTATION

- Hypotension in neonates can have numerous causes (Box 11.3).
- Very preterm infants frequently develop hypotension because the immature left ventricle is unable to mount the dramatic increase in output needed to adapt to the sudden increase in systemic vascular resistance with the removal of the low-resistance placental circuit.
- Symptoms manifest as tachycardia, prolonged capillary refill time, acidosis, elevation of the serum lactate level, and decreased urinary output.
- Near-infrared spectroscopy (NIRS) can be used to detect changes in tissue oxygenation of the cerebral and renal vascular beds.
  - Hypotension will result in downtrends of the NIRS.

TREATMENT

- Target the underlying cause!
- Volume resuscitation with isotonic saline at 10 to 20 mL/kg can be used.
  - Hypovolemia is a relatively rare cause of hypotension in neonates, apart from the relative hypovolemia caused by vasodilation in sepsis.
  - Aggressive volume resuscitation should be avoided because it increases morbidity and mortality.
  - Blood transfusion should be carried out if hypovolemia is secondary to blood loss.
- Vasoactive support
  - Dopamine is most commonly used to treat hypotension in preterm neonates.
  - Epinephrine, dobutamine, and vasopressin can be utilized to help with cardiac contractility.
  - Norepinephrine can be utilized in septic shock with alpha effects on peripheral vasoconstriction.
  - Milrinone (phosphodiesterase III [PDE-III] inhibitor) can be utilized in cardiac dysfunction to increase cardiac efficiency through contractility, lusitropy, and vasodilation.
  - A balance of vasoactive support is imperative, as high doses of each medication have side effects that can be counterproductive.
- Steroids
  - Hydrocortisone can be used in inotropic-resistant hypotension.

Box 11.3 Causes of Hypotension

Inflammatory response

Sepsis
Necrotizing enterocolitis
Asphyxia
Major surgery
Myocardial dysfunction
Closure of the ductus in a systemically dependent, ductal-dependent congenital heart lesion
Coarctation
Aortic stenosis
Hypoplastic left heart syndrome
Use of afterload reduction agents
Milrinone
Prostaglandin E2

- In critically ill infants, the cardiovascular system can develop desensitization to catecholamines. Steroid administration attenuates this response and decreases the need for inotropes.
- Concurrent administration of hydrocortisone with indomethacin in the first postnatal week increases the risk of gastrointestinal perforation.
- Homeostasis
  - Maintenance of normal pH and calcium levels also helps maintain the cardiovascular sensitivity to catecholamines.

Hypertension

OVERVIEW

- Hypertension (HTN) is defined as blood pressure greater than the 95th percentile.
- Most common causes of neonatal hypertension are renal parenchymal disease and renal vascular disease (Box 11.4).
- Genetic factor association includes cytochrome p450 genotype *CYP2D6*.
- Other causes include maternal steroid exposure, history of extracorporeal membrane oxygenation (ECMO), and maternal substance abuse (cocaine).

Box 11.4 Causes of Neonatal Hypertension

Renal

Acute renal failure
Polycystic kidney disease
Renal cortical and medullary necrosis
Hypoplastic kidney
Pyelonephritis
Obstructive uropathy
Nephrolithiasis

Vascular

Renal artery thrombosis
Aortic thrombus
Coarctation of the aorta
Renal vein thrombosis
Renal artery thrombosis
Idiopathic arterial calcification

Endocrine

Pheochromocytoma
Neuroblastoma
Hyperthyroidism
Adrenal disorders

Iatrogenic

Corticosteroids
Theophylline
Pancuronium
Phenylephrine eye drops

Other

Bronchopulmonary dysplasia
Patent ductus arteriosus
Increased intracranial pressure
Fluid overload

- Umbilical arterial catheter is a risk factor for developing hypertension.
  - Thromboembolic events occur at the time of placement secondary to endothelial injury.
  - The resultant decrease in kidney perfusion results in sodium and water retention.
- Chronic lung disease is a significant risk factor for HTN and can present after discharge from the neonatal intensive care unit.

CLINICAL PRESENTATION

- Hypertension is frequently asymptomatic.
- Signs and symptoms include tachypnea, tremor, lethargy, feeding difficulties, seizures, apnea, hypertonicity, hypertensive retinopathy, cerebral edema, and intracranial hemorrhage.
- The severity of the blood pressure elevation is not correlated to the presence or severity of signs and symptoms.
- Infants can develop congestive heart failure symptoms if left ventricular function is decreased due to HTN.

DIAGNOSIS

- Obtain a history of any prenatal exposures or procedures, such as prior umbilical artery catheters and review current medications.
- A full examination should include palpation for flank masses and auscultation for an epigastric bruit (renal artery stenosis).
- Labs include serum electrolyte, creatinine, and blood urea nitrogen levels.
- Urinalysis
- Renal ultrasound can detect renal vein thrombosis, renal artery stenosis, and renal parenchymal abnormalities.
- Echocardiograph can detect left ventricular hypertrophy and decreased left ventricular wall motion function and rule out coarctation of the aorta.

TREATMENT

- Asymptomatic infants with blood pressures between the 95th and 99th percentiles and no end-organ dysfunction can be observed.
- Infants with blood pressure readings greater than the 99th percentile or with end-organ involvement should be treated.
- Five classes of antihypertensives used in the neonatal population are diuretics, beta-blockers, ACE inhibitors, calcium channel blockers, and direct peripheral vasodilators (Table 11.1).
  - ACE inhibitors are very effective in neonates because of the high renal vascular resistance, but they should not be used until renal vascular disease is ruled out.
  - Diuretics are very effective in the treatment of lung disease–associated HTN.

Table 11.1   Oral Antihypertensives

Drug	Dose	Notes
Captopril (ACE inhibitor)	0.05–0.5 mg/kg/d tid	Monitor creatinine and potassium
Hydrochlorothiazide (thiazide diuretic)	2–4 mg/kg/d bid	Monitor electrolytes
Hydralazine (vasodilator)	0.75–7.5 mg/kg tid or qid	Tachycardia, fluid retention, lupus-like syndrome
Minoxidil (vasodilator)	0.1–0.2 mg/kg/dose bid or tid	Most potent vasodilator
Amlodipine (calcium channel blocker)	0.1–0.3 mg/kg/dose bid	Useful for chronic hypertension
Propranolol (beta-blocker)	1–8 mg/kg/d tid	Can cause bronchospasm and hypoglycemia; avoid in bronchopulmonary dysplasia

bid, Twice a day; *tid*, three times a day.

Table 11.2   IV Antihypertensives

Drug	Dose	Notes
Nicardipine (calcium channel blocker)	0.5–3 µg/kg/min	Tachycardia
Esmolol (beta-blocker)	100–300 µg/kg/min	Very short half-life
Hydralazine (vasodilator)	0.15–0.6 mg/kg	Tachycardia
Nitroprusside (vasodilator)	0.5–10 µg/kg/min	Thiocyanate toxicity when used for >72 hr or in renal failure

- Intravenous antihypertensives should be used in a neonatal hypertensive crisis with continuous blood pressure monitoring via an arterial line (Table 11.2).
  - Nicardipine is the drug of choice in a neonatal hypertensive crisis.
  - If the blood pressure is decreased too rapidly, cerebral ischemia and/or hemorrhage may result.

Suggested Readings

Colan SD. Classification of the cardiomyopathies. *Prog Pediatr Cardiol.* 2007;23:5–15.

Hill KD, Hamid R, Exil VJ. Pediatric cardiomyopathies related to fatty acid metabolism. *Prog Pediatr Cardiol.* 2008;25:69–78.

Jefferies JL, Towbin JA. Dilated cardiomyopathy. *Lancet.* 2010;375: 752–762.

Menn SC, Olson TM, Michels VV. Genetics of familial dilated cardiomyopathy. *Prog Pediatr Cardiol.* 2008;25:57–67.

Nugent AW, Daubeney PE, Chondos P, et al. Clinical features and outcomes of childhood hypertrophic cardiomyopathy: results from a national population-based study. *Circulation.* 2005;112(9):1332–1338.

12 Electrocardiography, Electrophysiology, and Dysrhythmias

KIMBERLY VERA

A normal electrocardiogram (ECG) reflects expected transit times through the conduction system. Abnormalities on an ECG can reflect an abnormality in conduction and rhythm, as well as an anatomic defect in the heart.

- Normal intervals (Fig. 12.1)
  - The PR interval measures the time of conduction from the sinoatrial (SA) node through the atrioventricular (AV) node and includes the depolarization time of the atria.
    - The PR interval is measured from the onset of the P wave to the onset of the QRS complex.
  - QRS duration measures the time of depolarization of the ventricles.
    - QRS duration is measured from onset to termination of the QRS complex.
  - The QT interval measures the time of ventricular depolarization and repolarization.
    - The QT interval is measured from onset of the QRS complex to the end of the T wave.
    - The QT interval must be corrected for heart rate (QTc interval).
    - Bazett's formula is used most often: $QTc = QT/(\sqrt{RR}\text{ interval})$.
  - The RR interval measures the time from one QRS complex to the next.
- Normal waveforms

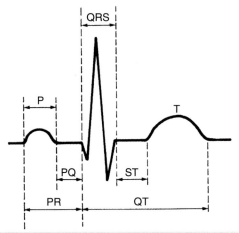

Fig. 12.1 Normal intervals on an electrocardiogram. (From Park MK. *Park's Pediatric Cardiology for Practitioners.* 6th ed. Philadelphia: Elsevier; 2014.)

- The P wave represents depolarization of the atria.
  - The normal P wave axis is 0 degrees to +90 degrees with a positive P wave in leads I and aVF.
- QRS represents depolarization of the ventricles.
  - The QRS axis represents the mean vector of the ventricular depolarization (Fig. 12.2).
  - Newborns have right axis deviation when compared to adults, with up to +180 degrees considered normal (Fig. 12.3).
  - An abnormal QRS axis is seen with ventricular hypertrophy, bundle branch block, and ventricular conduction disturbances.
- Q waves are produced by depolarization of the ventricular septum.
  - Q waves are common in leads I, II, III, and aVF and are nearly always present in V5 and V6.
- T waves represent the ventricular repolarization process.

Normal sinus rhythm originates from the SA node and is influenced by the autonomic nervous system, catecholamines, temperature, and blood pressure. Impulses from the SA node proceed through the AV node, where the impulse is slowed to allow atrial contraction to finish prior to ventricular contraction. Conduction then passes through the His bundle and into the bundle branches to initiate ventricular contraction.

- Sinus arrhythmia is phasic variation in heart rate with respiration.
  - Sinus arrhythmia is the most common cause of an irregular heart rate.
  - It occurs more frequently at lower heart rates and is often seen in infants who are sleeping or in infants with high vagal tone.
- Sinus bradycardia is defined as a heart rate originating from the sinus node with rates of less than 80 beats/min while awake or less than 60 beats/min while asleep.
  - A common cause is increased vagal tone seen with gastric distention, upper airway obstruction, increased intracranial pressure, pharyngeal stimulation, and Valsalva maneuver.
  - Other causes include hypoxia, hypothyroidism, drug therapy, hypothermia, and long QT syndrome.
- AV block represents a slowing or complete blockage of conduction at the AV node and can be described as first-, second-, or third-degree block.
- First-degree block describes a prolonged PR interval.

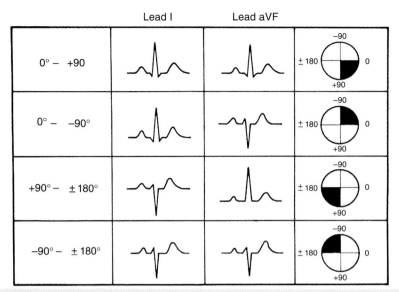

Fig. 12.2 Method of finding the QRS axis. (From Park MK. *Park's Pediatric Cardiology for Practitioners.* 6th ed. Philadelphia: Elsevier; 2014.)

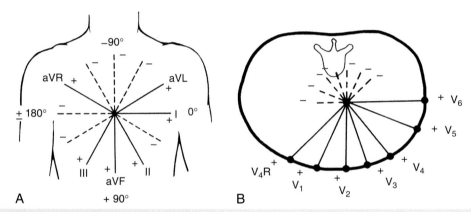

Fig. 12.3 Hexaxial reference system for electrocardiograms. (A) Frontal projection of vector loop. (B) Horizontal projection. Both parts A and B constitute the electrocardiogram. (From Park MK. *Park's Pediatric Cardiology for Practitioners.* 6th ed. Philadelphia: Elsevier; 2014.)

- The PR interval should be 160 ms or less on the first day of life and 140 ms or less after the first day of life.
- Causes include medication, especially digoxin, and surgical trauma from cardiac surgery.
- Treatment is not necessary.
■ Second-degree AV block is an intermittent loss of AV conduction and is further classified into Mobitz type I and Mobitz type II (Fig. 12.4).
  - Mobitz type I block, or Wenckebach, is a gradual prolongation of the PR interval, followed by a P wave with no following QRS complex.
    - Grouped QRS complexes are seen in Mobitz type I block.
    - Wenckebach is seen during sleep and in infants with high vagal tone.
    - No treatment is necessary.
  - Mobitz type II is intermittent loss of P wave conduction, without prior PR prolongation.
    - If every other P wave is conducted, it is a 2:1 block.
    - If more than one consecutive P wave fails to conduct, it is a high-grade (e.g., 3:1) block.

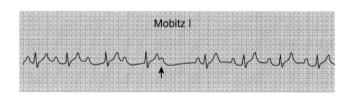

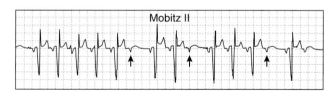

Fig. 12.4 Second-degree atrioventricular block. *Arrows* demonstrate P waves that are not followed by a QRS complex. (From Keane JF. *Nadas' Pediatric Cardiology.* 2nd ed. Philadelphia: Saunders; 2006.)

- High-grade block may progress to complete AV block.
- It is seen in infants born to mothers with connective tissue disease, in infants with congenital heart disease with L-looped ventricles, and in infants who have had cardiac surgery.

- A pacemaker may be needed, especially if a wide QRS is present.
- Third-degree AV block or complete heart block occurs when no atrial impulses are conducted to the ventricle.
  - P waves are completely disassociated from the QRS complexes.
  - QRS can be narrow or wide, depending on whether the escape rhythm originates near the AV node (narrow) or distal to the bundle of His (wide).
  - Atrial rates are normal for age and vary with stimuli.
  - Ventricular rates are regular, with minimal variability, with typical rates of 60 to 80 beats/min.
  - The most common cause is transplacental passage of SSA/Ro autoantibodies in mothers with connective tissue disease affecting the fetus.
  - Mothers often have no signs or symptoms of connective tissue disease.
  - The fetus can develop hydrops with signs of congestive heart failure at birth.
  - Neonates with congenital heart block are often asymptomatic due to compensated increased stroke volume.
    - Infants born with congestive heart failure or who develop signs of inadequate cardiac output require emergent transvenous and transcutaneous pacing.
  - Isoproterenol can be used medically to increase the ventricular rate in symptomatic infants.
  - Permanent pacemaker placement is indicated for congestive heart failure, cardiomegaly, ventricular dysfunction, premature ventricular contractions, prolonged QTc interval, and a wide ventricular escape complex.
  - Complete heart block can also occur in infants with complex congenital heart disease, such as those with congenitally corrected transposition and left atrial isomerism heterotaxy, as well as in infants after cardiac surgery.
- Sinus tachycardia is notable for fast heart rates, up to 240 beats/min in a neonate with a normal P wave axis.
  - Sinus tachycardia has some variability in rates.
  - Common causes include hypovolemia, fever, hypoxia, anemia, inadequate sedation, and pain.
  - Treatment should be directed at the underlying cause.
- Premature atrial contractions (PACs) occur when an ectopic atrial focus depolarizes earlier than the sinus node, creating an early P wave on the ECG (Fig. 12.5).
  - The early P wave may be a different morphology than the sinus P waves and may be buried in the preceding T wave.
  - The premature P wave may be followed by a normal narrow QRS complex or a wide QRS complex.
  - A wide QRS complex is produced when the early P wave is conducted aberrantly because a bundle branch is still refractory from the prior ventricular depolarization.
  - Very early PACs can be blocked because the AV node is still refractory from the prior ventricular depolarization.
  - Frequent blocked PACs can cause bradycardia.
  - PACs are common and usually have no specific etiology.

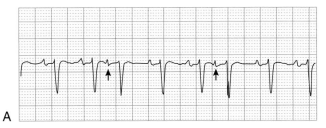

A

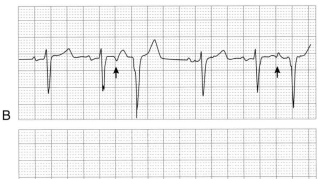

B

C

Fig. 12.5 Variations of premature atrial contractions (PACs). (A) PAC with a normal QRS complex. (B) PAC with a widened QRS complex. (C) PAC with no subsequent QRS complex (blocked PAC). (From Keane JF. *Nadas' Pediatric Cardiology.* 2nd ed. Philadelphia: Saunders; 2006.)

- Iatrogenic causes include intracardiac lines, caffeine, isoproterenol, dopamine, and epinephrine.
- Rare causes are electrolyte disturbances, cardiac tumors, and myocarditis.
- Even frequent PACs do not cause symptoms and do not require treatment.
- They usually resolve spontaneously by the third month of life.
- Supraventricular tachycardia (SVT) is the most common arrhythmia in infants and children.
- Accessory mediated tachycardia accounts for 75% of SVT in infants who have accessory pathways of anomalous tissue bands that connect the atria to the ventricle, which allow conduction between the atria and ventricle outside of the AV node.
  - In Wolff-Parkinson-White (WPW) syndrome, the accessory pathway conducts antegrade (from the atrial to the ventricle) during sinus rhythm, creating preexcitation, or a delta wave, on the ECG.
  - It occurs because normal conduction through the AV node is slowed, but the conduction across the accessory pathway is not, thus allowing some of the ventricle to depolarize early (Fig. 12.6).
    - Up to one-third of patients with WPW syndrome have only intermittent preexcitation on the ECG.
  - Concealed accessory pathways can only conduct retrograde (from the ventricle to the atria), and the baseline ECG is often normal.
    - It is the mechanism in more than half of infants with reentrant SVT.

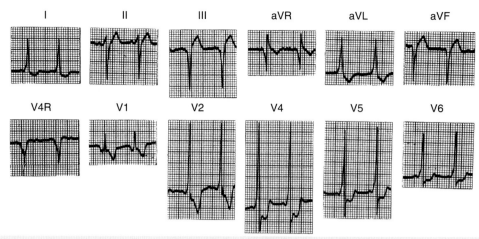

Fig. 12.6 Electrocardiogram demonstrating delta waves. (From Park MK. *Park's Pediatric Cardiology for Practitioners.* 6th ed. Philadelphia: Elsevier; 2014.)

- Orthodromic reciprocating tachycardia occurs when an impulse, often a PAC, is conducted through the AV node and then is conducted retrograde from the ventricle back to the atria.
- This impulse then goes back down the AV node, creating a self-perpetuating circuit.
- Accessory mediated SVT has rates of greater than 250 beats/min, with minimal variability.
- Onset and termination of the tachycardia are abrupt.
- QRS complexes are typically narrow, and P waves are often not visible.
- Infants typically tolerate these rates for 36 to 72 hours before signs of congestive heart failure develop.
- Accessory mediated SVT can be acutely terminated by measures that cause temporary block of the AV node.
  - Vagal maneuvers are first-line treatment.
  - Ice slurry applied to the patient's forehead, eyes, and nose bridge for 10 to 20 seconds is an option.
  - If vagal maneuvers fail, rapidly push adenosine at 0.1 mg/kg via a three-way stopcock.
  - A short period of asystole should be seen after administration.
  - Repeat the dose at 0.2 mg/kg if the short asystolic period is not seen with the lower dose.
  - For hemodynamically unstable SVT, synchronized direct current (DC) cardioversion should be performed as the first intervention.
  - The initial energy dose of 0.5 J/kg may be increased to 1 to 2 J/kg if there is no response.
- Prophylactic antiarrhythmic treatment is often indicated because the recurrence rate of neonatal SVT is high.
  - Beta-blockers are often used.
  - Digoxin may be used as prophylaxis but is contraindicated in patients with preexcitation.
- Permanent junctional reciprocating tachycardia
  - This occurs with a concealed accessory pathway that conducts in a slow retrograde fashion.
  - Heart rates are generally slower than typical SVT, 180 to 200 beats/min, with more rate variability.

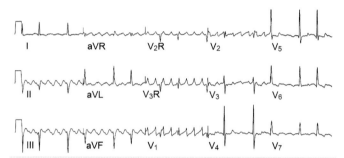

Fig. 12.7 Atrial flutter. (From Keane JF. *Nadas' Pediatric Cardiology.* 2nd ed. Philadelphia: Saunders; 2006.)

- It is more resistant to typical SVT antiarrhythmic therapy and may require ablation.
- Atrial flutter
  - A reentrant circuit forms within the atria only, leading to very rapid atrial rates of 375 to 500 beats/min.
  - AV block is common at these high rates.
  - Atrial flutter leads to variable ventricular response rates frequently at 2:1 or 3:1.
  - The ECG will show flutter waves, which appear sawtooth-like (Fig. 12.7).
  - This can be difficult to see on a baseline ECG, but the flutter waves are easy to see after the administration of adenosine.
  - Adenosine is helpful in the diagnosis but will not terminate the rhythm because this arrhythmia is not dependent on the AV node.
  - Atrial flutter can be terminated by DC cardioversion or overdrive pacing via a transesophageal lead.
  - Recurrence of atrial flutter in a structurally normal heart is rare so prophylactic treatment is typically not required.
- Ectopic atrial tachycardia is automatic tachycardia caused by atrial cells, which depolarize independently and more rapidly than the sinus node.
  - P-wave morphology is different from that of the sinus P waves.
  - The onset and termination of tachycardia are gradual.

- Infants are typically asymptomatic initially but can develop congestive heart failure symptoms after several days.
- A dilated cardiomyopathy can develop if the infant goes untreated for weeks to months.
- Adenosine does not terminate the rhythm but can transiently slow the rate, allowing for mechanism delineation.
- Treatment is focused on rate control and involves the use of beta-blockers.
- Ectopic atrial tachycardia often resolves spontaneously.
- Refractory cases can be treated with ablation.
- Premature ventricular contraction (PVC) (Fig. 12.8) is an early depolarization of the ventricle, not preceded by a P wave.
  - The QRS complex is typically wider than the sinus QRS complex.
  - Uniform PVCs have the same QRS morphology.
  - Multiform PVCs have multiple QRS morphologies.
  - Multiform PVCs are much more likely to represent significant underlying pathology.
  - It is important to evaluate for metabolic abnormalities, myocarditis, cardiac tumors, and structural heart disease.
  - The most common cause is idiopathic, and no treatment is needed, with resolution in the first few months of life.

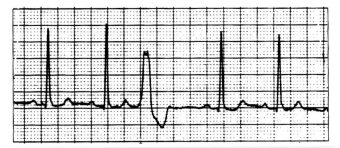

Fig. 12.8 Premature ventricular contraction. (From Keane JF. *Nadas' Pediatric Cardiology.* 2nd ed. Philadelphia: Saunders; 2006.)

- Ventricular tachycardia is a wide complex rhythm that often results from reentry within the ventricle.
  - The rates should be at least 20% greater than the sinus rate.
    - A wide complex rhythm at less than 20% of the sinus rate is an accelerated idioventricular rhythm.
  - Nonsustained ventricular tachycardia lasts less than 30 seconds.
  - Sustained ventricular tachycardia lasts longer than 30 seconds.
  - P-wave complexes are disassociated from the ventricular complexes.
  - Torsades de pointes is a type of ventricular tachycardia where QRS complexes continually change but spiral around the baseline (Fig. 12.9).
  - Magnesium sulfate is used in torsades de pointes.
  - Causes include electrolyte and metabolic abnormalities, myocarditis, drug toxicity, myocardial tumors, and myocardial ischemia.
  - Sustained ventricular tachycardia is a critical emergency requiring prompt treatment because infants are hemodynamically unstable.
    - Patients in shock should undergo DC cardioversion at 1 to 2 J/kg.
    - The energy can be doubled for a second shock if the first shock is unsuccessful.
    - If the patient is responsive with reasonable vital signs, amiodarone (5 mg/kg) or procainamide (15 mg/kg) can be given.
- Electrolyte abnormalities can be reflected on the ECG (Figs. 12.10 and 12.11)
  - Hypocalcemia prolongs the QTc.
  - Hypercalcemia shortens the QTc.
  - Hypokalemia can produce a U wave, prolonged QTc, flat or biphasic T waves, and depressed ST segments.
  - Hyperkalemia is first seen on the ECG with peaked T waves.
  - The QRS then becomes prolonged, followed by the PR interval.
  - The P waves then disappear, and the QRS complexes become biphasic, like a sine wave.

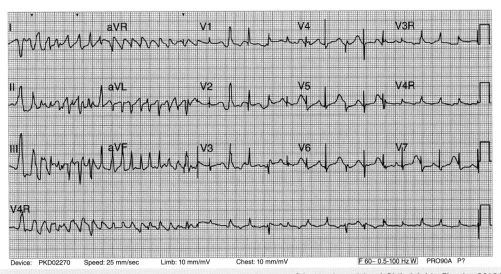

Device: PKD02270   Speed: 25 mm/sec   Limb: 10 mm/mV   Chest: 10 mm/mV   F 60~ 0.5-100 Hz W   PRO90A P?

Fig. 12.9 Torsades de pointes. (From Gleason CA. *Avery's Diseases of the Newborn.* 9th ed. Philadelphia: Elsevier; 2012.)

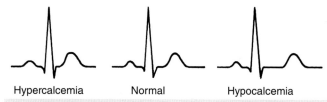

Fig. 12.10 Electrocardiographic changes in hypocalcemia and hypercalcemia. (From Park MK. *Park's Pediatric Cardiology for Practitioners.* 6th ed. Philadelphia: Elsevier; 2014.)

SERUM K

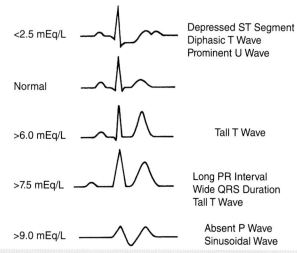

Fig. 12.11 Electrocardiographic changes in hypokalemia and hyperkalemia. (From Park MK. *Park's Pediatric Cardiology for Practitioners.* 6th ed. Philadelphia: Elsevier; 2014.)

Suggested Readings

Buyon JP, Clancy RM, Friedman D. Cardiac manifestations of neonatal lupus erythematosus: guidelines to management, integrating clues from the bench to bedside. *Nat Clin Pract Rheumatol.* 2009;5(3):139–148.

Chun KK, Van Hare GF. Advances in the approach to treatment of supraventricular tachycardia in the pediatric population. *Curr Cardiol Rep.* 2004;6(5):322–326.

McDaniels GM, VanHare GF. Catheter ablation in children and adolescents. *Heart Rhythm.* 2006;3(1):95–101.

Texter KM, Kertesz NJ, Friedman RA, et al. Atrial flutter in infants. *J Am Coll Cardiol.* 2006;48(5):1040–1046.

Tortoriello TA, Snyder CS, Smith EO, et al. Frequency of recurrence among infants with supraventricular tachycardia and comparison of recurrence rates among those with and without preexcitation and among those with and without response to digoxin and/or propranolol therapy. *Am J Cardiol.* 2003;92(9):1045–1049.

13 Pharmacologic Therapy of Heart Disease

KIMBERLY VERA

- *Digoxin* is a cardiac glycoside used as an inotropic agent.
  - Its primary mechanism of action is inhibition of Na$^+$/K$^+$-ATPase activity in the sarcolemma, resulting in increased intracellular sodium. This affects the sodium–calcium exchange, leading to increased intracellular calcium. The increased calcium available to the contractile proteins increases contractility.
    - Secondary effects of digoxin include slowing of cardiac conduction and heart rate.
  - The primary indication for digoxin use is for patients in heart failure with poor systolic cardiac function.
    - Digoxin is also used as an antiarrhythmic.
  - Digoxin is primarily given enterally, and clearance depends on renal excretion.
  - Dosage must be altered in infants with renal impairment.
  - Serum digoxin levels can be measured, but they are generally used in cases of suspected toxicity and not for routine monitoring.
  - Toxicity is manifested by symptoms of poor feeding, vomiting, atrioventricular block, and cardiac arrhythmias.
    - Prolongation of the PR interval is an expected consequence of usage and is not considered a sign of toxicity.
    - Hypokalemia can promote digoxin toxicity, so diuretics should be used with care in conjunction with digoxin use.
    - Amiodarone reduces the elimination of digoxin, so concurrent use should be done with a decreased dose of digoxin.
    - Digoxin toxicity is treated with normalization of potassium levels, antiarrhythmic therapy for arrhythmias, cardiac pacing for atrioventricular block, and Fab antibody fragments for severe toxicity.
- Adrenergic agonists mediate their effects via specific receptors (Table 13.1).

Table 13.1 Receptors Stimulated by Adrenergic Drugs

Drug	Predominant Receptors Affected
Dopamine	Beta-1, dopamine receptor 1 (DA1)
Dobutamine	Beta-1
Epinephrine	Beta-1, beta-2, alpha-1
Isoproterenol	Beta-1, beta-2
Norepinephrine	Alpha-1

- Beta-1 receptors in the myocardium mediate increases in heart rate, contractility, and increased cardiac conduction.
- Beta-2 receptors in the lung mediate bronchodilation and pulmonary vasodilation.
- Beta-2 receptors in skeletal muscle cause vasodilation.
- Alpha-adrenergic receptors in the vasculature mediate vasoconstriction.
- Dopaminergic receptors in the renal and splanchnic vascular beds mediate vasodilation.
- All adrenergic agents require close and continuous hemodynamic monitoring to titrate the dose appropriately.
- Adrenergic agents should be administered through a central venous catheter because extravasation from a peripheral IV can cause significant tissue damage.
- *Dopamine* acts via both beta-adrenergic receptors and alpha-adrenergic receptors.
  - Dopamine also promotes the release of norepinephrine within the myocardium, causing additional stimulation of the beta-1 receptors.
  - At high doses, dopamine stimulates alpha-1 adrenergic receptors, causing vasoconstriction.
  - At low doses, dopamine stimulates dopaminergic receptors in the renal vasculature, promoting renal vasodilation in animal studies.
  - Considerable variability is seen in response at similar doses (some neonates demonstrate an increase in left ventricular output and others a larger increase in mean airway pressure [MAP]).
  - Echocardiography studies show that the predominant mechanism of action is via peripheral vasoconstriction with little increase in left ventricular output (LVO) or superior vena cava (SVC) flow.
  - Sustained high doses of dopamine can lead to gangrene from severe vasoconstriction, tachycardia, and arrhythmias.
  - Dopamine clearance is delayed in the presence of liver or renal dysfunction. Metabolism and clearance of dopamine are decreased in preterm neonates.
  - Dopamine is inactivated when given with sodium bicarbonate.
- *Dobutamine* acts via both beta-adrenergic receptors and alpha-adrenergic receptors.
  - At typical doses, the primary response is via the beta-1 receptors, resulting in an increase in contractility, with minimal effect on heart rate and pulmonary vascular resistance.
  - In the peripheral circulation, the β2-mediated vasodilation and α1-mediated vasoconstriction negate each

other with minimal impact on systemic blood pressure (BP) and afterload.

- The chronotropic effect occurs early after initiation of infusion. After the first 10 to 60 minutes of infusion, the inotropic properties dominate.
- In animal studies, it has been shown to increase cardiac output via both an increase in heart rate and stroke volume.
- As the dose of dobutamine increases, the heart rate and myocardial oxygen demand increase.
- Dobutamine is less effective at increasing blood pressure when compared to dopamine, but it is more effective at improving systemic blood flow.
- The primary use is in infants with heart failure due to poor systolic ventricular function.

- *Epinephrine* is an endogenous catecholamine, with very potent effects on both alpha- and beta-adrenergic receptors.
  - At low doses, beta-1 effects are predominant, with increased heart rate, blood pressure, and contractility.
  - As the dose increases to moderate, a beta-2 receptor effect is seen, with a mild decrease in the diastolic blood pressure.
  - At high doses, the alpha-adrenergic effects are predominant, leading to significant vasoconstriction.
  - In a piglet model, doses <1.6 µg/kg/min of epinephrine increased cardiac output (CO) and lowered both pulmonary vascular resistance (PVR) and systemic vascular resistance (SVR), whereas doses >1.6 µg/kg/min may lower CO and increase SVR and PVR.
  - Comparative studies have shown increases in stoke volume, cardiac output, cerebral blood flow, and systemic vascular resistance to a greater degree for epinephrine than for dopamine.
  - Epinephrine increases myocardial oxygen demand and can lead to ventricular arrhythmias (myocardial β1 activation), myocardial ischemia and tissue ischemia, hyperglycemia, and lactic acidosis (hepatic β2 activation).

- *Isoproterenol* is a synthetic catecholamine with effects on both beta-1 and beta-2 receptors.
  - Isoproterenol increases cardiac contractility and heart rate via beta-1 effects and promotes systemic vasodilation via beta-2 effects.
  - The beta-2 effect also makes this drug a potent pulmonary vasodilator.
  - The primary indication for isoproterenol is bradycardia due to either sinus node dysfunction or atrioventricular block.
  - The major side effects of isoproterenol are tachycardia and arrhythmias.

- *Norepinephrine* (NE) is an endogenous catecholamine that predominantly arises due to release from sympathetic nerve terminals with a minor component released from the adrenal medulla.
  - NE is a potent nonselective α-agonist with some effect at the β1 receptor.
  - It is used as a first-line therapy in pediatric vasodilator shock such as sepsis.
  - It is associated with an increase in systemic vascular resistance and systemic arterial pressure with little or no change in heart rate or cardiac output.

- Limited experience suggests that it may be effective in some term neonates with shock refractory to dopamine and dobutamine.

- *Milrinone* is a selective phosphodiesterase-3 (PDE-3) inhibitor that increases intracellular 3′,5′-cyclic adenosine monophosphate (cAMP) by blocking the enzyme pathway for its degradation and results in an increase in nitric oxide (NO) signaling, which decreases intracellular calcium and causes vasodilation.
  - Milrinone leads to a reduction in systemic blood pressure; therefore, caution is advised in hypotensive patients.
  - It has a half-life of ~4 hours, which is prolonged in organ dysfunction, prematurity, and hypoxic–ischemic encephalopathy (HIE).
  - It improves hemodynamics by using indices of right and left ventricular function in post-cardiac surgery, congenital diaphragmatic hernia, and persistent pulmonary hypertension of newborn.
  - Milrinone prophylaxis is associated with a lower risk of postoperative instability after ligation of hemodynamically significant patent ductus arteriosus (PDA).
  - An improvement in oxygenation and right ventricular function has been documented in extremely low-birthweight (ELBW) infants with pulmonary hypertension.

- *Vasopressin* is an endogenous neuropeptide secreted from the posterior pituitary gland.
  - In major organs in the systemic circulation (e.g., skin, liver, pancreas), vasopressin is a potent vasoconstrictor via V1 receptors located in vascular smooth muscle; thus, it increases systemic vascular resistance and blood pressure.
  - It affects regulation of plasma osmolarity, circulating blood volume, and vascular tone via V2 receptors in the collecting duct of the kidney and water reabsorption via regulation of aquaporins.
  - Vasopressin stimulates central nervous system V3 receptors, resulting in a reduction in heart rate.
  - It has a theoretical benefit in hypotensive infants with left ventricular diastolic dysfunction.
  - Vasopressin is associated with septal hypertrophy/hypertrophic obstructive cardiomyopathy.
  - Adrenocorticotropic hormone (ACTH), in conjunction with vasopressin, leads to an increase in adrenal cortisol secretion and may act synergistically with catecholamines.
  - It can improve hemodynamics and short-term physiologic endpoints in severe sepsis and catecholamine-resistant shock. Caution should be used in neonates with higher risk for impaired myocardial performance due to potential decrease in cardiac output.

Diuretics

- Diuretics are indicted in infants with congestive heart failure and fluid overload.
- *Furosemide* is a loop diuretic that acts via inhibition of chloride–sodium–potassium cotransport in the thick ascending limb of the loop of Henle. The reduction of absorption of chloride, sodium, and potassium leads to the increased excretion of free water.
  - Furosemide is renally excreted, and dose adjustment is required in those with renal impairment.

- The half-life of furosemide is 20 hours in preterm infants and 8 hours in term infants.
  - Adverse effects include dehydration, hypokalemia, hypochloremic metabolic alkalosis, and ototoxicity.
- *Spironolactone* is a potassium-sparing diuretic that inhibits aldosterone in the distal tubule.
- *Thiazide diuretics* act by inhibiting sodium and chloride transport in the distal convoluted tubule.
  - Adverse effects of thiazide diuretics include hypokalemia, hyperuricemia, and hypercalcemia.
- *Spironolactone* is a relatively weak diuretic, so it is often used in combination with other diuretics to lessen the hypokalemic effect of most diuretics.
  - The primary adverse effect of spironolactone is hyperkalemia.

Prostaglandins

- Prostaglandin E1 (PGE1) is used to maintain the patency of the ductus arteriosus or dilate a closed or closing ductus arteriosus in an infant with ductal-dependent congenital heart disease.
- It must be infused continuously, given its short half-life.
- Intravenous access is preferred, but PGE1 can be given through an umbilical arterial line.
- PGE1 dilates both systemic and pulmonary venous vasculature.
- Side effects include hypotension, apnea, fever, irritability, edema, and cutaneous flushing.

Maternal Drugs in Pregnancy

- Fetal exposure to numerous maternal drugs (Table 13.2) and maternal diseases can result in fetal heart disease.

Table 13.2 Maternal Drugs Associated With Fetal Cardiac Abnormalities

Drug	Cardiac Lesion
Carbamazepine	ASD, PDA
Cocaine	ASD, VSD, congenital heart block, TGA
Coumadin	VSD
Cyclophosphamide	TOF
Daunorubicin	TOF
Ethanol	VSD, ASD, DORV, PA, dextrocardia, PDA, TOF
Methotrexate	Dextrocardia
Lithium	Ebstein anomaly
Phenytoin	VSD, pulmonary stenosis, aortic stenosis, coarctation of the aorta
Retinoic acid	VSD, HLHS, TGA, TOF
Thalidomide	TOF, truncus arteriosus, septal defects
Trimethadione	TGA, TOF, HLHS
Valproic acid	TOF, VSD, aortic stenosis, PDA
Vitamin D	Supravalvar aortic stenosis, pulmonary stenosis

ASD, Atrial septal defect; *DORV*, double-outlet right ventricle; *HLHS*, hypoplastic left heart syndrome; *PA*, pulmonary atresia; *PDA*, patent ductus arteriosus; *TGA*, transposition of the great arteries; *TOF*, tetralogy of Fallot; *VSD*, ventricular septal defect.

Suggested Readings

Latifi S, Lidsky K, Blumer JL. Pharmacology of inotropic agents in infants and children. *Prog Pediatr Cardiol.* 2000;12(1):57–79.

Lowrie L. Diuretic therapy of heart failure in infants and children. *Prog Pediatr Cardiol.* 2000;12(1):45–55.

Noori S, Seri I. Neonatal blood pressure support: the use of inotropes, lusitropes, and other vasopressor agents. *Clin Perinatol.* 2012;39(1):221–238.

Shekerdemian L. Perioperative manipulation of the circulation in children with congenital heart disease. *Heart.* 2009;95:1286–1296.

Ward RM, Lugo RA. Cardiovascular drugs for the newborn. *Clin Perinatol.* 2005;32:979–997.

Neurology and Neurodevelopment

NIRANJANA NATARAJAN, ANGELA K. TYSON, LAURA PRICE, JENNIFER BURNSED, SONIA LOMELI BONIFACIO, ANGELINA S. JUNE, JUSTIN ROSATI, JULIE RICCIO, LAURA PRICE, JONATHAN RYAN BURRIS, ALLISON H. PAYNE and GAL BARBUT

14 *Neurologic Evaluation*

NIRANJANA NATARAJAN

The examination of the preterm or term neonate varies based on gestational age. Neurologic examination of the neonate should include evaluation of mental status (alertness, etc.), cranial nerves, motor strength and tone, response to sensory stimulation, and primitive reflexes. These aspects evolve during development and are often state dependent in a neonate. Much of the exam is performed with observation of the unswaddled newborn.

Physical Examination

- Head shape, circumference, and assessment of fontanelle
- Level of alertness: response to touch, ability to spontaneously open eyes to exam
- Cranial nerve: use of brainstem reflexes to aid assessment
- Primitive reflexes
- Motor: degree of spontaneous movement, presence or absence of patterned movements, tone by gestational age
- Deep tendon reflexes
- Sensory: response to touch

Mental Status

Mental status in the neonate may often be determined first by observation, followed by attempts to interact with the neonate. This portion of the exam is "state dependent." Neonates are optimally examined during the time when they are awake and in a calm state. Neonates examined immediately after or during a feed may be sleepy, thus limiting the examination. Key observations help determine the neonate's mental status:

- Does the neonate arouse easily with unswaddling or light touch?
- If crying with the examination, does the infant soothe easily by containment or pacifier (if appropriate for postmenstrual age [PMA])?
- Can the neonate stay awake for the exam, or is stimulation required to maintain an awake state?

Encephalopathy

Altered mentation is referred to as *encephalopathy*. The modified Sarnat scale has helped categorize the varying degrees of encephalopathy into mild, moderate, and severe. The scale incorporates motor posture and tone, as well as primitive reflexes. As discussed elsewhere in this section, the differential diagnoses of neonatal encephalopathy are broad, with hypoxic–ischemic encephalopathy as the most frequent cause.

- Mild encephalopathy: Infant is hyperalert or irritable. Tone is frequently increased, with a hyperactive Moro response. Sympathetic tone predominates.
- Moderate encephalopathy: Infant is lethargic, with decreased spontaneous movements. Tone is typically decreased with weak or incomplete primitive reflexes. Parasympathetic tone predominates.
- Severe encephalopathy: Infant has a stuporous appearance or no responsiveness. There is no spontaneous activity seen, and tone is flaccid with absent primitive reflexes.

Cranial Nerves

To test cranial nerves (CNs) in the neonate, knowledge of brainstem reflexes and the age when they appear is necessary.

- Optical blink reflex (dazzle reflex): CN II (optic) and CN VII (facial). By 26 weeks' PMA, neonates consistently blink to light stimulus. By 32 weeks, blink will remain as long as light remains present.
- Pupillary response: CN II and CN III (oculomotor). Pupillary reaction to light begins at 30 weeks' PMA, and a consistent reaction is present by 32 to 35 weeks' PMA.
- Visual tracking and optokinetic reflex: By term, a neonate should be able to visually fixate on a face and briefly track it at a distance of approximately 1 foot. By 34 weeks' PMA, the infant should be able to follow a bright red object. Optokinetic nystagmus to a rotating drum is present by 36 weeks and is consistent by term.
- Oculomotor functions, controlled by CN III, CN IV (trochlear), and CN VI (abducens), can be evaluated by oculocephalic reflex by 25 weeks' gestation. Eye position at rest (such as dysconjugate gaze) should be evaluated.
- Facial strength can be evaluated with observation. A neonate with hypotonic facies, as noted by a "carp" appearance with mouth open or by decreased nasolabial folds, may suggest a neuromuscular disorder. Neonates with asymmetric facies present only when crying should be closely evaluated for hypoplasia of the depressor anguli oris muscle, which can occur in isolation but also can be associated with renal or cardiac defects; this is not a disorder of the facial nerve or central nervous system.
- Gag reflex: tests CN IX (glossopharyngeal) and CN X (vagus).

Primitive Reflexes

- The Moro response is obtained by sudden dropping of neonate's head in comparison to the torso. This is best elicited by holding the neonate at an inclined position with one hand holding the trunk and a second hand prepared to catch the neonate's head behind it. The neonate is gently dropped back, and the falling head is captured by the examiner. Alternatively, with the neonate lying flat, the infant's torso is gently raised by their hands a few inches from the mattress with the back of the head still touching the mattress, and then the hands are released. The hands should open and the arms first abduct then flex.
  - The Moro response is present by 28 weeks.
  - It is well formed by 37 weeks.
  - It disappears by 6 months.
  - An asymmetric Moro reflex raises suspicion of a brachial plexus injury. Asymmetry is rarely, if ever, secondary to focal brain injury.
- The Palmar response is elicited by placing a finger or object in the palm. Normal response is complete hand closure.
  - The Palmar response is present by 28 weeks and strong by 32 weeks.
  - It disappears by 2 months of age when voluntary grasp arises.
  - Asymmetric absence of palmar response is worrisome for peripheral injury.
  - Persistent fisting with thumb tucked interiorly is suggestive of cerebral injury.
- The tonic neck reflex is flexion of the arm contralateral to head movement.
  - The tonic neck reflex is present by 35 weeks.
  - It is strongest near 44 weeks.
  - It disappears by 6 months of age.
  - Obligatory tonic neck reflex is concerning for a focal cerebral injury.
- The rooting reflex of turning toward a stimulus when touched near the lips starts near 28 weeks and serves to help a neonate find the breast for nursing.

Motor Tone and Strength

Strength in the neonate can be determined by observation, assessing for frequency of spontaneous movements. Tone develops caudal to rostral, with increasing flexor tone to the extremities with increasing maturity to term gestation.

- Tone can be estimated on examination by observing posture. Frog legging is indicative of hypotonia, whereas persistent leg extension can indicate high tone in the term neonate.
- Degree of head lag, ventral suspension, scarf sign, shoulder slip-through, popliteal angle, and ankle flexion can help determine tone.
- Assessments such as the Dubowitz neurologic exam or the Ballard exam can help assess tone for gestational age.

Deep Tendon Reflexes

- Deep tendon reflexes are easiest to elicit in the pectoralis, biceps, brachioradialis, patella, and achilles.
- Head should be maintained midline, as head positioning can alter tone and reflexes.
- Between 4 and 6 beats of clonus is normal in neonates.
- Extensor response on plantar stimulation (Babinski) is normal.
- Abnormal responses include asymmetry of reflexes with head midline, unilateral sustained clonus, unilateral extensor plantar response, or obligate extensor plantar response.

Abnormalities Suggesting Increased Intracranial Pressure

When examining neonates with risk or presence of hydrocephalus, certain findings may clue the clinician to increasing intracranial pressure:

- Splaying of sutures
- Bulging fontanelle
- Skew deviation of eyes in primary gaze
- Tight popliteal angle
- Increased or unexplained apnea and bradycardia events

Suggested Readings

Dubowitz L, Ricciw D, Mercuri E. The Dubowitz neurological examination of the full-term newborn. *Ment Retard Dev Disabil Res Rev.* 2005;11(1):52–60.

Mercuri E, et al. Neurologic examination of preterm infants at term age: comparison with term infants. *J Pediatr.* 2003;142(6):647–655.

Volpe JJ. Neurological examination. In: Volpe JJ, et al, ed. 5th ed. Philadelphia: Saunders; 2008. *Neurology of the Newborn.* xiv:1094.

15 Development of the Nervous System

ANGELA K. TYSON and LAURA PRICE

Table 15.1 summarizes central nervous system (CNS) developmental stages, timing of development, and anomalies associated with maldevelopment at each developmental stage.

Neural Tube Defects

MYELOMENINGOCELE

- Definition
  - Herniation of the spinal cord and meninges through an opened defect in the spinal canal resulting in exposed meninges and spinal cord

Table 15.1 CNS Developmental Stages and Associated Anomalies

Aspect/Stage of Development	Timing of Development	Associated Abnormalities
Primary neurulation (neural tube formation)	3–4 weeks	Encephalocele
		Myelomeningocele
		Anencephaly
		Myeloschisis
		Craniorachischisis
Secondary neurulation (canalization)	4–7 weeks	Tethered cord
		Meningocele
		Spinal cysts
		Teratoma
		Lipoma
Prosencephalic development	2–3 months	Holoprosencephaly
		Septo-optic dysplasia
		Agenesis of corpus callosum
		Agenesis of septum pellucidum
Neuronal/glial proliferation	2–4 months	Microcephaly
		Macrocephaly
		Holoprosencephalies
Neuronal migration	3–5 months	Schizencephaly
		Lissencephaly (e.g., Miller-Dieker syndrome, Walker-Warburg syndrome)
		Polymicrogyria (e.g., Zellweger syndrome)
		Pachygyria
		Heterotopia
Neuronal organization	3 months–2+ years	Fetal alcohol syndrome
		Aneuploidy (e.g., trisomy 13, 18, 21)
Myelination	Term–years	Malnutrition
		White-matter hypoplasia

- Usually no skin covering, can have leakage of cerebral spinal fluid (CSF)
  - Alpha-fetoprotein may be detected from CSF leak in utero in both the amniotic fluid and maternal circulation
  - Leakage of CSF from the lesion may be visible at birth
- Etiology
  - Disorder of primary neurulation (failure of posterior neural tube closure)
  - Occurs at 3 to 4 weeks' gestation
- Epidemiology
  - 0.8 to 1 per 1000 live births worldwide
  - 0.2 to 0.4 per 1000 live birth in the United States
- Ultrasound diagnosis
  - Direct visualization of the spinal defect
  - "Lemon sign"—concave shape of frontal calvarium
  - "Banana sign"—posterior convexity of the cerebellum (seen in Chiari II malformation)
- Maternal risk factors
  - Previously affected neonate with the same partner (highest risk)
  - Low folic acid intake, vitamin B12 deficiency
  - Use of valproate, carbamazepine, alcohol, and/or isotretinoin
  - Obesity, diabetes
  - Hyperthermia
- Prevention
  - Initiation of folic acid 30 days prior to gestation (400 µg daily)
    - Reduces the risk by 70% in the first child
  - If the mother had a prior child with myelomeningocele, then 4000 µg daily is recommended
- Treatment
  - Prenatal management
    - Associated with genetic anomalies; obtain a karyotype
    - In utero surgical repair at <26 weeks' gestation has been studied in a randomized control trial (Management of Myelomeningocele Study [MOMS])
      - Benefits of prenatal surgery
        - Decreased risk of in utero demise and neonatal demise
        - Decreased need for CSF shunt placement postnatally
        - Improved motor function and ambulation
        - Improved neurocognitive function
      - Risks of prenatal surgery
        - Higher risk of uterine rupture (due to surgical site with possible thinning), rupture of membranes (ROM), oligohydramnios, placental abruption, and resultant prematurity

- Delivery management
  - Observational studies of C-section versus vaginal delivery show overall equivocal outcomes
  - Route of delivery is per obstetric indications or if significant hydrocephalus develops
- Initial postnatal management
  - Keep warm, saline-soaked sterile gauze over the lesion and cover with sterile plastic dressing; no latex material
  - Avoid direct pressure on the lesion by placing infant side-lying or prone
  - Antibiotics for meningitis prophylaxis prior to repair
  - Neurosurgical consultation—obtain magnetic resonance imaging (MRI) of the brain and spine
  - Expedited surgical repair of the lesion and possible ventriculoperitoneal shunt will be necessary if significant hydrocephalus develops
- Associated findings
  - Chiari II (majority of cases)
  - Hydrocephalus (80–90% of cases)
  - Agenesis of the corpus callosum
  - Diffuse microstructural anomalies/hypoplasia of cranial nerve nuclei
- Long-term outcomes
  - Bowel and bladder dysfunction in virtually all children
  - Among those affected, 30% to 50% will develop a latex allergy; keep on latex allergy precautions
  - Secondary renal injury due to obstructive hydronephrosis and recurrent urinary tract infections (UTIs) can occur
  - The majority of affected infants have a normal IQ; however, many present with learning disabilities
  - Neuromotor function is associated with the level of lesion (see Table 15.2)

ENCEPHALOCELE

- Definition
  - Herniation of the brain parenchyma and meninges through an opened defect in the skull due to a lack of bone fusion (extracranial meninges ± brain parenchyma)

Table 15.2 Level of Myelomeningocele Lesion and Neuromotor Prognosis

Level of Myelomeningocele Lesion	Neuromotor Prognosis
Above T12 (cervical/thoracic/cervicothoracic)	Minimal motor function, unlikely to ambulate, wheelchair bound
T12–L2 (thoracolumbar)	Minimal to no ambulation abilities, need for full braces and/or wheelchair
L2–L4 (lumbar)	If + knee jerk reflex → ambulation likely with braces and ambulatory devices
L5–S1 (lumbosacral)	If + ankle and knee jerk reflexes → can ambulate; likely to require ankle braces
S2 – S4 (sacral)	If + anal wink, ankle and knee jerk reflexes → full ambulation; unlikely to require braces

- Etiology
  - Disorder of primary neurulation (failure of rostral neural tube closure)
  - Occurs at 3 to 4 weeks' gestation
- Epidemiology
  - 0.8 per 10,000 live births worldwide
  - Higher risk of occurrence with family history of other neural tube defects
- Prenatal findings
  - Maternal serum alpha-fetoprotein
    - If open defect, will be elevated; if closed defect, will be normal
  - High risk of spontaneous abortion
  - >80% located in the occipital region
- Delivery
  - Large > small defect leads to cesarean section > vaginal delivery indications
- Treatment
  - If open: antibiotic prophylaxis and repair at <24 hours of age
  - If closed and stable airway: delayed repair depending on anatomy
  - Obtain karyotype; it may be associated with other syndromes
- Associated findings
  - Hydrocephalus requiring shunt in minority of cases
  - Microcephaly
  - Often with other neural tube defects
- Long-term outcomes
  - Frontal encephaloceles (better prognosis)
  - Occipital lesions (higher risk of hydrocephalus and seizures)
  - The more brain tissue in the defect, the worse the long-term prognosis

ANENCEPHALY

- Definition
  - Neural tube defect resulting in failure of scalp and skull closure (open skull + forebrain degeneration)
  - Results in absent forebrain, loss of most of the cerebrum and cerebellum
  - May spare degeneration of the brainstem
- Etiology
  - Disorder of primary neurulation (failure of anterior neural tube closure)
  - Occurs at 3 to 4 weeks' gestation
- Epidemiology
  - 1 per 50,000 live births in the United States after folic acid supplements began to be added to grains per the US Food and Drug Administration (rate was previously higher)
  - Females > males
  - Higher risk in Hispanic population
- Maternal risk factors
  - Maternal folic acid, zinc, and copper deficiencies
- Prevention
  - Initiation of folic acid 30 days prior to gestation (400 μg daily)
  - If the mother had a prior child with a neural tube defect, then 4000 μg daily

- Prenatal findings
  - Polyhydramnios
  - Elevated alpha-fetoprotein
  - 80% without other defects but should still consider chromosomal analysis
  - Defect is visible on prenatal ultrasound by 3 months of gestation
- Treatment
  - Palliative care
- Long-term outcomes
  - Demise within the first few days to weeks of life

Embryologic Prosencephalon (Forebrain) Defects

FORMATION DEFECTS (APROSENCEPHALY, GARCIA-LURIE SYNDROME)

- Definition
  - No cerebral cortex development due to absent telencephalon and diencephalon formation
  - Caudal structures, including the mesencephalon (midbrain) and rombencephalon (hindbrain), are normal to mildly maldeveloped
- Etiology
  - Prosencephalon (forebrain) defect; occurs later in gestation
  - Suspected inheritance pattern is autosomal recessive
- Epidemiology
  - Extremely rare
- Prenatal findings
  - Ultrasounds findings with microcephaly and smaller facial features with abnormalities of the eyes, limbs, and genitalia
- Associated findings
  - Microcephaly, microphthalmia, microstomia, anal atresia, malformed external genitalia, limb abnormalities (particularly the radius), nasal and throat malformations
  - Intact skull, hair, and scalp/dermal coverings
- Long-term outcomes
  - Lethal, usually with fetal demise

CLEAVAGE DEFECTS (HOLOPROSENCEPHALY)

- Definition
  - Forebrain defect resulting in the improper cleavage of the right and left hemispheres of the brain
  - Four types, from most to least severe: alobar, semilobar, lobar, middle interhemispheric variant (MIHV)
- Etiology
  - Cleavage defect of the prosencephalon
  - ~50% of cases from 14 known genetic defects, high association with trisomy 13
- Epidemiology
  - 1 per every 250 embryos; most die early in utero
  - 1.2 per every 10,000 births
  - Higher risk with familial reoccurrences
- Maternal risk factors
  - Maternal diabetes

- Associated findings (the more severe the type, the more severe the clinical features)
  - Facial and eye abnormalities
    - Unusual facial and skull shape, cleft lip and/or palate, teeth malformations (particularly solitary midline maxillary central incisor), microphthalmia to anophthalmia or cyclopia, coloboma, choanal atresia, abnormal nares and/or nasal bridge
  - Neurological abnormalities
    - Abnormal nervous system morphology, absent or underdeveloped corpus callosum, microcephaly unless hydrocephalus develops, vertebral body formation abnormalities, anterior pituitary gland malfunction, spinal dysraphism and neural tube defects
  - Cardiovascular and pulmonary abnormalities
    - Aortic arch and pulmonary valve malformations, lung hypoplasia, arrythmias, congenital diaphragmatic hernia, Tetralogy of Fallot, ventricular septal defects
  - Gastrointestinal, renal, and genitourinary abnormalities
    - Splenic and renal malformations, urinary tract anomalies, omphalocele
  - Limb abnormalities
    - Polydactyly, talipes
- Long-term outcomes
  - Developmental delays, decreased IQ; many with dystonia and seizures, apnea, and endocrine dysfunction due to anterior pituitary malfunction
  - Prognosis and long-term survival are poor

MIDLINE DEFECTS (AGENESIS OF THE CORPUS CALLOSUM)

- Definition
  - Defect in midline development of the forebrain responsible for the connection of cerebral hemispheres
- Etiology
  - Inherited
  - Autosomal recessive trait
  - X-linked dominant trait
  - Fetal exposure
    - Infectious exposure (cytomegalovirus [CMV], toxoplasmosis, rubella, influenza) during the second trimester
    - Intrauterine alcohol exposure
  - Idiopathic
- Epidemiology
  - All etiologies: 7 per every 1000 births
- Maternal risk factors
  - Alcohol consumption
- Management postnatally
  - MRI of the brain to confirm the diagnosis (standard of care)
  - Chromosomal analysis
  - Care of the infant depends on the severity of presentation.
- Associated syndromes
  - Neurologic: Dandy-Walker malformation, neural tube defects, hydrocephalous

- Metabolic/genetic: Zellweger syndrome; Aicardi syndrome; trisomy 8, 13, and 18; pyruvate dehydrogenase deficiency
- Fetal alcohol syndrome
- Other infectious and congenital heart disease–associated syndromes
- Long-term outcomes
  - From normal life to global developmental delay, seizures, and hydrocephalous (requiring shunt placement)
  - All have increased risk of seizures later in life

Hydrocephalus

- Definition
  - Excessive CSF within the ventricles of the brain
- Etiology
  - In neonates, hydrocephalus is generally a result of abnormal CSF circulation or absorption
- Epidemiology
  - 0.8 per 10,000 live births in the United States
- Important associated diagnoses
  - Aqueductal stenosis (X-linked with adducted thumbs, or nonfamilial)
  - Intraventricular hemorrhage (higher risk with bilateral and higher grade bleeds)
  - Chiari type II malformation (in the setting of myelomeningocele)
  - Dandy-Walker malformation (posterior fossa cysts)
  - Intrauterine infection (toxoplasmosis, CMV)
  - Tumors
  - Ex vacuo (developmental anomalies, ischemic volume loss)
- Clinical presentation
  - Apnea/bradycardia episodes
  - Lethargy
  - Restricted upgaze/abnormal ocular movement
- Treatment
  - Early shunt placement in anatomic/congenital obstruction
    - Ventriculoperitoneal shunt
    - Ventriculoatrial shunt if abdominal scarring or infection
    - Ventriculosubgaleal shunt (VSG)
  - Serial lumbar puncture (LP) in communicating hydrocephalus, although it may become ineffective, as this often evolves to obstructive hydrocephalus
  - Other potential treatments
    - Ventricular access device (VAD) has the same outcomes and complications as the VSG.
    - Endoscopic third ventriculostomy (ETV) has controversial neonatal efficacy.
    - Acetazolamide and furosemide have both been shown to worsen outcomes
- Prognosis is best predicted by two variables:
  - Cerebral mantle thickness prior to shunting
  - Etiology of the hydrocephalus
    - Better in communicating hydrocephalus and myelomeningocele
    - Poor in aqueductal stenosis and Dandy-Walker malformation

Microcephaly

- Definition
  - Occipitofrontal circumference more than 2 standard deviations (SD) below the mean
- Causes
  - Microcephaly vera, which is genetic (typically autosomal recessive) or environmental
  - Early developmental malformations include:
    - Anencephaly, holoprosencephaly
    - Schizencephaly, lissencephaly, polymicrogyria
    - Septo-optic dysplasia
- Aneuploidies
  - Trisomies 13, 18, and 21
- Syndrome-associated examples
  - Smith-Lemli-Opitz syndrome
  - Williams syndrome
  - Cornelia de Lange syndrome
  - Prader-Willi syndrome
- Developmental disruptions
  - Infections: toxoplasmosis, rubella, CMV, herpes simplex virus (HSV), Coxsackieviruses
  - Maternal: diabetes mellitus, uremia, phenylketonuria (PKU), hyperthermia, radiation, cocaine, ethanol, phenytoin
  - Vascular events, stroke, hypoxic–ischemic encephalopathy (HIE), intraventricular hemorrhage (IVH), periventricular leukomalacia (PVL)
  - Neurodegenerative and metabolic disorders
- Multisuture craniosynostosis

Macrocephaly

- Definition
  - Occipitofrontal circumference more than 2 SD above the mean
- Causes
  - Isolated and familial macrocephaly
  - Hydrocephalus disorders
- Growth/overgrowth syndromes
  - Achondroplasia
  - Beckwith-Wiedemann syndrome
  - Sotos syndrome
  - Simpson-Golabi-Behmel syndrome
- Chromosomal disorders
  - Fragile X syndrome
  - Klinefelter syndrome
- Neurocutaneous disorders
  - Neurofibromatosis type I
  - Tuberous sclerosis
  - Sturge-Weber syndrome
- Degenerative and metabolic disorders
  - Tay-Sachs disease with neonatal macrocephaly
- Mass effects
  - Tumors, vascular anomalies, hematomas, effusions

Neonatal Neurotransmitter Effects

- Excitatory amino acids such as *glutamate* dominate in fetal/early neonatal life.
  - Topiramate, a glutamate receptor blocker, is a promising neonatal antiseizure drug.

Table 15.3   Moderators of Cerebral Blood Flow

Increase in This Factor	Effect on Cerebral Blood Flow	Mechanism/Notes
Dopamine	Increases	MAP increase in pressure-passive perfusion.
		β-adrenergic receptor activation
Indomethacin	Decreases	Prostaglandin inhibition
Ibuprofen	No effect	No significant CNS prostaglandin inhibition
Methylxanthine (aminophylline, caffeine)	Decreases	Antagonist to adenosine
Arterial blood pressure	Increases	When pressure-passive perfusion
Venous blood pressure	Decreases	Sudden/significant increase in RA pressure
		Germinal matrix bleed → venous congestion
⇑ $PaCO_2$	Increases	Hypercarbia: ⇑ perivascular H^+
⇓ $PaCO_2$	Decreases	Hypocarbia: ⇓ perivascular H^+
⇑ PaO_2	Decreases	Hyperoxia: increased Ca^+ vasoconstriction
⇓ PaO_2	Increases	Hypoxia: ⇑ H^+, K^+, adenosine, + prostaglandin
Hgb	Decreases	Increases CaO_2 (until significant polycythemia)

Cerebral blood flow is regulated by changes in vascular resistance (primarily arteriolar diameter) affected by local chemical factors. The chemical factors resulting in vasodilation include: H^+, K^+, adenosine, prostaglandins, nitric oxide, and osmolarity. Ca^+ increase results in vasoconstriction.

CaO₂, Arterial oxygen content; *CNS*, central nervous system; *Hgb*, hemoglobin: *MAP*, mean arterial pressure; *PaCO₂*, arterial partial pressure of CO_2 (carbon dioxide); *PaO₂*, arterial partial pressure of oxygen; *RA*, right atrial.

- *Adenosine* is elevated in the fetal CNS; it suppresses fetal respiration and decreases O2 consumption.
  - Theophylline and caffeine are adenosine antagonists which can reduce neonatal apnea
- *Gamma-aminobutyric acid* (GABA) receptor activation opens chloride channels.
  - GABA is initially excitatory in the fetus due to a high chloride content in the nerve cells, which leads to depolarization.
  - GABA then transitions to inhibitory when neurons change from high to low chloride content.
  - Phenobarbital and benzodiazepines are GABAergic:
    - Inhibitory in adults
    - Often excitatory in fetal or early neonatal neurons

Table 15.3 summarizes various factors that can affect cerebral blood flow in neonates.

Suggested Readings

Chu A, Heald-Sargent T, Hageman JR. Primer on microcephaly. *NeoReviews.* 2017;18(1):e44–e51.

Craig A, Lober RM, Grant GA. Complex fetal care: implications of fetal ventriculomegaly: a neurosurgical perspective. *NeoReviews.* 2015;16(4): e254–e259.

Greisen G. Autoregulation of cerebral blood flow. *NeoReviews.* 2007;8(1): e22–e31.

Onley AH. Macrocephaly syndromes. *Semin Pediatr Neurol.* 2007;14:128–135.

Shankaran S. Complications of neonatal intracranial hemorrhage. *NeoReviews.* 2000;21(3):e44–e47.

Verity C, Firth H, French-Constant C. Congenital abnormalities of the central nervous system. *J Neuro Neurosurg Psychiatry.* 2003;74(suppl I):i3–i8.

16 *Neonatal Encephalopathy*

JENNIFER BURNSED

Neonatal Encephalopathy

OVERVIEW

- Neonatal encephalopathy (NE) is defined as an alteration in consciousness or neurologic exam in a neonate.
- The possible etiologies of NE are broad (Table 16.1), but it is most commonly caused by hypoxic–ischemic encephalopathy (HIE).

Hypoxic Ischemic Encephalopathy

OVERVIEW

- HIE is a common cause of neonatal encephalopathy and is defined by its pathophysiology as a mismatch between cerebral blood flow and oxidative metabolism resulting in injury and encephalopathy.

PATHOPHYSIOLOGY

- Phases of injury include:
  - Primary energy failure (onset minutes to hours) characterized by
    - Decreased cerebral ATP and membrane depolarization
    - Increased excitotoxic neurotransmitter release and neuron damage
  - Latent phase (onset hours to days) characterized by
    - Oxidative stress, excitotoxicity, and inflammation
  - Secondary energy failure (onset days) characterized by
    - Mitochondrial dysfunction, oxidative stress, and excitotoxicity
    - Irreversible neuronal death
  - Tertiary phase (onset months to years) characterized by inflammation, impaired neuroregeneration and repair, and epigenetic changes

CLINICAL PRESENTATION

- Depends on duration, timing, and severity of event or insult and may evolve over hours to days
- Risk factors are listed in Table 16.2.

DIAGNOSIS AND EVALUATION

- Diagnosis of encephalopathy or suspected HIE is based on biochemical criteria, perinatal events, and exam criteria.
- History may include evidence of perinatal distress raising suspicion of hypoxic–ischemic insult, including abnormal fetal heart tracing, meconium-stained amniotic fluid, cord prolapse, uterine rupture, fetomaternal hemorrhage, and difficult extraction.
- Perinatal resuscitation also encompasses aspects of
  - Need for resuscitation (required assisted ventilation, chest compressions, medications)
  - Low Apgar scores persisting beyond 5 minutes
- Neurological exam criteria for evaluating encephalopathy are based on the standardized Sarnat staging shown in Table 16.3.
  - Assessment includes altered level of consciousness, abnormal tone, jitteriness, apnea, abnormal cry, assessment of anatomic nervous systems (bradycardia, pupillary reflex), reflexes (Moro), and seizures.
    - Seizures are often seen in the first 6 to 12 hours, usually with an onset within the first 24 hours.
  - Electroencephalogram (EEG) is useful for monitoring for seizures.
    - Electrographic seizures without clinical correlate are common (especially after administration of antiepileptic medication).
    - EEG background is useful for determining the severity and evolution of encephalopathy and outcome.

Table 16.1   Causes of Neonatal Encephalopathy

Hypoxic–ischemic encephalopathy

Perinatal stroke

Kernicterus

Metabolic derangements (inborn errors of metabolism, hypoglycemia)

Intracranial hemorrhage

Sinovenous thrombosis

Infection

Maternal toxins

Table 16.2   Risk Factors for Neonatal Encephalopathy

Preconception	Antepartum	Intrapartum
Fertility treatments	Multiple gestation	Induction of labor
Insulin-dependent diabetes mellitus	Placental abruption	Maternal fever
Thyroid disease	Intrauterine growth restriction	Emergency cesarean section
Advanced maternal age	Severe preeclampsia	Instrumented delivery
Nulliparity	Antepartum hemorrhage	Cord prolapse
	Postterm gestation	Malpresentation
		Lack of trained personnel

Table 16.3   Clinical Staging of Hypoxic–Ischemic Encephalopathy (Sarnat Criteria)

Finding	Stage 1	Stage 2	Stage 3
Level of consciousness	Alert	Lethargic	Comatose
Muscle tone	Normal	Hypotonic	Flaccid
Tendon reflexes	Normal/increased	Increased	Depressed/absent
Myoclonus	Present	Present	Absent
Complex reflexes			
Sucking	Active	Weak	Absent
Moro	Exaggerated	Incomplete	Absent
Grasp	Normal/exaggerated	Exaggerated	Absent
Oculocephalic "doll's eyes")	Normal	Overreactive	Reduced/absent

- Neuroimaging
  - Magnetic resonance imagining (MRI) is the gold standard.
  - Computed tomography (CT) scan is *not* recommended for diagnosis or prognosis.
  - Ultrasound may be helpful to visualize cerebral edema and severe injury but is not an ideal modality.
  - MRI is sensitive for diagnosis and prognosis.
    - Abnormal signal in the posterior limb of the internal capsule is associated with an adverse motor outcome.
    - MRI is helpful in predicting outcome at 18 months.
  - Patterns of injury seen on MRI:
    - Global usually occur in the context of severe/prolonged insult.
    - Basal ganglia/thalamus injury pattern is often associated with an acute event.
    - Watershed/white matter injury pattern is associated with prolonged or partial injury in arterial watershed zones.

TREATMENT

- Supportive care is the mainstay of treatment, as injury has already occurred.
  - ABCs (airway, breathing, circulation)
  - Monitor for and treat seizures appropriately (amplitude-integrated EEG or EEG monitoring, antiepileptic medications).
  - Treat and support other end-organ dysfunction (e.g., myocardial dysfunction, pulmonary hypertension, hepatic dysfunction, renal injury, coagulopathy).
  - There is no consensus regarding the treatment of cerebral edema (steroids, hyperventilation, furosemide, and mannitol have not been shown to be helpful and may be harmful).
  - Maintain normoglycemia, normotension, and normal blood gases.
  - Avoid hyperthermia, which has been linked to worse neurologic outcomes.
- Therapeutic hypothermia
  - Routine care for moderate to severe HIE; whole body and selective head cooling are equally effective
  - Initiate therapeutic hypothermia in the first 6 hours of age, as soon as possible (earlier onset associated with improved outcomes).

- Multimechanistic (decreases cerebral metabolic rate, decreases cerebral edema, anti-inflammatory, decreases free radical production)
- Improved 18- to 21-month neurodevelopmental outcomes, with the number needed to treat being ~7

PROGNOSIS AND OUTCOMES

- Outcomes are variable, depending on the severity of the insult and pattern of injury.
- Delayed return of spontaneous respirations, need for chest compressions, seizures, and base deficit > −16 are associated with a poor outcome.
- Mild encephalopathy outcomes were once thought to be normal; however, there is growing evidence that this is not the case. Ongoing research is investigating best practices and treatments for neonates with mild encephalopathy. Patients with severe encephalopathy are at high risk of severe impairments (spastic quadriplegia, epilepsy, cortical visual impairment) or death; moderate encephalopathy outcomes are highly variable.
- Injury to deep gray matter or posterior limb of internal capsule is often associated with adverse motor outcomes.

Metabolic Encephalopathies

OVERVIEW

- Encephalopathies from metabolic causes include severe hypoglycemia, kernicterus, and inborn errors of metabolism (organic acidurias, urea cycle defects, amino acidopathies, peroxisomal disorders, mitochondrial disorders, and glycogen storage disorders).

CLINICAL PRESENTATION

- Seizures, encephalopathy, vomiting, abnormal tone
- May mimic HIE or infection but history often does not support an acute event or infectious risk factors.
- Depending on the disorder, the patient may have an asymptomatic period at birth and then present with encephalopathy in the coming hours to days as toxic metabolites accumulate.

Table 16.4 Classic Magnetic Resonance Imaging Findings in Metabolic Disorders

Disorder	Magnetic Resonance Imaging Findings
Nonketotic hyperglycinemia	Early delayed myelination, agenesis of corpus callosum, atrophic basal ganglia, progressive cerebral atrophy
Molybdenum cofactor deficiency/sulfite oxidase deficiency	Edema in white matter and caudate, cystic changes, cortical/white matter/basal ganglia injury consistent with asphyxia
Pyridoxine-dependent seizures	Cerebellar hypoplasia, generalized atrophy, thin corpus callosum
Zellweger syndrome	Subependymal cysts, profound hypomyelination, cortical malformations
Pyruvate dehydrogenase deficiency	Delayed myelination, agenesis of corpus callosum, atrophy
Maple syrup urine disease	Delayed myelination, generalized edema
Urea cycle disorders	Resemble asphyxia: gray/white matter edema (subacute), cortical/white matter injury (chronic)

Adapted from Ibrahim M, et al. Inborn errors of metabolism: combining clinical and radiologic clues to solve the mystery. *AJR Am J Roentgenol*. 2014;203:W315–W327.

- May have metabolic lactic acidosis and/or hyperammonemia
- MRI may reveal a pattern of injury inconsistent with HIE.

DIAGNOSIS AND EVALUATION

- Blood gas, electrolytes, creatinine, BUN, liver function tests, ammonia, lactate, plasma amino acids, urine organic acids, and cerebral spinal fluid (CSF) studies (lactate, pyruvate) are useful for diagnosis.
- MRI is valuable in assessing changes in brain matter (see Table 16.4 for the characteristic patterns of injury for metabolic conditions).

TREATMENT

- Holding enteral feeds (NPO) versus adaptation of nutritional diet to meet metabolite deficit or accumulation
- Intravenous (IV) dextrose containing fluids, no protein initially
- Avoid catabolic state.
- Obtain a genetic/metabolic consultation.

- More focused treatment depends on the specific disorder (may need emergent dialysis or IV alternative waste therapy, such as sodium benzoate or sodium phenylacetate).
- Goal is treatment of the underlying disorder with a tailored diet, fluids, enzyme replacement, or possible drug therapy.

Suggested Reading

Badawi N, et al. Antepartum risk factors for newborn encephalopathy: the Western Australian case-control study. *BMJ*. 1998;317(7172):1549–1553.

Bonifacio S, Gonzalez F, Ferriero D. Neuroprotection strategies for the newborn. In: Gleason C, Juul S, eds. *Avery's Diseases of the Newborn*. 11th ed. Philadelphia: Saunders; 2018:910–921.

Ibrahim M, Parmar HA, Hoefling N, Srinivasan A. Inborn errors of metabolism: combining clinical and radiologic clues to solve the mystery. *AJR Am J Roentgenol*. 2014;203:W315–W327.

Molloy EJ, El-Dib M, Juul SE, et al. Neuroprotective therapies in the NICU in term infants: present and future. *Pediatr Res*. 2022;93(7):1819–1827.

Rutherford MA, Pennock JM, Schwieso JE, et al. Hypoxic ischaemic encephalopathy: early magnetic resonance imaging findings and their evolution. *Neuropediatrics*. 1995;26(4):183–191.

Sarnat HB, Sarnat MS. Neonatal encephalopathy following fetal distress. A clinical and electroencephalographic study. *Ann Neurol*. 1976; 33(10):696–705.

17 *Intracranial Hemorrhage and Vascular Injury*

SONIA LOMELI BONIFACIO

Subdural Hemorrhage

OVERVIEW

- Subdural hemorrhage is an injury that occurs between the dura mater and the arachnoid tissue that surrounds the brain. The dura mater contains bridging veins and the major venous sinuses.
- Risk factors include macrosomia, use of forceps, cephalopelvic disproportion, and shoulder dystocia.
- It is the most common intracranial hemorrhage in term newborns.
- Incidence is 2.9/100,000 live births; it doubles with vacuum or forceps use and is 10 times higher if both vacuum and forceps are used.
- Hemorrhage results from compression or stretching forces causing tearing of the falx cerebri or the cerebellar tentorium (both extensions of the dura mater).
  - Injury of the superficial veins leads to hemorrhage over the surface of the brain.
  - Injury of the straight sinus or vein of Galen leads to hemorrhage at the base of the brain into the posterior fossa.

CLINICAL PRESENTATION AND DIAGNOSIS

- Subdural hemorrhage is the suspected etiology with a history of traumatic or difficult delivery and the neonate has neurologic signs such as unequal pupils, eye deviation, or hemiparesis.
- Neonates may present with bulging anterior fontanelle, pallor, irritability, lethargy, and/or decreased Moro reflex, encephalopathy, and sometimes seizures.
- Posterior fossa bleeds can present differently with apnea and bradycardia, encephalopathy (altered mental status), seizures, or opisthotonos.
- Magnetic resonance imaging (MRI) is the diagnostic test of choice over computed tomography (CT) due to radiation. Ultrasound (US) is inadequate for diagnosis.

TREATMENT

- No treatment is needed if the neonate is asymptomatic.
- Symptomatology (signs of increasing intracranial pressure, neurologic deterioration, seizures) requires neurosurgical involvement. Evacuation of posterior fossa bleed may be needed.

Subarachnoid Hemorrhage

OVERVIEW

- Subarachnoid hemorrhage is bleeding of bridging veins in the subarachnoid space.
- It is the second most common intracranial hemorrhage in term neonates.

CLINICAL PRESENTATION AND DIAGNOSIS

- Most neonates are asymptomatic but can have symptoms similar to those with subdural hemorrhage.
- Symptoms present at 24 to 48 hours after birth with apnea and seizures (due to irritation from blood overlying the meninges and cortex).
- MRI is the diagnostic test of choice over CT due to radiation.

TREATMENT

- The injury usually self-resolves.
- Secondary hydrocephalus can develop due to impaired resorption of cerebral spinal fluid.
- Injury progression with signs of herniation requires immediate neurosurgical consultation. Secondary hydrocephalus can develop due to impaired resorption of cerebral spinal fluid.

Epidural Hematoma

OVERVIEW

- Epidural hematoma is injury to the middle meningeal artery resulting in bleeding between the dura and skull; it is associated with an overlying skull fracture.
- There is a higher incidence with instrumented deliveries.

CLINICAL PRESENTATION AND DIAGNOSIS

- May present with hypotonia, seizures, bulging fontanelle, and encephalopathy
- Diagnose with MRI or CT.

TREATMENT

- Close observation is necessary, but it usually resolves without intervention.
- Monitor for signs of herniation; if present, consult neurosurgery emergently.

Intraventricular Hemorrhage

OVERVIEW

- Intraventricular hemorrhage (IVH) most commonly occurs in premature neonates, with the highest incidence in those born at <29 weeks' gestation.
- The incidence has decreased over the last two decades, but it still occurs in about 20% of the highest risk patients.
- There are two common grading systems: Papile and Volpe.
  - Grade 1 IVH, germinal matrix hemorrhage ± ventricular enlargement < 10%
  - Grade 2 IVH, 10% to 50% of ventricle with blood, not distending ventricle
  - Grade 3 IVH, >50% of ventricle with blood, usually with distension
  - Grade IV IVH was previously described as an extension of a hemorrhage into the parenchyma but it is now commonly referred to as a *periventricular hemorrhagic infarction* (PVHI); it is thought to represent a venous infarction.
- Pathogenesis is multifactorial and related to
  - Fragile subependymal germinal matrix (site of origin of IVH)
  - Pressure passive state due to poor cerebral autoregulation
  - Lack of supporting basement membrane of the germinal matrix
  - Fluctuations in cerebral blood flow and increased cerebral venous pressure
  - Endothelial injury
  - Coagulopathy
- IVH can be seen in term infants in association with sinovenous thrombosis.

CLINICAL PRESENTATION AND DIAGNOSIS

- Injury is rarely present at birth; IVH presents within day 3 to 4 of life, and the vast majority by the first week of life.
- Presentation depends on the severity of the hemorrhage.
  - Grades I and II are usually clinically silent.
  - Grade III and PVHI may present with sudden deterioration, tachycardia, hypotension, decreasing hematocrit, and a full fontanelle.
- A low-grade hemorrhage can extend to a higher-grade hemorrhage over the course of several days.
- Diagnosis is made by cranial US.
- Screening US should be done on neonates born at <32 weeks or <1500 g.
  - Scans done by 72 hours will detect 90% of bleeds and nearly all by 7 days of age.

TREATMENT

- The best treatment for IVH is the prevention of preterm births.
  - Antenatal steroids and magnesium sulfate also reduce the incidence of IVH.
  - Postnatal interventions include delayed cord clamping and use of care bundles in the first 72 hours after—gentle ventilation, minimal handling, midline head positioning, and maintenance of normal carbon dioxide levels.
- Treatment is supportive care and maintenance of homeostasis to avoid secondary brain injury.
  - Maintain blood pressure in the normal range for gestational age.
  - Slow-volume resuscitation to avoid rapid changes in cerebral blood flow.
  - Avoid hypoglycemia, swings in carbon dioxide, hypoxia, and hypothermia.
- Monitor large-grade hemorrhages for development of obstructive hydrocephalus.
  - These hemorrhages occur in about 29%.
  - Follow head circumference closely.
  - Obtain serial US to monitor for ventricular dilation. Ventricular dilation typically develops 2 to 6 weeks post hemorrhage.
  - Serial lumbar punctures are done in some centers to avoid placing reservoirs or drains.
  - Ventriculoperitoneal (VP) shunts may be needed but carry significant risk of infection and malfunction.

OUTCOME

- Grade I and II may be clinically silent and involute over time.
- Severe Grade III and PVHI:
  - 50% to 75% of survivors will develop cerebral palsy, cognitive and/or motor impairments, or hydrocephalus.
  - Follow-up imaging for signs of periventricular leukomalacia is warranted.
  - Developmental pediatrics, physical therapy, and occupational therapy will likely be needed.

Intraparenchymal Cysts, Echodensities, Periventricular Leukomalacia

OVERVIEW

- Periventricular white matter is an area vulnerable to injury in preterm neonates.
- Echodensities in the periventricular white matter are common and can be transient or prolonged or progress to cyst formation.
  - Prevalence ranges from 18% to 40% and is dependent on gestational age at birth.
  - Outcomes are favorable for echodensities that resolve.
  - The impact of echodensities that persist on neurodevelopment is unknown.
- Intraparenchymal cysts are thought to be due to hypoxia–ischemia and/or inflammatory insults.
  - In preterm neonates they appear in the periventricular region.
- Periventricular leukomalacia (PVL) refers to white matter injury (WMI), characterized by focal cystic necrotic lesions in the area around the ventricles.

- PVL and periventricular WMI are thought to be due to hypoxia–ischemia, inflammation, infection, and abnormal oligodendrocyte maturation.

CLINICAL PRESENTATION AND DIAGNOSIS

- WMI identified by US is clinically silent in the neonatal period.
- Neurologic exam at discharge and evaluation of generalized movements may identify subtle abnormalities in neonates with significant PVL or WMI.
- PVL and more diffuse periventricular WMI increase the risk for development of spastic diplegia cerebral palsy (tightness and stiffness affecting lower extremities more than upper extremities).
- PVL screens can be done by serial cranial US at 4 to 8 weeks and by MRI at term corrected gestational age.

TREATMENT

- Infants with PVL benefit from early childhood development intervention.

Cerebellar Hemorrhage

OVERVIEW

- The cerebellar hemorrhage injury pathogenesis is multifactorial and similar to IVH.
- Risk factors include very low birth weight, significant resuscitation at birth, low APGAR scores, hemodynamic instability, patent ductus arteriosus, and prolonged mechanical ventilation.
- Hemorrhage can be isolated or seen in conjunction with IVH or white matter injury.
- Postmortem studies have shown that hemorrhages are found in 25% of low-birth-weight infants.
- Cerebellar hemorrhage is increasingly recognized in premature neonates due to improved US technology and higher utilization of MRI.

CLINICAL PRESENTATION AND DIAGNOSIS

- Cerebellar hemorrhage is clinically silent in the neonatal period.
- Several studies have shown an association with increased neonatal morbidity and mortality, as well as cognitive, motor, and behavioral abnormalities.

TREATMENT

- The mainstay of treatment is supportive care.

Prenatal Vascular Injury

OVERVIEW

- Prenatal vascular injury is a neurologic vascular injury prior to birth that can result in significant disruption of normal brain development dependent on the gestational age at which the insult occurs.
- Pathogenesis includes emboli, hemorrhage, vasoconstriction, and disseminated intravascular coagulation (DIC).
- Risk factors include demise of a co-twin, infection with cytomegalovirus (CMV), maternal diabetes, cocaine exposure, maternal abdominal trauma leading to fetal vascular changes, and certain hereditary conditions.

CLINICAL PRESENTATION AND DIAGNOSIS

- Depending on the gestational age and mechanism, prenatal vascular injury may be identified prior to birth with routine US surveillance of pregnancy.
- Obtain fetal MRI to identify the pathophysiology and extent of injury.
- Fetus may be identified as microcephalic.
- Destruction of brain tissue and resultant encephalomalacia or intracranial hemorrhage can be seen.
- Schizencephaly (fluid-filled cavity in the fetal brain) may also result from antenatal vascular injury (usually diagnosed after 28 weeks).
- Symptoms depend on the extent of brain injury and timing of insult during pregnancy relative to when the infant is born.
- There may be abnormal tone (low or high) and possibly contractures, poor feeding, and abnormal mental status.

TREATMENT

- The mainstay of treatment is supportive care.
- There is long-term risk for abnormal motor and cognitive development, as well as seizures.

Perinatal Cerebral Infarction

OVERVIEW

- Cerebral infarction (stroke) refers to conditions where there is a focal disruption of cerebral blood flow secondary to arterial or cerebral venous thrombosis, or embolization that occurs from 20 weeks of gestation through the 28th postnatal day and confirmed by neuroimaging or neuropathology studies.
- The etiology of infarction can be ischemic or hemorrhage.
- Cerebral infarction is classified as
  - Perinatal cerebral infarction, which occurs between 28 weeks' gestation and 7 days after birth
  - Neonatal cerebral infarction, which occurs between 0 and 28 days of life
  - Presumed perinatal infarction, which presents at >28 days of age
- Stroke occurs in 1/2300 to 1/4000 births.
- The etiology is multifactorial with a complex interplay of neonatal, maternal, genetic, and delivery factors.

CLINICAL PRESENTATION AND DIAGNOSIS

- Arterial ischemic stroke tends to be left-sided in distribution of the middle cerebral artery (MCA) and has a slight male predominance.

- Usually occurs by 24 hours after birth with clinical seizures (focal motor or apnea without bradycardia) in an otherwise well-appearing infant
  - May show mild encephalopathy and mild hypotonia
  - Rare to have focal motor deficits or asymmetry on exam
  - Seizures are repetitive and increase in frequency in the first hours after onset.
- Cerebral sinovenous thrombosis (CSVT) involves the large sinuses/veins (superior sagittal sinus) often traumatized during delivery.
  - Clinical presentation differs from an arterial stroke.
  - CSVT presents after several days of age in the setting of dehydration or sepsis.
  - Patients are more encephalopathic than those with focal arterial stroke.
- Presumed perinatal arterial ischemic strokes tend to present with signs of
  - Early handedness at 3 to 11 months of age
  - Seizures at 5 to 14 months of age
  - Abnormal gait at 12 to 21 months of age

TREATMENT

- Currently there are no therapeutic treatments for stroke.
- Supportive care is the mainstay of treatment, with hydration and avoidance of hyperthermia in the acute phase and monitoring and treatment of seizures.

- Hypothermia has not been trialed for stroke.
- Erythropoietin is effective in animal models but has not yet been tested in human randomized controlled trials (RCTs).
- Anticoagulation has been used in the treatment of CSVT but is not considered standard of care.
- Follow-up after discharge should include occupational therapy, developmental pediatrics, and child neurology.
- Epilepsy in early childhood may occur in up to two-thirds of patients.
- Outcomes are dependent on size and location.
  - 40% will be normal.
  - 57% will have cognitive or motor impairments.
  - 3% may die.
- There is a low risk of stroke recurrence.

Suggested Readings

Back SA. Brain injury in the preterm infant: new horizons for pathogenesis and prevention. *Pediatr Neurol*. 2015;53(3):185–192.

de Vries LS, Benders MJ, Groenendaal F. Imaging the premature brain: ultrasound or MRI? *Neuroradiology*. 2013;55(suppl. 2):13–22.

de Vries LS, Benders MJ, Groenendaal F. Progress in neonatal neurology with a focus on neuroimaging in the preterm infant. *Neuropediatrics*. 2015;46(4):234–241.

Guo T, Duerden EG, Adams E, et al. Quantitative assessment of white matter injury in preterm neonates: association with outcomes. *Neurology*. 2017;88(7):614–622.

Kirton A, deVeber G. Advances in perinatal ischemic stroke. *Pediatr Neurol*. 2009;40(3):205–214.

Caput Succedaneum

OVERVIEW

- Caput succedaneum represents swelling of the scalp secondary to pressure of the scalp and fetal head against the uterine and vaginal walls or cervix during labor and delivery.
- Pressure results in the accumulation of blood and serum in the tissue above the periosteum but below the skin.
- Caput succedaneum can cross suture lines due to its location above the periosteum.

CLINICAL PRESENTATION AND DIAGNOSIS

- Swelling of the scalp observed after birth
- Natural history and complications:
  - Benign with infrequent complications
  - Caput succedaneum resolves within several days to a week after birth.
  - Abrasions of the skin overlying the area of caput can develop a secondary infection.
  - If the caput is large in size or enlarges after birth and a vacuum was used, consider an iatrogenic encephalocele. Imaging should be performed if there are neurologic deficits or hemodynamic instability.

Cephalohematoma

OVERVIEW

- Cephalohematoma represents a collection of blood underneath the periosteum.
- Commonly occurs in instrumented or non-instrumented deliveries.

CLINICAL PRESENTATION AND DIAGNOSIS

- Cephalohematoma is a swelling or mass on the cranium that does *not* cross suture lines; they are usually unilateral (see Fig. 18.1).
- Natural history and complications:
  - Cephalohematoma is most prominent on postnatal day 3 of life.
  - Monitor for development of hyperbilirubinemia.
  - Involute over the course of several weeks.
  - Palpable nodules can form that resolve over the course of months; some calcify and can be felt longer.

- Rare complications include secondary infections of the cephalohematoma and osteomyelitis of the underlying skull.

Subgaleal Hemorrhage

OVERVIEW

- Subgaleal hemorrhage represents bleeding (rupture of the emissary veins) that occurs in the unrestricted space beneath the epicranial aponeurosis and above the periosteum.
- Hemorrhage can be large, with the potential to steal 40% or more of the newborn's intravascular blood volume (125 mL, assuming a weight of 3.5 kg and blood volume of 90 mL/kg).
- Each 1-cm increase in occipital frontal circumference (OFC) represents 30 to 40 mL of bleeding into the space.
- The incidence is 4/10,000 non-instrumented deliveries and 64/10,000 vacuum-assisted deliveries.

CLINICAL PRESENTATION AND DIAGNOSIS

- Boggy fluctuant cranium with distention that crosses suture lines and may have a fluid wave to touch (see Fig. 18.1).
- Bleeding is circumferential and thus extends down toward the orbits, along the temporal and occipital regions, and to the nape of the neck. Ears may appear to be protuberant.
- Signs and symptoms include tachycardia, pallor and poor perfusion, a decreasing hematocrit, and increasing head circumference.
- Large hemorrhages can result in hemorrhagic shock within hours following birth.
  - Mortality rates are high (14%) due to shock and consumptive coagulopathy.
- Diagnosis can be made with high clinical suspicion with addition of imaging such as ultrasound (US) and/or magnetic resonance imaging (MRI).
- MRI can be performed to confirm the location of hemorrhage and to rule out secondary hypoxic–ischemic injury in the setting of significant hemorrhage and shock.

MONITORING AND TREATMENT

- Frequent repeated exams, measurement of occipital–frontal head circumference, vital signs, and hematocrit are required.

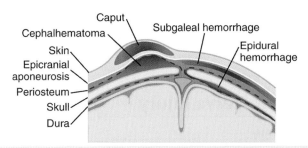

Fig. 18.1 Sites of extracranial (and extradural) hemorrhages in the newborn. Schematic diagram of important tissue planes from skin to dura. (From Kliegman MD, et al., eds. *Nelson Textbook of Pediatrics.* 19th ed. Philadelphia: Elsevier; 2011, Fig. 93.1.)

- The period of highest risk for extension of bleeding is the first 24 to 48 hours after birth.
- Hemodynamic instability and falling hematocrit warrant admission to the intensive care unit.
- Establish venous access for volume resuscitation, blood transfusion, and monitoring of blood pressure and signs of coagulopathy.
- Mainstay of treatment is supportive measures. Appropriate and timely volume resuscitation with normal saline, transfusion of packed red blood cells, and replacement of clotting factors and platelets as indicated by laboratory studies.
- Closely follow for indirect hyperbilirubinemia secondary to bleed and red blood cell breakdown.

Skull Fractures

OVERVIEW

- Skull fractures can occur during unassisted and assisted deliveries most commonly located in the frontal and parietal regions as depressed or linear injuries.
- Fractures can be due to compression of the skull against the pelvic bones or to assisted forceps.

CLINICAL PRESENTATION AND DIAGNOSIS

- Linear skull fractures by definition are not depressed and usually do not require intervention.
  - They are rarely associated with an intracranial injury.
  - Linear skull fractures may not be detected at birth.
  - If they are detected and there are no additional neurologic signs or symptoms, follow-up x-rays can be performed to document healing and to rule out the development of a leptomeningeal cyst.
- Depressed skull fractures are associated with prolonged second-stage labor and instrumented deliveries (forceps).
  - They tend to occur over the parietal region, and there may be associated intracranial bleeding.
  - Small, <1-cm depressed skull fractures can be managed with close observation.
  - Larger fractures (>1 cm) should be followed closely for the development of neurologic sequelae such as subdural bleeding and seizures.
  - Obtain MRI or computed tomography (CT) to characterize the injury, and obtain a neurosurgical consultation within 12 to 24 hours of birth. Treatment is determined by neurosurgery.

Treatment

- Linear skull fractures rarely require intervention, and they heal on their own.
- Depressed skull fractures with neurologic sequelae require consultation and evaluation by neurosurgery with treatment to be determined by their team.

Spinal Cord Injuries

OVERVIEW

- Spinal cord injuries tend to occur in full-term infants in deliveries that are complicated by breech vaginal deliveries or shoulder dystocia and require assistance (forceps or vacuum application).
- They occur in 0.14/10,000 live births.
- Injuries can range from a spinal epidural hematoma to full transection.
- Fetuses with hypotonia may have an increased risk of spinal cord injury during delivery due to decreased muscle tone, which allows the spine to be stretched and flexed more than the cord can accommodate.
- Postnatal spinal cord injury can be secondary to hemorrhagic compression or ischemia due to spinal stroke.
- Injury has also been seen in the setting of umbilical arterial catheters or extravasation of parenteral fluids from a central venous catheter.

CLINICAL PRESENTATION AND DIAGNOSIS

- Presentation and prognosis are dependent on the extent of injury to the cord and the level of the cord at which the injury occurs.
- At birth, patients can present with significant respiratory depression, hypotonia, and paraparesis.
- Urinary retention and abdominal distention may occur.
- Transection of the spinal cord represents the worst injury and results in complete paralysis below the level of transection.
- High cervical spine and brainstem injuries are associated with rotation and longitudinal traction of the head and neck during delivery. They carry a very high mortality rate due to compromise of the respiratory system.
- Lower cervical lesions still carry significant morbidity and mortality.

TREATMENT

- Secure the airway with intubation, and immobilize the head and neck.
- Obtain x-rays of the spine, and utilize MRI to visualize the spinal cord.
- Involve neurosurgical expertise.
- In rare cases, the use of therapeutic hypothermia has been reported.

Brachial Plexus Injury

OVERVIEW

- Brachial plexus injury occurs due to lateral traction of the fetal head and is due to compression of the nerve within the nerve sheath from hemorrhage or edema.
- It is associated with macrosomic infants, prolonged labors, and reduction of shoulder dystocia.
- Severe cases may involve avulsion of the nerve from the cord.
- Injury is usually unilateral and can involve C5, C6, and sometimes C7; occasionally, it can include from C5 through T1 with clinical manifestations related to the injured nerve roots.

CLINICAL PRESENTATION AND DIAGNOSIS

- C5/C6 injury (Erb-Duchenne palsy): The arm is held in adduction and is internally rotated with extension and pronation of the forearm.
- C7 injury (Waiter's tip deformity): The wrist is held in a flexed position due to weakness of the extensor muscles. Physical exam shows asymmetric Moro reflex, absent on the affected side; biceps reflex will be weak or absent.
- C8/T1 injury (Klumpke paralysis): Weakness of the flexor muscles of the wrist and intrinsic muscles of the hand is observed. Grasp reflex will be absent, and there may be a loss of sensation. This is the least frequent brachial plexus injury.
- Horner syndrome is an injury involving cervical sympathetic nerves and unilateral miosis.
- Complete brachial plexus injury results in complete paralysis of the arm.

TREATMENT

- Supportive and physical therapy to prevent contractures
- Obtain chest x-ray to assess for clavicular fracture.
- Position the arm in a natural position.
- Recovery is dependent on severity.
- Mild injuries improve over a course of 1 to 2 weeks.
- Complete brachial plexus injury and Klumpke carry a poor prognosis.
- Follow-up is recommended as an outpatient with orthopedics and physical therapy.

Facial Nerve Injury

OVERVIEW

- Facial nerve injury is the most common cranial nerve injury due to birth trauma.
- Most common site is at the exit of the nerve from the stylomastoid foramen, resulting in a lower motor neuron lesion.
- Facial nerve injury results from compression of a nerve against the maternal sacrum.

CLINICAL PRESENTATION AND DIAGNOSIS

- Infant is unable to close eyes; there is loss of the normal nasolabial fold, with asymmetric crying facies syndrome.
- Forehead is spared, as it is innervated by the opposite nerve.

TREATMENT

- None, as it usually self-resolves after 1 week.
- Moisturizing eye drops may be needed.

Phrenic Nerve Injury

OVERVIEW

- Phrenic nerve injury involves C3 to C5 and is associated with brachial plexus injuries that result in paralysis or poor movement of the diaphragm on the affected side.
  - Remember "C3 to C5 keeps the diaphragm alive."
- Extreme traction of the neck and shoulders during delivery may transect and or injure the phrenic nerve and brachial plexus.
- Risk factors include macrosomia and use of forceps.
- Neonates with congenital heart disease who have surgery in the newborn period are also at risk of phrenic nerve injury.
- Consider phrenic nerve injury as a diagnosis in patients who have had surgery involving the chest or neck and cannot be weaned off mechanical ventilation.

CLINICAL PRESENTATION AND DIAGNOSIS

- Neonates present with respiratory distress and tachypnea and may have cyanosis.
- Physical exam may show reduced rib cage movement on the side of the injury and exaggerated movement on the unaffected side.
- There may be paradoxical movement of the diaphragm.
- Chest x-ray shows an elevated hemidiaphragm.
- Echocardiogram or fluoroscopy can be utilized to evaluate diaphragmatic movement.

TREATMENT

- Treatment is supportive with suspected palsy and use of respiratory support as needed (continuous positive airway pressure [CPAP] or mechanical ventilation).
- Injuries with lack of improvement despite interventions may require surgical plication of the diaphragm.

Laryngeal Nerve Injury

OVERVIEW

- Laryngeal nerve injury can result in vocal cord dysfunction and/or paralysis.

CLINICAL PRESENTATION AND DIAGNOSIS

- Symptoms include stridor; respiratory distress; a hoarse, faint, or absent cry; and feeding difficulties, including dysphagia and aspiration.
- Otolaryngology involvement for evaluation is warranted.
- Diagnosis is by direct laryngoscopy.

TREATMENT

- Injury can be monitored and has the potential to self-resolve.
- Intervention by an otolaryngologist depends on injury severity, whether it is unilateral or bilateral, and if there are associated respiratory issues.

Suggested Readings

Akangire G, Carter G. Birth injuries in neonates. *Pediatr Rev.* 2016; 37(11):451–462.

Brand MC. Part 1: recognizing neonatal spinal cord injury. *Adv Neonatal Care.* 2006;6(1):15–24.

MacKinnon JA, Perlman M, Kirpalani H, et al. Spinal cord injury at birth: diagnostic and prognostic data in twenty-two patients. *J Pediatr.* 1993;122(3):431–437.

Menticoglou SM, Perlman M, Manning FA. High cervical spinal cord injury in neonates delivered with forceps: report of 15 cases. *Obstet Gynecol.* 1995;86(pt 1):589–594.

19 *Neonatal Seizures*

JENNIFER BURNSED and ANGELINA S. JUNE

Overview

- The neonatal period is one of the most common times for seizures in one's lifetime.
- Premature infants are more likely than term infants to have seizures.
- Causes are diverse and broad (Table 19.1).
- The most common cause is hypoxic–ischemic encephalopathy (HIE).
- Electrographic versus clinical:
  - Electrographic seizures occur on EEG without obvious behavioral manifestations and are common in the encephalopathic neonate.
  - Clinical seizures can be difficult to diagnose (behaviors may be normal, state-specific behaviors or non-epileptic abnormal behaviors in a sick neonate) and should be confirmed with electroencephalogram (EEG).
  - Electroclinical dissociation—surface electrodes used for monitoring are unable to pick up activity of "deep" neurons that may be producing clinical events (may be caused by antiepileptic medications or use of neuromuscular blockade).

Table 19.1 Differential Diagnoses of Neonatal Seizures

Electrolyte Abnormalities
- Hypoglycemia
- Hypocalcemia
- Hypomagnesemia
- Hypernatremia
- Hyponatremia
- Hypomagnesemia

Metabolic
- Nonketotic hyperglycinemia
- Ketotic hyperglycinemia
- Galactosemia
- Glycogen storage disease
- Urea cycle defects
- Neonatal adrenoleukodystrophy
- Zellweger syndrome

Infectious
- Bacterial meningitis
- Viral encephalitis
- Congenital infection (HSV, CMV, toxoplasmosis)
- Brain abscess

Injury/Cerebrovascular
- Hypoxia–ischemia
- Intraventricular hemorrhage
- Subarachnoid hemorrhage
- Epidural/subdural hematoma
- Cerebral infarct
- Ischemic or hemorrhagic lesions
- Cortical vein thrombosis

Structural/Anatomic Abnormality
- Cerebral dysgenesis

Genetic
- Autosomal dominant neonatal seizures
- Benign familial seizures
- Neurocutaneous syndromes

Medication/Toxin
- Prenatal exposures/withdrawal
- Local anesthetics
- Prescribed medications (isoniazid)

CMV, Cytomegalovirus; *HSV*, herpes simplex virus.
Modified from Gleason CA, Sawyer TA, eds. *Avery's Diseases of the Newborn.* 11th ed. Philadelphia: Elsevier; Table 65.2.

Seizure Classes and Characteristics

Seizure class is determined by the predominant clinical feature.

- Motor
  - Automatisms (or subtle seizures) are the most commonly observed type.
    - Examples include repetitive tongue or lip movements, eye movements, "bicycling" of legs, and autonomic changes (blood pressure, heart rate, desaturations, apnea).
  - Clonic seizures exhibit rhythmic rapid flexion followed by slow extension; they can be focal, multifocal, or bilateral.
  - Tonic seizures exhibit sustained flexion or extension of the limbs, trunk, or neck.
    - EEG correlation is important, as up to 30% of these movements are nonepileptic with either "brainstem release" or tonic posturing.
  - Myoclonic seizures exhibit rapid, isolated jerking movements that are focal, multifocal, and bilaterally symmetric or asymmetric.
    - They differ from clonic seizures by lacking the slow return phase.
    - A subtype includes benign neonatal sleep myoclonus, characterized as nonepilectic; movement stops when the infant is aroused to waking state.
  - Epileptic spasms are sudden flexion, extension, or mixed extension–flexion; they are less sustained than a tonic movement.
    - They are more sustained than a myoclonic movement.
    - They can be unilateral or bilateral symmetric or asymmetric.
- Non-motor
  - Autonomic seizures are a distinct change in autonomic nervous system function.
  - Examples include heart rate, thermoregulation, and pupillary exams.
  - Behavior arrest is an arrest of normal activity.
  - Sequential presentation:
    - No predominant feature, with a variety of clinical signs and symptoms
    - EEG findings occur in sequence, frequently with changing lateralization.
    - Commonly seen in epilepsies with a genetic basis

CLINICAL PRESENTATION

- Seizure type dictates presentation (Table 19.2).
- Seizure activity should be confirmed by EEG.

Table 19.2 Classification and Clinical Characteristics of Neonatal Seizures

Seizure Class	Characterization
Focal clonic	■ Repetitive, rhythmic contractions of muscle groups (limbs, face, trunk) ■ Unifocal or multifocal ■ May be synchronous or asynchronous in muscle groups on one side of body ■ May be simultaneous but asynchronous on both sides of body ■ Cannot be suppressed by restraint ■ Epileptic
Focal tonic	■ Sustained posturing of single limbs ■ Sustained asymmetric trunk posturing ■ Sustained eye deviation ■ Cannot be provoked with stimulation or suppressed by restraint ■ Epileptic
Generalized tonic	■ Sustained symmetric posturing of limbs, trunk, neck ■ May be extensor, flexor, or mixed ■ May be provoked or intensified by stimulation ■ May be suppressed by restrained or repositioning ■ Nonepileptic
Myoclonic	■ Random, single rapid contractions of muscle groups of limbs, face, trunk ■ Not repetitive or may recur at slow rate ■ Generalized, focal, or fragmented ■ May be provoked with stimulation ■ Epileptic or nonepileptic
Spasms	■ May be flexor, extensor, or mixed ■ May occur in clusters ■ Cannot be provoked or suppressed ■ Epileptic

Modified from Gleason CA, Sawyer TA, eds. *Avery's Diseases of the Newborn*. 11th ed. Philadelphia: Elsevier; Table 65.1.

- Nonepileptic behaviors may be mistaken for seizures.
  - Examples include jitteriness, benign sleep myoclonus, and neonatal dyskinesia.
  - Signs that the behavior may not be epileptic include being provoked by sensory stimulation, able to be stopped with touch/restraint, no autonomic changes, and no gaze abnormalities.
- Neonatal epilepsy syndromes include:
  - Benign familial neonatal seizures ("third day fits"):
    - Classically begin on day 3 of age
    - Most often resolve in first 1 to 4 months of life
    - May be focal or generalized tonic–clonic seizures
    - Mutations in the genes encoding for KCNQ potassium channels
  - Benign idiopathic neonatal seizures ("fifth day fits"):
    - Classically begin on day 5 of age.
    - Clonic seizures ± apnea
    - Often resolve in first weeks to months of life
- Physical exam may give clues helpful for diagnosis.
  - Encephalopathy
    - Heterogeneous clinical syndrome of disturbed consciousness, respiratory drive, neuromuscular tone, and reflexes
    - Seen with hypoxia–ischemia, inborn error of metabolism, and infection
  - Congenital anomalies
    - Facial port-wine stain in V1/V2 distribution indicates Sturge-Weber syndrome.
    - Cardiac rhabdomyomas ± hypopigmented skin lesions indicate tuberous sclerosis.
    - Congenital deafness + cardiac arrhythmias indicate an ion channel mutation (such as Jervell and Lange-Nielsen syndromes).

DIAGNOSIS AND EVALUATION

- History is crucial in determining etiologies and further evaluation.
  - Birth history to assess for possibility of HIE
  - Prenatal concern for structural brain abnormality
  - Maternal factors that may lead to electrolyte or metabolic abnormalities (hypoglycemia or hypocalcemia in the infant of a diabetic mother)
  - Maternal drug use or intoxication
  - Family history of seizures/epilepsy or neurologic problems
- Timing of seizure presentation
  - Fetal (may be observed as frequent "hiccups" by mother): nonketotic hyperglycinemia (classically)
  - <24 hours of age: HIE, infection (meningitis/sepsis), pyridoxine dependent seizures, maternal drug administration, intracranial hemorrhage or injury ante- or peripartum (subarachnoid hemorrhage, intraventricular hemorrhage), hypoglycemia
  - 24 to 72 hours: infection, neonatal abstinence syndrome/withdrawal, neurocutaneous syndrome, inborn error of metabolism (particularly urea cycle defects), cerebral infarction, cerebral hemorrhage
  - 72 hours to 1 week: familial seizures, cerebral dysgenesis, kernicterus, inborn errors of metabolism (methylmalonic aciduria, propionic acidemia, urea cycle defects), cerebral hemorrhage or infarct
  - 1 week to 1 month: cerebral dysgenesis, herpes simplex virus (HSV) encephalitis, inborn errors of metabolism, tuberous sclerosis
- Laboratory evaluation
  - Blood gas and electrolytes
  - Acidosis may be associated with HIE or inborn errors of metabolism, although it is necessary to differentiate between respiratory acidosis versus lactate acidosis and to correct the underlying cause.
  - Derangements such as hypoglycemia, hyponatremia, hypernatremia, or hypocalcemia may be a primary cause of seizure.
  - Metabolic studies
    - Lactate and pyruvate levels, plasma amino acids, urine organic acids, and ammonia are useful in inborn errors of metabolism (e.g., urea cycle defect, pyruvate dehydrogenase deficiency).
  - Genetic studies, if there is concern for benign familial neonatal seizures or channel gene mutations
  - Cerebrospinal fluid analysis is useful for infectious and metabolic workups.
  - Cell count, culture, Gram stain, glucose, and protein to assess for infection
  - HSV polymerase chain reaction (PCR) if there is concern for HSV infection
  - Lactate, pyruvate, and amino acids for metabolic workup

- Electroencephalography
  - Synchronized video monitoring is ideal to correlate behavior.
  - Prolonged monitoring is ideal in order to record events concerning for seizures, as well as baseline background of EEG.
  - EEGs may help identify a "seizure focus" based on EEG channels and locations with abnormalities.
  - Identification of interictal electroencephalographic abnormalities may help with prognosis and outcome.
- Imaging
  - Magnetic resonance imaging (MRI) is the ideal modality for diagnosing anatomic abnormality, intracranial hemorrhage (intraventricular, subarachnoid, subdural), venous infarction, perinatal ischemic stroke, or hypoxic–ischemic injury.
  - Head ultrasound may be useful for some diagnoses if unable to obtain MRI.

TREATMENT

- Identify and correct reversible causes such as metabolic abnormalities, electrolyte derangements, or neonatal abstinence syndrome/withdrawal.

- Antiepileptic drugs
  - The most used medication is phenobarbital.
  - Others utilized include benzodiazepines, levetiracetam, phenytoin, and valproic acid.
  - Medication choice and length of treatment are dependent on the center and clinician, as the efficacy and safety data in neonates are mixed.

Suggested Reading

Natarajan N, Ionita C. Neonatal seizures. In: Gleason C, Sawyer TA, eds. *Avery's Diseases of the Newborn*. 11th ed. Philadelphia: Saunders; 2018:961–970.

Pressler RM, Cilio MR, Mizrahi EM, et al. The ILAE classification of seizures and the epilepsies: modification for seizures in the neonate. Position paper by the ILAE Task Force on Neonatal Seizures. *Epilepsia*. 2021;62:615–628.

20 *Central Nervous System Infections*

JUSTIN ROSATI

Bacterial Meningitis

OVERVIEW

- The incidence of neonatal meningitis is approximately 0.3/1000 live births, with a mortality rate of 10% to 15% in term infants, approximately twice that in preterm.
- Bacterial meningitis is more common in the first postnatal month than at any other age.
- Early-onset meningitis occurs in the first week (usually first 72 hours); it is vertically transmitted and associated with complications of labor and delivery.
- Late-onset meningitis is due to community or nosocomial transmission.
- There is a poor correlation between blood and cerebrospinal fluid (CSF) cultures.
- Meningitis occurs in 23% of neonates with sepsis; 20% of neonates with group B *Streptococcus* (GBS) meningitis have negative blood cultures.

PATHOGENS

- GBS remains the most common in term infants; early-onset decreases with GBS screening protocols but no change in frequency of late-onset GBS meningitis.
- Other organisms include gram-negative enteric bacilli (30–40% of cases) and *Listeria* spp.
  - 50% of gram negatives are *Escherichia coli* (most with K1 polysaccharide capsular antigen), the most common pathogen in preterm infants.
  - Also encountered are *Klebsiella*, *Enterobacter*, *Citrobacter*, and *Serratia*.
- Nosocomial pathogens include *Staphylococcus*, *Candida*, and *Pseudomonas*.

CLINICAL PRESENTATION

- Clinical presentation is similar to sepsis, with temperature instability (60%), irritability, lethargy, decreased tone, seizures, poor feeding, respiratory distress, apnea, diarrhea, and full (but not bulging) fontanelle.
- Outcomes/prognosis:
  - Mortality has decreased to 10% to 20%, although it is higher in preterm infants.
  - Neurologic sequelae include developmental delay, seizures, hydrocephaly, subdural effusions, ventriculitis, brain abscess (especially *Citrobacter* spp.), cerebral palsy, blindness, and hearing loss.

- Morbidity is correlated with initial severity; predictors of severity include prolonged seizures, coma, need for inotropes, and decreased white blood cell count.
  - 21% to 38% of survivors with mild deficits
  - 24% to 29% of survivors with severe deficits

DIAGNOSIS AND EVALUATION

- Blood culture, complete blood count (CBC) with differential, urine culture
- Lumbar puncture (LP), preferably before initiation of antibiotics
- CSF interpretation is based on gestational age, chronologic age, and birth weight (Table 20.1).
  - Cell counts are similar regardless of gestational age; counts drop more slowly in preterm infants than in term infants, and cell counts decrease with increasing chronologic age.
  - 1% to 10% of infants with meningitis have normal CSF cell counts.
  - 20% of Gram stains are "no organisms seen."
  - In *Listeria* meningitis, there is a predominance of mononuclear cells.
  - CSF protein and glucose concentrations are highly variable.
- LP should be repeated in 24 to 48 hours if results are not definitive in a symptomatic infant and repeated in 2 to 3 days after the start of treatment to assess for sterilization of CSF.

TREATMENT

- Initial therapy includes ampicillin and an aminoglycoside; add cefotaxime if a gram-negative organism is suspected; adjust when the organism is identified (Table 20.2).
- Neuroimaging may be considered to exclude parameningeal foci and/or abscess.
- There is no evidence that steroids improve outcome (except in tuberculosis meningitis).

Other Pathogens

HERPES SIMPLEX

- Herpes simplex presents a higher risk of perinatal transmission during initial maternal episode (57% vs. 2%).
- There are three categories of disease:
  - Skin, eyes, mouth (SEM): 45%
  - Disseminated: 25%
  - Central nervous system (CNS): 30%

Table 20.1   Cerebrospinal Fluid Reference Ranges

Postnatal Age		Median WBC/mm³ (IQR)	Median Protein mg/dL (IQR)	Median Glucose mg/dL (IQR)
TERM INFANTS[a]				
≤7 days		3 (1–6)	78 (60–100)	50 (44–56)
8 days–6 months		2 (1–4)	57 (42–77)	52 (45–64)
PRETERM INFANTS (<37 WEEKS' GESTATIONAL AGE)[a]				
≤7 days		3 (1–7)	116 (93–138)	53 (43–65)
8 days–6 months		3 (1–4)	93 (69–122)	47 (40–58)
VERY LOW-BIRTH-WEIGHT INFANTS (24–33 WEEKS' GESTATIONAL AGE)[b]				
BW ≤1000 g				
	≤7 days	3 (1–8)	162 (115–222)	70 (41–89)
	8–28 days	4 (0–14)	159 (95–370)	68 (33–217)
BW 1001–1500 g				
	≤7 days	4 (1–10)	136 (85–176)	74 (50–96)
	8–28 days	7 (0–44)	137 (54–227)	59 (39–109)

BW, Body weight; *IQR*, Interquartile range; *WBC*, white blood cell.
[a]Srinivasan L, et al. Cerebrospinal fluid reference ranges in term and preterm infants in the neonatal intensive care unit. *J Pediatr.* 2012;161(4):729–734.
[b]Rodriguez AF, et al. Cerebrospinal fluid values in the very low birthweight infant. *J Pediatr.* 1990;116(6):971–974.

Table 20.2   Treatment Regimens for Bacterial Meningitis

Organism	Initial Treatment	Subsequent Treatment	Duration	Additional Comments
GBS	Ampicillin + aminoglycoside	Ampicillin or penicillin alone	14 days	Consider repeat LP at end of treatment.
Gram-negative	Cefotaxime + aminoglycoside	Cefotaxime alone after negative cultures	21 days	Consider 14 days of treatment from negative culture.
Citrobacter *Enterobacter* *Serratia* *Pseudomonas*	Fourth-generation cephalosporin (cefepime) or carbapenem (meropenem) + aminoglycoside	—	21 days	Meropenem may be toxic at lower gestational ages and may result in seizures.
				Consider repeat LP before stopping antibiotics.
Coagulase-negative staphylococci	Vancomycin	—	14–21 days after negative culture	Remove foreign body if possible.
Listeria *Enterococcus*	Ampicillin + aminoglycoside	Ampicillin alone	14 days from negative culture	—

GBS, Group B *Streptococcus*; *LP*, lumbar puncture.

- Presentation of CNS herpes simplex includes nonspecific signs and symptoms plus bulging fontanelle and generalized or focal seizures, which appear approximately 16 to 17 days after birth, compared to symptoms presenting on average 9 to 11 days after birth for the other two categories. It may not present with skin lesions.
- Treatment markedly reduces mortality (from 50% to 15% or less) and morbidity.
  - Acyclovir 60 mg/kg/d, in three divided doses for at least 21 days
  - Suppressive therapy for 6 months

CANDIDA

- Risk of invasive disease is inversely related to birth weight, as is mortality.
- At least 15% of infants with invasive disease have CNS involvement.
  - Because CSF parameters, cultures, and imaging are unreliable, infants with invasive disease should be presumed to have CNS involvement and be treated accordingly.
- Invasion of CNS results in meningoencephalitis, cerebral abscesses, and ventriculitis with obstructive hydrocephalus.

- The choice of therapeutic agent is guided by the presence or absence of renal involvement; it should be continued for at least 21 days.
  - Use antifungal dosing adequate to treat hematogenous meningoencephalitis.
    - Amphotericin B-d (AmB-d): 3 to 5 mg/kg/dose IV every 24 hours
    - Fluconazole: 12 mg/kg/d; consider loading dose of 25 mg/kg

Suggested Readings

de Vries LS, Volpe J. Bacterial and fungal intracranial infections. In: Volpe J, Inder T, Darras B, et al., eds. *Volpe's Neurology of the Newborn.* 6th ed. Philadelphia: Elsevier; 2017:1050–1089.

de Vries LS, Volpe J. Bacterial and fungal intracranial infections. In: Volpe J, Inder T, Darras B, et al., eds. *Volpe's Neurology of the Newborn.* 6th ed. Philadelphia: Elsevier; 2017:973–1049.

James SH, Kimberlin DW. Neonatal herpes simplex virus infection: epidemiology and treatment. *Clin Perinatol.* 2015;42:47–59.

Kelly MS, Benjamin Jr DK, Smith PB. The epidemiology and diagnosis of invasive candidiasis among premature infants. *Clin Perinatol.* 2015;42:105–117.

Ku LC, Boggess KA, Cohen-Wolkowiez M. Bacterial meningitis in infants. *Clin Perinatol.* 2015;42:29–45.

Wilson CB, Nizet V, Maldonado Y, et al., eds. *Remington and Klein's Infectious Diseases of the Fetus and Newborn Infant.* 8th ed. Philadelphia: Elsevier; 2016.

21 Neonatal Abstinence Syndromes and Substance Exposure In Utero

JULIE RICCIO and LAURA PRICE

Abstinence Syndromes After Opiate, Benzodiazepine, Barbiturate, and Cocaine Exposure

OVERVIEW

- Neonatal opioid withdrawal syndrome (NOWS) is the preferred term if the withdrawal is known to be specifically from opioids.
- The modified Finnegan scoring system has been the American Academy of Pediatrics (AAP)-recommended opiate abstinence scoring system.
- It is utilized for the evaluation of infants withdrawing from opiates, but it is not a tool for diagnosis.
- Newer tools (e.g., Eat, Sleep, Console) have been created to assess withdrawal symptoms from opioids by focusing on the functional aspects of newborn well-being, including evaluating feeding, sleeping, and the ability to console.
- Management of withdrawal symptoms should focus on optimizing nonpharmacological interventions but may require treatment with opioid medications.
- It is often difficult to predict the course of abstinence syndromes in neonates, and it is further complicated by the frequency of polysubstance or polypharmacy exposure.
- See Table 21.1 for details of each exposure.

Alcohol

FETAL EFFECTS

- Increased risk of spontaneous abortion, abruption, breech, poor growth/small for gestational age (symmetric), microcephaly
- Alcohol is a known teratogen associated with anomalies in all organs, including:
    - Central nervous system (CNS) anomalies and neural tube defects
    - Orofacial clefts, skeletal anomalies
    - Cardiac defects (ventricular septal defect [VSD], arterial septal defect [ASD]), transposition, tetralogy of Fallot (TOF)
    - Renal agenesis or dysplasia

- Hypoplastic nails, abnormal fingerprint, hockey-stick palmar creases
- Abnormal hair whorls

NEONATAL EFFECTS

- Dose-dependent spectrum of effects ranging from "alcohol effects" to fetal alcohol syndrome (FAS)
- FAS is a severe disorder affecting growth, IQ, behavior, and appearance.
- Phenotype characteristics include:
    - Smooth philtrum
    - Thin upper-lip vermillion border
    - Short palpebral fissures

WITHDRAWAL

- Rarely recognized and likely underreported
- Symptoms include irritability, tremors, seizures, and opisthotonos.
- Long-term effects include attention-deficit/hyperactivity disorder (ADHD), IQ reduction, and behavioral changes.

TREATMENT

- Provide environmental support, such as frequent feedings and holding and decreased stimulation.
- No cure

Selective Serotonin Reuptake Inhibitors

FETAL EFFECTS

- Selective serotonin reuptake inhibitors (SSRIs) readily cross the placenta and fetal blood–brain barrier.
- Medication inhibition affects fetal 5-hydroxytryptamine (5-HT) levels, too.
- SSRIs are associated with increased rates of congenital anomalies (very low absolute numbers):
    - Right-sided cardiac outflow tract defects (paroxetine)
    - Potential neuro defects: anencephaly (paroxetine), craniosynostosis, Arnold-Chiari I (controversial)
- Absolute risks of SSRIs are low and should not prevent necessary maternal treatment.

Table 21.1   Neonatal Abstinence Syndromes

Exposure	Fetal Effects	Withdrawal	Treatment
Opiates	Placental transfer increases with advancing GA Methadone crosses placenta more readily than buprenorphine Fetal dependence increases with methadone Decreased fetal growth Increased fetal distress	Timing: peaks 3–4 days after methadone/buprenorphine CNS: hyperactivity, hypertonia, irritability, tremor, myoclonic jerks, sneezing, fever, and seizure Respiratory: tachypnea GI: hyperphagia, increased/poor suck, emesis, diarrhea, weight loss Vasomotor: nasal congestion, flushing, sweating, mottling Cutaneous: chin/knee excoriation, facial scratches, diaper dermatitis	Environmental: maternal rooming-in, swaddling, holding, decreased stimulation Breastfeeding (minimal transfer methadone or buprenorphine) Morphine PO Q 3–4 hours, or Methadone every 12–24 hours ± Phenobarbital adjuvant Buprenorphine, clonidine therapy being studied
Benzodiazepines	Placental transfer Significant chronic exposure results in fetal dependence Acute late third-trimester diazepam treatment results in "floppy infant syndrome" at birth	Timing: at or after the end of the first week of life and may be prolonged Symptoms: hypertonia, tremors, irritability, sucking, emesis, diarrhea, and seizures Seizures are more common than in opiate withdrawal	Environmental support Low-dose phenobarbital
Barbiturates	Placental transfer Chronic maternal use results in fetal dependence	Timing: later; median 6 days Symptoms: hypertonia, hyperactivity, irritable, myoclonic jerks, emesis, diarrhea, and seizures	Environmental support Low-dose phenobarbital
Cocaine (amphetamines similar effects, limited data)	Placental transfer Growth restriction Microcephaly Fetal stroke Möbius syndrome Gastroschisis, NEC Fetal distress, demise Prematurity Abruption	Timing: shortly after birth Neonatal symptoms are thought to be from toxicity, *not* withdrawal. Symptoms: hypertonia, irritability, tremors, tachycardia, arrhythmia, and seizure	Environmental support Phenobarbital for seizure

CNS, Central nervous system; *GA*, gestational age; *GI*, gastrointestinal tract; *NEC*, necrotizing enterocolitis; *PO*, per os (orally).

NEONATAL EFFECTS

- Persistent pulmonary hypertension (PPHN) was initially thought to be associated with SSRI use, but subsequent data are contradictory.
- Neonatal symptoms may be due to toxicity and/or withdrawal; they present in the first day and resolve by days 2 to 6.
- Symptoms include tachypnea, irritability, tremors/jitteriness, temperature instability, poor feeding, and seizures.
- No reduction in neonatal symptoms is seen with maternal SSRI discontinuation 2 weeks prior to birth.
- Breastfeeding is the preferred nutrition, as sertraline has the lowest concentrations in breast milk.

TREATMENT

- Environmental supports, including frequent feeds, holding, and breastfeeding and limited stimulation

- Pharmacologic therapy
  - Usually is not indicated
  - In extreme cases, consider phenobarbital or benzodiazepine.

Suggested Readings

Bondi DS, Khan OA, Hageman J. Maternal selective serotonin reuptake inhibitor use and neurologic effects on the neonate. *NeoReviews.* 2016;17(7):e356–e365.

Grossman MR, Lipshaw MJ. A novel approach to assessing infants with neonatal abstinence syndrome. *Hosp Pediatr.* 2018;8(1):1–6.

McQueen K, Murphy-Oikonen J. Neonatal abstinence syndrome. *N Engl J Med.* 2016;375(25):2468–2479.

Patrick SW, Barfield WD, Poindexter BB. Neonatal opioid withdrawal syndrome. Committee on Fetus and Newborn, Committee on Substance Use and Prevention. *Pediatrics.* 2020;146(5):e1–e18.

Tran H, Robb AS. SSRI use during pregnancy. *Semin Perinat.* 2015;39(7):545–547.

22 Hypotonia and Other Aspects

NIRANJANA NATARAJAN

Hypotonia and Weakness

OVERVIEW

- Hypotonia can be secondary to specific genetic causes or secondary to disorders affecting the central or peripheral nervous systems. Key features on the history and examination may help distinguish these causes, along with further diagnostic evaluation.
- Syndromic or genetic disorders can also cause neonatal hypotonia.
- Central nervous system (CNS) causes are broad and include brain malformations or genetic syndromes.
- Peripheral nervous system causes include disorders of the motor neuron, neuromuscular junction, and primary muscle diseases, such as muscular dystrophies and myopathies.

CLINICAL PRESENTATION

- Clinical manifestations of hypotonia and/or neuromuscular disorders include:
  - Facial hypotonia/facial diplegia, with open-mouth appearance
  - Decreased spontaneous movement and decreased tone for gestational age
  - Respiratory failure, with or without a bell-shaped chest, without respiratory disease
  - Muscle contractures
- Evaluation of deep tendon reflexes can help the clinician distinguish central causes from peripheral causes of weakness. The presence of increased reflexes localizes to the CNS, whereas the absence of reflexes raises concern for a motor neuron or muscle process.
- Evaluation for signs of neonatal encephalopathy or presence of seizures may suggest a CNS abnormality. Neuromuscular conditions may also predispose the neonate to difficulty in the birthing process, thus hypoxic–ischemic encephalopathy may coexist.
- The presence of dysmorphic features, cardiac disease, or other multiorgan involvement can indicate various genetic causes of hypotonia or inborn errors of metabolism.
- Pregnancy history should include questions regarding fetal movement, history of prior pregnancy losses, and family history of neurologic disorders.
- Examination of the mother, including assessment of facial weakness and myotonia, may indicate specific causes of neonatal hypotonia and weakness to the clinician.

DIFFERENTIAL DIAGNOSES

- Central hypotonia accounts for 60% to 80% of causes of neonatal hypotonia. Assessment for dysmorphisms and early consideration of genetic testing and neuroimaging are warranted.
- Congenital muscular dystrophies present with significant hypotonia and weakness, along with significant elevation of creatine phosphokinase (CPK), a muscle breakdown product.
- Alpha-dystroglycanopathies may also involve the eye and brain with congenital brain malformations.
- Congenital myotonic dystrophy presents differently in the neonate as compared to the child or adult. Clinical features include facial diplegia, bell-shaped chest, and talipes equinovarus. Respiratory failure is common secondary to pulmonary hypoplasia and poor intercostal muscle development. The history often reveals polyhydramnios and reduced fetal movement. This disorder displays genetic anticipation; a parent (typically the mother) is affected with facial diplegia, grip myotonia, and cardiac conduction defects.
  - Presence of grip myotonia in the mother should raise suspicion of this disorder.
  - Genetic testing of the *DMPK* gene on chromosome 19 and CTG repeat in the 3′ noncoding region should be performed. CTG repeats greater than 1000 are typically seen.
  - Mortality rates for congenital myotonic dystrophy are as high as 25% to 40%; however, infants surviving the neonatal period can survive into early adulthood, with close respiratory and cardiac follow-up. Survivors typically have cognitive delays.
- The term *congenital myopathies* refer to a group of muscle diseases that do not result in dystrophic changes on muscle biopsy. Affected individuals may present with hypotonia and weakness and respiratory failure due to weak intercostal muscles and diaphragm. Electromyography (EMG) demonstrates myopathic changes, and muscle biopsy may help drive the genetic workup.
- Spinal muscular atrophy (SMA) is a disorder of the motor neuron that occurs in approximately one in 10,000 live births. Neonates with SMA may have severe hypotonia and weakness affecting lower extremities more than upper extremities and proximal muscles more than distal muscles. The face is spared; tongue fasciculations are often present. Reflexes are absent. When suspected, it is imperative to test for the *SMN1* gene on chromosome 5, which is absent, as well as *SMN2*, a modifier gene. Historically, treatment has been supportive, with death often in the first year of life without aggressive respiratory

management. However, there are now three approved treatments that have shown significant improvement in outcomes: two antisense oligonucleotides, nusinersen and risdiplam, and gene therapy with onasemnogene abeparvovec-xioi. In response to the availability of treatment, nearly all states in the United States have included SMA on the newborn screen.

- Congenital myasthenic syndromes are a heterogeneous group of disorders characterized by defects in neuromuscular transmission at the neuromuscular junction. Neonates may present with hypotonia, bulbar weakness, and/or respiratory failure. CPK values and muscle biopsy are typically normal or nonspecific. Repetitive nerve stimulation obtained with nerve conduction studies suggests the diagnosis, prompting further genetic testing.
- Congenital peripheral neuropathies are a rare cause of neonatal hypotonia. Findings on examination include the absence of reflexes and distal more than proximal weakness, typically with feet abnormalities. The CPK level is normal. If EMG demonstrates neuropathic findings, further genetic evaluation is indicated.
- Congenital brain malformations can result in hypotonia. The examination may indicate normal to increased reflexes, sustained clonus, encephalopathy, or seizures.
- Hypotonia with encephalopathy may be a feature in the presentation of inborn errors of metabolism. Workup and management are discussed elsewhere.
- The presence of specific dysmorphic features or multisystem involvement should raise concern for specific syndromes, which include trisomy 21, Smith-Lemli-Opitz syndrome, Pompe disease, and congenital disorders of glycosylation.

DIAGNOSIS AND EVALUATION

Although the diagnostic evaluation should be tailored to the clinical presentation, the following testing may be considered in all neonates with hypotonia. The increasing availability of clinical exome and whole genome sequencing may alter the need for routine use of more invasive procedures such as EMG or muscle biopsy. Several proposed algorithms for workup have been proposed (and are included in the Suggested Readings).

- CPK—significantly elevated levels (five times normal) can be seen in muscular dystrophies; mildly elevated levels may be seen in congenital myopathies.
- Magnetic resonance imaging (MRI) of the brain
- SMN1/SMN2 testing if the newborn screen is positive for SMA, if the newborn is in a state where SMA is not on the newborn screen and hypotonia is present, or if there is a high index of suspicion.
- Genetic testing—the landscape and availability of genetic testing continue to evolve. Early consideration of clinical exome sequencing is warranted, recognizing its limitations with regard to disorders with trinucleotide repeats.
- EMG and nerve conduction studies can used useful when a peripheral cause of weakness is suspected; these can help distinguish between a myopathic or neuropathic process. Repetitive nerve stimulation can determine a neuromuscular junction disorder.
- Muscle biopsy can be helpful in determination of a primary muscle disorder.

In neonates with multisystem involvement, the following should also be considered:

- Genetic testing with karyotype should be considered in individuals with dysmorphic features consistent with trisomy 21 (e.g., facial features, including up-slanting palpebral fissures and flat nasal bridge; brachycephaly; single palmar crease; and a short neck).
- Chromosomal microarray analysis in patients with dysmorphic features
- DNA methylation analysis of the 15q11.2-q13 region for Prader-Willi syndrome
- For cardiac enlargement on chest x-ray or cardiac failure with associated elevation in CPK seen in Pompe disease, confirmatory testing should be done. Reduced or absent alpha-glucosidase (GAA) enzyme activity by dried blood spot, lymphocytes, or fibroblasts confirm disease. Enzyme replacement therapy is available for infant-onset disease.
- Where available, give early consideration to clinical exome sequencing, given the expanding spectrum of genetic disorders.

TREATMENT

- Management is largely supportive, with early involvement of pulmonary services for respiratory support.
- Physical therapy and rehabilitation services, as well as consultation with neurology, should be implemented early in the evaluation.
- Early identification of SMA, Pompe disease, or congenital myasthenic syndromes may allow for early initiation of treatment to alter the disease course.

Arthrogryposis

OVERVIEW

- The term *arthrogryposis multiplex congenita* (AMC) refers to fixed joint contractures affecting two or more limbs that are congenital and apparent at birth. This is distinguished from isolated talipes equinovarus, or dislocated hips, for example.
- AMC is a descriptive term; further evaluation is necessary to determine the cause.

PATHOGENESIS

- Over 400 causes of specific disorders associated with AMC have been described. AMC develops secondary to decreased fetal movement, termed *fetal akinesia*.
- AMC causes can be separated into intrinsic, extrinsic, and environmental factors to aid the clinician in determining the cause.
    - Intrinsic factors include myopathic, neuropathic, central nervous system, or neuromuscular transmission disorders. Numerous genes have been associated with arthrogryposis.
    - Environmental causes include maternal illnesses or infections affecting the fetus, maternal medications, or drug exposures.
    - Extrinsic causes include disorders resulting in compression of the fetus, such as Potter syndrome, or limitation of the in utero space by any cause, such as large uterine fibromas.

EVALUATION

- History is geared toward determining factors related to pregnancy, such as maternal infection or fever, trauma, and medication exposure, as well as fetal movements in utero. Earlier onset of fetal akinesia is associated with increased severity.
- Pay close attention to which joints are affected, whether distribution is more proximal or distal, flexor versus extensor muscles. The neonate's position at rest and degree of spontaneous movement may indicate a neuromuscular cause.
- Physical examination should be done for other associated anomalies, facial involvement, renal anomalies, or other organ involvement. Associated anomalies or dysmorphisms may help with determining causative factors.
- Imaging evaluation should include radiography of bony abnormalities or if there is concern for dislocated joints. MRI of the brain and spinal cord may be appropriate to evaluate for CNS involvement.
- If there is a concern for neuromuscular weakness, obtain CPK levels. EMG and nerve conduction studies with repetitive nerve stimulation can be performed; if abnormal, muscle biopsy of affected and unaffected tissue and/or genetic testing should be pursued.
- Genetic testing should be considered.

TREATMENT AND OUTCOMES

- Management is geared toward determination of the cause, as well as orthopedic, rehabilitation, and multidisciplinary care.
- Outcome is based on the underlying cause; most patients have normal intelligence.
- Orthopedic complications include scoliosis, osteoporosis, and fractures; these require close monitoring to optimize outcomes.

Vascular Malformations

VEIN OF GALEN MALFORMATION

- The vein of Galen malformation is the most common congenital arteriovenous (AV) shunt in the neonate.
- Although named for the vein of Galen, this malformation stems from an embryonic precursor, the median vein of the prosencephalon, which typically regresses by the 11th week of gestation and is replaced by internal cerebral veins. The large AV shunt has feeder veins.
- A vascular steal phenomenon is caused by an absence or reversal of diastolic flow due to the large size of the venous malformation, resulting in brain ischemia.
- High-output heart failure results from a decrease in cerebrovascular resistance and increased venous return to the heart. This cardiac failure may add to brain ischemia.
- It is prenatally detected in some neonates by imaging, whereas others may present in the neonatal intensive care unit (NICU) with high-output cardiac failure secondary to AV shunting. Typically, an asymmetric systolic–diastolic bruit can be auscultated over the anterior fontanelle or eyeballs.

- Potential neurologic complications include worsening vascular steal phenomena, thrombosis of the vein of Galen, and hemorrhagic rupture of the vein.
- Systemic complications include worsening or refractory cardiac failure with multiorgan involvement.
- Management includes early involvement of neurosurgery/interventional neuroradiology, with embolization of feeder vessels to decrease the vascular steal phenomenon.

STURGE-WEBER SYNDROME

- Port-wine birthmarks (PWBs) are a common finding in newborns. The best predictor for Sturge-Weber syndrome is a PWB involving any part of the forehead, including the midline frontonasal prominence and the upper eyelid.
- The classic triad of Sturge-Weber syndrome includes facial hemangioma, ipsilateral increased intraocular pressure or glaucoma, and leptomeningeal involvement with vascular malformation.
- Somatic mutations in *GNAQ* are causative of Sturge-Weber syndrome, and these mutations can be found in the affected skin of patients.
- Routine neuroimaging is not indicated for newborns with a high-risk PWB and no history of seizures or neurologic symptoms, but it can be considered in select cases.
- Any child with a high-risk PWB should be referred for a baseline ophthalmologic exam and follow-up by a pediatric ophthalmologist.

PHACES SYNDROME

- PHACES syndrome stands for *p*osterior fossa abnormalities, *h*emangiomas, *a*rterial malformations, *c*ardiac abnormalities/coarctation of the aorta, *e*ye abnormalities, and *s*ternal defects syndrome. First described in 1996, consensus-derived diagnosis and care recommendations have been proposed. Infants with a large segmental hemangioma affecting the head, infants with a less characteristic hemangioma but additional lesions concerning for PHACES, or infants with other characteristic anomalies for PHACES without hemangioma should be screened for PHACES syndrome with physical examination, MRI, and MR angiography of the brain, neck, and aortic arch, as well as an ophthalmologic examination.

Congenital Cerebral Neoplasms

- Neonatal brain tumors are relatively uncommon, representing 0.5% to 1.5% of all pediatric brain tumors.
- Congenital brain tumors have a predilection for the supratentorium rather than the infratentorium, which is more common in childhood.
- The most common type of congenital tumor in the central nervous system is a teratoma. Of all teratomas, 20% emerge from the lateral ventricles, and another 10% to 20% are estimated to arise from the third ventricle.

- Other congenital tumors include medulloblastomas or other primitive neuroepithelial tumors, choroid plexus tumors (papilloma or carcinoma), astrocytomas (which include subependymal giant cell tumors and glioblastoma multiforme), and craniopharyngiomas.
- The most common presentation may be incidental on fetal ultrasound or may be due to the presence of hydrocephalus found pre- or postnatally. Other common presentations include irritability and stillbirth. Neonates may also present with seizures, although the incidence of this is low.

TREATMENT

- If there is concern for a tumor seen on prenatal imaging, further imaging evaluation is imperative to aid in diagnosis because a fetal biopsy is not feasible.
- It is necessary to formulate a birth plan to address potential complications from hydrocephalus and associated macrocrania during delivery.
- Early consultation with neurosurgery is recommended to determine potential interventions.
- Radiotherapy is used infrequently due to the potential for long-term cognitive and motor effects.

PROGNOSIS

- The prognosis of congenital brain tumors depends on several factors, including lesion histology and location and degree of fetal development. Tumors compressing the brainstem are surgically challenging to access and may result in brainstem compromise. In these cases, mortality can be high; patients with choroid plexus papillomas or astrocytomas fare better because these tumors generally can be accessed more easily and do not cause brainstem compression.

Neurocutaneous Disorders

- Neurocutaneous disorders, also referred to as *phakomatoses*, are disorders that have CNS, dermatologic, and often ocular findings. Many of these are thought to stem from the common origin of these organ systems from the ectoderm.

INCONTINENTIA PIGMENTI

- This can affect the skin, teeth, hair, nails, eyes, and CNS.
- It has four stages that occur over a span of years.

- The initial vesicular stage typically presents prior to 6 months of age and can be present in the neonatal period.
- Vesicular lesions typically are linear and are on the body with facial sparing. They can initially appear as erythema only.
- It is an X-linked disorder. Deletion in *IKBKG* is causative and is de novo in 65% of patients.
- The diagnosis can be made genetically; however, affected males may require a skin biopsy for determination.
- Evaluation should include brain MRI and ophthalmology consultation, as patients are at risk for retinal detachment.

HYPOMELANOSIS OF ITO (PIGMENTARY MOSAICISM)

- Decreased pigmentation (hypomelanosis) following the lines of Blaschko is associated with intracranial abnormalities.
- Multiple chromosomal abnormalities have been associated with pigmentary mosaicism, but no distinct cause is known.
- Cell mosaicism is known to occur with the various abnormalities. Cases are thought to be sporadic in nature.

TUBEROUS SCLEROSIS COMPLEX

- Tuberous sclerosis complex (TSC) occurs in as many as one in 5800 live births. It is caused by a mutation in the gene hamartin or tuberin; inheritance is autosomal dominant.
- Neurologically, TSC can present in infancy or childhood with seizures. Although this presentation is reported in neonates, most affected newborns are found prenatally to have cardiac rhabdomyomas. Subependymal giant cell tumors, neuronal migration defects, and/or cortical tubers may occur.
- Although it is a neurocutaneous disorder, classic ash leaf spots, or hypopigmented macules, may be difficult to visualize in the newborn. Use of a Wood's lamp (ultraviolet lamp) may help elucidate skin lesions.

Suggested Readings

Hall JG. Arthrogryposis (multiple congenital contractures): diagnostic approach to etiology, classification, genetics, and general principles. *Eur J Med Genet*. 2014;57(8):464–472.

Mercuri E, Pera MC, Brogna C. Neonatal hypotonia and neuromuscular conditions. *Handb Clin Neurol*. 2019;162:435–448.

Sabeti S, Ball KL, Bhattacharya SK, et al. Consensus statement for the management and treatment of Sturge-Weber syndrome: neurology, neuroimaging, and ophthalmology recommendations. *Pediatr Neurol*. 2021;121:59–66.

Sugimoto M, Kurishima C, Masutani S, Tamura M, Senzaki H. Congenital brain tumor within the first 2 months of life. *Pediatr Neonatol*. 2015;56(6):369–375.

23 Neurodevelopmental Impairments

ALLISON H. PAYNE and JONATHAN RYAN BURRIS

Overview of Neurodevelopmental Impairment

- Neurodevelopmental impairment (NDI) is a composite outcome including any one of the following:
  - Cerebral palsy (CP)
  - Cognitive disability (generally IQ < 70–85; <–1 to 2 standard deviations [SD])
  - Most common disability in preterm infants
  - Severe hearing impairment (requiring at least amplification)
  - Severe visual impairment (visual acuity < 20/200, despite correction)
- Adverse developmental outcomes can impact daily function, including:
  - Global or specific learning disabilities
  - Language delay
  - Behavioral and attention issues
    - Preterm infants 2 × to 6 × more likely to have problems compared with term infants.
  - This may not be associated with hyperactivity or conduct issues in preterm infants.
  - Minor neuromotor dysfunction
  - Executive function disorders
  - Autism spectrum disorders
  - Seen in approximately 5% of preterm infants, 3 × the general population
  - Anxiety
  - Depression
  - Sensory impairments include:
    - Retinopathy of prematurity leading to vision impairment
    - Myopia and strabismus
    - Hearing impairment (1–10%)

Demographics of NDI

- Rates of childhood neurodevelopmental disabilities increase with the number and severity of neonatal morbidities.
- A higher incidence is seen in association with abnormal findings on neuroimaging and neonatal neurodevelopmental assessment.
- There is an inverse association of NDI with gestational age and/or birth weight.
- Breakdown of NDI incidence by gestational age:
  - Full term: 2%
  - Late preterm (34–36 weeks' gestational age [GA]): 2% to 3%

- Incidence: cerebral palsy 0.4% (~3 × term) and severe cognitive impairment 0.8% (~2 × term).
- They have lower scores than term-born peers in school readiness, reading, math, and expressive language testing and a higher risk for testing below grade level.
- Differences seen between late preterm infants and term peers in learning disabilities or attention issues may disappear by late adolescence.
- Moderately preterm (31–34 weeks' GA): 3% to 4%
  - Incidence:
    - Cerebral palsy: ~1%
    - Developmental delay: ~30% to 35%.
  - They have increased behavioral and emotional concerns, preform poorer on cognitive testing and neuropsychological functioning. Specific areas include: visuospatial reasoning, attention control, inhibition, and executive function.
- Very preterm (26–30 weeks' GA): 10%
  - Incidence:
    - Cerebral palsy: ~4%
    - Developmental delay: ~40%
    - Mild cognitive impairment: ~20%
    - Severe cognitive impairment: ~10%.
- Extremely preterm (25–26 weeks' GA): 40%
- Periviable infants (22 to <25 weeks' GA): up to 70%
  - Any disability (cognitive, motor, sensory):
    - Moderate–severe, 33%
    - Mild, 33%
    - None, 33%.
- Further specific incidences include the following:
  - Moderate cognitive impairment, 19% (~9 × risk at term)
  - Severe cognitive impairment, 11% (~30 × risk at term)
  - Cerebral palsy, 7% to 10% (~20 × –40 × risk at term)
  - Blindness, 1% to 2%
  - Hearing impairment, 1% to 2%
  - Special education needs, ~60%
  - Increased risk of neurobehavioral issues (attention, attention-deficit/hyperactivity disorder [ADHD], anxiety, autism), and subject-specific learning issues, such as math, spelling, and written language

Risk Factors for NDI

- Prematurity and severe growth restriction are the primary risk factors for NDI.

- Those with NDI may experience:
  - Severe asphyxia
  - Intraventricular hemorrhage (grade III or higher)
  - Periventricular leukomalacia
  - Chronic lung disease (days on mechanical ventilation, tracheostomy)
  - Sepsis or meningitis (bacteremia, necrotizing enterocolitis)
  - Malnutrition (poor postnatal growth trajectories, bowel loss)
  - Neonatal seizures
  - Postnatal dexamethasone exposure, especially early (<8 days of age) or repeated courses

Protective and Mitigating Factors for NDI in Prematurity

- Antenatal steroids prior to delivery serve as a key driver in reducing the risk of NDI.
  - Antenatal steroids indirectly reduce the risk of intraventricular hemorrhage, duration of mechanical ventilation, and bronchopulmonary dysplasia (BPD).
- Antenatal magnesium sulfate is utilized for fetal neuroprotection to reduce the risk of severe motor dysfunction, including cerebral palsy.
- Delivery at a regional perinatal center with maternal–fetal medicine (MFM) and a level III/IV NICU equipped to handle high-risk deliveries and neonates delivered 22 weeks' GA to term improves time to resuscitation following delivery, reducing mortality and morbidity.

Clinical Conditions at High Risk for NDI

MONOCHORIONIC DIAMNIOTIC TWINS

- Monochorionic diamniotic (MCDA) twins represent 20% of all twin gestations where fetuses share a common placenta. The placental vascular anastomoses present confer a risk for:
  - Twin–twin transfusion syndrome (TTTS)
  - Twin anemia polycythemia sequence (TAPS)
  - Twin reversed arterial perfusion (TRAP)
  - Selective intrauterine growth restriction
- In the case of spontaneous fetal demise of one fetus, the co-twin may exsanguinate through the placental vascular anastomoses to the deceased twin.
  - The co-twin is at risk of death (15%) or severe cerebral injury (34%).
  - In survivors, there is a risk of multicystic encephalomalacia (20%); cerebral palsy (10%); other neurologic injury such as porencephaly or intraventricular hemorrhage (IVH) (10%); and multiorgan damage.
- Overall, MCDA twins have higher rates of poorer neurodevelopmental outcomes compared to dichorionic diamniotic (DCDA) twins. Differences are largely attributable to prematurity and TTTS. Non-TTTS MCDA twins have outcomes similar to those for DCDA twins of similar gestational ages.

TWIN–TWIN TRANSFUSION SYNDROME

- Condition affects 10% to 15% of monochorionic pregnancies, but rarely in the setting of fused dichorionic placentation.
- Mortality is 80% to 90% if untreated, decreasing to 20% to 40% for both twins in spite of aggressive therapy.
- Two-thirds of cases of a single intrauterine fetal death in TTTS involve the demise of the donor twin.
- Ischemic brain lesions may result from intrauterine cardiac dysfunction or hemodynamic instability, including:
  - Leukoencephalopathy, IVH, hydranencephaly, porencephaly
- The rates of abnormality on neurologic imaging are ~7% with fetoscopic laser treatment and 17% with amnioreductions. Long-term outcomes have not shown significant differences, but studies have been limited.
- In cases diagnosed at <28 weeks' gestation, ~25% of both donor and recipient twins have abnormal findings on cranial ultrasound:
  - Severe IVH, ventricular dilation, cerebral echogenic foci, cerebral cysts, periventricular leukomalacia (PVL)
  - ~10% of abnormalities are PVL with a high association with CP.
- Long-term outcomes in TTTS:
  - Amnioreduction cohorts
    - ~25% of survivors following serial amnioreduction with CP
      - Risk of CP decreased to ~5% in cohorts with later diagnosis (<33 weeks).
    - ~20% of survivors without CP or significant cognitive impairment have mild speech delays or special education requirement.
  - Fetoscopic laser photocoagulation cohorts
    - 6% to 13% with significant neurologic deficits (e.g., CP, hemiparesis, spastic quadriplegia); many of these cases also with increased prematurity
    - 7% to 11% with minor neurologic deficits (e.g., strabismus, minor motor delays, mild speech impairments)

FETAL GROWTH RESTRICTION

- Fetal growth restriction (FGR) was previously referred to as intrauterine growth restriction (IUGR).
- Brain-sparing size does not equal normal brain development.
- Characteristics include:
  - Decreased total cerebral volume and total number of brain cells
  - Thinner cortical thickness and abnormal gyration
  - Reduced structural complexity of gray and white matter
  - Delay in myelination
  - Reduced posterior white matter volume
- Neurodevelopmental outcomes are influenced by timing of onset, severity of growth restriction, and gestational age at delivery.
- Early-onset FGR
  - Increased risk of motor, cognitive, and behavioral concerns at age 2 years and at school age
    - Outcomes reported may be confounded by preterm birth.

- Late-onset FGR
  - Increased risk of abnormal neurobehavior in the neonatal period and at age 2 years
- If FGR is associated with abnormal Doppler studies,
  - Poorer motor and cognitive outcomes at 2 years old and school age.
- FGR is a risk factor for perinatal brain injury.
  - Association with IVH is variable in clinical studies.
  - Abnormal umbilical artery Dopplers in the setting of placental insufficiency are associated with increased risk for IVH.
  - In early to moderate preterm infants, IVH rates are lower in FGR infants compared to appropriate for gestational age (AGA) preterms at given gestational age.
  - In late preterm births (>34 weeks), IVH rates for FGR infants are elevated compared to AGA late preterms.
- Neurodevelopmental outcomes:
  - Cognitive deficits
    - Occurred in 15% of a FGR brain-sparing cohort with IQ < 85 (−1 SD). At school age, abnormal umbilical artery Dopplers are associated with a 9-point drop in IQ compared to those with normal Dopplers.
  - Gross and fine motor deficits
    - 22% of spastic CP cases may be attributed to IUGR.
  - Reduced memory performance
  - Reduced visuomotor function
  - Associated with increased risks of attention-deficit/hyperactivity disorder (ADHD), anxiety, depression, poor social skills, behavioral concerns, and autism spectrum disorder.
  - Similar developmental and behavioral outcomes as birth weight–matched controls (i.e., more preterm, AGA, not growth restricted)
  - Early preterm birth (<28 weeks): AGA and small for gestational age (SGA) infants have similar incidences of cognitive deficits, attention deficits/hyperactivity, and school difficulties.
  - Preterm birth (29–32 weeks)—SGA infants have an increased risk compared to their AGA peers for cognitive deficits, ADHD, and school difficulties.
  - Risk of poor outcome increases with perinatal acidosis and male gender.

BRONCHOPULMONARY DYSPLASIA

- Increased risk for cognitive, language, motor, hearing, and vision deficits and CP.
- It is difficult to ascertain a direct association of BPD with NDI outcomes because of confounding factors of prolonged illness and hospitalization, sepsis, increased exposure to repeated doses of corticosteroids, sedatives, and poor nutrition, as well as variation in lung maturity at birth based on gestational age, weight, early premature rupture of membranes prior to delivery, and antenatal steroids.
- Those with ongoing BPD concerns have the following associations:
  - Those 3 years of age have a 2 × risk of NDI.
  - Those 8 years of age are 1.5 × more likely to require special education classes compared to very low birth weight (VLBW) infants without BPD.

- In the middle school years, there are higher rates of subtle neurologic deficits, perceptual motor integration, motor coordination, processing speeds, and behavioral difficulties.
- Adults experience deficits in problem solving, behavior awareness, and organization.

CONGENITAL HEART DISEASE

- Among children with complex congenital heart disease (CHD) requiring surgical repair, approximately 50% have later signs of neurodevelopmental disability.
  - May include one or more of the following:
    - Cognitive impairment
    - Learning difficulties
    - Expressive speech and language abnormalities
    - Visual–spatial and visual–motor impairments
    - Motor delays
    - ADHD
    - Deficits in executive function
- The spectrum of disability ranges from mild to moderate in severity but may occur in multiple domains and have a significant impact on academic and social functioning.
  - 33% have an increased need for special education and therapeutic support.
  - 33% of operative CHD patients have an underlying genetic disorder that may contribute to worse neurodevelopmental outcomes.
- Fetal brain development may be abnormal or injured due to abnormal fetal blood flow or increased cerebral vascular resistance associated with the CHD, leading to:
  - Immaturity of central nervous system (CNS) development.
  - Microcephaly (~25% incidence in complex CHD cohorts)
  - White matter injury, stroke, hemorrhage.
- Postnatal cerebral ischemia may occur before, during, and after surgical repair.
- White matter injury is the predominant injury pattern detected on MRI.
  - PVL occurs in ~25% of preoperative and >50% of postoperative cases.
  - Those with immature brain morphology have an increased risk.
- Brain immaturity predicts early neurodevelopmental outcome. Preoperative and postoperative injuries do not.
- Characteristics in those with CHD are as follows:
  - Infancy and toddler years
    - Generalized hypotonia, delayed motor milestones
    - Motor scores tend to improve over first 3 years, but there is a continued risk for fine motor and visuomotor impairments.
    - CP occurs in ~2% of complex CHD cases.
  - School-age children
    - Language impairments (particularly expressive), memory, and slower processing speeds
    - Most children without genetic disorders have cognitive IQ scores in the normal range; as a group, there is an ~5- to 10-point decrease in mean IQ.
    - Learning difficulties may be identified only with increased cognitive demand with increasingly complex tasks at later school ages.

- There are problems with peer interaction and emotional symptoms and executive function disorders; difficulties may persist into adolescence and adulthood.
  - Repairs using circulatory arrest show particular issues with motor and speech functioning.
  - Repairs using bypass show worse scores for impulsivity and behavior.

PERSISTENT PULMONARY HYPERTENSION OF THE NEWBORN

- Infants may experience acute persistent pulmonary hypertension of the newborn (PPHN) following birth with failure to drop pulmonary pressures due to conditions of: sustained asphyxia, meconium aspiration, severe RDS, sepsis, and/or surfactant deficiencies. Pulmonary hypertension can also be a result of chronic lung disease due to prematurity.
- PPHN confers a higher risk of neurodevelopmental impairment (25%) and hearing impairment (23%), despite early inhaled nitric oxide (iNO).

CONGENITAL DIAPHRAGMATIC HERNIA

- Improved respiratory and surgical management of patients with congenital diaphragmatic hernia (CDH) has improved survival rates (up to 70–90%).
- There are multiple risk factors for neurodevelopmental impairment:
  - Prenatal adverse impact on CNS development, with cerebral circulation changes
  - Postnatal hypoxia–ischemia, emboli, reactive oxygen species, acidosis, sedation, inflammatory microvasculopathy (may affect white matter maturation)
  - Increased risks for IVH, PVL, and seizures compared to term normal peers
- Severity of illness, prenatal intrathoracic liver, need for extracorporeal membrane oxygenation (ECMO), and continued oxygen requirement at 28 days of life are associated with developmental delays.
- Cognition and language development:
  - Normal range, 50% to 60%
  - Borderline/mild range, 25% to 35%
  - Severe range, 15% to 25%
  - Categorization is relatively stable over time.
- Motor development:
  - Most prominent domain for developmental delays.
  - 30% to 50% have motor dysfunction (mild to severe).
    - May present as persistent hypotonia, delayed motor coordination.
- Hearing:
  - 17% to 30% sensorineural hearing loss (SNHL), with about 66% of those infants having delayed onset
  - Risk factors for impairment include need for ECMO, increased duration of mechanical ventilation, duration of loop diuretics, and aminoglycosides.
  - Hearing deficits impact language acquisition, social development, and academic achievement.
- Behavioral:
  - Increased risk for emotion and behavior regulation, as well as poor attention, peer interaction, and development of social skills; associated with lower acquisition of higher level academic skills and school failure
  - Emerging concerns for associations of CDH and autism

HYPOXIC–ISCHEMIC ENCEPHALOPATHY

- Hypoxic–ischemic encephalopathy (HIE) is one of many causes of neonatal encephalopathy.
- Historically, the outcome is strongly associated with Sarnat staging.
  - Mild (stage 1): ~5% of survivors with >6-month gross motor delay
  - Moderate (stage 2): 4% mortality, ~16% of survivors with >6-month gross motor delay, 21% to 33% of survivors with a handicap (e.g., CP, cognitive delay, severe vision or hearing impairment, severe seizures)
  - Severe (stage 3): 75% mortality, 100% of survivors with handicap
- The outcome for infants with concerns of moderate to severe signs of encephalopathy and concerns for HIE can be favorably altered by the use of therapeutic hypothermia.
- Therapeutic hypothermia for moderate or severe encephalopathy initiated at <6 hours of life and continued for 72 hours reduces the risk for NDI or death. A meta-analysis of major randomized cooling trials has shown the following:
  - 24% reduction in risk of death or NDI at 2 years
  - 32% to 38% reduction in risk of major disability, CP, or developmental delay
  - ~44% reduction in risk of blindness
  - Nonsignificant decrease in deafness
  - Survival without neurologic abnormality is ~1.6 times more likely if cooled (24% controls, 40% cooled).
  - For cooled infants, the decrease in death did not lead to an increase in neurologic abnormality among the survivors.
- Therapeutic hypothermia has the greatest impact on the outcomes of infants with moderate encephalopathy.
  - Moderate: 33% reduction in risk of death or NDI
  - Severe: 17% reduction in risk of death or NDI

Suggested Readings

Cheong JLY, Doyle LW. An update on pulmonary and neurodevelopmental outcomes of bronchopulmonary dysplasia. *Semin Perinatol.* 2018;42(7):478–484.

Danzer E, Hoffman C, D'Agostino JA, et al. Neurodevelopmental outcomes at 5 years of age in congenital diaphragmatic hernia. *J Pediatr Surg.* 2017;52:437–443.

Laptook AR, McGowan EC. Outcomes in the era of therapeutic hypothermia. *NeoReviews.* 2014;15(9):e3860.

Patel T, Ilardi D, Kochilas L. Neurodevelopmental outcomes in children with congenital heart disease: ten years after the American Heart Association statement. *Clin Perinatol.* 2023;50(1):53–66.

Pierrat V, Marchand-Martin L, Marret S, et al. Neurodevelopmental outcomes at age 5 among children born preterm: EPIPAGE-2 cohort study. *BMJ.* 2021;373:n741.

Sacchi C, Marino C, Nosarti C, Vieno A, Visentin S, Simonelli A. Association of intrauterine growth restriction and small for gestational age status with childhood cognitive outcomes: a systematic review and meta-analysis. *JAMA Pediatr.* 2020;174(8):772–781.

Woythaler M. Neurodevelopmental outcomes of the late preterm infant. *Semin Fetal Neonatal Med.* 2019;24(1):54–59.

Yan S, Wang Y, Chen Z, Zhang F. Chorionicity and neurodevelopmental outcomes in twin pregnancy: a systematic review and meta-analysis. *J Perinatol.* 2023;43(2):133–146.

24 Causes and Effects of Environment on Neurodevelopmental Impairment

ALLISON H. PAYNE and JONATHAN RYAN BURRIS

Nutrition and Neurodevelopment

- Nutrition plays a role in supporting the structural and functional development of the brain from conception into adulthood.
- Both the nutritional status of the mother during pregnancy and the postnatal diet of the infant have a long-term impact.
- Prenatal maternal factors:
  - Maternal nutrition and health during pregnancy may influence fetal growth restriction (FGR) and subsequent outcomes.
  - Maternal risk factors for FGR, previously known as intrauterine growth restriction (IUGR), include nutritional deficiency, severe anemia, smoking, toxins/medications (e.g., warfarin, anticonvulsants, caffeine), and assisted reproductive technology.
  - Socioeconomic influences on maternal access to health resources and diet have associated disparities in IUGR and subsequent neonatal outcomes. Public health policy to reduce inequity is invaluable.
- Prenatal nutrition
  - Dietary quality, beyond caloric intake, is vital because specific nutrients are required during sensitive and critical periods of development.

Overview of Dietary Nutrients and Their Impact In Utero

- Folate is found in green leafy vegetables and yeast extract. In the synthetic form, it can be found in breads, cereals, and supplements.
  - Folate is critical in first trimester neural tube development, neural cell proliferation and differentiation, and maintenance of DNA synthesis.
  - Deficiencies in the first trimester are associated with anencephaly and spina bifida.
  - Its role in the second and third trimesters is less understood, and there is an active area of research regarding potential roles in fetal growth and autism spectrum disorders.
- Choline is found in animal products or plant foods, including nuts, legumes, and cruciferous vegetables.
  - Choline plays roles in neural tube closure and is a precursor for phospholipids and acetylcholine and methyl donors.
  - It is important in epigenetics and membrane formation, including in the gray and white matter.
- Vitamin B_{12} is found in meat, eggs, and dairy products. Supplementation may be required in vegetarian or vegan diets.
  - Vitamin B_{12} is essential for cellular processes, including as cofactors in enzymatic reactions, and it plays roles in the synthesis and regulation of neurotransmitters, neuronal structure and myelination, and fat and protein metabolism. Deficiency can lead to disruption of these processes and, along with folate deficiency, neural tube defects.
  - Maternal consequences of Vitamin B_{12} deficiency can lead to pernicious anemia.
- Zinc is found in meat, fish, seafood (highest in oysters), eggs, dairy products, beans, nuts, and whole grains.
  - Strict vegetable and non–whole grain cereal diets can lead to significant deficiency.
  - Zinc modulates neurogenesis and neuronal apoptosis.
- Tryptophan is found in poultry, canned tuna, dairy products, oats, nuts, and seeds.
  - Tryptophan is the sole precursor of serotonin; it plays roles in corticogenesis and neuronal migration.
- Polyunsaturated fatty acids (PUFAs; omega-3s, docosahexaenoic acid [DHA]) are found in fish (salmon, tuna), nuts and seeds (e.g., flaxseed, chia, walnuts), and plant oils.
  - PUFAs account for approximately a third of the total lipid content in the brain. The fetus is not able to make PUFAs de novo and is reliant on maternal intake.
  - PUFAs contribute to phospholipid membrane bilayers.
  - Accumulation of DHA in the second half of gestation is associated with rapid gray matter increases, as well as with cognitive and behavioral development.
- Iodine is found in iodized salt, fish, and grains. It is essential for thyroid hormone production.
  - Thyroxine (T4) supports neuronal migration, synaptogenesis, and myelination in the developing brain.
  - Globally, iodine deficiency is the leading cause of preventable mental impairments, including motor, cognitive, and behavioral function.
- Iron—heme iron is found in meats, seafood, and poultry. Non-heme iron is found in leafy greens, whole grains, nuts, seeds, and legumes.

- Iron promotes neurogenesis and myelination and is critical to hemoglobin formation and the delivery of oxygen to developing tissues.
- Deficiencies are associated with decreased hippocampal development and functions (memory and cognition) and increased risk of low birth weight.
- Adequate iron stores at birth are essential, as infants cannot regulate gut absorption of iron for the first 6 to 9 months of life.
- Fetal iron stores begin to accumulate in the second trimester and peak during the third trimester.
- Vitamin D is endogenously produced in skin by ultraviolet light exposure; it is found exogenously in cod liver oil, salmon, swordfish, tuna, egg yolk, fortified milks, and cereals.
  - Vitamin D contributes to neuronal differentiation, axonal connectivity, development of dopaminergic pathways, and transcription control of genes.
  - Deficiency is associated with lower cognitive and language development.
- Retinoic acid (vitamin A derivative) is found in beef, calf, chicken liver, eggs, fish oils, and dairy products.
  - It plays a role in molecular signaling pathways in the brain and promotion of cellular differentiation; it is also important in dopamine-regulated cognitive and motor activity.
- Thiamine (vitamin B_1) is found in pork, fish, lentils, enriched breads, cereals, noodles, and rice.
  - Thiamine acts as a mitochondrial enzyme cofactor; it plays a role in the metabolism of carbohydrates and amino acids, and it is required in the synthesis of nucleic acids, myelin, and neurotransmitters.
  - Deficiency is associated with specific language impairments (syntax and lexical retrieval).

Postnatal Nutrition and Impact on the Neonate

- Maternal breastfeeding and milk
  - The duration of breastfeeding is associated with IQ in some but not all studies for both term and low-birth-weight infants.
  - The magnitude of the effect of human milk on neurodevelopment seems to be dose dependent in premature infants, with sustained effects into toddler ages.
  - Maternal–infant bonding is enhanced with breastfeeding.
    - Oxytocin serves as a neurotransmitter and directly affects maternal nurturing behaviors and maternal–infant social interactions.
    - Human bonding studies suggest an increased impact on secure attachment that is lasting throughout childhood.
- Specific nutrients
  - Iodine deficiency is associated with decreased cognitive performance.
  - Iron influences psychological functioning; deficiency in early infancy may lead to sustained poor cognitive performance, affects development of auditory processing and executive function, and contributes to poor academic achievement and behavior issues.

- Zinc deficiency is associated with reduced cognitive and motor performance, as well as a higher incidence of attention-deficit/hyperactivity disorder (ADHD) and depression.
- Significant deficiency can manifest as acrodermatitis enteropathica with the triad of diarrhea, hair loss, and periorificial rash in a poorly growing infant.
- Infants who have short gut and have lost jejunum (highest rate of absorption in intestine) are also at risk.
- Folate—there is a positive association between folate intake and academic achievement.
- Protein deprivation results in reduced brain weight, altered formation of the hippocampus, and impairment of neurotransmitters.
  - Kwashiorkor is characterized by severe malnutrition with symptoms of fluid retention, distended abdomen, low muscle mass, and fatigue. It is most commonly seen in developing countries; however, it has been observed in those with severe poverty with lack of access to resources.
- Copper deficiency is extremely rare, but it can manifest as anemia, neutropenia, fatigue, difficulties walking, deficiency in learning ad memory, and osteoporosis/bone fractures.
- Highest risk infants are those with short gut syndrome.

Non-Nutritional Maternal–Infant Factors

- Maternal (prenatal) inflammation
  - Proinflammatory cytokines damage oligodendrocytes and their progenitors, potentially affecting downstream myelination.
  - Chorioamnionitis in preterm infants is associated with gray matter developmental impairments.
  - Breast milk is an important protective factor against sepsis and necrotizing enterocolitis.
- Maternal–infant bonding
  - The development of attachment between the parent and infant begins well before birth, perhaps as early as prepregnancy planning.
  - Influences include the parent's own childhood experiences, previous pregnancy experiences or losses, relationship status with partner, and availability of support systems.
  - Fetal exposure to maternal anxiety, depression, and stress is associated with cognitive delays, ADHD, poor executive function, dysregulation of stress responses, internalizing and externalizing problems, and greater negative emotionality in infancy and childhood.
  - Positive factors include:
    - Early skin to skin contact
    - Early suckling at breast (within first hour)
    - Rooming-in
    - Parent–infant synchrony (recognition of and response to infant needs)
  - Risk factors for poor attachment include:
    - Poor maternal–fetal bonding during pregnancy
    - Perinatal depression
    - Congenital malformations

- Disruption in maternal–infant interaction in the immediate postnatal period
- Infant requiring neonatal intensive care unit (NICU) care can lead to anxiety and stress.
- Postpartum depression
- Outcomes of poor bonding and attachment:
  - Breastfeeding failure
  - Child abuse, abandonment, neglect
  - Failure to thrive
  - Developmental delays
  - Increased risk of anxiety or depression in the child later in life

Potential Interventions to Improve Maternal–Infant Bonding and Neonatal Outcomes

- Kangaroo care demonstrates:
  - Improved physiologic stability of infant, including heart rate, respiratory rate, and temperature
  - Improved lactation success
  - Sustained group differences to 6 months and beyond
  - Improved infant emotional and cognitive outcomes
- Parent involvement in care:
  - Parent behavioral intervention programs help parents recognize infant stress and readiness for interaction cues.
    - Reduction in maternal depression and anxiety, increased confidence in parental roles, and reduction in length of stay.
- Positioning of the neonate demonstrates:
  - Infants requiring neonatal intensive care, especially premature infants, are more prone to positional plagiocephaly and dolichocephaly.
  - Midline positioning of the head in preterm infants <32 weeks may be associated with decreased incidence of intraventricular hemorrhage (IVH).
    - Turned head may lead to occlusion of the jugular venous drainage system and venule leakage in the germinal matrix
  - The Back to Sleep campaign, although reducing the risk of sudden infant death syndrome (SIDS), has increased rates of plagiocephaly and torticollis.
  - Regular changes in posture for preterm infants at rest promote normal neuromuscular and osteoarticular function and permit development of spontaneous and functional motor activity.
    - Prone-only positioning in the 31- to 36-week gestational age (GA) range was associated with dominance of extensor muscles, hyperabduction and flexion of the arms, and global neuromuscular rigidity.
  - Neuromotor problems in preterm infants are caused by imbalances between active and passive muscle power in the extrauterine environment.
  - Prone positioning for very low-birth-weight (VLBW) infants has been associated with better physiologic stability:
    - Improved gas exchange (increased arterial partial pressure of oxygen [PaO_2], decreasing partial pressure of carbon dioxide [PCO_2])

- Decreased respiratory rate
- Improved chest wall synchrony
- Increased overall sleep state and decreased energy expenditure
- More rapid gastric emptying and less reflux
- Utilize Eat, Sleep, Console in infants with neonatal withdrawal symptoms.
  - It has been demonstrated to improve maternal–infant bonding with active engagement of the mother following birth, reduce separation, reduce the need for pharmacologic intervention, and reduce hospitalization.

Family Risk Factors for Neurodevelopmental Impairment

- Social and environmental risk factors adversely affect child development and parent well-being, in addition to medical risk factors for the infant. These include the following:
  - Separated families
  - Low socioeconomic status
  - Low caregiver educational level
- Infants with increased social risk factors may demonstrate more benefit from interventional services than infants with fewer social risks.
- The combination of medical and social-environmental risk factors is associated with particular vulnerability for poor neurodevelopmental outcome.

Early Intervention and Its Impact on Infant and Toddler Development

- Early intervention is a nonspecific term referring to a range of interventions including, but not limited to, family support, physical therapy, occupational therapy, and speech and language therapies; it is introduced typically by age 3 years in the hope of taking advantage of developmental windows and neuroplasticity to optimize global and/or specific neurodevelopmental outcomes.
- Eligibility for early intervention services varies from state to state and internationally.
- Although early intervention has not been proven to prevent neurodevelopmental disability, there are many studies that demonstrate the benefit of early intervention programs.
  - There may be particular benefits of early interventions in the setting of severe hearing (hearing aids, sign language) and severe visual impairment to promote foundations of communication, daily functioning, and quality of life.
  - Educational interventions for preterm infants have shown beneficial effects on cognition, behavior, and motor outcomes through preschool ages, but significant differences have not been seen at school age and beyond.
- Studies of early intervention, particularly of long-term effects, are difficult. Such longitudinal studies are not only costly but also heavily influenced by individual differences and social and environmental factors.

- Interventions aimed at an infant's family, such as targeting maternal anxiety or depression and family coping, may improve parent functioning and outcomes and subsequently influence infant outcomes.

Other Developmental Influences

- Vision
  - Vitamin A deficiency is the leading cause of childhood blindness.
  - Causes of congenital blindness or poor vision include the following:
    - Leber congenital amaurosis
    - Retinal dystrophies
    - Congenital cataracts
      - Significant cataracts must be removed by 6 to 8 weeks of age to prevent vision loss from dense amblyopia.
      - Cataracts can be caused by galactosemia, with symptoms of poor feeding, lethargy, and hyperbilirubinemia.
  - Glaucoma
    - In neonates, this is a disease requiring prompt surgical intervention. Vision loss is generally irreversible.
  - Optic nerve abnormalities
  - Uveal colobomas
  - High refractive errors
  - Congenital infections
  - Hyphema
  - Cerebral (cortical) visual impairment—normal eye, visual impairment secondary to neurologic cause.
    - Greatest cause of visual impairment in children in developed countries, most often associated with neurologic deficit (e.g., cerebral palsy [CP], epilepsy)
    - Perinatal causes include intrauterine infections, cerebral dysgenesis, asphyxia, hypoglycemia, intracranial hemorrhages, periventricular leukomalacia (PVL), hydrocephalus, trauma, meningitis, and encephalitis.
- Retinoblastoma is the most common ocular malignancy of childhood.
  - Untreated, it is nearly uniformly fatal.
  - Five-year survival is >90% with timely recognition and treatment.
  - It is typically diagnosed between 1 and 2 years of age.
- Retinopathy of prematurity (ROP):
  - ROP is generally first diagnosed at 31 to 32 weeks' postmenstrual age, with progression over the next 2 to 5 weeks. Most VLBW infants (<1500 g) will have some degree of ROP.
  - Stages 1 to 3 most often spontaneously regress.
  - Stages 4 and 5 are likely to have poor or no functional vision, despite surgical intervention.
  - Among preterm infants, myopia and strabismus are common outcomes.

Suggested Readings

Demauro SB, Hintz SR. Risk assessment and neurodevelopmental outcomes. In: Gleason CA, Sawyer T, eds. *Avery's Diseases of the Newborn*. 11th ed. Philadelphia: Elsevier; 2023:287–305.

Heland S, Fields N, Ellery SJ, Fahey M, Palmer KR. The role of nutrients in human neurodevelopment and their potential to prevent neurodevelopmental adversity. *Front Nutr*. 2022;9:992120.

Melnyk BM, Feinstein NF, Alpert-Gillis L, et al. Reducing premature infants' length of stay and improving parents mental health outcomes with the Creating Opportunities for Parent Empowerment (COPE) neonatal intensive care unit program: a randomized controlled trial. *Pediatrics*. 2006;281:e1414.

Sandman CA, Glynn LM, Davis EP, et al. Neurobehavioral consequences of fetal exposure to gestational stress. In: Kisilevsky B, Reissland N, eds. *Advancing Research on Fetal Development*. New York: Springer; 2015:229–265.

Spittle A, Orton J, Anderson PJ, et al. Early developmental intervention programs provided post-hospital discharge to prevent motor and cognitive impairment in preterm infants. *Cochrane Database Syst Rev*. 2015;11:CD005495.

Spittle AJ, Treyvaud K, Lee KJ, et al. The role of social risk factors in an early preventative care programme for infants born very premature: a randomized controlled trial. *Dev Med Child Neurol*. 2018;60(1):54–62.

25 *Clinical Features of Neurodevelopmental Impairment*

ALLISON H. PAYNE and GAL BARBUT

Developmental Assessments

Corrected gestational age (age from original due date), not chronological age (from date of birth), should be used for all assessments of milestones, cognition, language, and motor development until at least 2 years' chronological age. All ages mentioned in this section refer to corrected gestational age.

- Timing
  - Assessments before 1 year of age are limited to detection of major motor and sensory disabilities.
  - Reliable assessment of neurodevelopmental outcome improves at ≥2 years.
    - Most transient neurologic abnormalities resolve by 18 to 24 months.
    - Language may be difficult to assess before the age of 3 years.
  - 4 to 5 years: Cognitive and language function testing is more precise.
  - >6 years: Subtle neurologic abnormalities, behavioral outcomes, and academic performance may be assessed.
  - Assessment at younger ages is likely to overestimate neurodevelopmental impairment (NDI) rates.
  - Assessment at school age or adolescence will more accurately reflect long-term outcome.
- Tools
  - There is no true gold standard in developmental assessment.
  - The Bayley Scales of Infant and Toddler Development is the most commonly used tool for cognitive and motor developmental assessment in high-risk infants up to 3 years of age. Direct comparisons of cohorts tested with different Bayley editions are difficult.
    - Norm-referenced: mean = 100, standard deviation = 15
    - First and second editions include:
      - Mental Developmental Index (MDI), a composite outcome of cognitive and language areas
      - Psychomotor Developmental Index (PDI), a composite outcome of fine and gross motor skills
    - The third edition (2006) and fourth edition (2019) include a core battery of five domains:
      - Cognitive
      - Language
      - Motor
      - Socioemotional
      - Adaptive behavior

- Cognitive assessment tools:
  - Cognitive assessment tools report on intelligence (a component of cognition), processing, memory, reasoning abilities, and strengths and weaknesses in specific areas of learning.
  - They are intended to be descriptive of functioning at the time of testing, not predictive of future functioning.
  - Infant cognitive testing has poor long-term validity due to
    - Measurement error and testing cooperation
    - Variance of educational exposures and environmental factors experienced among children
  - Cognitive testing may be affected by visual, hearing, attention, or behavioral issues
- Parental reports of development (e.g., Ages and Stages Questionnaire) can be very valuable in screening high-risk infants who may qualify for further evaluation or services.

Transient Neurologic Abnormalities

- Abnormalities of
  - Muscle tone (hypotonia or hypertonia)
  - Posture
  - Primitive reflexes
- High incidence in high-risk infants (40–80%)
- Peak prevalence for transient neurologic abnormalities is between 4 and 7 months' corrected age.
- Abnormalities generally resolve by 12 months' corrected age.
- Preterm children with a history of transient neurologic abnormalities and subsequent normalized neurologic examination have
  - Increased risk for lower cognitive and academic skills compared to preterm children with consistently normal neurologic examination
  - Better outcomes than preterm children with persistently abnormal neurologic examinations

Developmental Coordination Disorder

Developmental coordination disorder (DCD), also known as *dyspraxia*, was previously referred to as *mild functional motor impairment* or *minor neuromotor dysfunction*.

- DCD is a common neuromotor condition that

- Affects ~5% to 6% of all school-age children
- Affects ~one-third of all preterm children (~6 × –8 × increased risk compared to term children)
- Affects boys > girls (2–3:1)
- Non–cerebral palsy motor impairment:
  - Motor (fine or gross) coordination (e.g., issues with balance, coordination, dexterity) is worse than expected for chronologic age.
  - It is unrelated to a known medical condition (e.g., cerebral palsy, muscular dystrophy, visual impairment, or intellectual disability).
  - It interferes with academic achievement or activities of daily living.
  - It is in excess of what would be expected for IQ if intellectual disability is present.
  - Child is typically described as "clumsy."
  - Child may also show slowness and inaccuracy in motor skill performance.
  - Previous motor delays are not a prerequisite for diagnosis but may be present in history.
- Risk factors:
  - Prematurity, particularly <32 weeks' gestation
  - Small for gestational age
  - Late independent walking (≥15 months)
  - Postnatal steroid exposure
  - Intraventricular hemorrhage (IVH) and periventricular leukomalacia (PVL) do not independently increase the risk for DCD.
- Assessment:
  - Developmental Coordination Disorder Questionnaire (DCDQ)
  - Movement Assessment Battery for Children (MABC-2)
  - Bruininks-Oseretsky Test of Motor Proficiency
- Frequent comorbidities include attention-deficit/hyperactivity disorder (ADHD), autism spectrum disorders, or specific learning disabilities.
- Children are at risk for being overweight/obese, having physical injuries, experiencing psychosocial difficulties, having compromised physical fitness, and decreased participation in daily living, as well as in physical and social activities.
- Long-term outcomes suggest that DCD may be associated with increased depression and anxiety rates and a lower quality of life:
  - Motor skills (e.g., driving, handwriting) and executive functioning (planning ahead, multitasking) may continue to be problematic in adulthood.

Cerebral Palsy

- Cerebral palsy (CP) is a clinical description of a group of permanent disorders of the development of movement and posture affecting motor function.
  - CP has no specific pathologic or radiographic correlates.
  - CP is due to nonprogressive disturbance of fetal or infant brain development (injury or malformation).
- CP is the most common physical disability in childhood:
  - Prevalence is 1–4/1000 live births, increased in high-risk populations.

- Approximately half of all children with CP are born at term; half are preterm.
- Males are at higher risk than females.
- Term: 0.9–1.5/1000 (~0.15%)
- Multiples: 7/1000 (~0.7%)
- Fetal growth restriction (>35 weeks): 3–5/1000 (~0.4%)
- Preterm birth
  - <1000-g birth weight: 50/1000 (~5%)
  - 27–32 weeks' gestational age (GA): 60–80/1000 (6–8%)
  - <28 weeks' GA: 82/1000 (~8%)
  - <25 weeks' GA: 100–120/1000 (10–12%)
- Preterm infants are at risk.
- Postnatal risk factors confer greatest risk:
- Additional risk factors include maternal infection, multiple gestation, exposure to postnatal steroids, need for high-frequency ventilation, pneumothorax, sepsis, necrotizing enterocolitis (NEC), African American ethnicity, and low socioeconomic status.
- With abnormality on head ultrasound (HUS):
  - With any IVH and without PVL
    - Infants <26 weeks have worse outcomes than infants 27 to 32 weeks.
    - <25 weeks: normal HUS, ~10% CP; any IVH, ~20% CP
    - Week by week, stable rates of CP at 27 to 32 weeks for same HUS finding
    - If a ventriculoperitoneal (VP) shunt is needed for post-hemorrhagic hydrocephalus, risk increases.
  - If PVL or intraparenchymal hemorrhage:
    - CP risk, 40–60%
    - GA does not affect CP risk
- Term infants at risk
  - In utero factors confer greater risk in outcome of CP than perinatal or postnatal factors
    - Congenital malformations (particularly of the central nervous system [CNS]), stroke, fetal growth restriction
  - Maternal factors: infections, hypothyroidism, severe proteinuria
  - Perinatal and postnatal risk factors:
    - Ischemic stroke
    - Neonatal encephalopathy
    - 5-minute Apgar <3: 5% to 7% risk of CP
    - Severe hyperbilirubinemia
- Motor aspects of CP are frequently accompanied by difficulties with cognition, communication, sensation, perception, behavior, and musculoskeletal abnormalities.
- CP has a nonprogressive cause, but secondary impairments may change over time.

DIAGNOSIS

- Onset occurs during perinatal or infancy period, but diagnosis is reserved until at least 2 to 3 years of age to establish permanent nature.
- In infants with significant risk factors for CP and severe motor impairment on assessment, provisional diagnosis of CP can occur within first 2 years.

- Examination may show
  - Hyper- or hypotonia
  - Difficulty with oral feeds
  - Hand preference
  - Hands held in fist position with thumb adducted
  - Asymmetric crawling
  - Persistent primitive reflexes
  - Ankle clonus
  - Leg scissoring
- May also show behavioral abnormalities
  - Excessive crying, jitteriness, abnormal sleep patterns, irritability
- Underlying cause is not progressive, but clinical presentation of a child with CP may change over time with brain maturity.

CLASSIFICATION

See Fig. 25.1.

- Spastic CP accounts for 85% of all cases (up to 90% in preterm infants) and includes increased tone with velocity-dependent resistance to passive movement and pathologic reflexes (hyperreflexia, positive Babinski reflex).
  - Spastic diplegia (~35% of overall CP)
    - Affects the lower extremities with no or minimal upper extremity involvement
      - Often first noted with a persistent commando crawl (uses arms but drags legs behind)
      - Often seen with leg scissoring and toe walking
    - Predominant type for preterm infants
      - One-third have cognitive impairment.
      - Most common cause is PVL.
    - Strongly associated with damage to the immature white matter
    - Most will walk but may require assistance or devices; they can achieve independent care with bowel and bladder control.
  - Spastic hemiplegia (~25% of overall CP)
    - Affects unilateral upper and lower extremities and trunk
      - Arm is often involved more than leg.
      - Typical difficulty with hand manipulation
      - Circumduction gait
    - Most common in cases of
      - Unilateral stroke
      - Vascular malformations
      - Unilateral IVH or PVL
    - Typically, child is able to walk by 3 years of age.
    - Approximately two-thirds have cognitive and learning impairments.
  - Spastic quadriplegia (20% of overall CP)
    - Most severe form of CP
    - Causes include PVL, ischemia, and infection.
    - Low likelihood of ambulation
    - Often with flexion contractures at knees and elbows
    - High association with intellectual, speech, and visual disabilities and seizures
- Extrapyramidal (athetoid) CP (15% of overall CP)
  - Characteristically hypotonic, with poor head control and head lag; progresses over years to variable increased tone with rigidity
  - Upper extremities are affected more than lower extremities.

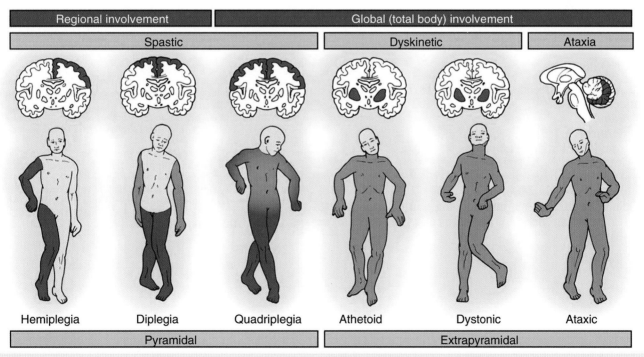

Regional involvement	Global (total body) involvement	
Spastic	Dyskinetic	Ataxia

Hemiplegia	Diplegia	Quadriplegia	Athetoid	Dystonic	Ataxic
Pyramidal			Extrapyramidal		

Fig. 25.1 Classification of cerebral palsy. Although overlaps in terminology exist, cerebral palsy can be classified according to distribution (regional vs. global involvement, hemiplegic, diplegic, quadriplegic), physiologic type (spastic, dyskinetic or dystonic, dyskinetic or athetoid, ataxic), or presumed neurologic substrate (pyramidal or extrapyramidal). (From Canale ST, Beaty JH, eds. *Campbell's Operative Orthopaedics.* 11th ed. Philadelphia: Elsevier; 2008.)

■ Feeding and speech may be difficult.
■ Seizures are uncommon.
■ Seen in cases of basal ganglia and thalamus injury:
  ▫ Asphyxia—symmetric scars of the putamen and thalamus
  ▫ Kernicterus—scars in globus pallidus and hippocampus
  ▫ Mitochondrial genetic disorders

FUNCTIONAL CLASSIFICATION

■ Wide spectrum of severity for cerebral palsy:
  ▫ Some children will achieve ambulation (~60% independent, ~10% assisted).
    ▫ More common if head control by 9 months, suppression of primitive reflexes by 18 to 24 months, and sitting by 2 years (corrected GA)
    ▫ Independent ambulation achieved by 3 years of age is likely to be sustained through adulthood.
  ▫ ~30% of children will not achieve ambulation.
■ The Gross Motor Function Classification System (GMFCS) is often used to describe mild, moderate, and severe status and better delineate prognosis.
  ▫ Five non-overlapping categories:
    ▫ Level 1, most able → level 5, least able
    ▫ Criteria for categories are separated into ages (infant, early child, school age).
  ▫ Levels 1 and 5 are usually stable over time.
  ▫ Levels 2 to 4 are less stable over time (level may change based on age-specific criteria).
  ▫ Levels 1 and 2 typically ambulate without assistance; they may run, jump, and climb stairs.
  ▫ Level 3 children tend to ambulate independently with assistance (walkers, crutches, braces).
  ▫ Levels 4 and 5 children are typically wheelchair bound; they vary in their ability to control the wheelchair independently.

PROGNOSIS

■ CP may have associated comorbidities related to the underlying cause:
  ▫ Pain
  ▫ Seizures
  ▫ Growth or nutrition failure
  ▫ Incontinence
  ▫ Sleep and behavioral problems
  ▫ Autism spectrum disorders
■ Children with CP require ongoing multidisciplinary care, including neurology, orthopedics, development and rehabilitation, ophthalmology, speech, audiology, and occupational and physical therapies to optimize outcome.
■ Interventions should be started as early as possible (when there are any concerns, even before the ability to diagnose CP definitively) to take advantage of brain plasticity and developmental windows for language, cognition, and motor development.
■ Possible treatments include the following:
  ▫ Assistive or adaptive devices to achieve mobility
  ▫ Communication technology, sign language
  ▫ Baclofen (botulinum toxin) or surgical interventions for spasticity
■ The goals of treatment are to prevent deformity, optimize motor function, and improve the child's quality of life.

Quality of Life

■ Parents of preterm adolescents report poorer health, behavior, and physical functioning.
  ▫ However, the self-reporting adolescent shows no differences compared to term peers.
■ In young adulthood, physical functioning and cognition are reported as lower than peers, but subjective quality of life is no different.
■ Discrepancies may indicate differing definitions of quality of life or adaptation over time.

Suggested Readings

Acharya K, Pellerite M, Lagatta J, et al. Cerebral palsy, developmental coordination disorder, visual and hearing impairments in infants born preterm. *NeoReviews.* 2016;17(6):e325–e331.

Harmon HM, Taylor HG, Minich N, et al. Early school outcomes for extremely preterm infants with transient neurologic abnormalities. *Dev Med Child Neurol.* 2015;57(9):865–871.

Harris SR, Mickleson ECR, Zwicker JG. Diagnosis and management of developmental coordination disorder. *CMAJ.* 2015;187(9):659–665.

Johnston MV. Encephalopathies. In: Kleigman RM, Stanton BF, Steme JW, Schor NF, eds. *Nelson Textbook of Pediatrics.* 20th ed. Philadelphia: Elsevier; 2016:2896–2909.

Oskoui M, Shevell MI, Swaiman KF. Cerebral palsy. In: Swaiman KF, Ashwal S, Ferriero DM, et al., eds. *Swaiman's Pediatric Neurology.* 6th ed. Philadelphia: Elsevier; 2017:734–740.

Riddle A, Miller SP, Back SA. Brain injury in the preterm infant. In: Gleason CA, Sawyer T, eds. *Avery's Diseases of the Newborn.* 11th ed. Philadelphia: Elsevier; 2023:809–826.

Stavsky M, Mor O, Mastrolia SA, et al. Cerebral palsy: trends in epidemiology and recent development in prenatal mechanisms of disease, treatment and prevention. *Front Pediatr.* 2017;5(21):1–10.

Wilson-Costello DE, Payne AH. Early childhood neurodevelopmental outcomes of high-risk neonates. In: Martin RJ, Fanaroff AA, Walsh MC, eds. *Fanaroff and Martin's Neonatal-Perinatal Medicine.* 11th ed. Philadelphia: Saunders; 2015:1018–1031.

Immunology and Infectious Diseases

KRISTIN SCHEIBLE and GEOFFREY A. WEINBERG

26 Development of the Immune System

KRISTIN SCHEIBLE

Development of Solid Organs of the Immune System

THYMUS

- The thymus is a mediastinal structure that originates from the bilateral third and fourth pharyngeal pouches during the seventh week of gestation.
- Thymic tissue remnants can be found along the migratory tract in conditions with absent thymic development.
- This is the location of T lymphocyte maturation from a common lymphoid progenitor to a naïve T cell.
- T-cell precursors (CD4$^-$, CD8$^-$) populate the thymus by week 8.
- Fully mature naïve T cells present in the thymus by week 12 (CD4, CD8, $\gamma\delta$ T cells, T regulatory cells) and egress to the circulation by 12 weeks.
- Antigen-presenting cells in the thymus express autoimmune regulator (AIRE) transcription factor, which allows the transcription and presentation of self-antigens to test for (and eliminate) self-reactive T-cell clones.
- Immune cells in the thymus do not communicate directly with circulating antigens or cytokines, enabling tight control over positive and negative selection and the prevention of autoimmunity.

SPLEEN

- The spleen buds from the dorsal mesogastrium by 5 weeks and hilar vessels from 8 weeks.
- Hematopoietic cells by 7 to 8 weeks secrete lymphotoxin, which stimulates structural organization of the spleen (red pulp, white pulp, venous sinuses).
  - Red pulp contains phagocytic monocytes, which remove senescent red blood cells and opsonized (antibody-coated) bacteria and cells; it develops at 13 weeks' gestation.
  - White pulp contains T cells and B cells poised to react against bloodborne pathogens; it develops late in the second trimester.
  - The marginal zone is the interface between the red and white pulp, where pathogens and other antigens are presented to T and B cells; it is not fully developed until 1 to 2 years postnatally.
    - The marginal zone contains specialized B cells that react against bacterial cell wall components and macrophages that bind bacterial polysaccharides—an important defense against *Streptococcus pneumoniae*, *Staphylococcus aureus*, and *Escherichia coli*.

LYMPH NODES

- Lymph nodes serve as sites for antigen concentration and presentation carried by antigen-presenting cells through the local lymphatic network.
- They bud off jugular and cardinal veins to form reticular networks at 8 to 13 weeks.
- Specialized lymphoid tissue inducer (LTi) cells infiltrate and secrete lymphotoxin, which stimulates structural organization.
- An influx of naïve T and B cells into the lymph nodes occurs between 12 and 14 weeks; they are then ready to be primed by infection.
  - B-cell follicles are detectable by 17 to 22 weeks but no germinal centers until stimulated by infection or other antigen, usually postnatally.
  - T-cell zones are detectable by 16 weeks.
- Lymphadenopathy (palpable lymph nodes) occurs in roughly one-third of healthy newborns, usually in the inguinal and cervical regions.
  - Supraclavicular lymphadenopathy is atypical.
  - This can also indicate the presence of a congenital infection, such as cytomegalovirus.

PEYER PATCHES (GUT-ASSOCIATED LYMPHOID TISSUE)

- Peyer patches are an interface between the gut lumen and immune system; they are concentrated in the distal ileum.
- They are biased toward an anti-inflammatory response.
- T-cell and B-cell clusters form at 11 weeks, visible structures by 22 weeks.
- Follicular dendritic cells are seen by 24 weeks; they take up and present antigen to T cells.
- Peyer patches increase postnatally with commensal colonization.

Development of the Cellular Immune System

HEMATOPOIESIS

- This is a process whereby immune and blood cells arise from stem cells (Fig. 26.1).
- Hematopoietic stem cells (HSCs) originate in the yolk sac, then the liver and bone marrow.
  - This self-renewing pluripotent cell population gives rise to multiple cell types, with increasing lineage commitment in response to specific environmental signals and internal cell-specific molecular programs.
    - Common myeloid progenitors

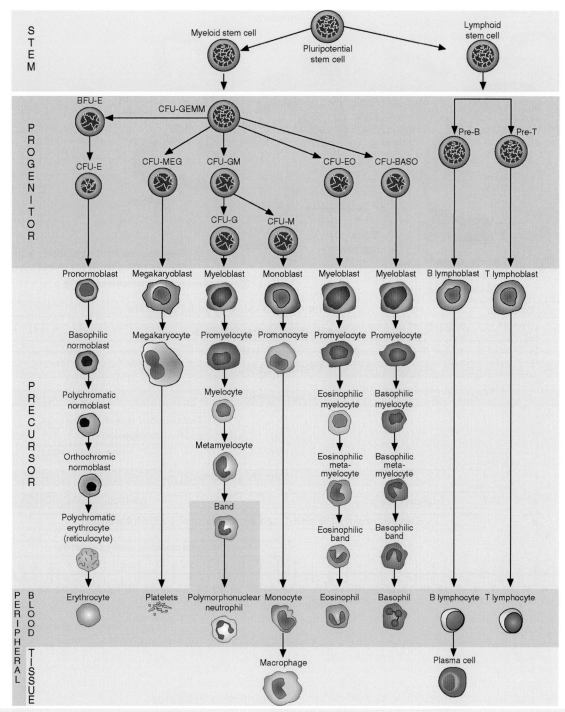

Fig. 26.1 Human hematopoiesis. *CFU-E*, Colony-forming units–erythroid; *BFU-E*, burst-forming units–erythroid. (From Rodak BF, Carr JH. *Clinical Hematology Atlas.* 5th ed. Philadelphia: Elsevier; 2009:11–16.)

□ Erythroid and myeloid lineages (granulocytes and monocytes)
▪ Common lymphoid progenitors
  □ Lymphoid lineages (T cells, B cells, innate lymphoid cells [ILCs])
▪ The layered immune system hypothesis states that sequential events of embryonic hematopoiesis result in varying progenitor sources and functional potential of immune cells during early human development (Fig. 26.2).
▪ The innate immune system develops first; embryonic adaptive cells share some characteristics with innate

cells (higher fractions of T and B cells with lower specificity compared to adults).
▪ Immune responses in premature newborns, and in some full-term infants, may be shaped by cells remaining from early fetal development.
  ▪ Primitive hematopoiesis (2–6 weeks' gestation)—blood islands located in the yolk sac produce only erythroid and myeloid progenitors.
    ▪ Primitive monocytes are the only monocytes capable of differentiating into long-lived, self-renewing microglial cells.

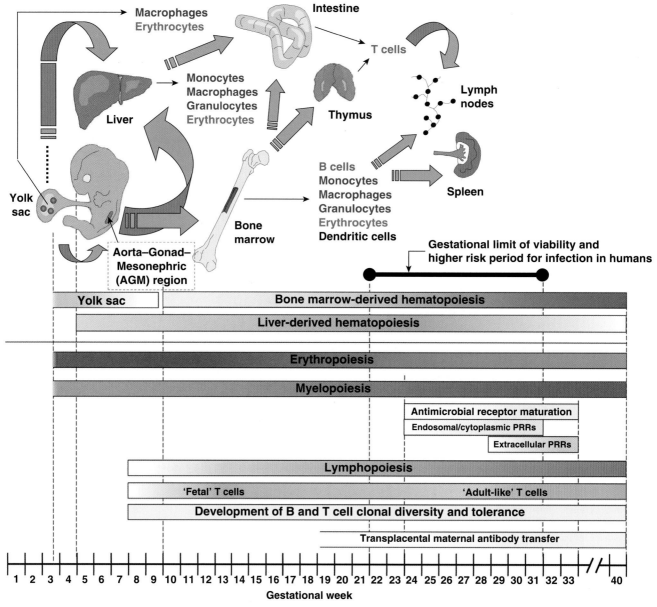

Fig. 26.2 Immune development during gestation. *PRRs,* Pattern recognition receptors. (From Kan B, Razzaghian HR, Lavoie PM. An immunological perspective on neonatal sepsis. *Trends Mol Med.* 2016;22(4):290–302.)

- Definitive hematopoiesis (beginning at 5 weeks' gestation) occurs in two overlapping stages based on the origin of the HSCs.
  - Aorta–gonad–mesonephros and liver (5–22 weeks) generate myeloid, erythroid, and some lymphoid (γδ T cells, natural killer [NK] cells, and CD5+ B cells) progenitors.
    - Contribute to organ development, including specialized kidney and alveolar macrophages
  - Bone marrow (after 11 weeks) generates myeloid, lymphoid, and erythroid progenitors and contributes to the final mature circulating pool of myeloid and lymphoid cells.
- Individual components of the immune system are described in the next chapter.

Suggested Readings

Farley AM, Morris LX, Vroegindeweij E, et al. Dynamics of thymus organogenesis and colonization in early human development. *Development.* 2013;140(9):2015–2026.

Heinig K, Sage F, Robin C, Sperandio M. Development and trafficking function of haematopoietic stem cells and myeloid cells during fetal ontogeny. *Cardiovasc Res.* 2015;107(3):352–363.

Kan B, Razzaghian HR, Lavoie PM. An immunological perspective on neonatal sepsis. *Trends Mol Med.* 2016;22(4):290–302.

Mebius RE, Kraal G. Structure and function of the spleen. *Nat Rev Immunol.* 2005;5(8):606–616.

Ygberg S, Nilsson A. The developing immune system: from foetus to toddler. *Acta Paediatr.* 2012;101(2):120–127.

27 Components of the Immune System

KRISTIN SCHEIBLE

Cellular Components of the Immune System

White blood cell levels vary by age and many clinical conditions. Normal levels and conditions affecting specific cell populations can be found in Table 27.1.

MYELOID LINEAGE IMMUNE CELLS

- Monocytes
  - Monocytes phagocytose, present antigen, produce cytokines and chemokines, participate in wound repair, tissue remodeling, and homeostasis.
  - Development
    - Monocytes exist in circulation and then differentiate into macrophages, dendritic cells, histiocytes, or other tissue-specific resident cells when localized.
    - Granulocyte-macrophage colony-stimulating factor (GM-CSF) is secreted by macrophages, T cells, mast cells, natural killer cells, endothelial cells, and fibroblasts and functions as a cytokine, major growth factor.
  - Multiple subtypes of monocytes are categorized based on the source of the progenitor, resident location, and function.
    - Primitive monocytes originate in the yolk sac, are a minor transient population in circulation, and are able to differentiate into self-renewing microglia.
      - Prune synapses, scavenge and maintain neural tissue homeostasis
  - Definitive monocytes originate in the liver and then the bone marrow.
    - Liver-derived monocytes are able to differentiate into self-renewing resident macrophages in the lung (alveolar macrophages), skin (histiocytes), heart (cardiac macrophages), kidney (macrophages and dendritic cells), and liver (macrophages, Küpffer cells). They present antigen to T cells and participate in tissue homeostasis.
    - Bone marrow- and liver-derived monocytes contribute to the circulating pool of mature monocytes that differentiate into macrophages and serve immune functions, including phagocytosis, antigen presentation, and cytokine production.
  - Three activation pathways:
    - Innate—Toll-like receptor stimulation increases nitric oxide synthase (NOS) and reactive oxygen species (ROS).
    - Classic—interferon-γ (IFN-γ) and lipopolysaccharide (LPS) enhance antigen presentation, inflammatory cytokines, and microbicidal activity.
    - Alternate—interleukin-4 (IL-4) and IL-13 increase cell growth, tissue repair, and parasite killing.

Table 27.1 White Blood Cell Indices at Birth

Cell Type	Mean × 10³/mL (Range)	No. Present (%)	Postnatal Peak	Increase	Decrease
Total white blood cells	18.1 (9–30)		12 hours	Infection; leukemoid response to stress; steroids; congenital leukemia; transient myeloproliferative disease of the newborn	Preeclampsia; prematurity; infection
Neutrophils	11 (6–26)	61	12 hours	Infection; steroids; congenital leukemia; transient myeloproliferative disease of the newborn	Prematurity; preeclampsia; infection; Rh hemolytic disease; bone marrow failure; syndromes organic acidemias; glycogen storage disease; copper deficiency; maternal anti–HNA-1b antibodies; drug-induced
Lymphocytes	5.5 (2–11)	31	6–12 months	Congenital syphilis; cytomegalovirus; *Bordetella pertussis*; phenytoin	Prematurity; infection; severe combined immunodeficiency; 22q11.2 deletion; steroids
Monocytes	1.1	6	12 hours	Prematurity; infection; candidal infection; congenital syphilis; steroids	Prematurity; infection
Eosinophils	0.4	2	2–4 weeks	Candidal infection; allergic sensitization; furosemide	Prematurity; infection

Adapted from The Johns Hopkins Hospital, Kahl L, Hughes HK. *The Harriet Lane Handbook*. 21st ed. Philadelphia: Elsevier; 2017.

- Granulocytes
  - Neutrophils represent the highest fraction of granulocytes and are present in the liver by 5 weeks' gestation.
    - Development
      - Neutrophils mature in the liver and bone marrow (myeloblast → promyelocyte → myelocyte → metamyelocyte → banded neutrophil → segmented neutrophil).
      - Production is stimulated by granulocyte-colony stimulating factor (G-CSF) >> IL-6 > IL-3.
      - Neutrophils increase in circulation during the third trimester, peak at 12 to 24 hours of life from a G-CSF surge, and rise to adult levels by 4 weeks.
    - Activation
      - Neutrophils attach to endothelial tissue until activated, then migrate directionally to sites of inflammation in response to chemical signals (chemoattractants such as IL-8).
      - Neutrophils function through phagocytosis and bactericidal activity of intracellular respiratory burst and secreted mediators.
        - Phagocytosis activity preterm < term < adult due to lower CR3 and Fc receptor activity (poor recognition of opsonized pathogens).
        - Respiratory burst is diminished in preterms, enhanced in full-term infants.
        - Higher IL-6 and IL-10 levels and lower IL-1β, tumor necrosis factor-α (TNF-α), and IFN-γ levels compared to adults
        - Reduced neutrophil extracellular trap (NET) activity (extrusion of chromatin and antimicrobial material that mechanically and chemically neutralizes bacteria at mucosal surfaces; NET inactivated by deoxyribonuclease)
        - Reduced chemokine-directed localization to infected sites
  - Eosinophils
    - Eosinophils are present in liver at 5 weeks.
    - Eosinophils are higher in neonates but lower in preterm compared to full-term infants.
    - They increase over the first 1 to 2 months postnatally in response to Th2 cytokines (IL-4, IL-5, IL-13).
    - They are located mainly at mucosal surfaces.
    - Eosinophils are key cells in allergic and antiparasite responses.
      - Activate in response to cytokines and cross-linking of surface-bound immunoglobulin E (IgE)
      - Release of allergy-related cytokines (IL-4, IL-5), toxic granules, collagenases, chemoattractants, leukotrienes, platelet-activating factor
  - Mast cells and basophils
    - Cord blood mast cells and basophils release higher amounts of histamine and IL-4 compared to adults when stimulated by IgE.
    - They are activated through cytokines and cross-linking of surface-bound IgE.
    - Mast cells are implicated in neonatal lung disease (hyperoxia-induced animal models and human lung tissue).
    - Mast cells may participate in tissue remodeling, including early follicular development in the ovary.

LYMPHOID LINEAGES

- T lymphocytes
  - T lymphocytes are important for recognizing and clearing cells infected with intracellular pathogens (e.g., viruses, *Listeria monocytogenes*, *Chlamydia*, *Salmonella*).
  - T lymphocytes provide cytokine signals to stimulate B cells to mature and secrete appropriate antibody isoforms, orchestrate immune response.
  - Development
    - Progenitors originate in liver, then bone marrow, during embryonic development; they circulate as double-negative (CD4- and CD8-antigen negative) common lymphoid progenitors, localize to the thymus, and mature into double-positive, when they are released as single-positive naïve T cells.
    - They undergo terminal deoxynucleotidyl transferase (TdT)–dependent somatic DNA rearrangement of VDJ segments during thymic maturation that enables production of random T-cell receptor sequences; the loop of DNA excised during rearrangement is detectable in recent thymic emigrants as a T cell excision circle (TREC).
    - TREC content is measured by dried blood spot as part of a newborn screening program to detect severe combined immune deficiency (SCID). TRECs increase with gestational age; therefore, preterm infants have a higher risk for false-positive SCID screening.
    - Two checkpoints during T-cell receptor development in the thymus prevent autoreactivity: positively selected (survive) when able to recognize self–major histocompatibility complex (MHC); negatively selected (deleted) when they react too strongly to self-antigen presented in self-MHC.
  - Activation
    - Each T cell recognizes a single peptide sequence when presented within an MHC molecule on another cell. Expansion of a pathogen-specific T-cell clone after initial priming results in a higher number of antigen-specific memory cells able to respond more rapidly on secondary exposure.
    - Each CD4 T-cell clone recognizes a unique short peptide sequence presented within the pocket of MHC II on infected antigen-presenting cells (monocytes, dendritic cells, macrophages, B cells) and polarizes toward unique functions:
      - Th1 (IFN-α, IFN-γ, TNF-α, IL-2) → antiviral, intracellular pathogen killing
      - Th2 (IL-4, IL-5, IL-13) → antiparasite, allergen, antibody production
      - Th17 (IL-17, IL-9, IL-23) → antibacterial, antifungal
      - T regulatory—IL-10, suppressive receptor activity, dampens inflammatory response
    - Each CD8 T-cell clone recognizes specific peptide sequences presented within the MHC (expressed on most nucleated cells) and matures into cytotoxic cells.
      - Produces inflammatory cytokines, granzyme, perforin, executes Fas-mediated killing

- The γδ T cells recognize patterns on antigen-presenting cells, behave in a more innate-like fashion, and localize primarily to mucosal sites.
  - Neonatal T cells have several unique properties:
    - They require multiple reinforcing signals in addition to peptide–MHC binding to activate.
    - They require multiple exposures to establish protective memory.
    - They are prone to differentiating into T regulatory cells and short-lived cytokine producers rather than long-lived memory T cells.
    - They have higher CD4/CD8 ratios and higher IL-8 and TNF-α cytokine production.
    - IFN-γ production is suppressed by promoter site hypermethylation.
- B lymphocytes
  - B lymphocytes produce and secrete antibody and present antigen to T cells in the lymph node.
  - Development
    - B-cell receptor (BCR) undergoes a DNA rearrangement similar to T cells, as well as a second somatic hypermutation event during active infection that increases binding affinity of BCRs.
    - Secreted antibody is a soluble B-cell receptor and heavy chain isotype; it switches from IgM, IgD → IgG, IgA, and IgE (isotype functions listed in Table 27.2).
    - Progenitors (pro–B cells) and precursors (pre–B cells) are detected in liver by 8 weeks' gestation and transition to bone marrow by 12 weeks.
      - Naïve B cell matures in lymph node, becomes plasma cell (antibody-secreting) or memory B cell (more rapidly differentiates into plasma cells on secondary infection).
      - Two major subsets of B cells:
        - B-1 (CD5+) B cells are a minor population present during fetal development; they only secrete IgM spontaneously, do not fully differentiate into memory, recognize carbohydrate antigens, and are enriched in fetal omentum.
        - B-2 B cells are major subclass; they undergo class switching and affinity maturation and then differentiate into memory B cells.
  - Activation: can be T-independent (against polysaccharides and haptens) or T-dependent (against protein or peptide antigens)

- T-dependent activation occurs when B cells present peptide antigen to T cells, which then provide reinforcement signals to mature the B cell response.
  - Newborn B cells have diminished splenic marginal zone B cells, which recognize polysaccharide antigens and protect against T-independent (nonprotein) antigens.
  - *Haemophilus influenzae* type B (HiB) and pneumococcal vaccines include a polysaccharide capsular antigen linked to a peptide antigen. T cells recognize the peptide and provide cytokine signals that induce antibody class switching and affinity maturation.
- Innate lymphoid cells
  - Innate lymphoid cells are present in fetal liver at 6 weeks; they recognize pathogens via patterned recognition receptors and function through cytokine production and receptor-mediated cytotoxic activity.
  - Interest is growing in this newly identified cell population that bridges innate and adaptive immune functions.
  - Innate lymphoid cells are grouped by cytokine function and marker expression:
    - Group 1 produces IFN-γ and TNF-α and includes NK cells (dominant lymphoid cells in fetal lung and liver, diminished function in newborns).
    - Group 2 produces IL-4, IL-5, IL-9, and IL-13.
    - Group 3 produces IL-17 and IL-22.

Development of Humoral and Soluble Components of the Immune System

CYTOKINES

- Cytokines are small proteins secreted by cells to signal behavior to receptor-expressing cells in an autocrine, paracrine, or systemic fashion.
- They can be inflammatory, antiinflammatory, or both, depending on the receiving cell type and presence of other cytokines.
- IFN-γ is critical for protection against intracellular pathogens; its production and activity are blunted in newborns.
- Newborns produce higher levels of innate-type inflammatory cytokines (IL-1, IL-2, IL-6, IL-8, TNF-α) and

Table 27.2 Antibody Isoforms

Isoform	Major Functions	Location	Placental Transfer	Age When Adult Levels Are Achieved
IgM	Complement activation	Circulation, mucosal sites	No	1 year
IgG1	Opsonization, neutralization, complement activation	Circulation, extravascular space	Yes; active transport during third trimester	Higher at birth than adult (in term gestation due to maternal antibody), nadir at 6–8 months, then comparable to adult by 3–4 years
IgG2	Neutralization	Circulation, extravascular space	Some	
IgG3	Complement activation, neutralization, opsonization	Circulation, extravascular space	Yes	
IgG4	Neutralization	Circulation, extravascular space	Some	
IgA	Neutralization	Mucosal sites, extravascular space	No	4–6 years
IgE	Mast cell activation	Circulation, extravascular space	No	Varies by genetic predisposition to atopy

regulatory cytokines (TGF-β, IL-10) compared to adults and lower levels of adaptive-type responses (IFN-γ, IL-4, IL-17).
- The balance of the cytokines instruct the immune system to respond appropriately to a given antigen (e.g., Th1, Th2, Th17; see above).

COMPLEMENT

- Complement is a collection of proteins that interact to augment, and sometimes inhibit, immunity through multiple pathways (Tables 27.3 and 27.4).
- Complement proteins enhance antibody function, recruit leukocytes, prime and mature adaptive immune cells, and lyse microbial membranes.
- They are activated through three overlapping pathways that have variable functions during fetal and neonatal development.
- They are produced in liver, except C7, which is secreted by neutrophils.

- They are measured by the CH50 assay (measures lysis of sheep erythrocytes in serial dilutions of human sera).
- Most components are diminished in newborns, with the exception of C7 and factor D. C9 (terminal element) is neurotoxic; low levels may protect newborns against hypoxia-induced brain injury.

ANTIMICROBIAL PEPTIDES AND PROTEINS

- Antimicrobial peptides and proteins (APPs) are soluble cationic molecules that neutralize infections, recruit and modulate immune cell activity at sites of infection, opsonize, and enhance phagocytosis.
- They are produced by many cell types (e.g., epithelial, immune); concentrations usually increase during normal gestation and postnatally.
- They can be constitutive or induced by inflammation.
- Human breast milk is an important source of APP in neonates.
- Common peptides and proteins listed in Table 27.5.

Table 27.3 Complement Pathways During Fetal and Neonatal Development

Pathway	Mechanism of Activation	Components	Preterm vs. Full Term	Full Term vs. Adult
Classic	Antibody + antigen, CRP	C1	↓	↓
		C2	→	↓
		C3	↓	↓
		C4	↓	↓
Lectin	Lectin + pathogen, carbohydrate, IgA	C2	→	↓
		C3	↓	↓
		C4	↓	↓
		Mannose-binding lectin	↓	↓
		Ficolins	↓	↓
		MASP-2	↓	↓
Alternative	Spontaneous hydrolysis of C3, foreign surfaces	C3	↓	↓
		Factor B	→	↓
		Factor D	→	↑
		Properdin	→	↓

CRP, C-reactive protein; *IgA*, immunoglobulin A; *MASP-2*, mannose-binding lectin-associated serine protease 2.

Table 27.4 Terminal and Regulatory Complement Components and Neonatal Development

Role	Component	Preterm vs. Full Term	Full Term vs. Adult
Terminal	C5	↓	↓
	C6	↓	↓
	C7	→	→
	C8	↓	↓
	C9	↓	↓↓
Regulator or role	Factor I; cleaves C4b, C3b	→	↓
	C1 inhibitor or binds C1r/s protease, inactivates MASP-1, MASP-2	Unknown	↓
	Factor H binds C4b, C3b	→	↓

MASP-1 and *MASP-2*, mannose-binding lectin-associated serine protease 1 and 2.

Table 27.5 Selected Antimicrobial Peptides and Proteins Found in Neonates

Peptide or Protein	Detected in Tissue	Function(s)	Preterm vs. Full Term	Full Term vs. Adult
C-reactive protein	Blood	Opsonization of bacteria and apoptotic cells	→	→
Defensins	Blood, breast milk, gut, trachea, vernix, amniotic fluid	Bactericidal; recruit innate and adaptive cells to sites of inflammation	↓	↓
Cathelicidins	Blood, breast milk, gut, trachea, skin, vernix	Bactericidal; recruit innate and adaptive cells to sites of inflammation	→	↑
Bactericidal, permeability-increasing protein	Blood, trachea	Opsonization of gram-negative bacteria	↓	↓
Lactoferrin	Breast milk, skin, vernix	Iron chelation; enhances immune cell adhesion and ROS production	→	↑
Lysozyme	Vernix, amniotic fluid	Bacterial lysis	↓	→
Collectins (mannose-binding protein surfactants A and D)	Gut, lung	Bind to nonhuman bacterial surface carbohydrates; opsonize bacteria and apoptotic cells	↓	→

ROS, Reactive oxygen species.

Suggested Readings

Battersby AJ, Khara J, Wright VJ, Levy O, Kampmann B. Antimicrobial proteins and peptides in early life: ontogeny and translational opportunities. *Front Immunol.* 2016;7:309.

McGreal EP, Hearne K, Spiller OB. Off to a slow start: underdevelopment of the complement system in term newborns is more substantial following premature birth. *Immunobiology.* 2012;217(2):176–186.
Murphy K, Travers P, Walport M, Janeway C. *Janeway's Immunobiology.* 8th ed. New York: Garland Science; 2012.

28 Abnormal Immune System Development

KRISTIN SCHEIBLE

Inflammation

- Inflammation is broadly defined as innate and adaptive immune activation triggered by pathogen invasion or tissue damage.
  - Molecular events vary based on initiating event, specific mediators activated, and location.
    - Consistent event: vasodilation, vascular permeability facilitates recruitment of proteins, fluids, leukocytes into damaged tissue
  - It involves collateral damage to the host (primary target is pathogen, but host tissue sustains secondary injury).
    - Often the inflammatory component causes more damage than the pathogen or injury.
      - Especially maladaptive if inflammation occurs in immunologically privileged sites (e.g., eye, brain, uterus, testicle, ovary)
    - Many canonical diseases in the preterm infant are thought to have an inflammatory component, including bronchopulmonary dysplasia, necrotizing enterocolitis, and periventricular leukomalacia.
- Characterized by four components: pain, swelling, heat, and redness.
- Can be infectious (viral, bacterial, fungal invasion), sterile (trauma, ischemia), or both (e.g., ventilator-induced lung injury, mucosal colonization)
- Three phases:
  - Recognition and activation
    - With infection, there is immediate recognition of the invading organism by the innate system through pathogen-associated molecular patterns (PAMPs).
      - Bind to cell surface pattern recognition receptors (PRRs) and Toll-like receptors (TLRs)
    - With tissue injury, there is recognition of damaged tissue or noxious exposure through damage-associated molecular patterns (DAMPs).
      - Bind to TLRs and intracellular nucleotide-binding and oligomerization domain (NOD)-like receptors (NLRs)
    - Many PAMPs and DAMPs signal transcription of inflammatory mediators through the nuclear factor kappa B (NF-κB) transcription factor pathway.
    - DAMP and PAMP pathways activate the complement system.
  - Isolation and clearance
    - Transcription and release of inflammatory mediators, such as interleukin-1β (IL-1β), tumor necrosis factor-α (TNF-α), IL-6, and chemoattractants

(IL-8), as well as upregulation of costimulatory molecules
  - Recruitment of effector cells (activated immune cells that kill and clear infected cells and pathogen)
    - Neutrophils and monocytes phagocytose infectious particles, releasing reactive oxygen and reactive nitrogen species (form purulent fluid).
  - Production of proinflammatory eicosanoids (e.g., histamine, prostaglandins, thromboxane, leukotrienes)
  - Recruitment of adaptive system (delayed if novel infection)
    - Coordinates immune response by programming appropriately polarized cytokine bias
      - Th1 (interferon-α [IFN-α], IFN-γ, TNF-α, IL-2) → antiviral, intracellular pathogen killing
      - Th2 (IL-4, IL-5, IL-13) → antiparasite, allergen, antibody production
      - Th17 (IL-17, IL-9, IL-23) → antibacterial, antifungal
    - Establishes memory cells that can respond more rapidly on secondary challenge
  - Proinflammatory cytokine release causes temperature instability in newborn (hyper- or hypothermia).
  - Increased metabolic rate results in increased glucose consumption, somnolence, lactic acidosis, and increased CO_2 production.
- Restoration of homeostasis
  - Critical step that prevents ongoing collateral injury, chronic inflammatory disease, and autoimmunity
  - Switch from proinflammatory eicosanoids to anti-inflammatory lipoxins, resolvins, and protectins
    - Blocks further neutrophil influx and recruits monocytes for wound healing
  - Release of anti-inflammatory hormones, including cortisol
  - Release of suppressive mediators
    - T regulatory cells secrete suppressive IL-10 and transforming growth factor-β (TGF-β) cytokines and shut down inflammatory cells through receptor engagement.
    - Innate cells secrete adenosine and IL-10.
  - Tissue repair
    - Recruitment of monocytes to clear damaged tissue and promote scar formation
    - Tissue-resident macrophages assist in wound healing and the removal of apoptotic immune cells and other cellular debris remaining following acute inflammatory process.

Newborn Susceptibility to Infection (Normal Immune System)

- Skin provides a physical barrier and is a rich source of specialized resident antigen-presenting cells, including histiocytes; stratum corneum (outer keratinized skin surface) is incomplete until 34 weeks' gestation and is more easily penetrated by bacteria.
- Mucosal epithelium includes internal surfaces that interface with the external environment (gut, airway, genital tract).
  - Mucosal integrity varies by site, with poor mechanical barrier function at earlier gestational ages.
  - Diminished mucus production
  - Poor airway clearance
- Tears contain high concentrations of antibody but are not fully mature until postnatal months 1 to 3.
- Gastric pH is higher in neonates and changing microbial environment.
- Blood–brain barrier is more permeable in newborns, allowing passage of pathogens and inflammatory mediators.
- Medications commonly used in sick newborns to suppress the immune system are shown in Table 28.1.

Primary Immunodeficiencies

OVERVIEW

- Can affect the solid organs, innate or adaptive immune system
- Differential can be directed by observing clinical stigmata (Table 28.2) or sentinel infections (Table 28.3).
- Often X-linked genetic inheritance pattern
- Concern for primary immune deficiency should be raised if:
  - Two or more serious bacterial infections
  - Two or more serious respiratory or soft tissue infections within 1 year
  - Unusual pathogens
  - Usual pathogens with severe illness or in unusual sites
- Failure to thrive is a common presenting sign.

ABNORMAL ORGAN DEVELOPMENT

- Asplenia and hyposplenia
  - Presentation
    - Can be isolated or associated with syndrome
      - Ivemark syndrome: bilateral right-sidedness, cardiac anomalies (transient global amnesia [TGA], Pulmonary stenosis or atresia, total anomalous pulmonary venous return [TAPVR]), intestinal malrotation
      - Smith-Fineman-Myers syndrome: mental retardation, short stature, cryptorchidism
      - Heterotaxy syndrome: left-sided (polysplenia) or right-sided (asplenia or hyposplenia) isomerism
      - Familial: autosomal dominant, isolated anomaly
  - Risk for severe infections with encapsulated bacteria (e.g., *Streptococcus pneumoniae*, *Haemophilus influenzae* b [Hib], *Neisseria meningitidis*, *Staphylococcus aureus*, *Salmonella*)

Table 28.1 Immunomodulating Medications

Medication	Interaction With Immune System
NSAIDs (indomethacin, ibuprofen)	Inhibit COX1/COX2 activity: diminished eicosanoid production and immune cell activation
G-CSF	Stimulates neutrophil survival, proliferation, and activity
GM-CSF	Stimulates granulocyte and monocyte survival, proliferation, and activity
Steroids	Demargination of bands and PMNs (increase in CBC), decreased monocytes, lymphopenia, reduced endothelial adhesion, downregulation of antigen-presenting molecules (MHC), suppression of eicosanoids, suppression of NF-κB
IVIG	Binds to and inhibits Fc-receptor, activation of anti-inflammatory pathways through complement-binding, blocks phagocytosis of desired cells, inhibition of T-cell cytotoxicity
Macrolides	Inhibit release of arachidonic acid and inflammatory eicosanoid production, inhibit NF-κB pathways, increase IL-10 and decrease TNF-α/IL-8/IL-1β production

CBC, Complete blood count; *G-CSF*, granulocyte colony-stimulating factor; *GM-CSF*, granulocyte–macrophage colony-stimulating factor; *IL-8*, interleukin-10; *IL-8*, interleukin-10; *IL-1β*, interleukin-1β; *IVIG*, intravenous immunoglobulin; *MHC*, major histocompatibility complex; *NF-κB*, nuclear factor kappa B; *NSAIDs*, nonsteroidal anti-inflammatory drugs; *PMNs*, polymorphonuclear leukocytes; *TNF*, tumor necrosis factor.

Table 28.2 Stigmata of Primary Immunodeficiencies

Clinical Presentation	Syndrome
Petechiae	Wiskott-Aldrich
Telangiectasias	Ataxia–telangiectasia
Eczematoid rash	Wiskott-Aldrich, hyper IgE
Seborrhea behind ears	Chronic granulomatous disease
Generalized seborrhea	Langerhans histiocytosis, T cell deficiencies
Nose tip dermatitis	Chronic granulomatous disease
Poor scar formation, delayed cord separation	Leukocyte defects
Rachitic rosary, bone in bone	ADA (AR-SCID)

ADA, Adenosine deaminase deficiency; *AR-SCID*, autosomal recessive severe combined immunodeficiency; *IgE*, immunoglobulin E.

Table 28.3 Sentinel Infections Associated With Primary Immunodeficiencies

Infection	Syndrome
Nocardia, Aspergillus spp.	Chronic granulomatous disease
Burkholderia cepacia pneumonia	Chronic granulomatous disease
Recurrent *Neisseria* spp.	Terminal complement deficiency
Escherichia coli bacteremia	Galactosemia
Pneumocystis carinii	T lymphocyte deficiency
Recurrent *Streptococcus pneumoniae* bacteremia	Asplenia, hemoglobinopathy, agammaglobulinemia, Kartagener
CMV, HSV	Hyper IgE, SCID, HIV
Gingivostomatitis	Neutrophil abnormalities

CMV, Cytomegalovirus; *HIV*, human immunodeficiency virus; *HSV*, herpes simplex virus; *IgE*, immunoglobulin E; *SCID*, severe combined immunodeficiency.

Table 28.4   Selected Syndromes With Severe Congenital Neutropenia

Syndrome	Gene Defect	Presentation (in Addition to Neutropenia)	Management
Autoimmune primitive neutropenia	(Autoantibody against FcRgIIIb)	Most frequent chronic neutropenia in children; late arrest of neutrophils; macrophagia of intramedullary PMNs	Conservative
Elastase mutation (severe congenital cyclic neutropenia)[a]	ELANE (AD)	Maturation arrest of neutrophils, no extrahematopoietic findings	G-CSF, sulfamethoxazole-trimethoprim (Bactrim)
Kostmann	HAX1 (AR)	Arrest of neutrophils at promyelocytes; cognitive delay and epilepsy	G-CSF, Bactrim, BMT
Cartilage hair hypoplasia	RMRP (AR)	Short-limbed dwarfism, fine hair, lymphopenia	Bactrim
Wiskott-Aldrich	WAS (X-linked)	Eczema, thrombocytopenia	IVIG, Bactrim, BMT
Shwachman-Diamond	SDBS (AR)	Exocrine pancreas insufficiency, anemia, thrombocytopenia	G-CSF (cautious), Bactrim erythropoietin, growth hormone, supportive treatment for pancreatic insufficiency
Barth	G4–G5 (X-linked)	Cardiomyopathy and fibrosis, acidopathy	G-CSF, Bactrim
Chédiak-Higashi	LYST (AR)	Oculocutaneous albinism, bleeding	Bactrim, BMT

[a]Most frequent primary neutropenia.
AD, Autosomal dominant; *AR*, autosomal recessive; *BMT*, bone marrow transplant; *G-CSF*, granulocyte-colony stimulating factor; *IVIG*, intravenous immunoglobulin; *PMNs*, polymorphonuclear leukocytes.

- Neonates with asplenia are at highest risk for *Klebsiella* and *Escherichia coli* infections.
- Persistent thrombocytosis and Howell-Jolly bodies remain in circulation.
- Male predominance (60%)
  - Evaluation
    - Genetic testing
    - Screening imaging to assess cardiac and abdominal anatomy
    - Complete blood count (CBC)
  - Treatment and prophylaxis
    - PCV13 (pneumococcal polysaccharide), Hib conjugate, and meningococcal (Menveo) vaccines are indicated in infancy; household contacts are encouraged to receive age-appropriate vaccines.
    - Antibiotic prophylaxis with oral penicillin VK from birth until 5 years of age
- Athymia
  - Presentation
    - Compromised T-cell maturation, can be complete or partial
      - Complete causes T-negative (T⁻), B-positive (B⁺), and NK-positive (NK⁺) deficiency
    - Usually found as part of DiGeorge anomaly; criteria are two of the three following features:
      - Cellular immunodeficiency with absence of part or all of thymus
      - Parathyroid deficiency
      - Congenital heart disease
    - 55% have 22q11 deletion.
      - Facial features include hypertelorism, hooded eyelids, short philtrum, micrognathia, and low-set ears.
    - Athymia is also found in CHARGE association and FOXN1 deficiency.
  - Evaluation
    - Serum ionized calcium levels
    - CBC; consider flow cytometry subset analysis
    - Testing for 22q11 deletion
    - Screening imaging for cardiac anomalies

- Transplantation (of mature T cells or thymus) is indicated for complete athymia.
- Bone marrow failure, impaired hematopoiesis
  - Heterogeneous group of diseases with variable presentation
    - Short stature, severe diarrhea, physical anomalies
    - Due to defects in hematopoiesis; syndromes affect more than one blood cell subset
    - High risk for malignant transformation of myeloid lineages
      - Malignant transformation may be associated with granulocyte-colony stimulating factor (G-CSF) treatment in these patients.
  - Immunodeficiencies from bone marrow failure presenting in newborn period:
    - Fanconi aplastic anemia (autosomal recessive or X-linked)—poor growth, severe anemia, thrombocytopenia, neutropenia
    - Shwachman-Diamond syndrome (autosomal recessive)—predominant neutropenia, pancreatic insufficiency

INNATE SYSTEM—NEUTROPHILS

- Primary neutropenias are rare; neutropenias are usually secondary to viral infection or autoimmune disorders (Table 28.4).
- Defined as persistent neutropenia (<1500 neutrophils/mL); can also be cyclic
- Present with infections of skin, mucosa (especially ear–nose–throat, gingivostomatitis, lungs)
- Benign ethnic neutropenia is a mild neutropenia common in individuals of African or Middle Eastern descent; it is the most common chronic form.
- Can occur as a primary neutrophil defect or as minor feature of other hematopoietic deficiencies
- Many neutropenia syndromes respond to high-dose G-CSF.
- Severe, chronic neutropenia is an indication for antimicrobial prophylaxis (e.g., sulfamethoxazole–trimethoprim [Bactrim]) and/or G-CSF.

Table 28.5 Specific T- and B-Cell Deficiencies

Cell Type (All T⁻ or T Low)	Gene Defect (Inheritance)	Cell Activity Impaired	Management
T-CELL DEFICIENCIES (SCID)			
B⁺, NK⁺	IL-7rα, IL-7rγ (X-linked)	T-cell maturation, survival, and differentiation	Isolation; avoid live vaccines; sulfamethoxazole-trimethoprim (Bactrim)
	CD3 complex defects (AR)	T-cell signaling and T-cell regulation	IVIG; immune replacement therapy (transplantation), ideally prior to first infection
	PTPRC (CD45) (AR)	T-cell receptor-signaling regulation	
	CORO1A (variable)	T-cell thymic egress and actin dynamics, calcium release	
B⁺, NK⁻	IL-2RG (X-linked)	IL-2cγr–mediated T and NK survival (shared receptor for IL-2, IL-4, IL-7, IL-9, IL-15 and IL-21), antibody maturation in B cells	
	JAK3 (AR)	IL-2cγr signal transduction (see above)	
B⁻, NK⁻	ADA (AR)	Purine salvage and clearance (purines are toxic to lymphocytes, induce apoptosis)	
	AK2 (reticular dysgenesis; AR)	Regulation of adenosine diphosphate (accumulation causes apoptosis in myeloid and lymphoid precursors)	
B⁻, NK⁺	RAG1 (Omenn) (AR)	V(D)J recombination	
	RAG2 (Omenn) (AR)	V(D)J recombination	
	DCLRE1C (Artemis)	V(D)J recombination, double-stranded DNA repair	
B-CELL DEFICIENCIES			
Transient hypogammaglobulinemia of infancy		Exaggerated physiologic nadir beyond 6 months (excellent prognosis)	None (conservative)
X-linked agammaglobulinemia		BTK deficiency causes failure of B-cell maturation—good prognosis	IVIG
X-linked hyper IgM		Absence of CD40L on T cells causes failure of antibody class switching—poor prognosis	Transplantation, IVIG
IgA deficiency (AD with variable penetrance)		Impaired class switching isolated to IgA isotype—most common PID, good prognosis	Symptomatic, avoid IVIG (host anti-IgA antibodies can react against donor IgA)
Hyper IgE (AD)		STAT3 signaling defect causes dysregulated cytokine production, with secondary preference for IgE class switching	Skin care, Bactrim, immunomodulators (IFN-γ, IVIG)

AD, Autosomal dominant; AR, autosomal recessive; IFN-γ, interferon-γ; IgA, immunoglobulin A; IgE, immunoglobulin E; IL, interleukin; IVIG, intravenous immunoglobulin; PID, primary immunodeficiency; SCID, severe combined immunodeficiency; STAT3, signal transducer and activator of transcription 3.

ADAPTIVE IMMUNE SYSTEM

- T-cell deficiencies (severe combined immunodeficiency [SCID]) (Table 28.5)
  - B- and/or natural killer (NK)-cell subsets can also be affected due to shared mechanisms of cell maturation.
  - Presentation
    - Early detection is possible by newborn screening (NBS) programs and, when present, is considered a pediatric emergency.
      - NBS with low T-cell receptor excision circle (TREC) can be false positive.
      - 50% of false positives for primary immunodeficiency are secondary to prematurity; 50% are due to secondary lymphopenias in full-term infants.
      - NBS with absent TRECs is highly specific for SCID.
    - If not detected by NBS, it can present with nystatin-resistant thrush, recurrent infections, absent lymph nodes or lymphadenopathy, rash, and/or atypical or severe infections.
    - There is a family history of immunodeficiency or early death in a maternal uncle.
  - Laboratory evaluation
    - CBC with differential
    - T-cell proliferative response, lymphocyte subsets (by flow cytometry)
    - Genetic testing
    - Serum immunoglobulins (after 6 months)
      - Antibody affinity maturation and class switching dependent on T-cell activity; B-cell and immunoglobulin levels may be normal but may not be protective without T-cell help.
    - Chest radiography
  - Diagnosed by genetic testing or HIV-negative status plus one of two criteria:
    - Absent or low T cells or low T-cell proliferation with mitogen stimulation testing
    - T cells of maternal origin (lack of fetal adaptive immune response enables maternal cell engraftment)
  - Management
    - Isolation
    - *Pneumocystis* prophylaxis and aggressive, prolonged treatment of infections
    - Intravenous immunoglobulin (IVIG)
    - Avoidance of live vaccines in patient and household contacts

Table 28.6 Functional Leukocyte Immunodeficiencies

Function	Syndrome, Inheritance	Presentation	Diagnosis	Management
Adhesion	Leukocyte adhesion deficiency (types I–III) (AR)	Neutrophilia, delayed cord separation, omphalitis, gingivitis, peritonitis, absence of abscess formation or pus accumulation	Low CD18 and CD11b	Oral hygiene, stem cell transplantation, fucose supplementation (LAD II)
Respiratory burst	Chronic granulomatous disease (X-linked)	Recurrent pneumonia, abscesses, *Aspergillus* infection	Abnormal NBT test	Antimicrobial prophylaxis, BMT
	Myeloperoxidase deficiency (compound heterozygous)	May be asymptomatic, *Candida albicans* infection	Normal NBT, absent MPO staining	Treatment of infections
Antigen presentation	MHC II deficiency (AR)	Hypogammaglobulinemia, CD4 lymphopenia, severe, recurrent infections (SCID phenotype)	Absent MHC II on B cells	Avoid live vaccines, transplantation
	MHC I deficiency (unknown)	Necrotizing granulomatous skin lesions, frequent respiratory infections, bronchiectasis	Absent MHC I on cells	Avoid live vaccines, transplantation

AR, Autosomal recessive; *BMT*, bone marrow transplant; *LAD II*, leukocyte adhesion deficiency type II; *MHC*, major histocompatibility complex; *MPO*, myeloperoxidase; *NBT*, nitroblue tetrazolium; *SCID*, severe combined immunodeficiency.

- ▫ Avoidance of ionizing radiation in T⁻, B⁻, and NK⁺ subtypes (impaired double-stranded DNA [dsDNA] repair)
- ▫ Poor prognosis without bone marrow transplantation or if transplantation occurs after first serious infection
- ■ Humoral deficiencies (B cell and antibody)
  - ▫ Presentation
    - ▫ Severe respiratory tract infections with encapsulated bacteria (e.g., *S. pneumoniae*, *H. influenzae*)
    - ▫ Poor growth, chronic diarrhea, recurrent fevers, chronic enteroviral infections
  - ▫ Laboratory evaluation
    - ▫ Total serum immunoglobulin (after 6 months)
      - ▫ Antibody subclass levels
    - ▫ Antibody titers to vaccine or isohemagglutinins in incompletely vaccinated infants
    - ▫ Genetic testing
    - ▫ CBC with differential, lymphocyte subsets
  - ▫ Management and prognosis depend on specific deficiency.

LEUKOCYTE FUNCTION DEFECTS

- ■ Can affect function shared by more than one cell type
- ■ Presentation and management depend on cell and function affected (Table 28.6).

Suggested Readings

Chinn IK, Shearer WT. Severe combined immunodeficiency disorders. *Immunol Allergy Clin North Am.* 2015;35(4):671–694.

Davies EG. Immunodeficiency in DiGeorge syndrome and options for treating cases with complete athymia. *Front Immunol.* 2013;4:322.

Picard C, Al-Herz W, Bousfiha A, et al. Primary immunodeficiency diseases: an update on the classification from the International Union of Immunological Societies Expert Committee for Primary Immunodeficiency 2015. *J Clin Immunol.* 2015;35(8):696–726.

Skokowa J, Dale DC, Touw IP, Zeidler C, Welte K. *Severe congenital neutropenias. Nat Rev Dis Primers.* 2017;3:17032.

Wilson C, Nizet V, Maldonado Y, Remington J, Klein J, eds. *Remington and Klein's Infectious Diseases of the Fetus and Newborn Infant.* 8th ed. Philadelphia: Saunders; 2016.

29 Infections of Organ Systems

GEOFFREY A. WEINBERG

Sepsis

OVERVIEW OF SEPSIS

- Sepsis is a clinical syndrome characterized by systemic signs of infection, leading to morbidity and mortality.
  - Sepsis may result from bacterial, fungal, or viral pathogens.
  - Systemic inflammatory response syndrome (SIRS) is the physiologic characterization of the sepsis syndrome.
  - SIRS can be caused by sepsis itself or by proinflammatory cytokines resulting from inflammation.
- *Early-onset sepsis* (EOS) traditionally is defined as having its onset at <7 days of life, although some experts use the definition of <3 days (72 hours) of life; most signs and symptoms of EOS develop in the first 3 days of life.
- *Late-onset sepsis* (LOS) is then defined as sepsis occurring from 7 to 90 days of life.
- Sepsis caused by group B streptococci (GBS) with onset >90 days of life has been termed *very late-onset sepsis*; with prolonged long hospital stays of extremely premature infants, some definitions of LOS sepsis include 7 days until discharge from the neonatal intensive care unit (NICU).
- Proven sepsis occurs with positive bacterial, fungal, or viral diagnostic tests from clinically relevant body sites.
- Probable sepsis includes a spectrum of definitions that occur with signs of sepsis or SIRS with either improvement after antibiotics or serially elevated nonspecific markers of inflammation such as serum C-reactive protein (CRP) or procalcitonin assays, or by some clinical risk assessment system.

EPIDEMIOLOGY OF SEPSIS

- EOS remains a major cause of global morbidity and mortality. Estimated EOS incidence is 50 to 150 cases per 1000 live births annually in lower income countries and 0.5 to 5 cases per 1000 live births annually in the United States and Western Europe.
- Gestational age has a major effect on EOS incidence; recent US EOS incidence for all newborns is ~1/1000 live births/year, but it is 10-fold greater among those newborns <30 weeks' gestational age at birth.
- Estimated LOS incidence is difficult to ascertain because LOS may depend on variable definitions, nosocomial outbreaks, and the distribution of birth weights in a particular nursery.
  - GBS LOS rates were lower than those of EOS GBS infection until recently; GBS EOS rates have decreased with peripartum antibiotic prophylaxis, but GBS LOS rates have not, so that now US GBS EOS rates approximate GBS LOS rates.
- The leading causes of bacterial sepsis in US neonates have changed over time, for uncertain reasons.
  - Before the 1950s: *Staphylococcus aureus* and *Streptococcus pyogenes* were the most common.
  - Late 1950s–1960s: Gram-negative enteric bacilli, especially *Escherichia coli*, increased.
  - Late 1960s to the present day: Group B beta-hemolytic streptococci (*Streptococcus agalactiae*) emerged to be the most common.
  - With the advent of GBS peripartum antibiotic prophylaxis in the United States, the incidence of GBS EOS has decreased, but GBS remains an important LOS pathogen. In LOS, *E. coli*, coagulase-negative staphylococci (CONS; most often *S. epidermidis*), and group D enterococci are prominent.
  - Both EOS and LOS may also be caused by *Listeria monocytogenes* in certain areas, particularly in Western Europe, although its incidence seems to have decreased in most of the United States, likely from better agricultural infection control and possibly also from effects of peripartum antibiotic prophylaxis against GBS.

RISK FACTORS AND ROUTES OF TRANSMISSION

- Risk factors for sepsis, especially EOS, can be those that facilitate pathogenesis of EOS or those that facilitate recognition of evolving EOS (e.g., maternal fever, fetal tachycardia, neonatal clinical illness).
- Maternal risk factors include maternal urinary tract infection; chorioamnionitis; colonization or past infection with GBS, *Neisseria gonorrhoeae*, or herpes simplex virus; membrane rupture at >18 hours; preterm delivery; complications in delivery; site of delivery (community, hospital); and consumption of *Listeria*-contaminated food.
- Infant risk factors include immaturity of immunologic mechanisms (e.g., neutrophil function, complement and immunoglobulin levels); congenital malformations (e.g., cardiac, neural tube, gastrointestinal disease); metabolic disease (galactosemia); and indwelling medical devices (e.g., endotracheal tubes, umbilical arterial or venous catheters, central venous catheters, ventricular drainage systems).
- Routes of transmission of infection:
  - EOS generally occurs from ascending bacteria entering the uterus following membrane rupture, from exposure to microbes during passage through the birth canal, from chorioamnionitis, or, less commonly, from transplacental infection.

- LOS more often occurs from environmental sources such as indwelling catheters, endotracheal tubes, hand contamination of hospital personnel and family members, contaminated formula, and equipment. Notably, however, LOS GBS or *Candida* infection may result from colonization at birth or shortly thereafter, yet present only later, for reasons that remain to be determined.
- Causes (see also Chapter 30):
  - Gram-positive bacteria—GBS, *S. aureus*, *L. monocytogenes*, *Enterococcus faecalis*, *S. epidermidis* (and other CONS); rarely, *S. pneumoniae*
  - Gram-negative bacteria—*E. coli*, *Klebsiella* spp., *Enterobacter* spp., *Pseudomonas aeruginosa*; rarely, *N. gonorrhoeae* and nontypeable *Haemophilus influenzae*
  - Fungi—*Candida albicans*, non-*albicans* candidal species
  - Viruses—enterovirus; herpes simplex virus (HSV) types 1 and 2; rarely, human parechovirus, adenovirus
  - In US full-term newborns, GBS remains more commonly recovered from babies with EOS than does *E. coli* (40% vs. 12%, respectively), but in preterm newborns this is reversed (GBS EOS, 12%; *E. coli*, EOS 30–40%).

CLINICAL PRESENTATION

- Signs and symptoms may vary and be nonspecific in neonates with sepsis, particularly EOS.
  - These include fetal tachycardia, foul-smelling amniotic fluid, low Apgar scores, temperature instability (either hyper- or hypothermia), poor feeding, lethargy, irritability, apnea, tachypnea, tachycardia, hypotension, poor peripheral perfusion, emesis, diarrhea, abdominal distention, jaundice, and cyanosis.
  - Symptoms and signs of sepsis may mimic those of other neonatal conditions (e.g., congenital heart disease, respiratory distress syndrome, bowel malformations, intraventricular hemorrhage).
  - EOS tends to be more systemic, whereas focal infections (e.g., cellulitis, meningitis, urinary tract infections [UTIs]) are more common with LOS.
  - The neonate with EOS presents more often with hypothermia than with fever, especially with very premature neonates.

DIAGNOSIS AND EVALUATION (SEE ALSO CHAPTER 30)

- *Empiric diagnostic approaches* are commonly used to diagnose and manage neonates with possible GBS EOS; all are based on the fact that the strongest predictors of GBS EOS are gestational age, intra-amniotic infection, and neonatal clinical illness. Those suggested by the American Academy of Pediatrics (AAP) are reviewed below.
  - Infants >35 weeks gestational age (see Fig. 29.1)
    - *Categorical risk assessment* approach (Fig. 29.1A) uses threshold values to identify infants at risk for GBS disease. Examples of categories reviewed are signs of clinical illness, maternal intrapartum temperature, and whether GBS prophylaxis was given to the mother intrapartum (all pregnant women in the United States are to be screened for GBS

vaginal-rectal colonization at 36 0/7 to 37 6/7 weeks' gestation, and initial intrapartum penicillin or ampicillin prophylaxis is given to those women who are colonized; see Chapter 31). Advantages of this approach include years of clinician experience and familiarity with it; limitations include poor discrimination of categorical risk factors, and higher rates of empiric antibiotics given.
    - *Multivariate risk assessment* (such as with the Kaiser Neonatal EOS calculator) (Fig. 29.1B) uses the individual infant's combination of risk factors and clinical status, along with current US EOS incidence rates, to produce an estimate of risk based on a validated Bayesian mathematical model. Advantages are more individualized estimates of risk, clear definitions, and reduction in empiric antibiotics given; limitations include restrictions of models excluding very preterm infants, need for local incidence data on sepsis.
    - *Clinical condition assessment* (Fig. 29.1C) is based on newborn clinical conditions. Advantages include more individualized estimates of risk and a reduction in empiric antibiotics given. Limitations include the need for repeated structured serial newborn evaluations, high staffing levels to perform these, and the need for development of local metrics for structured exams and care.
  - Infants <35 weeks gestational age
    - Infants born at <35 weeks gestational age are at greater risk for GBS EOS than are term infants. However, the risk varies and is dependent upon several maternal, peripartum, and neonatal factors. Suggested management is shown in Fig. 29.2.
    - Characteristics being studied in models for low risk of EOS caused by organisms other than GBS are similar. They include mode of delivery, rupture of membranes at delivery, and absence of clinical chorioamnionitis, among others.
- *Blood cultures* are the gold standard for the determination of the presence of bacterial or fungal (candidal) sepsis. Blood culture sensitivity is heavily dependent on the volume of blood cultured, which may be limiting in very low birth weight neonates; specificity is heavily dependent on the fidelity of the aseptic technique with which cultures are obtained.
  - *Methods*: Modern automated, continuously monitored blood culture machinery (e.g., BACTEC, BacTAlert systems) is now standard in larger hospitals and allows better and faster organism recovery due to advances in culture media and growth detection. Most relevant pathogens will have growth recognized in 36 to 48 hours, often by 24 hours; identification of antimicrobial susceptibility is often semiautomated by additional laboratory machinery and may take only another 24 to 36 hours. Some institutions use blood culture bottles containing resins to inactivate antimicrobials in the blood and improve recovery; it is uncertain whether any increase in pathogen recovery is outweighed by the extra expense of such techniques.
  - *Volume*: Blood culture pathogen recovery is directly correlated with the volume of blood cultured, with studies in adults showing increased recovery at 40 mL

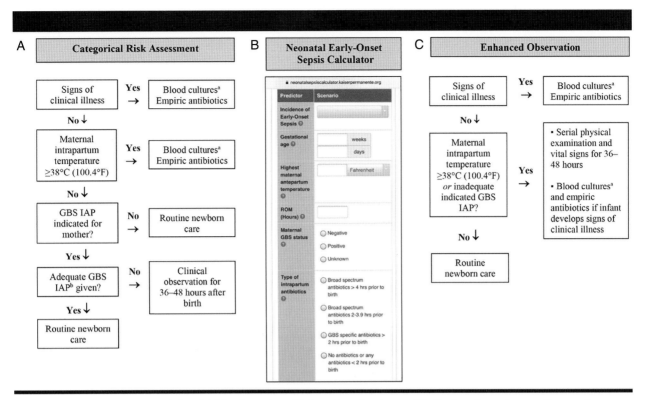

Reproduced from Puopolo KM, Lynfield R, Cummings JJ; American Academy of Pediatrics, Committee on Fetus and Newborn, Committee on Infectious Diseases. Management of infants at risk for group B streptococcal disease. *Pediatrics.* 2019;144(2):e20191881. The screenshot of the Neonatal Early-Onset Sepsis Calculator (**https://neonatalsepsiscalculator.kaiserpermanente.org/**) was used with permission from Kaiser-Permanente Division of Research.

[a]Consider lumbar puncture and CSF culture before initiation of empiric antibiotics for infants who are at the highest risk of infection, especially those with critical illness. Lumbar puncture should not be performed if the infant's clinical condition would be compromised, and antibiotics should be administered promptly and not deferred because of procedure delays.

[b]Adequate GBS IAP is defined as the administration of penicillin G, ampicillin, or cefazolin ≥4 hours before delivery.

Fig. 29.1 Risk assessment for early-onset group B streptococcal disease among infants born at ≥35 weeks of gestation. (Reused with permission from Puopolo KM, Lynfield R, Cummings JJ. American Academy of Pediatrics, Committee on Fetus and Newborn, Committee on Infectious Diseases. Management of Infants at Risk for Group B Streptococcal Disease. *Pediatrics.* 2019;144(2):e20191881.)

of blood taken per culture set versus 10 to 20 mL per set. In young children, infants, and especially premature infants, such volumes clearly are untenable.

- In full-term neonates, 1 to 2 mL of blood should be cultured per bottle, for a total of 2 to 4 mL per two-bottle (aerobic and anaerobic) set.
- In smaller premature infants, 0.5 to 1 mL per bottle should be obtained (total blood 1–2 mL per two-bottle set).
- In extremely premature infants who have very low total blood volumes, the minimum useful blood culture volume of 0.5 mL can be placed entirely in one aerobic bottle only.
- Ideally, two sets of blood cultures from different anatomic sites are obtained; each set consists of an aerobic media bottle and anaerobic media bottle. This technique increases the sensitivity by increasing volume and allows some estimate of contamination to be made (see contamination, below).
- *Contamination*: In general, true bacteremia occurs with recognized pathogens and is present throughout

the body, so that both blood culture sets will be positive. If one set is positive but the other is not, growth in the one set may represent growth of a low inoculation with a skin flora contaminant. Obviously, if only one culture set at a time is obtained, this distinction cannot be made. Selected pathogens (e.g., *S. aureus, Candida*) are unlikely to be contaminants, and growth should not be ignored even if obtained in only one set.

- *Lumbar puncture*: Examination of cerebrospinal fluid (CSF) is the gold standard for the diagnosis of meningitis.
  - Indications—all ill newborns should be considered for lumbar puncture.
    - In LOS, meningitis is commonly associated with bacteremia and sepsis; for example, meningitis is present in 33% of newborns with GBS LOS.
    - In EOS, meningitis is less common in babies with EOS but does occur; meningitis is present in about 10% of GBS EOS.
    - Positive CSF cultures are sometimes found in the absence of detectable bacteremia with both EOS and LOS (~10–20% of cases of GBS meningitis).

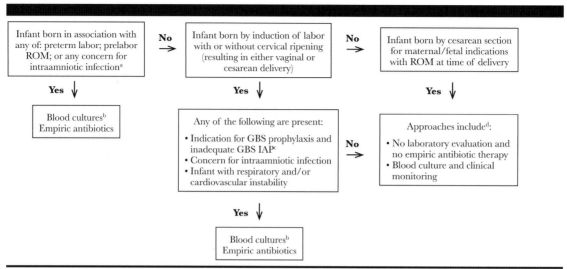

Fig. 29.2 Risk assessment for early-onset group B streptococcal disease among infants born at <35 weeks of gestation. (Reused with permission from Puopolo KM, Lynfield R, Cummings JJ. American Academy of Pediatrics, Committee on Fetus and Newborn, Committee on Infectious Diseases. Management of Infants at Risk for Group B Streptococcal Disease. *Pediatrics.* 2019;144(2):e20191881.)

- Contraindications—lumbar puncture may need to be deferred in critically ill neonates who cannot be safely positioned for the procedure due to cardiorespiratory compromise or in those with severe bleeding diatheses.
- Interpretation—the interpretation of the Gram-stained smear and culture are the same as in older children, but the cell content and protein content of neonatal CSF differ from those of older children and adults. Nevertheless, generalizations may be made from reported data. The ratio of CSF to blood glucose in neonates is similar to that in older infants and children, although the absolute CSF glucose content may appear low because neonates may be hypoglycemic relative to older infants.
  - Mean CSF white blood cell (WBC) counts in healthy neonates of any postmenstrual age are <10 cells/µL (range, 1–44), with <10% polymorphonuclear leukocytes (PMNs) in the differential.
  - Mean CSF protein in healthy neonates—60 to 80 mg/dL full term; 150 mg/dL preterm (range, 54–360)
  - Mean CSF glucose—46 to 51 mg/dL full term; 64 mg/dL preterm (range, 33–217)
- *Urine culture*: In distinction to meningitis, it is very rare for neonates younger than 72 hours of age being evaluated for EOS to have an ascending urinary tract infection; thus, urine cultures are not required at <72 hours of age. Urine should be obtained in neonates with possible sepsis who are 72 hours of age or older by either catheterization or suprapubic aspiration.
- *Laboratory aids to diagnosis*: Many biomarkers have been utilized, including components of the complete blood count (CBC), CRP, procalcitonin, various cytokines, acute-phase reactants, and neutrophil membrane markers; none has high enough sensitivity and specificity to predict neonatal sepsis accurately, although repeatedly high serial levels are concerning. A better use of many

of these markers, especially CRP, is the exclusion of sepsis (allowing antibiotics to be discontinued after empiric therapy has begun) when serial measurements are normal over a 24- to 48-hour duration, because of the high joint negative predictive value of serial testing.
- CBC components—after birth, PMNs and immature WBC forms are released from the bone marrow, producing a relative leukocytosis and left shift; however, it is variable enough that using high or low WBC counts, total neutrophil counts, or total band counts are not sensitive or specific enough for routine diagnostic assistance, except in the following cases:
  - WBC < 5000 cells/µL is somewhat more predictive of sepsis.
  - An immature-to-total neutrophil ratio ([band plus metamyelocyte plus myelocyte count]/[all immature forms + band + absolute neutrophil count]) > 0.2 is somewhat more predictive of sepsis, with ~75% sensitivity and ~75% specificity.
- CRP—a CRP > 10 mg/L has a modest predictive value for sepsis; however, serial levels of CRP < 10 mg/L at 8 and 24 hours of age may exclude sepsis, with a high (>99%) negative predictive value.
- Procalcitonin levels normally rise up to ~10 ng/mL in the first 36 hours of life; in several studies, it was found that procalcitonin > 2 ng/mL after 48 hours of life is more predictive of sepsis (or >10 ng/mL at any time after birth).

THERAPY (SEE ALSO CHAPTER 30)

- Antimicrobial agents
  - Duration of therapy is generally 10 days for uncomplicated bacterial sepsis, 14 to 28 days with concurrent meningitis (pathogen-dependent length of therapy).

- Antibacterials:
  - In EOS, the combination of ampicillin and an aminoglycoside (e.g., gentamicin) remains the cornerstone of EOS empiric therapy for potency against GBS, coliforms, enterococci, and *Listeria*. For definite or highly suspected meningitis (abnormal CSF profile), the combination of ampicillin and a third-generation cephalosporin (e.g., cefotaxime or, sometimes, the fourth-generation agent cefepime or a carbapenem) is preferred. Definitive therapy may be tailored after pathogen identification.
  - In LOS, the combination of vancomycin and an aminoglycoside (gentamicin) is preferred, rather than ampicillin and gentamicin, to broaden activity against *S. aureus* and coagulase-negative staphylococci while maintaining potency against GBS and gram-negative rods. If meningitis is suspected, vancomycin plus a third-generation cephalosporin (or carbapenem) is preferred. Tailoring of definitive therapy may be done after pathogen identification.
- Antifungals (duration often 21 days for *Candida* sepsis):
  - Amphotericin B deoxycholate is preferred for empiric therapy of high-risk infants with severe illness and possible fungal sepsis.
  - Fluconazole is a less toxic alternative in less ill neonates but will not be potent against several non-*albicans* candidal yeasts. Fluconazole does have good central nervous system (CNS) and urinary tract penetrance, however, and may be used for susceptible yeasts.
  - Echinocandins (e.g., micafungin) have good antifungal activity against yeasts but do not penetrate the CNS or urinary tract well.
- Antivirals:
  - HSV infection requires therapy with high-dose systemic acyclovir for 14 to 21 days at minimum, depending on the extent of disease.
  - Enteroviral sepsis of the newborn is treated with supportive therapy, but there are no current anti-enteroviral agents available. Anecdotal data have suggested that infusion of intravenous immunoglobulin might be effective.
  - There are no current antiviral agents active against parechoviruses or Zika virus.

Central Nervous System Infections

OVERVIEW

- CNS infections are more often associated with LOS (>7 days of age) than with EOS.
- Causes
  - GBS—serotypes of late-onset GBS meningitis often differ from those causing GBS EOS.
  - *E. coli*, other coliforms
  - *L. monocytogenes*
  - Rarely, *C. albicans*, *S. aureus*
  - Enterovirus, parechovirus, and HSV all may cause systemic sepsis with aseptic meningitis in the neonate

CLINICAL PRESENTATION

- Symptoms and signs may be subtle or masked by comorbid conditions (e.g., heart or lung disease, abdominal disease).
- They may overlap those of sepsis (see earlier); unlike the case in older infants, nuchal rigidity or meningeal signs are rarely seen in neonates.
- A bulging anterior fontanel may be present.
- Development of a brain abscess should be anticipated with selected unusual gram-negative pathogens (e.g., *Citrobacter* spp., *Cronobacter* [formerly *Enterobacter*] *sakazakii*).

DIAGNOSIS AND EVALUATION

- Blood and CSF cultures as for sepsis (see above); lumbar puncture should be performed if at all possible in all critically ill neonates suspected of sepsis and/or meningitis.

THERAPY

- Empiric (<7 days of age)
  - Ampicillin and a third- or fourth-generation cephalosporin (e.g., cefotaxime or cefepime) or ampicillin and a carbapenem (e.g., meropenem)
  - The highly protein-bound, third-generation cephalosporin ceftriaxone is generally avoided in neonates < 30 days of age because of possible displacement of bilirubin from albumin, risking kernicterus, and because of possible interactions with intravenous calcium supplementation often required by neonates.
- Empiric (>7 days of age)
  - Vancomycin and a third- or fourth-generation cephalosporin (e.g., cefotaxime, cefepime) or ampicillin and a carbapenem (e.g., meropenem)
- Definitive therapy (any age)
  - GBS: ampicillin, 14- to 21-day course. Some experts recommend that a second lumbar puncture be performed ~24 to 28 hours after therapy initiation to assist in management and prognosis.
  - *E. coli*, other gram-negative rods: as per susceptibility testing; cefotaxime, cefepime, or meropenem, 21- to 28-day course. Neonates with gram-negative meningitis should undergo repeat lumbar puncture to ensure CSF sterility after ~24 to 48 hours of therapy. If repeat CSF cultures remain positive, the choice and doses of antibacterial agents should be reevaluated, and another lumber puncture performed after another 24 to 48 hours of therapy.
  - *L. monocytogenes*: ampicillin, 14- to 21-day course
  - HSV: acyclovir, 21 days minimum for CNS infection; repeat lumbar puncture performed at end of therapy to ensure that HSV is no longer detectable by polymerase chain reaction (PCR) assay (if positive, additional therapy recommended)
  - Enterovirus, parechovirus: supportive management
- Additional evaluations after antibiotics—all neonates surviving meningitis need to have hearing evaluations and close attention paid in follow-up for attainment of developmental milestones.

- Rates of all neurodevelopmental sequelae (including deafness, blindness, hydrocephalus, functional abnormalities, developmental delays) after gram-negative meningitis are 15% to 30% for mild to moderate sequelae and 5% to 10% for major sequelae; those after GBS meningitis are 25% mild to moderate and 25% major.

Cutaneous and Soft Tissue Infections

OVERVIEW

- Neonatal rashes and skin abnormalities may reflect:
  - Cutaneous infections (e.g., impetigo, bullous impetigo)
  - Soft-tissue infections (e.g., boils, abscesses)
  - Toxin-induced infectious disease (e.g., *S. aureus* scalded skin syndrome)
  - Cutaneous manifestations of systemic infection (e.g., listeriosis, syphilis, neonatal invasive *Candida* infection, neonatal HSV infection)

CLINICAL PRESENTATION

- Impetigo, boils, cutaneous or soft tissue abscesses present similarly to those in older infants and children, generally after 5 to 10 days of life, often in diaper area or skinfolds; bullae not as closely grouped as HSV vesicles.
- *S. aureus* scalded skin syndrome includes tender scarlatiniform erythema of skin, with superficial (stratum granulosum layer of epidermis) desquamation of sheets of skin on gentle pressure or traction in affected and other areas (Nikolsky sign); rarely bacteremic, but dehydration and superinfection may result.
- *Listeria* infection: In severe early-onset listeriosis, granulomatosis infantisepticum is uncommonly seen, with small pale papules scattered across the skin. Biopsy and histology show granulomata.
- Congenital syphilis may present with dry peeling skin (similar to what is seen with post-dates babies), moist nasal and mucous membrane lesions, or moist lesions on hands and feet (moist lesions can be very infectious); chancres are not seen in neonates.
- Neonatal candidiasis: Rash may appear as simple oral or genital thrush or as part of a more invasive form of dermal candidiasis, with angry red plaque-like lesions over buttocks.
- HSV: Typical grouped or single dewdrop vesicles on an erythematous base may be seen in skin, eye, or mouth form of neonatal HSV disease and in disseminated or CNS disease, especially at sites of iatrogenic breaks in the skin (e.g., scalp electrode monitor, circumcision).

DIAGNOSIS AND EVALUATION

- Impetigo, boils, abscesses: bacterial cultures of infected area
- Syphilis: nontreponemal and treponemal serologic assays (e.g., rapid plasma reagin [RPR] assay, enzyme immunoassay, *Treponema pallidum* particle agglutination [TPPA])
- *Listeria*: blood cultures.
- HSV: viral PCR assay of scrapings from lesion (or culture if PCR assay not available)

THERAPY

- Impetigo, boils, abscesses
  - For minor impetiginized skin, therapy for group A beta-hemolytic streptococci (*S. pyogenes*) and *S. aureus* with a first-generation cephalosporin (cephalexin, cefazolin) or amoxicillin-clavulanic acid may suffice
  - For more extensive bullous or invasive lesions or in more ill neonates, methicillin-resistant *S. aureus* (MRSA) also must be a consideration; thus, clindamycin or vancomycin is indicated.
- *S. aureus* scalded skin syndrome: clindamycin or vancomycin (or cefazolin if MRSA excluded)
- *Listeria*: ampicillin, initially with gentamicin added
- *Candida*: for thrush, topical nystatin or an azole cream or ointment; for invasive candidiasis, fluconazole, micafungin, or amphotericin B deoxycholate
- HSV: acyclovir

Gastrointestinal Infections

OVERVIEW

- Diarrheal illness (acute gastroenteritis) is a major source of morbidity and mortality in older infants in lesser income countries but generally not in the NICU.
- Globally, the most commonly identified causes of severe acute gastroenteritis are rotavirus, norovirus, *Shigella*, enterotoxigenic and enteroaggregative *E. coli*, and *Cryptosporidium*, but many other viruses and bacteria can cause acute gastroenteritis.
- Colitis or gastroenteritis in the neonate in a US (or other high-income country) NICU is more likely to be related to necrotizing enterocolitis (NEC), which may be caused by a combination of bacterial or viral infections, gut ischemia, and other unknown factors.
- In a neonate < 1000 g birth weight and younger than 10 days of age, spontaneous intestinal perforation may occur in the absence of NEC; often, coagulase-negative staphylococci and *Candida* are recovered from abdominal fluid cultures, but their role in causing the perforation is uncertain.

CLINICAL PRESENTATION

- Both NEC and spontaneous intestinal peroration may present with poor feeding, abdominal distention, abdominal discoloration, emesis, diarrhea, and/or sepsis.

DIAGNOSIS AND EVALUATION

- Abdominal radiographs may show distended loops of bowel, pneumatosis of the bowel, portal venous air, or free air in the peritoneum.

THERAPY

- For so-called medical NEC (i.e., signs of NEC without evidence of perforation), an antibiotic with potency against bowel aerobic gram-positive and gram-negative bacteria and anaerobic bacteria is used, such as piperacillin–tazobactam (a single drug alternative to the combination of ampicillin + clindamycin + gentamicin) or sometimes meropenem.
- If perforation or severe sepsis is present, exploratory surgery with bowel resection and possible creation of an ostomy is performed, along with antibacterial therapy.

Genitourinary Infections

BASIC INFORMATION

- An ascending UTI or pyelonephritis (as opposed to simply recovering the same organism in urine from a neonate with bacteremic sepsis) is rare in the first 3 to 7 days of life.
- Fungal UTI with *Candida* may occur in very premature infants, with development of fungal balls leading to obstructive uropathy.

CLINICAL PRESENTATION

- Generally similar to presentation of sepsis; uncommonly, foul-smelling urine is identified.

DIAGNOSIS AND EVALUATION

- Urinalysis, with urine culture obtained by catheterization or suprapubic aspiration
- If *Candida* UTI is present, renal and bladder ultrasonography

THERAPY

- Therapy is organism dependent. For fungal UTI, fluconazole has the best urinary penetration of available systemic antifungals; a prolonged course of therapy may be required but rarely is urologic surgery needed to relieve obstruction.

Ocular Infections

OVERVIEW

- Ophthalmia neonatorum is purulent conjunctivitis occurring within the first month of life. It is often thought of as conjunctivitis being caused by either *N. gonorrhoeae* or *Chlamydia trachomatis.*
- However, early neonatal conjunctivitis may also be caused by skin, vaginal, and gastrointestinal pathogens, such as *S. aureus, S. pneumoniae, H. influenzae, Moraxella catarrhalis, S. pyogenes,* GBS, *E. coli, Klebsiella* spp., and *P. aeruginosa.*

- Chemical conjunctivitis may occur in the first day or two of life if silver nitrate is used for the prevention of ophthalmia neonatorum (Credé prophylaxis); in the United States, the vast majority of birth centers now use erythromycin ointment instead of silver nitrate.

CLINICAL PRESENTATION

- Gonococcal ophthalmia has an incubation period of 2 to 7 days and generally results in severe conjunctivitis, with purulent discharge.
- Chlamydial ophthalmia has an incubation period of 5 to 14 days and is less severe, with minimal watery discharge or crusting.
- Conjunctivitis caused by other microbes is of variable severity, often in the neonate older than 5 to 7 days of age.
  - Neonatal HSV may cause conjunctivitis as well, particularly in the skin, eye, and mouth form of HSV, generally at 6 to 14 days of life.
  - *P. aeruginosa* may cause conjunctivitis in older neonates with chronic sedation and mechanical ventilation.

DIAGNOSIS AND EVALUATION

- Maternal culture for gonococci, *Chlamydia*
- Cultures of conjunctival exudate (or PCR if HSV is suspected)

THERAPY

- Gonococcal ophthalmia or asymptomatic baby with exposure to maternal gonorrhea: ceftriaxone, one dose intramuscularly (IM); if disseminated gonococcal infection is suspected in the neonate, cefotaxime 7 days intravenously (IV); may need to irrigate eyes with saline.
- Chlamydial ophthalmia: oral azithromycin or erythromycin
- Conjunctivitis due to other infectious agents: topical antimicrobials, possibly with additional systemic antibiotics
- HSV: parenteral acyclovir, sometimes with additional ocular topical antivirals

Omphalitis

OVERVIEW

- Infection of the umbilical structures, with or without cellulitis of the abdominal wall
- Common causative organisms: *S. aureus, S. pyogenes,* GBS, *E. coli* and other gram-negative coliforms, *P. aeruginosa*
  - Rarely, causative anaerobes include *Clostridium perfringens* and *Clostridium tetani,* especially in low-income countries where contaminated instruments or traditional medicines (some of which are contaminated with soil or dung) are applied to the umbilical stump
  - Rarely, syphilis may cause funisitis alone.

CLINICAL PRESENTATION

- May progress through four stages:
  - Stage 1 (least serious)—funisitis (wet, possibly purulent inflammation of the umbilical cord only)
  - Stage 2—cellulitis of the insertion of the umbilical cord
  - Stage 3—abdominal wall cellulitis
  - Stage 4—necrotizing fasciitis of the abdominal wall
  - Neonatal tetanus may have few local signs at the umbilicus despite systemic paralytic toxemia.

DIAGNOSIS AND EVALUATION

- Cultures of the umbilical cord and affected areas should be done.
- Consider serologic testing for syphilis antibodies if isolated funisitis.

THERAPY

- Empiric therapy
  - For mild to moderate umbilical cellulitis, an agent with gram-positive and gram-negative potency, such as cefazolin; clindamycin if MRSA is suspected or common in the NICU, with gentamicin for gram-negative coverage
  - For more severe cellulitis, a broad-spectrum antibiotic combination such as piperacillin–tazobactam plus vancomycin for MRSA or a carbapenem + vancomycin
  - For syphilis: parenteral penicillin

Otitis Media

OVERVIEW

- Neonatal otitis media is uncommon; it is caused by sinopulmonary pathogens as in older infants (e.g., *S. pneumoniae*, *H. influenzae*) but also gram-negative bacteria (e.g., *E. coli*).

CLINICAL PRESENTATION

- May have nonspecific symptoms requiring otoscopy for diagnosis

DIAGNOSIS AND EVALUATION

- Otoscopy; tympanocentesis for culture of middle ear fluid traditionally recommended for otitis media occurring in the first 6 weeks of life

THERAPY

- Organism dependent; empiric therapy in hospitalized neonates could include a third- or fourth-generation cephalosporin.

Osteoarticular Infections

OVERVIEW

- Generally occur in late-onset time frame

- GBS, *S. aureus*, and *Candida* each can cause primary bone or joint infections or can be associated with bone or joint relapse after previous bacteremia or fungemia.
- Syphilis osteitis may present as early-onset or later-onset failure to move a limb (pseudoparalysis of Parrot).

CLINICAL PRESENTATION

- Septic arthritis: warmth, redness, swelling, tenderness, and limitation of range of motion of joint; often fever
- Osteomyelitis: possible warmth, redness over infected site on bone; fever; point tenderness, failure to move the extremity if a long bone
- Pseudoparalysis of Parrot: may or may not have swelling over the affected bone or fever; can mimic Erb's palsy

DIAGNOSIS AND EVALUATION

- Inflammatory markers include CRP, erythrocyte sedimentation rate (ESR), CBC, and differential.
- Radiography: Plain radiography is insensitive during first 2 to 4 weeks of infection but is useful to exclude fractures or periostitis from congenital syphilis. MRI is the most sensitive modality, next most is technetium-99 bone scintigraphy.
- Arthrocentesis or bone biopsy with Gram staining and culture of material obtained
- Blood cultures

THERAPY

- Empiric therapy
  - Targeted against GBS and *S. aureus*: first-generation cephalosporin (cefazolin) or antistaphylococcal penicillin (oxacillin or nafcillin); third- or fourth-generation cephalosporin such as cefotaxime or cefepime also may be considered, especially if prior sepsis with gram-negative bacteria
  - Empiric fluconazole, micafungin, caspofungin, or amphotericin B deoxycholate or lipid amphotericin B products if prior fungemia is documented
- Definitive therapy is organism dependent.
- Adjunctive surgical therapy may be necessary for both diagnosis and therapy, especially in septic arthritis or periosteal abscess.

Pneumonia

OVERVIEW

- Difficult to distinguish from neonatal sepsis, acute respiratory distress syndrome, aspiration, or bronchopulmonary dysplasia.
- Causative organisms and presentation are similar to neonatal sepsis (EOS or LOS).
- Occasionally, late-onset pneumonia may be caused by less common organisms acquired during birth (e.g., *C. trachomatis*) or from visitors or caretakers in the NICU (e.g., as respiratory syncytial virus, influenza virus, *Bordetella pertussis*).

CLINICAL PRESENTATION

- Respiratory distress, including apnea, tachypnea, cyanosis, grunting, retractions, rales, and desaturation (some or all of these)

DIAGNOSIS AND EVALUATION

- Blood cultures
- Endotracheal tube aspirate for Gram stain and cultures is difficult to interpret, because endotracheal colonization with many types of potentially pathogenic bacteria is both common and nonspecific (not necessarily indicative of deeper respiratory tract infection).
- Chest radiograph

THERAPY

- Empiric: as for sepsis (either EOS or LOS, depending on the age of the neonate)
- Definitive is organism dependent.

Suggested Readings

Flannery DD, Puopolo KM. Neonatal early-onset sepsis. *NeoReviews.* 2022;23:756–770.

Flannery DD, Edwards EM, Coggins SA, Horbar JD, Puopolo KM. Late-onset sepsis among very preterm infants. *Pediatrics.* 2022;150:e2022058813.

Nizet V, Klein JO. Bacterial sepsis and meningitis. In: Wilson CB, Nizet V, Maldonado Y, Remington JS, Klein JO, eds. *Remington and Klein's Infectious Diseases of the Fetus and Newborn Infant.* 8th ed. Philadelphia: Saunders; 2016:1132–1146.

Pappas PG, Kauffman CA, Andes DR, et al. Clinical Practice Guideline for the Management of Candidiasis: 2016 update by the Infectious Diseases Society of America. *Clin Infect Dis.* 2016;62:e1–e50.

Puopolo KM, Benitz WE, Zaoutis TE. AAP Committee on Fetus and Newborn; Committee on Infectious Diseases. Management of neonates born at ≥35 0/7 weeks' gestation with suspected or proven early-onset bacterial sepsis. *Pediatrics.* 2018;142:e20182894.

Puopolo KM, Benitz WE, Zaoutis TE. AAP Committee on Fetus and Newborn; Committee on Infectious Diseases. Management of neonates born at ≤34 6/7 weeks' gestation with suspected or proven early-onset bacterial sepsis. *Pediatrics.* 2018;142:e20182896.

Puopolo KM, Lynfield R, Cummings JJ. AAP Committee on Fetus and Newborn; Committee on Infectious Diseases. Management of infants at risk for group B streptococcal disease. *Pediatrics.* 2019;144:e20191881.

Shane AL, Sánchez PJ, Stoll BJ. Neonatal sepsis. *Lancet.* 2017;390:1770–1780.

30 Causative Agents of Infections

GEOFFREY A. WEINBERG

BACTERIA

Group B Streptococci (GBS; *Streptococcus agalactiae*)

OVERVIEW

- GBS is a major cause of perinatal infections in mothers and neonates, including early-onset sepsis (EOS) and late-onset sepsis (LOS).
- Gram-positive aerobic cocci in pairs or short chains
- GBS commonly colonize gastrointestinal and genitourinary tracts, rarely the pharynx; colonization during pregnancy can be constant or intermittent, ranging from 15% to 35% of pregnant women.
- GBS are transmitted from the mother to the neonate shortly before birth, during delivery, or after delivery; if after delivery, GBS are uncommonly transmitted from others (e.g., family members, caregivers, health care professionals).
- Routine screening for GBS during pregnancy and chemoprophylaxis of colonized pregnant women at labor and delivery have significantly reduced the incidence of GBS EOS infection; for unknown reasons, the incidence of GBS LOS is unaffected by chemoprophylaxis (see Chapter 31).

CLINICAL PRESENTATION

See also Chapter 29.

- Maternal infections: urinary tract infections, bacteremia, endometritis, chorioamnionitis
- Neonatal infections caused by GBS: EOS (<7 days of age), LOS (7–90 days of life), focal infections
  - EOS: respiratory distress, apnea, hypotension, pneumonia, and sometimes neutropenia; meningitis in ~5% to 10%. It typically presents in first 24 hours of life (range, 0–6 days).
  - LOS: bacteremia, hypotension, meningitis (~30%); presents around 3 to 4 weeks of age (range, 7–89 days; interquartile range, 20–49 days)
  - Focal infections: cellulitis, pneumonia, lymphadenitis, bone or joint infections
- Late late-onset or very late-onset GBS infection presents beyond 90 days of life, often as focal infection.
- GBS meningitis has high morbidity: ~45% overall morbidity, with 25% mild to moderate sequelae and 25% major sequelae (e.g., blindness, bilateral sensorineural hearing loss, cerebral palsy, profound developmental delay).

- Recurrence of GBS infection may be seen in 1% to 3% of infants despite appropriate treatment of first episode, from 3 to 60 days after completion of therapy.

DIAGNOSIS

- Gram stain and by recovery of organisms in culture of blood, cerebrospinal fluid, urine, or infected tissue

THERAPY

For prevention, see Chapter 31.

- GBS infection is best treated by beta lactams (ampicillin or penicillin G); some synergy is thought to be afforded by aminoglycosides (e.g., gentamicin), and gentamicin is often continued for the first 3 days of therapy.
  - Presumptive treatment of GBS EOS includes intravenous (IV) ampicillin + gentamicin.
  - Presumptive treatment of GBS LOS includes IV ampicillin + gentamicin or ampicillin + cefotaxime; vancomycin + gentamicin for LOS of unknown etiology (see Chapter 29).
- Definitive therapy when GBS identified: IV ampicillin or penicillin G
  - For GBS meningitis, high-dose ampicillin or penicillin G (plus an initial 3 days of aminoglycoside) administered for 14–21 days; if significant ventriculitis or delayed sterilization of the cerebrospinal fluid (CSF) occurs, some experts would treat for 28 days.
  - For GBS bacteremia or cellulitis without meningitis, 10 days of ampicillin or penicillin G may suffice.
  - Treatment of septic arthritis or osteomyelitis may require 3 to 4 weeks.

Staphylococcus aureus

OVERVIEW

- *Staphylococcus aureus* causes a number of localized and invasive suppurative infections, as well as three toxin-mediated syndromes: scalded skin syndrome and, in older children, toxic shock syndrome and food poisoning.
- Gram-positive cocci in pairs or grapelike clusters; coagulase-positive, in contrast to coagulase-negative staphylococci such as *Staphylococcus epidermidis*
- Ubiquitous human flora that colonizes skin and mucous membranes of 30% to 50% of healthy children and adults (especially anterior nares, throat, axilla, perineum, rectum)

- Second to coagulase-negative staphylococci as cause of health care–associated infection
- Transmitted by direct contact
- Unique clones of *S. aureus* have acquired beta-lactam resistance genes, rendering them resistant to antistaphylococcal penicillins such as methicillin, oxacillin, and nafcillin, as well as most cephalosporins; they are referred to as methicillin-resistant *S. aureus* (MRSA) as opposed to methicillin-susceptible *S. aureus* (MSSA)

CLINICAL PRESENTATION

- Localized infections include cellulitis, skin and soft tissue abscesses, pustulosis, impetigo (bullous and nonbullous), mastitis, furuncles, carbuncles, omphalitis, and wound infections.
- Staphylococcal scalded skin syndrome (SSSS) is a toxin-mediated infection in neonates and young children who likely have less immunity to the toxins that cause cleavage of the skin at the superficial stratum granulosum layer of the epidermis.
  - Presents with red, painful skin, which peels in sheets on gentle pressure or traction (Nikolsky sign)
  - Intravenous antibiotics (or if child not ill, sometimes oral antibiotics) are used to clear the causative organisms of SSSS, which are nearly always susceptible to methicillin (MSSA).
- Invasive infections include bacteremia (especially associated with foreign bodies such as intravascular catheters or cerebrospinal fluid shunts), septicemia, osteomyelitis or septic arthritis, endocarditis, pneumonia with or without pleural empyema, and visceral abscesses; septic thrombophlebitis of intravenous catheter sites may also be seen. These infections require parenteral therapy.

DIAGNOSIS

- Gram stain and recovery of organisms in culture of blood, infected tissue, or infected sites

THERAPY

- For localized infections, an antistaphylococcal penicillin such as oxacillin, nafcillin, or methicillin is used; a first-generation cephalosporin such as cefazolin, or clindamycin is given intravenously for neonates with MSSA infections. If the isolate is already known to be MRSA (or the child is known to be previously colonized or infected with MRSA), vancomycin is used instead. Oral antibiotics may be appropriate for localized superficial infections such as impetigo.
- For more serious skin and soft tissue wound infections or any invasive infections, IV therapy is used for both MSSA and MRSA.
  - Empiric therapy uses agents active against both MSSA and MRSA, such as IV vancomycin.
  - Definitive therapy is tailored according to antimicrobial susceptibility test results; for most MSSA infections, oxacillin, nafcillin or cefazolin are more potent than vancomycin.

Coagulase-Negative Staphylococci

OVERVIEW

- Coagulase-negative staphylococci (CONS), the most common cause of health care–associated infections, most commonly appear as bacteremia associated with intravascular catheters.
- Gram-positive cocci in pairs or grapelike clusters; upon laboratory testing, coagulase-negative, in contrast to *S. aureus*
- Ubiquitous human and environmental flora that commonly colonizes skin and mucous membranes
- Many species of CONS exist; not all hospital laboratories independently speciate them, but *S. epidermidis, S. haemolyticus, S. schleiferi, S. lugdunensis,* and *S. saprophyticus* are most often associated with infection in humans.
- CONS can generate a biofilm that allows them to adhere to both native and prosthetic surfaces and leads to difficulty in clearing infection, despite their relatively low virulence.
- CONS may be transmitted by direct contact, but most infection is likely from one's own flora.
- Most strains of CONS are resistant to antistaphylococcal penicillins and cephalosporins and often other antibiotics such as clindamycin, but they remain susceptible to vancomycin.

CLINICAL PRESENTATION

- Most common is late-onset bacteremia or sepsis in extremely low-birth-weight and very low-birth-weight infants
- Also common in neonates with intravascular catheters or indwelling foreign bodies (e.g., cardiac grafts, shunts, or valves; ventriculoperitoneal shunts)
- Recovery of CONS from blood cultures can indicate infection but may also reflect contamination of a blood culture with skin flora; this can make it difficult to interpret culture results. Repeated recovery of CONS from multiple cultures correlates with true infection, as does rapid time to positivity of growth in automated blood culture systems.

DIAGNOSIS

- Gram stain and recovery of organisms in culture of blood, infected tissue, or infected sites

THERAPY

- For CONS isolates thought to be causing true infection, the therapy of choice is vancomycin, unless the isolate is demonstrated to be susceptible to cefazolin or nafcillin (or methicillin or oxacillin) upon testing.

Listeria monocytogenes

OVERVIEW

- *Listeria monocytogenes* is an uncommon cause of infection in pregnant women and neonates

- Gram-positive, nonsporulating rod can be variable in shape (and misidentified as "diphtheroids," especially with older microbiology instrumentation); this intracellular pathogen can also grow extracellularly at colder temperatures.
- It is predominantly a foodborne-transmitted illness in adults; neonates acquire it vertically.
  - Common food sources contaminated with *L. monocytogenes* include deli-style ready-to-eat meats, poultry, unpasteurized milk, and soft cheeses.
  - In the past 20 years, the incidence of listeriosis in the United States has decreased, largely due to more rigorous agricultural screening and food-processing regulations.

CLINICAL PRESENTATION

- Pregnancy-associated infections may cause spontaneous abortion, fetal death, chorioamnionitis, and preterm delivery.
- Rarely, a serious congenital infection characterized by an erythematous, small papular rash (granulomatous papules under histologic examination), referred to as *granulomatosis infantisepticum*, is seen.

DIAGNOSIS

- Recovery of organisms in culture of blood or CSF
- Gram stains of CSF in neonates with *Listeria meningitis* frequently may be negative, in contrast to the usual positive CSF Gram stain examination in neonatal meningitis; *Listeria* organisms are intracellular and tend to adhere to the meninges.

THERAPY

- IV ampicillin plus an aminoglycoside (e.g., gentamicin), until clinical improvement is noted; many experts would continue combination therapy for the entire treatment course.
- Cephalosporins (including advanced generation cephalosporins) are not active against *L. monocytogenes*.
- For bacteremia, a 14-day treatment course is used; for meningitis, 21 days or longer (e.g., if brain abscess is present).

Escherichia coli and Other Gram-Negative Bacilli

OVERVIEW

- *Escherichia coli, Klebsiella* spp., *Enterobacter* spp., *Proteus* spp., *Pseudomonas aeruginosa, Serratia* spp., *Citrobacter* spp., and *Acinetobacter* spp. can all cause neonatal bacteremia, sepsis, and (particularly for *E. coli*) meningitis.
- Some gram-negative rods may have the ability to ferment lactose (e.g., *E. coli*); others do not (e.g., *Pseudomonas*).
- Neonatal infections caused by *E. coli*, especially meningitis, are often members of clones of K1 capsular serotypes, which are distinctly different from uropathogenic or diarrheagenic *E. coli*.

CLINICAL PRESENTATION

- Early signs of sepsis and/or meningitis can be subtle and similar to signs observed in GBS EOS or GBS LOS.
- Gram-negative sepsis may also be associated with necrotizing enterocolitis, with or without intestinal perforation.

DIAGNOSIS

- Gram-stain and recovery of organisms in cultures of blood or CSF
- Antimicrobial susceptibility testing is important, as many gram-negative bacteria have acquired multidrug resistance elements (e.g., extended spectrum beta-lactamases and carbapenemases).

THERAPY

- Ampicillin plus an aminoglycoside (e.g., gentamicin) is the traditional empiric therapy for sepsis possibly caused by gram-negative bacteria.
- For gram-negative rod meningitis, many authorities now favor combination therapy with ampicillin plus an advanced generation cephalosporin, such as cefotaxime or cefepime (or ampicillin plus a carbapenem) over ampicillin plus gentamicin, to take advantage of both the improved pharmacokinetics and pharmacodynamics of cephalosporins in the CSF, as well as their antimicrobial resistance spectrum.
- Suspected *Pseudomonas, Acinetobacter,* and other non–lactose-fermenting gram-negative bacteria require empiric therapy with an antipseudomonal penicillin such as piperacillin–tazobactam or a carbapenem such as meropenem; antimicrobial susceptibility testing should guide definitive therapy.

Syphilis (*Treponema pallidum*)

OVERVIEW

- Intrauterine infection with *Treponema pallidum* may cause congenital syphilis, which can cause stillbirth, hydrops fetalis, or premature birth, resulting in symptomatic or asymptomatic infants.
- Untreated congenital syphilis causes significant, crippling morbidity throughout childhood and adulthood; however, adequate treatment of early infant infection will prevent this.
- Thin, motile spirochetes are unable to be cultured in clinical laboratories and are difficult to identify under a microscope without darkfield optics. Thus, the diagnosis is made by serologic testing.
- Intrauterine transmission may occur throughout pregnancy but increases with the gestational age and is most common between 16 and 28 weeks' gestation. Early transmission during pregnancy causes fetal death in utero, stillbirth, or premature infants with symptoms of congenital syphilis. Transmission during the third trimester very often results in an infected but asymptomatic or only mildly symptomatic infant.

- The stage of maternal syphilis infection also affects transmission risk; mothers with early primary or secondary syphilis are more likely to transmit the infection than those with late latent or tertiary infection.

CLINICAL PRESENTATION

- Syphilis is asymptomatic in 50% to 60% of infected infants at birth, but illness may appear in the ensuing first few weeks of life.
- Symptoms of congenital syphilis include radiographic bone changes (osteochondritis and periostitis); hepatomegaly with or without splenomegaly; a desquamative generalized rash, sometimes with blistering or moist skin over the palms and soles and also the mucocutaneous junctions; jaundice; lymphadenopathy; disuse of a limb mimicking Erb's palsy (pseudoparalysis of Parrot); or persistent rhinitis ("snuffles").

DIAGNOSIS

- All pregnant women should be screened serologically for syphilis early in pregnancy and again near delivery, preferably at 28 to 32 weeks' gestation to allow early diagnosis and therapy.
- Two serologic assay types, as well as two testing algorithms, are commonly used (see Fig. 30.1):
  - Antibody assays
    - Nontreponemal antibodies detect nonspecific immunoglobulin G (IgG) antibody to cardiolipin; these include the rapid plasma reagin (RPR) assay, which has mostly replaced the older Venereal Disease Research Laboratory (VDRL) test, and others. These antibodies are positive in primary, secondary, and latent syphilis and decrease over time; importantly, they should revert to negative with successful treatment of syphilis. The RPR test results are reported as titers; for example, 1:8 means an eightfold dilution of serum was positive in the assay. This is a greater number than 1:2 (which implies antibodies detected only up to twofold dilution of serum; the titers are not arithmetic fractions). Some labs report the reciprocal titer (i.e., 1:8 is reported simply as 8).
    - Treponemal antibodies are often combined IgG and IgM antibodies tested by automated chemiluminescent or enzyme immunoassay (CIA or EIA) or by *T. pallidum* particle agglutination (TPPA) or fluorescent treponemal antibody absorption (FTA-ABS) assays. These antibody tests may become positive earlier in infection than the RPR, and, once reactive, are reactive for life, even after successful treatment of syphilis.
    - Both nontreponemal and treponemal antibodies are passed through the placenta and are found in neonatal serum, confounding detection of neonatal antibodies (i.e., both exposure of the neonate but no infection, as well as true infection, result in positive antibodies in neonatal blood).
  - Testing algorithms
    - In the traditional algorithm, nontreponemal tests (RPR) are performed first, and positive results are confirmed with more specific treponemal tests. If both assays are positive, syphilis is diagnosed. This algorithm is more familiar to clinicians but is less sensitive and may miss early syphilis in pregnant women.
    - In the newer "reverse algorithm" performed by many laboratories, the sensitive screening treponemal enzymatic antibody test is used; if positive, results are confirmed by a second treponemal test (such as the TPPA). An RPR is then performed. This algorithm has increased sensitivity but may be positive even after syphilis has been adequately treated, so it may be more difficult for quick decision-making (e.g., in labor and delivery units).
- Other tests that are frequently used in the evaluation for congenital syphilis include chest x-ray, long bone radiography, lumbar puncture, complete blood count and differential, and hepatic transaminases (Fig. 30.1).

THERAPY

- Penicillin is the therapy of choice for congenital syphilis; the route and extent of the therapy depend on the certainty of the diagnosis and the presence of symptoms of infection (see Fig. 30.1).
- Therapy of pregnant women with syphilis is also best achieved with penicillin. If therapy is begun more than 30 days before delivery, it is considered adequate to prevent congenital syphilis. However, therapy within 30 days of delivery, undocumented therapy, therapy associated with failure of response (e.g., a ≥ fourfold increase in maternal RPR) even if given more than 4 weeks before delivery, and therapy comprised of an antimicrobial other than penicillin are considered not adequate to prevent congenital syphilis (see Fig. 30.1).

Tuberculosis

OVERVIEW

- Although tuberculosis likely infects 2 billion people globally, congenital tuberculosis is very rare (although perhaps underdiagnosed, especially in developing countries).
- Vertical transmission of tuberculosis may occur from the hematogenous spread from an infected placenta or by aspiration or ingestion of infected amniotic fluid or genital secretions; genital tuberculosis in women frequently causes sterility, which might in turn be partly responsible for the rarity of congenital infection.

CLINICAL PRESENTATION

- Tuberculosis mimics sepsis or other congenital infections; it often causes prematurity, respiratory distress, hepatomegaly with or without splenomegaly, and irritability.

DIAGNOSIS

- This is best made by the recovery of organisms in blood culture, endotracheal aspirates (or gastric aspirates), CSF, or maternal placenta, or genital specimens.
- Chest x-ray and the tuberculin skin test may be useful, as well, although the tuberculin skin test may not be reactive for 6 weeks or more even in infected infants.

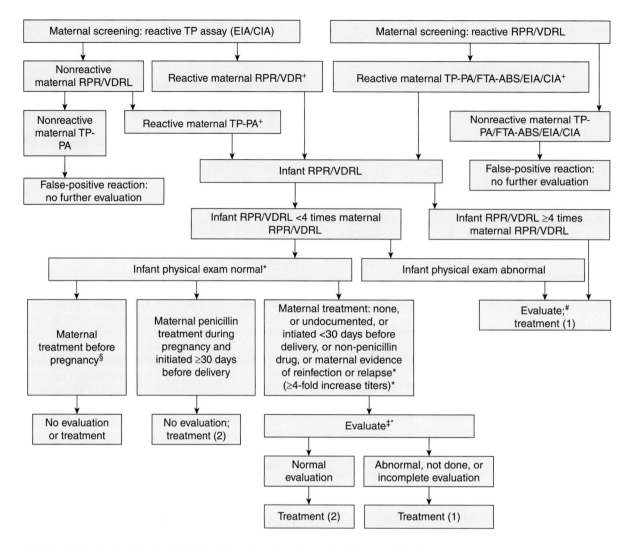

+ Test for HIV-antibody. Infants of HIV-infected mothers do not require different evaluation or treatment.

* If the infant's RPR/VDRL is nonreactive AND the mother has had no treatment, undocumented treatment, treatment initiation
<30 days before delivery, or evidence of reinfection or relapse (≥4-fold increase in titers),
THEN treat infant with a single IM injection of benzathine penicillin (50,000 U/kg). No additional evaluation needed.

§ Women who maintain a VDRL titer ≤1 : 2 (RPR ≤1 : 4) beyond 1 year following successful treatment are considered serofast.

Evaluation consists of CBC, platelet count; CSF examination for cell count, protein, and quantitative VDRL.
Other tests as clinically indicated: long-bone x-rays, neuroimaging, auditory brainstem response, eye exam,
chest x-ray, liver function tests.

‡ CBC, platelet count; CSF examination for cell count, protein, and quantitative VDRL; long-bone x-rays.

TREATMENT:
(1) Aqueous penicillin G 50,000 U/kg IV q 12 hr (≤1 wk of age), q8 hr (>1 wk), or procaine penicillin G 50,000 U/kg
 IM single daily dose, x 10 days
(2) Benzathine penicillin G 50,000 U/kg IM x 1 dose

Fig. 30.1 Algorithm for evaluation and treatment of infants born to mothers with reactive serologic test results for syphilis. *CBC,* Complete blood cell; *CIA,* chemiluminescence immunoassay; *CSF,* cerebrospinal fluid; *EIA,* enzyme immunoassay; *FTA-ABS,* fluorescent treponemal antibody absorption; *HIV,* human immunodeficiency virus; *IM,* intramuscular/intramuscularly; *IV,* intravenously; *RPR,* rapid plasma reagin; *TP, Treponema pallidum;* *TP-PA, Treponema pallidum* particle agglutination; *VDRL,* Venereal Disease Research Laboratory. (Modified from Michaels MG, Sanchez P, Lin PL. Congenital toxoplasmosis, syphilis, malaria, and tuberculosis. In: Gleason CA, Sawyer T, eds. *Avery's Diseases of the Newborn,* 11th ed. Philadelphia: Elsevier; 2024, Fig. 35.5.)

Similarly, the sensitivity of peripheral blood interferon gamma release assays is low in infancy.

THERAPY

- Multidrug therapy for an extended duration is the standard of care, although clinical trials in neonates have not been performed; an infectious disease or tuberculosis expert should be consulted.

Chlamydia trachomatis

OVERVIEW

- *Chlamydia trachomatis* is a very common cause of symptomatic and asymptomatic urogenital infections in men and women and can be transmitted from pregnant women to their neonates, causing neonatal conjunctivitis or pneumonia.
- Transmission from infected mothers is ~50% in vaginal births, less after cesarean section; infants may remain infected for much of the first year of life.
- Topical ophthalmia neonatorum prophylaxis given at birth is targeted at the prevention of gonococcal infection, but it does not fully prevent chlamydial conjunctivitis and is ineffective against preventing chlamydial pneumonia.

CLINICAL PRESENTATION

- Neonatal conjunctivitis (nongonococcal ophthalmia neonatorum)
  - Ocular congestion, edema of the eyelids, and conjunctival discharge develop in days to a few weeks (usually 5–14 days) after birth. Symptoms may last for 1 to 2 weeks if untreated.
- Neonatal pneumonia
  - Presents insidiously, typically with afebrile, staccato cough, tachypnea, and rales, at a few weeks to 5 to 6 months of life (typically around 4–6 weeks of age). Chest radiograph may show hyperinflation and infiltrates. It is sometimes accompanied by peripheral blood eosinophilia.

DIAGNOSIS

- Nucleic acid amplification tests (NAATs) are superior to culture techniques for the diagnosis of *C. trachomatis* in urogenital infection at all ages, but they are not yet approved for use in the United States for the diagnosis of neonatal conjunctivitis or pneumonia (eye or nasopharyngeal specimens).
- Recovery of organisms by culture of conjunctival or nasopharyngeal samples is less sensitive than the NAAT but may be done; if not easily available, a clinical diagnosis of neonatal chlamydial infection may be made in the appropriate clinical scenario.

THERAPY

- A macrolide, such as erythromycin (14-day course) or azithromycin (3-day course), is used for neonatal conjunctivitis or pneumonia.

- Azithromycin is preferred because of the association of erythromycin and infantile hypertrophic pyloric stenosis.
  - Mothers of infected infants, and the mother's sexual partners, should receive therapy for *C. trachomatis*, as well.
- Systemic therapy rather than topical therapy is used for neonatal chlamydial conjunctivitis to prevent subsequent pneumonia.
- Routine preventive therapy generally is not suggested for infants of mothers known to have untreated chlamydial infection at birth, but it may be done if adequate clinical follow-up cannot be ensured.

Genital Mycoplasma and Ureaplasma

OVERVIEW

- *Mycoplasma genitalium*, *M. hominis*, *Ureaplasma urealyticum*, and *U. parvum* are small, pleomorphic bacteria lacking cell walls; they are identified best by polymerase chain reaction (PCR) assays or less so by culture.
- They cause nongonococcal, nonchlamydial urethritis in men and women and endometritis in women; they have been associated in some studies but not in others with pregnancy loss, preterm birth, and development of bronchopulmonary dysplasia.
- *Ureaplasma* spp. have been isolated from blood and CSF of neonates, but their contribution to clinical outcome is uncertain.
- Therapy is not well defined; resistance to macrolides, fluoroquinolones, and even doxycycline has been described.

Anaerobic Bacteria

OVERVIEW

- Anaerobic bacteria such as *Bacteroides* spp. and *Clostridium* spp. are uncommonly recovered from the bloodstream of infants with bacteremia or sepsis, most often in neonates with necrotizing enterocolitis, postoperative abdominal infections, or fasciitis or after maternal chorioamnionitis.
- They are best treated with an anaerobe-active beta-lactam such as piperacillin–tazobactam, or meropenem or an agent such as clindamycin or metronidazole.
- *Clostridioides* (formerly *Clostridium*) *difficile* is a very common colonizer of neonatal and infant gastrointestinal tracts but is thought not to cause pseudomembranous colitis in infants younger than 1 to 2 years; in general, diagnostic studies for *C. difficile* should not be carried out in an infant younger than 1 to 2 years.

FUNGI

Candida albicans and Non–albicans spp.

OVERVIEW

- Invasive fungal infection with *Candida* spp. occurs in up to ~2% of all US neonatal intensive care unit (NICU) admissions.

- The risk of infection rises dramatically with decreasing gestational age and birth weight.
- *Candida* spp. are ubiquitous, colonizing the skin, mouth, gastrointestinal tract, and genitourinary tract, but are an uncommon cause of infection in pregnant women and neonates; they are acquired in utero (rare), during birth, or postnatally.
  - Budding yeast, some species of which form long buds or chains of buds, are referred to as pseudohyphae.
  - *C. albicans* causes about 50% of neonatal yeast infections, with other species comprising the balance.

CLINICAL PRESENTATION

- Local infections
  - Congenital candidiasis is a very rare form of dermal infection seen in the first day of life; deeply erythematous skin soon desquamates.
  - Diaper dermatitis (thrush) is a common, erythematous dermatitis in the perianal area or groin, with papular or pustular satellite lesions.
- Invasive (disseminated) infections
  - Candiduria, UTI: Renal candidiasis may be a local infection but is often associated with upper tract disease and possible systemic infection. It is characterized by the presence of yeast in catheterized urine samples, often with cortical abscesses or collections of fungal material in the collecting system demonstrable on renal ultrasound; may lead to urinary obstruction.
  - Peritonitis, as a consequence of bowel perforation, either from spontaneous intestinal perforation in the first week of life in neonates <1000 g or later from necrotizing enterocolitis.
  - Candidemia associated with central venous catheters
  - Candidemia associated with disseminated organ system candidiasis—for example, with pneumonia, septic arthritis, hepatosplenic lesions, or meningitis

DIAGNOSIS

- Made by recovery of organisms in culture of urine, blood, CSF, or peritoneal fluid
- Retinitis present in ~5% of cases of disseminated candidiasis; ophthalmologic examination may assist in looking for sites of disease in addition to renal ultrasound and lumbar puncture

THERAPY

- Antifungal choice
  - Amphotericin B remains the most potent agent, with the longest clinical experience. Amphotericin B deoxycholate is given intravenously and is well tolerated by neonates. It is significantly less expensive than liposomal amphotericin B used in older children and adults; however, liposomal amphotericin B is also effective.
  - Fluconazole has excellent penetration into the CSF and urinary tract and may be used if the yeast is identified as *C. albicans* or a fluconazole-susceptible, non-albicans *Candida*. It is the antifungal azole with the most experience in neonates, and it may be administered as an oral or intravenous drug.
  - Echinocandins such as micafungin or caspofungin are active against *Candida* spp. and may be used intravenously, especially for azole-resistant isolates (e.g., *C. krusei*).
- For catheter-associated fungemia, a 14-day treatment course is most often recommended; for disseminated disease or meningitis, 21 days or longer is recommended.
- For prevention of candidiasis with prophylactic fluconazole, see Chapter 31.

Other Fungal Infections

OVERVIEW

- Uncommonly, neonatal infection occurs from the cutaneous lipophilic yeast *Malassezia furfur*. *Malassezia* spp. cause tinea versicolor in older children and adults but may invade the bloodstream of infants with central venous catheters who are receiving total parenteral nutrition, especially parenteral lipid alimentation. Removal of the catheter, with interruption of the total parenteral nutrition for a few days, may suffice for therapy, but some experts recommend additional therapy with amphotericin B for 7 to 10 days.
- Other infections (e.g., other yeasts such as cryptococcosis; mold infections such as aspergillosis or fusariosis; endemic mycoses such as histoplasmosis, blastomycosis, or coccidioidomycosis) are very rare in the NICU.

VIRUSES

- General comments on viral infection
  - Viral infections in the neonate are likely more common than is currently recognized or able to be diagnosed with current diagnostic tests.
  - Transmission can occur prenatally (in utero), in the peripartum or intrapartum period, or in the immediate postpartum period.
  - Important prenatal (in utero) viral infections include cytomegalovirus (CMV), rubella virus, parvovirus B19, human immunodeficiency virus (HIV), lymphocytic choriomeningitis virus (LCMV), and varicella-zoster virus (VZV)
  - Important peripartum viral infections include hepatitis B virus (HBV), HIV, herpes simplex virus (HSV), enterovirus, and VZV.
  - Important postpartum viral infections include respiratory syncytial virus, influenza virus, VZV, and CMV.
  - Important, but less common, infections also include human parechovirus type 3 (HPeV 3) (mostly postpartum), Zika virus (in utero)
- Some general clinical findings suggest a specific diagnosis (Table 30.1).

Cytomegalovirus

OVERVIEW

- CMV infection is present at birth in 0.5% to 1% of all liveborn infants; it is the most common congenital viral infection in the United States.

Table 30.1 Clinical Findings Suggesting a Specific Congenital Viral Infection

Congenital Infection	Findings
Rubella	Congenital cataracts, pigmented retina, petechiae with blueberry muffin rash, bone defects with longitudinal bands of demineralization ("celery stalking"), cardiovascular malformations (patent ductus arteriosus, pulmonary artery stenosis), sensorineural hearing loss, fetal hydrops
Cytomegalovirus	Microcephaly with periventricular calcifications, chorioretinitis, petechiae with thrombocytopenia, jaundice, sensorineural hearing loss
Herpes simplex virus	Skin vesicles, keratoconjunctivitis, acute central nervous system findings (seizures), hepatitis, pneumonitis, sepsis-like picture
Parvovirus B19	Fetal hydrops, ascites, hepatomegaly, ventriculomegaly, hypertrophic myocardiopathy, anemia
Varicella zoster virus	Limb hypoplasia, dermatomal scarring in cicatricial pattern
Lymphocytic choriomeningitis virus	Hydrocephalus, chorioretinitis, intracranial calcifications; negative studies for cytomegalovirus, toxoplasmosis

Modified from Schleiss MR, Marsh KJ, Patterson JC. Viral infections of the fetus and newborn and HIV infection during pregnancy. In: Gleason CA, Juul SE, Sawyer T, eds. *Avery's Diseases of the Newborn*. 10th ed. Philadelphia: Elsevier; 2018, Table 37.1.

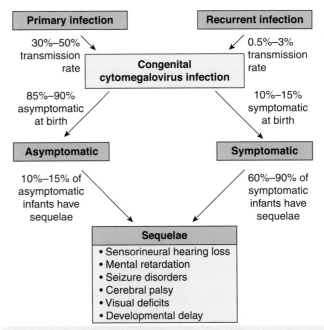

Fig. 30.2 **Profiles of congenital cytomegalovirus (CMV) epidemiology, infection, and outcome.** (Modified from Stokes C, Melvin AJ. Viral infections of the fetus and newborn infant. In: Gleason CA, Sawyer T, eds. *Avery's Diseases of the Newborn*. 11th ed. Philadelphia: Elsevier; 2024, Fig. 34.2.)

- In utero fetal infection can occur in women with no preexisting CMV immunity (maternal primary infection) or in women with preexisting antibody to CMV (maternal non-primary infection), either from reactivation of an existing maternal infection or infection with a new viral strain.
- Congenital infection and associated sequelae can occur irrespective of the trimester of pregnancy when the mother is infected.
- Primary maternal infection, although less common, is associated more with severe neonatal sequelae, especially if maternal infection is acquired during the first half of gestation (see Fig. 30.2).
- Congenital CMV infection is the leading nongenetic cause of sensorineural hearing loss (SNHL) in US children; ~20% of all hearing loss at birth and 25% of all hearing loss at 4 years of age can be attributed to congenital CMV infection.
- CMV is a member of the herpesvirus family; it is found only in humans, is ubiquitous across the globe, and exhibits extensive genetic diversity, allowing nonprimary reinfection.

CLINICAL PRESENTATION

- Congenital CMV infection has a wide spectrum of clinical manifestations, from asymptomatic to life-threatening disease. Symptoms and signs at birth include intrauterine growth retardation, microcephaly, periventricular intracranial calcifications, jaundice, hepatosplenomegaly, retinitis, and extramedullary dermal hematopoiesis ("blueberry muffin" rash). Sequelae are mostly neurologic (Fig. 30.2). When none of these findings is present, the neonatal infection is classified as asymptomatic.

DIAGNOSIS

- Neonates with congenital CMV shed CMV in saliva and urine; either fluid may be subjected to PCR amplification for timely diagnosis. Positive salivary CMV PCR should be confirmed with a urinary PCR however, as CMV in breast milk may be detected in salivary samples from breastfed babies (i.e., salivary CMV PCR is sensitive but not specific for true congenital infection but is a convenient starting point as it is easier to obtain than urine).
- A positive CMV urine (or blood) PCR during the first month of life is diagnostic for congenital CMV infection; after 4 to 6 weeks of age, positive results could represent postnatal infection (from breast milk, transfusions, or other contact).
- Many US states are now requiring CMV testing for newborns who fail audiologic screening in the nursery. Although such testing (with confirmatory PCR) may detect those truly CMV-infected newborns with neonatal hearing loss, infants with congenital CMV infection who have not yet developed sensorineural hearing loss will be missed. In addition, some newborns with congenital CMV infection who show apparent early hearing loss will have normal auditory function documented on formal repeat testing. It remains to be demonstrated whether universal CMV newborn screening will be superior on a population level to current CMV screening only after audiologic screening failure.

THERAPY

- Controlled clinical trials have shown that neonates with symptomatic congenital CMV disease have improved audiologic and neurodevelopmental outcomes at 2 years of age when treated with oral valganciclovir (an orally bioavailable prodrug of ganciclovir).

- Valganciclovir is administered orally or by gastrostomy tube for 6 months.
  - For infants unable to tolerate enteral feeding, intravenous ganciclovir provides similar systemic ganciclovir exposure but may have increased adverse effects.
  - Significant neutropenia occurs in ~20% of infants treated with oral valganciclovir and in ~67% of infants treated with parenteral ganciclovir; absolute neutrophil counts should be performed frequently (along with monthly serum aminotransferase concentrations to exclude uncommon hepatitis).
- In contrast, infants with asymptomatic congenital CMV infection should not receive antiviral treatment, because currently the drug risks appear to outweigh theoretic benefits.
- It is not yet certain whether very mildly symptomatic congenital CMV infection (e.g., isolated hearing loss but otherwise asymptomatic; isolated SGA but otherwise asymptomatic) benefits from valganciclovir therapy.

Herpes Simplex Virus

OVERVIEW

- Herpes simplex virus-1 (HSV-1) and HSV-2 are members of the herpesvirus family that may cause recurrent mucocutaneous disease and, in neonates (and older immunocompromised hosts), more severe invasive disease.
- HSV-1 and HSV-2 persist for life in latent form after causing the primary infection. Either may cause neonatal HSV infection.
- Neonatal HSV is acquired vertically, usually during birth through an infected maternal genital tract and uncommonly from an ascending infection through ruptured amniotic membranes. Rarely, postnatal transmission from a parent or other caregiver, usually from a nongenital infection (e.g., herpetic whitlow or herpes labialis lesion), has been reported. Rare cases of neonatal HSV infection also have followed certain ultra-religious circumcision practices involving direct orogenital suction of the infant circumcision site.
- The overall incidence of neonatal HSV infection in the United States is ~1 in 3000 to 10,000 annual births.
- Most cases of neonatal HSV occur in women who have had a recent primary or recurrent nonprimary infection, although most maternal infections are asymptomatic or subtle enough to escape diagnosis; thus, the history of past maternal HSV lesions is not clinically useful in the diagnosis of neonatal HSV.
  - The transmission rate of HSV among women who already have recurrent HSV in the first half of pregnancy is ~2%; after primary HSV infection is acquired late in pregnancy, it is ~33% to 50%. Thus, the relative risk of HSV transmission is high in primary infection, but the incidence of neonatal HSV infection is lower than this would suggest, because most pregnant women with HSV have recurrent infection.

CLINICAL PRESENTATION

- Neonatal HSV presents in three clinical forms, which may overlap to some extent.
  - Disseminated disease is a sepsis-like condition involving multiple organs, most prominently liver and lungs but also the central nervous system (CNS); it represents about 25% of all neonatal HSV infections.
  - CNS disease, with or without skin involvement, occurs in about 30% of neonatal HSV infections.
  - Skin, eye, and/or mouth (SEM) disease is localized to the skin, eyes, and/or mouth and occurs in about 45% of neonatal HSV infections.
- The onset of disease is generally around 2 weeks of age—during the first or second week of life for disseminated or SEM disease and between the second and third weeks for CNS disease.
- More than 80% of neonates with SEM disease and ~67% of those with CNS disease or disseminated HSV infection will have skin vesicles at some point in the illness, but these lesions may not be present at the time of onset of symptoms in CNS disease or disseminated forms.
- Disseminated and CNS diseases often are severe, with attendant high mortality and morbidity rates, even when antiviral therapy is administered.
  - Disseminated disease—30% mortality, 20% of survivors with sequelae
  - CNS disease—10% mortality, 70% of survivors with sequelae

DIAGNOSIS

- Neonatal HSV should be considered in neonates with culture-negative sepsis, severe liver dysfunction, or consumptive coagulopathy.
- For the diagnosis of neonatal HSV infection, the following specimens should be obtained: (1) swab specimens from the mouth, nasopharynx, conjunctivae, and anus ("surface specimens") for HSV PCR amplification assay (or viral culture, if PCR unavailable); (2) specimens of any visible skin vesicles for HSV for PCR; (3) CSF sample for HSV PCR; (4) whole-blood sample for HSV PCR; and (5) whole-blood sample for measuring alanine aminotransferase (ALT).

THERAPY

See Chapter 31 for preventive therapy algorithms after neonatal exposure.

- Parenteral acyclovir should be administered to all neonates with HSV disease, regardless of manifestations and clinical findings, for 14 days in SEM disease and for a minimum of 21 days in CNS or disseminated disease.
- All infants with neonatal HSV disease, regardless of disease classification, should have an ophthalmologic examination and neuroimaging studies.
- All infants with CNS involvement should have a repeat lumbar puncture performed near the end of therapy to document that the CSF is negative for HSV DNA by a PCR assay.
- In the uncommon event that the PCR result remains positive near the end of a 21-day treatment course,

acyclovir therapy should be extended, with a repeat CSF PCR assay performed near the end of the extended treatment period.

■ Oral acyclovir suppressive therapy for the 6 months following treatment of acute neonatal HSV disease improves neurodevelopmental outcomes and prevents skin recurrences; it should be administered in all cases of neonatal HSV infection.

Varicella-Zoster Virus

OVERVIEW

■ VZV is another member of the herpesvirus family; it causes chickenpox and herpes zoster (shingles) in older children and adults and, rarely, infection in neonates.
  ▦ Neonatal varicella may occur if a nonimmune pregnant women has varicella near the time of delivery.
  ▦ In contrast, congenital varicella syndrome is a very rare complication of maternal varicella earlier in the first 20 weeks of gestation (only ~100 cases reported).

CLINICAL PRESENTATION

■ Congenital varicella syndrome results in an embryopathy with cicatricial limb rashes and asymmetric muscular atrophy, limb hypoplasia, and other CNS, eye, and gastrointestinal tract anomalies; these infants have a significant infant mortality rate and also may develop early herpes zoster in infancy.
■ Maternal varicella in the last month of pregnancy or immediately postpartum may lead to neonatal varicella (chickenpox).
  ▦ If the mother's varicella develops during the period from 5 days before delivery to 2 days after delivery, the neonate may have severe disease, with high morbidity and mortality, developing at 5 to 10 days of life, similar to varicella in an immunosuppressed host, with fever, hemorrhagic rash, and visceral dissemination.
  ▦ Conversely, maternal varicella with onset of rash >5 days before delivery is less consequential for the infant, with mild disease developing, presumably because transplacental antibody has had time to begin to protect the fetus (assuming that it is >28 weeks' gestational age), and maternal viral replication has lessened.
■ Neonates born to women who have never had varicella or varicella immunization or those born at <28 weeks' gestation in whom transplacental antibody may not have begun to cross into the fetal circulation are susceptible to airborne varicella infection from other babies, visitors, or health care workers who have chickenpox or adults with herpes zoster.

DIAGNOSIS

■ VZV infection is best diagnosed from specimens taken from vesicular lesions by PCR assay.

THERAPY

See Chapter 31 for preventive therapy with immune globulin after exposure.

■ Parenteral acyclovir should be administered to all neonates with VZV disease whose mothers had onset of their varicella between 5 days prepartum and 2 days postpartum.
■ Neonates with milder infection from maternal varicella >5 days prepartum or those infected when >2 days old may be given oral or intravenous acyclovir, if a decision to provide therapy is made.

Human Parvovirus B19

OVERVIEW

■ Human parvovirus B19 is a small DNA virus that causes erythema infectiosum (fifth disease) in older immunocompetent children and fetal hydrops (hydrops fetalis) if a pregnant woman is first infected before 20 weeks' gestation.
  ▦ Approximately 50% of US women of childbearing age are susceptible to parvovirus B19 infection; transmission in the household is generally <50%, with even lower transmission to the fetus.
  ▦ Thus, only a minority of neonates are affected by parvovirus, with an annual seroconversion rate of susceptible women estimated at 1.5%; however, in documented seroconversion before 20 weeks' gestation, the rates of fetal hydrops or death are ~5%.

CLINICAL PRESENTATION

■ The major clinical presentation of parvovirus B19 in the fetus is nonimmune hydrops fetalis.
■ Fetal demise is very rare in the absence of fetal hydrops, and no birth defects among surviving neonates have been confirmed.

DIAGNOSIS

■ Parvovirus B19 is best detected by PCR amplification in blood, as well as by IgG and IgM assays.

THERAPY

■ No specific antiviral therapy
■ Intrauterine fetal transfusions for hydrops fetalis and neonatal anemia of parvovirus infections

Enterovirus

OVERVIEW

■ Enteroviruses include the small RNA viruses, polioviruses, coxsackieviruses, and echoviruses. The related human parechoviruses are discussed separately below.
■ Non–polio enteroviruses can cause a neonatal sepsis syndrome, particularly after late in utero or intrapartum transmission, when the neonate may become ill in the first weeks of life.

CLINICAL PRESENTATION

- Uncommonly, infection presents as culture-negative sepsis in the neonate < 7 days of age born to a mother with a febrile respiratory or nonspecific illness. Some cases of neonatal enterovirus infection are associated with severe morbidity and mortality.
- More commonly, enteroviruses cause a nonspecific febrile illness in an older neonate or infant.

DIAGNOSIS

- Enteroviruses may be detected by PCR amplification or, less often, viral culture in nasopharyngeal, blood, CSF, or stool samples; stool is least preferred because excretion may last for several weeks.

THERAPY

- Supportive therapy alone

Human Parechovirus Infections

OVERVIEW

- The human parechovirus (HPeV) is a small RNA virus once classified as an echovirus, along with other enteroviruses; there are several numbered serotypes. HPeV3, in particular, is a cause of sepsis and sometimes meningoencephalitis in infants <6 months of age; HPeV1 has been implicated in respiratory and gastrointestinal infections in infants and young children. Transmission is likely fecal–oral, as with other enteroviruses.
- HPeV3 sepsis occurred at a mean age of 6 weeks (range, 1 week to 7 months) in one large US children's hospital study. However, few cases have been identified in neonates not yet discharged from the hospital (most cases are in infants who presumably are infected at home post-discharge).

CLINICAL PRESENTATION

- Clinical signs and symptoms of HPeV3 infection are those of "hot, angry, and red babies"; that is, they demonstrate fever, irritability, and erythematous maculopapular or morbilliform rashes (which can be diffusely distributed or sometimes limited to the hands and feet).
- HPeV3 also may cause an unusual aseptic meningitis syndrome, with a distinctly normal cell count and protein, but positive PCR assay in CSF. Seizures, apnea, and encephalitis with white matter changes on MRI reminiscent of hypoxic ischemic encephalopathy have been reported. Many children appear to recover fully, although some have developed neurologic sequelae; exact rates of sequelae are likely confounded by diagnostic and reporting biases.

DIAGNOSIS

- HPeV3 may be detected by PCR amplification in CSF samples.

THERAPY

- Supportive therapy alone

Rubella Virus

OVERVIEW

- Rubella virus is an RNA virus infecting humans only.
- It causes rubella (formerly known as German measles), a mild illness with low-grade fever and exanthema.
- Congenital rubella syndrome (CRS), a serious embryopathy, occurs if maternal rubella occurs at <17 weeks' gestation; it is completely preventable by maternal immunization against rubella virus before childbearing.

CLINICAL PRESENTATION

- Infants with CRS typically are born with low birth weight and are small for gestational age (SGA), often with congenital cataracts, microphthalmos, glaucoma, hearing loss, and congenital heart defects (usually peripheral pulmonary artery stenosis or patent ductus arteriosus).
- The presence of extramedullary dermal hematopoiesis produces a so-called blueberry muffin appearance (similar to CMV infection); long-bone radiographs show irregular radiolucency (so-called celery stalking).
- Late manifestations of CRS in older infants and children include thyroid disease, diabetes mellitus, and immunodeficiency.

DIAGNOSIS

- The classic triad of congenital cataracts, hearing loss, and congenital heart disease should suggest the diagnosis of CRS.
- Rubella virus may be detected by PCR amplification of throat, blood, urine, or CSF specimens during the first year of life.

THERAPY

- None—CRS is preventable by ensuring that all pregnant women are screened for immunity to rubella by serologic testing.
- Pregnant women found not to be immune to rubella should be immunized during the immediate postpartum period.

Human Immunodeficiency Virus

OVERVIEW

- HIV infection in a pregnant woman may be transmitted to the child during pregnancy (~30% of overall transmission in the era before antiretroviral therapy), peripartum period (~60% of transmission in the pre-antiretroviral therapy era), or breastfeeding (~10% of transmission in the pre-antiretroviral therapy era). Breastfeeding is thus generally contraindicated for HIV-infected mothers in developed countries with clean water.

- The overall vertical transmission rate for HIV in the untreated mother–infant pair is ~25% in the absence of breastfeeding and up to 35% with breastfeeding. With successful virologic suppression, including a tripartite treatment regimen of combination antiretroviral therapy for the pregnant women, a short course of antiretroviral prophylaxis for the neonate, and in general, prevention of breastfeeding, mother to child transmission rates of 0.1% to 0.5% are achievable (see Chapter 31 for details).
- There are no symptoms or signs of in utero or perinatal HIV infection (i.e., there is no embryopathy).
- Diagnosis of perinatal HIV infection must be performed by PCR amplification.
  - HIV-exposed infants are seropositive for antibody at birth, whether truly infected or not, due to transplacental acquisition of maternal antibody (which can persist as long as 18 months after birth).
  - HIV RNA PCR or DNA PCR assays are sensitive and specific, but only ~40% of infected newborns will be diagnosed at birth; nearly 100% of infected infants can be diagnosed by 4 to 6 months of age, because test sensitivity increases greatly with age.
  - At minimum, serial PCR assays should be performed at 2 weeks, 1 month, and 4 to 6 months of age to diagnose HIV infection; most experts also test at birth and at additional intervals for those infants judged to be at greatest risk of HIV acquisition (e.g., those born to women without antiretroviral therapy or with less than ideal virologic suppression).
- See Chapter 31 for preventive therapy in the HIV-exposed neonate. Expert consultation should be obtained for women with HIV infection who are contemplating pregnancy or who are pregnant already, as well as for HIV-exposed neonates. Consultation is available with local or regional HIV experts, or with the National Perinatal HIV Hotline (1-888-448-8765), or at the AIDS Info website (a service of the US Department of Health and Human Services; https://clinicalinfo.hiv.gov/en/guidelines.

Hepatitis B Virus

OVERVIEW

- Perinatal transmission of the DNA virus, HBV, from infected mothers to neonates is highly efficient (>90%) and usually occurs from infected blood or body fluid exposures during labor and delivery. In contrast to peripartum transmission, in utero transmission accounts for less than 2% of all vertically transmitted HBV infections.
- Chronic HBV infection occurs in up to 90% of infants infected with hepatitis B at birth; chronic HBV is life-threatening later in adulthood (~25% risk of fatal hepatocellular carcinoma or cirrhosis).
- Postexposure prophylaxis with HBV vaccine or HBV vaccine and hepatitis B immune globulin (HBIG) is highly effective; see Chapter 31 for discussion of universal vaccination of neonates.
- HBV infection in neonates and infants is asymptomatic; diagnosis is established by detecting HBV surface antigen (HBsAg) serologically in the blood.

- Breastfeeding by an HBV-positive mother poses no additional risk of acquisition of HBV infection by the infant, with the appropriate administration of hepatitis B vaccine and HBIG.

Hepatitis C Virus

OVERVIEW

- In contrast to the highly efficient vertical transmission of HBV from infected mothers (in the absence of neonatal immunization) and the modest vertical transmission of HIV (in the absence of combination antiretroviral therapy), vertical transmission of the RNA virus HCV is distinctly uncommon (~5%).
- Vertical transmission of HCV may be elevated to ~10% to 15% if the mother is dually infected with HIV and HCV.
- There is no available postexposure HCV prophylaxis for the neonate.
- HCV infection in neonates and infants is asymptomatic; diagnosis is established by positive HCV antibody testing at 18 months of age (by which time the high levels of maternal transplacental antibody should have been cleared) or, if earlier diagnosis is desired, by a positive PCR amplification test for HCV at ~3 to 4 months of age.
- Maternal HCV infection is not a contraindication to breastfeeding, although HCV-infected mothers should consider abstaining if their nipples are cracked or bleeding.

Zika Virus

OVERVIEW

- Zika virus is a newly emergent RNA virus in the *Flavivirus* genus; it is related to dengue virus, yellow fever virus, and West Nile virus. Most human Zika infections are asymptomatic or are associated with mild fever, maculopapular rash, and conjunctivitis. However, Zika virus infection in a pregnant woman can lead to severe consequences of congenital Zika virus infection.
- Congenital Zika virus infection can cause fetal loss, microcephaly, severe neurologic anomalies (subcortical calcifications, ventriculomegaly despite microcephaly, abnormal cortical migration and hypoplasia), ocular anomalies (microphthalmia, cataracts, chorioretinal atrophy), and musculoskeletal disease (arthogryposis).
- Zika virus is transmitted by bites of *Aedes aegypti* and *A. albopictus* mosquitoes, both of which are found in the southern United States and throughout Central and South America. These vectors also transmit dengue, yellow fever, and chikungunya viruses. Less commonly, sexual transmission or blood transfusion can transmit Zika virus infection.
- A very large epidemic of Zika virus in Central and South America from 2015 to 2017, especially in Brazil, led to >5000 newborns born with microcephaly and neurodevelopmental defects. Maternal infection during the first trimester appeared to be most dangerous to the fetus, with 1% to 10% congenital microcephaly rates.

- Laboratory diagnosis of Zika virus infection is complex and should be done in consultation with experts in pediatric infectious diseases. Virus-specific RNA can be detected by PCR of serum and urine but only transiently; serologic testing is complicated by cross-reactivity with other more common flaviviruses (e.g., dengue, yellow fever, West Nile viruses).
- No specific treatment is available for Zika virus infection. Avoidance of travel to high-risk areas is the only prevention strategy for men and women of reproductive age; use of insect repellents by travelers (especially if pregnant) is recommended as well (see Chapter 31).

SARS-CoV-2 (COVID-19)

- Pregnant mothers can become quite ill with the SARS-CoV-2 virus which causes COVID-19, and vaccination is strongly recommended.
- Maternal COVID-19 can result in severe respiratory compromise, sometimes necessitating preterm delivery to allow sufficient respiratory function in the mother.
- Rarely, COVID-19 can be transmitted from mother to fetus. The newborn can also become infected shortly after birth. Providing breast milk is recommended, even when the mother is COVID-19 positive. Although there is no evidence that COVID-19 is spread in breastmilk, it is important to use precautions when a COVID-19+ mother is providing breast milk by:
  - Breastfeeding after hand hygiene using a mask
  - Providing pumped breast milk
- Immunoglobulins to COVID-19 are present in the breastmilk of previously infected people for up to 5 months after infection.
- Most newborns with COVID-19 have mild or no symptoms, but there have been some reports of severe symptoms, including fever, apnea, pneumonia, tachypnea, hypoxia, vomiting, and diarrhea.

PROTOZOA

Toxoplasmosis

OVERVIEW

- *Toxoplasma gondii* is an obligate intracellular parasite with worldwide distribution; it infects a wide range of mammals (cats are the definitive host), birds and, globally, up to ~30% of humans.
- Congenital toxoplasmosis occurs when a mother sustains a primary infection during pregnancy; conversely, immunocompetent women who have been infected prior to pregnancy (i.e., are seropositive already at the diagnosis of pregnancy) virtually never transmit toxoplasmosis to their neonate.
  - The seropositivity rate in US women of childbearing age is ~6% to 11%, with higher rates in those born overseas or living on farms (thus most US women of childbearing age are susceptible to primary infection during pregnancy).
  - The estimated overall vertical transmission rate of toxoplasmosis is ~25%.

- The current estimated incidence of acute primary infection among pregnant women in the United States is 0.2–1.1/1000 pregnant women, but a lower incidence of congenital toxoplasmosis in neonates has been reported (~0.2–0.9/10,000 live births).
- The probability of fetal infection increases as the gestational age at primary maternal infection increases.

CLINICAL PRESENTATION

- Congenital toxoplasmosis is a severe disease, although it is thought that perhaps 60% of newborns are asymptomatic at birth; visual or hearing impairment, learning disabilities, or developmental delays will become apparent in a large proportion of congenitally infected children in several months to years of age.
- The major clinical signs of congenital toxoplasmosis include chorioretinitis, cerebral calcifications (throughout the brain, in contrast to the periventricular distribution of those from congenital CMV infection), and hydrocephalus, alone or in combination.
  - The classic triad of chorioretinitis, parenchymal brain calcifications, and hydrocephalus rarely is seen at birth but is highly suggestive of congenital toxoplasmosis; eventually, if untreated, most infants will eventually develop all of the findings: >90% chorioretinitis, 80% calcifications, ~70% hydrocephalus, and ~60% complete triad of findings.
  - Cerebral calcifications can be demonstrated (in increasing order of diagnostic sensitivity, lowest to greatest) by plain radiography, ultrasonography, or computed tomography (CT) imaging of the head.
- Additional signs of congenital toxoplasmosis at birth include microcephaly, seizures, hearing loss, strabismus, a maculopapular rash, generalized lymphadenopathy, hepatomegaly, splenomegaly, jaundice, pneumonitis, diarrhea, hypothermia, anemia, petechiae, and thrombocytopenia.

DIAGNOSIS

- Congenital toxoplasmosis should be considered in infants born to the following women: (1) women suspected of having or who have been diagnosed with primary *T. gondii* infection during gestation; (2) women infected within 3 months of conception; (3) immunocompromised women (HIV-infected or otherwise) with serologic evidence of past infection with *T. gondii*; or (4) any infant with clinical signs or laboratory abnormalities suggestive of congenital infection.
- Serologic tests are the primary means of diagnosing primary and latent infection in women and congenital infections in neonates; PCR testing of amniotic fluid may also be carried out.
- Neonatal diagnosis:
  - Congenital infection is confirmed serologically by persistently positive IgG titers beyond the first 12 months of life; transplacental IgG antibody to *T. gondii* usually becomes undetectable by 6 to 12 months of age.
- Maternal diagnosis:
  - IgG-specific antibodies peak 1 to 2 months after infection and remain positive indefinitely, but the vast

majority will have decreased to low-positive levels by 6 months after the acute infection; the lack of *T. gondii*–specific IgM antibodies in a person with low-positive titers of IgG antibodies indicates infection of at least 6 months' duration.

- A positive IgM test in a pregnant woman should be followed up by confirmatory testing at a laboratory with special expertise in *Toxoplasma* serology (e.g., the Dr. Jack S. Remington Laboratory for Specialty Diagnostics at Sutter Health, Palo Alto, CA), because false-positive reactions do occur or persist for unexpectedly long periods.
- In pregnant women, the timing of the infection is critical (i.e., long-standing infection denotes little risk, but primary infection denotes greater risk of transmission); specialized tests such as an IgG avidity test, acetone [AC]/formalin [HS] or differential agglutination test, or IgA- and IgE-specific antibody tests also may be done to better define the timing of the infection. Consultation with an expert and use of an expert reference laboratory are advised.
- Congenital toxoplasmosis can also be definitively diagnosed prenatally by detecting parasite DNA in amniotic fluid by PCR assay.
  - Serial fetal ultrasonographic examinations should be performed in cases of suspected congenital infection to detect any increase in the size of the lateral ventricles of the CNS or other signs of fetal infection, such as brain, hepatic, or splenic calcifications.

THERAPY

See Chapter 31 for prevention.

- For both symptomatic and asymptomatic congenital infections, oral pyrimethamine combined with sulfadiazine (supplemented with folinic acid) is recommended as initial therapy.
- The duration of therapy is usually 1 year; the optimal dosage and duration have not been established definitively, and drug toxicity may occur—therapy of congenital toxoplasmosis should be pursued in consultation with a pediatric infectious diseases specialist.
- Maternal infection in pregnant women is best pursued in consultation with an expert. Infection early in pregnancy is treated with spiramycin, which blocks placental transmission but does not treat infection in the fetus. Spiramycin has limited availability in the US. Toxoplasmosis in mid-to late-pregnancy is treated with pyrimethamine combined with sulfadiazine (supplemented with folinic acid), which has some degree of fetal toxicity.

Malaria

OVERVIEW

- Congenital malaria is rare; ~0.5% of babies born to pregnant women with malaria in endemic areas become infected. Pregnant women who are less immune to malaria (Western travelers to malarious areas) have rates of congenital malaria up to 5%.
- *Plasmodium falciparum* is the most dangerous of the five species that infect humans.

CLINICAL PRESENTATION

- Congenital malaria may present at 2 to 8 weeks of age.
- Symptoms mimic sepsis, with fever in ~90%, anemia in 36%, splenomegaly in 30%, hepatomegaly in 20%, and thrombocytopenia, jaundice, irritability, and vomiting in ~10% each.

DIAGNOSIS

- Thin blood smears and rapid *Plasmodium* antigen detection tests; PCR testing is becoming more available and is highly sensitive and specific

THERAPY

- Congenital *P. falciparum* disease may be severe and chloroquine resistant.
- If chloroquine susceptibility is expected (non–*P. falciparum* disease or *P. falciparum* from nonresistant geographic areas), chloroquine is used as in older infants.
- *P. falciparum* congenital malaria therapy requires quinine and clindamycin, artemether–lumefantrine, or other specialized medications; consultation with an expert in pediatric infectious diseases is advised.

Suggested Readings

Committee on Infectious Diseases; Committee on Fetus and Newborn. Elimination of perinatal hepatitis B: providing the first vaccine dose within 24 hours of birth. *Pediatrics.* 2017;140(3):e20171870.

Flannery DD, Puopolo KM. Neonatal early-onset sepsis. *NeoReviews.* 2022;23:756–770.

Flannery DD, Edwards EM, Coggins SA, Horbar JD, Puopolo KM. Late-onset sepsis among very preterm infants. *Pediatrics.* 2022;150:e2022058813.

Kimberlin DW, Baley J. American Academy of Pediatrics, Committee on Infectious Diseases. Guidance on management of asymptomatic neonates born to women with active genital herpes lesions. *Pediatrics.* 2013;131(2):e635–e646.

Maldonado YA, Read JS. Committee on Infectious Diseases. Diagnosis, treatment, and prevention of congenital toxoplasmosis in the United States. *Pediatrics.* 2017;139(2):e20163860.

Nizet V, Klein JO. Bacterial sepsis and meningitis. In: Wilson CB, Nizet V, Maldonado YA, Remington JS, Klein JO, eds. *Remington and Klein's Infectious Diseases of the Fetus and Newborn Infant.* 8th ed. Philadelphia: Saunders; 2016:1132–1146.

Pappas PG, Kauffman CA, Andes DR, et al. Clinical Practice Guideline for the Management of Candidiasis: 2016 update by the Infectious Diseases Society of America. *Clin Infect Dis.* 2016;62:e1–e50.

Shane AL, Sánchez PJ, Stoll BJ. Neonatal sepsis. *Lancet.* 2017;390:1770–1780.

Wilson CB, Nizet V, Maldonado Y, Remington JS, Klein JO, eds. *Remington and Klein's Infectious Diseases of the Fetus and Newborn Infant.* 8th ed. Philadelphia: Saunders; 2016.

31 Prevention of Infections and Immunization

GEOFFREY A. WEINBERG

Immunization

- Immunization of infants <37 weeks' gestation or <2500 g birth weight generally follows the identical, routine, universal immunization recommendations for term infants, with few exceptions.
  - Immunizations for premature infants should be given at appropriate chronologic ages and with full doses of recommended vaccines.
  - Medically stable preterm infants who remain in the hospital at 2 months of chronologic age should be given all inactivated vaccines recommended for that age. Medically stable is defined as an infant who does not require ongoing management for serious infection, metabolic disease, or acute renal, cardiovascular, neurologic, or respiratory tract illness and who demonstrates a clinical course of sustained recovery and a pattern of steady growth.
  - The only immunization to consider deferring in a premature neonate in the neonatal intensive care unit (NICU) or nursery is oral rotavirus vaccine to prevent the potential nosocomial spread of this live vaccine virus.
    - Premature infants can receive rotavirus vaccine at the time of hospital discharge if they are between 6 and 15 weeks, 0 days of chronologic age and are medically stable.
    - Research is ongoing to determine the degree to which rotavirus vaccine virus actually spreads from hospitalized infants, given standard infection prevention practices in the NICU and nursery. Many institutions now administer oral rotavirus vaccine to age-appropriate newborns in the NICU. This decreases missed opportunities for immunization which places premature neonates at risk for disease after discharge.

Prevention of Specific Bacterial Infection

- Group B streptococci (GBS; *Streptococcus agalactiae*) (see also Chapters 29 and 30)
  - Universal chemoprophylaxis (intrapartum antibiotic prophylaxis [IAP]) is recommended by both the Centers for Disease Control and Prevention (CDC) and the American Academy of Pediatrics (AAP) and has reduced the incidence of GBS early-onset sepsis by >75%.
  - Late-onset GBS infection is not prevented by IAP.
  - All pregnant women are screened at 36 0/7 to 37 6/7 weeks' gestation for vaginal–rectal colonization.

- IAP is given to the following pregnant women:
  - Those with a previous infant with invasive GBS disease (regardless of screening during current pregnancy)
  - Those with GBS bacteriuria or urinary tract infection (UTI) during the current pregnancy
  - Those with positive GBS vaginal–rectal screening (unless a cesarean delivery is performed before onset of labor with intact membranes)
  - Those with unknown GBS colonization status at onset of labor or rupture of membranes with gestation < 37 weeks, rupture of membrane ≥ 18 hours, or temperature ≥ 38.0°C
  - Those with an intrapartum nucleic acid amplification test positive for GBS, if such testing is available
- Adequate IAP is defined as ≥4 hours of intravenous (IV) penicillin G or ampicillin, or for penicillin-allergic women without a history of anaphylaxis, IV cefazolin.
- For women with a history of penicillin allergy but with a low risk of serious allergic reactions (i.e., a history of nonspecific reactions to penicillin, non-urticarial maculopapular or morbilliform rash, absence of systemic respiratory symptoms, family history of reactions, or no recollection of symptoms), cefazolin is preferred due to its spectrum of activity and very low risk of reactivity.
- For penicillin-allergic women with a history of anaphylaxis, angioedema, or respiratory distress and urticaria to penicillin or to cephalosporins or a history of severe non-immunoglobulin E (IgE)-mediated reactions such as Stevens-Johnson syndrome or toxic epidermal necrolysis, clindamycin may be used if the GBS isolate is known to be susceptible; vancomycin is used if the isolate is nonsusceptible or of unknown susceptibility.
- Dosing information (all IV): penicillin G, 5 million units initial loading dose, then 2.5 to 3.0 million units every 4 hours until delivery; ampicillin, 2 g initial dose, then 1 g every 4 hours until delivery; cefazolin, 2 g initially, then 1 g every 8 hours until delivery; clindamycin, 900 mg every 8 hours until delivery; vancomycin 20 mg/kg every 8 hours until delivery (vancomycin infusion time ≥1 hour; 2 g maximum single dose)
- Although adequate IAP is defined as ≥4 hours of IV antimicrobials, the Kaiser Neonatal Early-Onset Sepsis Calculator discussed in Chapter 29 and shown in Fig. 31.1 cites >2 hours of therapy, because multiple other factors in addition to IAP length are considered within the multivariate model.

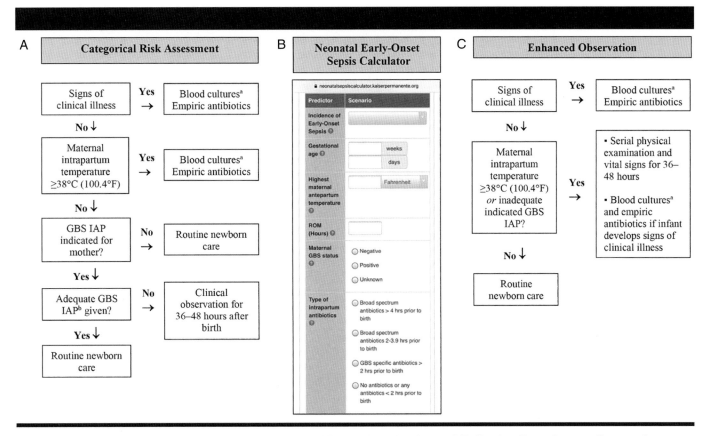

A Categorical Risk Assessment

B Neonatal Early-Onset Sepsis Calculator

C Enhanced Observation

Reproduced from Puopolo KM, Lynfield R, Cummings JJ; American Academy of Pediatrics, Committee on Fetus and Newborn, Committee on Infectious Diseases. Management of infants at risk for group B streptococcal disease. *Pediatrics.* 2019;144(2):e20191881. The screenshot of the Neonatal Early-Onset Sepsis Calculator (**https://neonatalsepsiscalculator.kaiserpermanente.org/**) was used with permission from Kaiser-Permanente Division of Research.

[a]Consider lumbar puncture and CSF culture before initiation of empiric antibiotics for infants who are at the highest risk of infection, especially those with critical illness. Lumbar puncture should not be performed if the infant's clinical condition would be compromised, and antibiotics should be administered promptly and not deferred because of procedure delays.

[b]Adequate GBS IAP is defined as the administration of penicillin G, ampicillin, or cefazolin ≥4 hours before delivery.

Fig. 31.1 **Risk assessment for early-onset group B streptococcal disease among infants born at ≥35 weeks of gestation.** *GBS,* Group B *Streptococcus; IAP,* intrapartum antibiotic prophylaxis. (From Kimberlin DW, et al., eds. *Red Book 2021: Report of the Committee on Infectious Diseases.* Itasca, IL: American Academy of Pediatrics; 2021, Fig 3.13.)

- Strategies for the evaluation and management of the newborn infant born to a woman receiving IAP are shown in Figs 31.1 and 31.2.

Prevention of Specific Fungal Infection

- *Candida albicans*
  - Several randomized clinical trials and retrospective cohort analyses have documented decreased invasive candidiasis among selected neonates who have been administered fluconazole prophylaxis, although doses, schedules, and target birth weights have varied across trials.
  - Fluconazole prophylaxis is recommended for the following:
    - Extremely low birth weight (ELBW; <1000 g) neonates in a NICU with historic rates of invasive candidiasis of ≥10%. Some authorities extend this prophylaxis to very low birth weight (VLBW; <1500 g) infants, as well.
  - Fluconazole administered IV, beginning at 48 to 72 hours of life for these neonates, at 6 mg/kg/dose twice weekly; when the infant can tolerate oral feeding, the same dose may be given orally.
  - Duration of prophylaxis is until 42 days of age or when IV lines are discontinued.

Prevention of Specific Viral Infection

- Hepatitis B virus (HBV)
  - About 1000 new cases of perinatal hepatitis B infection still occur annually in the United States, even though the overall case incidence has decreased by 90% since licensure of the vaccine in 1982.

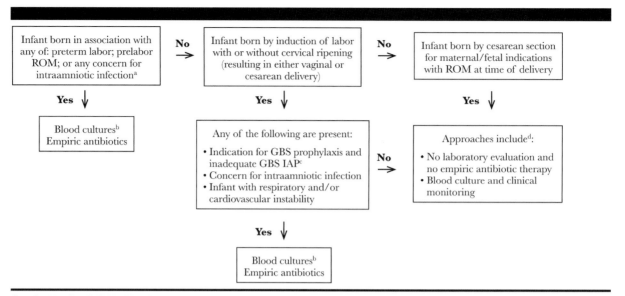

Reproduced from Puopolo KM, Lynfield R, Cummings JJ; American Academy of Pediatrics, Committee on Fetus and Newborn, Committee on Infectious Diseases. Management of infants at risk for group B streptococcal disease. *Pediatrics.* 2019;144(2):e20191881

[a] Intraamniotic infection should be considered when a pregnant woman presents with unexplained decreased fetal movement and/or there is sudden and unexplained poor fetal testing.

[b] Lumbar puncture and CSF culture should be performed before initiation of empiric antibiotics for infants who are at the highest risk of infection unless the procedure would compromise the infant's clinical condition. Antibiotics should be administered promptly and not deferred because of procedural delays.

[c] Adequate GBS IAP is defined as the administration of penicillin G, ampicillin, or cefazolin ≥4 hours before delivery.

[d] For infants who do not improve after initial stabilization and/or those who have severe systemic instability, the administration of empiric antibiotics may be reasonable but is not mandatory.

Fig. 31.2 Risk assessment for early-onset group B streptococcal disease among infants born at <35 weeks of gestation. *GBS*, Group B *Streptococcus*; *IAP*, intrapartum antibiotic prophylaxis; *ROM*, rupture of membranes. (From Kimberlin DW, et al., eds. *Red Book 2021: Report of the Committee on Infectious Diseases.* Itasca, IL: American Academy of Pediatrics; 2021, Fig 3.14.)

- Prevention of perinatal HBV infection relies on the proper and timely identification of infants born to mothers who are hepatitis B surface antigen (HBsAg) positive or of unknown status to ensure the administration of appropriate postexposure immunoprophylaxis with HBV vaccine and hepatitis B immunoglobulin (HBIG) (Fig. 31.3).
- All newborn infants with a birth weight ≥ 2000 g born to HBsAg-negative mothers should receive HBV vaccine by 24 hours of age (birth dose). Those newborns with birth weight < 2000 g born to HBsAg-negative mothers are given HBV vaccine at 1 month of age or at hospital discharge, whichever is first.
- All newborns of all birth weights born to women who are HBsAg-positive are given HBV vaccine at birth plus HBIG by 12 hours of age. Those born to women of unknown HBsAg status are given HBV and HBIG if the mother's status cannot be confirmed to be negative (see Fig. 31.3).
- In addition, HBsAg-positive pregnant women with a high HBV viral load may be eligible for anti-HBV therapy with antiviral agents such as lamivudine and tenofovir; expert consultation is advised.
- Human immunodeficiency virus (HIV)
  - The most important risk factor for vertical transmission of HIV is the maternal plasma HIV RNA viral load.
  - Vertical transmission of HIV is best prevented by a three-part strategy, requiring communication with the clinicians caring for the pregnant woman and consultation with experts in HIV medicine:
    - Ensuring that the mother is receiving a combination antiretroviral therapy regimen and adhering to it
    - Ensuring that the woman receives intrapartum IV zidovudine during labor and delivery if indicated (IV zidovudine may be held if *all* of the following criteria are met for a pregnant woman with HIV infection: receiving antiretroviral therapy during pregnancy; has a plasma HIV RNA viral load of <50 copies/mL within 4 weeks of delivery, and is adherent to their antiretroviral regimen)
    - Providing antiretroviral prophylaxis for the HIV-exposed neonate with zidovudine (and possibly two additional antiretroviral agents such as lamivudine, nevirapine, or raltegravir, depending on the exact circumstances of the mother's therapy and the child's birth) beginning as soon as possible (preferably within 6–12 hours of birth) and lasting for 4 to 6 weeks (depending on the medications used). Expert consultation is strongly advised (see below).
  - Serial virologic testing with nucleic acid amplification tests is required for neonatal diagnosis in all HIV-exposed births because transplacental IgG antibodies will confound the interpretation of standard HIV antibody testing.
    - Virologic testing is performed for all infants three times at a minimum: at 2 to 3 weeks, 4 to 8 weeks, and 4 to 6 months of age. Infants who are at higher risk of HIV acquisition (those with mothers who did not receive prenatal care or antepartum antiretroviral therapy, or who had HIV RNA of >1000 copies/mL near delivery, or who had acute HIV infection during pregnancy) should be tested additionally at birth and at 8 to 10 weeks (i.e., five tests for high-risk infants).

Maternal HBsAg Status	Infant Birthweight (g)	Birth		Follow-up*
HBsAg positive	≥2000	HBV vaccine†HBIG	≤12 h	Complete a 3 dose HBV vaccine series
	<2000	HBV vaccine†HBIG	≤12 h	Complete a 4 dose HBV vaccine series
HBsAg negative	≥2000	HBV vaccine†	≤24 h	Complete a 3 dose HBV vaccine series
	<2000	HBV vaccine†	Hospital discharge or age 1 month	Complete a 3 dose HBV vaccine series
HBsAg unknown	≥2000‡	HBV vaccine†	≤12 h	Complete a 3 dose HBV vaccine series
	<2000	HBV vaccine†HBIG	≤12 h	Complete a 4 dose HBV vaccine series

Adapted from Schillie S, Vellozzi C, Reingold A, et al. Prevention of hepatitis B virus infection in the United States: recommendations of the Advisory Committee on Immunization Practices. *MMWR Recomm Rep.* 2018;67(No. RR-1):1–31. DOI: http://doi.org/10.15585/mmwr.rr6701a1

HBsAg, hepatitis B surface antigen; *HBIG,* hepatitis B immunoglobulin; *HBV,* hepatitis B virus

*4-dose vaccine series acceptable for infants with birth weight ≥2000 g when using combination vaccines to complete the series.

†single-antigen vaccine.

‡mother with unknown status should be tested for HBsAg status as soon as possible after delivery; if found to be HBsAg positive, infant should receive HBIG as soon as possible, no later than 7 days of age.

Fig. 31.3 Administration of birth dose of hepatitis B vaccine by birth weight and maternal HBsAg Status. *HBIG,* Hepatitis B immunoglobulin; *HBsAg,* hepatitis B surface antigen. (Table 3 modified from Schillie S, Vellozzi C, Reingold A, et al. Prevention of Hepatitis B Virus Infection in the United States: Recommendations of the Advisory Committee on Immunization Practices. *MMWR Recomm Rep.* 2018;67(No. RR-1):1–31. DOI: http://dx.doi.org/10.15585/mmwr.rr6701a1.)

- Replacement formula feeding eliminates the additional risk of neonatal HIV infection by breastfeeding. In the United States, where safe infant feeding alternatives are available and are free for women in need, it has long been recommended that HIV-infected women not breastfeed their infants. However, the risk of transmission through breastfeeding is very low, but not zero, for those women on antiretroviral therapy (ART) who have maintained an undetectable HIV viral load and are adherent with their antiretroviral therapy. In selected circumstances, breastfeeding HIV-exposed infants may be considered, in consultation with an expert in pediatric HIV infection (see below). Shared decision making about the nonzero risks of HIV transmission by breastfeeding, as well as possible risk reduction methods (which are reasonable but not yet proven, such as use of infant antiretroviral prophylaxis during breastfeeding and additional virologic monitoring for the mother and child), in addition to the standard antiretroviral prophylaxis recommended for all infants with perinatal HIV exposure, is required.
  - Expert consultation should be obtained for women with HIV infection who are contemplating pregnancy or who are pregnant already and for HIV-exposed neonates. Consultation is available with local or regional HIV experts, or with the National Perinatal HIV Hotline (1-888-448-8765), or at the AIDS Info website (a service of the US Department of Health and Human Services; https://clinicalinfo.hiv.gov/en/guidelines).
- Herpes simplex virus (HSV)
  - During prenatal evaluations, all pregnant women should be asked about past or current signs and symptoms consistent with genital herpes infection in themselves and their sexual partners, but it should be recognized that the absence of previous signs and symptoms of genital herpes infections has poor sensitivity in determining the risk of genital HSV in pregnancy.
  - If a pregnant woman has had active recurrent genital herpes, the American College of Obstetricians and Gynecologists (ACOG) recommends suppressive antiviral therapy at or beyond 36 weeks of gestation for the woman, generally with oral valacyclovir.
  - Neonates born to women with known recurrent genital infection, but no genital lesions at delivery, should be observed by the parents for signs of infection in the first 4 to 6 weeks of life (e.g., vesicular lesions of the skin, respiratory distress, seizures, signs of sepsis) but do not require surface testing by polymerase chain reaction (PCR) or cultures or empiric acyclovir prophylaxis.
  - The management of neonates born to a pregnant woman with active genital lesions is complex; the risk of transmitting HSV to the newborn infant during delivery is influenced directly by the mother's classification of HSV infection, including whether she has primary or recurrent genital HSV infection and perhaps also whether she has some cross-protective immunity from a previous nongenital HSV infection.
  - The risk of HSV transmission varies up to 30-fold more in primary infection than in semi-immune or recurrent infection.
  - If membranes are intact or ruptured for <4 hours, but active genital HSV lesions are seen at delivery, cesarean section is recommended to decrease the risk of HSV transmission.
  - Many experts also will use HSV-1– and HSV-2–specific serologic tests of the mother, in conjunction with surface cultures (performed at 24 hours of age) of the newborn's eyes, skin, mouth, and rectum in an attempt to help guide management of the neonate, with or without empiric prophylactic acyclovir for neonates judged to

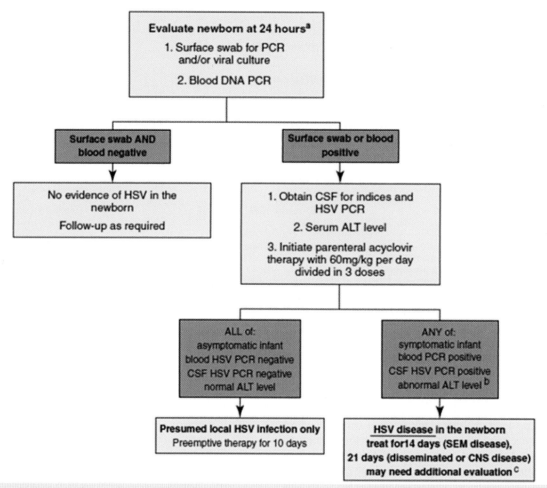

Fig. 31.4 Treatment of a newborn born to a woman with presumed active genital herpes simplex virus (HSV) lesions at delivery in the setting of recurrent genital HSV infection. [a]Awaiting period of 24 hours is currently recommended in this before HSV surface cultures and/or PCRs are obtained for HSV genome detection from the neonate. This approach aids in differentiation of contamination of neonatal skin from maternal secretions from true infection of the newborn. [b]ALT level greater than 2 times the upper limit of normal. [c]Additional evaluation may be required based on symptoms and response to therapy. *ALT*, Alanine aminotransferase; *CSF*, cerebrospinal fluid; *PCR*, polymerase chain reaction. (Modified from Stokes C, Melvin AJ. Viral infections of the fetus and newborn. In: Gleason CA, Sawyer T, eds. *Avery's Diseases of the Newborn.* 11th ed. Philadelphia: Elsevier, 2024, Fig 34.6.)

be at greatest risk of acquiring HSV (see Fig. 31.4 and further discussion in the AAP *Red Book 2021*, cited in the bibliography, for one such approach). Empiric acyclovir is often begun for newborns at 24 hours of age after diagnostic studies are performed. Reevaluation after PCR testing of the baby, as well as noting the clinical course, then determines further therapy (Fig. 31.4).

- Varicella-zoster virus (VZV)
  - Varicella infection (chickenpox) has a higher case-fatality rate in infants when the mother develops varicella from 5 days before to 2 days after delivery because there is little opportunity for the development and transfer of antibody from mother to infant, maternal viremia is recent, and the infant's cellular immune system is immature.
  - When varicella develops in a mother >5 days before delivery and gestational age is 28 weeks or more, the severity of disease in the newborn infant is modified by the transplacental transfer of VZV-specific maternal IgG antibody.
  - If zoster (shingles) develops in a pregnant woman, the infant will not be at risk, because of the transplacental transfer of VZV-specific IgG, unless the neonate is born at <28 weeks.

- Candidates for immunoprophylaxis with VariZIG (a licensed varicella-zoster hyperimmune globulin) or intravenous immunoglobulin (IVIG), if VariZIG is not available, include the following after a valid chickenpox exposure (e.g., household exposure or face to face exposure with a caretaker or staff in hospital):
  - Pregnant women without evidence of VZV immunity
  - Neonates born to women who develop chickenpox (but not zoster) within 5 days before delivery or within 2 days after delivery
  - Premature infants ≥ 28 weeks' gestation whose mother has no history of chickenpox or has no documented serologic immunity to VZV
  - Premature infants <28 weeks' gestation or ≤1000 g birth weight, regardless of maternal history or immunity
- Immunoprophylaxis, if used, should be given as soon as possible, within 10 days of the exposure.
- Airborne and contact precautions are recommended for neonates born to mothers with varicella and, if still hospitalized, should be continued until 21 days of life or until 28 days of age if VariZIG or IGIV was administered.

Transmission	Recommendations/Considerations
Meat and other edibles	• Meat should be cooked up to at least 63°C (145°F) for whole cut meat (excluding poultry), up to at least 71°C (160°F) for ground meat (excluding poultry), and up to at least 74°C (165°F) for all poultry (whole cuts and ground) (a food thermometer should be used) • Meat should be frozen at −20°C (−4°F) for at least 48 hours • Freezing and thawing at specific temperatures for specific time can kill *T gondii* tissue cysts • Infected meat that has been smoked, cured in brine, or dried may still be infectious • Contact with mucous membranes should be avoided when handling raw meat • Gloves should be worn when handling raw meat and hands should be thoroughly washed after handling raw meat • Kitchen surfaces and utensils should be thoroughly washed after contact with raw meat • Drinking unpasteurized goat milk should be avoided • Eating raw oysters, clams, or mussels should be avoided • Skinning or butchering animals without gloves should be avoided
Untreated water	• Drinking untreated water, including that from wells, or water with potential contamination by feces from domestic or wild cats should be avoided
Cat feces and soil	• Contact with material/soil potentially contaminated with cat feces, especially handling of cat litters or gardening, should be avoided. However, if not possible to be avoided, disposable gloves should be worn when gardening and during any contact with soil or sand and hands should be washed with soap and warm water afterward. • Cats should be kept indoors. Stray cats should not be handled or adopted while the woman is pregnant. • Cat litter box should be changed daily, because *T gondii* does not become infectious until 1 to 5 days after it is shed in a cat's feces. • Cats should be fed canned or dried commercial food, not raw or undercooked meats.

Fig. 31.5 Measures for the primary prevention of toxoplasmosis infection in pregnant women. (From Centers for Disease Control and Prevention. Toxoplasmosis (Toxoplasma infection). Available at: www.cdc.gov/parasites/toxoplasmosis/prevent.html. Accessed September 15, 2014.)

■ Zika virus
- ▪ Avoid travel to infected areas; use insect repellents (safe during pregnancy).
- ▪ Couples exposed to Zika virus or traveling from infected areas should avoid pregnancy for 3 months after possible exposure. Breastfeeding of infants may continue by exposed or infected mothers.

Prevention of Specific Parasitic Infection

■ Toxoplasmosis
- ▪ Whether or not to routinely screen all pregnant women for toxoplasmosis is controversial; the preventive effect of such screening depends on the incidence of maternal infection, risk of transmission at different times in pregnancy, whether the transmission to the neonate of the identified infection in the mother is preventable by medical therapy, and receiver–operator characteristics of serologic screening tests.
- ▪ Some European countries perform universal screening of pregnant women, but the lower incidence rates of maternal infection and conflicting data on the cost-effectiveness of screening have not led to a universally agreed-upon regimen in the United States.
- ▪ There are other approaches to the prevention of toxoplasmosis, aside from serologic screening (Fig. 31.5).
  - ▪ Antepartum education should be given about avoiding *Toxoplasma gondii*–related exposures during pregnancy.
  - ▪ Special attention should be paid to meat handling and cooking, in addition to avoidance of cat feces.
  - ▪ Diagnosis of toxoplasmosis in a pregnant woman is complex and may include serologic testing by specialized reference laboratories, PCR tests on amniotic fluid, and serial ultrasound monitoring (see

Chapter 30 and suggested readings below). Expert consultation is advised.
- ▪ Spiramycin is thought to prevent transmission of maternal toxoplasmosis to the fetus but it does not cross the placenta well, so it does not treat an infected fetus reliably; pyrimethamine–sulfadiazine does cross the placenta and treats the fetal infection, and leucovorin (folinic acid) is used to lessen hematologic adverse effects.
- ▪ If a pregnant woman is suspected or confirmed to have acquired toxoplasmosis before the 18th week of the current pregnancy, oral spiramycin is given to the mother to prevent transmission to the fetus; amniocentesis is performed for PCR testing of the amniotic fluid as soon as possible at or after 18 weeks' gestation, and fetal ultrasonography is performed every 4 weeks.
  - ☐ If the PCR test result of the amniotic fluid is negative and the ultrasonography remains normal, spiramycin is continued until delivery.
  - ☐ If the amniotic fluid PCR test result is positive and/or fetal ultrasonography is suggestive of congenital infection, then maternal therapy with oral pyrimethamine plus sulfadiazine plus leucovorin is given from ~18 weeks' gestation until delivery.
- ▪ If a pregnant woman is suspected or confirmed to have acquired toxoplasmosis after the 18th week of the current pregnancy, oral pyrimethamine plus sulfadiazine plus leucovorin is given to the woman through delivery.
- ▪ Spiramycin is not commercially available in the United States. It can be obtained at no cost (provided by Sanofi-Aventis) through consultation (with the Dr. Jack S. Remington Laboratory for Specialty Diagnostics at SutterHealth, 1-650-853-4828, or the US Food and Drug Administration, 1-301-796-1600). An Investigational New Drug application may be required.

Suggested Readings

Flannery DD, Puopolo KM. Neonatal early-onset sepsis. *NeoReviews*. 2022;23:756–770. doi:10.1542/neo.23-10-e756.

Flannery DD, Edwards EM, Coggins SA, Horbar JD, Puopolo KM. Late-onset sepsis among very preterm infants. *Pediatrics*. 2022;150:e2022058813.

Kimberlin DW, Barnett E, Lynfield R, Sawyer MH, eds. *Red Book 2021: Report of the Committee on Infectious Diseases*. Itasca, IL: American Academy of Pediatrics; 2021.

Puopolo KM, Benitz WE, Zaoutis TE. AAP Committee on Fetus and NewbornCommittee on Infectious Diseases. Management of neonates born at ≥35 0/7 weeks' gestation with suspected or proven early-onset bacterial sepsis. *Pediatrics*. 2018;142:e20182894.

Puopolo KM, Benitz WE, Zaoutis TE. AAP Committee on Fetus and NewbornCommittee on Infectious Diseases. Management of neonates born at ≤34 6/7 weeks' gestation with suspected or proven early-onset bacterial sepsis. *Pediatrics*. 2018;142:e20182896.

Puopolo KM, Lynfield R, Cummings JJ. AAP Committee on Fetus and NewbornCommittee on Infectious Diseases. Management of infants at risk for group B streptococcal disease. *Pediatrics*. 2019;144:e20191881.

Valentine GC, Wallen LD. Neonatal bacterial sepsis and meningitis. In: Gleason CA, Sawyer T, eds. *Avery's Diseases of the Newborn*. 11th ed. Philadelphia: Saunders; 2024:439–533.

NUTRITION

KENDRA HENDRICKSON and WILLIAM W. HAY, JR.

32 *Nutrition and Growth*

KENDRA HENDRICKSON and WILLIAM W. HAY, JR.

The Fetus

CHANGES IN BODY COMPOSITION

Growth of Fetal Size

- Fetal weight increases exponentially in the middle of gestation, then slows during the latter third of gestation.

Weight interval (g)	Growth rate (g/kg/d)
500–1000	20–23
1000–1500	17–20
1500–2000	14–17
2000–2500	12–14

Under usual conditions, the fetus grows at its genetic potential. Small fetuses of small parents or large fetuses of large parents do not reflect fetal growth restriction or fetal overgrowth, respectively; in fact, their rates of growth are normal for their genome.

- The smaller (generally, shorter) the mother, the more she limits fetal growth by "maternal constraint," which represents a limitation of uterine size. Uterine size is directly related to maternal height; thus, a shorter mother will have a smaller uterus with reduced endometrial surface area and the capacity for placental growth.
- Normal human fetuses grow at an average rate of 15 to 20 g/kg/d among different populations with a mean of ~17 g/kg/d from 24 to 36 weeks, with symmetrical growth of head and length.

Developmental Change of Fetal Body Composition

- Nonfat dry weight and nitrogen content (predictors of protein content and lean body mass) show a linear relationship with fetal weight and an exponential relationship with gestational age (GA).
- 80% of the nitrogen content of the fetus is in protein.
- With advancing gestation, fetal protein synthesis rate declines.
  - Skeletal muscle has a lower protein synthetic rate in late gestation than in earlier gestation.
- Fat production in the fetus begins at the start of the third trimester.
  - Rate of fetal fat accretion is linear between 36 and 40 weeks' gestation but can be increased or decreased by excess or reductions, respectively, of maternal sugar and fat dietary intakes.
  - By the end of gestation, fat accretion ranges from 1.6 to 3.4 g/kg/d.

- By term, fat content of the human fetus is 12% to 18% of body weight.
  - Fat content is <10% in severely intrauterine growth restriction (IUGR) fetuses.
  - Fat content is >20% in macrosomic infants of diabetic mothers.
- Rate of fetal fatty acid oxidation is low due to:
  - Plasma fatty acid concentrations are low.
  - The carnitine palmitoyl transferase enzyme system is not sufficiently developed to deliver long-chain fatty acids to the respiration pathway inside the mitochondria.
- Fetal water content increases directly with body weight (as fraction of body weight, it decreases with advancing gestation).
- Extracellular water decreases are greater than intracellular water as gestation advances due to increased cell number and increased cell size.
- Many tissues in the fetus (brain, liver, lung, heart, and skeletal muscle) produce glycogen over the second half of gestation.
  - Liver glycogen content is the most important store of carbohydrate (CHO) for systemic glucose needs immediately after birth.
    - Fetal liver glycogen concentration is ~80 to 120 mg/g at term, twice adult concentrations.
  - Skeletal muscle glycogen content increases during late gestation (source of glucose for glycolysis within the myocytes).
  - Lung glycogen content decreases in late gestation with:
    - Loss of glycogen-containing alveolar epithelial cells
    - Development of type II pneumocytes
    - Onset of surfactant production
  - Cardiac glycogen is essential for postnatal cardiac energy metabolism and function.
- Macrosomic fetuses of diabetic mothers have higher body and organ contents of glycogen.
- IUGR fetuses have normal to increased liver glycogen content, but this declines near term.

NUTRIENT REQUIREMENTS

Glucose

- Glucose is the principal substrate in the fetus for maintenance of energy production and expenditure, energy storage as glycogen in liver and skeletal muscle, and energy requirements of protein synthesis and growth.
- Glucose utilization rates (GURs) in the human fetus:

- Higher at mid-gestation: 7 to 9 mg/kg/min at 24 to 28 weeks' gestation when fetal brain size, fetal growth, and protein synthetic rates are twice that at term
- The GUR declines to 3 to 5 mg/kg/min at term as bone, fat, and muscle (which use less glucose than the brain and heart) increase as fractions of body weight.

Amino Acids

- Amino acids (AAs) are supplied to the fetus at 3.5 to 4 g/kg/d at 24 to 28 weeks' gestation (decreases to 1.5–2 g/kg/d at term).

Fatty Acids

- Fatty acid (FA) uptake rates by the human fetus have not been measured.
  - FAs are used for structural components of membranes and for growth of adipose tissue in later gestation.
  - FA oxidation rates are low in the fetus due to limited supply and lack of enzymes necessary for mitochondrial fatty acid uptake.

FACTORS THAT INFLUENCE INTRAUTERINE GROWTH

Hormonal Factors

- Insulin and insulin-like growth factors contribute to fetal growth by promoting cell replication earlier in gestation and hypertrophy later in gestation.
- Fetal insulin production begins at the start of the second trimester and increases in response to glucose and AAs as gestation progresses.
- Insulin and AAs promote the production of insulin-like growth factor 1 (IGF-1), which enhances growth.
- The predominant growth-regulating effect of insulin in the fetus is its capacity to enhance glucose utilization, but it also enhances AA utilization for protein synthesis.

Maternal, Placental, and Fetal Factors

- Fetal growth is regulated by placental size and the rate of placental transfer of oxygen and nutrients (AAs for protein synthesis, glucose for energy production) to the fetus.
- Fetal weight in late gestation correlates positively with placental weight.
- Oxygen transport to the fetus by the placenta is facilitated by increases in uteroplacental blood flow.
- Transport of glucose and AAs is determined by the trophoblast membrane exchange area, transporter concentrations, and activity in the trophoblast membranes.
- AAs are actively concentrated in the trophoblast intracellular matrix by Na^+/K^+–adenosine triphosphatase and H^+-dependent transporter proteins at the maternal-facing microvillus membrane of the trophoblast and then transported into the fetal plasma to concentrations higher than maternal levels.
- Net total fetal AAs uptake is 30% to 40% of the combined carbon requirements for oxidative metabolism and provides 100% of the fetal nitrogen requirements.

- AAs are directly transported from maternal to fetal plasma by the placenta or may be metabolized into other AAs, which then interact with metabolic pathways in the fetus that:
  - Recycle certain AAs to the placenta
  - Promote vascular development (arginine producing nitric oxide)
  - Promote oxidation (ketoisocaproic acid from leucine)
  - Promote protein synthesis (including synthesis of nonessential AAs)
- Skeletal muscle in later gestation is a major consumer of both essential and nonessential AAs from the circulation.
- Evidence for a relatively high rate of fetal oxidation of AAs comes from three observations:
  - AAs are taken up by the fetus in excess of their rate of deposition in fetal protein.
  - Fetal urea production rates are high.
  - Fetal infusions of carbon-labeled AAs in animal models demonstrate fetal production and excretion of labeled carbon dioxide.
- The rate of glucose transfer from maternal to fetal plasma is directly related to the maternal glucose concentration.
- Placental glucose transport increases progressively over gestation.
  - Reflecting growth of the surface area of the trophoblast
  - Reflecting increased numbers of glucose transporters
- The concentration of glucose in the fetal plasma declines relative to maternal plasma glucose in the second half of gestation.
- Three principal mechanisms are responsible for the increase in fetal glucose clearance:
  - The size, cellularity, and glucose metabolic rate of the brain increase relative to other fetal tissues and organs.
  - Progressive development of fetal insulin secretion by the expanding mass of pancreatic islets and beta cells
  - Increased growth of insulin-sensitive tissues (skeletal muscle, heart, adipose tissue)
- Free FAs are transported by concentration-dependent plasma membrane fatty acid transport/binding proteins and cytoplasmic fatty acid-binding proteins (FABPs).
  - Transport is increased when maternal concentrations are high.
  - Transport of essential long-chain polyunsaturated fatty acids (linoleic acid and its omega-6 product, arachidonic acid; linolenic acid and its omega-3 product, docosahexaenoic acid) involves specific transporters and binding proteins and is dependent on maternal diet.
- Normal variations in maternal nutrition have little effect on fetal growth. They do not alter maternal plasma concentrations of nutrients or the rate of uterine blood flow (determinants of nutrient substrate delivery to and transport by the placenta).
- Maternal diets lower in simple sugars, higher in complex carbohydrates, and limited in total lipid potentially prevent later life obesity in these offspring.
- Adequate maternal intake of omega-3 polyunsaturated FAs during pregnancy benefits fetal neurodevelopment.

Newborn Infants

CHANGES IN BODY COMPOSITION

- Significant portions of preterm infants have IUGR and tend to be small for gestational age (SGA).
- For the first few postnatal days, all newborn infants lose extracellular fluid and thus body weight.
- The more preterm the infant, the slower the growth of the body in all compartments.
- The majority of very preterm infants remain relatively growth restricted by term gestation.
    - A principal cause is insufficient nutrition (primarily of protein).
    - Other causes include intermittent hypoxia, stress with increased catabolic hormone secretion, and sepsis, as well as treatments such as steroids, catecholamines, diuretics, and ventilation.
- By term, preterm infants are shorter and lighter than term infants, with relatively more fat than lean mass.

ENERGY REQUIREMENTS

- Energy needs for preterm infants to achieve normal growth rates (Tables 32.1, 32.2)
    - Total energy intake must be sufficient to support basal metabolism (~50 kcal/kg/d).
    - Growth of lean mass requires additional energy (15 kcal/kg/d).
    - Growth of fat mass uses additional energy (20–30 kcal/kg/d).
    - Energy lost in stools increases with enteral feeding (5–15 kcal/kg/d).
    - Physical activity accounts for 0% to 5% of total energy expenditure in preterm infants.
    - Total energy needs are reduced to 0 to 10 kcal/kg/d for infants in incubators/radiant warmers.
    - Achieving recommended energy intakes in very preterm, very low-birth-weight infants during the first few postnatal days exclusively by the parenteral route with standard infusion rates of dextrose and lipid can result in hyperglycemia, which has been associated with increased morbidity and mortality.
- There is no evidence that energy intake above normal levels enhances neurological development or achieves appropriate growth and body composition.
- Higher energy intakes in preterm infants result in greater fat accumulation compared to normally growing fetuses of the same GA, but there is no evidence that this extra accumulation during the NICU period persists into infancy and childhood.

Table 32.1 Energy Requirements for Preterm Infants to Achieve Normal Growth Rates (kcal/kg/d)

Enterally Fed Infants		Intravenously Fed Infants	
Resting energy expenditure (REE)	40–50	Resting energy expenditure	40–50
Activity (0–5% of REE)	0–5	Activity	0–5
Thermoregulation	0–10	Thermoregulation	0–5
Thermic effect of protein synthesis	15	Thermic effect of protein synthesis	15
Fecal loss of energy	5–15	Fecal loss of energy	0
Energy storage (growth)	20–30	Energy storage (growth)	20–30
Total	80–125	Total	60–105

PROTEIN INTAKE IN NEWBORNS

Essential and Nonessential Amino Acids

- Essential AAs cannot be synthesized in body cells and must be obtained from exogenous sources for normal maintenance and growth; they are indispensable for growth.
    - Essential AAs include leucine, isoleucine, valine, lysine, threonine, tryptophan, methionine, phenylalanine, and histidine.
- Nonessential AAs can be synthesized in body cells.
    - Nonessential AAs are also fundamental for growth because they produce polyamines (specifically, spermidine synthase), which are required for the activation of protein synthesis.
- Conditionally essential AAs: At critical stages of development (in the fetus or preterm infant of similar GA), some AAs may not be synthesized sufficiently.
    - Conditionally essential AAs include tyrosine, glutamine, arginine, cysteine, glycine, and proline.

Protein Requirements of Newborns

- Protein requirement of the healthy term infant in the first month of life is 1.5 to 2 g/kg/d.
- Protein requirement of preterm infants is higher (2.5–4.5 g/kg/d), depending on gestational age.
    - Critical amount of AAs for preventing growth faltering in very preterm infants (<30–32 weeks) is ~1.5 g/kg/d.
    - AAs >3.5 to 4 g/kg/d parenterally or 4 to 4.5 g/kg/d enterally in very preterm infants offer no advantage.
- Protein accretion is linearly related to protein intake at any energy intake:
    - ~1.5 to 2 g/kg/d at term
    - 2.5 to 3 g/kg/d at ~30 to 36 weeks
    - 3.5 to 4 g/kg/d at ~24 to 30 weeks

Table 32.2 Nutrition and Growth

| Weight | PARENTERAL | | | | ENTERAL | |
| | Kcal/kg/d | | Protein (g/kg/d) | | Kcal/kg/d | Protein (g/kg/d) |
	Starting	Goal	Starting	Goal		Goal Intake
<1000 g	45–55	100–115	2.5–3	3.5–4	110–130	3.5–4
<2000 g	60–70	90–110	2.5–3	3.5	110–130	3.5–4
≥2000 g	45–70	90–110	2.5–3	3	105–125	2.5–3
Term	45–70	90–105	2.5–3	2.5–3	90–105	1.5–2.5

- Rates of protein synthesis and the requirements for AA and protein supply are the same in preterm infants as in normally growing fetuses of the same gestational age.
- Protein accretion increases directly with protein intake and sufficient energy for protein synthesis to maximal rates for gestational age.
- Excess protein intake can produce higher blood urea and ammonia concentrations (seldom to toxic levels).
  - Increased ammonia and urea are appropriate as protein intake is increased (suggests normally functioning amino acid oxidation, hepatic urea synthesis, and renal excretion).
  - Venous plasma concentrations of urea (>60 mg/dL) and ammonia (>100 μmol/L) are usually confounded by renal and liver failure.
  - Protein intake > carbohydrate (CHO) and lipid diets in preterm infants produce leaner infants by term.
  - Higher protein intake with adequate CHO and lipid intake increases weight gain with a higher percentage of lean body mass.

Protein Metabolism in Newborn Infants

- Protein digestion begins in the stomach and duodenum with acid hydrolysis.
- Basal and pentagastrin-stimulated acid secretion doubles from the first to fourth week after birth in preterm infants.
- Proteases (enterokinase) is produced in the upper small intestine in response to food.
  - Despite low gastrointestinal proteases in preterm infants, there is no evidence of insufficient protein digestion.
- Activation of trypsinogen, the key enzyme in initiating the cascade of protein digestion by proteases, is essential.
- Trypsinogen levels should be 6% at 25 to 30 weeks' gestation and 29% at term of older children.
- Hydrolyzed protein formulas increase amino acid absorption and reduce time to full enteral feeds.
  - They do not promote greater protein balance for the same protein intake.
  - They have lower total amino acid contents than nonhydrolyzed protein formulas.

FAT INTAKE IN NEWBORNS

Essential and Nonessential Fatty Acids

- Preterm infants have insufficient capacity for de novo synthesis of long-chain polyunsaturated fatty acids (LC-PUFAs), so they need to obtain them from their diet.
- Linoleic acid (18:2, omega-6) and α-linolenic acid (18:3, omega-3) are the only fatty acids known to be essential for complete nutrition.

Features of Essential Fatty Acid Deficiency

- Clinical cases of essential fatty acid (EFA) deficiency are relatively rare.
- EFA deficiency (severe and prolonged) can lead to a clinical syndrome consisting of:
  - Dermatitis (perianal region)
  - Thrombocytopenia
  - Infection

- Failure to thrive
- An increased triene/tetraene ratio
- Prevention of EFA deficiency includes enteral feeding of milk as soon as possible after birth.
- When intravenous nutrition is used, it must meet the minimum requirements for EFA with IV lipid emulsions:
  - 0.5 to 1 g/kg/d intake in the form of IV lipid from soybean oil or as 2 g/kg/d for multicomponent lipid emulsions such as Smoflipid emulsion, both given as 20% (0.2 g/mL) solutions
  - A minimum linoleic acid intake of 0.25 g/kg/d in preterm infants and 0.1 g/kg/d in term infants also supplies adequate amounts of linolenic acid.
- Preterm infants may benefit from LC-PUFA supplementation (important for growth and brain and visual development), but this has not been confirmed with longer term outcome studies.
  - Term and preterm formulas have added docosahexaenoic acid (DHA) and arachidonic acid (ARA).

Fat Requirements of Preterm and Full-Term Infants

- Human neonates have relatively high white fat content: 12% to 18% of body weight at term.
- Term infants also have stores of brown fat (necessary for neonatal thermogenesis).
- In utero fat deposition occurs predominantly during the last 12 to 14 weeks of gestation.
- Dietary fats are important to sustain growth, provide EFAs, and promote the absorption of fat-soluble vitamins.
- Fat intakes of 2 to 3 g/kg/d IV in the first few days of life provide sufficient LC-PUFAs and calories for basal metabolism and prevention of EFA deficiency.
- Recommended dietary fat intakes in infants consist of 40% to 55% of total calories (4.4–6.0 g/100 kcal) as provided by normal breast feeding.

Fat Metabolism in Newborn Infants

- Newborn infants digest fat and absorb fatty acids from the gastrointestinal tract less efficiently than older children.
- Preterm infants demonstrate even greater deficiencies in fat digestion and metabolism.
- Preterm infants have malabsorption of 10% to 30% of dietary fat due to a small bile acid pool and relative lack of pancreatic lipase.
  - Bile acids are essential to emulsify large fat globules of long-chain fatty acids and to facilitate lipid hydrolysis and are lower in preterm infants.
  - Bile-stimulated lipase activity is higher in milk of mothers delivering preterm than in those delivering at term.
  - Bile-stimulated lipase activity is decreased in pasteurized milk.
- Additional fat digestion occurs due to lingual and gastric lipases (lipase in human milk).
- Pancreatic lipases are less available for fat digestion and absorption.
- Preterm formulas and human milk fortifiers have high percentages of fat from medium-chain triglycerides (do not require bile acid emulsification).

CARBOHYDRATE INTAKE IN NEWBORNS

Carbohydrate Requirements

- Newborns exhaust the supply of stored glucose from the liver within 12 hours of birth if milk/formula or IV glucose is not provided.
  - The normal glucose utilization rate in the term newborn is 3 to 5 mg/kg/min.
  - Glucose is the primary energy source for brain metabolism.
- Maintenance of normal plasma glucose concentrations is fundamental.
  - Vital organs (brain and heart) take up glucose according to plasma glucose concentrations and not IV infusion rates or rates of hepatic glucose production.
  - When plasma glucose concentrations decline, the newborn brain may use ketone bodies as additional energy sources.
  - Glucose concentrations are limited in very preterm and SGA infants with IUGR.
- Provision of 40% to 50% of total caloric intake as CHO (10–12 g/kg/d) prevents accumulation of ketone bodies and hypoglycemia in the newborn.
  - This amount of CHO is supplied as lactose in human milk or formulas.

Carbohydrate Metabolism in Newborn Infants

- 50% of an infant's energy needs are normally provided by CHO metabolism.
- Glucose is largely derived from exogenous CHO sources when glycogenolysis has exhausted stored hepatic glucose.
  - Gluconeogenesis develops soon after birth and is not easily suppressed by increases in plasma glucose or insulin concentrations.
- Mechanisms for enteral CHO digestion and absorption mature in a defined sequence in the human fetus.
  - Sucrase, maltase, and isomaltase are fully active by 24 to 28 weeks' gestation.
  - Lactase is not fully active at birth until term, but lactose intolerance is uncommon.
  - Pancreatic amylase activity remains low until after term birth.
  - Salivary amylase activity is present even in very preterm infants.
- Other CHOs (e.g., mannose, inositol) and oligosaccharides (prebiotics) play important roles in nutrition and organ development for the preterm infant.
  - Mannose is an essential CHO for protein glycosylation and normal neural development.
  - Inositol is present in high concentrations in human milk and can be synthesized by newborn infants of ≥33 weeks' gestation.
- Predominant CHO in human milk is lactose (glucose + galactose).
  - Galactose provides 50% of the calories derived from lactose.
  - Galactose plays a major metabolic role in energy storage.
  - The newborn liver readily incorporates galactose from the portal circulation into hepatic glycogen.

- Digestion of complex CHO occurs in the lumen of the intestine, and nutrient absorption occurs at the enterocyte interface (microvillus membrane).
- CHO absorption is limited initially in neonates by a relative deficiency of lactase (splits lactose into glucose and galactose).
  - Lactase activity in an infant < 34 weeks' gestation is 30% of a normal term infant.
  - Lactase functional activity increases with feeding in preterm infants and approaches term levels by 10 days after birth.
  - 20% of dietary lactose reaches the colon in neonates, where it lowers pH.
  - It promotes colonic growth of *Bifidobacterium* and *Lactobacillus*.
- Preterm formulas have reduced lactose content (40–50% of the total CHO).
  - Milk fortifiers provide little or no lactose.
- If there are signs of lactose intolerance (frequent loose stools, abdominal distention, or positive stool reducing substances), a lactose-free infant formula may be considered.
- Helpful for calculations: energy from fat, 9 kcal/g; protein, 4 kcal/g; carbohydrate, 4 kcal/g

Large- and Small-for-Gestational-Age Infants

CLASSIFICATION OF FETAL GROWTH

- Small-for-gestational-age (SGA) infants have a birth weight < 10th percentile for gestational age.
- Appropriate-for-gestational age (AGA) infants have a birth weight between the 10th and 90th percentiles for gestational age.
- Large-for-gestational age (LGA) infants have a birth weight > 90th percentile for gestational age.
- Intrauterine growth restriction (IUGR) infants have a slower than normal rate of fetal growth at any gestational age.
- Macrosomic infants weigh >4500 g at term birth.
- Normal-birth-weight infants weigh >2500 g at term birth.
- Low-birth-weight (LBW) infants weigh <2500 g at any gestational age.
- Very low-birth-weight (VLBW) infants weigh <1500 g at any gestational age.
- Extremely low-birth-weight (ELBW) infants weigh <1000 g at any gestational age.

Postnatal Growth Patterns of SGA and IUGR Infants

- SGA infants are not growth restricted in utero; with small mothers and fathers, they tend to grow along the lower growth percentiles at which they were born.
  - They are constitutionally shorter later in life.
  - Head circumference growth increases in proportion to length and weight.
- SGA infants with recent IUGR due to nutritional deficiency from placental insufficiency tend to catch up in growth.
- IUGR refers to a slower than normal rate of fetal growth.

- Undernutrition from placental insufficiency is the leading cause of IUGR in developed countries.
- Maternal undernutrition is the leading cause in less developed countries.
- Chronically IUGR fetuses develop decreased capacity for amino acid synthesis into protein and for cell growth.
  - Leads to decreased muscle mass and glucose intolerance (reduced glucose uptake and utilization capacity)
  - Often have evidence of increased protein breakdown
  - Persistent slower growth is common.
  - Later-life shorter stature, smaller brains, reduced fat free mass, and reduced neurocognitive development

IUGR Infant Nutrition

- There is no consensus about the optimal amount of protein to feed SGA and IUGR infants.
  - Provide weight-appropriate amounts of milk and limit amino acid in total parenteral nutrition (TPN) to 3.0 to 3.5 g/kg/d.
  - Evidence for benefit or risk from restricting nutrition for these IUGR infants is lacking.
- IUGR infants characteristically develop both hyperglycemia (usually early after birth) and hypoglycemia (usually later).
- Initial hyperglycemia in IUGR neonates is due to decreased pancreatic insulin secretion from hypoxia-stimulated catecholamine suppression and reduced fetal pancreatic beta cell proliferation (response to reduced glucose, amino acid, growth factor stimulation, and hypoxia).
  - IUGR fetuses tend to produce glucose from their livers (which normal fetuses do not) by uniquely developed hepatic insulin resistance in response to glucocorticoids and hypoxia.
  - After birth (24–72 hours), hyperglycemia can occur due to continued stress, hypoxia, high catecholamine concentrations that suppress insulin secretion, and high rates of IV glucose infusion.
- Once stabilized, IUGR newborn infants often develop hypoglycemia, which can continue for days to weeks. Causes of hypoglycemia in IUGR infant:
  - IUGR infants with asymmetric growth restriction have higher brain-to-liver weight ratios and thus a higher body weight–specific glucose utilization rate.
  - Adjusting IV glucose infusion rates to a body weight more consistent with the head circumference often helps avoid insufficient glucose infusion rates for the brain, which is where most of the glucose is used in the body.
  - IUGR fetuses respond to chronically reduced glucose supply and concentrations by upregulating glucose transporters and the maintenance of glucose utilization by all organs (sustaining normal cellular metabolism).
  - As oxygenation improves, catecholamines diminish, reducing their suppression of insulin secretion.
- Frequent enteral feedings day and night are the best approach to treating mild to moderate hypoglycemia in IUGR infants.
  - Oral dextrose gel can be used up to several times to supplement enteral feeding if the infant is relatively stable and the glucose concentrations are increasing

into the normal range (54 mg/dL [3.0 mmol/L] to 108 mg/dL [6 mmol/L]).
  - Serious hypoglycemia involves severe clinical signs such as flaccid hypotonia with apnea, coma, and seizures, which should be treated immediately with IV dextrose infusions by a bolus (200 mg/kg)–constant infusion (5–7 mg/kg/min) approach with frequent (every 30 minutes until stable for 2–4 hours) follow-up plasma glucose concentration measurements and enteral feeding as soon as tolerated.
  - Rarely, diazoxide can be used to suppress insulin secretion when hypoglycemia is marked and persistent (more than 1–2 weeks); this agent has serious side effects, including pulmonary edema and pulmonary hypertension, requiring close clinical monitoring both in the hospital and at home.

Large-for-Gestational-Age Infants

- LGA infants can be normal, coming from large mothers and fathers, or they can be due to excess energy intake and fat production (macrosomia), the latter in infants of gestational diabetics and infants whose mothers were obese or with metabolic syndrome.
- Exposure to high glucose concentrations produces a common fetal and neonatal phenotype of excess adiposity and high insulin secretion rates, especially in response to sudden hyperglycemia, leading to rebound hypoglycemia.
- It is best to rely on frequent plasma/blood glucose concentration measurements to guide treatment, as there is little correlation between mild to moderate "symptoms" (signs) of hypoglycemia and actual glucose concentrations.
- Initiate enteral feeding as soon as possible after birth to diminish IV glucose stimulation of insulin secretion.
  - Oral dextrose gel can be used in otherwise stable term infants of diabetic mothers (IDMs). Up to several doses of oral dextrose gel can be used, along with enteral feeding and frequent glucose monitoring.
  - It has a modest risk of producing acute increases in glucose concentration that can stimulate insulin secretion and secondary or rebound hypoglycemia.
  - Smaller and more frequent feedings and often continuous enteral feeding via orogastric/nasogastric tubes can prevent hyperinsulinism.
- Term IDMs who are not acutely hypoglycemic have total GURs of only 3 to 4 mg/kg/min, considerably below the infusion rates many of these infants receive.
  - Contributing to this lower body weight–specific utilization rate is the larger fat mass in these infants.
  - Adjusting IV glucose infusion rates to a body weight more consistent with the head circumference in IDMs often helps avoid advancing to higher glucose infusion rates with the risk of stimulating excess insulin secretion.

FETAL ORIGINS OF ADULT-ONSET DISORDERS

- Fetal nutritional deprivation produces adaptive mechanisms to help ensure survival to birth.

- Programming: Adaptive mechanisms may persist after birth into adulthood.
  - Upregulation of glucose and insulin sensitivity from increased glucose transporters and insulin receptors
  - Diminished insulin secretion
  - Reduced muscle mass and lean body growth (includes bone and brain)
- Such programming allows later life insults ("second hits") such as excess glucose from high simple sugar diets and total energy to promote development of obesity, type 2 diabetes, and cardiovascular disorders (metabolic syndrome).
- Both IUGR and macrosomic infants are at increased risk to develop this common later life phenotype.
- The more preterm the infant at birth, the higher the prevalence of hypertension, obesity, metabolic syndrome, and fatty liver index in an adult who was born preterm versus an adult born at term.
- Rapid postnatal growth rate in the first to second year of life: weight gain > growth rates of length and head circumference, sign of excess energy intake and production of fat (risk of later obesity).

Suggested Readings

Hay Jr. WW. Growth and development: physiological aspects. In: Caballero B, ed. *Encyclopedia of Human Nutrition*. 4th ed. Cambridge, MA: Academic Press; 2023;4:66–82.

Hay Jr. WW. Nutritional support strategies for the preterm infant in the neonatal intensive care unit. *Pediatr Gastroenterol Hepatol Nutr.* 2018;21:234–247.

Hay Jr. WW. Optimal nutritional management for prevention and treatment of chronic lung disease (CLD, or BPD—bronchopulmonary dysplasia) in preterm infants. In: Kallapur SG, Pryhuber GS, eds. *Updates on Neonatal Chronic Lung Disease*. San Diego, CA: Elsevier; 2020:177–193.

Hay Jr. WW, Philip AGS, Stevenson DK. Intrauterine growth restriction. In: Stevenson DK, Benitz W, Sunshine P, Hintz S, Druzin M, eds. *Fetal and Neonatal Brain Injury*. 5th ed. Cambridge: Cambridge University Press; 2017:89–115.

Huff KA, Denne SC, Hay Jr. WW. Energy requirements and carbohydrates in preterm infants. In: Koletzko B, Cheah F-C, Domellöf M, Poindexter BB, Vain N, van Goudoever JB, eds. *Nutritional Care of Preterm Infants*. Basel: Karger; 2021:60–74.

33 Minerals, Vitamins, and Trace Minerals

KENDRA HENDRICKSON and WILLIAM W. HAY, JR.

Minerals

NEONATAL MINERAL REQUIREMENTS AT VARIOUS GESTATIONAL AGES

- Sodium (Na), chloride (Cl), and potassium (K) intakes are restricted to 0 to 2 mmol/kg/d after birth due to delayed urinary flow rates exacerbated by respiratory distress syndrome (RDS).
  - Avoid volume and sodium overload, and allow diuresis to occur.
- When urinary flow rates have been established, the requirements of Na, K, and Cl are between 2 and 4 mmol/kg/d (higher for preterm infants when their urinary flow rates are high, as well as for growth requirements).
- After this period, urinary excretion of electrolytes depends on intake.
- Cl intake is restricted when dilutional acidosis occurs.
- Cl is added when respiratory failure leads to CO_2 retention, with bicarbonate retention producing metabolic alkalosis.
- Typical urinary concentrations for Na are 20 to 40 mmol/L; for K, 10 to 30 mmol/L.
- For infants receiving diuretic therapy, urinary Na concentrations can reach up to 70 mmol/L.
- Insufficient Na intake impairs longitudinal growth and lean mass gain.

REQUIREMENTS OF MINERALS AT VARIOUS GESTATIONAL AGES

- Enteral absorption rates for both calcium (Ca) and phosphorus (P) are limited in preterm infants.
  - They are enhanced with calcium- and phosphorus-enriched preterm formulas.
- Adequate enteral intake for term infants in the first 6 months of life:
  - Calcium, 70 mg/kg/d
  - Phosphorus, ~100 mg/d
- Enteral requirements for preterm infants are much higher due to more active bone formation and remodeling:
  - Calcium, 150 to 220 mg/kg/d
  - Phosphorus, 60 to 140 mg/kg/d
  - The ideal enteral Ca:P ratio is 1.8:1 to 2:1 mg, weight basis.
- Fortification of human milk is used to ensure adequate intakes of Ca and P to preterm infants fed human milk (mother's milk and donor milk).
- Recommended intravenous (IV) intakes of Ca and P are lower than enteral requirements, as there is no or minimal stool loss with IV intakes:

- Calcium, 65 to 100 mg/kg/d
- Phosphorus, 50 to 80 mg/kg/d
- The ideal IV Ca:P ratio is 1.3:1 to 1.7:1 mg, weight basis.
- Risk factors in preterm infants for Ca and P deficiency (subsequent rickets) are:
  - Gestational age <27 weeks or birth weight <1000 g
  - Long-term parenteral nutrition (>4–5 weeks)
  - Severe BPD requiring diuretics
  - Fluid restriction
  - Long-term steroid treatment
  - History of necrotizing enterocolitis (NEC)
  - Intolerance to enteral formula or human milk
- Preterm infants that are intrauterine growth restriction (IUGR), small for gestational age (SGA), <30 weeks' gestation, or fed excess IV amino acids and energy after birth are at risk for refeeding hypophosphatemia.
  - The presence of two or more risk factors compounds the risk.
  - A molar ratio of 0.8 to 1:1 in the early days of total parenteral nutrition (TPN) is recommended.
  - Phosphorus levels should be monitored daily in the first days of life.
  - Severe hypophosphatemia can result in muscle weakness, respiratory failure, cardiac dysfunction, and death.
- Hypercalcemia
  - Hypercalcemia is due to excess delivery of calcium or vitamin D or inadequate phosphorus delivery.
  - Maternal disorders of hypoparathyroidism, parathyroid hyperplasia, abnormal renal function, and Williams syndrome can contribute.
  - Symptoms include lethargy, seizures, hypertension, constipation, abdominal pain from intestinal cramping.
- Hyperphosphatemia
  - Hyperphosphatemia is due to excess delivery of phosphorus.
  - Abnormal renal function, hypoparathyroidism
- Magnesium is an essential part of the bone matrix.
  - Enteral requirements are 8 to 15 mg/kg/d.
  - Supplementation during pregnancy
  - Maternal treatment is used in a setting of pre-eclampsia to prevent seizures.
  - Magnesium may be given for neuroprotection of the fetus to reduce rates of cerebral palsy.
  - Prenatal dosing may result in hypermagnesemia of the newborn; hypotonia is the most common clinical sign, but respiratory depression and hypotension are also possible.

Table 33.1 Recommended Vitamin and Trace Mineral Intakes for Enterally Fed Preterm and Term Infants

	Term (per 100 kcal)	Preterm (per 100 kcal)
Vitamin A (µg RE)	60–150	365–1000
Vitamin D (IU)	40–100	400–1000
Vitamin E (mg α-TE/100 kcal)	0.5–5	2–10
Vitamin K (µg RE)	1–25	4–25
Vitamin C (mg)	6–15	18–55
Pantothenic acid (mg)	0.3–1.2	0.5–1.9
Biotin (µg/kg)	1–15	1.5–15
Thiamine (vitamin B_1) (µg)	30–200	140–300
Riboflavin (vitamin B_2) (µg)	80–300	200–400
Niacin (vitamin B_3) (µg)	550–2000	900–5000
Pyridoxine (vitamin B_6) (µg)	30–130	50–300
Cobalamin (vitamin B_{12}) (µg)	0.08–0.7	0.1–0.8
Folic acid (µg)	11–40	35–100
Zinc (mg)	1.5–2	1.3–2.3
Manganese (µg)	1–100	6.3–25
Copper (µg)	60–160	100–250
Iodine (µg)	8–35	6–35
Selenium (µg)	1.5–5	1.8–5

RE, Retinol equivalents; *TE,* tocopherol equivalents.

Vitamins

REQUIREMENTS FOR VITAMINS IN NEWBORN INFANTS

- Vitamins are obtained from organic substances; they are present in trace amounts in natural food and are essential to normal metabolism.
- The biological roles of many vitamins in preterm infants are not completely understood.
- Vitamins generally are given on a weight-specific basis (not gestational age).
- Because vitamins play a central role in many metabolic processes, signs of vitamin deficiency are nonspecific: lethargy, irritability, and poor growth.
- Routine supplementation of vitamins above the recommended doses is not advised.
- Table 33.1 shows the recommended vitamin and trace mineral intake for enterally fed preterm infants.

MANIFESTATIONS OF WATER-SOLUBLE VITAMIN DEFICIENCIES

- Water-soluble vitamin deficiencies are uncommon in preterm and term infants.
- Vitamin B_1 (thiamine)
  - Deficiency leads to beriberi, a clinical syndrome with neurological and cardiac symptoms.
  - Seen with pyruvate dehydrogenase complex deficiency and maple syrup urine disease
- Vitamin B_2 (riboflavin)
  - Deficiency leads to dermatitis, cheilosis, and photophobia.
  - Seen with glutaric aciduria type I
- Vitamin B_3 (niacin)

- Deficiency leads to pellagra or the clinical syndrome with the classical "four D" conditions of dermatitis, diarrhea, dementia, and death.
- Vitamin B_4 (adenine)
  - Deficiency results in no known disorder in preterm or term infants.
  - Component of DNA, RNA, ATP, and the three coenzymes nicotinamide adenine dinucleotide (NAD), a reduced form of NAD (NADH), and flavin adenine dinucleotide (FAD)
  - It functions synergistically and closely with vitamins B_2 and B_3 to generate energy.
- Vitamin B_5 (pantothenic acid)
  - Deficiency is not seen in preterm infants.
- Vitamin B_6 (pyridoxine)
  - Deficiency conditions are not seen in preterm infants.
- Vitamin B_7 (biotin)
  - Deficiency leads to glossitis, scaling dermatitis, loss of appetite, or alopecia.
  - Seen with biotinidase deficiency, pyruvate dehydrogenase complex deficiency, propionic acidemia, beta-methylcrotonyl glycinuria
- Vitamin B_8 (inositol)
  - Deficiency: Vitamin B_8 is required for cranial neural tube closure of the fetus, but there are no known deficiency disorders in preterm or term infants.
  - Vitamin B_8 is a major component of human milk and is supplemented in infant formula. The benefits of inositol on rates of lung disease, retinopathy of prematurity, and hepatic disease have been suggested, but current evidence is insufficient to support additional supplementation.
- Vitamin B_9 (folate)
  - Deficiency leads to megaloblastic anemia, diarrhea, mouth ulcers, or peripheral neuropathy.
  - Vitamin B_9 deficiency is the most common vitamin deficiency in the United States (particularly in pregnant women); prenatal supplementation is effective in reducing the rate of neural tube defects in the embryo and fetus.
- Vitamin B_{12} (cyanocobalamin)
  - Deficiency leads to megaloblastic anemia and associated neurological dysfunction.
  - Deficiency states, although rare, can be seen in:
    - Breastfed infants whose mothers follow a strict vegan or vegetarian diet that is deficient in vitamin B_{12}
    - Infants with short bowel syndrome (SBS) where the terminal ileum is removed
- Vitamin C (ascorbic acid)
  - Deficiency leads to scurvy, characterized by sore, spongy gums, loose teeth, fragile blood vessels, swollen joints, and anemia (not seen in preterm infants).
  - Vitamin C promotes gastrointestinal iron absorption and serves as an antioxidant.

MANIFESTATION OF FAT-SOLUBLE VITAMIN DEFICIENCIES

- Infants with fat malabsorption due to cholestatic liver disease or SBS are at risk for developing fat-soluble vitamin deficiency.

- Fat-soluble vitamin supplementation may be necessary in these patients.
- Vitamin A is essential for growth and differentiation of epithelial tissues (includes the lung).
  - Deficiency leads to photophobia, conjunctivitis, and failure to thrive.
  - Preterm infants have low stores of vitamin A at birth.
  - Preterm infants with lung disease have lower plasma vitamin A levels than those without lung disease.
  - Deficiency may contribute to the development of bronchopulmonary dysplasia (BPD). Vitamin A supplementation has not become standard practice (due to the need for repeated intramuscular injections).
  - Recommended enteral intake ranges from ~200 to 1000 μg/kg/d (665–3340 IU/kg/d) for preterm infants and ~250 μg/kg/d for term.
- Vitamin D is essential for bone health.
  - Deficiency can result in rickets, pathologic fractures, or rachitic rosary.
  - Infants who require assisted ventilation, have no exposure to ultraviolet light in the hospital, and have limited exposure after discharge have minimal cutaneous synthesis of vitamin D.
  - Recommended enteral intake of vitamin D is 400 IU/d.
  - This dose maintains adequate serum concentrations of vitamin D (>50 nmol/L) and helps prevent rickets, which is associated with vitamin D deficiency.
  - Higher doses (800–1000 IU/d) have been recommended for infants with extreme prematurity, SBS, cholestasis, or long-term exposure to diuretics and/or steroids.
- Vitamin E is a major natural antioxidant that protects lipid-containing RBC cell membranes against oxidative injury, reduces hemolysis, and may prevent neonatal oxygen toxicity, such as retinopathy of prematurity (ROP) and intraventricular hemorrhage (IVH).
  - Deficiency can result in hemolytic anemia, reticulocytosis, thrombocytosis, or acanthocytosis.
  - Recommended enteral vitamin E intake is 3.3 to 16.4 IU/kg/d.
  - The dietary ratio of vitamin E to polyunsaturated fatty acids (PUFAs) should be ≥0.6 mg of D-α-tocopherol (0.9 IU) per gram of PUFA.
  - Recommended IV vitamin E is 2.8 IU/kg/d as α-tocopheryl acetate.
  - Fish oil in IV lipid emulsions provides more vitamin E than with soy oil emulsions.
- Vitamin K is essential for clotting factors II, VII, IX, and X and protein C and S. It prevents hemorrhagic disease of the newborn in the first weeks of life.
  - Deficiency can lead to hemorrhagic disease, prolonged prothrombin time, normal partial thromboplastin time, or normal platelet count.
  - A single dose of intramuscular vitamin K (1 mg for >1500 g, 0.3–0.5 mg for <1500 g) is sufficient.
  - Subsequent vitamin K supplementation helps prevent deficiency in critically ill infants who receive broad-spectrum antibiotics (reduces vitamin K synthesis by gut bacteria) and may have other abnormalities of hemostasis or hepatic function.

POTENTIAL ADVERSE EFFECTS OF PHARMACOLOGIC USE OF FAT-SOLUBLE VITAMINS

- Vitamin A: Acute toxicity can lead to liver damage and increased intracranial pressure (bulging fontanelle, vomiting, papilledema).
- Vitamin D: Excessive dosing results in hypercalcemia, constipation, muscle weakness, and vomiting.
  - Severe cases show damage to the bones and kidneys.
  - Usually seen in infants discharged on high-dose vitamin D
- Vitamin E: Excessive dosing is associated with increased incidence of hemolytic anemia, ROP, and BPD.
  - Increases risk of sepsis, NEC, and retinal hemorrhage in very low-birth-weight (VLBW) infants
- Vitamin K: Excessive dosing causes hemolytic anemia (results in hyperbilirubinemia).
  - Blocks the effects of oral anticoagulants

Trace Minerals

- The content of trace minerals in human milk is the gold standard for requirements in term infants.
  - Requirements for the preterm infant are estimated from in utero accretion rates.
  - Preterm infants are relatively lacking in some important minerals (e.g., iron, zinc).
  - Accumulation occurs mostly in the third trimester.
- Trace mineral supplementation of human milk or the use of an enriched preterm formula usually is necessary to achieve the recommended trace element requirements.
- Trace mineral deficiencies are most common in infants with excessive gastrointestinal losses from ostomy/fistula output or diarrhea.

IRON

- Iron deficiency causes short- and long-term genomic changes and negatively affects the growth and functioning of brain, muscle, and heart, as well as intestinal development. It can impair cell differentiation and neurodevelopment processes.
- Iron intake should be 2 to 3 mg/kg/d for both term and preterm enterally fed infants.
- Preterm infant with anemia of prematurity and on erythropoietin should receive 6 mg/kg/d.
- Risks of iron overload and toxicity increase with red cell transfusions.
- Decreased growth, impaired neurodevelopment, and increased infection are deficiency risks, as well as possible increased risks of ROP or BPD (potentiated by unbound iron and the generation of free radicals).
- Iron supplementation often is delayed for 2 weeks after a transfusion.
- Potential risks of excess IV iron in preterm infants include neonatal sepsis, iron overload, and anaphylaxis.
- Formula-fed infants should receive only iron-fortified formula.
- Iron content of human milk fortifiers varies between products.

ZINC (Zn)

- Zn deficiency can be acquired from prolonged maternal milk ingestion from mothers with low Zn levels. Symptoms include scaling erythematous plaques, diarrhea, slow growth, and hair loss.
- Acrodermatitis enteropathica is an inborn error of Zn metabolism.
  - Acrodermatitis enteropathica is inherited as an autosomal recessive disorder.
  - It is characterized by growth impairment and periorofacial and acral dermatitis with perianal inflammation and excoriation.
- SGA/IUGR infants and infants with intestinal resection are at greater risk for Zn deficiency.
- Human milk Zn content declines over the early months of lactation.
- Human milk fortifiers and formulas contain some Zn.
- Zn supplementation promotes growth (weight and length), neurodevelopment, and motor development.

COPPER (Cu)

- Cu deficiency can result in hypopigmentation of skin and hair, bone abnormalities, microcytic hypochromic anemia unresponsive to iron therapy, neutropenia, or leukopenia.
- Deficiency is rare and occurs when Cu is withheld from parenteral nutrition (PN) due to associated PN liver disease.
- Current recommendations are to remove Cu only if evidence of toxicity is present.
- Cu dosage may be increased to 10 to 15 μm/kg/d in infants experiencing abnormally high biliary or enterostomy drainage.
- High doses of enteral Zn and iron intake can contribute to Cu deficiency.

SELENIUM (Se)

- Deficiency leads to increased risk of sepsis, cardiac and skeletal muscle myopathies, abnormalities in hair and nails, microcytic anemia, and increased erythrocyte fragility.
- Se deficiency is more likely in infants with SBS.

MANGANESE (Mn)

- Mn deficiency is rare and limited to mucopolysaccharide and lipopolysaccharide formation.

CHROMIUM (Cr)

- Cr deficiency can lead to neuropathy and hyperglycemia but is rare in human infants.

IODINE

- Iodine is a major component of thyroid hormones triiodothyronine (T3) and thyroxine (T4).
  - Infants with high intestinal losses can develop hypothyroidism.
  - Even with human milk fortification, iodine content remains below intake recommendations for preterm infants.
- Parenteral iodine intake of 1 μm/kg/d is recommended for preterm infants.
- Intake recommendations account for iodine-containing antiseptics that are absorbed through the skin; however, current practice has moved to using chlorhexidine products.
- The current US neonatal parenteral trace mineral product does not contain iodine.

MOLYBDENUM (MO)

- Mo deficiency is not reported, except in molybdenum cofactor deficiency.
- Mo is not provided in parenteral multivitamins, infant formulas, or oral multivitamins.

POTENTIAL TOXICITIES OF TRACE MINERAL SUPPLEMENTATION IN NEONATES

- Zinc toxicity: potential Cu and iron deficiency
- Copper toxicity: potential hepatotoxicity
  - Acute Cu toxicity in preterm infants is rare, even with cholestasis.
  - Chronic excessive intake or reduced biliary excretion can result in hepatic cirrhosis and hepatotoxic cell injury (increased alanine aminotransferase).
- Manganese toxicity: potential neurotoxicity
  - Mn supplementation should be stopped with any signs of hepatic dysfunction or cholestasis.
  - Mn toxicity can still occur without hepatic dysfunction, because Mn is a common contaminant in PN solutions.
  - Parenteral calcium gluconate to prevent osteopenia contributes to Mn contamination and potential toxicity
- Chromium toxicity: potential nephropathy (reduced glomerular filtration rate [GFR]), evidence of renal tubular damage
- Selenium toxicity: hair loss, weakness in older children
  - Toxicity in neonates has not been documented.

Suggested Readings

American Academy of Pediatrics Committee on Nutrition. Nutritional needs of preterm infants. In: Kleinman RE, Greer FR, eds. *Pediatric Nutrition Handbook*. 8th ed. Itasca, IL: American Academy of Pediatrics; 2020:113–162.

Ballard O, Morrow AL. Human milk composition; nutrients and bioactive factors. *Pediatr Clin North Am*. 2013;60(1):49–74.

Bauer J, Gerss J. Longitudinal analysis of macronutrients and minerals in human milk produced by mothers of preterm infants. *Clin Nutr*. 2011;30(2):215–220.

Embleton ND, Moltu SJ, Lapillonne A, et al. Enteral nutrition in preterm infants (2022): a position paper from the ESPGHAN Committee on Nutrition and invited experts. *J Pediatr Gastroenterol Nutr*. 2023;76(2):248–268.

Finch CW. Review of trace mineral requirements for preterm infants: what are the current recommendations for clinical practice? *Nutr Clin Pract*. 2015;30:44–58.

Koletzko B, Cheah F-C, Domellöf M, Poindexter BB, Vain N, van Goudoever JB, eds. *Nutritional Care of Preterm Infants*. Basel: Karger; 2021.

Krebs NF, Hambidge KM. Zinc in the fetus and neonate. In: Polin RA, Abman SH, Rowitch DH, Benitz WE, Fox WW, eds. *Fetal and Neonatal Physiology*. Philadelphia: Elsevier; 2022:282–286.

McArdle HJ, Georgieff MK. Fetal and neonatal iron metabolism. In: Polin RA, Abman SH, Rowitch DH, Benitz WE, Fox WW, eds. *Fetal and Neonatal Physiology*. Philadelphia: Elsevier; 2022:257–264.

O'Callaghan KM, Roth DE. Fetal and neonatal calcium, phosphorus, and magnesium homeostasis. In: Polin RA, Abman SH, Rowitch DH, Benitz WE, Fox WW, eds. *Fetal and Neonatal Physiology*. Philadelphia: Elsevier; 2022:265–281.

34 *Enteral Nutrition*

KENDRA HENDRICKSON and WILLIAM W. HAY, JR.

Human Milk

- The ideal enteral diet for human neonates
  - Human milk provides sufficient energy, protein, fat, carbohydrate, micronutrients, and water for normal metabolism, growth, and development in term infants.
  - Supplements of protein and certain minerals for very to extremely preterm low-birth-weight infants weighing less than 1500 g at birth are necessary to meet estimated nutrient requirements for growth.
  - In more mature, late preterm infants, increased volumes of milk feeding (>180–200 mL/kg/d) can, if tolerated, provide sufficient nutrition without fortification to meet estimated nutrient requirements for growth.
- Contraindications to the use of human milk are rare.
  - Breastfeeding should be restricted in mothers with untreated maternal miliary tuberculosis or brucellosis, active herpes virus lesions on the breast, or acute varicella or human immunodeficiency virus (HIV) infection, as well as in infants with congenital galactosemia and in infants whose mothers are taking antimetabolites.
  - With maternal COVID, current evidence suggests that breast milk is not likely to spread the virus. While inpatient, options may include providing pumped milk, or, if a mother desires to co-room and direct breastfeed, strict hand washing and masking are recommended.
- Relative contraindications:
  - Breast feeding in mothers with drug abuse (e.g., narcotics, phencyclidine, cocaine, cannabis)
    - Mothers who test positive for such drugs should be enrolled in drug rehabilitation programs with follow-up to ensure participation rather than stopping breastfeeding, particularly among mothers with preterm infants for whom the advantages of mother's own milk (MOM) generally outweigh the risks of addiction and neurodevelopmental defects in the infant.
  - Maternal medications: chemotherapy, lithium, retinoids, iodine
    - For prescribed maternal medications that are concerning for breastfeeding adjustments can be made:
      - Work with the mother's provider to find a compatible substitution.
      - Time the dosage of medication to reduce exposure.
      - Give only partial volume as maternal milk to bring potential exposure to a safe level.
      - Pump and store milk; it can be used when metabolism and excretion capacity has improved with age.
- The development of a beneficial gastrointestinal (GI) flora, characterized by a large prevalence of bifidobacteria and lactobacilli, is supported by human milk feedings.

- Human milk provides a variety of antimicrobial factors such as secretory immunoglobulins (e.g., IgA), leukocytes, complement, lactoferrin, and lysozyme that protect against infections and necrotizing enterocolitis (NEC).
- Human milk contains hormones and growth factors such as epidermal and nerve growth factors, insulin-like growth factor (IGF)-1 and -2, erythropoietin, prolactin, calcitonin, steroids, thyrotropin-releasing hormone (TRH), and thyroxine, which promote gut development and function, as well as organ maturation, growth, and function.
- Several essential and conditionally essential amino acids (AAs) present in high concentrations in human milk promote gut growth and development.
- The protein and fat components of human milk are readily digestible, and human milk contains large numbers of enzymes that aid in nutrient digestion and processing (e.g., lipase).
- Exclusive human milk feeding of infants at high risk for allergies may reduce the risk for developing atopic disease or milk protein allergy in infancy.
- Human milk enhances neurodevelopment, including vision, mental scales (particularly cognition), motor scales, behavior, and hearing.
- Preterm infants who are breastfed at discharge have less subnormal neurodevelopment at 2 to 5 years.
  - These effects last into infancy, childhood, and adolescence.
- There are psychological benefits to a mother who provides her own milk to her infant:

"Mother's expressed milk for very low birth weight infants (≤1500 g) in the NICU provides short- and long-term health benefits, including reduction of necrotizing enterocolitis, late-onset sepsis, chronic lung disease, retinopathy of prematurity, and improved neurodevelopment. Mother's expressed milk should be considered medical therapy, with higher doses associated with maximal health benefits. The AAP recommends pasteurized donor human milk when a mother's milk is not available or is contraindicated. Fortification of mother's milk or donor milk with bovine or human milk-derived human milk fortifiers should be considered to optimize growth in the VLBW infant."

AMERICAN ACADEMY OF PEDIATRICS (AAP)

COMPOSITION OF BREAST MILK: MOTHERS OF PRETERM INFANTS AND MOTHERS OF FULL-TERM INFANTS

- Very to extremely preterm infants will not grow at the normal rate of fetal growth on mature human milk

Table 34.1   Major Nutrient Composition of Mature Human Milk and Preterm Formulas

	Mature Preterm Human Milk (Unfortified)	Enfamil Premature	Similac Special Care
Nutrient density (kcal/oz)	19–21	24	24
Protein (g/100 kcal)	2.2	3.3	3
% Total calories	8	13	12
Sources	Human milk	Bovine whey, protein concentrate, non-fat milk	Bovine whey, protein concentrate, non-fat milk
Fat (g/100 kcal)	5.4	5	5.4
% Total calories	44–52	44	47
Sources	Triglycerides	MCT oil, soy oil, high-oleic vegetable oil, DHA, ARA	MCT oil, soy oil, high-oleic vegetable oil, DHA, ARA
Carbohydrates (g/100 kcal)	10	11	10
% Total calories	40–44	43	41
Sources	Lactose	Lactose, corn syrup solids	Lactose, corn syrup solids

ARA, Arachidonic acid; *DHA,* docosahexaenoic acid; *MCT,* medium-chain triglyceride.

alone because of the greater needs for protein and salts to promote growth at in utero rates.

- Mean protein content is higher in preterm mother's colostrum and milk right after birth (1.5–2.5 g/dL) compared with term mother's milk (0.7–1.5 g/dL). There is marked variability of protein content of preterm mother's milk at and shortly after birth.
- Protein content in preterm mother's milk declines over 1 to 2 weeks of full lactation to the concentrations found in mature milk and donor milk (mean value of about 0.9 g/dL). Lactose and lipid contents of preterm mother's milk are similar to those of mature mother's milk.
- Milk from mothers of preterm infants has more sodium initially than milk obtained at term.
- Mother's milk can support adequate growth in larger and healthier preterm infants (e.g., late preterm infants) who have the capacity to take in larger volumes (usually >180–200 mL/kg/d).
  - Important when feeding preterm infants with donor human milk
  - Donor human milk has lower protein (mean of ~0.9 g/dL) and salt concentrations than early preterm mother's milk.

DIFFERENCES IN THE NUTRITIONAL COMPOSITION OF HUMAN MILK AND INFANT FORMULAS

- Unfortified mature preterm human milk is lower in nutrient density and protein content than commonly used preterm formulas.
- Major nutrient compositions for mature preterm milk and preterm formulas are shown in Table 34.1.
- Preterm formulas have higher concentrations of calcium, phosphorus, sodium, potassium, chloride, iron, zinc, and magnesium than mature, unfortified human milk.
- Standard fortifiers supplementing mature human and donor milk are necessary to approximate the estimated mineral compositions of preterm formulas and promote appropriate growth and development.
- Preterm formulas have higher concentrations of vitamins A, D, E, K, C, riboflavin, B_6, and folic acid than mature, unfortified human milk.

- A standard multivitamin is commonly used for preterm infants fed their own mother's milk or donor milk to meet the vitamin D intake requirements (400 IU/d).
  - These products contain water- and fat-soluble vitamins that, when combined with preterm fortifiers and formula, deliver an excess of some nutrients (manganese, vitamin A).
  - The multivitamin is not complete; therefore, provision of micronutrients such as molybdenum, selenium, and chromium may be below recommendations.
- Iron supplementation is needed until 6 to 12 months of age; intake may come from oral ferrous sulfate, iron-fortified formula, milk fortifier, or multivitamin products.
  - <2 kg weight: 2 to 3 mg/kg/d
  - >2 kg weight: 1 to 2 mg/kg/d

IMMUNOLOGICAL AND ANTI-INFECTIVE CONSTITUENTS IN HUMAN MILK AND THEIR EFFECTS

- Lactoferrin (LF) and its iron-binding capacity:
  - LF has bacteriostatic function in the intestinal mucosa of the newborn:
    - Chelates iron and prevents growth of various pathogens
    - Has a direct cytotoxic effect against bacteria, viruses, and fungi
    - Immunomodulatory functions
      - Assists to limit excessive immune responses:
        - Inhibits inflammatory cytokines, including interleukin (IL)-1β, IL-6, IL-8, and tumor necrosis factor alpha (TNF-α)
        - Stimulates activity and development of the immune system
  - Part of the activity of LF can be attributed to the formation of lactoferricin:
    - Potent cationic peptide with bactericidal activity formed during the digestion of LF
- Immunoglobulin A (IgA) is responsible for 80% to 90% of total immunoglobulins in human milk.
  - IgA acts locally on the intestine as a first line of defense directed at foreign antigens, which include:
    - Commensal or pathogenic microorganisms

- Toxins, viruses, and other antigenic materials (lipopolysaccharide)
  - IgA prevents their adherence to and penetration into the epithelium without triggering inflammatory reactions that could be harmful to the newborn (immune exclusion).
- High-affinity dimeric IgA antibodies inactivate viruses (e.g., rotavirus).
- IgM: High-affinity IgM antibodies react with viruses and bacteria to protect the mucosal surfaces of infants.
  - Acts via agglutination and complement activation
- IgG is found at low concentrations in human milk.
  - Neutralizing and opsonizing activity
    - IgGs activate the complement system and antibody-dependent cytotoxicity.
  - IgG1, IgG2, and IgG3 activate phagocytosis.
  - IgG4 is anti-inflammatory (responding to allergens).
- Lactoperoxidase: In the presence of hydrogen peroxide, it catalyzes the oxidation of thiocyanate (present in saliva), forming hypothiocyanite that can kill both gram-positive and gram-negative bacteria.
- Lysozyme enzyme activity is capable of degrading the outer wall of gram-positive bacteria.
  - Lysozyme has the ability to kill gram-negative bacteria in vitro (synergistically with LF).
  - Lysozyme may have antiviral activity.
- Human milk contains a variety of live cells, including:
  - Macrophages, T cells, stem cells, and lymphocytes with anti-infective and immunologically protective functions
- Human milk contains large amounts of human milk oligosaccharides (HMOs).
  - HMOs are prebiotic agents that encourage the growth of beneficial (probiotic) organisms.
- Human milk contains many hundreds to thousands of distinct bioactive molecules that protect against infection and inflammation and contribute to immune maturation, organ development, and healthy microbial colonization.

HUMAN MILK: EFFECTS OF DIFFERENT PROCESSING METHODS

- Mother's own milk can be produced at home or produced in the neonatal intensive care unit (NICU) and stored.
  - Varying degrees of nutrient loss may occur with long-term storage.
    - Depends on the nutrient and the storage methods
  - For the majority of human milk components, significant degradation occurs only with long-term storage and multiple freeze–thaw cycles (which reduce bactericidal capacity).
  - Vitamin C loss occurs rapidly, even in the process of feeding freshly expressed human milk using a bottle.
- Donor milk
  - Donated human breast milk can contain pathogenic microorganisms that could be transferred to infants, thus it requires sterilization procedures to ensure its safety.
  - Such procedures diminish or destroy many nutritional and immunologic components of milk.
- Heat treatment (pasteurization) of human milk is the most common approach for sterilization.

- It may reduce the concentration and functional capacity of many bioactive components.
- Holder pasteurization (62°C for 30 minutes):
  - Milk banks associated with the Human Milk Banking Association of North America use this method.
  - It does not adversely affect the protein content of donor milk.
  - Flash-heat treatment may preserve the bacteriostatic activity of donor milk more than the other methods.
- Retort processing is a high-temperature, short-time pasteurization method that uses pressure and agitation to create a sterile, shelf-stable donor milk.
  - Nutrient analyses are provided by the manufacturers.
  - Limited data are available from studies on the impact of retort processing on bioactive components; available studies did not replicate the proprietary methods employed by for-profit donor human milk companies.
- Pasteurization significantly reduces all classes of immunoglobulin.
  - IgA, lysozyme, LF, bile salt-stimulated lipase (BSSL), cytokines (most are anti-inflammatory), lipases, macrophage inflammatory protein, TGF-β, and growth factor proteins (insulin, adiponectin, and erythropoietin).
  - Overall there is considerable variability in biological activity both before and after pasteurization.
  - Total lipid generally is reduced (up to 60%), but free fatty acids (FFAs) are increased.
    - Pasteurization is damaging to the fat content of donor milk compared to multiple freeze–thaw cycles.
- No significant reductions in lactose have been noted.
- Higher heat sensitivity has been noted for water-soluble vitamins (e.g., vitamin C) but less so for fat-soluble vitamins.
- Zinc concentrations are unchanged but activity is impaired by denaturation of zinc-binding proteins.

HUMAN MILK FORTIFICATION

- Extremely low-birth-weight (ELBW) infants require greater nutrient supplies than are provided with mature maternal or donor milk alone at commonly tolerated feeding volumes to meet nutrient requirements for growth due to:
  - Lower minimal energy reserves (carbohydrate stores in glycogen, fat in adipose tissue, protein in muscle)
  - Intrinsically higher metabolic rate (greater relative mass of more metabolically active organs: brain, heart, liver)
  - Higher protein turnover rates (especially when growing)
  - Higher glucose needs for energy and brain metabolism
  - Higher lipid needs to match the in utero rate of fat deposition
  - Excessive evaporative rates (immature skin)
  - High urinary water and solute losses (depends on intake and renal maturation)
  - Low rates of gastrointestinal peristalsis
  - Limited production of gut digestive enzymes and growth factors

- Higher incidence of stressful events (hypoxemia, respiratory distress, sepsis)
- Metabolic effects of medications (steroids, antibiotics, sedatives, catecholamines)
- Abnormal neurological outcome if not fed adequately
- Recommended daily requirements for energy, protein, calcium, sodium, phosphorus, magnesium, iron, zinc, and several vitamins that are necessary to meet the normal rate of in utero growth are usually not achieved in the growing "healthy" ELBW, very to extremely preterm infant fed with unsupplemented human milk, unless feeding milk volume feeds >180 to 200 to as high as 250 mL/kg/d.
  - Preterm infants with respiratory distress, infection, excessive heat losses, GI disorders, or surgery have even greater nutritional needs.
- Most new formulations of commercially available fortifiers use hydrolyzed cow's milk protein, which may lead to less GI intolerance and less bovine protein–induced GI inflammation (possibly also actual bovine protein allergy).
- Hydrolyzed liquid protein fortifier can improve the growth of weight, length, and head circumference when protein and energy requirements are met using this product.
- Human milk–based fortification is available and could possibly reduce the potential for NEC; reduced growth is similar compared to bovine-based fortifier.

PHYSIOLOGY AND PATHOPHYSIOLOGY OF HUMAN MILK PRODUCTION AND SECRETION

- Anatomy and function
  - Mammary tissue includes alveoli (small sacs made of milk-secreting cells) and excretory ducts.
    - Milk collects in the lumen of the alveoli and ducts between feedings.
  - The alveoli are surrounded by myoepithelial cells that contract in response to tactile stimulation (suckling, manual expression) and oxytocin to produce milk flow along the ducts.
  - Each nipple has an average of nine milk ducts surrounded by muscle fibers and nerves
    - Montgomery glands within the pigmented areola surrounding the nipple secrete an oily fluid that protects the skin of the nipple and areola during lactation and produce the mother's individual scent that attracts her baby to the breast.
  - The ducts beneath the areola fill with milk and become wider during a feed (when the oxytocin reflex is active).
- Hormonal regulation of lactation
  - Prolactin secretion increases markedly during pregnancy and stimulates the growth and development of the mammary tissue.
  - Milk secretion is suppressed during pregnancy by the pregnancy hormones progesterone and estrogen.
  - After delivery, progesterone and estrogen decrease rapidly, allowing prolactin to stimulate milk secretion.
  - Suckling by the infant increases prolactin secretion and its stimulation of milk production in the alveoli.
  - Prolactin concentrations are highest about 30 minutes after suckling begins.

- Oxytocin is essential for establishing lactation by stimulating the myoepithelial cells around the alveoli to contract, thereby increasing milk flow through and out of the ducts.
  - The oxytocin reflex is referred to as the "letdown reflex" or the "milk ejection reflex."
  - Oxytocin is produced more quickly than prolactin.
  - It increases the flow of milk already in the breast alveoli and ducts, helping the infant to get the milk more easily.
  - Oxytocin also stimulates uterine contractions (contributing to uterine pain during early suckling).
- Prolactin and oxytocin secretion increases in response to gentle areolar and nipple tactile stimulation, enhanced by skin-to-skin contact and promoting breastfeeding and emotional bonding.
- A delay in breastfeeding of even 4 to 6 hours after birth may lead to breastfeeding failure, and early initiation of breast expression in mothers of preterm infants is equally important.
- Preterm birth and milk production:
  - Mammogenesis and lactogenesis are limited in mothers who deliver early.
  - Milk production is limited immediately after birth (regardless of gestation).
    - Lactogenesis I (pregnancy): The synthetic capability of the breast to produce milk-specific components (lactose, casein, and α-lactalbumin) develops; it begins by 22 weeks of pregnancy, with the production of unique milk components from the lactocytes.
    - Lactogenesis I (term delivery): Epithelial cells change into milk producing cells; it begins at delivery to 36 to 96 hours after.
  - First 48 hours after term birth: production of colostrum is 2–20 mL/feed.
    - Lactogenesis II is closure of the spaces between epithelial cells with increased milk secretion. Stimulation and milk removal result in increased growth and development of the alveoli and ducts (occurs between 30 and 72 hours after birth).
    - Lactogenesis II requires adequate levels of prolactin, insulin, and adrenocorticoid hormones; it is triggered by the withdrawal of progesterone following delivery of the placenta.
    - Lactogenesis III is the maintenance stage of lactation (usually occurs after about 9 days postpartum).
  - Any preterm infants can grasp the nipple with lips and tongue from 28 weeks' gestational age and often can suckle and remove some milk from the nipple as early as 31 weeks.
  - Coordination of suckling, swallowing, and breathing develops between 32 and 35 weeks.
  - Some preterm infants can fully breastfeed by ~36 weeks, although most infants born preterm will not be fully efficient at breastfeeding until term corrected age.
  - Preterm birth is stressful and may lead to unsuccessful milk production if supportive nursing care, lactation counseling, encouragement by physicians, and provision of a calm, quiet, private environment are not provided.
    - Many mothers delivering preterm infants have not breastfed previously and are not familiar with the sensations caused by the release of oxytocin.

- Inadequate milk production in some stressed mothers of very preterm infants can be caused by failure of milk ejection.

BREAST MILK PRODUCTION IN THE NICU

Strategies to Acquire and Feed Mother's Own Milk in the NICU

- Provide prenatal education to encourage breastfeeding and enhance knowledge and perception of lactation.
- Establish family-centered care, including a milk-friendly environment that promotes use of breast milk and breastfeeding.
- Integrate NICU-based lactation care providers to support and guide mothers throughout the hospital stay.
- Have processes in place to initiate breast pump use within 1 hour after birth.
  - Initiation at 3 to 6 hours after birth for very low-birth-weight (VLBW) infants has been shown to increase the frequency of expressions, thus supporting supply. This is possibly related to alleviating some stress associated with expressing immediately following a traumatic delivery.
- Promote kangaroo mother–baby care.
- Ensure access to effective and efficient hospital-grade electric pumps, double collection kits, and customized breast shield sizing.
- Promote frequent pumping to support milk production.
  - Encourage pumping in proximity to the infant.
  - Avoid exclusive hand expression in the early days after birth.
  - Monitor pumped milk schedules and volume during the critical first 2 weeks when breast-pump–dependent mothers are at risk for long-lasting milk volume problems.
  - Use lactation services to provide timely interventions to increase milk production.
- Incorporate tested lactation technologies (milk analysis and test weighing) to objectively manage growth on MOM feedings.
- Provide support to reduce maternal distress and anxiety.
  - Positively reinforce the mother's motivation.
  - Allow parents to take part in the care of their infants.
  - Aim patient- and family-centered interventions at reducing stress.
  - Encourage attention to a healthy diet and adequate sleep schedule for the mother.
  - Provide staff and resources for individual psychological and psychosocial support and peer-to-peer support.
- Promote and provide donor milk when MOM is not available and formula is not desired.
- Optimize counseling of mothers to avoid problems such as promoting discharge at the expense of breastfeeding and pumping breast milk emphasized over breastfeeding.

ADVANTAGES AND DISADVANTAGES OF THE USE OF DONOR HUMAN MILK

- Donor human milk is a pasteurized product from accredited milk banks and used when maternal milk is insufficient or unavailable.
- Donor milk is pasteurized to prevent infections in the infant. Pasteurization removes much of the anti-infective properties of milk; it reduces lipase activity, the content of live cells including microbes, and cytomegalovirus (CMV).

- Infection rates and NEC rates are much lower with MOM and pasteurized donor milk than formulas.
- Donor milk in the United States is low in docosahexaenoic acid (DHA) and arachidonic acid (ARA) content.
- Supplemented donor milk is an appropriate choice for extremely low-birth-weight (ELBW) and VLBW preterm infants whose mother's milk is unavailable.
- Donor milk provides >75% improvement in feeding tolerance compared with formulas.
- Rates of NEC and related sepsis may be lowest among very preterm infants fed with an exclusive human milk diet (compared with formula fed infants).

Formulas

DISTRIBUTION OF NUTRIENTS IN INFANT FORMULAS

- Nutrient composition of infant formula is modeled on the composition of human milk, but, due to the variability of human milk and reduced bioavailability of formula components, more extensive data are used to assess formula effects.
  - Content requirements of formulas are further supported by a comparison of their effects on growth patterns, biochemical markers, and functional outcomes.
- Standard minimum and maximum contents have been established for macronutrients:
  - Protein, 1.8 to 4.5 g/100 kcal
  - Formula fat, 3.3 to 6 g/100 kcal (30%–55% of energy)
  - Formula CHO, 9 to 14 g/100 kcal (40%–56% of energy)
  - Formulas for term infants contain 20 kcal/oz and are adequate to meet the needs of term infants with an intact GI tract and "normal" fluid requirements.
  - Preterm formulas are available in 20, 24, and 30 kcal/oz preparations, with similar osmolalities and renal solute loads.
- Common sources of macronutrients:
  - Cow's milk protein, soy protein isolates, hydrolyzed cow's milk protein, and soy
    - Goat's milk protein does not have US Food and Drug Administration (FDA) approval for use in infant formulas.
  - Glucose polymers or corn syrup solids
  - Common fat sources, such as palm oil, soy oil, coconut oil, sunflower oil, and safflower oil, in various combinations
- Recommendations provide the essential requirements of amino acids, fatty acids, and micronutrients.

BENEFITS AND RISKS OF FORMULAS THAT CONTAIN NONSTANDARD SOY PROTEINS

- Soy protein formulas are reserved for term infants:
  - With galactosemia, severe lactose intolerance, or hereditary lactase deficiency
  - Who are of vegan families (counseled on the need for a balanced protein diet in their infant)
  - With an immunoglobulin E (IgE)-mediated cow's milk protein allergy (CMPA)

- Soy-derived formulas are not used for preterm infants due to the poor quality of protein, lower digestibility and bioavailability, and lower calcium and zinc accretion rates.
- The concentrations of phytates, aluminum, and phytoestrogens that are in soy formulas make them less ideal for any infant.
- For term infants, formulas derived from protein hydrolysates are reserved for infants who have proven CMPA and are not breastfed.
- Soy formulas have no role in the prevention of atopic disease.
- Extensively hydrolyzed formulas have been used in the past to delay or prevent atopic dermatitis in infants at high risk and who are not breastfed. Recent research has called this practice into question without strong evidence for efficacy and potential harm.
- In families with a strong history of CMPA,
  - Breastfeeding is protective against development of CMPA.
  - Consider maternal restriction of cow's milk protein in the mother's diet if infant has clear clinical signs (e.g., eczema) after being breastfed.

MEDICAL INDICATIONS FOR NONSTANDARD INFANT FORMULAS

- Elemental and extensively hydrolyzed formulas
  - Are used in infants with malabsorption, severe liver disease, short bowel syndrome (SBS), dysmotility syndromes (e.g., in gastroschisis), or severe protein allergy
  - The protein source is derived from free AAs.
  - Fat source is derived from medium-chain triglyceride (MCT) oil (0%–55%).
  - Many are lactose free.
- Elemental or hydrolyzed formulas may be useful after a severe episode of infectious gastroenteritis with mucosal injury and resulting protein or lactose intolerance.
- Partially hydrolyzed whey preterm infant formula has not been shown to benefit feeding tolerance, enteral intake, or growth in the premature infant.

- Modified formulas are available for infants with special nutritional needs due to inherited enzyme deficiencies.
  - Lactose intolerance can be due to a congenital lactase deficiency, galactosemia, or phenylketonuria (PKU).
  - These formulas require multivitamin and mineral supplements (if used for preterm infants).
- Some preterm infants have apparent cow's milk protein "allergy" (feeding intolerance, intestinal dilation, and hematochezia without other signs of illness or NEC).
  - These infants may benefit from a reduction in maternal cow's milk protein diet or use of hydrolyzed cow's milk protein fortifiers (if the mother is breastfeeding) or use of hydrolyzed cow's milk protein formulas.

STANDARD INFANT FORMULA MODIFICATIONS FOR USE IN PRETERM INFANTS

- Preterm formulas are developed to meet the unique nutritional needs of preterm infants (though most were not specifically tested in ELBW infants).
- Preterm formulas contain whey-to-casein ratios of 60:40 and have higher protein contents than those of term formulas (2.4 g/100 mL in preterm formula vs. 2 g/100 mL in term formula or human milk).
- Lactose is reduced due to a concern for early lactase deficiency.
- The remaining carbohydrate is provided by glucose polymers (easily digested) and provide a lower osmolality (~300 mOsm/L).
- Fat blends include 20% to 50% MCTs to compensate for lower bile salts and lipases.
- Protein concentrations are increased to 2.7 to 3.3 g/100 kcal and are whey predominant.
- Calcium (Ca) and phosphorus (P) contents are increased, with a Ca:P ratio of 1.8–2:1, providing for improved bone mineralization.
- Carnitine is commonly added to aid in lipid oxidation.
- Other minerals and vitamins also are present in higher concentrations in preterm formulas.
- Increasing caloric density or goal volumes addresses most growth concerns, but it may also be necessary to

Table 34.2   Mineral and Vitamin Contents of Preterm Infant Formulas (Based on Similac Special Care Premature and Enfamil Premature)

MINERALS (PER 100 KCAL)		VITAMINS (PER 100 KCAL)			
		Fat Soluble		**Water Soluble**	
Calcium	165–180 mg	Vitamin A (IU)	1250–1350	Vitamin B$_6$ (μg)	150–250
Phosphorus	90–100 mg	Vitamin D (IU)	150–300	Vitamin B$_{12}$ (μg)	0.25–0.55
Sodium	43–70 mg	Vitamin E (IU)	4–6.3	Vitamin C (mg)	20–37
Potassium	98–129 mg	Vitamin K (μg)	9–12	Biotin (μg)	4–37
Chloride	81–106 mg			Niacin (μg)	4000–5000
Magnesium	9–12 mg			Pantothenic acid (mg)	1.2–1.9
Manganese	6–12 μg			B$_2$ riboflavin (μg)	300–620
Zinc	1.5 mg			B$_1$ thiamine (μg)	200–250
Copper	120–250 μg			Folic acid (μg)	37–40
Iodine	6–25 μg				
Iron	1.8 mg				
Selenium	2–5 μg				

provide additional individual nutrients (e.g., protein, minerals, zinc, sodium).

- Indications for use of high-protein ($\sim$3.5 g/100 kcal) preterm formulas include:
  - Birth weight < 1500 g
  - Infants who are fluid/volume restricted due to, for example, congenital heart disease and bronchopulmonary dysplasia (BPD)
  - Promotion of wound healing (postoperative)
  - Cumulative deficit of protein intake (early total parenteral nutrition weaning before full enteral feeding is established)
  - Inadequate growth in length and/or head circumference (treated with liquid protein supplements)
  - Unfortified human milk feeds (e.g., direct breastfeeding or use of donor milk)
- Mineral and vitamin content of preterm infant formulas are provided in Table 34.2.

Suggested Readings

American Academy of Pediatrics Committee on Nutrition. Nutritional needs of preterm infants. In: Kleinman RE, Greer FR, eds. *Pediatric Nutrition Handbook*. 8th ed. Itasca, IL: American Academy of Pediatrics; 2020:113–162.

Embleton ND, Moltu SJ, Lapillonne A, et al. Enteral nutrition in preterm infants (2022): a position paper from the ESPGHAN Committee on Nutrition and invited experts. *J Pediatr Gastroenterol Nutr*. 2023;76(2):248–268.

Fenton TR, Elmrayed S, Alshaikh B. Nutrition, growth and long-term outcomes. *World Rev Nutr Diet*. 2021;122:12–31.

Hay WW. Nutritional support strategies for the preterm infant in the neonatal intensive care unit. *Pediatr Gastroenterol Hepatol Nutr*. 2018;21:234–247.

Huff KA, Denne SC, Hay WW Jr. Energy requirements and carbohydrates in preterm infants. In: Koletzko B, Cheah F-C, Domellöf M, Poindexter BB, Vain N, van Goudoever JB, eds. *Nutritional Care of Preterm Infants*. 2nd ed. Basel: Karger; 2021:60–74.

Koletzko B, Cheah F-C, Domellöf M, Poindexter BB, Vain N, van Goudoever JB, eds. *Nutritional Care of Preterm Infants*. 2nd ed. Basel: Karger; 2021.

35 *Parenteral Nutrition*

KENDRA HENDRICKSON and WILLIAM W. HAY, JR.

Overview

- The more preterm and less developed the infant, the less body stores (protein, fat, glycogen) are available to provide nutrients for metabolic needs.
- Intravenous feeding is always indicated when metabolic needs are not met by enteral feeding.
- The metabolic and nutrient requirements of the newborn are equal to or greater than those of the fetus of the same gestational age.
- Intravenous feeding is essential, but it should not be a sole substitute for enteral nutrition unless the infant has absolutely no capacity for enteral feedings. These conditions are rare (usually short-term) and include:
  - Intestinal obstructions (atresia or totally obstructing bands), malformations (gastroschisis, severe omphalocele), or early gut infarctions and perforations
    - These infants may still be able to feed enterally in small amounts to stimulate maturation of the gastrointestinal tract.
- Parenteral nutrition is important to ensure full protein and energy supplies to maintain neuronal development.
  - Protein and energy intakes in the first week of life are associated with improved developmental outcomes in preterm infants at 18 months of age.
  - Protein and energy intakes in the first three weeks of life are associated with greater adult lean body mass and higher resting energy expenditure.

NUTRITIONAL COMPOSITION OF PARENTERAL SOLUTIONS

- Total parenteral nutrition (TPN) is a combination of nutrients—dextrose, crystalline amino acids, fat emulsion, sterile water, electrolytes, vitamins, and minerals—administered intravenously.
  - In neonates, fat emulsion is often administered in a separate syringe co-infused into the intravenous line, which allows for smaller micron filters for the lipids and easier visualization of particulate matter in dextrose solution.
- TPN calories are increased as tolerated to a goal caloric intake of 90 to 115 kcal/kg/d for extremely preterm (EPT), extremely low birth weight (ELBW) infants and 90 to 110 kcal/kg/d for more mature infants, obtained from macronutrients at the recommended intake rates.
  - Dextrose solutions are usually 5% or 10% dextrose weight/volume in solution, with other concentrations added as needed.

- Glucose infusion rates range from 3 to 10 mg/kg/min while maintaining normal plasma glucose concentrations.
- Crystalline amino acids (AAs) are provided in stock solutions ranging from 3% to 20%.
- Average daily AA intakes start at
  - 2.5 g/kg/d on days 0 to 1
  - 3.5 to 4 g/kg/d (goal by days 2–4) for ELBW/EPT infants
  - 3 to 3.5 g/kg/d (goal by day 2) for late preterm infants
  - 2.5 to 3 g/kg/d (goal for term infants)
- Pediatric formulations contain higher concentrations of branched-chain AAs (leucine, isoleucine, valine) and decreased amounts of methionine and phenylalanine.
- Cysteine is added at the time of compounding due to stability issues.
- Neonates have additional AAs that are considered conditionally essential. These are not always provided in sufficient amounts at lower TPN infusion rates, thus requiring enteral feeding of milk or formula for sufficiency.
- Nonessential AAs must be provided in sufficient amounts to ensure appropriate rates of protein synthesis and net protein balance (Table 35.1).
- Intravenous fat emulsions (IVFEs) should be a 20% solution (20 g/100 mL) to minimize phospholipid content and improve clearance.
- IVFEs are used to provide energy and essential fatty acids for TPN formulations.
  - They are initiated at 1 to 2 g/kg/d and increased to a goal of 3 to 3.5 g/kg/d by days 2 to 3.
  - In the United States, available IVFEs are 100% soybean oil or a combination product using several oil sources (soybean, olive, and fish oil).
- A 10% solution of pure fish oil is approved for use in conjunction with soybean emulsion for infants who are dependent on full TPN and are suffering from persistent or progressive TPN-associated cholestasis (maximum dose, 1 g/kg/d).
- Without IVFE, essential fatty acid deficiency can develop within days in infants who receive no enteral nutrition of milk or formula.
- Essential fatty acids include linoleic acid (LA) and alpha-linolenic acid (ALA).
  - LA produces arachidonic acid (ARA), and ALA produces docosahexaenoic acid (DHA) and eicosapentaenoic acid (EPA).
  - ARA is more inflammatory than DHA or EPA but is still essential for brain development. Multicomponent IV lipid emulsions should be infused at ≥2 g/kg/d to prevent ARA deficiency.

Table 35.1 Neonatal Amino Acid Requirements

Essential	Conditionally Essential	Non-essential
Phenylalanine	Cysteine	Alanine
Valine	Arginine	Glutamic acid
Tryptophan		
Threonine	Tyrosine	Aspartic acid
Isoleucine	Proline	Asparagine
Methionine	Glutamine	Serine
Histidine		
Leucine	Glycine	
Lysine		
Mnemonics		
PVT TIM HaLL	CATy PiGG	All GaAAsS

- Electrolytes are added as salts that also provide acetate, chloride, and phosphorus. Dosage is based on fluid status and laboratory values.
- Calcium is provided in the form of calcium gluconate.
- Carnitine, vitamins, trace elements, and some medications may also be added.
- TPN can contain up to 40 different nutrient components that impact stability and compatibility.

IMPORTANCE OF PROTEIN AND NONPROTEIN NUTRIENTS TO ACHIEVE OPTIMAL ENERGY

- Even at standard infusion rates, current TPN solutions with lower concentrations of certain essential amino acids (e.g., leucine, isoleucine, threonine, lysine) can limit protein accretion.
- The composition of current neonatal parenteral amino acid solutions is based on providing plasma concentrations similar to those of term, fully breastfed infants.
  - Preterm infants require considerably greater amounts of amino acids to achieve their higher gestational age–appropriate protein accretion rates.
- At lower (and suboptimal) nonprotein calorie intakes (<60–70 kcal/kg/d), increasing energy intakes promote net protein accretion rates. When adequate nonprotein calories (>80–90 kcal/kg/d) have been provided, the impact of energy on protein accretion is maximized; any additional energy is used for the deposition of fat in adipose tissue.
  - The total caloric goal is 90 to 115 kcal/kg/d for very preterm infants.
  - The goal is 90 to 110 kcal/kg/d for late preterm and term infants.
  - The relationship between energy intake and protein accretion is curvilinear.
    - In contrast, protein accretion at any caloric (energy) intake is directly dependent on protein intake (either as intact protein in enteral diets or as amino acids in TPN solutions).

CALCULATING THE CALORIC CONTENT OF PARENTERAL NUTRITION SOLUTIONS

- Protein concentrations in parenteral nutrition are ordered as g/kg/d.
  - Amino acids produce about 4 kcal/g of energy if totally oxidized.

- Therefore, the amount of amino acids (g/kg/d) received can be multiplied by 4 to determine the kcal/kg/d from protein.
- Glucose is ordered as a dextrose percent, which equates to g/dL (e.g., 12.5% = 12.5 g/100 mL).
- Glucose produces about 4 kcal/g of energy if totally oxidized; therefore, the total glucose energy supply in g/kg/d × 4 will provide the kcal/kg/d from glucose.
- Lipid emulsions are usually infused separately and ordered as g/kg/d.
  - Lipids produce about 10 kcal/g of energy if totally oxidized.
  - The ordered amount of g/kg/d × 10 provides the kcal/kg/d from fat.
- A standard parenteral infusion of 3 g/kg/d amino acids and 10% dextrose at 100 mL/kg/d and a lipid infusion of 3 g/kg/d would provide:
  - Total energy intake of 82 kcal/kg/d
  - 3 g amino acids × 4 kcal/g = 12 kcal/kg/d
  - 10 g of dextrose × 4 kcal/g = 40 kcal/kg/d
  - 3 g lipid × 10 kcal/g = 30 kcal/kg/d

Complications of Parenteral Nutrition

RELATIONSHIP BETWEEN THE CALCIUM AND PHOSPHORUS CONTENT OF TPN SOLUTIONS AND OSTEOPENIA

- Intravenous calcium (Ca) and phosphorus (P) supplementation should be started in high-risk infants soon after birth.
- The usual dosing range of parenteral calcium in the form of calcium gluconate is 0.6 to 2.5 mmol/kg/d (25–100 mg/kg/d of elemental calcium), and the dose is titrated based on either the total serum calcium level or ionized calcium level.
- Phosphorus is given as sodium phosphate with a dosing range of 0.75 to 2.5 mmol/kg/d (25–80 mg/kg/d of phosphate).
  - Phosphorus (and potassium) concentrations should be measured early after birth, especially in very preterm infants; if low, phosphorus should be given early to prevent refeeding syndrome (excessive use of phosphorus to support adenosine triphosphate [ATP] production with rapid administration of glucose and amino acids).
- The Ca:P ratio should preferentially be kept at 1.3 to 1:1 on a molar basis and 1.3 to 1.7:1 on a mg/mg basis to maximize accretion of both minerals.
  - Lower ratios may be used during refeeding hypophosphatemia.
- The solubility of calcium and phosphorus in TPN solutions is often the limiting factor in provision of these minerals. Care is needed to avoid precipitation of calcium phosphate by considering the following when ordering and preparing parenteral nutrition:
  - Acidity improves solubility. The addition of amino acids, cysteine (added separately due to stability), and glucose decreases pH.
  - The sequence of adding calcium and phosphorus to the solution affects the solubility.

- Calcium and phosphorus solubility product (the equilibrium constant for a solid substance dissolving in an aqueous solution)
- Caution should be taken if calcium is infused into a peripheral IV catheter, as severe tissue necrosis and sloughing can occur with extravasations and even minor leaks.
  - Some intensive care units avoid peripheral calcium administration entirely except in emergencies, such as hypocalcemic seizures or shock.
- Magnesium supplementation ranges from 0.12 to 0.4 mmol/kg/d (3–10 mg/kg/d).

ASSOCIATION OF CHOLESTASIS WITH TPN NUTRITION

- Cholestasis or intestinal failure–associated liver disease (IFALD) is more common in:
  - Extremely preterm infants
  - Infants with short gut syndromes (who receive parenteral nutrition exclusively and for prolonged periods).
- IFALD is first noticed by increased direct (conjugated) bilirubin concentrations, which should be measured weekly in infants on prolonged TPN (>14 days).
- IFALD is reduced by providing any enteral nutrition.
- IFALD is markedly reduced in frequency with the use of lipid emulsions that contain less soybean oil and may be reversed with lipid emulsions that contain fish oil or a combination of omega-3–rich oils.
  - These emulsions also contain anti-inflammatory DHA and vitamin E.
  - Phytosterols that are high in soybean oils have been shown independently to cause or worsen liver inflammation and cholestatic disease.

COMPLICATIONS FROM CATHETERS USED FOR PARENTERAL NUTRITION

- Peripheral IV lines can be used for parenteral nutrition at less than 900 to 1000 mOsm/L, which limits both dextrose (12.5%) and amino acid concentrations (3%) to prevent local skin and subcutaneous skin inflammation and necrosis with common extravasations.
  - Adding heparin limits clotting and prolongs catheter lifetime.
- Umbilical vein catheters (UVCs) are associated with air embolism during placement (rare), sepsis (if kept in >5–7 days), and hemorrhage (can dislodge).
- Percutaneously inserted central catheters (PICCs) are commonly used for long-term central venous access.
  - Major risk factors involve thrombosis and erosion of the catheter tips extravascularly, producing complications of pleural effusion with lung collapse and pericardial effusions with cardiac tamponade.
- Any prolonged IV line, more commonly with central lines (>5–7 days for UVCs), increases the risk of invasive bacterial infection and systemic sepsis.
  - Sepsis can be reduced by a common insertion and management protocol by only highly skilled and practiced caregivers with the use of meticulous sterile precautions for insertion and care.
  - Central lines should not be used for blood sampling or other drug infusions except during major life-threatening crises, although they often are used for essential medications such as antibiotics for proven sepsis in extremely small infants in whom peripheral subcutaneous IVs are not possible.
  - Central line–related sepsis is no longer compensated financially by public and private insurance unless it occurs when the central line is proven to be life-saving and alternative approaches are not available (rarely allowed).

METABOLIC COMPLICATIONS OF PARENTERAL NUTRITION

- The principal metabolic complication of parenteral nutrition is hyperglycemia.
  - This problem has increased in recent years and has been associated with increased rates of morbidity and mortality.
  - Most preterm infants, as well as term infants, continue to produce glucose from their livers at about 2 to 3 mg/kg/min even in the presence of normal to increased plasma concentrations of glucose and insulin, which normally inhibit hepatic glucose production.
  - If the parenteral dextrose infusion rate is >7 to 9 mg/kg/min, then total glucose utilization capacity will be exceeded, resulting in progressively increasing glucose concentrations.
  - Hyperglycemia from excessive dextrose infusion is compounded by stress with increased production of catecholamines, glucagon, and cortisol, which suppress or limit insulin secretion and action and increase hepatic glucose production.
  - Excessive dosing of IV lipids also aggravates hyperglycemia by providing competitive lipid carbon for oxidation and by producing co-factors in the liver from beta-oxidation of fatty acids that promote the regulatory enzymes in the gluconeogenic pathway.
- The principle metabolic complications of fat emulsions are hypertriglyceridemia and essential fatty acid deficiency (EFAD), but they also contribute to hyperglycemia by providing competitive carbon for oxidation.
  - Hypertriglyceridemia (>250 mg/dL) is increased by maturational deficiency of lipases, which are inversely related to gestational age; low levels of carnitine palmitoyltransferase (CPT), the protein necessary for transfer of longer chain fatty acids into the mitochondria for oxidation and energy production; and competition from glucose carbon (commonly associated hyperglycemic conditions).
  - Risks of hypertriglyceridemia can be diminished significantly by enteral feeding of milk or preterm formulas, which have natural or added carnitine, as well as lipases in human milk.
  - EFAD can develop within days when IVFEs are withheld from the TPN-dependent neonate. Minimal provision to prevent deficiency varies with the IVFE being used (0.5 g/kg/d of 100% soybean emulsion, 2 g/kg/d of a blended fat emulsion).
  - EFAD symptoms can include thrombocytopenia, dermatitis, hypertriglyceridemia, elevated transaminases, and failure to thrive.
  - The ratio of triene to tetraene (when using soybean emulsion) and full fatty acid profiles (when using the blended emulsion) are used to diagnose EFAD.

- The principal metabolic complication of IV amino acid solutions is lower than needed plasma concentrations of essential and some conditionally essential amino acids.
  - High amino acid concentrations generally are the result of excessive and unnecessary infusion rates (>4 g/kg/d) and limited urinary excretion, although caution should be used in giving high infusion rates to infants with clearly damaged liver function from hypoxic–ischemic injury.
  - Blood urea nitrogen concentrations and ammonia concentrations should increase by small amounts with increased amino acid infusion rates if the amino acids are appropriately oxidized and producing ammonia and the liver is functioning well to remove ammonia through the urea cycle.

POTENTIAL TOXICITIES ASSOCIATED WITH THE USE OF PARENTERAL NUTRITION

- Manganese (Mn) can produce potential neurotoxicity.
  - Mn supplementation should be discontinued with any signs of hepatic dysfunction or cholestasis.
  - Common TPN components have been shown to have Mn contamination.
  - Standard multi–trace element packages used in the United States contain significant Mn. Individual trace elements may be used as an alternative.
- Chromium (Cr) contamination is also prevalent in TPN components, and current recommendations are that supplementation is not necessary.
  - Standard multi–trace element packages used in the United States contain significant Cr. Individual trace elements may be used as an alternative.
- Aluminum contamination is found in albumin, blood products, certain medications, and TPN components.
  - Preterm infants are at high risk of aluminum accumulation and toxicity, as they often require TPN for many days and have immature kidneys incapable of excreting aluminum efficiently.

- Calcium gluconate and phosphate salts are high in aluminum content and are required by preterm infants in substantial amounts to promote bone mineralization.
  - The US Food and Drug Administration (FDA) has set limits for aluminum content of TPN components, but manufacturers are often unable to meet these restrictions. Health care providers should make a concerted effort to use the least contaminated products.
  - A readily available substitution is using sodium phosphate in preference to potassium phosphate.
- Phytosterols and low antioxidant factors (e.g., DHA, vitamin E) can lead to cholestasis.
- Peroxide formation occurs when lipids, amino acids, vitamins, and trace elements are exposed to ambient light and phototherapy at any point.
  - Complete photoprotection of the infusions, including tubing at the bedside, has been shown to reduce oxidative stress in preterm infants.
  - Oxidative stress contributes to the development of morbidities associated with prematurity.

Suggested Readings

American Academy of Pediatrics Committee on Nutrition. Nutritional needs of preterm infants. In: Kleinman RE, Greer FR, eds. *Pediatric Nutrition Handbook.* 8th ed. Itasca, IL: American Academy of Pediatrics; 2020:113–162.

Carnielli VP, Correani A, Giretti I, et al. Practice of parenteral nutrition in preterm infants. *World Rev Nutr Diet.* 2021;122:198–211.

Hendrickson K, Reilly AM, Bhatia J, Hay Jr. WW. Practical parenteral nutrition. In: Polin RA, Benitz W, eds. *Workbook in Practical Neonatology.* 7th ed. Philadelphia: Elsevier; 2019:84–98.

Olsen SL, Oschman A, Tracy K. Total parenteral nutrition. In: Gardner SL, Carter BS, Enzman-Hines M, Niermeyer S, eds. *Neonatal Intensive Care: An Interprofessional Approach.* 9th ed. St. Louis: Elsevier; 2021:459–479.

Patel P, Bhatia J. Total parenteral nutrition for the very low birth weight infant. *Semin Fetal Neonatal Med.* 2017;22:2–7.

van Goudoever JB, van den Akker CHP. Parenteral nutrition for critically ill term and preterm neonates: a commentary on the 2021 European Society for Paediatric Gastroenterology, Hepatology and Nutrition Position Paper. *J Pediatr Gastroenterol Nutr.* 2021;73:137–138.

Gastroenterology and Bilirubin

REBECCA ABELL, MEGAN E. GABEL and AARTI RAGHAVAN

36 *Gastrointestinal Development*

REBECCA ABELL and MEGAN E. GABEL

Esophagus

- Structure
  - By week 4 of gestation, the primitive foregut is formed by folding of the endoderm and splanchnic mesoderm into a tubular structure.
  - A complex process of infolding and fusion of the lateral sides of the proximal foregut gives rise to the respiratory tube (ventral) and esophageal tube (dorsal).
  - Incomplete fusion of the lateral grooves results in failure of separation of the dorsal and ventral tubes, leading to a tracheoesophageal fistula (TEF).
  - The esophageal lumen is reestablished by week 10 of gestation.
  - By the end of the first trimester, neuroblasts and circular muscle are present throughout the esophagus.
  - By week 16, stratified squamous epithelium is present.
  - The upper esophageal sphincter is present by week 32.
  - By 40 weeks, the esophagus is approximately 8 to 10 cm in length.
  - The structure of the esophageal musculature is divided into three segments:
    - Upper third—striated muscle
    - Middle third—striated and smooth muscle
    - Lower third—smooth muscle
- Function
  - Swallowing is first seen as early as week 16.
  - Non-nutritive sucking can be seen as early as gestation week 20.
  - Nutritive sucking does not appear until weeks 32 to 34.
  - Superficial glands are present in the esophageal mucosa by week 20.
  - Mucosal and lingual lipases are secreted by squamous cells by week 28.

Stomach

- The stomach arises from the embryonic foregut.
- By week 4, it is recognizable as a fusiform dilation.
- The endocrine chief, mucous, and parietal cells appear by week 12. By week 16, these cells secrete hydrochloric acid, intrinsic factor, pepsin, gastrin, and mucus.
- The stomach enlarges ventrodorsally and rotates 90 degrees clockwise on a longitudinal axis.
- The primitive gut is lined with endoderm.
- The mesoderm differentiates into smooth muscle layers.
- There are two functional zones of motor activity:
  - The proximal zone (fundus and proximal third of the body) is a reservoir that can distend to accommodate bolus feeding; it generates steady contractions stimulated by the vagus nerve.
  - The distal zone is responsible for mixing and breaking down food to allow food to empty into the duodenum.
- Gastric acid plays a protective role against bacteria entering into the gastrointestinal (GI) tract. Thus, it protects the upper aerodigestive tract and modulates the intestinal microbiome.
  - Term infants have a neutral gastric pH at birth, which decreases within the first 48 hours of life.
  - Premature infants have a prolonged period of alkaline pH.

Intestine

- This primitive gut tube forms by week 4, when a portion of the yolk sac incorporates into the embryo during craniofacial and lateral folding (Fig. 36.1).
- The lumen is occluded as a third epithelial layer rapidly proliferates, then recanalizes. Failure to recanalize results in intestinal atresia or stenosis.
- The intestine is divided into the foregut, midgut, and hindgut.
  - The caudal portion of foregut gives rise to the upper duodenum.
  - The midgut gives rise to lower duodenum, jejunum, ileum, appendix, ascending colon, and proximal two-thirds of the transverse colon.
  - The hindgut gives rise to one-third of the transverse colon, descending colon, sigmoid colon, rectum, and superior part of anal canal.
- The midgut loop herniates through the umbilical ring at week 6.
- Neuroblasts appear at week 7.
- During week 11, the midgut loop rotates counterclockwise around the superior mesenteric artery (SMA) as it returns to the abdominal cavity.
  - Failure of this loop to return to the abdomen results in omphalocele; gastroschisis results from a herniation through a defect in the abdominal wall musculature, typically to the right of the umbilical cord.
  - If there is only partial intestinal rotation, malrotation ensues.
- At week 24, lactase activity is <25% of activity at 40 weeks. Increase in lactase activity occurs during weeks 32 to 34.
- Myenteric muscle contractions are seen at week 32.

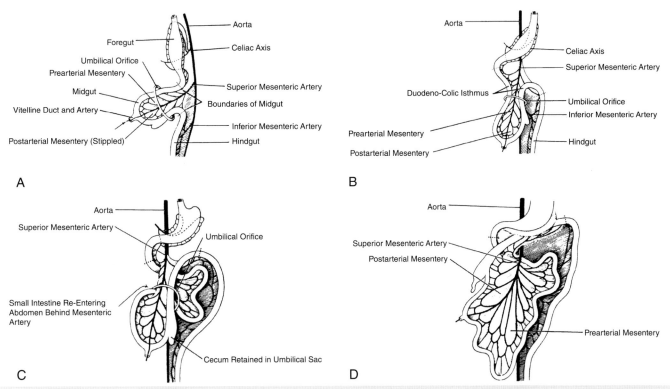

Fig. 36.1 Normal rotation of the alimentary tract. (A) Fifth week of intrauterine life, lateral view. The foregut, midgut, and hindgut are shown with their individual blood supply supported by the common dorsal mesentery in the sagittal plane. The midgut loop has been extruded into the umbilical cord. (B) Eighth week of intrauterine life, anteroposterior view. The first stage of rotation is being completed. Note the narrow duodenoocolic isthmus from which the midgut loop develops and the right-sided position of the small intestine and left-sided position of the colon. Maintenance of this position after birth is termed *malrotation*. (C) During the ~10th week of intrauterine life and the second stage of rotation, anteroposterior view. The bowel in the temporary umbilical hernia is in the process of reduction. The most proximal portion of the prearterial segment enters the abdomen to the right of the superior mesenteric artery and is held forward close to the cecum and ascending colon, permitting the bowel to pass under it. As the coils of small intestine collect within the abdomen, the hindgut is displaced to the left and upward. (D) During the 11th week of intrauterine life and the end of the second stage of rotation. From its original sagittal position, the midgut has rotated 270 degrees in a counterclockwise direction about the origin of the superior mesenteric artery. The essentials of the permanent disposition of the viscera have been attained. (Original figure was published in Gardner CE Jr, Hart D. Anomalies of intestinal rotation as a cause of intestinal obstruction: report of two personal observations; review of one hundred and three reported cases. *Arch Surg*. 1934;29(6):942–981. This image is reproduced in Gleason CA, Devaskar SU, eds. *Avery's Diseases of the Newborn*. 9th ed. Philadelphia: Elsevier; 2011:1072.)

- The small intestine typically measures between 200 and 300 cm at 40 weeks.
- Gut-associated lymphoid tissue (GALT) contributes significantly to the immune system.
  - Peyer patches are lymphoid follicles that are the sites of T- and B-cell activity.
  - Lamina propria lymphocytes are responsible for secreting immunoglobulin A (IgA), which binds and neutralizes intestinal bacteria.

Pancreas

- Dorsal and ventral pancreatic buds arise from the endoderm of the caudal foregut at weeks 4 to 5.
  - Each bud communicates with the foregut through a duct.
  - The duodenum rotates, resulting in movement of the ventral pancreatic bud posteriorly and inferiorly to the dorsal pancreatic bud.
- The two buds fuse to form the pancreas at week 7.
  - Ventral pancreatic bud forms the inferior part of the head of the pancreas and uncinate process.

- Dorsal pancreatic bud forms the superior part of the head, body, and tail of the pancreas.
- The ductal systems of the two buds join at week 8.
- Differentiation of endocrine and exocrine structures is present by week 14.
  - By gestational week 14, insulin and pancreatic zymogen granules are present.
  - By gestational week 16, amylase is present.
  - By gestational week 31, trypsin, lipase, and amylase are secreted.
- The concentration of pancreatic enzymes is lower in preterm infants at birth.

Liver/Hepatobiliary

- The liver is formed from the endoderm.
- The liver bud arises from the cranioventral portion of the endoderm.
- The liver grows and is encapsulated and lobulated, with bile ducts present by week 6.
- Hepatoblasts, precursors to hepatocytes, migrate into the septum transversum mesenchyme, with hematopoietic and endothelial precursors.

Table 36.1 Anatomic and Functional Maturation of the Gastrointestinal Tract

		POSTCONCEPTIONAL AGE (WEEKS)			
15	20	25	30	35	40
Mouth	Salivary glands	Swallow	Lingual lipase	*Sucking*	—
Esophagus	Muscle layers present	Striated epithelium present	*Poor lower esophageal sphincter tone*	—	—
Stomach	Gastric glands present	G cells appear	*Gastric secretions present*	*Slow gastric emptying*	—[a]
Pancreas	Exocrine and endocrine tissue differentiate	Zymogen present	*Reduced trypsin, lipase*	—	—[a]
Liver	Lobules form	*Bile secreted*	*Fatty acids absorbed*	—	—[a]
Intestine	Crypt and villus form	*Glucose transport present*	*Dipeptidase, sucrase, and maltase active*	*Lactase active*	—
Colon	—	Crypts and villi recede	—	*Meconium passed*	—

[a]Full functional maturation occurs postnatally. *Italics* indicate functional maturation.
From Berseth CL. Developmental anatomy and physiology of the gastrointestinal tract. In: Taeusch HW, Ballard R, Gleason C, eds. *Avery's Diseases of the Newborn.* 8th ed. Philadelphia: Elsevier; 2005:1071–1085.

- Bile acids are synthesized by week 12 and secreted by week 22.
- The bile acid pool size in preterm infants is one-third of that seen in term infants.
- Due to immature processing of bile salts, preterm infants are at increased risk of developing cholestasis, especially after chronic parenteral nutrition.
- The lymphatic system develops by week 15.

Gallbladder and Biliary Tree

- The hepatic diverticulum gives rise to the hepatic parenchyma, intrahepatic biliary tree, and common bile duct.
- The cystic diverticulum gives rise to the cystic duct and the gallbladder.
- The cystic duct fuses with the common bile duct.

- Hepatoblasts in the mesenchyme near the portal vein form a layered structure called the *ductal plate.* The ductal plate cells form bile ducts in the intrahepatic portal tracts.
- Canaliculi are formed when hepatocytes join.
- By week 4, the intrahepatic biliary tree is present.
- Table 36.1 summarizes the anatomic and functional maturation of the entire gastrointestinal tract.

Suggested Readings

Gleason CA, Sawyer T. *Avery's Diseases of the Newborn.* 11th ed. Philadelphia: Elsevier; 2024.
Huang J, Walker WA, eds. *Review of Pediatric Gastrointestinal Disease and Nutrition.* Hamilton, Ontario: BC Decker; 2005.
Martin RJ, Fanaroff AA, Walsh MC. *Fanaroff and Martin's Neonatal-Perinatal Medicine.* 11th ed. Philadelphia: Elsevier; 2015.
Wyllie R, Hyams JS, Kay M. *Pediatric Gastrointestinal and Liver Disease.* 5th ed. Philadelphia: Elsevier; 2015.

37 *Gastrointestinal Anomalies*

REBECCA ABELL and MEGAN E. GABEL

Oropharynx

- Epstein pearls
  - Small cystic lesions on the hard palate present in 80% of newborns
  - Typically disappear within 1 month of life
  - Larger cysts rarely require surgical excision.
- Tumors of the mouth
  - Epignathus
  - Extremely rare congenital teratoma of the upper jaw or palate
  - A benign tumor with associated morbidity because it can present with severe airway obstruction or feeding difficulty
  - Can present with other congenital malformations including cleft palate, bifid tongue, bifid uvula, congenital heart defects, and inguinal hernias
  - Treatment is surgical excision.
  - Congenital epulis
  - Rare congenital benign neoplasm, also known as *granular cell tumor* or *congenital gingival granular cell tumor*
  - Arises from upper or lower jaw
  - May interfere with respiration or feeding

Salivary Glands

- Hemangiomas and lymphangiomas are the most common tumors.
- Benign lesions are confined to the intracapsular portion of the gland.
- When a histologic diagnosis is confirmed, treatment is observation.

Esophagus

- Esophageal duplication cysts
  - Comprise 10% to 15% of all GI duplications
  - Can lead to esophageal obstruction
  - Neonates are typically asymptomatic but can present with respiratory or digestive symptoms.
  - Cysts are diagnosed by chest radiograph and computed tomography (CT) demonstrating a mediastinal mass.
  - Magnetic resonance imaging (MRI) is necessary to rule out a neurenteric cyst, which may have a connection to the pinal canal.
  - Treatment is surgical resection.

- Tracheoesophageal fistula (TEF) (Fig. 37.1)
  - Five common anatomic variants with type C (esophageal atresia/distal TEF) account for 85% of cases.
  - Develops before the eighth week of gestation as a result of abnormal division of the dorsal and ventral foregut
  - Incidence is 1/3000 to 1/4000 live births.
  - Up to 7% of neonates with TEF have a chromosomal abnormality.
  - Up to 70% have at least one other congenital anomaly.
  - Most commonly seen in association with vertebral, anorectal, cardiac, tracheal, esophageal, renal/genitourinary, and limb (VACTERL) association
  - Can be seen with CHARGE syndrome (coloboma, heart defect, atresia choanae, restriction of growth/development, genital hypoplasia, ear defect/deafness)
  - Diagnosis
    - Prenatal history of polyhydramnios in one-third of cases due to esophageal atresia
    - Shortly after birth, it presents with increased oral secretions, feeding difficulties, and respiratory distress.
    - Gasless abdomen is suggestive of isolated esophageal atresia.
    - Inability to pass nasogastric (NG) tube to the stomach suggests the diagnosis.
    - Distal fistula may present with significant abdominal distention.
    - H-type TEF may present outside of the newborn period with history of more mild respiratory issues associated with feeding or recurrent aspiration pneumonia.
  - Treatment
    - Nothing by mouth (NPO), acid suppression, and intravenous (IV) fluids
    - Decompression of esophageal pouch with a suction catheter
    - Preoperative evaluation of associated congenital anomalies is necessary.
    - Definitive treatment is corrective surgery.
  - Postoperative complications
    - Anastomotic leak in 10% to 15% of cases
    - Esophageal stricture
    - Gastroesophageal reflux (GER)
    - Recurrent fistula
    - Tracheal obstruction
- Gastroesophageal reflux
  - GER is a normal physiologic condition in the neonate due to a lower resting pressure of the lower esophageal sphincter (LES; 2–3 mm Hg).
  - Normal resting pressure (10–15 mm Hg) is obtained by 6 months of life.
  - 82% of cases are related to transient relaxation of the LES.

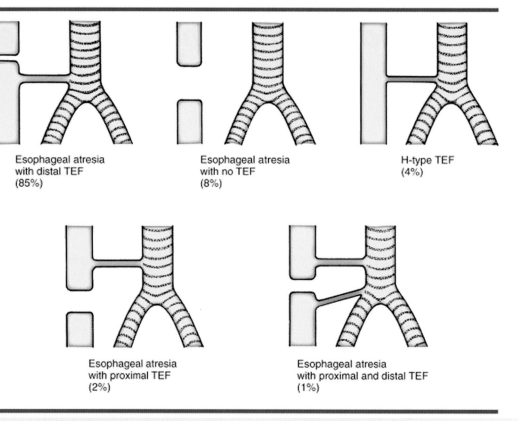

Esophageal atresia
with distal TEF
(85%)

Esophageal atresia
with no TEF
(8%)

H-type TEF
(4%)

Esophageal atresia
with proximal TEF
(2%)

Esophageal atresia
with proximal and distal TEF
(1%)

Fig. 37.1 Various types of tracheoesophageal fistulas (TEF) with relative frequency (%).

- Symptoms of pathologic gastroesophageal reflux disease (GERD) include poor weight gain, irritability, feeding aversion, and apnea/bradycardia.
- Barium swallow will rule out underlying anatomic abnormalities but has low yield to diagnose GERD.
- Gastric emptying studies may be helpful to identify delayed gastric emptying that may contribute to GER.
- Impedance studies can identify acid as well as nonacid reflux; however, a weak association exists between findings and the presence of clinically significant GERD.
- Treatment
  - Inclined positioning
  - Addition of rice cereal to formula
  - Acid blockade (H2 blocker or proton pump inhibitor) will not decrease physiologic reflux but will decrease mucosal acid exposure.
  - Prokinetic agents: erythromycin (risk of pyloric stenosis), metoclopramide (risk of irreversible tardive dyskinesia)
  - Surgical intervention: Nissen fundoplication in high-risk patients that are refractory to medical treatment

Stomach

- Microgastria
  - Very rare congenital anomaly
  - Associated with mega-esophagus, malrotation, biliary anomalies, situs inversus, skeletal anomalies/defects, asplenia, and GERD

- Presents with vomiting, failure to thrive, persistent diarrhea
- Diagnosed by upper GI (UGI) contrast study
- Treatment
  - Continuous enteral feeding with supplemental parenteral nutrition until gastric adaptation and ability to transition to bolus feeding
  - If surgical intervention is necessary, the standard approach includes gastric augmentation with roux-en-Y jejunal reservoir.
- Gastric volvulus
  - Results from inadequate mesenteric fixation
  - Often associated with other anomalies such as malrotation, diaphragmatic defect, or asplenia
  - Symptoms include emesis (bilious/nonbilious) and abdominal distention.
  - Abdominal radiograph demonstrates massive gastric dilation.
  - UGI shows transverse lie of the stomach and inversion of the greater curvature and pylorus.
  - Treatment requires emergent surgery.
- Pyloric stenosis
  - Idiopathic hypertrophy of pyloric muscle resulting in narrowing and elongation of pyloric channel
  - Results in gastric outlet obstruction
  - Incidence is 1/1000 to 3/1000 live births.
  - Male predominance (4:1)
  - Association between maternal and infant exposure to erythromycin
  - Typically presents between 3 and 6 weeks of age with progressive projectile vomiting

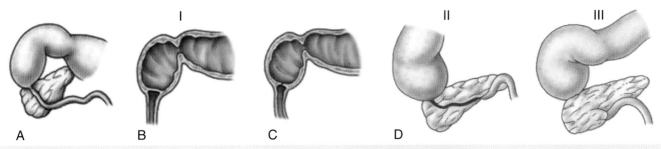

Fig. 37.2 **Duodenal and intestinal atresia and stenosis.**

- Hypochloremic hypokalemic contraction alkalosis is suggestive.
- Hypoglycemia and indirect hyperbilirubinemia may be present.
- Hallmark of physical exam is palpation of "olive" in the epigastrium.
- Diagnosis is confirmed with ultrasound.
- Treatment includes correction of metabolic derangements and surgical pyloromyotomy.
- Pyloric atresia
  - Incidence is 3/100,000.
  - Congenital partial or complete gastric obstruction involving the antrum or the pylorus
  - Associated with trisomy 21 and junctional epidermolysis bullosa
  - Presents in the first few days of life with nonbilious emesis, feeding difficulties, and abdominal distention
  - History of polyhydramnios common due to obstruction
  - Can lead to stomach rupture within first 12 hours of life
  - Diagnosis: upper GI contrast study
  - Treatment includes correction of metabolic derangement and gastric decompression, followed by gastroduodenostomy.

Small Intestine

- Duodenal atresia (DA) and stenosis (Fig. 37.2)
  - Atresia or stenosis occurs when the duodenal segment does not recanalize during the 8th to 10th weeks of gestation.
  - Most infants with DA have other associated anomalies (trisomy 21, congenital heart disease, intestinal malrotation, esophageal atresia, or imperforate anus).
  - History of polyhydramnios is common with DA.
  - Obstruction of the duodenal lumen can be complete, partial, intrinsic, or extrinsic.
    - Extrinsic forms include malrotation with obstruction from Ladd bands or from twisting on a small mesenteric base, compression by an anterior or preduodenal portal vein, gastroduodenal duplication, cysts or pseudocysts of the pancreatic–biliary tree, or annular pancreas.
  - Diagnosis: double bubble, polyhydramnios on fetal USG; after delivery, emesis, double bubble on KUB
  - Treatment: replogle, IV nutrition until surgical repair, evaluation for associated anomalies
- Annular pancreas

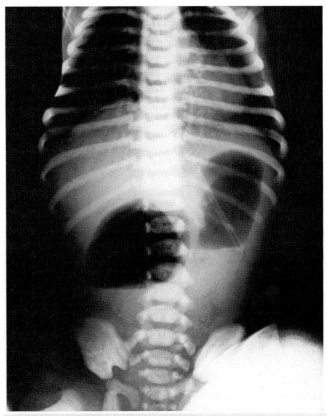

Fig. 37.3 **"Double bubble" sign seen with duodenal atresia.**

- Occurs when the ventral pancreatic bud does not rotate behind the duodenum, causing an extrinsic compression encircling the second portion of the duodenum
- Can be associated with other intrinsic duodenal anomalies
- Prenatal ultrasound may demonstrate two dilated, fluid-filled structures.
- Infant presents with bilious emesis within 24 hours of birth, without abdominal distention.
- Abdominal radiographs demonstrate classic "double bubble" sign (Fig. 37.3).
- Treatment involves placement of NG for decompression, fluid and electrolyte stabilization, and evaluation for associated anomalies prior to surgical correction.
- Duplications of the small intestine
  - Duodenal duplications are most common in the first or second portion and may be lined with gastric mucosa.

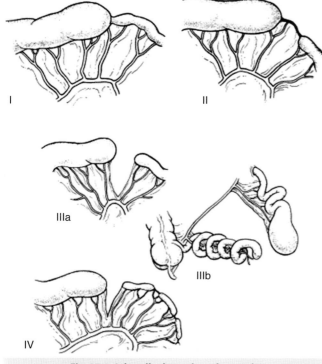

Fig. 37.4 Jejunoileal atresis and stenosis.

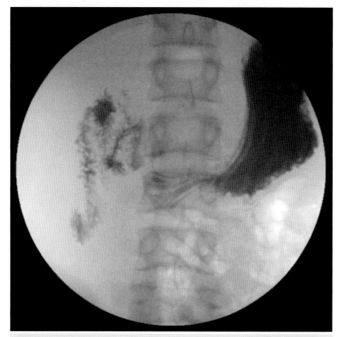

Fig. 37.5 Upper gastrointestinal series demonstrating malrotation.

- They can cause pancreatitis due to compression of pancreatic duct.
- Hemorrhage or perforation are indications for emergent surgery.
- May be detected with prenatal ultrasound as a right upper quadrant cystic mass
- UGI may demonstrate extrinsic compression, but ultrasound and CT are needed for definitive diagnosis.
- Treatment is surgical resection.

- Jejunoileal atresia (Fig. 37.4)
  - Occurs after 12th week of gestation
  - Due to mesenteric vascular disruption leading to ischemic necrosis
  - Classified into five subtypes:
    - Type I. Mucosal (membranous) web
    - Type II. Blind ends connected by a fibrous cord
    - Type IIIa. Blind ends separated by a V-shaped mesenteric defect
    - Type IIIb. Apple-peel or Christmas-tree deformity (blind ends; distal small bowel segment forms corkscrew around ileocecal artery terminus)
    - Type IV. Multiple atresias (string of sausages)
  - Prenatal ultrasound may show polyhydramnios and distended loops of fetal bowel.
  - Infants present with bilious emesis, abdominal distention, failure to pass meconium, and jaundice.
  - Abdominal radiographs demonstrate dilated, thumbsized loops of bowel.
  - Contrast enema is diagnostic with the presence of microcolon.
  - Treatment involves decompression of the stomach, fluid resuscitation, and subsequent surgical resection.
- Malrotation and/or volvulus
  - Occurs between the 6th and 12th weeks of gestation if counterclockwise rotation and fixation do not occur properly
  - Malrotation occurs in 1/100, but only 1/6000 are diagnosed.
  - 70% are not diagnosed in the newborn period because they are not symptomatic unless obstructed by Ladds bands or volvulus.
  - Volvulus presents with acute bilious emesis and clinical deterioration.
  - Upper GI is indicated to assess the position of ligament of Treitz, which will not cross the midline (Fig. 37.5).
  - Emergent surgical intervention is vital in volvulus to avoid significant bowel ischemia and necrosis. Malrotation without volvulus warrants nonemergent surgical intervention to avoid future volvulus.

Large Intestine

- Intestinal atresia
  - Less than 10% of intestinal atresia/stenosis occur in the colon.
  - Etiology is thought to be vascular compromise in utero, most likely along the vascular watershed area of the hepatic flexure.
  - Incidence is approximately 1/20,000.
  - Diagnosis is suspected with dilated bowel on prenatal ultrasound.
  - Abdominal distention occurs within 24 to 28 hours of birth, and there is often no passage of meconium.
  - Diagnosis is suggested by abdominal radiograph showing distended small bowel loops.
  - Water-soluble contrast enema can establish a diagnosis and differentiate among meconium plug syndrome, small left colon syndrome, and Hirschsprung disease.
  - Treatment involves gastric decompression, IV antibiotics, and surgical correction.

- In stable patients without peritonitis, primary anastomosis is possible.
- Size discrepancy between the dilated proximal colon and small distal colon may not allow for primary anastomosis; proximal ostomy and distal mucus fistula are created and reanastomosis is performed after the dilated portion of bowel has decompressed.
- Meconium plug syndrome (MPS)/small left colon syndrome
  - Functional immaturity of colon resulting in obstructive meconium plugs
  - MPS is thought to be related to transient colonic hypomotility; it is more frequent in preterm infants and infants of diabetic mother (IDMs) and when there is history of maternal eclampsia.
  - Hypomotility may be related to immaturity of myenteric plexus ganglia.
  - Maternal magnesium sulfate administration can lead to neonatal hypermagnesemia, which depresses the function of intestinal smooth muscle, contributing to MPS.
  - Neonatal hypoglycemia can also result in decreased intestinal motility.
  - Diagnosis is suggested by dilated loops of bowel on abdominal radiograph.
  - Water-soluble contrast enema is both diagnostic and therapeutic.
    - Contrast enema with multiple filling defects which represent meconium plugs
    - Obstruction is often resolved with contrast enema; infrequently, surgical intervention is required.
  - Further evaluation for cystic fibrosis or Hirschsprung disease may be indicated.
- Consequences of surgical resection of distal ileum, cecum, and large intestine
  - Primary role of the colon is absorption of water and electrolytes.
  - Terminal ileum is the only segment that reabsorbs bile salts actively.
  - If 50 cm or more of ileum are lost, bile salt synthesis by the liver cannot compensate for the decrease in enterohepatic circulation.
  - Bile acids are necessary for the digestion and absorption of fats and fat-soluble vitamins.
  - Inadequate lipid emulsification results and colonic fluid losses are increased.
  - Loss of the ileum/ileocecal valve accelerates gastric emptying and small bowel motility and further reduces absorptive capability.
  - It is thought to be mediated by peptide tyrosine tyrosine (PYY) and glucagon-like peptide 1 (GLP-1).

Rectum and Anus

- Imperforate anus
  - Incidence is 1/5000 births.
  - Slightly more common in males
  - Occurs when there is arrest of the caudal descent of the urorectal septum to the cloacal membrane during development

- Diagnosis
  - Based on good perineal exam
  - Females may pass meconium through a perineal, vestibular, or vaginal fistula or may present as cloaca (rectum, vagina, and urinary tract meet and fuse, creating a single common channel).
  - Males may have a cutaneous fistula that tracks midline toward the penis, which may present with meconium in the urine or air in the bladder.
  - X-ray may demonstrate progressive distal bowel obstruction.
  - Perineal ultrasound may be more helpful.
  - Consider VATER syndrome (VACTERL association).
- Treatment
  - Low defects can be managed with surgery to restore anorectal canal.
  - High and intermediate defects require colostomy and later elective repair.
- Hirschsprung disease
  - Occurs in 1/5000 births
  - Male to female ratio is 4:1.
  - Caused by agenesis of ganglion cells in the myenteric and submucosal plexuses; decreased expression of nitric oxide synthase gene also adds to dysmotility
  - Multiple gene mutations have been identified, but receptor tyrosine kinase (RET) is the most common.
  - 20% to 30% of cases are associated with congenital anomalies/syndromes. It is most commonly seen with trisomy 21, multiple endocrine neoplasia type 2 (MEN2), Waardenburg syndrome, Smith-Lemli-Opitz syndrome, and central hypoventilation syndrome.
  - It occurs when vagal neural crest cells do not migrate appropriately between weeks 5 and 12; the earlier this occurs, the longer the segment of aganglionic bowel.
  - Anus is always involved; the amount of intestine involved can vary.
  - Presenting symptoms vary.
    - Failure to pass meconium within first 24 to 48 hours of life
    - Bilious vomiting
    - Constipation with abdominal distention, often suppository dependent
    - Failure to thrive
  - Diagnosis
    - Rectal exam demonstrates tight anus with empty rectal vault.
    - Contrast enema demonstrates different caliber of small aganglionic segment and dilated proximal segment. This "transition zone" may not be apparent until 3 to 4 weeks of age.
    - Continued presence of contrast in rectosigmoid 24 hours later is very suggestive of Hirschsprung disease.
    - Contrast enema will not be diagnostic in total colonic aganglionosis.
    - Definitive diagnosis is obtained with rectal suction biopsy or full-thickness biopsy taken at 2 to 4 cm above the anal verge that demonstrates an absence of ganglion cells. The presence of acetylcholinesterase (AChE) with hypertrophic nerve fibers is diagnostic.

- Treatment includes surgical resection of aganglionic bowel and anastomosis of anus to ganglionic bowel proximally. There is a risk of enterocolitis persists, even after surgery.
- Hirschsprung-associated enterocolitis (HAEC)
  - Characterized clinically by fever, abdominal distention, bloody diarrhea, and sepsis
  - Leading cause of morbidity and mortality in children with Hirschsprung disease

Pancreas

- Pancreatic agenesis/hypoplasia
  - Rarely reported conditions that lead to endocrine/exocrine pancreatic insufficiency
  - Hypoplasia results from agenesis of the dorsal bud (typically provides 90% of pancreatic tissue).
  - Fatty replacement of the pancreatic tissue
  - Can lead to intrauterine growth restriction
  - Treatment is hormone and enzyme replacement.
- Schwachman syndrome
  - Triad of pancreatic insufficiency, bone marrow dysfunction, and poor growth
  - 89% of patients have mutations mapped to chromosome 7q11.
  - Defect involves enzyme secretion and acinar function.
  - Clinical presentation includes steatorrhea, neutropenia ± anemia or thrombocytopenia, and failure to thrive.
  - Skeletal anomalies can be present.
    - Progressive long-bone dysostosis or metaphyseal chondrodysplasia is seen in 50%.
    - Rib cage abnormalities are seen in one-third of patients.
  - Treatment is pancreatic enzyme replacement and close monitoring for infection.
  - Mortality is increased (30%) due to infections and increased risk of leukemia.
- Cystic fibrosis (CF)
  - CF is a genetic disease that can present in the newborn period with intestinal obstruction due to meconium plugs and meconium ileus.
  - CF can lead to peritonitis, volvulus, or bowel necrosis.
  - Microcolon may also occur due to in utero intestinal obstruction and subsequent underdevelopment of the colon.
  - Clinical manifestations also include prolonged jaundice, liver disease, and failure to thrive.
  - Respiratory symptoms typically develop outside of the newborn period.
  - CF is caused by mutation of the cystic fibrosis transmembrane regulator (CFTR) gene on chromosome 7.
    - This gene encodes a protein that forms a chloride channel.
    - More than 800 different mutations have been described, with F508 deletion being the most common.
    - Autosomal recessive
  - Prenatal diagnosis
    - Ultrasound showing hyperechoic fetal bowel pattern, meconium peritonitis, abdominal calcifications suggestive of CF

- Chorionic villus sampling or amniocentesis is diagnostic.
- Diagnosis is often made after birth by newborn screening.
- Confirmatory test is sweat testing for chloride concentration analysis; sweat chloride > 60 mEq/dL is diagnostic.
- Testing for pancreatic insufficiency (stool elastase) can also suggest the diagnosis.
- Management requires a multidisciplinary approach with pulmonology, gastroenterology, nutrition, and social work.
- GI care in infancy is centered on providing adequate calories for growth, appropriately dosing pancreatic enzymes, and addressing acute issues with meconium ileus.
- Prognosis has improved significantly, with half of individuals living past 40 years of age.

Meconium Syndromes

- Meconium ileus
  - Almost always associated with CF (occurs in 10–20% of patients with CF)
  - Inspissated meconium leads to obstruction in the distal small bowel.
  - Presents with signs of bowel obstruction within 24 to 48 hours of life
  - Signs include bilious emesis, abdominal distention, and failure to pass meconium.
  - If bowel necrosis has occurred in utero, a pseudocyst may develop and can present as a palpable mass.
  - Volvulus may also occur and present as an acute abdomen.
  - Diagnosis is determined by abdominal x-ray showing gaseous distension, and "soap-bubble appearance" due to air in meconium is suggestive.
  - Initial management includes hydration, gastric decompression, and antibiotics.
  - Nonoperative treatment is indicated for uncomplicated cases and involves enema.
  - Successful 50% of the time but associated with 11% perforation rate
  - Operative treatment includes enterotomy and bowel irrigation with N-acetylcysteine.
  - At times, it is necessary to divert the bowel to allow for continued bowel irrigation.
- Meconium peritonitis
  - Intestinal obstruction can lead to bowel necrosis and perforation during the fetal period.
  - Meconium in the peritoneal cavity leads to an inflammatory reaction.
  - Results in calcification and scarring, termed *fibroadhesive peritonitis*, which seals off the perforation
  - Meconium ascites occurs when perforation allows liquid meconium to fill the peritoneal cavity in the perinatal period.
  - Infants can be asymptomatic but can be diagnosed due to calcifications on radiograph.
  - If infants present with bowel obstruction, surgical intervention is indicated.

- Surgery often involves resection of necrotic bowel or intestinal diversion.
- Meconium plug syndrome (also covered in Large Intestine section)
  - Also termed functional inertia of prematurity or neonatal small left colon syndrome
  - Typically occurs in preterm infants, also seen in infants of diabetic mothers
  - Immature intestinal motility leads to meconium obstruction in the colon.
  - Contributing factors may be hypermagnesemia and hypoglycemia.
  - Presents with abdominal distention and failure to pass meconium
  - Abdominal radiograph shows multiple dilated loops of bowel.
  - Water-soluble contrast enema can be diagnostic and therapeutic.
  - Surgical treatment is rarely required.

Abdominal Wall Defects

- Gastroschisis
  - Herniation of abdominal contents through an abdominal wall defect
  - Etiology is thought to be intrauterine vascular accident.
  - Risk factors include young maternal age, lower socioeconomic status, and firstborn infants.
  - Defect is typically on the right side of the umbilicus.
  - Diagnosis can be made prenatally via ultrasound and elevated levels of maternal alpha-fetoprotein (AFP) and amniotic AFP.
  - Bowel is not protected by the peritoneal sac and is exposed to amniotic fluid leading to fibrous "peel" covering the exposed surface.
  - Intestinal atresia may also be present in 5% to 25% of cases.
  - Other associated anomalies are infrequent (15%) and not associated with increased risk of abnormal chromosomes, in contrast to omphalocele.
  - Consider ruptured omphalocele, given higher risk of other congenital anomalies.
  - At birth, the entire gastrointestinal tract may be eviscerated.
  - Abdominal defect can be restrictive, leading to significant risk of vascular compromise.
  - Initial treatment includes placing the infant's lower body in a sterile bag, positioning to maintain blood flow to extraabdominal intestines (care must be taken to avoid kinking mesenteric vessels), keeping bowel moist, Replogle decompression, adequate fluid and hydration to account for accelerated losses, and broad-spectrum antibiotics.
  - Primary closure of the defect is possible in 90% of cases.
  - For larger defects, a staged reduction via silo system is necessary to avoid respiratory failure and abdominal compartment syndrome.
  - Infants typically have prolonged ileus and are at increased risk for NEC.

- Long-term consequences include poor motility, feeding intolerance, need for prolonged parenteral nutrition, and short bowel syndrome.
- Survival rate is 90% to 95%.
- Omphalocele
  - Congenital defect in the central abdominal wall
  - Results from failure of lateral body folds and craniocaudal folds to converge and close the ventral abdominal wall
  - Typically occurs around the 10th week of gestation
  - Eviscerated intestinal contents are covered by mesenchymal membrane and are protected from amniotic fluid.
  - Membrane rupture may appear to be a gastroschesis.
  - Liver may herniate through the abdominal wall defect.
  - Omphalocele can be associated with other congenital abnormalities in 50% to 75% of cases, including congenital heart disease, VACTEL association, Beckwith-Wiedemann syndrome, and trisomies 13,18, and 21.
  - Diagnosis can be made by ultrasound at 19 weeks' gestation.
  - Due to association with cardiac and chromosomal disorders, amniocentesis and fetal echocardiogram are recommended.
  - Initial treatment includes wrapping bowel in sterile saline-soaked gauze, Replogle decompression, adequate fluid and hydration, and broad-spectrum antibiotics.
  - Operative repair is performed as soon as possible after birth.
  - For larger defects, a staged reduction via silo system is necessary to avoid respiratory failure and abdominal compartment syndrome.
  - Survival rate is 30% to 80%, largely due to associated anomalies.

Syndromes Associated With Gastrointestinal Malformation

- Pentalogy of Cantrell: sternal, diaphragmatic, and pericardial defects, upper abdominal omphalocele, ectopia cordis
- Beckwith-Wiedemann syndrome: macrosomia, visceromegaly, hemihypertrophy, hypoglycemia, renal pathology
- EEC syndrome: ectodermal dysplasia, cleft palate, ectrodactyly
- OEIS complex: omphalocele, exstrophy, imperforate anus, spinal defect

Suggested Readings

Gleason C, Sawyer T, eds. *Avery's Diseases of the Newborn.* 11th ed. Philadelphia: Elsevier; 2024:897–924.

Martin R, Fanaroff A, Walsh M, eds. *Fanaroff and Martin's Neonatal-Perinatal Medicine, Diseases of the Fetus and Infant.* 11th ed. Philadelphia: Elsevier; 2019.

Wyllie R, Hyams J, eds. *Pediatric Gastrointestinal and Liver Disease: Pathophysiology, Diagnosis, Management.* 3rd ed. Philadelphia: Saunders; 2005; Chapters 21 and 22.

38 Acquired Disorders of Gastrointestinal Tract

REBECCA ABELL and MEGAN E. GABEL

Gastrointestinal Bleeding

See Table 38.1.

NECROTIZING ENTEROCOLITIS

- Necrotizing enterocolitis (NEC) is the most common acquired gastrointestinal (GI) condition in premature infants.
- Clinical presentation: lethargy, tachycardia, hypotension, increased apnea and bradycardia that may progress to respiratory failure, tachypnea due to abdominal distention and metabolic acidosis, pallor/poor perfusion, feeding intolerance, abdominal distention and tenderness, abdominal wall erythema, hypoactive bowel sounds, bloody stools
- Clinical features
  - 90% of infants with NEC are premature; NEC occurs in ~12% of very low-birth-weight (VLBW) infants (<1500 g at birth).
  - Postnatal age of onset and incidence are inversely related to birth weight and gestational age.
  - Term and late preterm infants infrequently develop NEC; risk factors (associated with bowel ischemia) include intrauterine growth restriction (IUGR) and small for gestational age (SGA), birth asphyxia, congenital heart disease, gastroschisis, polycythemia, hypoglycemia, sepsis, and exchange transfusion.

Table 38.1 Causes of Gastrointestinal (GI) Bleeding in the Neonate

Upper GI Bleeding	Lower GI Bleeding
Swallowed maternal blood	Milk protein allergy, allergic colitis
Vitamin K deficiency	Hirschsprung disease
Stress gastritis or ulcer	Necrotizing enterocolitis
Acid peptic disease	Intussusception
Vascular anomaly	Gastrointestinal duplication
Coagulopathy	Duodenal web
Mallory-Weiss tear	Anal fissure
Bowel obstruction	Coagulopathy
Milk protein allergy	Volvulus
	Infectious colitis
	Meckel diverticulum
Presentation of Upper GI Bleeding	**Presentation of Lower GI Bleeding**
Hematemesis	Bright red blood in the stool
Coffee ground emesis	Tarry stools
Melena	

- NEC can occur in epidemics.
- It occurs more frequently in African American infants than in white infants.
- NEC is more common following initiation of enteral feeds.
- Breast milk and established feeding guidelines are protective factors.
- Overall, up to 50% require surgery or drainage tube.
- NEC is a predictor of neurodevelopmental morbidity.
- One-third have positive blood cultures.
- Multiple risk factors are likely, including bowel ischemia, immaturity of immune system, and enteral feeding.
- Diagnosis (Table 38.2)
  - Suspect with clinical features; laboratory values can reveal neutropenia, thrombocytopenia, hyponatremia, metabolic acidosis from lactate accumulation
  - Abdominal x-ray findings vary depending on severity and may include dilated loops of bowel, stacked loops, fixed loop (concerning for necrotic bowel), pneumatosis intestinalis (when extensive can appear as "tram tracks"), portal venous gas (later two pathognomonic for NEC), and perforation (football sign with outline of falciform ligament from air demonstrates massive extraluminal air; left lateral decubitus can help identify more subtle free air layered against the liver). Ultrasound may detect early pneumatosis or portal venous air.
- Treatment
  - Supportive care includes bowel rest, decompression of the GI tract, fluid resuscitation, treat hypotension, avoid dopamine (can worsen bowel necrosis from vasoconstriction), broad-spectrum antibiotics, respiratory support if needed.
  - Operative management includes all of the above plus surgical resection of necrotic bowel; consider peritoneal drain as an alternative based on clinical condition.

SHORT BOWEL SYNDROME

- Short bowel syndrome may occur following bowel resection to treat NEC (most commonly), midgut volvulus, omphalocele, aganglionosis, jejunal or ileal atresia, and gastroschisis.
- Symptoms usually develop after >2/3 bowel is removed.
- An infant is more likely to survive if >15 cm bowel remains with intact ileocecal valve or 40 cm bowel remains in the absence of the ileocecal valve.
- Most frequent cause of intestinal failure in neonates
- Complications
  - Malabsorption of nutrients
  - Gastric hypersecretion
  - Small bowel bacterial overgrowth

Table 38.2 Stages of NEC and Examples of NEC Imposters

Name of Entity	Major Diagnostic Criteria	Treatment	Pitfalls
Stage 1 NEC	Clinical signs in baby: feeding intolerance, vomiting, abdominal distension, gastric residuals	Observation, but often NPO, antibiotics, frequent blood monitoring, radiographs	Seen very commonly in extremely preterm infants, those on nasal or mask ventilation, or those being monitored for gastric residuals
Stage 2 NEC	Clinical signs can be similar to those above but also include radiographic criteria such as pneumatosis intestinalis and/or hepatic portal venous gas.	NPO, gastric suction, antibiotics for 7–10 days, frequent lab and radiographic monitoring	Benefits of antibiotics and length of antibiotic treatment are unknown. Radiographic signs can be misleading, especially a bubbly appearance in the bowel where a radiographic reading is "cannot rule out NEC."
Stage 3 NEC	Abdominal distension, pneumoperitoneum on radiograph, necrosis diagnosed at laparotomy or autopsy	Usually surgical emergency, with drain placement and/or exploratory laparotomy with resection of diseased bowel	It may be readily confused with spontaneous intestinal perforation or congenital bowel disease if bowel is not directly visualized. This is common when only a drain is placed without direct examination of the bowel.
Spontaneous intestinal perforation (SIP)	As above with stage 3 NEC but minimal bowel necrosis	Surgical emergency with drain placement and/or exploratory laparotomy Resection is usually not required.	As above; often confused with surgical NEC, but treatment and prognosis are different Pathophysiology is also different, with high level of inflammation.
Ischemic bowel due to cardiac anomalies	Abdominal distention, most commonly associated with low left ventricular output such as seen in hypoplastic left heart, aortic atresia, interrupted aortic arch	As with stage 2 or 3 NEC	Complexities associated with heart disease may cause hesitation to do abdominal surgery.
Variants of food protein intolerance syndrome (FPIES)	Abdominal distention can be seen but is not pathognomonic; often presents with bloody stools and may have eosinophilia.	Responds well to highly elemental diet	Does not have good biomarkers to differentiate from other intestinal injuries

NEC, Necrotizing enterocolitis; *NPO*, nil per os.
Data from Lure AC, et al. Using machine learning analysis to assist in differentiating between necrotizing enterocolitis and spontaneous intestinal perforation: a novel predictive analytic tool. *J Pediatr Surg.* 2021;56:1703–1710. Lueschow SR, et al. A critical evaluation of current definitions of necrotizing enterocolitis. *Pediatr Res.* 2022;91:590–597.

- Intestinal adaptation difficulties
- Cholestatic liver disease from chronic parenteral nutrition, possible liver failure
- Catheter-related complications
- Enterocolitis
- Management
  - Parenteral nutrition to support growth, including SMOF (fish oil) for fat component
  - H2 blockers or proton pump inhibitors to suppress acid secretion
  - Intermittent treatment with antibiotics for bacterial overgrowth
  - Enteral feeds to help with intestinal growth and adaptation—small volumes of elemental formula with medium-chain triglycerides
  - If the ileocecal valve is missing, infant is at high risk for diarrhea and fat and vitamin B_{12} malabsorption and will need vitamin B_{12} supplementation.
  - Surgical management includes bowel-lengthening procedures or intestinal transplantation.

NEONATAL INTUSSUSCEPTION

- Extremely rare
- Often missed diagnosis and confused with NEC

- Most cases involve small bowel.
- Clinical presentation includes abdominal distention, feeding intolerance, vomiting, and bloody stools.
- Diagnosis
  - Ultrasound is the gold standard.
  - X-rays may be unremarkable or show dilation of bowel loops or gas–fluid levels.
  - Contrast enema if colonic involvement

ALLERGIC ENTERITIS AND COLITIS—MILK PROTEIN ALLERGY

- Caused by immunologic hypersensitivity to milk protein
- The frequency is 2% to 6%, but only 0.5% in breastfed infants.
- 30% to 60% can also have allergy to soy protein.
- Acute gastroenteritis is a risk factor.
- Clinical presentation
  - 50% to 60% have gastrointestinal or skin symptoms.
  - Excessive spits, cramping, bloody stools, or urticaria
  - 30% have respiratory symptoms, such as wheezing.
- Diagnosis is based on clinical improvement with a milk-free diet or recurrence of symptoms with the reintroduction of milk.
- There are no diagnostic biochemical tests.

- The most sensitive and specific test to predict if a reaction to cow's milk will occur is a cow's milk–specific immunoglobulin E (IgE) and an index of lymphocyte stimulation with beta-lactoglobulin.
- Biopsies are not needed for diagnosis but demonstrate partial or total villous atrophy, with an increase in eosinophils.
- Treatment is removal of cow's milk protein.
  - Formulas containing hydrolyzed proteins or amino acid–based formulas can be used.
  - Breastfed infants require removal of dairy from the mother's diet.
  - 28% of children can tolerate milk protein by the age of 2 years and 78% by 6 years.

Malabsorption Syndromes

DISORDERS OF CARBOHYDRATE ABSORPTION

- Enterocytes lining the small intestine produce enzymes that convert disaccharides and oligosaccharides into monosaccharides.
- Enzymes are maltase–glucoamylase (MGA), sucrose–isomaltase (SI), and lactase phlorizin hydrolase.
- Monosaccharides are absorbed via transport proteins.
- Carbohydrate malabsorption can occur due to deficiency of these enzymes or a defect in a transport protein involved in absorption.
- Patients present with severe, watery, osmotic diarrhea.
- Diarrhea regresses when the infant receives nutrition NPO.
- Diagnosis is often made based on the age of the patient and what foods are present in the diet (Table 38.3).

ENZYME DEFICIENCIES

Congenital Sucrase–Isomaltase Deficiency

- Congenital sucrase–isomaltase deficiency (CSID) is most common.
- Mapped to chromosome 3
- Presents around age 3 to 6 months when baby is introduced to foods containing sucrose
- Severe watery diarrhea, acidosis, abdominal distention, cramping, failure to thrive (FTT)
- Stool pH is <7 due to fermentation of sugars by colonic bacteria.
- Reducing substances negative (sucrose is nonreducing sugar)

Table 38.3 Age of Onset of Different Malabsorption Syndromes

Age of Onset	Disorder
Immediate neonatal period	Glucose–galactose malabsorption (GGM)
	Congenital lactase deficiency
Weaning age	Glucoamylase deficiency
	Congenital sucrose–isomaltase deficiency (CSID)

Adapted from Martin RJ, Fanaroff AA, Walsh MC, eds. *Fanaroff and Martin's Neonatal-Perinatal Medicine.* 11th ed. Philadelphia: Elsevier; 2020.

- Endoscopy with biopsy for disaccharidase activity is the gold standard for diagnosis.
- Treatment: avoidance of sucrose

Congenital Lactase Deficiency

- Very rare diagnosis
- Autosomal recessive; most cases have been described in Finland
- Presents with introduction of lactose (breast milk, lactose-based formula)
- Severe watery diarrhea, vomiting, FTT, lactosuria, aminoaciduria, lethargy
- Diagnosis made by failure of blood glucose to rise after administration of lactose
- Gold standard is endoscopy with biopsy for disaccharidase activity.
- Treatment: lactose-free diet

Maltase–Glucoamylase Deficiency

- Very rare condition
- 60% homology to SI
- Not uncommon to see MGA and CSID concurrently
- Presents with diarrhea and distention
- Symptoms begin with introduction of starch into diet.
- Endoscopy with biopsy for disaccharidase activity is the gold standard for diagnosis.
- Treatment: lactose-free formula and starch elimination

Transport Defects

GLUCOSE–GALACTOSE MALABSORPTION

- Very rare condition
- Autosomal recessive, chromosome 22
- Leads to defect in sodium–glucose linked cotransporter (SGLT) protein
- Severe watery diarrhea in newborn period can lead to death.
- Occurs when infant is fed breast milk or glucose-containing formula
- Diagnosis made by stools positive for reducing substances.
- Oral glucose test does not lead to rise in serum glucose.
- Diarrhea stops when NPO.
- Intestinal biopsies are normal.
- Treatment: formula with fructose as carbohydrate component

Disorders of Protein Absorption

PRIMARY INTESTINAL ENTEROPEPTIDASE DEFICIENCY

- Very rare
- Enteropeptidase converts trypsinogen to trypsin, which then activates other pancreatic enzymes.
- Presenting symptoms: diarrhea, FTT, protein-losing enteropathy, significant serum hypoalbuminemia
- Diagnosis by biopsy with enzyme quantification or measurement of enzyme level in duodenal fluid
- Treatment: protein–hydrolysate formula

Disorders of Fat Absorption

HYPOBETALIPOPROTEINEMIA AND ABETALIPOPROTEINEMIA

- Autosomal dominant disorder
- Low or absent plasma concentrations of apolipoprotein B lipoproteins and low-density lipoprotein (LDL) cholesterol
- In heterozygotes, typically clinically asymptomatic
- Homozygous patients have complete absence of beta-lipoproteins; they present with fat malabsorption, acanthocytosis, retinitis pigmentosa, and neuromuscular degeneration.
- Abetalipoproteinemia (autosomal recessive [AR]) presents with the same symptoms due to absence of beta-lipoproteins.
- Treatment: low-fat diet, fat-soluble vitamin supplementation

CHYLOMICRON RETENTION DISEASE (ANDERSON DISEASE)

- Autosomal recessive disorder of lipoprotein assembly
- Presenting symptoms: hypocholesterolemia, fat malabsorption, FTT
- Clinical presentation is similar to abetalipoproteinemia, but extra intestinal manifestations are less severe.
- Treatment: low-fat diet, fat-soluble vitamin supplementation

PRIMARY BILE ACID MALABSORPTION

- Due to disruption in enterohepatic circulation of bile
- Presenting symptoms: diarrhea, steatorrhea, decreased serum cholesterol
- Treatment: cholestyramine, low-fat diet

Disorders of Electrolyte Absorption

CONGENITAL CHLORIDE DIARRHEA

- Congenital chloride diarrhea (CCD) is the most common cause of congenital secretory diarrhea with intact mucosal histopathology.
- AR transmission, defect in intestinal brush border chloride–bicarbonate exchange
- Severe watery diarrhea high in chloride beginning in immediate neonatal period

- Persists when NPO
- Patients have hyponatremia, hypokalemia, hypochloremia, and metabolic alkalosis.
- Treatment: oral chloride, potassium supplements, suppression of gastric acid

CONGENITAL SODIUM DIARRHEA

- AR transmission
- Exceedingly rare
- Due to defect in sodium–hydrogen exchanger in jejunal brush border
- Presents similarly to CCD but with high sodium content in diarrhea
- Can also present with abdominal distention and failure to pass meconium
- Laboratory tests will show hyponatremia, metabolic acidosis, and hypokalemia.
- Treatment: fluid and electrolyte replacement

Disorders of Villous Architecture

MICROVILLUS INCLUSION DISEASE

- Microvillus inclusion disease (MVID) is a congenital defect of the intestinal brush border.
- Presents with severe diarrhea (up to 500 mL/kg/d)
- Persists when NPO
- Diagnosis is made via duodenal biopsy specimens that show villous atrophy.
- Treatment options include lifelong parenteral nutrition or small bowel transplantation.

TUFTING ENTEROPATHY

- Presents in first weeks of life with severe life-threatening diarrhea
- Duodenal biopsy shows epithelial shedding.
- Treatment options are lifelong parenteral nutrition or small bowel transplantation.

Suggested Readings

Gleason CA, Sawyer T, eds. *Avery's Diseases of the Newborn.* 11th ed. Philadelphia: Elsevier; 2024.

Huang J, Walker WA, eds. *Review of Pediatric Gastrointestinal Disease and Nutrition.* Hamilton, Ontario: BC Decker; 2005.

Martin RJ, Fanaroff AA, Walsh MC. *Fanaroff and Martin's Neonatal-Perinatal Medicine.* 11th ed. Philadelphia: Elsevier; 2020.

Wyllie R, Hyams JS, Kay M. *Pediatric Gastrointestinal and Liver Disease.* 5th ed. Philadelphia: Elsevier; 2015.

39 Liver Disease, Abdominal Masses, and Ascites in the Newborn

REBECCA ABELL and MEGAN E. GABEL

Cholestasis of the Neonate

- Obstruction of bile from the liver cells into the intestine
- Generally considered a direct (or conjugated) bilirubin greater than 2.0 mg/dL or more than 20% of the total bilirubin
- May be caused by viruses, metabolic disease, rare diseases that affect the function of the liver, or congenital malformations of liver and bile ducts
- Presence is suggested with clinical jaundice and confirmed with elevated direct bilirubin noted when obtaining a fractionated serum bilirubin.
- See Table 39.1 for causes, clinical presentation, and diagnosis.

Congenital Malformations of the Liver and Bile Ducts

CHOLEDOCHAL CYSTS

- Cystic dilation of hepatobiliary tree
- Incidence is 1/100,000 to 1/150,000 in Western countries.
- They are more common in Asian countries.
- They are four times more common in females.
- Proposed etiology: regurgitation of pancreatic secretions into the biliary tree at the time of pancreaticobiliary duct fusion, resulting in weakening and dilation of the duct
- Can coincide with biliary atresia
- Clinical presentation
  - Jaundice
  - Elevated liver enzymes
  - Direct hyperbilirubinemia and elevated gamma-glutamyltransferase (GGT)
  - Obstructive symptoms such as cholangitis, pancreatitis, hepatitis, cirrhosis, and/or portal hypertension if not treated
- Diagnosis
  - Ultrasound
  - Can be diagnosed prenatally
  - Classified (types I–VI) based on Todani criteria, presence of multiple saccular or cystic dilations of the intrahepatic ducts (known as Caroli disease)
  - 80% are diagnosed before age 10.

- Treatment
  - Surgical resection
  - Risk of malignancy if not removed

INTRAHEPATIC BILIARY HYPOPLASIA: ALAGILLE SYNDROME

- Autosomal dominant
- Paucity of intralobular ducts
- Occurs in 1/30,000 live births
- Mutations in the *JAG1* and *NOTCH2* genes
- Clinical presentation
  - Triangular facies
  - Posterior embryotoxon (iris strands)
  - Butterfly vertebrae
  - Renal disease
  - Cardiac defects (peripheral pulmonic stenosis, tetralogy of Fallot)
  - Direct hyperbilirubinemia
  - May have acholic stool
  - Elevated alanine aminotransferase (ALT)
  - Elevated bile acids
  - Very elevated GGT—may be up to 20 times the normal value
- Diagnosis is made by liver biopsy.

EXTRAHEPATIC BILIARY ATRESIA

- Occurs in 1/15,000 to 1/18,000 live births
- Most common cause of prolonged conjugated hyperbilirubinemia in neonates
- Progressive fibroinflammatory cholangiopathy leads to obliteration of extrahepatic biliary tree, resulting in obstruction and cirrhosis of liver.
- Clinical presentation
  - Appear well at birth
  - Direct bilirubin is typically <7 mg/dL.
  - Hepatosplenomegaly
  - GGT elevated
- Pathogenesis
  - Defect in morphogenesis of biliary tract
  - Defect in fetal or prenatal circulation
  - Environmental toxin exposure
  - Viral infection
  - Immunologic or inflammatory dysregulation

Table 39.1 Metabolic and Genetic Causes of Neonatal Cholestasis

Disease Process	Presentation	Diagnosis
Biliary atresia	Dark urine, acholic stools	Ultrasound, HIDA scan, liver biopsy, intraoperative cholangiography
Alagille syndrome	Characteristic facies, cardiac findings, vertebral anomalies	Chest x-ray (butterfly vertebrae), ophthalmology, echo, GGT, cholesterol level increased, decreased levels of fat-soluble vitamins, liver biopsy
Choledochal cyst	Abdominal mass	Cyst seen on ultrasound, ERCP, MRCP
Caroli disease, syndrome	Bacterial cholangitis, portal hypertension	Ultrasound of liver and kidneys, ERCP, MRCP if >1 year old, *PKHD1* gene (ARPKD)
Gallstones or biliary sludge	May have acholic stools	Ultrasound, ERCP, GGT, LFTs elevated
Idiopathic neonatal giant cell hepatitis	Prolonged jaundice	Histologic diagnosis after other causes excluded
Neonatal sclerosing cholangitis	Dark urine, acholic stools	GGT often > 800 IU/L, ERCP, liver biopsy with small duct destruction, intraoperative cholangiogram shows pruning of small bile ducts
PFIC	Severe cholestasis, intractable pruritus, possible coagulopathy	GGT decreased or normal in types 1 and 2, GGT increased in type 3, liver biopsy, genetic testing
A1AT deficiency	Neonatal jaundice	GGT often high, A1AT level low, A1AT PI phenotype analysis (ZZ, SZ, MZ)
Cystic fibrosis	Jaundice and hepatomegaly, steatorrhea, failure to thrive, meconium ileus	Newborn screening with high IRT, stool elastase low, sweat test with elevated sweat chloride, genetic testing
Gaucher disease	Splenomegaly, hepatomegaly, thrombocytopenia, anemia, bleeding, osteopenia	β-Glucocerebrosidase decreased, chitotriosidase increased, alkaline phosphatase increased; bone marrow biopsy with "crinkled paper" cytoplasm, glycolipid-laden macrophages, foam cells
Niemann-Pick type C	Splenomegaly	Filipin-positive reaction (detection of cholesterol in fibroblasts), increase in chitotriosidase, genetic testing
Wolman disease, LAL deficiency	Hepatomegaly, neonatal liver failure	Hyperechoic liver, lysosomal lipase acid decreased in peripheral blood mononuclear cell
Mitochondrial disorders	Lethargy, vomiting, hypotonia, seizures, hypoglycemia, coagulopathy, lactic acidosis	Genetic testing, fasting and postprandial lactate, INR, plasma lactate-to-pyruvate ratio > 20
Tyrosinemia	Cholestasis and coagulopathy, Fanconi-related nephropathy or seizures	Newborn screening, urinary excretion of succinylacetone is increased, 4-hydroxy-phenylketones and γ-aminolevulinic acid increased, genetic testing
Galactosemia	Vomiting, diarrhea, renal tubular acidosis, cataracts, FTT, coagulopathy	Newborn screening, presence of reducing substances in urine, galactose-1-phosphate uridyltransferase activity in red blood cells decreased
Congenital disorders of glycosylation	Dysmorphic facies, DD, seizures, dystrophy, hepatomegaly, cyclic vomiting, diarrhea, hypoalbuminemia, protein-losing enteropathy	Triglycerides increased, ATIII decreased, factor XI decreased, proteins C and S decreased
Hypothyroidism	Jaundice	Newborn screening, TSH and free T_4 elevated
Panhypopituitarism	Hypoglycemia, prolonged jaundice, micropenis	Glucose, cortisol, TSH, free T_4, IGF-1, and IGF-BP decreased, hypercalcemia, liver biopsy with bile duct paucity; MRI may show microadenoma or absent sella
ARC syndrome	Limb contractures, arthrogryposis multiplex congenita, facial dysmorphia, rental tubular acidosis, cholestasis, platelet dysfunction, ichthyosis	Genetic testing

A1AT, Alpha-1-antitrypsin; *ARC,* arthrogryposis–renal dysfunction–cholestasis syndrome; *ARPKD,* autosomal recessive polycystic kidney disease; *ERCP,* endoscopic retrograde cholangiopancreatography; *FTT,* failure to thrive; *GGT,* gamma-glutamyltransferase; *HIDA,* hepatobiliary iminodiacetic acid scan; *IGF-1,* insulin-like growth factor 1; *IGF-BP,* insulin-like growth factor binding protein; *INR,* international normalized ratio; *IRT,* immunoreactive trypsinogen; *LAL,* lysosomal acid lipase; *LFT,* liver function test; *DD,* developmental delay; *MRCP,* magnetic resonance cholangiopancreatography; *PFIC,* progressive familial intrahepatic cholestasis; *T₄,* thyroxine; *TSH,* thyroid-stimulating hormone.

- Diagnosis
  - Ultrasound: Absence of gallbladder is suggestive, but the presence of gallbladder does not rule it out; triangular cord sign is suggestive of biliary atresia.
  - Scintigraphy, or hepatobiliary iminodiacetic acid (HIDA) scan:
    - Ensures hepatic uptake and excretion of analogues of iminodiacetic acid into intestines
    - Pretreatment includes phenobarbital 5 mg/kg/d for 5 days prior to study.
  - Liver biopsy demonstrates bile plugging, proliferated ducts, edema, and fibrosis.
  - Exploratory laparotomy with cholangiography for definitive diagnosis
- Treatment
  - Kasai procedure
  - Roux-en-Y jejunostomy
  - Best prognosis if done before 60 days of age

Box 39.1   Neonatal Abdominal Masses

Retroperitoneal—Kidney

- Hydronephrosis
- Multicystic dysplastic kidney
- Autosomal recessive polycystic kidney disease
- Autosomal dominant polycystic kidney disease
- Mesoblastic nephroma
- Renal vein thrombosis

Retroperitoneal—Other

- Adrenal abscess
- Fetus in fetu

Pelvic

- Hydrometrocolpos
- Ovarian cyst

Gastrointestinal

- Intestinal duplication
- Malrotation
- Obstruction
- Sacrococcygeal teratoma

Table 39.2   Neonatal Ascites

Type of Ascites	Features
Chylous	Clear or milky fluid; high triglyceride level and leukocyte count; protein content variable
Urinary	Urine: elevated urea, creatinine, and potassium; low or normal sodium and chloride
Biliary	Bilirubin > 4 g/dL
Pancreatic	May have elevated amylase, fat, and protein
Other	Neonatal hydrops; congestive heart failure; rupture of large ovarian cyst

Abdominal Masses

See Box 39.1 for type and location of neonatal abdominal masses.

NEONATAL ASCITES

See Table 39.2. for type and clinical features.

- Chylous ascites
  - Most common type
  - Occurs more frequently in males
  - Most often due to congenital failure of lymphatic channels to communicate
  - May accompany intestinal malrotation and incomplete volvulus
  - Often refractory to therapy; can lead to malnutrition and immunodeficiency due to extravasation of protein and lymphocytes
  - Treatment includes paracentesis and formula containing medium-chain triglycerides (MCTs).
- Urinary ascites
  - 25% of neonatal ascites
  - Caused by obstructive uropathy
  - Most commonly due to posterior urethral valves but can also be from ureteroceles, urethral atresia, bladder neck obstruction, neurogenic bladder, or bladder hematoma
  - Need to evaluate patient for abnormalities in urinary tract and collecting system
  - Treatment includes surgical decompression or correction of underlying issue.
- Biliary ascites
  - Caused by spontaneous perforation of biliary tree
  - In 68%, perforation is in the main biliary tree.
  - Two forms:
    - Acute—abdominal distention, vomiting, lack of bowel signs, may not have jaundice
    - Chronic form—early jaundice, gradual abdominal distention
  - Diagnosis is confirmed by scintigraphy or ultrasound.
  - Treatment is laparotomy with biliary drainage.
- Pancreatic ascites
  - Extremely rare
  - May be due to pancreatic duct anomaly
  - Only symptom is abdominal distention.
  - Urine and serum amylase levels can be normal.
  - Treatment requires surgical drainage.
- Ruptured ovarian cyst presents with hemoperitoneum in addition to ascites.
- Ascites is associated with hydrops in utero, such as from severe fetal anemia (Rh incompatibility, parvovirus).

Suggested Readings

Fawaz R, Baumann U, Ekong U, et al. Guideline for the evaluation of cholestatic jaundice in infants: Joint Recommendations of the North American Society for Pediatric Gastroenterology, Hepatology, and Nutrition and the European Society for Pediatric Gastroenterology, Hepatology, and Nutrition. *J Pediatr Gastroenterol Nutr.* 2017;64(1):154–168.

Gleason CA, Sawyer T, eds. *Avery's Diseases of the Newborn.* 11th ed. Philadelphia: Elsevier; 2024:940–955.

Götze T, Blessing H, Grillhösl C, Gerner P, Hoerning A. Neonatal cholestasis: differential diagnoses, current diagnostic procedures, and treatment. *Front Pediatr.* 2015;3:43.

Huang JMD, Walker WA, eds. *Review of Pediatric Gastrointestinal Disease and Nutrition.* 4th ed. Hamilton, ON: BC Decker; 2005; Sections 1, 2, 3.

Ronnekleiv-Kelly, Soares KC, Ejaz A, Pawlik TM. Management of choledochal cysts. *Curr Opin Gastroenterol.* 2016;32:225–231.

40 Bilirubin Biochemistry Metabolism and Measurement

AARTI RAGHAVAN

Bilirubin Biochemistry

- Life span of red blood cells (RBCs) in the newborn is 1.5 to 3 months.
- Bilirubin is a yellow–orange pigment (4Z, 15Z, bilirubin; IX, alpha isomer) formed by the degradation of hemoglobin in mammals. This provides 80% of the bilirubin in neonates.
- Other sources include degradation of myoglobin from muscles, cytochromes, and catalase activity.
- Biliverdin is formed as an intermediate step, and carbon monoxide is a by-product.
- Due to the shorter life span of RBCs, bilirubin production in neonates is 8.5 mg/kg/d compared with 4 mg/kg/d in adults.
- Other factors leading to increased bilirubin production in newborns compared with adults:
  - Increased cytochrome turnover
  - Increased enterohepatic circulation

Bilirubin Physiology, Pathways of Synthesis, Transport, and Metabolism in the Newborn

BILIRUBIN PRODUCTION

- Heme is produced by the degradation of RBCs in the reticuloendothelial system.
- Heme breaks down into biliverdin (IX alpha) by the action of heme oxygenase, with iron and carbon monoxide produced as by-products. Carbon monoxide combined with hemoglobin forms carboxyhemoglobin, which is released through the lungs.
- Heme oxygenase 1 is induced by inflammatory mediators leading to increased heme breakdown in neonates with comorbidities such as respiratory distress syndrome or bronchopulmonary dysplasia.
- Biliverdin is converted into bilirubin (IX alpha) by the action of bilirubin reductase.
- The degradation of 1 g of hemoglobin = 34 g of bilirubin.

TRANSPORT AND PROTEIN BINDING

- Unconjugated bilirubin is water insoluble and is transported in plasma bound to albumin.
- 7 to 8 mg/dL of bilirubin binds to one molecule of albumin.
- Binding occurs via two sites: primary high-affinity binding site and secondary low-affinity binding site. Other binding sites exist but are not clinically significant.
- Due to tight binding with albumin, bilirubin only occurs in its free unbound form in a low nanomolar range, even in cases of hyperbilirubinemia.
- When the molar concentration of bilirubin exceeds the albumin-binding capacity, levels of free unbound bilirubin increase.
- Bilirubin binding to albumin increases with postnatal age and decreases in sick infants and in the presence of binding competitors such as ampicillin, sulfa drugs, ceftriaxone, free fatty acids, and benzyl alcohol.

UPTAKE AND CONJUGATION

- The bilirubin–albumin complex travels to hepatocytes via plasma.
- Bilirubin is transported into the hepatocytes by carriers such as ligandin or glutathione S-transferase.
- Increased uptake of bilirubin occurs when ligandin concentrations are increased.
- Ligandin concentrations reach adult levels 1 to 2 weeks after birth. Concentrations are also increased by drugs such as phenobarbital.
- Glucuronyl transferase (uridine diphosphate [UDP]–glucuronyl transferase) catalyzes the binding of glucuronic acid to bilirubin, resulting in water-soluble bilirubin glucuronide (polar form) that can be excreted in bile.
- Bilirubin monoglucuronide is formed in the endoplasmic reticulum of microsomes (25%); diglucuronide formation occurs at the cell membrane (60%).
- Conjugation of bilirubin converts water-insoluble to water-soluble molecules, resulting in decreased intestinal absorption because hydrophilic molecules do not get absorbed easily.

EXCRETION

- Conjugated bilirubin is excreted into bile by an energy-dependent mechanism against a concentration gradient.
- Due to this energy-dependent mechanism, the clearance of bilirubin from the hepatocyte is a saturable process and is a rate-limiting step after the first week of postnatal life.
- Bile is secreted into the intestines and is then reduced to stercobilinogen and urobilinogen and excreted into stool.
- Alternatively, deconjugation in the small intestine is mediated by beta-glucuronidase in the brush border of the intestine. Unconjugated bilirubin is reabsorbed into the circulation. This cycle of conjugation, excretion, deconjugation, and absorption is known as *enterohepatic circulation*.

- Relatively low levels of bacterial flora also prevent conversion to urobilinogen, increasing intestinal absorption.
- Enterohepatic circulation in neonates is slightly slower due to decreased nutrient intake and decreased intestinal transit time.

BILIRUBIN PHYSIOLOGY IN THE FETUS

- Fetal bilirubin production is approximately 150% that of adults.
- Heme degradation results in the formation of bilirubin IX alpha, heme oxygen, and biliverdin.
- The rate-limiting step in bilirubin metabolism is the reduced levels of UDP–glucuronyl transferase, which is at low levels until 30 weeks' gestation and increases to 1% of adult levels at term.
- Bilirubin appears in the fetus from 14 weeks' gestation.
- At 16 weeks, unconjugated bilirubin IX alpha appears in bile.
- By 38 weeks' gestation, the primary isomer is bilirubin IX alpha.
- Although amniotic fluid does contain bilirubin in early gestation, it is not seen near term.
- Unconjugated bilirubin in the fetus is eliminated by crossing the placenta or via the liver into bile.
- Biliverdin and bilirubin conjugates do not cross the placenta.
- Conjugation and excretion into bile are confirmed by the accumulation of bilirubin in meconium, up to 5 to 10 times the daily neonatal production.
- Beta-glucuronidase activity in the meconium converts conjugated bilirubin to its unconjugated form, allowing absorption into the portal circulation.
- Reabsorbed bilirubin may be reconjugated in the liver or may cross the placenta into the maternal circulation.
- Due to the efficient elimination of unconjugated and conjugated bilirubin from the fetus, the fetal bilirubin level rarely rises to severe levels, even with hemolytic disease, where anemia is the overriding concern.

Measurement

- Principle of traditional method: reaction with the diazo agent, resulting in colored bilirubin derivatives, which are quantified by spectrophotometry
  - Directly reacting bilirubin (direct bilirubin)—Conjugated bilirubin reacts directly with the diazo agent to yield colored derivatives.
  - Indirectly acting bilirubin (indirect bilirubin)—When the reaction is catalyzed by caffeine or dimethylsulfoxide (DMSO), unconjugated bilirubin is energized to react with the diazo agent, forming colored derivatives.
  - Total bilirubin = Indirect derivatives + Direct bilirubin derivatives.
  - Other, less reliable methods used for measurement include fluorimetry and high-pressure liquid chromatography.
  - Spectrophotometry is most commonly used.
  - Other methods are often influenced by the products of bilirubin and glucuronide metabolism, which are found in an age-dependent and subject-dependent manner.
    - The administration of drugs, nutrition, and treatments such as phototherapy or exchange transfusions affect the concentration of bilirubin.
- Measurement of free bilirubin (i.e., unbound to albumin)
  - This method is not widely available for clinical use.
  - It is of interest due to the neurotoxic potential of free bilirubin.
  - Most bilirubin is bound to albumin, so free levels are expected to be low.
  - When bilirubin levels are high, levels exceed albumin-binding sites, resulting in high free bilirubin levels.
  - Because free bilirubin measurement tools are not well established, the serum bilirubin-to-albumin ratio is used as a surrogate marker.
- Noninvasive measurement of bilirubin
  - Transcutaneous measurement of yellow–orange pigment in the skin using optical technology
  - Provides an index of total bilirubin
  - Useful for serial measurements and measurement of trends
  - Serves as a screen; need confirmatory blood sampling and testing

How to Use Predischarge Bilirubin Measurement to Predict Risk of Severe Hyperbilirubinemia

- Bilirubin rises in an hourly fashion over the first few days of life, typically peaking at 4 to 5 days of life.
- Infants discharged at approximately 48 hours of life have only started to demonstrate increasing bilirubin.
- For this reason, all newborns must have follow-up soon after discharge (1–3 days after discharge).
- The timing of discharge should be determined based on risk factors such as feeding history, race and ethnicity (East Asian ethnicity at higher risk), previous sibling with hyperbilirubinemia, cephalohematoma, and bruising.
- The American Academy of Pediatrics recommends routine screening for bilirubin and risk evaluation based on hours of life prior to discharge.
- Predischarge bilirubin level and gestational age are the most sensitive factors to assess risk.
- Complete absence of hyperbilirubinemia is highly predictive of low-risk infants.

Suggested Readings

Hansen TWR. Core concepts: bilirubin metabolism. *NeoReviews.* 2010;11(6):e316–e322.

Krediet TG, Cirkel GA, Vreman HJ, et al. End-tidal carbon monoxide measurements in infant respiratory distress syndrome. *Acta Paediatr.* 2006;95(9):1075–1082.

Maisels MJ, Bhutani VK, Bogen D, Newman TB, Stark AR, Watchko JF. Hyperbilirubinemia in the newborn infant ≥ 35 weeks' gestation: an update with clarifications. *Pediatrics.* 2009;124(4):193–1198.

Martin RJ, Fanaroff AA, Walsh MC. *Fanaroff and Martin's Neonatal-Perinatal Medicine.* 11th ed. Philadelphia: Elsevier; 2020.

May C, Patel S, Peacock J, Milner A, Rafferty GF, Greenough A. End-tidal carbon monoxide levels in prematurely born infants developing bronchopulmonary dysplasia. *Pediatr Res.* 2007;61(4):474–478.

41 *Bilirubin Toxicity*

AARTI RAGHAVAN

Overview

- Severe jaundice in the newborn can cause bilirubin toxicity.
- In most patients, elevated serum bilirubin has no long-term sequelae.
- Elevated free unbound bilirubin can cross the blood–brain barrier and affect the brain.
- Typical areas of brain that are affected include the *basal ganglia*, *cranial nerve nuclei*, and *hippocampus*, which are stained yellow on pathologic examination.
- Staining correlates with neuronal necrosis and loss and gliosis.
- The level of free bilirubin is determined by its binding to serum albumin.
- Factors affecting bilirubin binding to albumin are detailed in Table 41.1.

Acute Bilirubin Encephalopathy

Acute bilirubin encephalopathy is an acute manifestation of bilirubin-induced neurologic dysfunction (BIND).

CLINICAL PRESENTATION

- Elevated serum bilirubin
  - Early bilirubin toxicity is transient and reversible.

Table 41.1 Factors Decreasing Bilirubin Binding to Albumin

Condition	Mechanism
Low serum albumin ■ Preterm infant ■ Sick infant	Low albumin-binding site availability
Drugs ■ Sulfisoxazole ■ Moxalactam ■ Ceftriaxone ■ Indomethacin ■ Salicylates ■ Ampicillin (rapid infusion)	Competitively displaces bilirubin from albumin
Acidosis (pH < 7.4)	Increases movement of bilirubin into tissues, including brain
Increased free fatty acids (e.g., intravenous lipid infusion, hypoxemia)	Displaces bilirubin
Benzyl alcohol	Inhibits albumin–bilirubin binding

- Increasing lethargy with a concomitant increase in serum bilirubin concentrations, with reversal of lethargy following interventions such as double-volume exchange transfusion

DIAGNOSIS AND EVALUATION

- The exact bilirubin level to cause BIND is unknown, although the risk appears greater with other risks such as prematurity and concomitant illness.
- Serum bilirubin should be used as part of a dynamic process of monitoring over time because bilirubin metabolism varies over time.
- The brainstem auditory evoked response (BAER) demonstrates changes in wave latency and magnitude, especially prolongation of latencies of waves III and IV–V and interpeak I–III and I–V, suggestive of brainstem conduction interference.
- BAER findings at this stage are typically reversible.
- An abnormal BAER may be due to cranial nerve VIII injury.
- Because cochlear function may be normal, otoacoustic emission (OAE) tests are not sufficient to screen for neuropathy.
- Magnetic resonance imaging (MRI) scans show focal changes in the globus pallidus and hippocampus.

Kernicterus

OVERVIEW

- Worsening encephalopathy due to hyperbilirubinemia, with pathologic findings of yellow staining and necrosis of neurons in basal ganglia, hippocampus, subthalamic nuclei, and cerebellum, with subsequent gliosis in these areas
- Cerebral cortex is typically spared.
- Extraneural sequelae are seen in >50% of affected infants—necrosis of renal tubular cells, intestinal mucosa and pancreatic cells, and accumulation of bilirubin crystals.

PATHOGENESIS

- Bilirubin enters the brain because of any of the following reasons:
  - Increased production of bilirubin overwhelms normal conjugation mechanisms.
  - Low serum albumin or decreased albumin-binding capacity (seen in sick or preterm infants) results in

increased free serum bilirubin; other factors affecting bilirubin–albumin binding are detailed in Table 41.1.
- Disruption of blood–brain barrier
- Increased serum osmolarity, hypoxemia, and meningitis all contribute.

- Increased in situ production of bilirubin.
  - Hemeoxygenase-1 and -2 (HO1 and HO2) break down hemoglobin outside the reticuloendothelial system in the brain and are upregulated under stress.
  - Biliverdin reductase converts biliverdin to bilirubin, which is cleared by bilirubin oxidase and transported out of the central nervous system (CNS).
  - All of these enzymes are developmentally regulated.
  - The breakdown of transport increases in situ accumulation of bilirubin.

- Postulated theories of CNS neuronal injury include the following:
  - Passage through lipid moieties of cell membranes into subcellular organelle such as mitochondria, interfering with energy metabolism
  - Binding to cytoplasmic protein and inhibiting function
  - Interference with DNA function

CLINICAL PRESENTATION

- There are several phases.
  - Phase 1: jaundice, poor suck, hypotonia, drowsiness
  - Phase 2: hypertonia, fever, torticollis, with or without opisthotonos
  - Phase 3: reduced hypertonia, high-pitched cry, hearing and visual abnormalities, poor feeding, athetosis, seizures
- Typical duration of symptoms is 24 hours.
- Mortality is 50%.
- Long-term sequelae include choreoathetoid cerebral palsy, upward gaze palsy, sensorineural hearing loss, and dental dysplasia; infant may have normal intellect.
- Long-term sequelae may be seen in infants with no evidence of bilirubin encephalopathy or kernicterus.
- Presentation in preterm infants is less typical; bilirubin levels for risk may be lower.

RISK FACTORS FOR KERNICTERUS

- Prematurity
  - Less typical clinical presentation
  - May cross blood–brain barrier at lower levels
  - May not stain the brain like in a term infant due to difference in CNS permeability and bilirubin metabolism
  - Mortality due to kernicterus is higher than in term infants.
- Sepsis
- Rapid rate of rise of bilirubin, such as with hemolytic diseases
- Asphyxia
- Hyperosmolar states—hyperglycemia, hypernatremia, dehydration, uremia due to renal failure
- Hypoxia
- Hypercarbia
- Hypoalbuminemia

EVALUATION AND DIAGNOSIS

- Diagnosis is based on
  - Clinical evaluation, with findings as above
  - Extremely elevated serum bilirubin values
- Evaluation includes
  - Impact of kernicterus
    - MRI of the brain
    - BAER (serial)
- Assessment of the cause of kernicterus includes the following:
  - Infant blood type and Coombs test
  - Maternal blood type
  - Complete blood count with reticulocyte count
  - Liver function tests (with total and fractionated bilirubin)
  - Peripheral smear (assess hemolysis)
  - Osmotic fragility
  - Glucose-6-phosphate dehydrogenase levels
  - Blood cultures (sepsis increases risk of direct hyperbilirubinemia)
  - Thyroid function tests

TREATMENT

- Phototherapy
  - Mechanism of action
  - Light energy converts subcutaneous bilirubin (4Z–15Z bilirubin) to photoisomers (E configuration instead of Z configuration = lumirubin), which are also unconjugated but less lipophilic and can be excreted in urine or bile.
  - Efficacy depends on the following:
    - Wavelength (420–490 μm, blue range)
    - Surface area for exposure
    - Distance to baby (more effective when closer)
    - Irradiation (at least 30 μW/cm²)
  - Side effects
    - Dehydration
    - Rash
    - Retinal injury
    - Gonadal injury
  - Contraindications
    - Bronze baby syndrome (bronzing of skin and urine) when phototherapy is used in patients with conjugated hyperbilirubinemia
    - Acute intermittent porphyria can cause bullae formation and death.
- Intravenous immunoglobulin
  - Useful in ABO and Rh incompatibility when response to phototherapy is suboptimal
  - More useful with ABO incompatibility than Rh incompatibility
  - Competitively binds to antigen and prevents antibody binding, preventing hemolysis
  - Dose: 500 to 1000 mg/kg intravenous (IV) over 2 to 4 hours
  - May reduce the need for exchange transfusion
  - Higher dose may be given again if limited response is seen.
- Double-volume exchange transfusion
  - Indications

- Are based on American Academy of Pediatrics (AAP) recommendations for management of hyperbilirubinemia in infants older than 35 weeks
- Bilirubin levels in combination with risk factors such as postnatal age, gestational age, glucose-6-phosphate dehydrogenase deficiency, asphyxia, and acidosis
- Consider double-volume exchange transfusion after failed IV hydration, phototherapy, intravenous immunoglobulin (IVIG), corrected hypoalbuminemia unless indirect bilirubinemia is critically elevated or there is a rapid rate of rise (>0.5 mg/dL, which can be seen in Rh incompatibility).
- Exchange transfusion should be considered at bilirubin levels of 20 to 25 mg/dL. Exact level should be based on AAP recommendations (which are reassessed as new data become available) and the patient's clinical condition.
- Technique
  - Red blood cells (RBCs) are reconstituted with 5% albumin or fresh-frozen plasma.
    - Citrate used as an anticoagulant in the blood increases the risk for hypocalcemia.
- Side effects
  - Umbilical and portal vein thrombosis
  - Thrombocytopenia
  - Necrotizing enterocolitis
  - Hypocalcemia
  - Respiratory and metabolic acidosis
  - Graft-versus-host disease
  - Infections such as human immunodeficiency virus (HIV) or hepatitis C (very low risk)
  - Risk is relatively lower when performed in an intensive care unit by experienced, trained professionals.

Suggested Readings

Gleason CA, Sawyer T, eds. *Avery's Diseases of the Newborn*. 11th ed. Philadelphia: Elsevier; 2024.

Maisels MJ, Bhutani VK, Bogen D, Newman TB, Stark AR, Watchko JF. Hyperbilirubinemia in the newborn infant ≥ 35 weeks' gestation: an update with clarifications. *Pediatrics*. 2009;124(4):1193–1198.

Watchko JF. Hyperbilirubinemia and bilirubin toxicity in the late preterm infant. *Clin Perinatol*. 2006;33(4):839–852.

42 Physiologic and Breast Milk Jaundice

AARTI RAGHAVAN

Hyperbilirubinemia

OVERVIEW

- Normal serum bilirubin levels in children and adults are <0.9 mg/dL unconjugated bilirubin and <0.4 mg/dL conjugated bilirubin.
- Almost every newborn has a serum bilirubin above these values.
- This can occur due to various factors, such as newborn physiology (increased red blood cell [RBC] turnover, shortened RBC life span, immature hepatic function), race, inadequate feeding leading to dehydration, and age.
- Such forms of exaggerated physiology resulting in hyperbilirubinemia are known as *physiologic hyperbilirubinemia.*
- Factors influencing the severity of physiologic jaundice include:
  - Gestational age
  - Effectiveness of feeding
  - Polycythemia
  - Maternal medications such as diazepam
- Risk factors for developing clinically significant hyperbilirubinemia include:
  - Lower gestational age
  - Jaundice in first 24 hours
  - Predischarge bilirubin (serum and transcutaneous concentration) close to phototherapy levels
  - Phototherapy before discharge
  - Parent or sibling requiring phototherapy or exchange transfusion
  - Family history of inherited RBC disorders
  - Exclusive breastfeeding with suboptimal intake
  - Scalp hematoma or bruising
  - Down syndrome
  - Macrosomia

Breastfeeding Jaundice

OVERVIEW

- Hyperbilirubinemia occurs due to insufficient breastfeeding, typically within the first 2 weeks of life.
- Jaundice is the most common etiology for indirect hyperbilirubinemia in term infants that may require therapy.

INFLUENCING FACTORS

- Maternal factors include ineffective technique, insufficient milk production, cracked nipples, and fatigue.
- Infant factors include poor latch and poor suck.

MECHANISM

- Inadequate infant intake, resulting in dehydration
- The effects of gestational age, race, and ethnicity can additionally influence serum bilirubin.

PATHOGENESIS

- Maternal and neonatal factors as mentioned above may reduce the oral intake of breast milk in the first weeks.
- This is particularly significant during the first few days, when colostrum is produced in small volumes.
- Reduced latch or breast milk let-down reduces stimulation and milk production, resulting in a further decrease of oral intake.
- Early formula supplementation may further lead to reduced breast milk production due to reduced let-down and stimulus.
- Poor oral intake may lead to delayed meconium passage and intestinal stasis, leading to increased enterohepatic circulation and increased bilirubin load to the liver exceeding its conjugation capacity.

CLINICAL PRESENTATION

- Signs of dehydration include history of poor oral intake, decreased urine output, delayed capillary refill time, poor skin turgor, sunken fontanel, dry mucosa, and weight loss.
- Physical activity is decreased.
- Icterus may or may not be present.

DIAGNOSIS AND EVALUATION

- Physical examination, weight loss, fluid status (urine output [UOP], stooling), and reported inadequate intake/difficulty feeding concerning for dehydration
- Screening with transcutaneous bilirubin or serum bilirubin
- Other laboratory analyses may be conducted, such as serum electrolytes and urinalysis (may show increased specific gravity).
- Elevated indirect serum bilirubin

TREATMENT

- Prevention
  - Frequent breastfeeding, initiating within 1 hour of birth, 8 to 12 times per day
  - Evaluation of breastfeeding technique and providing maternal access to a lactation consultant

- In instances of inadequate breast milk production, supplementation with formula may be needed until the breast milk supply is established. Breast pumping can help establish supply. Of note, women who have had breast reduction surgery are at higher risk of inadequate milk production due to ductal transection.
- Close monitoring of exclusively breastfed neonates for signs of dehydration, decreased urination or passage of meconium, development of jaundice, inappropriate weight loss, or poor weight gain prior to discharge
- Close follow-up post discharge
- Therapy
  - Phototherapy for indirect bilirubin levels above light level
  - Intravenous rehydration, as indicated

Breast Milk Jaundice

OVERVIEW

- Indirect hyperbilirubinemia is typically seen after first 7 days in breastfed infants.
- Incidence is 10% to 30% in breastfed infants.

INFLUENCING FACTORS

- Breast milk intake

MECHANISM

- Various substances have been implicated in the development of breast milk jaundice. They include the following:
  - Presence of high concentrations of beta-glucuronidase in maternal milk, which deconjugates bilirubin and increases enterohepatic reabsorption of bilirubin, resulting in increased bilirubin delivery to the liver
  - Factors in breast milk such as metal ions, steroids, and nucleotides could control uridine diphosphate glucuronyl transferase, which could reduce bilirubin excretion and cause hyperbilirubinemia.
  - Serum elevation of bile acids or taurine–glycine conjugates may be related to the cause.

CLINICAL PRESENTATION

- Breastfed or breast milk bottle-fed infants
- Typically infants are vigorous and healthy with normal weight gain and gastrointestinal elimination.
- Peak presentation is 5 to 15 days.

- Most peak at levels of 5 to 10 mg/dL; some more pronounced cases may reach 25 to 30 mg/dL.
- Duration to resolution is weeks to months (mean, 9 weeks).
- There is no identifiable disease that causes hyperbilirubinemia, except its association with breast milk.

DIAGNOSIS AND EVALUATION

- Although transcutaneous bilirubin can be used for screening, care should be exercised, given the narrow range of sensitivity.
- Elevated levels should be confirmed by serum fractionated bilirubin level measurement.
- Total and direct bilirubin should be measured to rule out conjugated hyperbilirubinemia.
- For very elevated bilirubin (>20 mg/dL) the following should be considered: complete blood count to rule out a hemolytic process; blood culture, urinalysis, and urine culture to rule out urosepsis; and thyroid function test to rule out thyroid dysfunction as clinically indicated.

TREATMENT

- Observation and close monitoring are essential.
- Phototherapy is typically not indicated for isolated breast milk jaundice in a well-appearing newborn. It can be considered for elevated bilirubin above light level based on phototherapy guidelines, hydration status, ability to ensure follow-up, etc.
- For very high levels of serum bilirubin, interruption of breastfeeding with formula supplementation for 24 hours can lower serum bilirubin levels quickly and confirm the diagnosis.
- Management of hyperbilirubinemia in newborns 35 weeks' gestation or more:
  - Risk stratification for assessment and treatment of hyperbilirubinemia should be based on the latest recommendations from the AAP.
  - The goal of management of indirect hyperbilirubinemia is to reduce the risk of bilirubin encephalopathy and neurotoxicity.

Suggested Readings

Gleason CA, Sawyer T, eds. *Avery's Diseases of the Newborn*. 11th ed. Philadelphia: Elsevier; 2024.

Kemper AR, Newman TB, Slaughter JL, et al. Clinical practice guideline revision: management of hyperbilirubinemia in the newborn infant 35 or more weeks of gestation. *Pediatrics*. 2022;150(3):e2022058859.

Martin RJ, Fanaroff AA, Walsh MC. *Fanaroff and Martin's Neonatal-Perinatal Medicine*. 11th ed. Philadelphia: Elsevier; 2020.

Maternal-Fetal Medicine

J. CHRISTOPHER GLANTZ and LISA M. GRAY

43 *Pregnancy*

J. CHRISTOPHER GLANTZ and LISA M. GRAY

Maternal Adaptation to Pregnancy

- Hemodynamic
  - Plasma volume increases 50% while red blood cell (RBC) mass expands 20%; physiologic anemia of pregnancy.
  - Heart size increases 10% (hypertrophy and increased diastolic filling).
  - Stroke volume and heart rate increase; there is a 50% increase in cardiac output.
  - When supine and ≥20 weeks, uterine compression of the vena cava lowers venous return and cardiac output, causing hypotension.
  - Uterine blood flow increases 10-fold to ~1 L/min.
  - Systemic vascular resistance declines (progesterone, prostaglandin, angiotensin resistance, and shunting through low-resistance placenta).
  - Diastolic blood pressure (BP) declines 10 mm Hg by 20 weeks and then gradually increases back to baseline.
- Renal
  - Renal blood flow and the glomerular filtration rate increase by 50%.
  - Serum urea nitrogen and creatinine levels decrease by 40%.
  - Glucose load exceeds loop reabsorption, causing glycosuria.
  - Dilation of renal calyces and ureters occurs; "physiologic" hydronephrosis is common (right > left due to uterine dextrorotation).
  - Glycosuria plus urine stasis increase the risk of pyelonephritis.
- Respiratory
  - There is minimal change in the respiratory rate, but an increase in tidal volume causes increased minute ventilation, with no change in forced expiratory volume in 1 second (FEV_1) or forced vital capacity.
  - Hyperventilation raises PO_2 (partial pressure of oxygen) and lowers PCO_2 (partial pressure of carbon dioxide), improving maternal–fetal gradients.
  - Compensatory increased renal bicarbonate excretion maintains pH and avoids respiratory alkalosis.
  - Decreased functional reserve capacity increases susceptibility to hypoxia.
- Hematologic
  - Increased thrombogenesis + decreased thrombolysis = hypercoagulable.
  - Venous thromboembolism (VTE) risk increased fivefold.
  - White blood cell (WBC) count increases; mild thrombocytopenia is common.
- Endocrine
  - Placental hormones alter maternal metabolism; increased fatty acid metabolism + insulin resistance = more glucose available to fetus.
  - Steroid hormone synthesis increases.
  - Estrogen induces production of thyroid-binding globulin; total thyroid hormone levels increase, but free levels are unchanged.
- Gastrointestinal
  - Gastrointestinal motility is slowed, increasing nutrient and water absorption.
  - Nausea, vomiting, and constipation are common.
- Changes in laboratory values
  - Increased—steroid hormones, prolactin, total T_4, WBC, alkaline phosphatase (from placental production), lipids, coagulation factors, PO_2
  - Decreased—hematocrit (Hct), platelets, creatinine, blood urea nitrogen (BUN), glucose, sodium, calcium (total but not ionized), bicarbonate, PCO_2
  - No change—free thyroxine (T_4), transaminases, bilirubin, prothrombin time (PT), partial thromboplastin time (PTT), bleeding time

THE PLACENTA

- Morphology and development
  - Trophoblast derived from extraembryonic cells in blastocyst
    - Cytotrophoblast cells extend into the decidua to anchor villi and invade maternal spiral arteries, dilating them to improve flow.
    - Syncytiotrophoblast is a "shell" of fused cytotrophoblasts.
  - Progressive placental growth increases cross-sectional vascular area and lowers placental vascular resistance.
  - Hemochorial architecture
    - Maternal blood is in direct contact with fetal chorion (not fetal blood).
    - Villi containing fetal blood vessels project into intervillous spaces.
- Respiratory gas exchange
  - Efficient transfer of respiratory gases is due to simple diffusion along gradients.
  - Fetal hemoglobin has higher affinity for O_2 than maternal hemoglobin and preferentially offloads O_2 to the fetus.
  - Transfer is flow dependent; gas exchange is limited by maternal uterine vascular disease, hypotension, hypovolemia, infection, placental infarction, abruption, or hypoplasia.

- Placental transport—substances cross via different mechanisms based on size, lipid solubility, protein binding, and presence of transporters.
  - Simple diffusion of respiratory gases and small nonpolar molecules
  - Facilitated diffusion of glucose and some glucocorticoids
  - Channels: water and some ions
  - Active transport of sodium, potassium, amino acids, and proteins
  - Receptor-mediated endocytosis of low-density lipoproteins (LDLs) and iron
- Metabolism and endocrine function
  - Fetus has limited gluconeogenesis; most glucose is maternally derived.
  - Human placental lactogen and placental growth hormone stimulate maternal lipolysis and gluconeogenesis, increasing glucose levels for fetal use.
- Abnormal placentation
  - Poor trophoblast invasion is associated with fetal loss and preeclampsia.
  - Excessive or abnormal trophoblast invasion causes placenta accreta/percreta.

MULTIFETAL GESTATIONS

- Zygosity (number of ova fertilized):
  - Monozygous = one ovum that splits (30% of multiple gestations)
  - Multizygous = more than one ovum (70% of multiple gestations)
- Chorionicity (number of placentas) and amnionicity (number of sacs) are determined by zygosity and/or time of conceptus split.
  - Multizygous—each fetus will have its own placenta and sac.
  - Monozygous with splitting in:
    - 1 to 3 days: each fetus has its own placenta and amniotic sac
    - 3 to 8 days: shared placenta (monochorionic) but two amniotic sacs
    - 8 to 13 days: shared placenta and sac (monoamniotic)
    - >13 days: conjoined twins
- Multifetal gestations are associated with adverse infant outcomes.
  - Anomalies, aneuploidy, stillbirth, preterm delivery (PTD), fetal (intrauterine) growth restriction (IUGR), preterm premature rupture of membranes (PPROM), perinatal death, intraventricular hemorrhage (IVH), and periventricular leukomalacia

ASSISTED REPRODUCTIVE TECHNOLOGY (ASSISTANCE WHEN INFERTILITY IS IMPAIRED)

- Ovulation induction
  - Medications are used to improve ovulation when egg quality is normal.
  - Use of clomiphene citrate or letrozole has 8% to 10% twinning risk.
  - Use of injectable gonadotropins has increased risk of high-order multiples.

- Intrauterine insemination (partner or donor)
  - Bypasses cervix in cases of abnormal semen analysis
  - Is not independently associated with increased risk of multifetal gestation
  - Unrelated donor is used in cases of male factor infertility or to avoid inherited disease.
- In vitro fertilization (IVF)
  - Process:
    - Injectable gonadotropins stimulate multiple ovarian follicles.
    - Eggs are harvested via ultrasound-guided transvaginal aspiration.
    - Eggs and sperm are mixed in vitro.
    - Conceptus is incubated and then transferred into the uterus.
    - Prenatal genetic diagnosis is an option prior to transfer.
  - May use unrelated egg donor to address premature ovarian failure or poor egg quality or to avoid inherited disease
  - IVF is an independent risk factor for
    - Multifetal gestation risk related to number of embryos transferred
    - Aneuploidy, fetal anomalies, hypertensive disorders of pregnancy, IUGR, PTD, abnormal placentation, cesarean delivery

Prenatal Care

PRECONCEPTION CARE

- Maternal health optimization before pregnancy improves perinatal outcomes.
  - Control chronic medical conditions; discontinue teratogenic medications.
  - Screen for relative contraindications to pregnancy (e.g., severe renal insufficiency, certain cardiac conditions).
- Reproductive planning
  - Avoid short interpregnancy interval (delivery to next conception <18 months).
  - Recommend use of contraception until health is optimized.
- Testing and immunization
  - Screen and treat for sexually transmitted infections (STIs).
  - Update needed immunizations.
  - Expand genetic carrier screening for high-risk groups (e.g., Ashkenazi Jews, French Canadian, Mediterranean, Southeast Asian); can be considered in all patients although it is of limited benefit unless the partner is known and is willing to be tested.
- Substance use and teratogens
  - Counsel on smoking cessation.
  - Recommend avoiding teratogens and illicit substance use (refer for treatment).
- Nutrition and dietary supplementation
  - Reduce excess body weight through a healthy diet (refer for nutrition consultation), regular exercise, or bariatric surgery (if appropriate).
  - Start 400 μg folic acid 1 month before conception to reduce the rate of open neural tube defects (ONTDs); 4 mg daily for women with prior defect.

- Assess diet and consider supplementation to achieve recommended daily doses of calcium, vitamin D, iron, and other vitamins and minerals, as needed.

INITIAL PRENATAL VISIT

- Establish prenatal care in the first trimester.
- Perform a complete history and risk assessment.
  - Medical, obstetrics and gynecology (OB/GYN), family, genetic, and social history
  - Medication use, substance use and abuse, domestic violence
- Determination of gestational age (GA) and estimated due date (EDD)
  - Menstrual history, uterine size, and ultrasound (if discrepant findings)
  - Accurate GA is vital, especially if at risk for PTD, IUGR, or postdates.
- Physical examination and routine prenatal laboratory tests
  - Complete blood count (CBC)
  - Blood typing and antibody screening
  - STI screening includes serology for rubella, syphilis, hepatitis B surface antigen, and human immunodeficiency virus (HIV); chlamydia and gonorrhea testing.
  - Urinalysis and culture
- Possible additional laboratory tests
  - Cystic fibrosis and spinal muscular atrophy (SMA) carrier testing, hemoglobin electrophoresis (if at risk for hemoglobinopathy), fragile X premutation testing (if suggested by personal/family history)

SUBSEQUENT PRENATAL VISITS

- Monthly until 28 weeks, then every other week to 36 weeks, then weekly
  - Weight, BP, urine protein and glucose levels (if indicated), fundal height, and fetal heart rate (FHR)
  - Assess for signs and symptoms of labor, hypertensive disorders, or abnormal fetal growth

OTHER ROUTINE ASSESSMENTS AND INTERVENTIONS

- Aneuploidy screening/testing
  - Low-risk patients—first-trimester, screen at 11 to 13 weeks (nuchal translucency plus serum human chorionic gonadotropin [hCG] and pregnancy-associated plasma protein A [PAPP-A]), or do a second-trimester serum screen (usually four analytes) at 15 to 22 weeks.
  - High-risk patients (maternal age ≥35 years, prior aneuploidy, abnormal serum screening or ultrasound)—cell-free DNA analysis at ≥10 weeks
  - Diagnostic testing—chorionic villus sampling (CVS) at 10 to 13 weeks and amniocentesis at ≥15 weeks (both have become infrequent after cell-free DNA became available)
- Maternal serum alpha-fetoprotein (AFP) screening at 15 to 22 weeks
  - For open defects or placental dysfunction, although less helpful as ultrasound has improved

- Fetal anatomy ultrasound at 18 to 20 weeks
- Gestational diabetes (GDM) screening at 24 to 28 weeks
- Repeat antibody screen at 28 weeks if Rh-negative; Rh immune globulin administration
- Immunizations
  - Hepatitis B for all susceptible women
  - Hepatitis A if hepatitis B or C positive (+)
  - Influenza for all women in every pregnancy
  - COVID-19 for all women in accordance with Centers for Disease Control and Prevention (CDC) guidelines
  - Tdap for all women after 27 weeks in every pregnancy
  - Pneumococcal or meningococcal for HIV+, sickle cell disease, or asplenia
- Group B *Streptococcus* (GBS) cervical culture at 35 to 37 weeks

Pregnancy Complications

MATERNAL HEALTH CONDITIONS

- Obesity—prevalence in women of reproductive age is ~30%; another ~30% are overweight.
  - Confers increased maternal risk proportional to body mass index
  - Maternal effects include hypertension, GDM, cesarean delivery (intraoperative and postoperative complications), and VTE.
  - Fetal effects include miscarriage, stillbirth, birth defects (particularly neural tube and cardiac), and macrosomia.
  - Management
    - Weight loss (or bariatric surgery) prior to conception
    - Early screening for GDM
    - Fetal surveillance to monitor growth (fundal heights are unreliable)
- Diabetes mellitus (DM)
  - Complicates ~6% to 10% of pregnancies (90% are GDM)
  - Pregestational DM
    - May have comorbid renal, cardiovascular, or neurologic disease that worsens perinatal outcome
    - Risk of complications is proportional to the degree of glycemic control and comorbid conditions.
  - Gestational DM
    - Lower risk of complications than pregestational DM
    - Early screening diagnoses likely represent previously undiagnosed type 2 DM (although still characterized as gestational).
  - Maternal effects of DM
    - Hypertension, delivery lacerations, hemorrhage, cesarean delivery
  - Fetal effects of DM
    - Pregestational DM only—miscarriage, stillbirth, and birth defects (especially heart and ONTDs)
    - Any DM—fetal growth disorders (usually macrosomia), cardiomyopathy, birth injury, neonatal metabolic abnormalities, respiratory distress syndrome (RDS)

- Management
  - Nutritional counseling to attempt dietary control
  - Achieve glycemic control through blood glucose (BG) checks—qid
    - Fasting BG <95 mg/dL
    - 1-hour postprandial BG <140 mg/dL
    - Metformin or insulin if diet fails (insulin is considered first-line, but metformin is more acceptable to many patients; glyburide is no longer commonly used).
- Fetal evaluation
  - Targeted anatomic ultrasound; echocardiography for pregestational diabetics
  - Fetal surveillance (ultrasound to monitor growth and antepartum testing to monitor fetal oxygenation; note that this will be referred to as "fetal surveillance" from now on)
  - Delivery timing determined by degree of glycemic control
    - Gestational with good control: 40 weeks
    - Pregestational with good control: 39 weeks
    - Poor control: typically 37 to 38 weeks
  - Cesarean if estimated fetal weight (EFW) ≥4500 g; there is twice the risk of shoulder dystocia compared with the same EFW without DM.
- Hypertensive disease
  - Complicates ~10% of pregnancies
  - Chronic hypertension (CHTN)
    - Hypertension preceding conception or noted before 20 weeks
    - At risk for superimposed preeclampsia
    - Comorbid renal disease or diabetes worsens outcomes
  - Management
    - Baseline laboratory evaluation of renal and liver function
    - BP monitoring; antihypertensive management (goal now is BP <140/90)
    - Meds most often include a beta-blocker or calcium channel blocker.
    - Fetal surveillance; delivery at term (38–39 weeks)
  - Gestational hypertension
    - Asymptomatic high BP is first noted after 20 weeks of pregnancy.
    - May progress to preeclampsia, so close follow-up is required
    - Note that BP ≥160/110 is considered preeclampsia with severe features, regardless of other findings.
    - Management is the same as for CHTN, but only start antihypertensives for severe-range BP, and deliver slightly earlier (37–38 weeks).
  - Preeclampsia syndromes
    - Preeclampsia—hypertension associated with proteinuria (>300 mg/d), laboratory abnormalities, or symptoms at >20 weeks of pregnancy
    - Eclampsia—new-onset seizures in a woman with preeclampsia
    - HELLP syndrome is a severe subtype of preeclampsia with abnormal laboratory profile.
      - Hemolysis—elevated lactate dehydrogenase (LDH) level, low Hct, abnormal smear
      - Elevated liver enzyme levels—transaminases ≥2 × normal
      - Low platelets—thrombocytopenia (<100 K)
    - Signs and symptoms usually resolve rapidly in postpartum period but some diagnoses are not made until after delivery.
    - Gestational age and severity of disease dictate management; severity is often inversely proportional to gestational age at onset.
    - Severe features are defined by the presence of any of the following:
      - Persistent systolic BP ≥160 or diastolic BP ≥110 mm Hg
      - Persistent symptoms are headache, visual disturbances, upper abdominal pain, and dyspnea (pulmonary edema).
      - Laboratory abnormalities include those seen with HELLP or serum creatinine ≥1.1 mg/dL (or doubling from baseline).
  - Management
    - Maternal hospitalization; close outpatient observation can be considered for mild disease
    - Steroids for fetal maturity (if preterm)
    - Serial BP, laboratory testing, and fetal monitoring
    - Antihypertensive management (if required)
    - Intrapartum magnesium sulfate for maternal seizure prophylaxis (and/or for fetal neuroprotection if <32 weeks)
  - Delivery timing
    - Immediate for eclampsia, pulmonary edema, refractory hypertension, abruption, fetal demise, non-reassuring fetal status, or if any severe features at ≥34 weeks
    - Expectant management is appropriate when <37 weeks and no severe features, or in some cases <34 weeks if severe features are present but stable and hypertension is controlled.
    - In the latter cases, give steroids for lung maturation and attempt to delay delivery ≥48 hours if otherwise stable.
    - Antihypertensive therapy (for severe-range hypertension to prevent maternal stroke)
    - First line: intravenous labetalol or hydralazine; enteral (PO) nifedipine
    - Other beta- or calcium channel blockers may be used, but their safety is less clear.
    - Methyldopa has been historically used due to its fetal safety profile but is less effective than first-line agents.
    - Diuretics counteract the normal expansion of blood volume; they are not usually started during pregnancy (although may be continued if used preconceptionally for CHTN).
    - Angiotensin-converting enzyme inhibitors (ACEIs) and angiotensin receptor blockers (ARBs) are contraindicated in pregnancy due to decreased fetal renal perfusion and skull ossification.
  - Maternal effects of HTN include stroke, seizures, renal dysfunction, hemorrhage, and death.
  - Fetal effects of HTN include IUGR, PTD, placental abruption, hypoxia, and perinatal death.
- Cardiac disease
  - Complicates 1% to 4% of pregnancies and is a leading cause of maternal mortality
  - Preconception consultation to:

- Optimize prepregnancy maternal medical or surgical therapy.
- Provide contraception until maternal health is optimized.
- Discuss pregnancy contraindications (high maternal mortality).
  - New York Heart Association heart failure class III or IV symptoms include severe mitral or aortic stenosis, aortic root dilation >4.5 cm, severe pulmonary hypertension, ejection fraction ≤30%, prior peripartum cardiomyopathy with persistent dysfunction, or symptomatic coronary artery disease.
- Most conditions are managed similarly to those in the nonpregnant state, but
  - There is a higher risk of decompensation (increased cardiovascular demands).
  - Some medical therapy is contraindicated (e.g., ACEIs, ARBs).
  - Surgical interventions may carry unacceptable fetal risks.
    - Fetal loss is a risk with maternal cardiopulmonary bypass.
  - Maternal effects include cardiac arrhythmias, functional decompensation (may be permanent), heart failure, VTE, and death.
  - Fetal effects include IUGR, PTD, death, and CHD (up to 15% if maternal CHD).
- Management
  - Serial assessment of maternal cardiac function (with echocardiography)
  - Multidisciplinary maternal care
  - Fetal echocardiography (if maternal CHD) and fetal surveillance
  - Delivery planning
    - Timing of delivery is determined by maternal cardiac status.
    - Vaginal delivery is preferred for most diseases; may be assisted delivery if patient cannot tolerate Valsalva.
    - Epidural is recommended to decrease catecholamine release.
- Pulmonary disease
  - Risks are related to the degree of maternal hypoxia and ability to tolerate physiologic changes in pregnancy.
  - Maternal effects include worsening hypoxia, respiratory failure, and death.
  - Fetal effects include IUGR and PTD.
  - General management
    - Multidisciplinary maternal care
    - Supplemental O_2 to keep O_2 saturation >95%
    - Fetal surveillance
    - Preterm delivery for refractory respiratory insufficiency
      - Vaginal delivery with epidural preferred
  - Asthma
    - No alterations in care from nonpregnant state
    - Most pregnancies have good outcome.
    - Increased risk of PPROM and PTD if steroid dependent
  - Cystic fibrosis (CF)
    - High risk of serious complications: maternal malnutrition, need for mechanical ventilation,

infection, diabetes (gestational effects + pancreatic insufficiency), PTD; 1% maternal mortality
- Respiratory infections
  - Increased risks due to relative immune suppression
    - High attack rates and hospitalization rates; worse outcomes
  - Pneumonia
    - 25% of cases require hospitalization
    - 2% intubation; 2% maternal mortality
    - Care is similar to that for nonpregnant patients.
  - Influenza
    - 10 × rate of hospitalization and intensive care unit (ICU) admission
    - Universal immunization is recommended.
    - Prompt antiviral treatment of pregnant women reduces ICU and hospital admission, mechanical ventilation, and death.
  - COVID-19
    - Pregnancy increases the likelihood of severe disease (but absolute risk is low).
    - COVID vaccination during pregnancy is safe.
    - Pregnancy does not alter treatment (exception: molnupiravir is not recommended).
    - Extracorporeal membrane oxygenation (ECMO) can be used in critical respiratory failure during pregnancy.
    - Maternal risks of hemorrhage, thrombosis, stroke, infection, preterm labor, and delivery
    - Neonatal survival is reported to be approximately 70%.
- Renal disease
  - Risk of complications is proportional to the degree of renal insufficiency.
  - Maternal effects include hypertensive disorders and declining renal function.
  - Fetal effects include PTD (usually indicated), IUGR, and perinatal mortality.
  - Concurrent hypertension or diabetes worsens perinatal outcomes.
  - Serum creatinine level of >2.5 mg/dL is a relative contraindication to pregnancy; there is a high probability of end-stage renal disease with low live birth rate.
  - Dialysis confers a high risk of fetal loss and ~100% risk of PTD and IUGR.
  - Renal transplant recipients can have successful pregnancies if >1 year post-transplantation, no signs of rejection, and minimal residual insufficiency.
  - Management includes laboratory and fetal surveillance.
  - Term or near-term delivery if stable (although PTD is commonly indicated)
- Hematologic disease
  - Anemia (hemoglobin [Hgb] <11 g/dL)
    - Iron deficiency is the most common cause; universal supplementation decreases maternal anemia and iron deficiency at term.
    - Fetal effects: usually good perinatal outcome with adverse effects (e.g., IUGR, PTD, perinatal death) only in severe cases
  - Hemoglobinopathies
    - Severity of disease depends on gene carriage.

- Fetal risks include inheritance, miscarriage, IUGR, or stillbirth.
- Sickle cell disease (SCD)
  - Sickle cell trait has favorable pregnancy outcome, but there is a 25% risk of SCD in offspring if both partners have the trait.
  - Maternal effects include pain crisis (75%), infection, acute chest syndrome, blood transfusion, VTE, and death (1%).
  - Management
    - Genetic counseling, maternal vaccination, high-dose folic acid supplementation (4 mg daily)
    - Laboratory and fetal surveillance—most can deliver at term.
  - Alpha-thalassemia
    - Pregnancy outcome and degree of anemia depend on the number of normal alpha genes (four = normal, zero = lethal)
    - Most affected pregnancies occur in silent carriers or those with mild anemia (two or three functional alpha genes); most have a favorable pregnancy outcome.
    - Management includes laboratory screening and genetic counseling; *cis* mutations (Southeast Asians) confer risk of lethal anemia.
- Thromboembolic risk: Personal and family history and thrombophilia test results determine the need for antepartum or postpartum anticoagulation.
  - Heparins do not cross the placenta, thus lack direct fetal effects.
  - Warfarin crosses the placenta and confers 6% risk of embryopathy.
  - No obstetric safety data are available for other anticoagulant medications.
  - Mechanical heart valves pose high risk of thrombosis.
  - Heparin is less effective than warfarin in this context; the maternal benefits of warfarin may outweigh fetal risks.
- Immunologic disease
  - Lupus
    - Outcomes depend on periconception disease status and presence of comorbid conditions; best outcomes are for quiescent disease more than 6 months before conception.
    - Maternal effects include hypertension, renal insufficiency, and VTE.
    - Fetal effects
      - Miscarriage, stillbirth, IUGR, PTD
      - Fetal marrow suppression (if on immunosuppressants)
      - Congenital heart block (anti-Ro, anti-La antibodies)
      - Transient neonatal lupus syndrome (maternal antibodies)
    - Management
      - Most treatments are compatible with use in pregnancy; outcomes are improved with hydroxychloroquine.
      - Laboratory and fetal surveillance; term delivery if stable

- Antiphospholipid antibody syndrome
  - Increased risk of VTE: recommend prophylaxis with heparins, low-dose aspirin.
  - Fetal effects: IUGR and stillbirth
- Idiopathic thrombocytopenia purpura (antiplatelet antibodies)
  - Antibodies cross the placenta; may cause neonatal thrombocytopenia.
  - Maternal platelet counts do not correlate well with neonatal counts.
  - Spontaneous vaginal delivery is acceptable; operative vaginal delivery is relatively contraindicated.
- Malignancy
  - Gestational age at diagnosis may alter management and prognosis.
    - Tumor growth is generally not affected by pregnancy.
  - Pregnancy termination
    - Consider with first-trimester diagnosis if needed to expedite definitive maternal therapy.
    - Advised for lethal fetal conditions (e.g., moles)
  - Most chemotherapy agents can be used after first trimester.
    - Main exception is folate inhibitors (methotrexate).
    - Maternal benefits of prompt treatment usually outweigh fetal risks of therapy.
    - Surgery is usually acceptable, but radiation is contraindicated.
  - Fetal effects include IUGR, PTD (to pursue more aggressive maternal therapy), and hematologic suppression (delivery should be timed several weeks after last chemotherapy course to minimize risk).
    - Fetal metastases (rare, most common with melanoma)
- Phenylketonuria
  - Fetal effects include fetal inheritance, low birth weight, cardiac defects, microcephaly, cognitive impairment
  - Management
    - Genetic counseling
    - Maternal dietary management is best if phenylalanine level <6 mg/dL before and during pregnancy (diet unpleasant; compliance is poor).
    - Fetal evaluation by targeted anatomy survey and echocardiography
    - Term delivery
- Neurologic disease
  - Epilepsy
    - 90% of women have a healthy pregnancy.
    - Planned conception and optimization of antiepileptic drugs (AEDs) result in fewer seizures and fetal anomalies.
    - If seizure free for 6 to 12 months and the neurologist agrees, consider stopping AEDs several months before conception.
    - If possible, discontinue potentially teratogenic AEDs.
      - Phenytoin: skull, facial, brain anomalies; IUGR
      - Valproic acid: neural tube, facial, cardiac defects; hypospadias; poor cognition
      - Topiramate: facial clefts
      - Carbamazepine: facial clefts
    - Management includes serum AED monitoring, high-dose folic acid (although benefit is uncertain with

AEDs), targeted anatomy survey (consider echocardiography), and term labor and delivery. Goal is the lowest effective dose of monotherapy.

- Spinal cord injury
  - Fertility is not compromised.
  - Maternal effects include urinary tract infections, pressure ulcers, altered mobility, VTE, and autonomic dysreflexia.
  - Fetal effects include unattended birth (maternal non-awareness of labor).
  - Management
    - Serial urine cultures; antibiotic suppression for recurrent urinary tract infections (UTIs)
    - Serial cervical examinations and maternal education on symptoms of labor (e.g., abdominal tension, lower extremity cramping and spasticity, dyspnea)
    - Delivery planning
      - Minimize autonomic dysreflexia by early epidural, Foley catheter, and frequent vital sign monitoring.
      - Assisted vaginal delivery if unable to push
- Multiple sclerosis
  - Remission in pregnancy is typical; postpartum flares are common.
  - Treatment with disease-modifying drugs:
    - Reassuring but limited fetal safety information is available.
    - Decreases the risk of postpartum flare
    - Some providers discontinue during pregnancy because outcomes are generally favorable without treatment.
  - Fetal effects include IUGR.
- Myasthenia gravis
  - Management generally is similar to that for the non-pregnant state.
  - Myasthenia is usually stable during pregnancy. Perinatal outcome is good; flares are most common in the first trimester.
  - Transient neonatal myasthenia: 10% to 20% risk from passage of antiacetylcholine receptor antibodies; may persist for 3 months
  - Some commonly used medications may precipitate myasthenic crisis and should be avoided, including antibiotics (aminoglycosides, vancomycin, clindamycin), beta blockers, and magnesium sulfate.
- Infectious disease
  - For HIV, universal prenatal testing is recommended.
    - Main obstetric risk is perinatal transmission.
      - Proportional to maternal viral load
      - Greatest risk with initial seroconversion
    - Reduction in perinatal transmission
      - Antiviral treatment reduces risk from 25% to <1% (antepartum, intrapartum, neonatal prophylaxis).
      - Most antiretrovirals are acceptable for use.
      - Avoid fetal exposure to maternal blood (invasive testing, rupture of membranes, fetal scalp electrode placement).
    - Vaginal delivery is appropriate unless viral load >1000, in which case cesarean delivery is scheduled at 38 weeks.
- Hepatitis B

- Universal prenatal testing is recommended.
- Main obstetric risk is perinatal transmission.
  - Proportional to maternal viral load and e-antigen positivity
  - Reduction in perinatal transmission
    - Universal neonatal vaccination and hepatitis B immunoglobulin (HBIG) prophylaxis markedly reduce risk.
    - Antivirals are acceptable for use in pregnancy; treatment is recommended for log viral load ≥5.
    - Avoid fetal exposure to maternal blood.
    - No benefit to cesarean delivery
- Hepatitis C
  - Universal prenatal testing is recommended.
  - Main obstetric risk is perinatal transmission.
    - Avoid fetal exposure to maternal blood.
    - No benefit to cesarean delivery
- Herpes
  - If positive history, begin acyclovir at 36 weeks to minimize shedding at birth.
  - Cesarean if active lesion while in labor
- Acute pyelonephritis
  - Maternal effects include sepsis, acute respiratory distress syndrome (ARDS), and respiratory failure.
  - Fetal effects include PTD or fetal death.
  - Prompt antibiotic treatment improves outcomes.
- Psychiatric illness
  - Pregnancy risks of untreated disease include poor engagement with prenatal care, suicide, poor maternal weight gain, IUGR, and neonatal neurodevelopmental impairment.
  - Adequate mental health care improves maternal self-care, function, and compliance with prenatal care and lowers the risk of self-harm.
  - Risks of untreated disease generally outweigh risks of medication.
    - Selective serotonin reuptake inhibitors (SSRIs)
      - Commonly used with relative safety
      - Sertraline is preferred first-line agent.
      - Paroxetine has inconsistent association with fetal cardiac defects; consider echocardiography if used.
      - Neonatal effects include withdrawal signs/symptoms.
    - Antipsychotics increase the risk of diabetes.
    - Benzodiazepines: small increase in facial clefts; neonatal hypotonia and withdrawal signs/symptoms
    - Mood stabilizers: Lamotrigine is first line, and lithium has been associated with Ebstein anomaly (newer data dispute this risk). Consider fetal echocardiography.
- Trauma
  - Falls, motor vehicle accidents, domestic violence, penetrating trauma
  - Perinatal risks include uterine rupture/trauma, placental abruption, fetal hypoxia, fetal injury, PTD, and perinatal death.
  - Maternal stabilization is first priority, then:
    - Establish gestational age, obtain an ultrasound/fetal survey, and monitor FHR.
    - Expedite delivery for fetal indications if the mother is stable or perimortem.

- Nonobstetric surgery
  - Surgery indicated for essential maternal indications should be performed.
    - Fetal risks of untreated maternal disease outweigh those of surgery.
  - If possible, nonurgent (but indicated) surgery should be deferred to the second trimester because miscarriage and preterm contractions are less likely.
  - Elective surgery should be postponed until after delivery.
  - Risk of PTD is increased after surgery during pregnancy; may be due to the condition that necessitates the surgery or to the surgery itself.
  - Anesthesia
    - No currently used general anesthetics are teratogenic.
    - Physiologic changes in pregnancy raise risks of general anesthesia (remains relatively safe if no concurrent cardiorespiratory disease).
      - Airway changes can complicate intubation.
      - Susceptibility to hypoxia is increased.
      - Gastric emptying is delayed, with increased risk of aspiration.
    - Regional anesthesia may be appropriate and minimizes maternal risks and fetal drug exposure.
  - Intraoperative optimization
    - Avoid hypotension by avoiding supine positioning (use left lateral tilt); anticipate and aggressively treat hemorrhage.
    - Avoid hypoxia by preoxygenating before anesthesia induction and maintaining normal ventilation.
    - FHR monitoring during surgery is controversial; it may depend on the procedure, gestational age, and feasibility.

FETAL CONDITIONS

- Aneuploidy
  - Diagnosed by karyotype or microarray via amniocentesis, CVS, or umbilical cord blood sampling (cell-free DNA is a screen, not definitive)
  - High rate of structural anomalies and fetal loss
  - Multidisciplinary care is recommended for ongoing gestations.
- Anomalies
  - Fetal anomalies may be isolated or multiple as part of a syndrome.
  - Prognosis is highly variable and depends on the type and number of anomalies.
  - Certain anomalies may dictate delivery timing or management.
    - Cesarean delivery is recommended for
      - Bulky external defects (hydrocephalus, large omphalocele)
      - Defects at risk of rupture (myelomeningocele, although outcome data on planned cesarean delivery are conflicting)
      - Defects with risk of hemorrhage (sacrococcygeal teratoma)
      - Defects that require immediate postnatal intervention (e.g., cyanotic congenital heart disease with restricted trial septum)

- The ex utero intrapartum treatment (EXIT) procedure is applied for conditions associated with severe airway obstruction (e.g., large epignathus or severe micrognathia).
  - Fetal head delivered during cesarean done under deep general anesthesia, placental circulation maintained, airway placed, delivery completed
  - Carries increased maternal operative risks
- Vaginal delivery following spontaneous labor is appropriate for most other anomalous fetuses (including gastroschisis).
- Alloimmunization (also known as isoimmunization)
  - Red blood cell alloimmunization, isoimmunization
    - Maternal sensitization to RBC antigens from fetal–maternal hemorrhage or maternal blood transfusion
    - Maternal antibodies cross the placenta and cause immune-mediated destruction of fetal RBCs.
    - Severe fetal anemia may lead to hydrops or death.
    - Fetus is at risk if positive maternal antibody screen titer is >1:8 or prior affected fetus and father is positive for RBC antigen; paternal antigen testing can stratify risk.
    - Management includes serial antibody titers and serial ultrasound screening for fetal anemia (if at risk by titer or by history).
  - Fetal middle cerebral artery peak systolic velocity (MCA-PSV) correlates with the degree of fetal anemia (PSV >1.5 multiples of the median [MoM] = high risk of severe anemia).
    - If anemia is confirmed by percutaneous umbilical blood sampling (PUBS), provide fetal transfusion through the cord or fetal peritoneal cavity.
    - Fetal or neonatal alloimmune thrombocytopenia
    - Maternal sensitization to fetal platelet antigens
    - Maternal antibodies cross the placenta and cause immune-mediated destruction of fetal platelets; confers high risk of IVH
    - Diagnosis (suspected if prior affected neonate or current finding of prenatal intracranial hemorrhage)
      - Parental platelet antigen typing with evidence of maternal–paternal mismatch; maternal anti-platelet antibodies
    - Management includes prenatal maternal intravenous immunoglobulin (IVIG) and steroids; avoid vaginal delivery if fetal cord platelet count <100,000/μL.
- Fetal hydrops
  - Immune hydrops
    - Fetal cardiac failure secondary to severe anemia from maternal RBC alloimmunization
    - Incidence is decreased with the use of anti-D immunoglobulin; other RBC antigens are now relatively more common (e.g., Kell, MNS, Jka, C/c, E/e)
  - Nonimmune hydrops
    - Fetal cardiac failure from other causes
    - Broad differential diagnosis
      - Cardiac: heart defects or arrhythmias; high-output failure
      - Aneuploidy and genetic syndromes
      - Structural anomalies: skeletal, thoracic, urinary tract
      - Other: anemia, infection, metabolic defects

- Evaluation includes ultrasound, amniocentesis for genetic and microbiologic analyses, and maternal antibody screen, parvovirus serology, and Kleihauer-Betke.
- Some cases are treatable (e.g., fetal anemia or arrhythmias), but most are not.
- Prognosis is poor and depends on gestational age, degree of hydrops, and presumptive cause.
- Fetal growth restriction (FGR, aka intrauterine growth restriction [IUGR])
  - Defined as sonographic EFW or abdominal circumference (AC) <10th percentile (but most fetuses <10th percentile are constitutionally small, not growth restricted)
  - Distinguish from low birth weight (BW <2500 g).
  - Note that the accuracy of sonographic EFWs is ±10% to 15%.
  - Pathologic causes of small for gestational age fetus
    - Uteroplacental insufficiency (most common)
      - Lagging abdominal circumference may be an early sign.
      - Confirmed by oligohydramnios, abnormal Doppler, and/or poor interval growth
    - Structural anomalies, aneuploidy, and genetic syndromes
      - Consider amniocentesis, which is recommended for karyotype and microarray.
    - Fetal infection is suspected with concurrent calcifications, microcephaly, ventriculomegaly, and brain abnormalities.
      - Diagnosed by amniotic fluid culture or polymerase chain reaction (PCR) assay
      - Maternal serologies most helpful when negative.
    - Management
      - Twice-weekly non-stress tests (NSTs)
      - Weekly ultrasound for amniotic fluid volume and umbilical artery Doppler
      - Serial assessment of fetal growth (every 2–4 weeks)
      - Early delivery may be indicated for nonreassuring testing, Doppler findings, or lack of interval growth.
- Macrosomia
  - Variably defined as EFW >4000 g or >4500 g
  - Increases the risk of cephalopelvic disproportion and shoulder dystocia
    - Cesarean delivery should be considered for EFW >4500 g (diabetic) or EFW >5000 g (nondiabetic) because shoulder dystocia risk is >50%.
  - Management is hampered by the inaccuracy of sonographic EFW estimates leading to cesarean deliveries that in retrospect were unnecessary.
- Fetal infections
  - Transplacental: rubella, cytomegalovirus (CMV), herpes simplex virus (HSV; generally primary), parvovirus, toxoplasmosis, listeria, syphilis
  - Intrapartum: HIV, varicella, hepatitis B and C, GBS, HSV
  - Maternal symptoms are often mild or absent, but there may be sonographic signs of fetal infection (most often IUGR, calcifications, or hydrops).
  - Diagnosis and treatment

- Maternal serology (may be difficult to determine time of exposure)
- Amniotic fluid culture or PCR (specific for fetal infection but may lack sensitivity if done early; repeat testing may be required)
- Antibiotic treatment is available for some maternal and fetal infections (e.g., toxoplasmosis, syphilis)
- Intrauterine transfusion may be indicated (and lifesaving) with severe fetal anemia due to parvovirus
- Universal GBS screening and intrapartum antibiotic prophylaxis of GBS-positive women decrease early-onset GBS sepsis.
- Complications of twins
  - Conjoined twins are rare (~1% of monozygotic twins).
    - Prognosis is poor and depends on the number and nature of shared organs.
  - Dichorionic twins
    - Most common type of twinning
    - Maternal risks include gestational DM, preeclampsia, anemia, acute fatty liver, cesarean delivery, and postpartum hemorrhage.
    - Fetal risks include miscarriage, stillbirth, structural and genetic anomalies, growth disturbances, PTD, malpresentation, PROM, umbilical cord prolapse, and abruption after delivery of first twin.
    - Delivery is generally at 38 weeks, with the route depending on presentation (trial of labor is acceptable if presenting twin is cephalic, irrespective of twin B presentation).
  - Monochorionic twins
    - Approximately 20% of all twin pregnancies
    - Risks include those of dichorionic twins, with additional risks:
      - Twin–twin transfusion syndrome (TTTS), where vascular anastomoses result in unbalanced blood flow between twins
        - Donor twin: anemia, IUGR, and oligohydramnios ("stuck twin" if severe)
        - Recipient: polycythemia, large EFW, polyhydramnios
        - Affects 15% of monochorionic twin pregnancies
        - Less frequent when monoamniotic
      - Staged I to V based on sonographic features (I = least affected, V = worst)
        - Second trimester is most common time for severe TTTS.
        - Consider laser therapy if <28 weeks and stage II or more.
        - There is a high risk of perinatal loss with untreated severe TTTS.
  - Twin anemia–polycythemia sequence (TAPS)
    - A form of TTTS resulting in disparate fetal hematocrits without amniotic fluid discrepancies
    - Caused by fewer or smaller caliber anastomoses
  - Twin reversed arterial perfusion (TRAP)
    - One normally developed twin and one acardiac twin
    - "Pump" twin's heart is responsible for circulation through both fetuses; at risk for high-output failure.

- Treated with selective umbilical cord occlusion of the acardiac twin
- Monoamniotic twins
  - High risk of cord entanglement and fetal demise
  - Close fetal surveillance starting at viability
  - Cesarean delivery at 32 to 34 weeks
- Co-twin death
  - Dichorionic: slight increase in risk of death for surviving twin
  - Monochorionic: ~20% risk of death; 25% neurodevelopmental injury if second twin survives (from acute hypotension/exsanguination into low-resistance dead co-twin)
  - Expectant management (close sonographic and FHR monitoring with delivery by 36 weeks) following co-twin death
  - Expedited delivery is unlikely to improve outcome.

OBSTETRIC COMPLICATIONS

- Placenta previa
  - Placenta touching or covering the internal cervical os
  - Risk factors include prior cesarean delivery or uterine surgery, prior placenta previa, multifetal gestation, multiparity, and smoking.
  - Diagnosis
    - Commonly found if transvaginal ultrasound is done in second trimester
    - Repeat ultrasound at 32 to 35 weeks to rule out persistence
    - Most previas resolve by term.
    - Uterus grows, and the placental edge draws away from os.
  - Maternal–fetal complications
    - Hemorrhage (two-thirds have antepartum bleeding), placenta accreta, PTD, hysterectomy, maternal or fetal death
  - Management
    - Pelvic rest; cesarean at 36 to 38 weeks (depending on stability)
- Low-lying placenta (within 2 cm of but not covering os)
  - Hemorrhage risk is increased with proximity to os.
  - Cesarean delivery is often done if <1 cm from os.
- Vasa previa
  - Rare complication of velamentous cord: fetal vessels traverse cervical os
    - Fetal exsanguination can occur when membranes rupture.
  - Diagnosed by transvaginal color Doppler ultrasound
  - Management
    - Consider antepartum admission for fetal surveillance and proximity to obstetric and neonatal ICU services.
    - Cesarean delivery at 34 to 37 weeks
- Placenta accreta, increta, and percreta (abnormal trophoblast invasion)
  - Risk factors include prior cesarean delivery, uterine surgery (risk proportional to number of surgeries) or placenta accreta, placenta previa, submucous fibroid, age ≥35 years, and smoking.
  - Diagnosis by ultrasound in second or third trimester

- Multiple placenta lacunae ("moth-eaten" appearance)
- Bulge and/or increased vascularity at bladder interface
- Lack of normal retroplacental hypoechoic zone
- Classification
  - Accreta: villi adherent to (but do not invade) myometrium
  - Increta: villi invade myometrium
  - Percreta: villi extend to uterine serosa or into adjacent structures
- Maternal–fetal complications include hemorrhage, disseminated intravascular coagulation (DIC), PTD, IUGR, hysterectomy, and maternal or fetal death.
- Management
  - Planned 34- to 36-week cesarean delivery via fundal incision to avoid placenta; placenta left in situ, and hysterectomy done
  - Preparation for potential massive blood product transfusion and/or bowel-bladder resection
- Placental abruption
  - Partial or complete detachment of the placenta from the uterine wall prior to delivery of the fetus; may be chronic or acute
  - Signs and symptoms include abdominal pain, vaginal bleeding (but may be concealed), uterine hypertonus or tachysystole, and FHR abnormalities.
  - Risk factors (but most cases occur without risk factors) include smoking, hypertension, trauma, cocaine use, polyhydramnios, twins, and rupture of membranes (ROM).
  - Maternal risks include hemorrhage, coagulopathy, cesarean delivery, hysterectomy, and death.
  - Fetal risks include PTD, asphyxia, and perinatal death.
  - Management depends on gestational age and degree of hemorrhage.
    - When preterm, expectant management should be considered as long as bleeding is not excessive, vital signs are stable, and the fetal status is reassuring.
    - Inpatient hospitalization until bleeding resolves
    - Steroids for fetal maturity if preterm
    - Close maternal and fetal surveillance
    - Delivery at 36 to 37 weeks
- Antepartum and intrapartum hemorrhage
  - Differential diagnosis of vaginal bleeding
    - First trimester: miscarriage (up to 60% are due to aneuploidy)
    - Second and third trimesters: preterm labor (PTL), placenta or vasa previa, abruption, PROM
  - Maternal risks include coagulopathy, hypovolemia, shock, and death.
  - Fetal risks include PTD, IUGR, nonreassuring fetal status, and perinatal death.
- PPROM
  - Risk factors include smoking, antepartum hemorrhage, polyhydramnios, multifetal gestations, trauma, and invasive procedures.
  - Maternal risks include infection, sepsis, abruption, and cesarean delivery.
  - Fetal risks include PTD, fetal infection, sepsis, IUGR, umbilical cord prolapse, and perinatal death.

- Management
  - Hospitalization (close outpatient observation can be considered in select patients); most patients deliver within 7 days of PPROM
  - Steroids, GBS prophylaxis, latency antibiotics (increase time from PPROM to delivery), and serial maternal–fetal assessment
  - Optimal timing of delivery is uncertain; delivery is usually initiated at 34 to 36 weeks.
- Preterm labor
  - Of patients admitted with threatened PTL, 50% ultimately deliver at term.
  - Risk factors
    - Maternal risk factors include uterine anomalies, trauma, infection, maternal illness, low socioeconomic status, and Black race.
    - Obstetric risk factors include multifetal gestations, PPROM, antepartum hemorrhage/abruption, and cervical insufficiency.
    - Fetal risk factors include anomalies, genetic syndromes, and IUGR.
  - Maternal risks vary by underlying cause.
  - Fetal risks include PTD, infection, sepsis, malpresentation, umbilical cord prolapse, and perinatal death.
  - Management
    - Hospitalization, GBS prophylaxis, steroids
    - Tocolysis for 48 hours to complete steroid course; long-term tocolysis not beneficial

SERIAL MATERNAL–FETAL ASSESSMENT

- Oligohydramnios
  - Variably defined as an amniotic fluid index (AFI) or four-quadrant technique <5 cm or single deepest vertical pocket (SDP) <2 cm
  - SDP technique results in equivalent perinatal outcome but fewer inductions and cesarean deliveries.
  - Differential diagnoses: rupture of membranes, fetal urinary tract anomalies, uteroplacental insufficiency
  - Management depends on underlying cause; rupture of membranes and uteroplacental insufficiency may prompt indicated PTD.
- Polyhydramnios
  - Variably defined as AFI ≥24 cm or SDP ≥8 cm
  - Differential diagnoses
    - Idiopathic (most common), DM, aneuploidy, TTTS, fetal hydrops, fetal neuromuscular disorder (impaired fetal swallowing), structural anomalies that obstruct fetal swallowing (e.g., GI obstruction, facial clefts, restrictive skin defects)
  - Maternal risks include hemorrhage, dyspnea, and cesarean delivery.
  - Fetal risks include malpresentation, PTD, cord prolapse, and placental abruption.
  - Management depends on cause.
  - Amnioreduction for maternal symptoms
  - Most cases can deliver at term.
- Postterm pregnancy (pregnancy progressing into the 42nd gestational week)
  - Uncommon because earlier spontaneous or induced delivery is likely

- Increasing evidence indicates that labor induction after 39 weeks avoids fetal risks of ongoing pregnancy without increased maternal risk.
- Fetal effects include dysmaturity, hypoxia, meconium, macrosomia, and stillbirth.
- Management:
  - Fetal surveillance with NST and AFI assessment after 40 weeks; delivery preferable before 42 weeks

DRUG AND ENVIRONMENTAL EXPOSURES

- Teratogenic effects are related to agent, dose, duration, and time of exposure.
  - Before 6 weeks: "all or none" effect (embryo death vs. no effect)
  - Between 6 and 9 weeks: organogenesis may be affected
  - After 9 weeks: organ development and maturation may be impaired
- Medication exposures
  - Commonly used in obstetric management
    - Calcium channel blockers (e.g., nifedipine): no adverse effects
    - Beta blockers (e.g., labetalol): some may increase IUGR
    - Beta agonists (e.g., terbutaline): tachycardia, neonatal hypoglycemia
    - Nonsteroidal anti-inflammatory drugs (e.g., indomethacin, ibuprofen)
      - Short courses in second trimester are well tolerated.
      - Use at >32 weeks can cause premature ductus constriction.
      - Prolonged use can lead to fetal renal injury.
    - Magnesium sulfate can result in poor neonatal tone and respiratory effort.
    - Steroids
      - Fluorinated steroids (e.g., betamethasone, dexamethasone) readily cross the placenta; nonfluorinated steroids (e.g., prednisone, methylprednisolone) are largely inactivated.
      - Beneficial effects for fetal maturity include increased surfactant production and decreased risk of IVH, necrotizing enterocolitis, and perinatal death.
      - Adverse fetal effects with chronic or repeated use include facial clefts, decreased growth and head size, and adrenal suppression.
- Radiation exposures
  - Teratogenic effects are unlikely if 5 to 10 mGy (this is more than most diagnostic tests).
  - High-dose exposure has an "all or none" effect in early first trimester, but later exposure is associated with IUGR, smaller head size, and cognitive impairment.
  - Therapeutic procedures
    - Radiation therapy is contraindicated in pregnancy.
    - Radioactive iodine (to treat maternal Graves' disease)
      - ≤12 weeks: generally no observed fetal effects
      - >12 weeks: concentrated in fetal thyroid (hypothyroidism)

- Drugs of abuse
  - Tobacco (~10% use during pregnancy in the United States) is associated with PPROM, abnormal placentation, IUGR, PTD, and sudden infant death syndrome.
  - Marijuana (~6–8% use during pregnancy in the United States) is associated with low birth weight, neurocognitive impairment, and sudden infant death syndrome.
  - Alcohol: Fetal alcohol syndrome (FAS) is associated with IUGR, microcephaly, and facial dysmorphism (short palpebral fissures, thin upper lip, smooth philtrum).
    - Common cause of neurocognitive impairment
    - Dose–response effect but no known threshold for a safe intake
  - Cocaine and amphetamines are associated with increased risk of miscarriage, hypertension, placental abruption, PTL, PPROM, and maternal cardiac arrest.
    - Fetal and neonatal effects include ischemic malformations (cocaine), PTD, IUGR, perinatal death, and neurocognitive impairment.
    - Neonatal withdrawal signs include irritability, tremor, hyperactivity, high-pitched crying, and continual sucking.
  - Heroin and opioids are associated with increased risk of infectious sequelae of IV drug use (e.g., hepatitis, HIV, bacteremia, endocarditis, other STIs), miscarriage, IUGR, placental abruption, PTD, and stillbirth.
    - Neonatal opioid withdrawal affects 60% to 70% of exposed neonates.
    - Breastfeeding decreases the duration and severity and is advised if no illicit use.
    - Complications are lower with opioid agonist therapy (methadone or buprenorphine), with a lower rate of relapse than detoxification.
- Environmental exposures
  - Lead: Sources of exposure include drinking water, flaking house paint, workplace exposure, jewelry, cosmetics, dishes from outside the United States, and herbal supplements.
    - Fetal effects include miscarriage, IUGR, PTD, and cognitive impairment.
  - Mercury: Sources of exposure include large fish, dental amalgams, thermometers, cosmetics and ceramics from outside the United States, and industrial waste.
    - Fetal effects include cognitive impairment or Minamata disease.

Suggested Readings

American Academy of Pediatrics and American College of Obstetricians and Gynecologists. *Guidelines for Perinatal Care.* 8th ed. Washington, DC: American College of Obstetricians and Gynecologists; 2017.

American College of Obstetricians and Gynecologists Task Force on Hypertension in Pregnancy. Washington, DC: American College of Obstetricians and Gynecologists; 2013.

Berghella V, ed. *Maternal-Fetal Evidence Based Guidelines.* 4th ed. Boca Raton, FL: CRC Press; 2022.

Landon MB, Galan HL, Jauniaux ERM, et al, eds. *Gabbe's Obstetrics: Normal and Problem Pregnancies.* 8th ed. Philadelphia: Elsevier; 2021.

Lockwood CJ, Moore TR, Copel J, et al, eds. *Creasy & Resnik's Maternal-Fetal Medicine: Principles and Practice.* 8th ed. Philadelphia: Saunders; 2018.

44 Fetal Assessment and Treatment

J. CHRISTOPHER GLANTZ and LISA M. GRAY

Genetic Screening and Testing

- Fetal aneuploidy screening
  - First-trimester screening: ultrasound for nuchal translucency measurement + maternal blood for human chorionic gonadotropin (hCG) and pregnancy-associated plasma protein A (PAPP-A)
    - Performed at 11 to 13 weeks; set 5% screen-positive rate
    - ~85% detection rate for trisomy 21 (lower for T18)
  - Second-trimester (quad) screening: maternal blood test for serum hCG, alpha-fetoprotein (AFP), estriol, and inhibin
    - Performed at 15 to 22 weeks; set 5% screen-positive rate
    - ~80% detection rate for trisomy 21 (lower for T18)
  - Cell-free DNA screening: Free DNA in maternal blood is analyzed for chromosomal imbalances.
    - Performed at ≥10 weeks
    - >99% sensitivity for trisomy 21
    - >90% sensitivity for trisomy 13 and 18, monosomy X
    - More expensive than first and second trimester screening
    - 1% to 8% risk of screen failure typically due to insufficient fetal fraction; increased risk of aneuploidy with these "no-call" results
  - Maternal serum AFP (MSAFP) is a maternal blood test that screens for open fetal defects (e.g., neural tube, ventral wall).
    - Performed at 14 to 22 weeks
    - High MSAFP indicates increased risk for open fetal defects; 95% sensitivity (ultrasound also sensitive for these defects).
    - MSAFP is also associated with placental dysfunction, fetal growth restriction, multiple gestation, fetal demise, and underestimated gestational age.

Invasive/Diagnostic Genetic Testing

- Common indications for genetic testing (amniocentesis or chorionic villus sampling [CVS]):
  - Advanced maternal age (≥35 years at delivery), abnormal genetic screening, fetal anomalies, maternal or previous fetal aneuploidy, history of metabolic disease or hemoglobinopathy
  - Requires culture of amniocytes or villi so is subject to culture failure

- Karyotype detects large duplications, deletions, and aneuploidy with 99.9% accuracy.
- Microarray can detect microduplications and microdeletions.
  - Can be performed on nonviable tissue
  - May detect variants of uncertain clinical significance that require comprehensive genetic counseling
- Chorionic villus sampling
  - Performed at 11 to 13 weeks for karyotype and microarray
  - Not always successful (cells do not always grow)
  - Samples placental villi; 1% chance of confined placental mosaicism (aneuploid cells make up part of the placenta but not in the fetus)
  - 0.5% to 1% risk of pregnancy loss
- Amniocentesis
  - Performed at ≥15 weeks (later than CVS)
  - Allows genetic testing and/or assessment for fetal infection
  - Karyotype, microarray, PCR, cultures
  - Carries 1/200 to 1/1000 risk of pregnancy loss
- Fetal blood sampling (cordocentesis)
  - Performed at ≥18 weeks (limited by size and accessibility of fetal vessels)
  - Allows genetic testing, assessment of blood type, hematocrit, platelet count, and fetal transfusion
  - Carries 1% risk of fetal loss

Specific Genetic Testing

- Carrier screening is testing to identify carriers of autosomal or X-linked recessive conditions. Couples who are both carriers have a 25% risk of having an affected child/son.
  - Carrier frequencies vary by race and ethnicity.
  - Expanded screening panels are available, but they increase the risk of variants of uncertain significance.
  - For cystic fibrosis, maternal blood is sent for targeted gene mutation analysis.
    - Highest incidence in Caucasians
    - Universal screening is offered to mother; paternal testing is offered if the mother is a carrier.
  - For Tay-Sachs, maternal blood is sent for targeted gene mutation analysis.
    - Highest incidence in Ashkenazi Jews
    - Maternal screening is offered in this population; paternal testing is offered if the mother is a carrier.
    - Expanded carrier screening panels are available for Ashkenazi Jews.

- For spinal muscular atrophy, maternal blood is sent for targeted gene mutation analysis.
  - Universal screening is offered to the mother; paternal testing offered if the mother is a carrier.
- Sickle cell disease and thalassemia
  - Sickle cell and beta-thalassemia trait are identified by hemoglobin electrophoresis.
  - The beta-thalassemia trait can be identified by mild anemia with low mean corpuscular volume (MCV) on maternal complete blood count (CBC); hemoglobin electrophoresis and genetic testing may be necessary to confirm the finding.
  - Targeted screening is recommended in at-risk ethnic groups (African American, Mediterranean, Southeast Asian)
- Fragile X syndrome
  - Fragile X premutation carrier screening is recommended for those with:
    - Family history of Fragile X
    - Family history of intellectual disability suggestive of Fragile X
    - Unexplained premature ovarian insufficiency
- Infections
  - Group B *Streptococcus* (GBS)
    - 20% of pregnant women carry GBS in the vagina; it can be transmitted to the fetus at birth
    - Without intrapartum treatment, 1% of colonized neonates develop early-onset GBS sepsis.
    - Maternal risk factors for neonatal GBS sepsis include PTL, preterm premature rupture of membranes (PPROM), intrapartum fever, previous GBS sepsis in a newborn, and GBS cystitis.
    - A universal screening protocol (rectovaginal culture at 35–37 weeks) with routine intrapartum prophylaxis has reduced the incidence of early-onset neonatal sepsis.
      - Does not affect late-onset GBS sepsis
  - Rubella
    - Congenital infection can cause fetal anomalies or death.
    - Universal screening for immune status is performed to identify at-risk women; postpartum vaccination is offered.
  - Hepatitis B
    - Vertical transmission is possible; infection is endemic in many parts of the world.
    - Universal screening (with hepatitis B surface antigen testing) is performed to identify the following:
      - Infected women for fetal risk assessment and possible antiviral treatment (tenofovir when maternal viral loads > 6–8 log10 copies/mL)
      - At-risk women to offer antepartum vaccination
  - Hepatitis C
    - Vertical transmission is possible but infrequent.
    - Universal screening (with hepatitis C antibody testing) is performed to identify:
      - Infected women who may benefit from postpartum antiviral treatment
      - At-risk fetuses who require neonatal assessment
  - Human immunodeficiency virus (HIV)
    - Vertical transmission is possible; infection is endemic in some parts of the world.
    - Diagnosed by a combination of antigen/antibody testing; viral load can be assessed using the polymerase chain reaction (PCR) assay
    - Universal screening is recommended to identify infected women to offer antiviral treatment for maternal health preservation and prevention of neonatal transmission.

Ultrasound Screening

- Gestational age determination
  - Due date determination by last menstrual period (LMP) may be imprecise (variation in menstrual cycle length and uncertain day of conception).
  - Sonographic fetal measurements can estimate gestational age.
    - First trimester (most accurate)—fetal crown-rump length is used.
      - Estimated due date (EDD) is changed if ultrasound (US) dating differs by >5 to 7 days from LMP dating.
    - Second and third trimesters—composite biometry (combination of head, abdominal, and femur measurements) is used.
      - Second-trimester US accuracy is ±10 to 14 days.
      - Third-trimester US accuracy is ±2 to 3 weeks.
- Anomaly detection
  - Rationale is that prenatal anomaly detection may do the following:
    - Inform parental decisions about abortion and avoidance of maternal morbidity from delivery procedures, and to clarify care goals.
    - Optimize fetal and neonatal care.
    - Allow transfer to a higher level of care as indicated, engage needed specialists, permit fetal testing and interventions, and allow postnatal planning.
  - Ability to detect anomalies depends on
    - Type of the anomaly
      - High detection—neural tube defects, abdominal wall defects
      - Low detection—small atrial septal defect (ASD)/ ventricular septal defect (VSD), cleft palate without cleft lip
    - Number of fetuses due to limited resolution in multifetal gestations
    - Maternal body habitus (e.g., limited resolution with obesity)
    - Gestational age at examination
      - First trimester—limited by small fetal size
      - Second trimester—optimal age for anomaly detection
      - Third trimester—limited by fetal ossification, crowding
    - Experience of the ultrasound laboratory; quality of equipment, index of suspicion
- Aneuploidy detection
  - Rationale is that fetal aneuploidy often has visible anomalies or markers.
  - Fetuses with structural anomalies have increased risk of aneuploidy (varies by the anomaly).

- First-trimester detection by nuchal translucency (NT) screening
  - Nuchal edema is associated with aneuploidy (risk proportional to NT measurement) and congenital heart disease.
  - Risk is modified by concurrent maternal serum analyte testing.
  - If NT >3.0 mm,
    - >10% risk of aneuploidy
    - Justifies diagnostic testing or cell-free DNA screening
    - Increased risk of fetal heart defects (need echo)
- Second-trimester detection by genetic sonogram to look for anomalies and sonographic markers (normal variants that are associated with fetal aneuploidy)
  - Absent nasal bone, nuchal fold ≥ 6 mm, echogenic bowel
  - Minor markers include choroid plexus cysts, echogenic intracardiac focus, short femurs/humeri, and pyelectasis.
  - Sonographic detection rates are 60% for trisomy 21 and up to 90% for trisomy 13 and 18.
- Anemia surveillance
  - Anemia lowers blood viscosity; the velocity of blood flow is inversely proportional to blood viscosity.
  - Middle cerebral artery (MCA) peak systolic velocity (PSV) is measured with Doppler and converted to multiples of the median (MoM)
    - Weekly MCA-PSV surveillance with isoimmunization and high antibody titer
    - MCA-PSV >1.5 MoM is associated with moderate to severe fetal anemia; consider intrauterine transfusion.
- Growth assessment
  - Fetal growth can be monitored with serial US.
  - Fetal biometric measurements (head circumference, biparietal diameter, abdominal circumference, femur length) are used to determine estimated fetal weight (EFW).
    - Growth restriction is defined as EFW or abdominal circumference below the 10th percentile (although most such fetuses are constitutionally small, not growth restricted).
    - Large for gestational age = EFW > 90th percentile
  - Accuracy of fetal weight estimates is ±10% to 15%.
  - Reassess at ≥14-day intervals (results unreliable if done more frequently).

Evaluation of Fetal Status

- Fetal movement surveillance
  - Rationale is that the fetus requires oxygen for physical activity; there is an increased risk of stillbirth with decreased fetal movement.
  - Mother counts fetal movements; ≥10 within 2 hours is normal.
    - Decreased fetal movement should prompt antenatal testing.
  - Poor discriminator of adverse outcomes
    - Most periods of decreased fetal movement are due to fetal sleep, normal variation, or lack of maternal perception.
    - Fetus may already be dead when lack of movement is noted.
- Nonstress test (NST)
  - Rationale is that normal oxygenation is required for normal autonomic nervous system function and cardiac response (detectable by fetal heart rate [FHR] monitoring).
  - Consists of ≥20 minutes of FHR and uterine activity monitoring
  - Reactive NST is defined by
    - Normal FHR baseline: 110 to 160 beats/min
    - Moderate FHR variability: variation of 5 to 25 beats/min around baseline
    - Presence of two or more accelerations in FHR: ≥10 beats/min (<32 weeks) or ≥15 beats/min (≥32 weeks) above the baseline, lasting ≥10 or ≥15 seconds, respectively
    - Absence of late decelerations
  - Widely used for initial assessment of fetal status; loss of reactivity is an early indicator of hypoxemia
  - A reactive NST predicts a high likelihood of survival for the following week.
    - Less predictive in conditions in which acute decompensation may occur (e.g., diabetes, intrauterine growth restriction [IUGR])
  - Nonreactive NSTs often are false positive but they still should prompt further evaluation (usually biophysical profile); 85% of these will be normal.
- Biophysical profile (BPP)
  - Rationale is that the fetus requires oxygen for physical activity; amniotic fluid volume is indirectly related to placental function.
  - Based on ultrasound parameters (30 minutes of observation) plus NST
  - Five parameters are evaluated (2 points if present and 0 points if absent).
    - Fetal heart rate reactivity on NST
    - Fetal breathing: at least 30 seconds of fetal breathing movements
    - Fetal tone: one episode or more of fetal extension, with return to flexion
    - Gross fetal movement: three or more discrete body movements (e.g., rolling)
    - Amniotic fluid volume: deepest vertical pocket ≥ 2 cm
  - Parameters have differing sensitivity to fetal hypoxemia.
    - NST > breathing > body movements > tone
    - Oligohydramnios is a marker of chronic hypoxemia caused by redistribution of flow and decreased renal perfusion.
  - BPP parameters can be influenced by factors other than hypoxemia, such as the following:
    - Prematurity, drugs, sleep cycles, ruptured membranes (oligohydramnios), certain fetal anomalies
  - Management is based on score and gestational age
    - 8 to 10/10: no asphyxia present, no need for further intervention

- 6/10: equivocal test, fetal asphyxia cannot be excluded
  - At term, repeat BPP in 8 hours and deliver if persistent.
  - Preterm, repeat BPP in 8 to 24 hours; if persistent, consider delivery based on gestational age.
- 4/10: fetal hypoxemia likely, close monitoring or delivery
- 0 to 2/10: fetal hypoxemia highly likely, delivery indicated

- Contraction stress test (CST)
  - Rationale is that contractions squeeze arteries perfusing the placenta, reducing O_2 transfer; with poor placental reserve, fetal hypoxemia elicits late FHR decelerations.
  - FHR monitoring is performed during induced or spontaneous contractions; repetitive late decelerations indicate uteroplacental insufficiency.
  - CST is not affected by gestational age, sleep cycles, or medications, but it cannot be done when labor is contraindicated (e.g., placenta previa).
  - CST is more time and labor intensive than BPP; thus, it is infrequently performed.
  - A negative CST (i.e., no late decelerations) has a similar predictive value for good fetal outcome as does a normal BPP score.

- Ultrasound Doppler velocimetry
  - Used to evaluate fetal anemia and placental function
  - Umbilical artery Doppler
    - Placenta normally has low vascular resistance; dysfunction increases resistance, decreasing passive diastolic flow more than systolic.
    - Ratio of systolic-to-diastolic flow (S/D ratio) is elevated with uteroplacental insufficiency; progressive placental resistance causes absent or reversed end diastolic flow (worsening prognosis).
    - Umbilical artery Doppler in suspected IUGR lowers perinatal mortality and cesarean and induction rates.
  - Middle cerebral artery (MCA) Doppler
    - Fetal anemia causes MCA peak systolic velocity to increase due to decreased blood viscosity.
    - So-called brain-sparing adaptation to hypoxemia by increasing cerebral flow through lower MCA resistance (lowers pulsatility index)

- Fetal lung maturity testing
  - Rarely done because unindicated early delivery is avoided and testing is unnecessary if delivery is clearly indicated
  - Multiple amniotic fluid testing methods are available, including the lecithin-to-sphingomyelin ratio, phosphatidyl glycerol, and lamellar body counts, among others.
    - All have similar accuracy; a positive result is highly predictive of maturity, but a negative result is a poor predictor of lung immaturity.

Fetal Therapy

- Fetal transfusion
  - Indication: severe fetal anemia or thrombocytopenia
  - It is a lifesaving procedure, but has 1% fetal mortality from umbilical cord puncture; may result in emergent cesarean delivery.
  - Procedure
    - Ultrasound guidance to insert needle into umbilical vein
    - Blood sent for CBC; if severe anemia or thrombocytopenia, transfusion volume is calculated and infused and CBC rechecked
    - May need to repeat within several weeks
- Treatment of twin–twin transfusion syndrome (TTTS)
  - Amnioreduction (mild or late TTTS)
    - Up to several liters of amniotic fluid may be aspirated.
    - Reduced fluid volume and pressure may improve intertwin flow.
    - If no improvement, refer for laser therapy.
  - Laser therapy (up to 26 weeks)
    - Endoscopic laser to photocoagulate unbalanced vascular anastomoses and normalize intertwin blood flow
    - Not always successful, as some placentae and anastomoses are inaccessible
    - Improved survival for moderate-to-severe TTTS
    - Delivery at 34 to 35 weeks for successfully treated cases
    - Risks include PPROM, infection, preterm delivery (PTD), fetal death, and intertwin membrane rupture (managed as monoamniotic gestation).
  - Selective reduction
    - Selective feticide by endoscopic occlusion of one twin's cord
    - Considered when laser therapy is not feasible or when the anticipated outcome for one fetus is particularly poor
    - Carries risks similar to those for laser therapy
- Fetal surgery
  - Some fetal anomalies (e.g., myelomeningocele, sacrococcygeal teratoma) are amenable to surgical amelioration prior to birth.
  - Extremely invasive, with maternal surgical risks (including need for cesarean delivery in all future pregnancies) and high risk of PTD
  - Candidates are evaluated on a case-by-case basis at a fetal therapy referral center.

Suggested Readings

American College of Obstetricians and Gynecologists' Committee on Genetics. Carrier screening for genetic conditions. Committee Opinion No. 691. *Obstet Gynecol.* 2017;129:e41–e55.

Landon MB, Galan HL, Jauniaux ERM, et al., eds. *Gabbe's Obstetrics: Normal and Problem Pregnancies.* 8th ed. Philadelphia: Elsevier; 2021.

Lockwood CJ, Moore TR, Copel J, et al., eds. *Creasy & Resnik's Maternal-Fetal Medicine: Principles and Practice.* 8th ed. Philadelphia: Saunders; 2018.

45 *Labor and Delivery*

J. CHRISTOPHER GLANTZ and LISA M. GRAY

Normal Labor and Delivery

- Labor is the physiologic process of coordinated uterine contractions that lead to delivery of the fetus and placenta.
  - First stage: onset of contractions to full cervical dilation
  - Second stage: delivery of the fetus (pushing)
  - Third stage: delivery of placenta
- Most women will enter spontaneous labor between 38 and 42 weeks.
- The precise mechanism controlling the onset of labor is unknown.
- Uterine blood flow decreases during contractions due to myometrial compression on branch uterine arteries.
  - Placental perfusion is intermittently lowered, limiting gas exchange.
  - Uncompromised fetuses tolerate these perfusion changes but, with low placental reserve, the fetus may become progressively hypoxemic.
- Intrapartum fetal heart rate (FHR) monitoring
  - Used in virtually all pregnancies to limit fetal morbidity and mortality
  - For low-risk pregnancies, intermittent auscultation is acceptable.
  - For high-risk pregnancies, continuous electronic FHR monitoring is advised.
    - External (Doppler-based; may not trace well) or internal (fetal scalp electrode; more accurate but invasive)
  - Features of FHR tracing used to assess fetal status:
    - FHR baseline is normally 110 to 160 beats per minute (bpm).
      - Tachycardia (>160 bpm) is seen with infection, fetal anemia, acidosis, arrhythmia, or prolonged fetal activity.
      - Bradycardia (<110 bpm) is associated with drug effects, fetal arrhythmia, maternal hypotension/hypothermia, fetal hypoxia and acidosis.
    - Variability (variation in FHR from measured baseline):
      - Absent—if prolonged, may indicate severe acidosis
      - Minimal—1 to 5 bpm; most often fetal sleep cycle but possible acidosis if persistent
      - Moderate—6 to 25 bpm; reliably excludes acidosis
      - Marked—>25 bpm; possible early hypoxemia
    - Accelerations are elevations in FHR with fetal movement.

- Decelerations can be
  - Early—shallow FHR depressions that begin with onset of contraction, nadir at contraction peak, and end as contraction ends (mirror image of contraction); caused by head compression and considered benign
  - Variable—abrupt depressions in FHR that are variable in shape, duration, and association with contractions; caused by cord compression, which may cause hypoxia if prolonged or recurrent
  - Late—shallow FHR depressions that begin after contraction starts, nadir after contraction peak; resolve after contractions ends; caused by uteroplacental insufficiency; indicative of at least transient hypoxemia
  - Category I tracings indicate normal fetal acid–base status and require no intervention.
    - Normal baseline and moderate variability with or without accelerations or early decelerations
  - Category III tracings are ominous; they require immediate evaluation and usually expedited delivery.
    - Bradycardia, sinusoidal, or absent variability plus repetitive variable or late decelerations
  - Category II tracings (most common) are those with any pattern that is not category I or III; they require evaluation and possible intrauterine resuscitation, and delivery may be indicated.
- Labor analgesia
  - Narcotics provide transient and variable labor pain relief; can cause neonatal respiratory depression.
  - Epidural provides long-acting and highly effective analgesia for labor or cesarean; minimal fetal effects if no maternal hypotension, and small amounts of epidural or intrathecal narcotic rarely cause depression.
  - Spinal provides 2 to 3 hours of surgical-level analgesia but may cause more profound maternal hypotension than epidural.
  - General anesthesia provides continuous and effective analgesia for surgical delivery; it requires intubation and can cause neonatal respiratory depression.
- Routine delivery procedures:
  - Active management of placental delivery (e.g., uterotonics, gentle cord traction, uterine massage) decreases the risk of postpartum hemorrhage.
  - Delayed umbilical cord clamping increases neonatal iron stores.
    - Preterm infants have less need for transfusion and less necrotizing enterocolitis and intraventricular hemorrhage (IVH) but increased neonatal jaundice.
    - Term infants have improved iron stores at 4 months but have an increased risk of neonatal jaundice.

Labor and Delivery Complications

- Dystocia ("difficult labor"; abnormally slow progress)
  - Prolonged or protracted labor; arrest of dilation or descent
  - Oxytocin augmentation if suboptimal contraction pattern or intensity and if no evidence of cephalopelvic disproportion
  - May require instrumental or cesarean delivery
- Meconium-stained amniotic fluid
  - Common, affecting 10% to 20% of pregnancies
  - Usually benign, but also associated with fetal hypoxemia, pulmonary hypertension, and meconium aspiration syndrome; warrants closer FHR monitoring and consideration of pediatric evaluation at delivery
  - Postdelivery DeLee suctioning of meconium is no longer recommended.
- Maternal hypotension
  - Causes maternal hemorrhage, dehydration, supine position (with aortocaval compression), and epidural-related sympathetic blockade
    - Less common are uterine rupture, sepsis, and hepatic–splenic rupture.
  - Management includes treating the underlying cause and maintaining uterine perfusion.
    - Position change, intravenous fluid bolus, phenylephrine (or ephedrine) for refractory postepidural hypotension; manage hemorrhage
- Chorioamnionitis/intra-amniotic infection
  - Clinical diagnosis with maternal fever, maternal–fetal tachycardia, uterine tenderness, elevated white blood cell count (WBC), and foul-smelling or purulent amniotic fluid
  - Considered with any intrapartum fever (epidural analgesia and prostaglandin administration also are associated with fever)
  - Risk factors include prolonged labor or ruptured membranes, internal monitor placement, and frequent digital cervical examinations.
  - Maternal effects include sepsis, dysfunctional labor, endomyometritis, and abscess.
  - Fetal effects include sepsis, hypoxia, organ injury, and death.
  - Treatment includes antibiotics and delivery (regardless of gestational age).
- Management of nonreassuring intrapartum FHR tracings
  - Tachycardia: Identify and treat the cause of tachycardia (maternal fever, infection, hypovolemia, fetal anemia).
  - Variable decelerations: position change, vaginal examination (rule out cord prolapse), amnioinfusion if persistent and low amniotic fluid volume
  - Late decelerations or absent variability: uteroplacental blood flow improvement and IV fluid bolus; position change; prompt delivery if unresolved late decels
  - Note that supplemental maternal O_2 is often administered, but it is no longer recommended (no evidence of benefit).
  - Bradycardia: Identify and treat the cause of bradycardia (e.g., maternal drugs, heart block, acidosis); prompt delivery if unresolved acute episode.

- Normal FHR monitoring predicts a non-acidotic, non-asphyxiated fetus, but abnormal monitoring is a poor predicator of fetal compromise.
  - Little or no evidence of hypoxia in most babies born by cesarean for abnormal FHR tracings
  - Umbilical cord blood gases usually normal or just respiratory acidosis
- Prolonged second stage
  - Defined as a second stage lasting >2 hours without epidural or >3 hours with epidural
  - Can be expectantly managed if reassuring maternal and fetal status
  - Management
    - Operative vaginal delivery with use of forceps or vacuum extractor
      - Cervix should be completely dilated and the vertex engaged.
      - Maternal risks include lacerations, hemorrhage, and need for emergent cesarean delivery if unsuccessful.
      - Fetal risks include shoulder dystocia, cephalohematoma or subgaleal hemorrhage, IVH, fractures, or nerve injury.
      - Contraindications include incomplete dilation, high station, non-vertex presentation, uncertain fetal position, fetal bleeding, or bone mineralization disorder.
    - Cesarean delivery—Cesarean in the second stage is associated with increased maternal–fetal complications (more difficult fetal extraction, hemorrhage).
- Breech vaginal delivery
  - Risk of head entrapment requiring maneuvers for delivery
  - Risk profile may be acceptable in certain candidates.
    - Multiparous patient with normal estimated fetal weight (EFW)
    - Second twin when concordant fetal growth and cephalic first twin
    - Nonviable fetus
    - Excess maternal risk with cesarean delivery
  - Fetal risks include fractures (including neck), asphyxia, neurodevelopmental impairment, and perinatal death.
- Shoulder dystocia
  - It is an obstetric emergency when the fetal shoulder is impacted behind the maternal pubic symphysis.
  - Risk factors include macrosomia, maternal diabetes, operative vaginal delivery, precipitous delivery, and prior shoulder dystocia.
  - Management
    - Stop maternal pushing and call for assistance.
    - McRoberts position—Flex maternal hips to widen pelvic outlet.
    - Apply suprapubic pressure to change shoulder angle.
    - Posterior arm delivery reduces fetal bisacromial diameter.
    - Rotational maneuvers rotate the fetus by applying pressure to fetal shoulders to alleviate impaction.
    - Intentional clavicular fracture—Collapse shoulder medially.
    - Cephalic replacement (Zavanelli maneuver)—Push fetus back into the uterus and perform emergent cesarean delivery.

- Maternal–fetal complications
  - Maternal hemorrhage and pelvic floor lacerations
  - Fetal brachial plexus injury (most are transient), clavicular or humerus fracture, asphyxia, and perinatal death
- Neonatal complications from cesarean delivery
  - Fetal hormonal changes during labor facilitate transition to extrauterine life
  - Cesarean delivery is associated with fetal lacerations and, when scheduled, increased frequency of transient tachypnea and respiratory distress syndrome (RDS).

Breastfeeding

- Confers many maternal–fetal benefits
- Contraindicated with
  - HIV, active untreated tuberculosis, illicit drug use, heavy alcohol use, or radioactive isotope therapy

- Some medications required for maternal health maintenance (sedatives, anxiolytics, angiotensin-converting enzyme [ACE] inhibitors/angiotensin receptor blockers [ARBs], cytotoxic drugs)

Suggested Readings

American Academy of Pediatrics and American College of Obstetricians and Gynecologists. *Guidelines for Perinatal Care.* 8th ed. Elk Grove, IL: American Academy of Pediatrics; Washington, DC: American College of Obstetricians and Gynecologists; 2017.

Berghella V, ed. *Maternal-Fetal Evidence Based Guidelines.* 4th ed. Boca Raton, FL: CRC Press; 2022.

Cunningham FG, Leveno KJ, Dashe JS, et al., eds. *Williams Obstetrics.* 26th ed. New York: McGraw Hill; 2022.

Landon MB, Galan HL, Jauniaux ERM, et al., eds. *Gabbe's Obstetrics: Normal and Problem Pregnancies.* 8th ed. Philadelphia: Elsevier; 2021.

Resuscitation and Stabilization

MELISSA CARMEN

46 Resuscitation, Stabilization, and Asphyxia

MELISSA CARMEN

Perinatal Asphyxia

OVERVIEW

- Asphyxia results in a series of changes in the fetus and newborn, corresponding to changes in the pH of the blood.
- Interruption in blood flow and oxygen supply will result in the fetus or newborn transitioning to anaerobic respiration, with a resultant buildup of lactic acid, leading to a decrease in the pH of the blood and an acidotic state.
- Chronic in utero asphyxia will result in a different presentation and constellation of symptoms in the neonate.
- The causes of asphyxia are listed in Box 46.1.

Acute Perinatal Asphyxia

CLINICAL PRESENTATION

Presentation varies in that asphyxia has effects on multiple organ systems with a variety of symptoms.

- Apnea
  - *Primary apnea* can result from acidosis secondary to decreased fetal circulation; it is often recoverable with stimulation.
    - It may progress into a period of gasping and, without intervention, may develop into secondary apnea.
  - *Secondary apnea* results after a more prolonged period of decreased oxygenation and will lead to a decreased heart rate, as well as additional cardiovascular compromise if not corrected.
    - Secondary apnea can only be corrected with improved ventilation, usually via positive-pressure ventilation (PPV) through a mask or endotracheal tube.
- Vascular redistribution
  - The hypercapnia, hypoxemia, and acidosis that result from asphyxia will initially cause a redistribution of blood flow to the heart, brain, and adrenal glands.
  - Persistent hypercarbia, hypoxemia, and/or acidosis may lead to decreased systemic blood pressure and loss of autoregulation of the cerebral blood flow.
  - Prolonged periods of decreased systemic blood pressure and perfusion can result in end-organ damage in other systems as blood is shunted away from some organs to maintain cerebral perfusion.
  - Acute kidney injury with increased creatinine levels and abnormal urine production (e.g., polyuria, oliguria, and/or anuria).

- Ischemic bowel injury can occur and may increase the risk of necrotizing enterocolitis in at-risk infants.
- Eventually, prolonged asphyxia results in decreased cerebral blood flow, which can lead to hypoxic–ischemic brain injury.

Hypoxic–Ischemic Brain Injury

- Cellular mechanism of injury (Fig. 46.1):
  - Injury occurs after a hypoxic or ischemic event resulting in asphyxia, shortly before or at the time of delivery.
  - Following the insult, there is a depletion of high-energy phosphates (adenosine triphosphate [ATP]), referred to as *primary energy failure.*
  - Energy failure results in immediate necrotic cell death, from which the brain metabolism may be able to recover. Necrosis occurring after cellular membrane breakdown (from lack of ATP) results in the leakage of cellular contents, resulting in inflammation and necrotic cell death.
  - If the injury is severe, after a brief period of attempted recovery the brain may enter a phase of *secondary energy failure.*
    - Secondary energy failure may occur hours to days after the initial insult (usually, 6–48 hours).
  - Glutamate, an excitatory amino acid, accumulates in the extracellular space due to increased production, as well as decreased reuptake by damaged cells.
  - This results in an increased Ca^{2+} influx and activation of degradative enzymes, as well as reactive oxygen species, which lead to delayed apoptotic cell death.
  - The goal of therapies, such as therapeutic cooling, is to prevent the onset or lessen the impact of secondary energy failure by decreasing cellular metabolism in the brain:
    - Suppress cell death by decreasing proapoptotic proteins and increasing antiapoptotic proteins and neurotropic factors.
    - Suppress inflammation by decreasing activated microglia and neutrophils, decreasing reactive oxygen species and proinflammatory cytokines.

CLINICAL PRESENTATION

- The definition of hypoxic–ischemic encephalopathy (HIE) due to perinatal asphyxia, as given by the American Academy of Pediatrics (AAP) and American College of Obstetrics and Gynecology (ACOG), includes the following:

Box 46.1 Causes of Perinatal Asphyxia

Category	Causes	Acute	Chronic
Maternal	Decreased uterine blood flow	√	√
	Maternal hypotension	√	
	Preeclampsia/eclampsia	√	√
	Abnormal uterine contractions	√	
Placental	Infarcts	√	√
	Premature separation (abruption)	√	√
	Inflammatory changes		√
Fetal	Cord compression (nuchal, prolapsed) or entanglement (twins)	√	√
	Breech presentation	√	
	Anemia	√	√
	Hypovolemia (in utero blood loss)	√	√
	Infection	√	√
Neonatal	Hypovolemia	√	
	Apnea related to drug-induced depression (narcotics, magnesium)	√	
	Congenital anomalies of the airway and lung	√	√
	Prematurity	√	√
	Hypoxic respiratory failure (e.g., persistent pulmonary hypertension of the newborn, meconium aspiration syndrome)	√	

- Significant metabolic or mixed acidosis in an umbilical arterial sample
  - pH < 7.00 or base excess (BE) > −12 presents a high risk for fetal compromise.
- Normative values:
  - Umbilical venous blood reflects blood supply from placenta to fetus: average pH, 7.20 to 7.40; PO_2, 30 mm Hg; PCO_2, 40 mm Hg; BE = −3.
  - Umbilical artery blood reflects blood returning from fetus to placenta: average pH, 7.15 to 7.35; PO_2, 16 mm Hg; PCO_2, 55 mm Hg; BE = −3.
- Neonatal neurologic abnormalities
  - Multiple organ involvement
  - Apgar score of <4 for longer than 5 minutes
    - See Table 46.1 for assigning Apgar scores.
    - Scores are assigned at 1 and 5 minutes after birth. If the score remains less than 7 at 5 minutes, the score should continue to be assigned every 5 minutes until 20 minutes of life.
    - Apgar scores were developed to provide a more consistent and objective way to describe the condition of an infant in the delivery room.
    - They are utilized to describe the infant's condition and response to delivery room interventions, but scores do not dictate the next step in resuscitation.

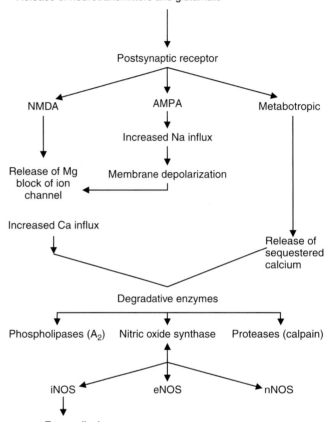

Fig. 46.1 Cellular mechanism of injury after hypoxic-ischemic insult. *AMPA,* Alpha-amino-3-hydroxy-5-methyl-4-isoxazoleproprionic acid; *ATP,* adenosine triphosphate; *eNOS,* endothelial nitric oxide synthase; *iNOS,* inducible nitric oxide synthase; *Mg,* magnesium; *Na,* sodium; *nNOS,* neuronal nitric oxide synthase; *NMDA,* N-methyl-D-aspartate. (From Gleason C, Devaskar SU, eds. *Avery's Diseases of the Newborn.* 9th ed. St. Louis: Elsevier; 2012;877 figure for a review book).

- Poor scores have been shown to be associated with increased mortality, but scores are not predictive of long-term neurologic outcomes.

TREATMENT

- Therapeutic cooling
  - Criteria for the diagnosis of HIE that qualify neonates for therapeutic cooling may vary slightly from the AAP and ACOG definition; the criteria are based on various studies of therapeutic head and whole-body cooling that have shown improved neurodevelopmental outcomes in infants with moderate to severe encephalopathy at birth.

Table 46.1 Apgar Scores

Parameter	Score		
Component assessed (points)	0	1	2
Heart rate (beats/min)	0	<100	>100
Respiratory effort	Apneic	Irregular, shallow, or gasping	Vigorous, crying, regular breathing
Color	Pale, cyanotic (central)	Pale or cyanotic extremities	Pink, well perfused
Muscle tone	Absent	Weak, passive tone	Active movement
Reflex irritability	Absent	Grimace	Active avoidance

- Criteria include clinical and biochemical components:
  - History of perinatal asphyxia event
  - Evidence of acute acidosis on umbilical artery gas
  - Apgar score of <5 at 10 minutes or continued need for mechanical ventilation at 10 minutes after birth
- Neurologic criteria:
  - Seizure
  - Evidence of moderate to severe encephalopathy on examination (must have at least three to six components in the moderate to severe category)
  - Sarnat staging criteria

Chronic Perinatal Asphyxia

OVERVIEW

- Causes of chronic perinatal asphyxia include preplacental and uteroplacental insufficiency.
- In preplacental insufficiency, both the mother and fetus are hypoxic in conditions such as:
  - High-altitude
  - Maternal cyanotic heart disease
  - Other maternal conditions/illnesses that cause hypoxia in the mother
- In uteroplacental insufficiency, maternal oxygenation is normal but uteroplacental circulation is impaired in conditions such as:
  - Pre-eclampsia
  - Placental defect/insufficiency (e.g., abnormal implantation, effects due to maternal disease such as diabetes)

CLINICAL PRESENTATION

- Chronic perinatal asphyxia increases the risk of preterm birth and/or fetal demise.
- Intrauterine fetal growth restriction
  - Growth usually slows at 25 to 31 weeks of gestation.
- Failure to reach genetically determined growth potential
- During initial stages of hypoxia, the fetus is able to adapt and preferentially direct blood flow to the brain, myocardium, and upper body (potentially away from kidneys, intestines, and lower body).
- Short-term complications at increased risk after birth may include:
  - Perinatal asphyxia
  - Meconium aspiration
  - Persistent pulmonary hypertension of the newborn (PPHN)
  - Hypothermia

- Hypoglycemia
- Polycythemia
- Thrombocytopenia
- Neutropenia
- Necrotizing enterocolitis
- Long-term complications at increased risk for after birth may include:
  - Poor growth/failure to thrive
  - Poor neurodevelopmental outcomes
  - Increased risk of cardiovascular disease later in life

Resuscitation

OVERVIEW

- Approximately 4% to 10% of infants will require resuscitation at birth, necessitating PPV, with <1% requiring significant resuscitative measures, such as chest compressions or medications to increase the heart rate.
- All deliveries should be attended by at least one person trained in the initial steps of newborn resuscitation, with the ready availability of a provider trained in more advanced techniques, such as intubation and obtaining vascular access.
- Timely and effective resuscitation can greatly affect an infant's chance for a meaningful recovery after the perinatal asphyxia.

AIRWAY AND VENTILATION

- Establishing a patent and secure airway that allows for adequate ventilation is crucial in the successful resuscitation of the neonate, because most episodes of bradycardia will respond to improved ventilation.
- Most infants can be effectively ventilated with a bag and mask device and do not require the placement of an advanced airway, such as a laryngeal mask airway or endotracheal intubation.
- Indications for PPV:
  - Apnea or gasping
  - Heart rate (HR) < 100 beats/min
  - Some infants who are spontaneously breathing but fail to maintain adequate ventilation may also benefit from PPV or from continuous positive airway pressure (CPAP) to help maintain functional residual capacity (FRC).

VENTILATION DEVICES AND PROCEDURES

- Flow-inflating bag
  - Requires a source of compressed air and secure seal of the mask on the face or endotracheal intubation

- Can provide CPAP when mask applied to face and bag is not deflated
- Self-inflating bag
  - Can deliver positive-pressure breaths without a compressed air source but cannot provide CPAP
  - If attached to an oxygen source, can deliver free-flow oxygen
- T-piece resuscitator
  - Requires a compressed air source
  - Can deliver consistent peak inspiratory pressure (PIP) and positive end-expiratory pressure (PEEP) by adjusting valves on the device to deliver desired pressures
  - Breaths are delivered by intermittently occluding the cap on the T-piece attached to the mask.
  - Can provide CPAP when mask is applied to the face and the dial on the T-piece cap is not occluded

Laryngeal Mask Airway

- A laryngeal mask airway (LMA) is a device that fits over the laryngeal inlet; it can be used to ventilate an infant without having to visualize the vocal cord and glottis directly for placement.
- It may be useful when attempts at endotracheal intubation are not successful or when abnormal airways make placement of an endotracheal tube difficult (e.g., Pierre Robin sequence, macroglossia, cleft palate).
- LMA is intended for babies > 2 kg, although many have used LMA for infants greater than 1.5 kg.

Endotracheal Intubation

- Should be considered when:
  - Mask ventilation is ineffective or is prolonged for more than a few minutes.
  - Chest compressions are being performed and a secure airway should already be established or be in the process of being established.
  - Congenital anomalies pose an increased risk of complications when air accumulates in the bowel due to positive pressure ventilation from a face mask (such as congenital diaphragmatic hernia); in this case, intubation should be done immediately.
  - It is determined that the infant requires surfactant to establish improved oxygenation. There has been a recent increase in the practice of alternative methods of surfactant delivery (e.g., via LMA, less invasive surfactant administration, nebulized formulation); however, these techniques are beyond the scope of this review.

Meconium

- Intubation for direct suctioning of meconium below the cords is no longer recommended by the Neonatal Resuscitation Program (NRP).

Oxygen

- Oxygen should be treated as a drug and used judiciously during resuscitation.

- Resuscitation of term infants should begin with 21% fraction of inspired oxygen (FiO_2) room air, with the level titrated up to maintain saturation in the target range noted by the NRP.
- There is no clear evidence regarding the best concentration at which to begin resuscitation of preterm infants, but some studies have shown that starting resuscitation with an oxygen concentration from 21% to 40% may allow for effective resuscitation while limiting exposure to oxygen free radicals and reactive oxygen species.
- Preterm infants are especially at risk for cellular damage with prolonged exposure to high concentrations of oxygen, and efforts should be made to titrate oxygen levels as soon as possible during resuscitation.

ASSESSMENT OF EFFECTIVENESS

- Effective ventilation is the most important step in the resuscitation of the newborn.
- Every effort should be made to assess for and ensure effective ventilation before moving forward in the resuscitation algorithm to chest compression or resuscitation medications.
- Effective ventilation can be assessed by noting good chest rise and rising heart rate with each administered breath.
- If an endotracheal tube is in place, end-tidal CO_2 monitors may be useful to assess whether the tube is in the correct position and able to provide adequate ventilation.
- Improvement in heart rate and oxygenation are also indicators that the neonate is being adequately ventilated.
- Remember the mnemonic *MR SOPA* when providing ventilation through a mask device to troubleshoot for areas that may be impeding ventilation:
  - *M* (mask): Check to make sure the mask is the appropriate size for the patient and that it makes a secure seal around the mouth and nose.
  - *R* (reposition): Reposition the infant's head and neck to ensure that the baby is in a proper sniffing position and that the head is not too hyperextended or flexed, both of which may occlude the airway.
    - Neonates may benefit from a shoulder roll to aid in proper positioning.
  - *S* (suction): A variety of fluids (e.g., blood, amniotic fluid, meconium) present at the time of delivery may obstruct an infant's airway.
    - Suction the nose before the mouth.
    - Routine suctioning of the stomach is not necessary unless PPV has been given for an extended period of time and there is a need to decompress the stomach for air.
  - *O* (open): Make sure that the infant's mouth is open by gently placing a finger in the mouth to open it, securing the mask, and continuing attempts at ventilation.
  - *P* (pressure): The infant may require various amounts of pressure to move the chest wall adequately.
    - Pressure should be increased until adequate chest rise is seen.
    - A preterm infant, especially one with surfactant deficiency, has decreased compliance in the lungs and may require increased pressure to open the alveoli adequately and properly ventilate.

▪ It is important not to use excessive pressure because this can lead to barotrauma and/or pneumothorax.

▪ *A (alternative airway)*: Mask ventilation is not always adequate to ventilate the lungs sufficiently.

▪ If the above steps have been attempted and there is still no improvement in ventilation and heart rate, the provider should move to placing a more secure airway, such as an LMA or endotracheal intubation.

CARDIOVASCULAR CONSIDERATIONS

▪ The goal of neonatal resuscitation is to keep the infant's HR > 100 beats/min.

▪ Adequate ventilation is the most effective intervention to return the HR to normal; however, there are cases where additional interventions, including chest compressions, fluid resuscitation, and/or vasoactive drugs, may be needed to allow for the return of spontaneous circulation.

Chest Compressions

▪ Chest compressions are indicated when the HR remains less than 60 beats/min after at least 30 seconds of PPV to inflate the lungs (effective ventilation).

▪ Chest compressions should be coordinated with ventilation breaths in a 3:1 compression-to-breath ratio.

▪ The goal is for 120 events in a 60-second period—that is, 90 compressions and 30 breaths.

▪ Electrocardiographic monitoring should be used when resuscitation is needed.

▪ Techniques
  ▪ *Two-finger technique*: The first and second fingers are placed perpendicular to the chest wall, on the sternum, just above the xyphoid process. Compress the chest one-third the anteroposterior (AP) diameter of the chest.
  ▪ *Two-thumb encircling technique* (recommended): Place the thumbs on the sternum, just above the xyphoid process, and encircle the torso with the remaining fingers. Compress the chest one-third the AP diameter of the chest.

▪ Complications include rib fractures and impediment of ventilation if not properly coordinated with breaths.

Volume Resuscitation

▪ The most common cause of hypovolemia at birth is due to fetal blood loss.

▪ This can be caused by placental abruption or laceration, fetal–maternal hemorrhage, cord avulsion, or cord prolapse.

▪ Signs of hypovolemia in the delivery room that may indicate the need for fluid resuscitation include pallor, decreased perfusion, and/or decreased pulses and acidemia.

▪ Fluid resuscitation should not be routinely used unless there is a known history of risk factors for hypovolemia.

▪ Administering fluid to a euvolemic infant whose cardiac function is diminished, either due to arrest or underlying cardiac disease, may actually worsen the infant's condition.

▪ Normal saline (0.9% NaCl solution) can be used at an initial dose of 10 mL/kg, usually over 5 to 10 minutes, but may be given faster.

▪ Packed red blood cells may also be needed if there is a history of significant fetal blood loss or suspicion of severe anemia.

Pharmacology and Drugs Used in Resuscitation

▪ Epinephrine in a 0.1-mg/mL concentration (1:10,000) is the only concentration that should be used in a neonatal resuscitation.

▪ The volume given during resuscitation is 0.02 mg/kg/dose intravenous (IV) or intraosseous (IO; equal to 0.2 ml/kg).

▪ Subsequent doses may be given in the range of 0.01 to 0.03 mg/kg (0.1–0.3 mL/kg).

▪ The dose should be given rapidly, followed by a 3-mL saline flush.

▪ IV dosing is the preferred route due to inconsistencies with administration and absorption via the endotracheal tube (ETT).

▪ An endotracheal dose of 0.1 mg/kg (equal to 1 mL/kg) can be considered while IV or IO access is being obtained (dose range, 0.05–0.1 mg/kg).

Principles of Palliative Care

OVERVIEW

▪ Palliative care aims to reduce pain and suffering, improve quality of life, assist with informed decision making, and coordinate care and communication among clinicians, families, and medical providers.

▪ Models of neonatal palliative care:
  ▪ Integrative
    ▪ Embedded in usual neonatal intensive care practice and plans
    ▪ Initiated early (possibly even via prenatal consult) in high-risk populations and may continue beyond the neonatal intensive care unit (NICU) admission
    ▪ Promotes the recognition of palliative care as a core element of intensive care
  ▪ Consultative
    ▪ Palliative care specialist provides consult on certain aspects of care for infants who are at high risk for poor outcomes.

ROLE OF PALLIATIVE CARE SERVICES IN THE NICU

▪ Prenatal palliative care consultation
▪ Management of pain and other symptoms
▪ End-of-life care
▪ Discharges to hospice from NICU
▪ Communication and conflict resolution
▪ Collaboration in care of the medically complex infant

Suggested Readings

American Academy of Pediatrics and American Heart Association; Weiner GM, Zaichkin J, et al. *Textbook of Neonatal Resuscitation*. 8th ed. Itasca, IL: American Academy of Pediatrics; 2021.

Bidegain M, Younge N. Comfort care vs palliative care: is there a difference in neonates? *NewReviews*. 2015;16(6):e333–e339.

Chalak L. Perinatal asphyxia in the delivery room: initial management and current cooling guidelines. *NeoReviews*. 2016;17(8):e463–e470.

Gleason C, Sawyer T, eds. *Avery's Diseases of the Newborn*. 11th ed. St. Louis: Elsevier; 2024: Chapters 15, 55.

Shankaran S, Pappas A, Laptook AR, et al. Outcomes of safety and effectiveness in a multicenter randomized controlled trial of whole-body hypothermia for neonatal hypoxic-ischemic encephalopathy. *Pediatrics*. 2008;122(4):e791–e798.

Genetics and Dysmorphism

LAURIE STEINER, JOTISHNA SHARMA and GEORGIANNE LEE ARNOLD

47 *Molecular Genetics*

LAURIE STEINER

Basics of Human Genetics

- Most cells in the human body contain 46 chromosomes, two copies of each of the autosomes (1–22) and two sex chromosomes (XX or XY).
- Notable exceptions include red blood cells, which do not contain nuclei or DNA, and gametes (sperm or oocyte), which contain 23 chromosomes.
- Each chromosome contains hundreds to thousands of genes, which are regions of DNA that encode for protein.
- Humans have two copies of most genes: one paternally intertied copy and one maternally intertied copy.
- Humans have 20,000 to 25,000 genes. The total genetic information contained within a cell is referred to as the genome.

Decoding the DNA Blueprint

- DNA is composed of four bases: A (adenine), T (thymine), G (guanine), and C (cytosine).
- The genetic information encoded in DNA is first transcribed to RNA, which is then translated into protein.
- Protein coding genes are made up of exons and introns.
  - Regions of genes that code for protein are *exons*.
  - The intervening sequences between exons are *introns*.
  - Regions of the genome that are between protein coding genes are *intergenic*.
  - Regions of DNA within intronic and intergenic regions often contain important regulatory sequences that determine how and when genes are expressed.

Three Different Types of RNA Participate in Protein Synthesis

- Messenger RNA (mRNA)
  - DNA is transcribed into RNA by RNA polymerase to generate mRNA.
  - Introns are removed from mRNA in a process referred to as *splicing*.
  - mRNA contains a series of three base-pair sequences (codons) that can code for a specific amino acid or code for termination of protein synthesis (stop codon).
  - The genetic code is degenerate, because an amino acid can be encoded by more than one codon.
- Transfer RNA (tRNA)
  - Each tRNA binds a specific amino acid and has a three base-pair sequence that can pair with the complementary sequence in the mRNA.
  - During the process of translating mRNA to protein, tRNA reads each codon and delivers the appropriate amino acid to the growing peptide.
- Ribosomal RNA (rRNA)
  - Ribosomes translate mRNA into protein.
  - Ribosomes are composed of proteins and rRNA.
- Other types of RNA
  - MicroRNA and long noncoding RNA are important regulators of gene expression and do not directly participate in protein synthesis.

Several Enzymes Play an Important Role in the Transmission of Genetic Information

- DNA polymerase is responsible for copying DNA during cellular replication.
- RNA polymerase transcribes DNA into RNA.
- Reverse transcriptase generates DNA from RNA.
  - It is important for the function of retroviruses, such as HIV.

Epigenetic Gene Regulation

- Epigenetics refers to heritable modifications to DNA or DNA-binding proteins that change how genes are expressed without changing the underlying DNA sequence.
- Epigenetic modifications are critical determinants of developmental and cell type–specific gene expression. Disruption of normal patterns of epigenetic gene regulation is associated with both developmental disorders and cancer.
- *DNA methylation* is the process by which a methyl group is added to a cytosine and is a common form of epigenetic gene regulation.
  - Cytosine is more likely to be methylated when it is adjacent to a guanine (CpG).
  - Areas of DNA rich in these regions are referred to as CpG islands.
  - Methylation of CpG islands is a common epigenetic mechanism of gene repression.
- Other common forms of epigenetic gene regulation include posttranslational modification of histone proteins and noncoding RNAs.

Uniparental Disomy and Disorders of Imprinting

- *Uniparental disomy* is the inheritance of two homologous chromosome regions from one parent, instead of inheriting one copy from the mother and one copy from the father.
- *Imprinting* is the epigenetic silencing of a gene based on the parent of origin.
- Prader-Willi and Angelman syndromes, which are caused by deletion or uniparental disomy of 15q11-13, are classic disorders of imprinting.
  - The genes on chromosome 15q11-13 are expressed based on parent of origin.
  - Maternal uniparental disomy or deletion of the paternally inherited chromosome 15q11-13 results in Prader-Willi syndrome.
  - Paternal uniparental disomy or deletion of the maternally inherited chromosome 15q11-13 results in Angelman syndrome.

Single-Gene Disorders and Mode of Inheritance

- Genetic disorders caused by a single gene with predictable patterns of inheritance are *Mendelian disorders*.
  - Examples are cystic fibrosis and sickle cell anemia.
- *Alleles* are variants of genes.
  - The most common allele is generally referred to as wild-type.

- Variants from the wild-type allele are referred to as mutant, although it is important to note that many variant (mutant) alleles do not cause disease.
- *Single-nucleotide polymorphisms* (SNPs) are sequence variants that commonly occur in the population (generally with a frequency of >1%).
  - A person's SNP profile generally varies based on his or her genetic/ethnic background.
  - SNPs generally do not cause disease.
  - SNPs are used as markers in genome-wide association studies to identify allelic variants associated with complex genetic disease (conditions generally not attributable to a single gene disorder).
- *Autosomal dominant* disorders occur following the inheritance of a single copy of a mutated allele.
  - Each generation of the family pedigree is affected, with each affected individual having an affected parent (Fig. 47.1A).
  - An affected individual has a 50% chance of having an affected child.
  - An example is Huntington disease.
- *Autosomal recessive* disorders occur following the inheritance of two mutated alleles.
  - In autosomal recessive disorders, the parents are often carriers (heterozygous for the mutant allele) but are not affected because one wild-type allele is sufficient to prevent the disease phenotype (see Fig. 47.1B).
  - If both parents are carriers, there is a 25% chance that their child will be affected.
  - An example is cystic fibrosis.
- Disorders with *mitochondrial inheritance* occur due to mutations in mitochondrial DNA.

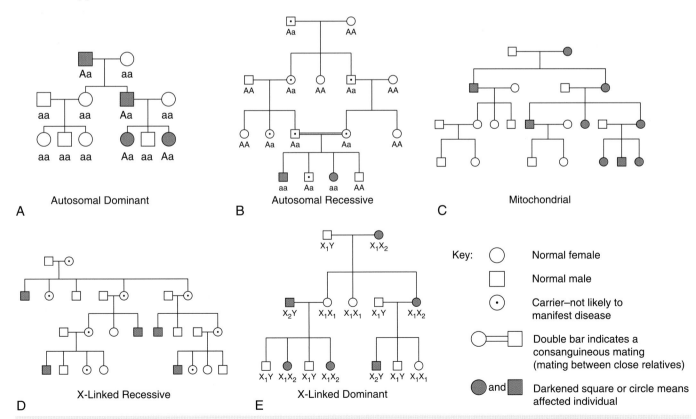

Fig. 47.1 (A–E) Pedigrees demonstrating different modes of inheritance. (Compiled from Figs. 4.3, 4.6, 4.8, 5.8, 5.12, and 5.15, in Jorde L, Carey J, Bamshad M. *Medical Genetics.* 5th ed. Philadelphia: Elsevier; 2016.)

- Mitochondria are organelles that generate energy for the cell by converting oxygen and nutrients into adenosine triphosphate (ATP).
- Mitochondria contain their own chromosome (mtDNA) that encodes for several genes essential for mitochondrial function.
- Disorders of mtDNA are inherited almost exclusively from the mother (see Fig. 47.1C).
- *X-linked recessive* disorders are caused by mutant alleles that reside on the X chromosome, and their inheritance pattern is affected by gender.
  - Females are generally not affected.
  - Males have a 50% chance of being affected if their mother is a carrier (see Fig. 47.1D).
  - In females, each cell contains two copies of the X chromosome; however, one copy is randomly silenced in a process known as *lyonization*.
  - In rare cases, females can be affected by an X-linked recessive disorder if the active X chromosome in the majority of their cells carries the mutant allele (i.e., they have silenced the majority of the X chromosomes that carry the wild-type allele).
  - An example is hemophilia A.
- *X-linked dominant* disorders are caused by mutant alleles that reside on the X chromosome, and both genders are affected.
  - Males are more severely affected, with some X-linked disorders being lethal in males.
  - Each offspring of an affected female has a 50% chance of being affected, whereas among offspring of affected males all daughters are affected but none of the sons (see Fig. 47.1E).

Structural Chromosomal Abnormalities That Contribute to Human Genetic Disease

- *Mitosis* is the process by which somatic cells divide to create two daughter cells that contain 46 chromosomes each.
- *Meiosis* is the process by which germ cells divide such that the daughter cells ultimately contain one copy of each autosomal chromosome and one copy of a sex chromosome (X or Y) for a total of 23 chromosomes.
- *Aneuploidy* refers to an abnormal number of chromosomes (i.e., more or less than the normal complement of 46 for somatic cells and 23 for germ cells).
  - Aneuploidy occurs due to *nondisjunction*, which is the failure of chromosomes to appropriately segregate during cell division.
  - An example is trisomy 21.
- Incomplete failure of chromosomal segregation during cell division or inappropriate crossover of genetic information between chromosomes (called recombination) can result in abnormalities of chromosomal structure or copy number variations (too many or too few copies of a given gene). These include the following:
  - Insertions and deletions, frequently referred to as *indels*, are the addition or deletion of base pairs to the DNA sequence.

- Large indels (5–10 megabases) can be detected by G-banding on a karyotype.
- Smaller indels are detected by fluorescence in situ hybridization (FISH) or comparative genomic hybridization microarray.
- Many indels are incidental findings and have no known clinical significance.
- Other indels can have a profound clinical impact because they change the copy number of a critical gene or set of genes.
- DiGeorge syndrome (22q11 deletion) is an example of a common deletion that results in human disease.
- *Translocations* are chromosomal rearrangements where genetic information is rearranged between two nonhomologous chromosomes. There are several types of translocation:
  - *Balanced translocations* result from an equal crossover of genetic information between nonhomologous chromosomes. In a balanced translocation, each daughter cell receives a complete complement of genetic information. Balanced translocations are often asymptomatic but can result in disease if:
    - The translocation disrupts an important genetic regulatory element or gene.
    - The translocation creates an abnormal fusion gene.
    - The translocation results in an unbalanced amount of genetic material being passed on to offspring. For example, carriers of a Robertsonian translocation of chromosome 21 are generally asymptomatic but have an increased risk of having a child with trisomy 21.
  - *Unbalanced translocations* are the consequence of unequal crossover of genetic information between nonhomologous chromosomes and can result in gain or loss of genetic information.
- An *inversion* is a section of chromosome that is in the reverse orientation relative to the reference sequence.
  - Inversions typically occur when there are two breaks in a chromosome and the intervening DNA sequence rotates 180 degrees before the breaks are repaired.
  - As inversions are not associated with loss or gain of genetic information, they are often asymptomatic.
  - Inversions can be deleterious if they disrupt a critical gene or genetic regulatory element.

Diseases Caused by Trinucleotide Repeat Expansion

- *Trinucleotide repeats* are a series of three nucleotides, consecutively repeated, that occur within a region of DNA.
- During DNA replication, trinucleotide repeats are prone to "expansion mutation," where the number of triplet repeats in a given sequence increases. Beyond a certain threshold (which is different for each gene), the trinucleotide repeats interfere with the expression or function of their associated gene.
- Expansion of trinucleotide repeat sequences underlies >20 human genetic diseases, most notably fragile X syndrome, myotonic dystrophy, and Huntington disease.

- *Fragile X syndrome*: Repeats occur in noncoding regions of the genome and affect the expression of their associated gene.
- *Huntington disease*: Repeats occur in the region of the gene that codes for protein, resulting in a dysfunctional and sometimes toxic protein.
- *Anticipation* is the process by which a disease has an earlier age of onset or increased severity with each successive generation of a family.
  - Anticipation occurs in trinucleotide repeat diseases because expanded (but not normally sized) trinucleotide repeats tend to be unstable, and their size increases with each subsequent generation.
- Expansion of trinucleotide repeats between generations can be impacted by the parent of origin.
  - For example, in fragile X syndrome and myotonic dystrophy, anticipation occurs primarily when the expanded trinucleotide repeat sequence is transmitted from the mother.

Commonly Used Genetic Tests

- A *karyotype* assesses the number and appearance of the chromosomes. *G-banding* is a method of staining the chromosomes to facilitate the detection of structural chromosome abnormalities, including translocations, inversions, and large insertions or deletions (indels). Karyotypes are readily available and fairly low cost, but they can only be done on actively dividing cells and do not have sufficient resolution to detect abnormalities smaller than ~5 Mb.
- *FISH* uses fluorescent probes to detect specific genes or regions of the genome and is commonly used to detect insertions or deletions (Fig. 47.2). For example, FISH for 22q11 is frequently used to diagnose DiGeorge syndrome. FISH can also be used to diagnose aneuploidy.

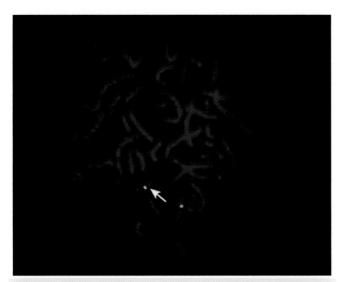

Fig. 47.2 Fluorescence in situ hybridization (FISH) assay demonstrating a microdeletion. Two fluorescent spots are visualized for the control probe (*green*), indicating that it is annealing to the control region on homologous chromosomes. The single fluorescent spot visualized with the experimental probe (*red*) indicates deletion of the test region on one chromosome (*arrow*). (From Gilner J, Kuller J, Valea F. *Reproductive Genetics in Comprehensive Gynecology.* 7th ed. Philadelphia: Elsevier; 2017:22–47.)

It often has a faster turnaround time than a karyotype because it does not require actively dividing cells.
- *Array comparative genomic hybridization* (aCGH; DNA microarray) is used to detect unbalanced copy number variations (indels) that are too small to be detected by karyotype. Many indels detected by aCGH are not associated with any known disease phenotype. The resolution of aCGH varies based on the specific type of microarray used, but, in general, aCGH can detect indels of ~200 kb or larger.
- *Targeted mutation* screening determines the sequence of a single gene or small group of genes. Targeted mutation screening is used when clinical findings suggest a specific Mendelian disorder with a known disease-causing allele. For example, if an infant has an elevated immunoreactive trypsinogen (IRT) on newborn screening, then targeted mutation screening can be done on the CFTR gene to evaluate for cystic fibrosis.
- *Gene panels* determine the sequence of a group of genes linked to a specific clinical presentation or phenotype.
- *Whole exome sequencing* (WES) uses next-generation sequencing technologies to determine the sequence of all of the protein-coding regions (exons) in the genome and can also detect variants as small as 1 bp. The goal of WES is to find variants in protein coding genes that may be responsible for a disease phenotype. In neonates, WES is most commonly used in critically ill infants suspected to have an underlying genetic disorder but that do not have an obvious unifying diagnosis.
- *Whole genome sequencing* (WGS) uses next-generation sequencing technology to determine the sequence of the entire genome. Depending on the laboratory performing the test, WGS can detect both copy number variations and sequence variants. Similar to WES, WGS is most commonly used in critically ill infants suspected of having an underlying genetic disorder.

Diagnostic Approach to the Infant With Suspected Genetic Disease

- A genetic workup should be considered in any infant that has more than one major and one minor abnormality that are not clearly attributable to environmental exposures such as fetal alcohol syndrome or diabetic embryopathy.
- A genetic workup should also be considered in any critically ill infant with failure of one or more organ systems without a clear underlying cause.
  - Major anomalies have a significant medical impact and are never part of normal variation (e.g., congenital heart disease).
  - Minor anomalies do not have a medical impact but are uncommon in the general population (e.g., single palmar crease).
- The first step in the genetic evaluation/consultation should be a detailed prenatal and birth history, family history, and physical examination. The initial diagnostic approach will be determined by the results of this evaluation.
  - If a specific genetic disorder is suspected, targeted genetic evaluation is indicated. For example, if an infant has clinical features consistent with trisomy 21, a karyotype or FISH for chromosome 21 would be the appropriate evaluation.

- If the initial evaluation does not reveal a causative exposure or strongly implicate a specific genetic diagnosis, the choice of further studies, such as targeted mutation screening, gene panels that assess a group of genes for a causative mutation, WES, or WGS, depends on clinical findings and status. When possible, testing should be done in consultation with a clinical geneticist.
- Recent studies have suggested that WGS and WES have a high diagnostic yield and are cost effective as first-line tests in critically ill infants where genetic disease is suspected.

Newborn Screening for Genetic Disorders

- All 50 states and the District of Columbia offer newborn screening. The goal of newborn screening is early identification of treatable genetic conditions.
- The majority of states use tandem mass spectrometry (MS/MS) on dried blood spots, often referred to as Guthrie cards, to screen for inborn errors of metabolism. MS/MS permits analysis of many different metabolites from a single sample. Newborn screening panels vary by state, but most include disorders of amino acid metabolism, organic acid metabolism, and fatty acid oxidation. Screening for endocrine disorders, including congenital hypothyroidism and congenital adrenal hypoplasia, is also included in most newborn screening panels.
  - A positive newborn screen in a well, term neonate requires referral to a clinical geneticist (if positive for inborn error of metabolism) or endocrinologist (if positive for endocrine disorder) for confirmatory testing and management.
  - Of note, samples from premature or critically ill neonates may be difficult to interpret and are more likely to generate false-positive and false-negative results.
- Newborn screening for cystic fibrosis is done in all 50 states and the District of Columbia and is done by measuring IRT on dried blood spots. Infants with an elevated IRT are referred for confirmatory testing via sweat testing and/or mutation analyses of the CFTR gene.
- Newborn screening for sickle cell disease and other hemoglobinopathies is also performed in all 50 states and the District of Columbia. Screening is done on dried blood spots using a combination of isoelectric focusing (IEF) and high-performance liquid chromatography (HPLC). Infants with a positive newborn screening result should be referred to a pediatric hematologist for confirmatory testing with hemoglobin electrophoresis.
- The majority of infants are also screened for hearing loss after birth. Hearing loss can be due to genetic, environmental, or infectious factors. Cytomegalovirus (CMV) infection is a notable cause of hearing loss due to congenital infection.

Suggested Readings

Cotton CM, Murry JC. The human genome and neonatal care. In: Gleason CA, Juul SE, eds. *Avery's Diseases of the Newborn*. 10th ed. Philadelphia: Elsevier; 2018:180–189.

Jorde L, Carey J, Bamshad M. *Medical Genetics*. 5th ed. Philadelphia: Elsevier; 2016.

Wagner T, Bhoj E. Contemporary evaluation of the neonate with congenital anomalies. *NeoReviews*. 2017;18(9):522–531.

Zin A. Inborn errors of metabolism. In: Martin R, Fanaroff A, Walsh M, eds. *Fanaroff and Martin's Neonatal-Perinatal Medicine*. 10th ed. Philadelphia: Saunders; 2015:1553–1615.

48 *Patterns of Congenital Disorders*

JOTISHNA SHARMA

Chromosomal Disorders

- Incidence: 1% to 2% of live births
- 2% of pregnancies in women > 35 years
- 50% of all spontaneous first trimester abortions
- 5% of couples with two or more miscarriages

Types of Chromosomal Abnormalities

- *Numerical*: alteration in the normal chromosomal number (46)
  - Aneuploidy
    - Loss (i.e., monosomy) or gain (i.e., trisomy) of individual chromosome from the diploid set
    - Monosomy
      - Autosomal monosomies are typically lethal early in pregnancy.
      - Survival is possible in mosaic forms.
    - Trisomy: presence of three chromosomes
      - Most common type of aneuploidy
      - May be mosaic
  - Polyploidy
    - Euploid cells with more than the normal diploid number of 46 (2n)—that is, 3n, 4n
    - Common abnormality in losses during first trimester of pregnancy losses
    - Triploidy: three haploid sets of chromosomes (3n)
    - Mosaicism: two or more cell lines in a single individual
- *Structural*: alteration in the structure of the chromosomes
  - Deletion: portion of chromosome missing or deleted
  - Inversion: portion of chromosome broken off, turned upside down, and reattached; results in genetic material inversion
  - Duplication: portion of genetic material is duplicated, resulting in extra genetic material
  - Translocation: two types
    - Balanced translocation
      - Equal exchange to chromosome segments between two chromosomes
    - Robertsonian translocation
      - One chromosome joins the end of another at the centromere.
      - Involves chromosomes 1, 14, 15, 21, and 22
      - Relatively common (1:1000)
      - Phenotypically normal
      - Increased risk for offspring of carriers
  - Rings: Portion of chromosome is broken off and reattached in the form of a ring/circle.
  - Isochromosomes: One arm of chromosome is missing (monosomy) and the other duplicated in a mirror image fashion (trisomy).

Trisomy 21 (T21) "Down Syndrome"

OVERVIEW

- Most common chromosomal abnormality, with an incidence of one per 700 live births

Etiology

- Meiotic nondisjunction (>90%) is associated with advanced maternal age (>35 years).
- Translocation (3–5%): two types
  - De novo arises from balanced translocation carrier parent and results in unbalanced trisomy offspring.
  - Translocated chromosome 21 rearranges with another acrocentric chromosome (usually chromosome 14), leading to Robertsonian translocation.
- Mitotic nondisjunction or mosaic (3%): Phenotype varies from normal to a typical T21.

Prenatal Assessment

- Karyotyping: amniocentesis and chorionic villus sampling (CVS) in first trimester
- Maternal serum quad screen test: decreased α-fetoprotein, decreased unconjugated estriol, increased total human chorionic gonadotropin (HCG), and increased inhibin A
- Ultrasound (US) findings include nuchal translucency/thickening, shortened long bones, underdeveloped/absent fetal nasal bone (70%), echogenic small bowel, and "double-bubble" sign (duodenal atresia).

CLINICAL PRESENTATION AND ASSOCIATED ANOMALIES

- *General*: hypotonia[a] (80%), joint hyperflexibility[a] (80%), poor Moro reflex[a] (85%)
- *Craniofacial and neurologic*: flat facial profile[a] (90%), brachycephaly, upslanting palpebral fissures[a] (80%), late closure of fontanelles, inner epicanthal folds, open mouth with protruding tongue, atlantoaxial instability (1–2%), seizures (5–10%; often manifest during

---

[a]Principle features in the neonate.

255

infancy), incomplete fusion of vertebral arches of lower spine (37%)
- *Developmental delay*: motor (worse in first 3 years of life), language delay
- *Cognitive impairment*: affected by genetic and environmental factors, autism (1%)
- *Dentition*: hypodontia and delayed dental eruption
- *Eyes*: Brushfield spots with peripheral hypoplasia of iris, fine lens opacities (59%) on slit-lamp examination, nystagmus (35%), strabismus (45%), cataract (15%), myopia (70%)
- *Ears*: hearing loss (75%), middle ear effusions (60–80%)
- *Neck*: excess skin on back of neck[a] (80%)
- *Hands and feet*: hypoplasia of midphalanx of fifth finger[a] (60%) with clinodactyly (50%), single palmer crease[a] (45%), palmar axial triradius (84%), wide gap with deep plantar groove between first and second toes
- *Cardiac* (40%): atrioventricular (AV) canal defects, ventricular septal defect (VSD), atrial septal defect (ASD), patent ductus arteriosus (PDA), tetralogy of Fallot (TOF)
- *Gastrointestinal anomalies* (12%): duodenal atresia (2–5%), diastasis recti, tracheoesophageal fistula (TEF), Hirschsprung disease, imperforate anus
- *Skin and hair*: cutis marmorata (43%), dry hyperkeratotic skin with time (75%)
- *Genitalia (male)*: micropenis, decreased testicular volume
- *Endocrine*: hypothyroidism (5%; association with thyroid autoantibodies or thyroid agenesis), short stature, fertility (primary gonadal failure results in infertility, rare cases of female fertility)
- *Hip and pelvis*: hip dysplasia/dislocation (6%), avascular necrosis, slipped capital femoral epiphyses
- Hematologic
  - Transient myeloproliferative disorder (TMD) (10%) regresses by 3 months of age.
    - Risk of later onset of leukemia (10–30%): *GATA1* gene mutation
  - Leukemia (1%)
    - Acute Megakaryoblastic leukemia (AMKL)
    - Acute lymphoblastic leukemia with Down syndrome (DS-ALL): mutations in the JAK/STAT pathway
  - Polycythemia (18–64%), neonatal thrombocytopenia, defects in T-cell maturation and function with increased infection risk
- *Others*: 11 ribs, tracheal stenosis, obstructive sleep apnea (50–75%)[a]

DIAGNOSIS AND EVALUATION

- Genetic test
  - Fluorescent in situ hybridization (FISH) identifies extra chromosome 21 but does not detect translocation.
  - Karyotype: high-resolution chromosomal analysis to confirm translocation
- Echocardiogram (echo)
- Gastrointestinal radiography and contrast studies, based on clinical concerns
- Hematologic: complete blood count (CBC) at birth and as needed
- Ophthalmologic exam: first month of life, then annually
- Hearing screen

- At birth with follow-up assessment by 3 months of life
- Age-appropriate testing at 6 months, then annually
- Screen for hypothyroidism
  - Within first 2 weeks of life (usually newborn screen)
  - Thyroid-stimulating hormone (TSH) and free thyroxine (fT_4) level
  - Follow-up screening at 6 and 12 months of life, then annually
- Growth
  - Parameters at birth, 10% to 25% percentile range
  - Postnatal growth restriction not uncommon

TREATMENT

- Genetic: Confirm diagnosis and provide genetic counseling.
  - One child with T21: Maternal recurrence risk of another affected child is 1% higher than her age-specific risk (more significant in younger mothers).
  - De novo translocation: Recurrent risk is less than 1%.
  - Mother with Robertsonian translocation
  - Risk for another translocation T21 fetus is 15% at amniocentesis and 10% at birth.
  - If the father is the translocation carrier, the recurrence risk is lower (1–2%).
- Surgical intervention (as needed)
- Treatment for hypothyroidism
- Early intervention and developmental therapy

PROGNOSIS

- Causes of mortality include congenital heart disease and infection (pneumonia).
- 50% survive to 60 years.
- When older than 40 years of age, neurodegenerative disease with features of Alzheimer disease occurs.

Trisomy 18 (T18) "Edward Syndrome"

OVERVIEW

- Second most common multiple malformation syndrome, with an incidence of one per 6000 live births
- Associated with a high rate of in utero demise; 5% of conceptuses survive to birth
- 3:1 female preponderance

Etiology

- Presence of extra chromosome 18 (complete, mosaic, or partial trisomy 18q)
- Most commonly nondisjunction: complete trisomy (94%)
- Associated with advanced maternal age (>35 years)

Prenatal Assessment

- Karyotyping: amniocentesis and CVS
- Maternal serum triple screen test: decreased α-fetoprotein, decreased unconjugated estriol, decreased total HCG
- US findings include growth restriction, oligohydramnios or polyhydramnios, limb anomalies, absence of nasal bone (55%), heart defects, and choroid plexus cyst.

CLINICAL PRESENTATION AND ASSOCIATED ANOMALIES

- *General*: small for gestational age (SGA),[b] single umbilical artery,[b] weak cry, one-third preterm and one-third post-term,[b] small placenta[b]
- *Craniofacial and neurologic*: microcephaly, prominent occiput,[b] wide fontanelles, cleft palate/lip, small mouth,[b] micrognathia,[b] hypotonia in newborn period, hypertonia beyond neonatal period,[b] seizures (25–50%), marked to profound psychomotor and intellectual disability,[b] Dandy-Walker malformation, agenesis of corpus callosum
- *Eyes*: short palpebral fissures,[b] inner epicanthal folds, colobomas of iris, cataract
- *Ears*: low-set malformed auricles[b]
- *Hands and feet*: clenched hands,[b] overlapping digits,[b] absence of distal crease on fifth finger,[b] hypoplastic nails,[b] hypoplastic/absent thumb,[b] "rocker bottom" feet, short hallux, syndactyly of second and third toes[b]
- *Hip and pelvis*: limited hip abduction,[b] small pelvis, dislocated hip[b]
- *Thorax and pulmonary*: short sternum (decreased number of ossification centers),[b] small nipples,[b] eventration of diaphragm
- *Cardiac (80–100%)*: VSD,[b] ASD,[b] PDA,[b] bicuspid aortic valve (AV), pulmonic stenosis (PS), coarctation of aorta (CoA), TOF
- *Gastrointestinal*: hernia (inguinal, umbilical),[b] diastasis recti,[b] Meckel diverticulum, omphalocele, tracheoesophageal fistula, extrahepatic biliary atresia
- *Skin and hair*: redundancy,[b] cutis marmorata,[b] hirsutism of forehead and back[b]
- *Genitourinary*: horseshoe kidney (66%), ectopic kidney, cryptorchidism and hypospadias (male), hypoplasia of labia majora with prominent clitoris (female)[b]

DIAGNOSIS AND EVALUATION

- Genetic test
  - FISH offers quicker time to diagnosis and may assist in plan of care.
  - Karyotype: high-resolution chromosomal analysis to confirm translocation
- Other investigations: echo, brain magnetic resonance imaging (MRI), ophthalmologic exam

TREATMENT

- Genetic: Confirm diagnosis and provide genetic counseling.
  - Maternal recurrence risk of T18 in future pregnancy is 1% greater than her age-specific risk.
- Infant care options include medical and surgical interventions or palliative care attained after discussion among medical providers and parents.

PROGNOSIS

- Very poor, with 50% mortality in first week of life
- >90% infants die in first 6 months of life.

---

[b]Abnormalities occur in ≥50% of patients.

- Only 5% are alive at 1 year; few have survived to childhood.
- Risk of kidney and liver cancer is increased in survivors.
- Causes of mortality include central apnea (early deaths), infection, and congestive heart failure.

Trisomy 13 (T13) "Patau Syndrome"

OVERVIEW

- Incidence is one per 5000 to 10,000 live births.
- There is a high rate of in utero demise, as only 2% to 3% of fetuses survive to birth.

Etiology

- Due to the presence of extra chromosome 13 (complete, mosaic, or partial trisomy 13q)
- Most commonly nondisjunction: complete trisomy
- Associated with advanced maternal age (>35 years)

Prenatal Assessment

- Karyotyping: amniocentesis and CVS
- US findings include increased nuchal translucency (21%), growth restriction, central nervous system and facial anomalies (64%), absence of nasal bone (35%), and heart defects (54%).

CLINICAL PRESENTATION AND ASSOCIATED ANOMALIES

- *General*: SGA,[c] microcephaly,[c] single umbilical artery[c]
- *Craniofacial and neurologic*: holoprosencephaly[c] (50%), cutis aplasia[c] (50%), sloping forehead,[c] wide fontanelles,[c] cleft lip[c] (60–80%) ± cleft palate, micrognathia, apnea, hypertonia/hypotonia, seizures (electroencephalogram [EEG] with hypsarrhythmia), agenesis of corpus callosum, cerebellar hypoplasia, myelomeningocele
- *Eyes*: colobomas of iris,[c] microphthalmos,[c] retinal dysplasia,[c] shallow orbital ridges, upslanting palpebral fissures, absent eyebrows, anophthalmos, cyclopia
- *Ears*: abnormal helices,[c] low-set ears,[c] hearing loss
- *Neck*: excess skin on back of neck
- *Hands and feet*: distal palmar axial triradii,[c] single palmer crease,[c] hyperconvex narrow fingernails,[c] flexion of fingers with/without overlapping,[c] camptodactyly,[c] postaxial polydactyly,[c] cleft between first and second toes, hypoplastic toenails, equinovarus
- *Hips and pelvis*: hypoplasia of pelvis with shallow acetabular angle[c]
- *Thorax and pulmonary*: thin posterior ribs with or without missing rib,[c] situs inversus of lungs diaphragmatic defect
- *Cardiac (80%)*: VSD,[c] PDA,[c] ASD,[c] dextrocardia,[c] PS, hypoplastic aorta, bicuspid AV
- *Gastrointestinal*: hernia (inguinal and umbilical),[c] omphalocele, Meckel diverticulum
- *Skin*: capillary hemangiomata (forehead)[c]
- *Genitourinary*: polycystic kidney (30%), hydronephrosis, horseshoe kidney, male (cryptorchidism,[c] abnormal

---

[c]Abnormalities occur in ≥50% of patients.

scrotum[c]), female (bicornuate uterus,[c] hypoplastic ovaries)

- *Hematologic*: increased frequency of nuclear projections in neutrophils ("drumstick" appearance),[c] persistence of embryonic and/or fetal hemoglobin[c]
- *Others*: flexion deformity of large joints, S-shaped fibula[c]

DIAGNOSIS AND EVALUATION

- Genetic test
  - FISH offers quicker time to diagnosis and may assist in plan of care.
  - Karyotype: high-resolution chromosomal analysis to confirm translocation
- Other investigations: echo, brain MRI, ophthalmologic exam

TREATMENT

- Genetic: Confirm diagnosis and provide genetic counseling.
  - Maternal recurrence risk of T13 in future pregnancy is 1% greater than her age-specific risk.
- Options for care of the infant, including medical and surgical interventions or palliative care, are determined after discussion among medical providers and parents.

PROGNOSIS

- Overall prognosis is extremely poor, with 80% mortality during the neonatal period.
- Median survival is 7 days of life.
- Rare childhood survivors have profound cognitive impairment and feeding difficulties.

Turner Syndrome (45,X)

OVERVIEW

- Phenotype is associated with loss of all or part of one copy of the X chromosome in a female conceptus.
- Incidence is one per 2500 female newborns.
- 0.1% of fetuses with a 45,X complement survive to term; more than 99% are spontaneously aborted.

Etiology

- Faulty chromosomal distribution leads to 45,X individual.
- In 80% of cases, it is the paternally derived X chromosome that is lost.
- 50% are due to the 45,X karyotype or loss of one entire X chromosome cases (monosomy).
- 50% are due to a variety of X chromosome anomalies, including deletions, isochromosomes, translocations, and mosaicism.
- *SHOX* gene is important for bone development and growth.
  - Loss of one copy of this gene is responsible for short stature and skeletal abnormalities in Turner syndrome.
- Advanced maternal age is *not* a risk factor.

Prenatal Assessment

- Karyotyping: amniocentesis and CVS
- US findings include cystic hygroma (26%), fetal hydrops (11%), increased nuchal translucency (13%), and heart defects (13%).

CLINICAL PRESENTATION AND ASSOCIATED ANOMALIES

- *General*: wide phenotype variability, short stature, webbed neck (50%)
- *Craniofacial and neurologic*: high arched palate (>80%), epicanthal folds (40%), hearing loss, anomalous auricles (>80%)
- *Neck*: low posterior hairline
- *Hands and feet*: lymphedema (>80%), nail hypoplasia, cubitus valgus (>70%), distal palmar axial triradii (40%), medial tibial exostosis (60%)
- *Hips and pelvis*: hip dislocation
- *Thorax and pulmonary*: shield chest, widely spaced nipples (>80%), pectus excavatum
- *Cardiac* (30–50%): bicuspid AV (30%), CoA (10%), aortic stenosis, mitral valve prolapse
- *Skin*: excessive pigmented nevi (>50%), loose skin
- *Genitourinary*: horseshoe kidney, double/cleft renal pelvis, gonadal dysgenesis

DIAGNOSIS AND EVALUATION

- Karyotype: chromosomal analysis
- Other investigations: echo

TREATMENT

- Genetic: Confirm diagnosis and provide genetic counseling.
  - Majority are due to a sporadic event: monosomy (non-disjunction) or mosaic.
  - No adequate data on recurrence risk
  - Partial deletion of X chromosome is rare and can be inherited.
- Growth issues (short stature) are a concern; offer growth hormone therapy at 4 to 5 years of age.
- Primary ovarian failure
  - Due to gonadal dysplasia (streak gonads) greater than 90%
  - Delay of secondary sexual characteristics and primary amenorrhea
  - Cyclic hormonal therapy is initiated at the age of puberty.
  - Infertility is common but may be treated with assisted reproductive therapy.
- Exploratory laparotomy
  - 6% of females with Turner syndrome have 45,X/46,XY mosaicism.
  - To remove any residual gonadal tissue (eliminate risk of gonadoblastoma)

PROGNOSIS

- Intellectual development: Most have normal intelligence but difficulties with spatial and perceptual reasoning.

- Increased risk for dissection of the aorta: aortic root dilation (8–42% prevalence)
- Morbidity is related to diabetes mellitus, hypertension, and ischemic heart disease.

Triploidy (69, XXX or 69, XXY)

OVERVIEW

- Karyotype containing three copies of each chromosome
- Occurs in 2% of conceptuses
- Majority of triploid fetuses spontaneously abort: live births are rare.
- 15% of chromosomally abnormal pregnancies

Etiology

- Extra set of chromosomes is paternally derived in 69% of cases.
- 60% of cases have been XXY.
- Mosaicism (combinations of diploid and triploid, mixoploid) has been documented.
- Advanced maternal age is not a risk factor.

CLINICAL PRESENTATION AND ASSOCIATED ANOMALIES

Malformations of the fetus and newborn

- Disproportionate prenatal growth deficiency
- Neural tube defects, hydrocephalus
- Holoprosencephaly, ocular and auricular malformations
- Cardiac defects
- Third and fourth syndactyly of fingers
- Abnormal placenta (large and cystic)
- Partial hydatidiform moles

PROGNOSIS

- No data to indicate increased risk of recurrence
- A triploid pregnancy sometimes is preceded or succeeded by a molar pregnancy.

Deletion Syndromes

- Partial monosomy of a chromosome can lead to a recognizable pattern of malformations.
- Deletion or loss of genetic material from the short (*p*) arm of chromosome

Chromosome 1p36 Deletion Syndrome (1p36)

OVERVIEW

- Incidence is one per 10,000 live births.
- Monosomy for the distal short arm of chromosome 1 or deletion of 1p36
- Most frequently occurring subtelomeric deletion

Etiology

- Majority of deletions arise de novo.

CLINICAL PRESENTATION AND ASSOCIATED ABNORMALITIES

- Microcephaly, frontal bossing, midface hypoplasia, orofacial cleft
- Hypotonia, seizures, infantile spasm, diffuse brain atrophy, hearing loss
- Cardiac: PDA, VSD, ASD, Ebstein anomaly, cardiomyopathy
- Brachydactyly, camptodactyly, scoliosis, delayed bone age
- Renal anomalies, cryptorchidism, micropenis, hypoplastic labia minora

DIAGNOSIS AND EVALUATION

- Genetic test
  - High-resolution karyotype may not detect all deletions.
  - Confirmatory test: FISH and array comparative genomic hybridization (CGH)
- Other investigations include echo, brain MRI, EEG, audiology, and ophthalmologic exam.

PROGNOSIS

- Feeding issues: poor suck and swallowing, auditory and visual impairment
- Intelligence quotient (IQ) generally less than 60 among those who survive to adulthood.

Wolf-Hirschhorn Syndrome (4p-)

OVERVIEW

- Incidence is one per 50,000 live births.
- Distal deletions of the short arm of chromosome 4

Etiology

- De novo mutation: >80% of 4p deletions
  - Deleted chromosome is paternally derived (80%); recurrence risk is very low.
- Translocation: 10% to 15%
  - 2:1 excess of maternally derived 4p deletions
  - Parental chromosomal analysis is indicated for recurrence risk counseling.

CLINICAL PRESENTATION AND ASSOCIATED ABNORMALITIES

- Intrauterine growth restriction (IUGR), microcephaly, cleft lip/palate, cutis marmorata, scoliosis
- "Greek warrior helmet" facies: hypertelorism, epicanthal folds, beaked nose, high forehead with prominent glabella
- Optic nerve defects, coloboma, hypotonia, seizures
- Cardiac: ASD, PS
- Cryptorchidism, hypospadias, clitoral hypoplasia

DIAGNOSIS AND EVALUATION

- Genetic test:
  - High-resolution karyotype may not detect small submicroscopic deletions.
  - Confirmatory test: microarray, cytogenetic analysis using 4p telomere probes
- Other investigations: echo, ophthalmologic exam

PROGNOSIS

- Feeding issues, failure to thrive, and developmental delay are common.
- One-third of infants die in the first year of life.

Cri du Chat Syndrome (5p-)

OVERVIEW

- Incidence is one per 50,000 live births.
- Partial monosomy of chromosome 5p

Etiology

- De novo mutation (>90% of 5p deletions)
  - Deleted chromosome is paternally derived (80%).
  - Recurrence risk is very low (<1%).
- Translocation: 10%
  - Malsegregation of balanced translocation in carrier parent
  - Recurrence risk is 10% to 15% of unbalanced translocation.
  - Parental chromosomal analysis is indicated for recurrence risk counseling.

CLINICAL PRESENTATION AND ASSOCIATED ABNORMALITIES

- Low birth weight, microcephaly, round face, hypertelorism, downward-slanting palpebral fissures, broad nasal bridge, short philtrum
- Hypotonia, agenesis of corpus callosum, cerebral atrophy, cerebellar hypoplasia
- Cardiac: ASD, VSD, TOF
- Unusual cry (cat-like cry): ascribed to abnormal laryngeal development
- Renal anomalies: renal agenesis, horseshoe kidney

DIAGNOSIS AND EVALUATION

- Genetic test: high-resolution karyotype
- Other investigations: echo, renal US, brain MRI

PROGNOSIS

- Feeding issues during infancy, intellectual disability, and developmental delay
- Most individuals have normal life expectancy.

Microdeletion Syndromes

- Disorders result from inappropriate dosage of crucial genes in a given genomic segment via structural mechanisms (deletion).

- In many of the microdeletion syndromes, there is a possibility that a reciprocal duplication of the exact same region may also occur.

22q.11.2 Deletion Syndrome (DiGeorge Syndrome)

OVERVIEW

- Incidence is one per 3000 live births.
- Most common microdeletion syndrome in humans

Etiology

- 90% of deletions occur de novo.
- Less than 10% are inherited from an affected parent (considered autosomal dominant).
- Interstitial deletion of chromosome 22q11.2
- Clinical phenotype is related to haploinsufficiency of one of these genes (*TBX1*).
  - *TBX1* encodes a T-box transcription factor.
- Reciprocal duplications of the 22q11.2 common deletions have been reported.
  - 70% inherited the duplication (usually from a normal parent).

CLINICAL PRESENTATION AND ASSOCIATED ABNORMALITIES

- Microcephaly (40–50%), hypertelorism, hooded eyelids, bulbous nasal tip
- Cleft lip/palate, conductive hearing loss, small mouth, micrognathia
- Hypotonia (70–80%), hyperextensible fingers/toes (63%)
- Cardiac (85%): interrupted aortic arch type B, truncus arteriosus, TOF
- Thymus and parathyroid: aplasia/hypoplasia, hypocalcemia
- Renal agenesis, hypospadias, abnormal T-cell function

DIAGNOSIS AND EVALUATION

- Genetic test: FISH or DNA microarray (80–90% detected)
  - Both parents of affected child should be tested to determine if they carry the deletion.
- Other investigations: echo, renal US, brain MRI

PROGNOSIS

- Developmental and learning disabilities: speech and language delay
- Death, usually due to cardiac defects

Single Gene (Mendelian) Disorders

- Familial: dominant, recessive, autosomal, or sex-linked
  - Autosomal dominant (AD) disorders
  - When affected individual has normal parents, it may be due to

- New mutation
  - Skipped generation (nonpenetrance of the genes)
  - Gonadal mosaicism (gene present in cells of gonad of one parent)
  - Autosomal recessive (AR) disorders
    - Risk is increased with consanguinity.
    - Each sibling of an affected individual carries a one-quarter risk of being affected and a two-thirds risk of being a carrier.
  - X-linked recessive and X-linked dominant disorders
- Pedigree analyses of families are useful to determine the inheritance pattern.
- Genetic heterogeneity: Two different genes cause the same phenotype.
  - It can be caused by more than one genetic mechanism.
  - Molecular diagnosis assists in defining mode of inheritance.

Fragile X Syndrome

OVERVIEW

- Incidence is one in 4000 males, one in 8000 females.
- Individuals have developmental delay, intellectual disability, and/or autism.
- 1% to 3% have a full mutation.
- Most common inherited cause of intellectual disabilities
- Most common known cause of autism
- The phenotype is identified most readily in males.
- Carrier mother has 50% chance of passing mutated gene to each of her children.
- Carrier father will pass permutation gene to all his daughters (become carriers), but not to his sons.
- Fragile X permutation can be passed silently through generations.

Etiology

- X-linked dominant inheritance
- Due to expansions of a trinucleotide repeat (CGG) in the 5′ untranslated region of the *FMR1* gene located at the Xq27.3
  - Normal individuals have from 6 to 54 repeats.
  - Male and female permutation carriers have 54 to 200 repeats.
  - Affected individuals (full mutation) have >200 repeats.

CLINICAL PRESENTATION AND ASSOCIATED ABNORMALITIES

- Macrocephaly, prominent forehead, elongated face, prognathism (puberty)
- Large ears, pale blue irides, epicanthal folds, high arched palate, cleft palate
- Hypotonia, pectus excavatum, mitral valve prolapse, aortic dilation
- Hand flapping or biting (60%), poor eye contact (90%), anxiety
- Hyperactivity/hyperarousal, aggression outburst, autism spectrum disorder (60%)

- Males: mild to profound intellectual disability (IQ, 30–55)
- Females with full mutation have IQ less than 70 (30–50%).
- Female permutation carriers have a 20% risk for premature ovarian failure.
- Fragile X–associated tremor/ataxia syndrome (FXTAS)
  - Deficits in executive function, atypical parkinsonism, cerebellar tremor, dementia
  - 46% of male and 17% of female permutation carriers develop symptoms after age 50.

DIAGNOSIS

- DNA analysis of the *FMR1* gene

PROGNOSIS

- Normal life span; sensory processing disorders are common.
- Infancy: feeding problems (e.g., gastroesophageal reflux [GER]), otitis media
- Growth rate is increased in the early years but with delayed motor milestones.

Mitochondrial Disorders

- Maternally inherited
- Result in dysfunction of the mitochondria with inadequate production of energy in critical tissue
- Clinically multisystem involvement:
  - Visual loss, progressive myopathy, seizures, encephalopathy, diabetes
- High spontaneous mutations
- Wide spectrum of severity (due to heteroplasmy)
- Affected females transmit disease to their offspring (male and female).
  - Risk approaches 100% (human egg is the source of all of the mitochondria of the offspring).
  - Clinical phenotype occurs when a threshold of abnormal to normal mitochondria is exceeded in the critical tissue.
  - Phenotypically unaffected daughters of affected women also have risk of vertical transmission.
  - Lack of clinical disease does not preclude that some of the daughter's mitochondria may harbor the mutation.
- Affected males have normal offspring.

Non-Mendelian Inheritance

PARENT OF ORIGIN EFFECTS

- Genomic imprinting
  - Only one copy of the normal two copies of genes (one each inherited from mother and father) is either active or "turned on."
  - The active copy depends on the parent of origin.
- Uniparental disomy (UPD)
  - The two copies of a chromosome pair or part of a chromosome come from the same parent.
  - UPD is associated with advanced maternal age.

ANGELMAN SYNDROME

- Maternally derived deletion chromosome 15q11-13 (60%)
- Paternal UPD (40%) chromosome 15

BECKWITH-WIEDEMANN SYNDROME

- 85% sporadic
- Less than 5% genetic, including paternal UPD—two copies of paternally derived chromosome 11p15.5

PRADER-WILLI SYNDROME

- Prevalence is one in 15,000.

Etiology

- Loss of activity on the long arm of chromosome 15 (15q11-13) due to
  - Imprinting (70%): paternally derived deletion of 15q11-13
  - Maternal UPD (25–30%): possesses two normal maternally derived chromosome 15
  - Mutation of the imprinting center or translocation (1–3%)

Clinical Presentation

- Central hypotonia, almond-shaped eyes, small down-turned mouth
- Small hands and feet, micropenis, hypoplastic scrotum, cryptorchidism

Diagnosis

- Methylation analysis detects all three molecular defects (deletion, UPD, mutation); abnormal findings in 99% of those affected.
  - If methylation pattern is abnormal, then perform:
    - FISH for detection of a deletion
    - Molecular assay to confirm maternal UPD
- An abnormal methylation analysis and normal FISH and UPD studies indicate an imprinting defect.
- Counseling
  - Recurrence risk is negligible for de novo deletions.
  - Recurrence risk without deletions is one in 1000.

PROGNOSIS

- Hypotonia improves in first year of life.
- Hypothalamic and primary gonadal dysfunction
- Developmental delay: speech and gross motor
- Intellectual disability is mild to moderate
- Feeding
  - Infancy: poor feeding and failure to thrive

Table 48.1 Recurrence Risk for Some Multifactorial Defects

Defect	RECURRENCE RISK FOR		
	Normal Parents of One Affected Child	Future Males	Future Females
Cleft lip with or without cleft palate	4–5%	—	—
Cleft palate alone	2–6%	—	—
Cardiac defect (common type)	3–4%	—	—
Pyloric stenosis	3%	4%	2.4%
Hirschsprung disease	3–5%	—	—
Clubfoot	2–8%	—	—
Dislocation of hip	3–4%	0.5%	6.3%
Neural tube defects (anencephaly, myelomeningocele)	3–5%	—	—
Scoliosis	10–15%	—	—

Adapted from Jones KL, Jones MC, del Camp M. *Smith's Recognizable Patterns of Human Malformation*. 8th ed. Philadelphia: Saunders; 2021.

  - Childhood: hyperphagia and obesity with subsequent diabetes risk
- Behavioral issues: temper tantrums, obsessive–compulsive disorder

Multifactorial Disorders

- Familial clustering is observed.
- Many common malformations have different birth frequencies in different populations.
- The risk of the majority of defects in offspring of normal parents with an affected child is 2% to 5% (Table 48.1), 20 to 40 times the frequency in the general population.
- Second-degree relatives (uncles, aunts) have a marked decrease in risk compared to first-degree relatives.
- As the number of affected family members increases, so does the risk for recurrence.
- Consanguinity: Inbreeding increases the number of "susceptibility genes" and risk.
- The more severe the malformation, the greater the risk for recurrence.
- Recurrence risk is increased for relatives of the least affected gender (if gender differences are noted).

Suggested Readings

Gleason CA, Sawyer T, eds. *Avery's Diseases of the Newborn*. 11th ed. Philadelphia: Elsevier; 2024.
Jones KJ, Jones MC, del Campo M. *Smith's Recognizable Patterns of Human Malformation*. 8th ed. Philadelphia: Saunders; 2021.

49 Nongenetic Etiologies for Congenital Defects

GEORGIANNE LEE ARNOLD

Overview

- Not all birth defects are genetic in origin.
- Nongenetic factors can cause malformations, deformations, and disruptions.

Malformations

- Permanent, abnormal development of a structure
- The defect occurs during early embryonic development.
- Examples of malformations:
  - Congenital heart defects
  - Neuronal migration defects
  - Unilateral or bilateral clefts
  - Limb agenesis

Deformations

- Abnormalities in a structure caused by an extrinsic force
- Timing is typically during later fetal development.
- Fairly common
- Often responsive to physical therapy
- Often the result of abnormal uterine shape, unusual fetal positioning, or secondary to a malformation in a sequence, including renal malformations resulting in oligohydramnios, leading to fetal compression with deformation of feet (club feet) and face (facial flattening) (i.e., Potter syndrome)
  - Examples of deformations:
    - Fetal akinesia sequence
    - Torticollis–plagiocephaly deformation sequence
    - Positional congenital hip subluxation
    - Positional scoliosis

Disruptions

- Abnormalities in a structure caused by interference with or breakdown of a normal developmental process
- Examples of disruptions:
  - Amniotic band sequence
    - Caused by amnion rupture
    - Amnion strings wrap around limbs, causing constriction rings/amputations.
    - Can cause facial clefts
    - Clubfoot is common.
    - Treatment is supportive.
  - Porencephaly secondary to cerebrovascular accident

- Basal ganglia cysts from energy deficiency disorders
- Teratogens, including maternal drugs of abuse, prescription medications, environmental exposures, metabolic disorders, infections, and assisted reproductive technology

Teratogens (see Table 49.1)

OVERVIEW

- Cause nongenetic birth defects through maternal exposure
- Vulnerable periods:
  - Embryogenesis (through 8 weeks): period of organogenesis when exposure is most likely to result in structural birth defects
  - Fetal period (9–40 weeks): fetal and brain growth most likely to be affected
- Examples of windows of greatest vulnerability:
  - Heart: first 8 weeks
  - Limbs: first 12 weeks
  - Palate: first 12 weeks
- Genetic effects may affect susceptibility to teratogens.

DRUGS OF ABUSE

- Alcohol: fetal alcohol spectrum disorders
  - Overview
    - Disrupt fetal development at all stages of pregnancy
    - Leading preventable cause of birth defects and neurodevelopmental abnormalities
  - Clinical presentation
    - Variable spectrum of structural and developmental anomalies
  - Diagnosis and evaluation: Institute of Medicine diagnostic categories
    - Fetal alcohol syndrome (FAS)
      - Evidence of prenatal alcohol exposure
      - Evidence of central nervous system (CNS) abnormalities
      - Facial abnormalities: short palpebral fissures, smooth philtrum, thin upper lip narrow
      - Growth deficits
    - Partial FAS (pFAS)
      - Some (but not all) features of FAS
    - Alcohol-related neurodevelopmental disorder (ARND)
      - Prenatal alcohol exposure and some CNS structural or functional abnormalities

Table 49.1 Partial List of Common Teratogens

Category	Teratogen	Time of Susceptibility	Fetal Effects
Drugs of abuse	Alcohol	Any	Fetal alcohol spectrum disorders (structural, CNS, growth, neurodevelopmental)
	Cocaine	Any	Low birth weight, microcephaly
	Nicotine	Any	Cleft lip/palate, low birth weight, microcephaly
Antiepileptic	(Categorical)		Heart, hypospadias, facial clefts
	Valproate	Any	Neural tube defects, anatomic and neurodevelopmental defects
	Phenytoin	Any	Fetal hydantoin syndrome (facial, skeletal [digital], neurodevelopmental)
ACE inhibitors	Various	First trimester	Cardiac, neural tube defects
		Trimesters 2–3	Renal dysplasia and failure, oligohydramnios
Cancer/Immune	Methotrexate	Any (highest 6–8 weeks)	Limb defects, CNS, GI, heart, neurodevelopmental
	Thalidomide	20–36 days	Limb defects, CNS, eye, ear, heart, GI, others
	Aminopterin	First trimester	Neural tube defects, facial clefts
	Retinoic acid	First trimester	CNS, neural tube defects, microcephaly, facial clefts, limb defects, others
Psychiatric	Lithium	First trimester	Cardiac, particularly Ebstein anomaly
Anticoagulant	Warfarin	Any	Facial (nasal hypoplasia), CNS, cardiac defects, fetal hemorrhage
Environmental	Mercury	Any	CNS defects, neurocognitive defects
	Radiation	2–18 weeks	Microcephaly, neurocognitive defects
	Temperature	Any	Neural tube defects, cardiac, facial defects
Maternal metabolic disorders	Diabetes	Preexisting	Caudal regression, renal, cardiac defects
		Gestational	Macrosomia
	PKU	Any	Cardiac, GI defects, microcephaly, neurocognitive defects
Infection	Toxoplasmosis	First trimester	Fetal death
		Second trimester	Hydrocephalus, intracranial calcifications, chorioretinitis
	Rubella	Trimesters 1–2	Hearing loss, cataract, retinopathy, cardiac defect

CNS, Central nervous system; *GI*, gastrointestinal; *PKU*, phenylketonuria.

- Alcohol-related birth defects (ARBDs)
  - One or more: heart, kidney, skeletal, immune
  - Seen in conjunction with FAS or pFAS
- Treatment
  - Symptomatic, early intervention services

MATERNAL PRESCRIPTION MEDICATIONS

- Antiepileptic medications
  - Overview
    - Two to three times increased risk of birth defects in various studies
    - Risk depends on specific drug and dose.
    - In general, risks are increased for heart, hypospadias, and oral clefts.
    - Polytherapy significantly increases risks.
  - Valproate
    - Significant risks of various anatomic and neurodevelopmental defects
    - 1% to 2% risk for neural tube defects
  - Phenytoin
    - Fetal hydantoin syndrome
    - Distal digital hypoplasia, intrauterine growth retardation, facial dysmorphism, intellectual disability
- ACE inhibitors
  - First trimester: increased risk for cardiac, neural tube, and other defects
  - Second and third trimesters: risk for renal dysplasia and failure, and oligohydramnios

- Cancer/immune drugs
  - Methotrexate
  - Most severe effects at 6 to 8 weeks postconception
  - Limb defects, CNS anomalies, gastrointestinal/cardiac defects, intellectual disability
- Thalidomide
  - Limb defects are prominent.
  - All organs and neurodevelopment can be affected.
  - Most severe risks are at days 20 to 36.
- Aminopterin
  - Neural tube defects, facial clefts
  - Interferes with folic acid
- Retinoic acid
  - CNS, neural tube defects, microcephaly, facial clefts, limb defects, others
- Lithium
  - Ebstein anomaly and other cardiac defects
  - Dose dependent
- Warfarin
  - Characteristic facial defects (nasal hypoplasia)
  - Cardiac, CNS defects, stippled epiphyses
  - Fetal hemorrhage

MATERNAL ENVIRONMENTAL EXPOSURES

- Mercury
  - Neural tube defects, neurocognitive defects
- Radiation
  - Microcephaly, neurocognitive defects

- Peak vulnerability 8 to 18 weeks
- High doses required (equivalent to 500 chest x-rays)
- Temperature (maternal fever >38.9°C)
  - Neural tube defects, cardiac defects, clefts

MATERNAL METABOLIC DISORDERS

- Diabetes
  - Prepregnancy diabetes
    - Up to nearly four times higher risk of birth defect
    - Related to prepregnancy glucose control and body mass index
    - Highest risks are caudal regression, renal, and cardiac.
  - Gestational diabetes
    - Occurs later in pregnancy
    - Structural birth defect risk not significantly elevated
    - Macrosomia, delivery issues, neonatal hypoglycemia
- Maternal phenylketonuria
  - Cardiac, gastrointestinal defects, microcephaly, neurocognitive defects
  - Outcome related to maternal phenylalanine level

MATERNAL INFECTIONS

- Toxoplasmosis
  - First trimester: fetal death
  - Second trimester: hydrocephalus, intracranial calcifications, chorioretinitis

- Rubella
  - Risk in trimesters one and two
  - Triad of deafness, eye abnormalities (cataract, retinopathy, microphthalmia), cardiac (pulmonary artery stenosis, patent ductus arteriosus

ASSISTED REPRODUCTIVE TECHNOLOGY (ART)

- 30% to 40% increase in nongenetic birth defects in some studies

  - Gastrointestinal and lower limb reduction defects are higher in ART.
  - Intracytoplasmic sperm injection is potentially associated with imprinting defects (specifically Prader-Willi and Beckwith-Wiedemann syndromes).

Suggested Readings

Alwan S, Chambers CD. Identifying human teratogens: an update. *J Pediatr Genet.* 2015;4(2):39–41 (reference for question 3).

Clinical Teratology website: http://depts.washington.edu/terisdb/terisweb/index.html.

Gilbert SF, Sunderland MA. *Developmental Biology.* 6th ed. Sunderland MA: Sinauer Associates; 2000.

Graham J, ed. *Smith's Recognizable Patterns of Human Deformations.* Philadelphia: Elsevier; 2007.

Hattori, et al. Association of four imprinting disorders and ART. *Clin Epigenetics.* 2019;11:21 (reference for question 2).

Hoyme HE, Kalberg WO, Elliott AJ, et al. Updated clinical guidelines for diagnosing fetal alcohol spectrum disorders. *Pediatrics.* 2016;138(2):e20154256 (reference for question 1).

50 *Evaluation of Infants With Congenital Anomalies*

JOTISHNA SHARMA

Overview

- 3% of newborns in the United States are affected by a major congenital anomaly.
- 1% of newborns have multiple congenital anomalies.
- Congenital anomalies are the fourth leading cause of neonatal mortality.
- Congenital anomalies are present in 10% of neonatal intensive care admissions.
- Major congenital anomaly presents a five times increased risk of morbidity.
- Major congenital anomaly identified prenatally presents a three times increased risk of death in utero.

CONGENITAL ANOMALY

- Structural defect identified at birth
    - Internal or external

MAJOR ANOMALY

- Defect with significant impact on individual function
- Requires medical, surgical, or cosmetic intervention

MINOR ANOMALY

- Defect without a significant impact on a person's overall function
- Usually does not require surgical, medical, or cosmetic intervention
- Incidence varies (14–41%).
- Pattern of minor anomalies may represent a genetic syndrome.

RELATIONSHIP BETWEEN MAJOR AND MINOR ANOMALIES

- 20% of patients with major anomalies have three or more minor anomalies.
- Among patients with one minor anomaly, only 4% have a major anomaly.

DYSMORPHISM

- Abnormal external physical features
- Clues to underlying developmental defect or normal variant

BASIS FOR CONGENITAL ANOMALY (SEE ALSO CHAPTER 49)

- Malformations
    - Structural defects in tissue formation or abnormal morphogenesis
    - Examples include neural tube defect, congenital heart defects, and cleft palate.
    - Causes
        - Genetic
        - Teratogenic
    - Recurrence risk is dependent on cause.
- Deformations
    - Defects are due to abnormal mechanical forces on morphologically normal tissue in utero.
    - Associated with
        - Multiple gestations
        - Uterine malformations
        - Oligohydramnios
    - Examples include club feet and hip dislocation.
    - Occur in 2% of births
    - Rarely genetic cause
    - 90% undergo spontaneous resolution.
    - Recurrence risk is low.
- Disruptions
    - Defects due to destruction or interruption of normal developmental process
    - Usually affect a body part, rather than a specific organ
    - Example: vascular interruption
        - Monozygotic twinning
        - Prenatal exposure to cocaine
    - Example: limb reduction defects from amniotic bands
        - Rarely genetic cause
        - Low recurrence risk
- Dysplasia
    - Defective morphology due to abnormal organization of cells within a specific tissue
    - Tissue specific—for example, skeletal dysplasia
    - Localized or generalized

MULTIPLE CONGENITAL ANOMALIES

- Definition
    - Two or more major malformations (example cardiac defect, tracheoesophageal fistula, imperforate anus)

    or

- Three or more minor malformations (example club foot, hypertelorism, low-set ears)
- Patterns
  - Sequence
    - Pattern of multiple anomalies
    - Due to a single cause
    - Examples include Potter sequence (oligohydramnios sequence) and Pierre-Robin sequence.
  - Association
    - Nonrandom occurrence of multiple malformations
    - No known cause
    - Example: VACTERL (vertebral defects, anal atresia, cardiac defects, tracheoesophageal fistula, renal anomalies, and limb abnormalities)
  - Syndrome
    - Recognized pattern of anomalies
    - Due to a specific cause (inherited)

Etiology of Congenital Anomalies

EVALUATION

- History
  - Prenatal history
  - Maternal health
    - Age: risk of nondisjunction chromosomal anomalies rises with maternal age
  - Maternal immunization: rubella, varicella
  - Maternal disease
    - Diabetes: three-fold increase in congenital anomalies
    - Obesity
    - Seizure disorder
  - Pregnancy and fetal health
    - Amniotic fluid volume
      - Polyhydramnios
      - Oligohydramnios
      - Anhydramnios
    - Premature labor
    - Premature rupture of membrane
    - Fetal movement
  - Type of conception
    - Natural
    - Assisted reproductive technology (ART)
      - Risk of major malformations is approximately 1.3 times greater in ART-conceived children, including:
        - Congenital heart defects
        - Neural tube defects
        - Facial cleft
        - Gastrointestinal malformations
        - Genitourinary malformations
        - Imprinting disorders
      - Overall malformation rates ARE similar for intracytoplasmic sperm injection (ICSI) and in vitro fertilization (IVF).
      - Increased urogenital defects (hypospadias) with ICSI
  - Exposures
    - In utero infections
    - Medications
    - Smoking
    - Substance abuse
    - Environmental agents (teratogens)
  - Prenatal testing
    - Maternal quad screen
    - Chorionic villus sampling (CVS)
    - Ultrasonography
    - Amniocentesis
  - Birth history
    - Gestational age at delivery
    - Fetal position at delivery (breech)
    - Length of labor
    - Type of delivery
    - Evidence of fetal distress such as meconium-stained amniotic fluid
    - Apgar scores
    - Need for delivery room resuscitation
    - Birth parameters
      - Weight
      - Length
      - Head circumference
    - Physical examination at birth, noting any malformations
  - Neonatal medical history
    - Medical status
      - Need for cardiorespiratory support
      - Growth pattern
      - Development
      - Review of systems (ROS)
- Family history
  - Critical to genetic evaluation
  - Pedigree analysis
    - Three-generation pedigree schematic diagram
  - Ethnicity of both sides of the family
  - Consanguinity
  - First-degree relatives with similar anomalies
  - Extended family history
    - Identify relatives with congenital anomalies and developmental abnormalities.
    - Photographs are helpful.
  - Reproductive history
    - Infertility
    - Miscarriages (having more than two first-trimester miscarriages increases the risk of a balanced translocation in one parent)
    - Stillbirths (~25% of stillbirths have malformations, and ~50% have a genetic cause)
    - For couples with more than two pregnancy losses, recommend chromosomal analysis or karyotyping.
- Physical examination (Tables 50.1 and 50.2)
  - Growth parameters
    - Weight
    - Length
    - Head circumference
  - Head and neck
    - Shape and size of head
    - Shape and size of fontanelles: anterior and posterior
    - Scalp defects
  - Eyes
    - Canthal measurements
    - Inner and outer canthal distances

Table 50.1   Physical Findings with Differential Diagnoses

Organ	Manifestation	Differential Diagnoses
Growth parameter	Small for gestational age (SGA)	Chromosomal abnormalities, genetic syndromes, congenital infections, multiple gestation
	Large for gestational age (LGA)	Infant of diabetic mother, Beckwith-Wiedemann syndrome, Sotos syndrome (cerebral gigantism)
Head	Macrocephaly	Familial (autosomal dominant), hydrocephalus, achondroplasia, neurocutaneous syndrome
	Microcephaly	Familial (autosomal dominant, autosomal recessive), chromosomal abnormalities, genetic syndrome, congenital infections
	Large fontanelle	Hypothyroidism; trisomies 21, 18, 13
		Zellweger syndrome, hypophosphatasia, cleidocranial dysostosis
	Small fontanelle	Craniosynostosis, hyperthyroidism, hyperparathyroidism, abnormal brain growth
	Dolichocephaly (increase AP skull diameter)	Premature infants, trisomy 18
	Brachycephaly (decrease AP skull diameter)	Trisomy 21, microdeletion syndromes, Crouzon syndrome
	Craniosynostosis	Apert syndrome, Pfeiffer syndrome, Carpenter syndrome, Crouzon syndrome
	Frontal bossing	Achondroplasia, rickets, hydrocephalus
Hair	Sparse	Ectodermal dysplasia, cartilage-hair hypoplasia, oculodentodigital syndrome
	Hirsutism	Cornelia de Lange syndrome, fetal hydantoin syndrome, fetal alcohol syndrome, trisomy 18, familial ethnic variation
	Abnormal scalp hair pattern	Microcephaly: lack of normal parietal whorl
		Turner and Noonan syndromes: low posterior hairline
		Trisomy 13: cutis aplasia (punched-out scalp lesions)
Eyes	Hypotelorism	Holoprosencephaly, trisomy 13, Parry-Romberg disease
	Hypertelorism	Cri-du-chat syndrome, Wolf-Hirschhorn syndrome, DiGeorge syndrome, achondroplasia, midline facial anomalies
	Epicanthal folds	Trisomy 21, fetal alcohol syndrome, Turner syndrome
	Upward slant of palpebral fissure	Trisomy 21
	Downward slant of palpebral fissure	Treacher Collins syndrome, Apert syndrome, mandibular dysostosis, Noonan syndrome
	Short palpebral fissure	Microphthalmia, fetal alcohol syndrome, trisomy 21, DiGeorge syndrome
	Coloboma	Treacher Collins syndrome, CHARGE syndrome, renal hypodysplasia
	Synophrys (fusion of eyebrows in midline)	Cornelia de Lange syndrome, microdeletion syndromes, familial
Ears	External anomalies	CHARGE syndrome, DiGeorge syndrome
	Low-set ears	Trisomy 21, 18, and 13; Turner syndrome; Noonan syndrome; DiGeorge syndrome; Cri-du-chat syndrome
	Preauricular pits/tags	Familial, branchiootorenal (BOR) syndrome
	Microtia	Infant of diabetic mother, prenatal exposure to isotretinoin, thalidomide, alcohol, Treacher Collins syndrome, Goldenhar syndrome
Nose	Hypoplastic alae nasi	Hallermann-Streiff and microdeletion syndromes
	Broad nose	Frontonasal dysplasia, microdeletion syndromes
	Depressed nasal bridge	Achondroplasia, trisomy 21
	Single nostril	Holoprosencephaly
Mouth	Microstomia	Trisomy 18, fetal valproate syndrome, Hallermann-Streiff, holoprosencephaly
	Macrostomia	Mandibular dysostosis, lateral facial cleft, Angelman syndrome, Noonan syndrome, Beckwith-Wiedemann syndrome, Treacher Collins syndrome
	Prominent full lip	Williams syndrome
	Thin upper lip	Fetal alcohol syndrome, Cornelia de Lange syndrome
	Median cleft lip	Holoprosencephaly
	Cleft lip and palate	Pierre-Robin sequence, Stickler syndrome, DiGeorge syndrome
	Hypertrophied alveolar ridges	Smith-Lemli-Opitz syndrome
	Macroglossia	Beckwith-Wiedemann syndrome, trisomy 21, hypothyroidism
	Micrognathia	Pierre Robin sequence, Stickler syndrome
Neck	Excessive skin folds	Turner syndrome, Noonan syndrome, trisomy 21

Table 50.1   Physical Findings with Differential Diagnoses—cont'd

Organ	Manifestation	Differential Diagnoses
Chest	Small thoracic cavity	Skeletal dysplasia: thanatophoric dysplasia, Jeune asphyxiating thoracic dystrophy
	Short sternum	Trisomy 18
	Pectus excavatum and carinatum	Skeletal dysplasia, connective tissue disorders
Abdomen	Hypoplasia of abdominal musculature (prune belly)	Eagle-Barrett syndrome (intrauterine bladder outlet obstruction)
	Omphalocele	Beckwith-Wiedemann syndrome, Trisomy 13
Anus	Imperforate	Caudal regression sequence, VACTERL
Genitalia	Hypogenitalism	Prader-Willi syndrome, Smith-Lemli-Opitz syndrome
	Ambiguous genitalia	Denys-Drash syndrome
	Virilization	21-Hydroxylase deficiency
Spine	Tufts of hair, sinuses	Spinal cord anomalies
Skin	Thick, coarse	Costello syndrome
	Cutis marmorata/livedo reticularis	Trisomy 21, hypothyroidism, Cornelia de Lange Familial: autosomal dominant
	Café-au-lait spots	NF1
	Hypopigmented macules	Tuberous sclerosis
	Irregular pigmented lesions in whorls	Incontinentia pigmenti
	>1 hemangioma	Possible internal hemangioma
	Edema, generalized	Trisomy 21, Turner syndrome, Noonan syndrome (RASopathies)

AP, Anteroposterior; *CHARGE,* coloboma of the eye, heart defects, atresia of the choanae, restriction of growth and development, and ear abnormalities and deafness; *NF1,* neurofibromatosis type 1; *VACTERL,* vertebral defects, anal atresia, cardiac defects, tracheoesophageal fistula, renal anomalies, and limb abnormalities.

- Interpupillary distances
- Palpebral fissure
- Lengths
- Upward or downward slanting
- Epicanthal folds
- Nares
  - Shape of nasal tip and ala nasi
  - Columella length
  - Choanal patency
- Mouth and throat
  - Shape of palate and uvula
  - Cleft lip or palate
  - Tongue deformities
  - Lip pits
  - Frenula
  - Natal teeth
- Chin
  - Retrognathic
  - Ears
  - Lengths
  - Placement
  - Folding
  - Preauricular and postauricular pits, tags
- Neck
  - Webbing or excess nuchal folds
- Thorax and chest
  - Inter-nipple distance
  - Chest circumference
  - Auscultation of lungs and heart
- Abdomen
  - Organomegaly
  - Ascites
  - Cord vessels (number)
  - Umbilical hernia
- Genitourinary
  - Hypospadias
  - Chordee
  - Cryptorchidism
  - Microphallus
  - Ambiguous genitalia
- Anus
  - Patent
  - Tags
  - Placement
- Back
  - Spine shape
  - Spine defects—meningomyelocele
  - Sacral dimple, tag, tuft of hair
- Extremities
  - Polydactyly (>five digits)
    - Preaxial
    - Postaxial
  - Syndactyly (fusion of digits)
  - Clinodactyly (incurving of the digits)
  - Extremity length
  - Hand and foot length
- Dermatoglyphics
  - Single transverse palmar crease—85% of patients with trisomy 21
  - Wide space between the great and second toes—50% of patients with trisomy 21
- Skin
  - Phakomatoses
    - Café-au-lait spots are associated with neurofibromatosis type 1.
    - Ash leaf spots (detected with use of Wood lamp) are associated with tuberous sclerosis.
  - Irregular pigmentation

Table 50.2 Minor Anomalies of Extremities-Associated Syndromes

Manifestation	Differential Diagnoses
Hypertrophy of limbs	Beckwith-Wiedemann syndrome, Klippel-Trenaunay-Weber syndrome
Hemiatrophy	Russell-Silver syndrome
Rhizomelia (proximal shortening of the limbs)	Achondroplasia
Mesomelia (shortening of the middle segment)	Thanatophoric dysplasia
Single palmar crease	Trisomy 21
Clinodactyly (incurving of the fifth digit)	Trisomy 21
Clinodactyly of fourth and fifth fingers radially and second finger in an ulnar direction	Trisomy 18 Trisomy 13
Lymphedema of hands and feet	Turner syndrome Noonan syndrome
Rocker-bottom feet	Trisomy 18
Acheiria (congenital absence of entire hand)	Amniotic band syndrome Cornelia de Lange syndrome Fetal hydantoin syndrome Incontinentia pigmenti
Acheiropodia (absence of both hands and feet)	Horn-Kolb syndrome
Radial (preaxial side of limb) deficiency	Fanconi anemia Thrombocytopenia (absent radius syndrome)
Polydactyly (partial or complete supernumerary digits)	Most common limb malformation Postaxial > preaxial in African Americans Isolated is autosomal dominant (AD) Postaxial: trisomy 13, chondroectodermal dysplasia, Meckel-Gruber syndrome, Bardet-Biedl syndrome Preaxial: Carpenter syndrome, Majewski short rib-polydactyly syndrome
Syndactyly (fusion of digits)	Minimal fusion of second and third toes common, benign Extensive syndactyly: trisomy 21, Smith-Lemli-Opitz syndrome, Pfeiffer syndrome, Apert syndrome
Brachydactyly (shortening of ≥1 digit due to anomalous development)	Skeletal dysplasia, Albright hereditary osteodystrophy, trisomy 21
Arachnodactyly (unusually long, spider-like digits)	Marfan syndrome Homocystinuria
Arthrogryposis (multiple congenital contractures)	Spinal muscular atrophy Sporadic Associated with oligohydramnios
Joint hypermobility	Marfan syndrome Ehlers-Danlos syndrome Kabuki syndrome
Camptodactyly (irreducible flexion of the digits)	Isolated AD Trisomy 8 Trisomy 10q Freeman-Sheldon syndrome

- □ Hypomelanosis of Ito suggests chromosomal mosaicism.
  - ▫ Hemangiomas
- ■ Neurologic examination
  - ▫ Neurologic status is usually the most reliable prognostic predicator.
  - ▫ Tone
  - ▫ Reflexes
  - ▫ Unusual movements
  - ▫ Feeding ability
  - ▫ Seizure activity
- ■ Adjunct studies for consideration based on physical exam findings
  - ▫ Evaluation of internal organ malformation
  - ▫ Chest x-ray/abdominal x-ray
    - ▫ Echocardiogram
    - ▫ Abdominal ultrasound (US)
  - ▫ Identification of organ system involvement
    - ▫ Ophthalmology examination
    - ▫ Skeletal survey
    - ▫ Electromyography (EMG)
  - ▫ Assessment of neurologic function
    - ▫ Magnetic resonance imaging (MRI) of brain
    - ▫ Electroencephalogram (EEG)
    - ▫ Nerve conduction studies
- ■ Specialized laboratory tests (see also Chapter 47)
  - ▫ Karyotype
    - ▫ Analysis of stretched and stained chromosome preparation
    - ▫ Confirm clinical diagnosis
    - ▫ May explain a set of major malformations not classically encountered together
  - ▫ Fluorescence in situ hybridization
    - ▫ Small deletions detected
  - ▫ DNA microarray
    - ▫ Detects copy number changes (smaller deletions or duplications not detectable by karyotype)
    - ▫ Performed in targeted or genome-wide fashion
    - ▫ Comparative genomic hybridization
    - ▫ Single-nucleotide polymorphism or oligonucleotide arrays
  - ▫ Molecular analysis
- ■ Diagnosis
  - ▫ May be no unifying diagnosis
  - ▫ Treatment and prognosis are based on organ involvement and degree of impairment.

Suggested Readings

Jones KL, Adam MP. Diagnosis of the dysmorphic infant. *Clin Perinatol.* 2015;42(2):243–261.

Leppig KA, Werler MM, Cann CI, Cook CA, Holmes LB. Predictive value of minor anomalies. I. Association with major malformations. *J Pediatr.* 1987;110(4):531–537.

Mitchell AL. Congenital anomalies. In: Martin RJ, Fanaroff AA, Walsh MC, eds. *Fanaroff and Martin's Neonatal-Perinatal Medicine.* 11th ed. Philadelphia: Elsevier; 2020:489–515.

Verma RP. Evaluation and risk assessment of congenital anomalies in neonates. *Children* (Basel). 2021;8:862.

Wild KT, Sheppard SE, Zackai EH. The dysmorphic infant. In: Gleason CA, Sawyer T, eds. *Avery's Diseases of the Newborn.* 11th ed. Philadelphia: Elsevier; 2024:335–346.

51 Inborn Errors of Metabolism

GEORGIANNE LEE ARNOLD

Overview

Inborn errors of metabolism are considerably more common than previously recognized (as many as 1:2000 births).

Metabolic Tests

- Three most commonly used basic metabolic tests are plasma amino acids, urine organic acids, and plasma acylcarnitine analysis (Table 51.1).
- It is critical to prioritize collecting samples in the acute setting when testing is most sensitive.
- Other clinical suspicion-directed specific tests might be indicated, as well.
  - Plasma amino acid analysis:
    - Typically identifies protein metabolic disorders.
    - Urine or cerebrospinal fluid (CSF) amino acid analysis may be required for some disorders.
  - Urine organic acid analysis:
    - Typically identifies organic acidemias and fatty acid oxidation disorders
  - Plasma acylcarnitine profile analysis (by tandem mass spectrometry):
    - Particularly sensitive for protein and fatty acid oxidation disorders
    - In some cases, can be done on dried blood spots (e.g., newborn screening)

Table 51.1 Common Metabolic Tests for Inborn Errors of Metabolism[a]

Test	Usual Sample	Secondary Samples[b]	Indication
Amino acid analysis	Plasma	Urine Cerebrospinal fluid	Suspected protein metabolism disorder (also to measure alanine in energy deficiency disorders)
Organic acid analysis	Urine	Vitreous humor (postmortem)	Suspected protein metabolism disorder, suspected energy deficiency disorder
Acylcarnitine analysis	Plasma	Blood spot card Urine	Suspected protein metabolism disorder or fatty acid oxidation disorder

[a]These should be performed in the acute state, if possible.
[b]In specific cases.

Metabolic Disorder Classification

- Metabolic disorders can be classified in three categories (Box 51.1): disorders of intoxication, energy deficiency, or complex molecules.
- All categories can present at any age, from prenatal onset to adulthood (Table 51.2).

DISORDERS OF INTOXICATION

Overview

- "Intoxication" with abnormally accumulating metabolite
- Most commonly from a defect in amino acid (protein) metabolism (Fig. 51.1), occasionally other substrates (e.g., galactose, fructose) (Fig. 51.2)
- Infant is usually well at birth (maternal–placental unit clears most metabolites) but becomes ill in hours to years.
  - Often presents with "newborn crash"
  - Well-appearing newborn develops poor feeding/vomiting, abnormal tone, altered mental status.
  - Symptoms are progressive and not improved with traditional management (fluid, antibiotics).
  - Other times for initial presentation include changing from breast to formula feedings (increasing dietary protein) or during an intercurrent illness (with catabolism).
- Made worse by ingestion of offending metabolite or fasting (when body increases metabolism of endogenous stores for energy)
- Prevention of catabolism and dietary restriction of the offending metabolite are the mainstays of treatment.
- Ketosis is always abnormal in the neonate and should prompt an evaluation for an inborn error of metabolism.
- Unexplained tachypnea and/or neurologic irritability should always prompt emergent measurement of ammonia.

Specific Disorders of Intoxication: Amino Acid Metabolism

- Phenylketonuria (PKU)
  - Overview
    - Relatively common (1/15,000 births)
    - Due to defect in changing the amino acid phenylalanine into tyrosine

- Phenylalanine accumulates and intoxicates the brain.
- Clinical presentation
  - If untreated: intellectual disability, fair complexion, eczema, and neurologic abnormalities
  - If treated early: relatively normal cognitive outcome
- Diagnosis and evaluation

Box 51.1 Common Inborn Errors of Metabolism Detected on Newborn Screening or Having Neonatal Presentation

Disorders of Intoxication

Protein
  Amino acidopathies
    Phenylketonuria
    Maple syrup urine disease
  Urea cycle defects
  Organic acidemias
Carbohydrate
  Galactosemia
  Hereditary fructose intolerance

Disorders of Energy Deficiency

Glucose metabolism disorders
  Glycogen storage disorders
  Disorders of gluconeogenesis
  Pyruvate carboxylase deficiency
  Fructose-1,6-bisphosphatase deficiency
  Pyruvate dehydrogenase deficiency
Mitochondrial disorders
Fatty acid oxidation defects

Disorders of Complex Molecules

Peroxisomal disorders
  Peroxisome assembly disorders
    Zellweger syndrome
  Single-enzyme disorders
    X-linked adrenoleukodystrophy
    Others
Lysosomal disorders
  Lysosomal storage disorders
  Lysosomal targeting disorder
    I-cell disease
Cholesterol synthesis disorders
  Smith-Lemli-Opitz syndrome

- Detectable on newborn screening but requires at least 24 hours for phenylalanine accumulation to become significant
- Diagnosis by plasma amino acid analysis, with significant elevation of phenylalanine and elevated ratio of phenylalanine to tyrosine
- Treatment
  - Restrict dietary phenylalanine (protein).
  - Replete tyrosine and other essential amino acids.
  - Affected women must be under excellent control during pregnancy to avoid teratogenic effects on the fetus, including fetal microcephaly, congenital heart and other structural defects, and intellectual disability.
- Maple syrup urine disease (MSUD)
  - Overview
    - Results from impaired metabolism of the branch chain amino acids valine, leucine, and isoleucine.
    - Pan-ethnic but more common in the Mennonite population
    - Name refers to the odor detectable in concentrated urine (also noted in earwax), but this odor is not often clinically prominent.
  - Clinical presentation
    - Acute intoxication with leucine leads to mental status changes, neurologic irritability, cerebral edema, and coma. Chronic intoxication results in intellectual disability.
  - Diagnosis and evaluation
    - Laboratory findings include ketosis, and plasma amino acid analysis reveals significant elevations of valine, leucine, isoleucine, and the pathognomonic metabolite alloisoleucine.
    - *Significant ketosis is always abnormal in the newborn* and should raise concern for a metabolic defect.
    - The disorder is detectable on newborn screening. The infant might be ill before the screening results are available.
  - Treatment
    - Acute treatment of the MSUD crisis follows the basic principles of protein metabolic crisis management (Box 51.2).
      - *Restrict* the offending metabolite (leucine).
      - *Reduce* abnormal metabolite production from metabolism of amino acids for energy (by forcing anabolism with high caloric supplementation).

Table 51.2 Classification of Inborn Errors of Metabolism

Disorder Class	Presentation	Treatable	Treatment Options
Intoxication	Prenatal: rare	Commonly	Restrict offending substrate.
	Postnatal: days to years		Reduce metabolite formation (prevent fasting/promote anabolism).
			Restore enzyme (vitamin cofactor, transplantation, etc.).
			Replete deficient products.
Energy metabolism	Prenatal: occasional (when severe)	Sometimes	Restrict offending substrate.
			Reduce metabolite formation and prevent energy deficiency.
	Postnatal: birth to years		Restore enzyme (vitamin cofactor, etc.).
			Replete deficient products.
Complex molecules	Prenatal: common	Rarely (but improving)	Enzyme replacement (some disorders)
	Postnatal: birth to years		Bone marrow transplant (some disorders)
			Supplement deficient products (some disorders).

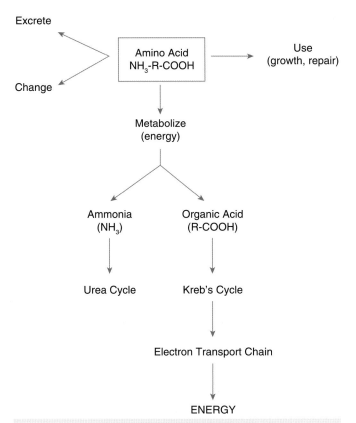

Fig. 51.1 Metabolism of protein.

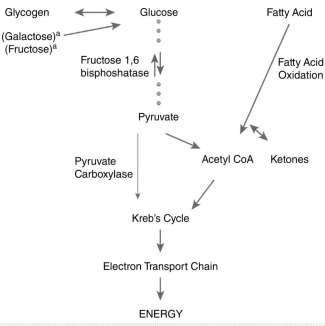

Fig. 51.2 Energy metabolism from glucose and fatty acid oxidation. [a]Galactosemia and hereditary fructose intolerance are considered disorders of intoxication.

Box 51.2 Principles of Acute Management of Metabolic Crisis in Intoxicating Protein Metabolism Disorders

1. Restrict offending substrate.
2. Reduce endogenous production of the abnormal metabolite by restoring anabolism.
   a. Intravenous glucose at 8–10 mg/kg/min in infants and children
   b. Intralipid if appropriate (except in fatty acid oxidation disorders)
   c. Non-offending amino acids (with metabolic nutritionist assistance)
   d. Enteral feeding when tolerated (with metabolic nutritionist assistance)
   e. Restore carefully calculated intake of protein after 24 hours (even if ammonia is still high).
3. Remove the abnormal metabolite.
   a. Ammonia scavenging medications, when indicated
   b. Dialysis if indicated
   c. Increase urinary excretion (carnitine, conjugation, etc. as indicated).
4. Restore enzyme function.
   a. Enzyme cofactors, if applicable
   b. Enzyme replacement, if applicable
5. Replete deficient products, if applicable.

□ *Remove* the abnormal metabolite (leucine), by dialysis if needed.
□ *Restore* enzyme function (some patients respond to thiamine).
□ *Replete* deficient products when indicated (valine and isoleucine supplementation are usually needed).
▪ Chronic management requires dietary leucine restriction and supplementation of other essential amino acids.
▪ Prevention of catabolism is a mainstay of chronic treatment.
▪ Liver transplantation can correct the hepatic genetic defect.
■ Urea cycle defects
  ▪ Overview
    ▪ Nitrogen is removed from amino acids (as ammonia) and detoxified in the urea cycle (see Fig. 51.1).
    ▪ Enzymatic defects can occur in any of the steps of the urea cycle and can appear at any age.
  ▪ Clinical presentation
    ▪ Commonly presents with "newborn crash" (but can present at any age, even adulthood).
    ▪ Presentation includes altered mental status, respiratory alkalosis/tachypnea, vomiting/poor feeding, neurologic irritability (initially clonus/hyperreflexia, later flaccidity/coma), and cerebral edema.
    ▪ Ketoacidosis is uncommon in urea cycle defects (but can occur).
    ▪ Ornithine transcarbamylase (OTC) deficiency is carried on the X chromosome. Carrier females are at risk for hyperammonemia during stress (including newborn stress) and particularly postpartum during uterine involution.
    ▪ Duration of hyperammonemia predicts outcome better than ammonia level.
  ▪ Diagnosis and evaluation
    ▪ Measure ammonia, plasma amino acids (particularly citrulline and arginine), and orotic acid (preferably in the acute state).
    ▪ The specific enzymatic defect can be confirmed by DNA or enzyme analysis.

- Newborn screening can identify some urea cycle defects but is not sensitive for the detection of OTC deficiency or other proximal defects. The infant might be ill before the screening results are available.
  - Treatment
    - Pillars of management of protein management disorders (see Box 51.2):
      - *Restrict* protein intake.
      - *Reduce* ammonia production by reversing catabolism with high calorie intake.
      - *Remove* ammonia by ammonia scavenging drugs (sodium phenylacetate, sodium benzoate, and dialysis, if necessary).
      - *Restore* enzyme activity (provide carglumic acid if *N*-acetylglutamate synthase [NAG-S] deficiency is suspected).
      - *Replete* deficient products (citrulline or arginine).
    - It is important to reinstitute carefully measured protein intake within 24 hours, or a negative nitrogen balance will worsen the crisis.
    - Chronic management includes careful regulation of protein intake, ammonia-scavenging drugs, and prevention of catabolism.
    - Liver transplantation can correct the metabolic defect.
    - After initial presentation, most crises are associated with conditions leading to catabolism, such as intercurrent infections and fasting.
- Organic acidemias
  - Overview
    - After the ammonia is removed from the amino acid, the remaining carbon skeleton is now an organic acid and is metabolized to produce energy, typically through the Krebs cycle (see Fig. 51.1).
    - Common disorders of organic acid metabolism (organic acidemias) include propionic acidemia, methylmalonic acidemia, or isovaleric acidemia.
  - Clinical presentation
    - The "newborn crash" is a common presentation, but can present at any age.
    - Systemic effects include ketoacidosis, bone marrow suppression, and secondary biochemical impairment of the urea cycle with hyperammonemia.
    - Hyperammonemia can be profound and in some cases difficult to distinguish from urea cycle defects.
    - Bone marrow suppression leads to varying degrees of neutropenia, anemia, and thrombocytopenia (which can resemble neonatal sepsis).
    - Acidosis with elevated anion gap and ketosis can occur.
  - Diagnosis and evaluation
    - *Ketoacidosis in the neonate is always abnormal*, and an organic acidemia should always be suspected in the differential diagnosis.
    - Plasma amino acid analysis typically notes elevated glycine. Urine organic acid analysis and plasma acylcarnitine analysis usually identify the specific disorder, and DNA or enzyme analysis can confirm.
    - The organic acidemias are generally detectable on newborn screening. The infant might be ill before the screen result is available.
    - Altered mental status and bone marrow suppression can resemble sepsis, but the presence of an elevated anion gap and ketosis shoul prompt evaluation for an inborn error of metabolism.
  - Treatment
    - Treatment of acute organic acidemias resembles acute urea cycle defects (see Box 51.2):
      - *Restrict* protein.
      - *Reduce* abnormal metabolite production with high calorie intake.
      - *Remove* abnormal metabolites; ammonia-scavenging agents can be controversial but can be instituted while waiting for studies that will differentiate urea cycle from organic acid disorders, and dialysis may be necessary.
      - *Restore* enzyme activity (vitamin B_{12}, the cofactor for methylmalonyl CoA mutase, should be supplemented acutely until a cobalamin responsive form of methylmalonic acidemia is ruled out).
      - *Replete* carnitine deficiency.
    - Chronic management includes careful regulation of protein intake and prevention of catabolism, along with carnitine and other supplements.
    - Liver transplant is partially corrective, but metabolic stroke risk remains.
    - Like other protein intoxication disorders, crises are often associated with poor oral intake and catabolism.
- Non-protein intoxication disorders (see Fig. 51.2)
  - Galactosemia
    - Overview
      - A defect in galactose metabolism (a sugar found in milk)
    - Clinical presentation
      - Findings in untreated patients include cataracts, liver disease, failure to thrive, *Escherichia coli*, and sepsis.
    - Diagnosis and evaluation
      - Detectable on newborn screening
      - Enzyme is assayed in red cells, so transfusion can reduce screening sensitivity.
      - Infant may already be ill by the time the screen is returned.
    - Treatment
      - Urgent medical evaluation of screen-positive infants
      - Galactose-free diet
      - Mild to moderate intellectual disability is common even with dietary treatment.
  - Hereditary fructose intolerance
    - Overview
      - A defect in fructose metabolism
      - Fructose is found predominantly in table sugar (sucrose) and fruit.
      - Some infant formulas (even elemental) and pacifier-dipping solutions contain sucrose/fructose.
    - Clinical presentation
      - Acute symptoms include hypoglycemia, hypophosphatemia, shock, and liver dysfunction.
      - Chronic symptoms include failure to thrive and liver dysfunction.
    - Diagnosis and evaluation
      - Diet history is critical, as problems generally begin after the introduction of fructose/sucrose in the diet.

- Diagnosis can be confirmed by DNA analysis.
- Newborn screening is not available for this disorder.
  - Treatment
    - Dietary restriction of sucrose and fructose.

DISORDERS OF ENERGY DEFICIENCY

- Overview
  - Disorders of energy deficiency result primarily from a direct block in energy production, usually in carbohydrate or fatty acid metabolism (see Fig. 51.2).
  - Glucose, the basic carbohydrate, is metabolized for energy via glycolysis, then the Krebs cycle, and ultimately the respiratory chain.
  - Fat oxidation also supplies its end products to the Krebs cycle and respiratory chain, as well as producing ketone bodies, which can be exported to distant tissues for metabolism.
  - The maternal–placental unit cannot compensate for intracellular energy deficiency. Thus, prenatal onset can occur, particularly in some of the most severe pyruvate metabolism disorders (see Table 51.2).
  - The most metabolically active regions of the brain (basal ganglia) are most vulnerable to cell death from acute energy deficiency, leading to cystic degeneration.
  - Newborn screening does not generally detect these disorders (except fatty acid oxidation disorders).
- Pyruvate dehydrogenase (PDH) deficiency
  - Overview
    - PDH deficiency is a rate-limiting step between glycolysis and the Krebs cycle (see Fig. 51.2).
    - It results in impaired ability to create energy from carbohydrates.
    - Severity can vary widely, from mild to neonatal lethal.
    - The most common neonatal severe presenting genetic defect is X-linked dominant; females can be as severely affected as males.
  - Clinical presentation
    - Neurologic abnormalities including hypotonia, intellectual disability, seizures, ataxia, and other symptoms.
    - Basal ganglia damage and/or metabolic strokes are seen or develop and progress over time; neonatal lactic acidosis can be profound.
  - Diagnosis and evaluation
    - Metabolic findings include lactic acidosis, as well high alanine on plasma amino acids.
    - Magnetic resonance imaging (MRI) findings can be helpful in raising clinical suspicion.
    - Diagnosis is by DNA or enzyme analysis.
    - The disorder is not diagnosed on newborn screening.
  - Treatment
    - This disorder is the exception to the general rule that metabolic crises should be treated with high-dose glucose. High-dose glucose should *not* be given in PDH deficiency.
    - Some cases respond to a ketogenic diet.
    - Some might respond to thiamine or lipoic acid cofactors.

- Pyruvate carboxylase deficiency
  - Overview
    - Pyruvate carboxylase deficiency is the first step in gluconeogenesis (the creation of glucose).
    - There is wide variation in severity, from neonatal lethal to milder forms.
  - Clinical presentation
    - Findings include ketosis and lactic acidosis (significant ketosis is always abnormal in the neonate).
    - Hypoglycemia is not a particularly common finding.
    - The infant can have profoundly altered mental status and abnormal tone.
  - Diagnosis and evaluation
    - In the most severe cases, there is secondary biochemical impairment of the urea cycle and hyperammonemia.
    - Plasma amino acids may reveal high plasma citrulline and alanine levels.
    - Diagnosis is by DNA or enzyme analysis.
    - The disorder is not diagnosed by newborn screening.
  - Treatment
    - Provide glucose (8–10 mg/kg/min) and protein calories to prevent activation of gluconeogenesis.
    - Chronic management includes a high-carbohydrate and high-protein diet and prevention of fasting.
- Fructose-1,6-bisphosphatase deficiency
  - Overview
    - A defect in gluconeogenesis (see Fig. 51.2)
    - Most infants do not become ill until liver glycogen stores are exhausted (thus might not present when on frequent feedings).
  - Clinical presentation
    - Fasting or poor feeding can precipitate hypoglycemia and ketoacidosis with lactic acidosis.
  - Diagnosis and evaluation
    - Urine organic acids may reveal glycerol (it is important to be certain the glycerol did not originate from skin-care products).
    - Diagnosis is primarily by DNA analysis.
    - The disorder is not detected by newborn screening.
  - Treatment
    - Avoidance of fasting and fructose
    - During acute episodes or when fasting, give high-dose glucose and intralipid similar to protein metabolic disorders (see Box 51.2).
- Mitochondrial disease (defects in oxidative phosphorylation)
  - Overview
    - Genes regulating mitochondrial function are encoded in both nuclear and mitochondrial DNA.
    - Neonatal-onset disease is more commonly associated with genetic defects in nuclear genes having Mendelian inheritance (dominant, recessive, X-linked).
    - Thirteen enzymes involved in oxidative phosphorylation (and their transfer RNA) are encoded within the mitochondrial DNA and show maternal inheritance.
    - Consider mitochondrial disease when two or more nonembryologically related organ systems are affected.
  - Clinical presentation
    - Can present at any age, with some of the most severe disorders presenting in the neonatal period

- Acute neonatal presentation typically includes significant lactic acidosis but can also include dysfunction in one or more high energy–requiring organs such as brain, liver, or heart.
  - Later presentations include intellectual disability, hypotonia, seizures and other neurologic dysfunction, endocrine disorders, and others.
- Diagnosis and evaluation
  - Elevated alanine is common in plasma amino acid analysis.
  - DNA analysis may be helpful in reaching a diagnosis.
  - Not diagnosed by newborn screening
- Treatment
  - Varies based on the specific defect
  - Avoid catabolism.
  - Diet should be tailored to the individual defect.
  - Some patients are treated with "mitochondrial cocktails," including coenzyme Q10, carnitine, and various enzyme cofactors such as thiamine, biotin, and others.
- Fatty acid oxidation defects
  - Fat oxidation provides 9 kcal/g (compared to ~4 kcal from protein or carbohydrates).
  - Fats are chains of carbons and hydrogens.
  - One (four-step) cycle of fatty acid oxidation removes two carbons that are metabolized to energy through the Krebs cycle or can be converted to a ketone that can be exported to other tissues (see Fig. 51.2).
  - Fatty acid oxidation enzymes have chain-length specificity.
    - Long-chain: 12 to 18 carbons
    - Medium-chain: 6 to 10 carbons
    - Short-chain: <6 carbons
  - There can be secondary effects from intoxication with accumulation of fatty acid oxidation intermediates.
  - After the neonatal period, absence of ketosis during hypoglycemia is an important diagnostic clue.
- Medium-chain acyl-CoA dehydrogenase (MCAD) deficiency
  - Overview
    - MCAD deficiency is the most common fatty acid oxidation disorder (approximately 1/15,000 births).
    - Neonatal presentation can be seen in the most severely affected infants or in those with inadequate calorie intake.
    - Infants become symptomatic when liver glycogen is exhausted, most commonly during fasting and intercurrent illnesses when oral intake is depressed.
  - Clinical presentation
    - Hypoglycemia, altered mental status or tone
    - Transient hepatomegaly
  - Diagnosis and evaluation
    - Diagnosis is confirmed by plasma acylcarnitine analysis and urine organic acid analysis.
    - This disorder is detectable by newborn screening. A screen-positive infant is a medical emergency until it can be determined that infant feeding is adequate.
  - Treatment
    - Treatment is avoidance of fasting.

- Administer glucose at 8 to 10 mg/kg/min during fasting or intercurrent illness.
- Disorders of long-chain fatty acid oxidation (very long-chain acyl-CoA dehydrogenase [VLCAD] deficiency and long-chain hydroxyl acyl-CoA deficiency [LCHAD]/ trifunctional protein [TFP] deficiency)
  - Overview
    - Variable severity, can present from neonatal to adulthood
    - Long-chain fatty acids require esterification to carnitine to pass into the mitochondria for oxidation.
    - Several additional defects occur in the process of carnitine esterification or passage through the mitochondrial membrane (not reviewed here).
  - Clinical presentation
    - Severe presentations include hypoglycemia, hypotonia, altered mental status, and hepatomegaly and can be fatal.
    - Later presentations can include myopathy and recurrent rhabdomyolysis.
  - Diagnosis and evaluation
    - Diagnostic metabolites are identified on urine organic acid analysis and plasma acylcarnitine analysis.
    - These disorders are diagnosable on newborn screen; a screen-positive child is a medical emergency until severe disease is ruled out.
    - Diagnosis can be confirmed with DNA, enzyme, or other metabolic testing.
  - Treatment
    - Restriction of dietary long-chain fat and supplementation with medium-chain fat
    - Prevention of catabolism, intravenous glucose during fasting (8–10 mg/kg/min)

DISORDERS OF COMPLEX MOLECULES (LYSOSOMES, PEROXISOMES, CHOLESTEROL BIOSYNTHESIS)

- Overview
  - These disorders are metabolic processes occurring in organelles.
  - Disorders of the peroxisome and the lysosome, as well as cholesterol metabolism, can have a neonatal phenotype and are reviewed here.
- Peroxisomal defects
  - Overview
    - Peroxisomes are responsible for cellular detoxification, oxidation of the longest-chain fats (>20 carbons), synthesis of plasmalogens (phospholipids involved in myelin/nerve cell integrity), production of bile acids, and other functions.
    - Two categories of defects exist:
      - Defect in peroxisome synthesis (peroxisomal assembly defects), in which all functions are affected
      - Single enzyme defects, in which only a single peroxisomal function is affected
- Peroxisomal assembly defects
  - Overview
    - Absent (or "ghost") peroxisomes

- Most severe is Zellweger (cerebrohepatorenal) syndrome.
- Milder presentations/later onset (neonatal adreno-leukodystrophy or infantile Refsum disease)
- Clinical presentation
  - Dysmorphic features (often resembling trisomy 21), hepatomegaly with liver dysfunction, bile acid deficiency, leukodystrophy, profound hypotonia, chondrodysplasia punctata, and other abnormalities
- Diagnosis and evaluation
  - Peroxisomal function testing (very-long-chain fatty acids, plasmalogens, phytanic acid, other peroxisomal testing)
  - Note that phytanic acid elevations are not seen until the child has ingested significant amounts of phytanic acid in dairy/food.
  - Diagnosis is confirmed by DNA testing.
  - These defects are not directly diagnosed by newborn screen but might be identified secondarily on screening for X-linked adrenoleukodystrophy.
- Treatment
  - Supportive/palliative only
  - Cholic acid, adrenal hormone replacement, gastrostomy feedings, and others
- Single-gene peroxisomal disorders
  - Overview
    - Peroxisomes are intact but lack a single enzyme.
    - Disorders include X-linked adrenoleukodystrophy, rhizomelic chondrodysplasia punctata, and bile acid deficiencies, among others.
    - Presentation and testing are specific to the individual disorder.
      - "Lorenzo's oil" may help delay the onset or may slow progression in X-linked adrenoleukodystrophy, but it is not curative.
- Lysosomal storage disorders (LSDs)
  - Overview
    - Site of cellular debris degradation
    - Some LSDs can present with prenatal/neonatal hydrops.
    - Disease categories include mucopolysaccharidoses, oligosaccharidoses, Fabry disease, and others.
    - Diagnosis is by enzyme assay or DNA analysis.
    - Some are treatable by enzyme replacement, substrate reduction therapies, or bone marrow transplant but are not curable.
    - Newborn screening is expanding for a number of LSDs.
- Mucolipidosis type II (I-cell disease)
  - Overview
    - Defect in targeting all enzymes for entry into the lysosome
  - Clinical presentation
    - Coarse features, hepatomegaly, dysostosis multiplex (resembles severe Hurler syndrome)
  - Diagnosis and evaluation
    - All lysosomal enzymes are elevated in blood (due to failure to enter the lysosome).
    - Diagnosis is confirmed by biopsy or DNA analysis.
    - I-cell disease is not detectable by newborn screening.

- Treatment
  - Supportive/palliative only
- Hurler syndrome
  - Overview
    - Caused by lack of alpha-iduronidase
  - Clinical presentation
    - Early: hepatomegaly, gibbus, coarse features, umbilical hernia, corneal clouding
    - Later: developmental delay, short stature, dysostosis multiplex
  - Diagnosis and evaluation
    - Elevated heparin and dermatan sulfate on urine MPS screen
    - Enzyme deficiency in blood or confirmation of DNA analysis
    - Now diagnosable on newborn screening in some states
  - Treatment
    - Hematopoietic stem cell transplantation improves many features and stabilizes cognitive function but does not improve joint and bony abnormalities.
    - Enzyme replacement therapy can improve many features but is not curative.
- Disorders of cholesterol synthesis
  - Overview
    - Cholesterol is a precursor for steroid hormones, bile acids, myelin, cell membranes, and embryogenesis.
    - A defect has been identified in nearly every step of cholesterol synthesis.
    - Common manifestations include multiple congenital and developmental anomalies, as well as skeletal and skin abnormalities.
    - Category includes disorders with chondrodysplasia punctata (e.g., Conradi-Hünermann syndrome, CHILD [congenital hemidysplasia with ichthyosiform erythroderma and limb defects] syndrome), skin abnormalities (CHILD syndrome), and others.
- Smith-Lemli-Opitz syndrome
  - Overview
    - Defect in the last step of cholesterol synthesis
  - Clinical presentation
    - Neuronal migration abnormalities, skeletal anomalies (including characteristic two to three toe syndactyly, genital undervirilization [in males]
    - Milder cases with more subtle features
  - Diagnosis and evaluation
    - Elevated 7-dehydrocholesterol (precursor to cholesterol)
    - Disorder is not detected by newborn screening.

METABOLIC ENCEPHALOPATHY

- Overview
  - Metabolic encephalopathy is associated with all three categories of metabolic defects (intoxication, energy deficiency, and complex molecules).
    - Acute encephalopathy is more likely to be associated with intoxication or energy deficiency disorders.
    - Intoxicating metabolites include ammonia, amino acids, organic acids, lactate, and other accumulated substances.

- Ammonia should always be measured early in the investigation of unexplained mental status changes, particularly in the presence of neurologic irritability, clonus, hyperreflexia, or coma, or when *unexplained tachypnea/respiratory alkalosis* occurs.
- Any patient undergoing lumbar puncture or toxicology analysis to look for occult causes of unexplained mental status changes should also have basic metabolic testing, including blood ammonia.
- Urine ketones should be assessed in the presence of concern for a metabolic disorder. Presence of ketones in a neonate is a metabolic disease until proven otherwise. Absence of ketosis after the neonatal period during hypoglycemia is also suspicious for a metabolic disorder.
- Metabolic causes of acidosis
  - The anion gap reflects the presence of unmeasured anions. Bicarbonate loss in urine or stool is typically accompanied by hyperchloremia, which maintains a normal anion gap. Elevated anion gap can be due to excess presence of an anion (e.g., lactate, ketones, organic acid).
    - Normal anion gap acidosis
      - Bicarbonate loss (renal or stool) is rarely metabolic except in the case of Fanconi-type renal tubular acidosis.
    - Elevated anion gap acidosis is frequently metabolic in the neonate (profound ketoacidosis is *always* abnormal in a neonate).
      - Organic acidemia
      - Energy deficiency or gluconeogenic disorders
      - Occasionally seen in severe urea cycle defect
- *Remember to think of metabolic causes of neonatal seizures.* Although these disorders are rare, they not routinely detected on "regular" metabolic testing (such as amino or organic acid analysis or newborn screening) and so must be specifically considered in the differential diagnosis.
  - Glycine encephalopathy (aka "non-ketotic hyperglycinemia")
    - Commonly burst-suppression, intractable
    - Check ratio of CSF to plasma glycine
  - Sulfite oxidase or molybdenum cofactor deficiency
    - Commonly burst-suppression, intractable
    - Look for low uric acid (low in molybdenum cofactor deficiency).
    - Dipstick fresh urine for sulfite.
    - Notify laboratory of suspected diagnosis when sending amino acid analysis.
    - Consider checking for S-sulfocysteine.
  - Pyridoxine, folinic acid, or pyridoxal 5′-phosphate–dependent epilepsies
    - Typically respond to vitamin B_6
    - Response is *not* always "instant."
    - Some require pyridoxal 5′-phosphate or folinic acid, or both.
  - Glut-1 deficiency
    - Abnormal glucose transport into the brain
    - Low ratio of CSF to plasma glucose
    - May respond to ketogenic diet

Suggested Readings

Adam MP, Feldman J, Mirzaa GM, et al., eds. *GeneReviews*® [Internet]. Seattle: University of Washington, Seattle; 1993–2023.

Saudubray JM, Baumgartner MR, García-Cazorla Á, Walter J., eds. *Inborn Metabolic Diseases*. Springer, Berlin, Heidelberg; 2022. https://doi.org/10.1007/978-3-662-63123-2_16.

Valle DL, Antonarakis S, Ballabio A, Beaudet AL, Mitchell GA. eds. *The Online Metabolic and Molecular Bases of Inherited Disease*. McGraw Hill; 2019. Accessed November 21, 2023. https://ommbid.mhmedical.com/content.aspx?bookid=2709&sectionid=225069716.

Water, Salt, Renal

ERIN RADEMACHER

52 *Water/Electrolyte Metabolism and Acid–Base Balance*

ERIN RADEMACHER

Water Metabolism

- Total body water (TBW) is expressed as a percentage of body weight in kilograms (kg). It decreases from ~95% of total weight at 16 weeks' gestation to 75% of total weight at 40 weeks (Fig. 52.1).
- TBW is divided into intracellular and extracellular water (ECW). ECW is further divided into interstitial space and intravascular space. The percentage of TBW contained in the ECW declines with gestational age (GA). At term birth, almost 50% of TBW is intracellular.
- ECW decreases after birth. Term infants typically lose ~5% to 10% of birth weight over the first 4 to 7 days. Preterm infants can lose 15% over the first 5 to 10 days. Failure to lose ECW is associated with increased risk of patent ductus arteriosus (PDA), necrotizing enterocolitis (NEC), and bronchopulmonary dysplasia (BPD).
    - Before delivery, fluid shifts from intravascular to interstitial space.
    - After birth, fluid shifts back into the intravascular space over the first few days, resulting in release of atrial natriuretic peptide (ANP), which in turn results in a loss of water and sodium from the kidney and loss of TBW.
- Maintenance water requirement = Urine volume + Other losses (stool, typically 5–10 mL/kg/d; emesis, drains) + Insensible water loss + Amount needed for tissue generation (10–15 mL/kg/d)
- The best indicators of appropriate fluid prescription are stable sodium levels and appropriate weight gain (or loss in the first week).
- See Table 52.1 for guidelines for water needs for different GAs and postnatal ages.
- Insensible water losses (IWLs) are comprised of water lost through the skin (2/3 total) and respiration (1/3 total).
- Preterm infants have increased skin losses due to an immature epithelial layer, increased body surface area–to–body weight ratio, and increased skin vascularity. Administration of steroids prenatally accelerates skin maturation and can decrease skin losses.
- IWLs will increase or decrease under different conditions (Table 52.2).
- Arginine vasopressin (AVP; antidiuretic hormone [ADH], vasopressin) is the major effector involved in water metabolism. It is synthesized in the hypothalamus and stored in the posterior pituitary gland.
- A rise in plasma osmolality (sensed by osmoreceptors in hypothalamus) or a fall in intravascular volume (detected by baroreceptors in the heart) leads to the release of ADH.

- Intravascular volume depletion trumps plasma osmolality if the two stimuli are in opposing directions.
- ADH acts on its receptor, vasopressin 2 receptor (V2R), which is located on the basolateral (blood side) of distal tubules and collecting duct cells in the nephron.
- Binding of ADH to V2R stimulates adenylate cyclase, leading to increased levels of cyclic adenosine monophosphate (cAMP) and fusion of vesicles containing the water channel aquaporin-2 (AQP2) to the apical membrane (urine side), allowing water to move from the urinary space into the cell
- When ADH levels fall, the AQP2 is recycled out of the apical membrane into vesicles.
- Two other effectors of water metabolism are thirst and angiotensin II, which stimulates thirst.
- Normal urine output (UOP) on postnatal day 1 is 1 to 2 mL/kg/h, but it increases to 3 to 5 mL/kg/h by days 3 to 5.
- Maximal urine concentrating ability is ~600 mOsm/kg in preterm and 800 mOsm/kg in term infants, reaching adult levels of 1200 mOsm/kg by 6 to 12 months.
- Preterm infants are unable to generate or maintain the countercurrent mechanism critical to concentrating urine due to immature tubules and short loops of Henle that do not reach the inner medulla.
- Full-term infants can maximally dilute urine (50 mOsm/kg). Preterm have slightly impaired dilution ability (70 mOsm/kg).

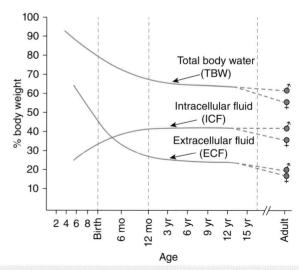

Fig. 52.1 Changes in total body water and its components with increasing age. (From Martin RJ, Fanaroff AA, Walsh MC, eds. *Fanaroff and Martin's Neonatal-Perinatal Medicine.* 11th ed. Philadelphia: Elsevier; 2020:1855, Fig. 92.1.)

Table 52.1   Fluid Requirements by GA

| Birth Weight (g) | Insensible Water Loss (mL/kg/d) | TOTAL WATER REQUIREMENTS BY AGE (ML/KG/D) | | |
		Days 1–2	Days 3–7	Days 8–30
<750	100+	100–200	120–200	120–180
750–1000	60–70	80–150	100–150	120–180
1001–1500	30–65	60–100	80–150	120–180
>1500	15–30	60–80	100–150	120–180

Adapted from data from Martin RJ, Fanaroff AA, Walsh MC, eds. *Fanaroff and Martin's Neonatal-Perinatal Medicine*, 11th ed. Philadelphia: Elsevier/Saunders, 2020:1857, Table 92.1.

Table 52.2   Factors That Affect Insensible Fluid Loss

Factors that Increase Losses[a]	% Increase	Factors That Decrease Losses[a]	% Decrease
Prematurity	100–300, depending on how low the gestational age is	Incubator	25–50
Radiant warmer	50–100	Humidified air	15–30
Phototherapy	25–50, depending on equipment[b]	Sedation	5–25
Increased activity	5–25	Decreased activity	5–25
Hyperventilation	20–30	Increased ambient humidity	—
Hyperthermia	>10 per °C	Plastic blanket, chamber, or heat shield[c]	30–70
Loss of skin integrity	Varies with extent of lesion	—	—

[a]Factors are additive in each column.
[b]Effects of fiberoptic blankets/pads are not known. LED phototherapy does not change insensible water losses.
[c]Plexiglass heat shield is not effective under radiant warmer.

Disorders of Water Metabolism

SYNDROME OF INAPPROPRIATE ANTIDIURETIC HORMONE (SIADH)

Overview

- ADH release is triggered by non-physiologic mechanism: perinatal asphyxia, pneumothorax, RDS, pneumonia, continuous positive airway pressure (CPAP), meningitis, intraventricular hemorrhage, and drugs (morphine, barbiturates, carbamazepine).

Clinical Presentation

- Hyponatremia with mild/moderate expansion of extracellular volume (ECV)

Diagnosis and Evaluation

- Urine osmolality > serum osmolality
- Urine sodium > 20 mEq/L
- Normal thyroid, kidney, adrenal function

Treatment

- Fluid restriction is of primary importance.
- Remove the stimulus to ADH release.
- Lasix 1 to 2 mg/kg/d + NaCl if first two measures are not successful

CONGENITAL NEPHROGENIC DIABETES INSIPIDUS (CNDI)

Overview

- X-linked mutation of V2R renders receptor unable to bind ADH (90% cases).
- Autosomal (usually recessive): mutation of AQP2

Clinical Presentation

- Polyuria, polydipsia, recurrent dehydration episodes, fevers, constipation, failure to thrive (FTT)

Diagnosis and Evaluation

- Hypernatremia
- Urine osm < serum osm
- No response to DDAVP (1-deamino-8-D-arginine vasopressin, also known as desmopressin, a synthetic analog of vasopressin)
- Genetic testing available

Treatment

- Ensure adequate water intake to normalize sodium (Na); may require nasogastric or gastrostomy tube for overnight fluid.
- Decrease solute load through a low-Na diet (low protein also when growth is completed).
- Thiazides: Induction of intravascular depletion leads to increased reabsorption Na/water in proximal nephron.

- Amiloride may augment thiazide effect and prevent hypokalemia.
- Nonsteroidal anti-inflammatory drugs (NSAIDs)

SECONDARY NEPHROGENIC DIABETES INSIPIDUS

Overview

- Kidney response to ADH is reduced but there is no mutation in V2R or AQP2.
- It is seen with hypokalemia, hypercalcemia, post urinary obstruction, or chronic kidney disease (CKD).

CENTRAL DIABETES INSIPIDUS

Overview

- Decreased secretion of vasopressin
- Can be seen with meningitis or disruption of pituitary gland
- Treatment: increased water intake, DDAVP ± thiazide diuretic

SODIUM METABOLISM

- Positive Na balance is required for growth.
- After first 24 to 48 hours, Na requirement is generally 1 to 2 mEq/kg/d for days of life 3 to 7, then increases after first week to 2 to 3 mEq/kg/d.
- Premature infants (GA < 28 weeks) may require much higher Na intake (4–10 mEq/kg/d) due to immature tubules leading to renal Na wasting.
- Fractional excretion of sodium (FENa) decreases with increasing GA: >5% in GA ≤ 26 weeks, around 1% by 30 to 32 weeks, and <0.5% by 38 weeks.
- Some trials suggest that Na supplementation is associated with better long-term neurodevelopment in preterm infants.
- Na is reabsorbed from tubular lumen via transporters or channels in the apical membrane (urine side) throughout the nephron and then pumped out of the cell via the Na,K-ATPase on the basolateral membrane (blood side). Na,K-ATPase is critical to this process. Activity is lower in neonates than adults (Fig. 52.2).
- In neonates, the proximal tubule reabsorbs ~50% to 60% (similar to adult capacity) of the filtered Na via Na/H exchanger or Na-X cotransporter (where X is glucose, amino acid, or phosphate). Na/H exchanger activity is lower in neonates than in adults.
- Thick ascending limb of loop of Henle (LoH) reabsorbs Na via the Na-K-2Cl channel (furosemide sensitive).
- Distal convoluted tubule (DCT) reabsorbs Na via the Na-Cl cotransporter (thiazide sensitive).
- Cortical collecting duct (CCD) reabsorbs Na via the epithelial Na channel (ENaC) under the control of aldosterone.
- Maturation of the nephron during fetal development and after birth allows increased reabsorption of Na from the distal LoH and distal segments.
  - Na,K-ATPase and the proximal tubule Na transporters are increased by thyroid hormone and glucocorticoid.
  - The LoH Na-K-2Cl channel and the DCT Na-Cl channel are increased by glucocorticoids.

DISORDERS OF SODIUM METABOLISM

Hyponatremia

- Hyponatremia is usually defined as Na < 130 mEq/L.
- It occurs in 30% of very low-birth-weight (VLBW) infants in the first week; 25% to 65% develop later.
- Three mechanisms lead to hyponatremia (Fig. 52.3):
  - Inability to excrete water load most common cause. This may be due to
    - Decreased effective blood volume providing a stimulus for ADH release
    - Decreased fluid delivery to distal nephron either from decreased glomerular filtration rate (GFR) in acute kidney injury (AKI) or from increased proximal Na and water reabsorption in volume-depletion states
  - Excessive Na loss
    - May be physiologic (i.e., high FENa in preterm)
    - Has pathologic causes; see sections on congenital adrenal hyperplasia, pseudohypoaldosteronism, and Bartter syndrome
  - Inadequate intake
- High maternal water intake during labor or oxytocin use may cause hyponatremia in the neonate.
- Correction is estimated by Na$^+$ deficit (mEq) = 0.7 × body weight (kg) × (Na$_{desired}$ − Na$_{current}$).
  - Usually replaced as 2/3 in first 24 hours, with the remainder over the next 24 hours
  - If Na < 120 mEq/L, consider using 3% saline (513 mEq/L Na) to correct serum Na to 120 mEq/L over 4 to 6 hours, then replace the remainder over 48 hours.

Hypernatremia

- Hypernatremia is usually defined a Na > 150 mEq/L.
- Occurs in 40% of preterm infants < 29 weeks
- Mechanisms (Fig. 52.4)
  - Increased water loss is the most common etiology; it is often due to underestimated IWL. Inadequate breast feeding and diarrhea are other common causes.
  - Excessive Na administration from medications (NaHCO$_3$ boluses), improperly prepared formula or total parenteral nutrition (TPN), or high Na in breast milk (can be seen when latching difficulty or decreased frequency of breastfeeds)
- Therapy
  - Need to provide the water deficit + maintenance water/Na need + any excessive losses.
  - H$_2$O deficit (L) = 0.7 × weight (kg) × [(Na current/Na desired) − 1]
  - Correction should be slow (0.5 mEq/h) in cases of chronic or unknown duration to avoid cerebral edema.
  - With Na > 175 mEq/L, may need to add 3% saline to normal saline to make a fluid with 10 to 15 mEq/L less Na than the current serum Na.

POTASSIUM METABOLISM

- Transported actively across placenta from mother to fetus

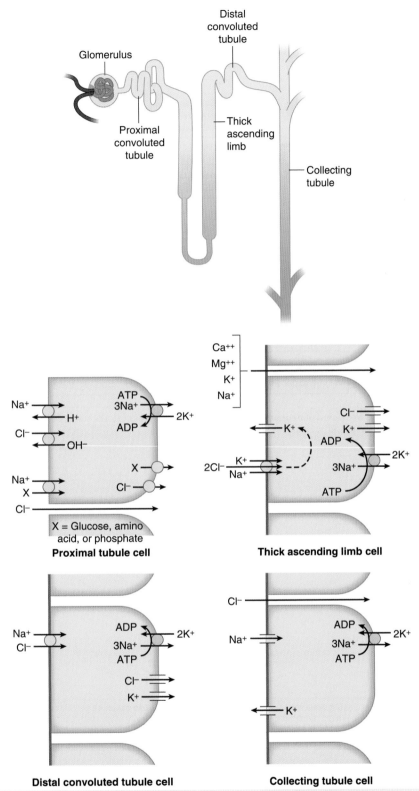

Fig. 52.2 . Na transport along the tubule. *ADP*, Adenosine diphosphate; *ATP*, adenosine triphosphate. (From Polin RA, Abman SH, Rowitch DH, Benitz WE, eds. *Fetal and Neonatal Physiology*. 6th ed. Philadelphia: Elsevier; 2022:986, Fig. 97.3.)

- Positive balance is required for growth; typically start 1 to 2 mEq/kg/d after the first 48 hours of life and when urine output is well established, then increase to 2 to 3 mEq/kg/d.
- Infants have higher plasma levels than adults (average 5 vs. 4 mEq/L).

- Potassium (K) shifts into/out of cells under certain conditions:
  - Into cell: insulin, β2 agonists, metabolic alkalosis
  - Out of cell: α-adrenergic agonists, metabolic acidosis, hyperosmolality

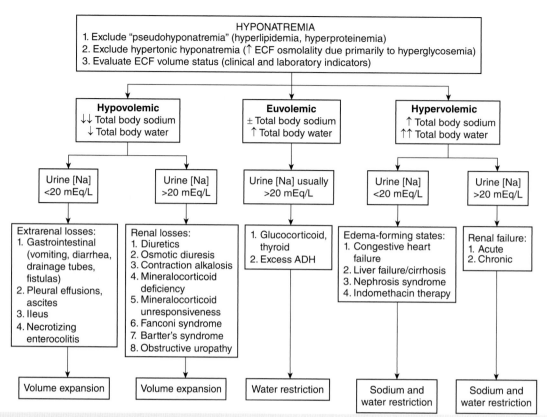

Fig. 52.3 **Algorithm for evaluation and treatment of neonatal hyponatremia.** *ADH,* Antidiuretic hormone; *ECF,* extracellular fluid. (From Gleason CA, Juul SE, eds. *Avery's Diseases of the Newborn*. 10th ed. Philadelphia: Elsevier; 2018:376, Fig. 30.5.)

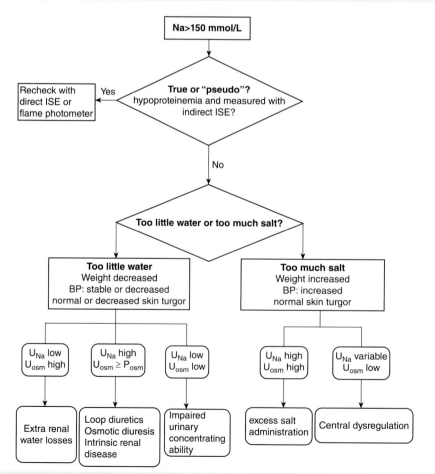

Fig. 52.4 **Algorithm to determine causes of hypernatremia.** *BP,* Blood pressure; *ISE,* ion-selective electrode; *U_Na*, urine sodium; *U_osm*, urine osmolality. (From Bockenhauer D, Zieg J. Electrolyte disorders. *Clin Perinatol.* 2014;41:575–590.)

- Metabolic acidosis caused by mineral acid (HCl or NH4$^+$Cl) causes much larger shifts than organic anion acidosis (lactic, acetoacetic, and β-hydroxybutyrate acids).
- Excretion is mainly via kidneys; gastrointestinal tract provides a lesser mechanism.
- K is freely filtered at glomerulus but is then reabsorbed along the tubule.
- Renal excretion is by secretion in the distal nephron, mainly cortical collecting duct (Fig. 52.5). K enters cells via Na,K-ATPase and then exits to urine space via K channels.
- Secretion is affected by
  - Rate of distal Na delivery and the transepithelial voltage:
    - When Na is avidly reabsorbed in proximal nephron due to intravascular volume depletion, less Na reaches the distal tubule. This results in deceased Na reabsorption via ENaC, which diminishes the electrochemical gradient that would favor K secretion into urine
  - Tubular flow rate: A high flow rate stimulates K secretion in a mature kidney, but neonates lack these maxi-K channels.
  - Plasma K level: Higher plasma levels allow a steeper gradient, favoring entry from blood into distal tubule cells and subsequently secretion into lumen.
  - Aldosterone stimulates ENaC and Na,K-ATPase to reabsorb Na, thus making lumen more negative, which favors K secretion from cell. Neonates are relatively insensitive to aldosterone.
  - Acid–base balance
    - Alkalosis stimulates K secretion via two mechanisms:
      - Stimulation of Na,K-ATPase and therefore K uptake into cell
      - Increases length of time K channels open on apical membrane to allow exit into urine

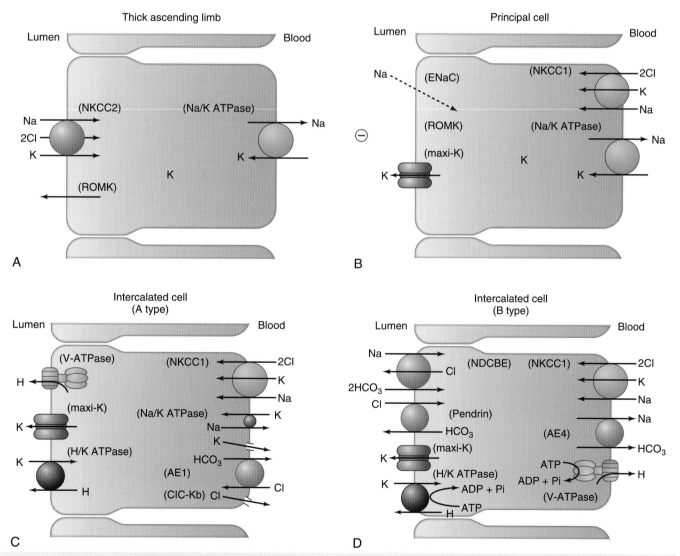

Fig. 52.5 Potassium handling along the nephron. *ENaC,* Epithelial sodium channel; *NKCC1,* Na-K-2Cl cotransporter-1; *ROMK,* renal potassium secretory channel. (From Gleason CA, Juul SE, eds. *Avery's Diseases of the Newborn.* 10th ed. Philadelphia: Elsevier; 2018:997, Fig. 98.4.)

□ Acute metabolic acidosis inhibits K secretion by inhibiting an apical K channel (renal potassium secretory channel [ROMK]).

□ Chronic metabolic acidosis has variable effects on secretion.

- Hypokalemia:
  - Usually defined as <3.5 mEq/L; rarely symptomatic until <2.5 mEq/L
  - Seen with diuretics, diarrhea, renal dysfunction, nasogastric drainage, alkalosis
  - EKG changes: flattened T waves, prolonged QT interval, U waves
  - Treatment: Correct alkalosis first. If mild, give enteral supplement or increase amount in TPN/fluids. If severe, IV KCl max of 0.3 mEq/kg given over 30 to 60 minutes.
- Hyperkalemia: K > 6.5
  - Seen with renal dysfunction, metabolic acidosis, cell breakdown
  - >50% of infants weighing <1000 g
  - EKG changes: peaked T waves, wide QRS, bradycardia, tachycardia, supraventricular tachycardia, ventricular tachycardia, ventricular fibrillation
  - Therapy centers on shifting K into cells and stabilizing the myocardium as acute temporizing measures and elimination from body (see Table 52.3).

ACID–BASE BALANCE

- Normal pH ranges between 7.35 and 7.45.
- Growth and development depend on the acid–base balance.
- Mechanisms to keep pH in the normal range include buffering systems that act acutely and compensatory systems to maintain balance chronically (Table 52.4).
- Extracellular buffering system: The carbonic acid–bicarbonate system is the most important. Carbonic anhydrase (CA) catalyzes the following reaction:

$$H^+ + HCO_3^- \leftrightarrow H_2CO_3 \leftrightarrow H_2O + CO_2$$

- Intracellular buffering systems:
  - Hemoglobin, intracellular proteins, intracellular phosphate
  - Require several hours to reach maximum capacity
  - Much of buffering is done in bones: chronic acidosis leads to increased bone resorption.
- Respiratory compensatory mechanism:
  - Immediate regulator of homeostasis by maintaining normal partial pressure of carbon dioxide in arterial blood (PaCO$_2$)
  - Chemoreceptors (central more than peripheral) are activated by changes in pH or PaCO$_2$.
  - Develops within minutes for respiratory acidosis but takes several hours to develop for metabolic acidosis

Table 52.3   Therapy of Hyperkalemia

Medication	Dosage	Onset	Length of Effects	Mechanism of Action	Comments and Cautions
Calcium gluconate	100 mg/kg intravenously over 2–5 min	Immediate	30 min	Protects the myocardium from toxic effects of potassium; no effect on total body potassium	Can worsen digoxin toxicity
Sodium bicarbonate	1–2 mEq/kg	Immediate	Variable	Shifts potassium intracellularly: no effect on total body potassium	Maximum infusion: mEq/min in emergency situations
Tromethamine	3–5 mL/kg	Immediate	Variable	Shifts potassium intracellularly: no effect on total body potassium	—
Insulin plus dextrose	Insulin 0.1–0.15 U/kg intravenously plus dextrose 0.5 g/kg intravenously	15–30 min	2–6 h	Shifts potassium intracellularly: no effect on total body potassium	Monitor for hypoglycemia
Albuterol[a]	0.15 mg/kg every 20 min for three doses then 0.15–0.3 mg/kg	15–30 min	2–3 h	Shifts potassium intracellularly: no effect on total body potassium	Minimum dose 2.5 mg
Furosemide	Per os: 1–4 mg/kg per dose once or twice per day Intravenously: 1–2 mg/kg per dose given every 12–24 h	15 min to 1 h	4 h	Increases renal excretion of potassium	—
Sodium polystyrene	1 g/kg rectally every 6 h	1–2 h (rectal route faster)	4–6 h	Removes potassium from the gut in exchange for sodium	Use with extreme caution in neonates, especially preterm neonates; contains sorbitol and may be associated with bowel necrosis and sodium retention.

[a]From Singh BS, Sadiq HF, Noguchi A, Keenan WJ. Efficacy of albuterol inhalation in treatment of hyperkalemia in premature neonates. *J Pediatr.* 2002;141:16–20. Gleason CA, Juul S, eds. *Avery's Diseases of the Newborn.* 10th ed. Philadelphia: Elsevier, 2018: 380, Table 30.4.

Table 52.4 Compensatory Mechanisms for Primary Acid–Base Disorders

Acid–Base Disorder	Primary Event	Compensation	Rate of Compensation
METABOLIC ACIDOSIS			
Normal anion gap	Decreased HCO_3^- concentration	Decreased PCO_2	For 1-mEq/L decrease in HCO_3^- concentration, PCO_2 decreases by 1–1.5 mmHg
Increased anion gap	Increased acid production Increased acid intake	Decreased PCO_2	For 1-mEq/L decrease in HCO_3^- concentration, PCO_2 decreases by 1–1.5 mmHg
Metabolic Alkalosis	Increased HCO_3^- concentration	Increased PCO_2	For 1-mEq/L increase in HCO_3^- concentration, PCO_2 increases by 0.5–1 mmHg
RESPIRATORY ACIDOSIS			
Acute (<12–24 h)	Increased PCO_2	Increased HCO_3^- concentration	For 10-mmHg increase in PCO_2, HCO_3^- concentration increases by 1 mEq/L
Chronic (3–5 days)	Increased PCO_2	Increased HCO_3^- concentration	For 10-mmHg increase in PCO_2, HCO_3^- concentration increases by 4 mEq/L
RESPIRATORY ALKALOSIS			
Acute (<12 h)	Decreased PCO_2	Decreased HCO_3^- concentration	For 10-mmHg increase in PCO_2, HCO_3^- concentration increases by 1–3 mEq/L
Chronic (1–2 days)	Decreased PCO_2	Decreased HCO_3^- concentration	For 10-mmHg decrease in PCO_2, HCO_3^- concentration decreases by 2–5 mEq/L

HCO_3^-, Bicarbonate; PCO_2, partial pressure of carbon dioxide.
Modified from Brewer ED. Disorders of acid-base balance. *Pediatr Clin North Am*. 1990;37:429–447. Gleason CA, Juul S, eds. *Avery's Diseases of the Newborn*. 10th ed. Philadelphia: Elsevier, 2018: 385, Table 30.5.

- Compensation for metabolic process is incomplete: pH does not normalize.
- Winters' formula predicts the respiratory response to a primary metabolic acidosis:

$$pCO_2 = (1.5 \times HCO_3^-) + 8 \pm 2$$

- Renal compensatory mechanism:
  - Starts within hours but takes days to reach its maximal effect
  - Secretion of H^+ is the primary mechanism of urine acidification.
  - Filtered bicarbonate is recycled back into cells as CO_2 where it is reformed into bicarbonate and transported back into blood.
- Urinary acidification process:
  - Proximal tubule
    - Adults reabsorb 70% to 90% of the filtered bicarbonate; neonates reabsorb less.
    - H^+ is secreted into the lumen via a Na/H exchanger and H^+-ATPase where it combines with the filtered bicarbonate via action of luminal CA to form CO_2, which then diffuses back into the cell. Cellular CA uses this CO_2 to regenerate bicarbonate, which is then transported to blood along with Na (Fig. 52.6).
    - Ammoniagenesis results in net acid secretion via generation of NH_4^+

$$Glutamine \rightarrow NH_4^+ + \alpha\text{-ketoglutarate}$$

    - NH_4^+ is secreted into lumen via the Na/NH_4^+ exchanger.

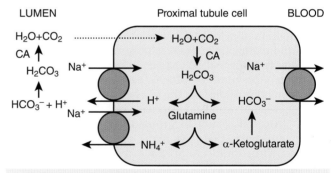

Fig. 52.6 Proximal tubule reabsorption of bicarbonate and secretion of ammonium. (From Martin RJ, Fanaroff AA, Walsh MC, eds. *Fanaroff and Martin's Neonatal-Perinatal Medicine*. 11th ed. Philadelphia: Elsevier; 2020:1864, Fig. 92.4.)

  - The α-ketoglutarate buffers intracellular H^+ and results in HCO_3^-, which is transported to blood via the Na/HCO_3^- transporter.
- The response of the fully mature tubule to systemic acidosis is to
  - Increase proximal tubule cell uptake of glutamine.
  - Increase the number of Na/H exchangers on the apical surface.
  - Increase citrate reabsorption from the lumen.
  - Decrease phosphate reabsorption.
- The thick ascending limb (TAL) and distal tubule
  - Reabsorb 20% of the filtered bicarbonate
  - TAL takes up secreted NH_4^+ by the proximal tubule to store in the medullary interstitium, where it can be secreted by a collecting duct.

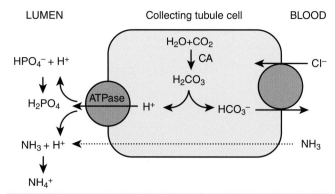

Fig. 52.7 Cortical collecting duct acid secretion. (From Martin RJ, Fanaroff AA, Walsh MC, eds. *Fanaroff and Martin's Neonatal-Perinatal Medicine.* 11th ed. Philadelphia: Elsevier; 2020:1864, Fig. 92.5.)

- Collecting duct (Fig. 52.7)
  - Type A intercalated cells have H^+-ATPase on the apical membrane to secrete H^+ into the lumen, where it combines with filtered anions (PO_4^- and sulfates) to form titratable acids.
  - Metabolic acidosis leads to increased insertion of preformed H^+-ATPase.
  - NH_3 is also secreted from the medullary interstitium and combines with secreted tyrosine hydroxylase–containing (TH^+) neurons to form NH_4^+.
  - Type B intercalated cells secrete HCO_3^- via the Cl^-/HCO_3^- exchanger.
  - Maximal urinary acidification in mature kidney results in a urine pH of 4.5 to 5; preterm kidney can only reach a urine pH of 6.
- Regulation of acid–base balance in neonates
  - Mild metabolic acidosis is normal shortly after birth due to maternal respiratory alkalosis (hyperventilation of pregnancy), which stimulates a compensatory metabolic acidosis in the mother.
    - Normal umbilical artery pH is 7.20 to 7.28.
    - Normal serum bicarbonate is 19 to 21 mEq/L full-term, 16 to 20 mEq/L preterm.
  - Growing children produce 1 to 2 mEq/kg/d of non-volatile acid.
  - Respiratory compensation effectiveness depends on the maturity of the central respiratory control system and lung function. Preterm infants have decreased sensitivity to changes in CO_2.
  - Renal compensation:
    - Immature tubules result in decreased ability to reclaim the filtered bicarbonate, which contributes to the lower serum bicarbonate levels seen in neonates.
    - Urinary excretion of titratable acid and NH_4^+ also increases with GA.
    - By 1 month after delivery regardless of GA, distal tubular H^+ secretion is present.
- Neonatal metabolic acidosis:
  - Causes increased non-volatile acid or decreased HCO_3 in extracellular fluid (ECF) (Box 52.1).
  - Categorized by high or normal anion gap (AG), where $AG = Na - (Cl + HCO_3^-)$
  - Normal values vary among labs but are usually 8 to 16 mEq/L.
  - For every decrease of 1 g/dL albumin, AG decreases by 2.5 mEq/L.

Box 52.1 Common Causes of Metabolic Acidosis in Neonates

Increased Anion Gap

Lactic Acidosis

- Hypoxemia, shock, sepsis
- Inborn errors of carbohydrate or pyruvate metabolism
- Pyruvate dehydrogenase deficiency
- Pyruvate carboxylase deficiency
- Mitochondrial respiratory chain defects
- Renal failure

Ketoacidosis

- Glycogen storage disease (type I)
- Inborn errors of amino acid or organic acid metabolism

Normal Anion Gap

- Bicarbonate loss: acute diarrhea; drainage from small bowel, biliary, or pancreatic tube; fistula drainage; bowel augmentation cystoplasty; ureteral diversion with bowel
- Renal tubular acidosis
- Mineralocorticoid deficiency
- Administration of Cl-containing compounds: arginine HCl, HCl, $CaCl_2$, $MgCl_2$, NH_4Cl hyperalimentation, high-protein formula
- Carbonic anhydrase inhibitors
- Dilution of extracellular fluid compartment

Adapted from Brewer E. Disorders of acid-base balance. *Pediatr Clin North Am.* 1990;37:429. From Martin RJ, Fanaroff AA, Walsh MC, eds. *Fanaroff and Martin's Neonatal-Perinatal Medicine.* 11th ed. Philadelphia: Elsevier. 2020:1866, Box 92.1.

- Increased AG may not be present in neonates with lactic acidosis.
- Treatment
  - Remove the inciting event.
  - Alkali (Na bicarbonate) use is controversial. It requires adequate ventilation; other complications include fluid overload, hypernatremia, cerebral vasoconstriction, decreased O_2 delivery to the brain due to a shift in the oxyhemoglobin dissociation curve, and intracellular acidosis due to CO_2 diffusion into cells.
  - Full correction = Base deficit (mEq/L) × Body weight (kg) × 0.3. Usually give 50% of calculated dose and reassess.
  - Na or K acetate may be used to treat chronic acidosis and can be added to TPN.
  - Monitor K, as it will drop intracellularly with rises in pH.
- Neonatal respiratory acidosis
  - Results from decreased excretion of CO_2 due to primary lung disease and ventilation–perfusion (V/Q) mismatch; may require mechanical ventilation to increase excretion of CO_2.
  - Preterm infants respond with increased respiratory rate with only a small increase in tidal volume; term infants respond with increased tidal volume.
  - Renal compensation is limited by the inability of immature tubules to reclaim more filtered bicarbonate.
  - Administration of alkali not indicated as increased serum HCO_3^- stimulates hypoventilation
- Neonatal metabolic alkalosis (Box 52.2)
  - Most commonly seen in neonatal intensive care units with prolonged diuretic use
  - Other causes include loss of H^+ from the gastrointestinal tract (vomiting, nasogastric suction) or kidneys,

Box 52.2 Common Causes of Metabolic Alkalosis in Neonates

- Acid loss: vomiting (e.g., pyloric stenosis), nasogastric suction
- Diuretics
- Chloride deficiency: chronic chloride-losing diarrhea, Bartter syndrome, low-chloride formula, loss via skin secondary to cystic fibrosis
- Administration of alkali: bicarbonate, lactate, acetate, citrate

From Martin RJ, Fanaroff AA, Walsh MC, eds. *Fanaroff and Martin's Neonatal-Perinatal Medicine*, 11th ed. Philadelphia: Elsevier; 2020:1866, Box 92.2.

exogenous bicarbonate, contraction of extracellular fluid volume (ECFV) around a fixed amount of HCO_3^- (have lost more Cl– than HCO_3^-).
- May be maintained by continued decrease in ECFV, which
  - Leads to decrease in GFR and less filtered bicarbonate
  - Stimulates avid proximal Na reabsorption which leads to HCO_3^- reabsorption
  - Stimulates the renin–angiotensin system (RAS), resulting in increased aldosterone, increased distal Na reabsorption, and excretion of H^+ and K^+
- K depletion stimulates renal ammoniagenesis and inhibits shift of H^+ out of the cell.
- Respiratory response: decreased rate and tidal volume
- Renal response: decrease in absorption of filtered HCO_3^- and distal net acid excretion
- Therapy: Remove inciting condition, restore ECFV, and correct low K^+ and Cl^-.
- Prolonged pH > 7.6 may increase the risk of sensorineural deafness.
- Neonatal respiratory alkalosis
  - Results from increased excretion of CO_2 and is typically secondary to fever or iatrogenic hyperventilation
  - Rare cause is urea cycle defect, where increased NH_4^+ may stimulate the central respiratory center.

PSEUDOHYPOALDOSTERONISM (PHA)

Overview

- Kidney is unresponsive to aldosterone.
- Autosomal dominant (AD) form = mutation in aldosterone receptor.
- Autosomal recessive (AR) form = mutation in subunit of ENaC.

Clinical Presentation

- Polyuria, dehydration, vomiting, FTT
- AR type is systemic, more severe, and lifelong (renal, sweat glands, salivary glands, nasal mucosa, lung, colon are involved).
  - Respiratory symptoms (cough, wheezing, tachypnea) from impaired mucociliary clearance; may mimic cystic fibrosis
  - Eczema/skin lesions
- AD type is renal limited, and symptoms usually resolve by age 2.

- Secondary or transient forms:
  - Medications
    - Amiloride, triamterene, trimethoprim, and pentamidine, which block ENaC
    - Spironolactone, a mineralocorticoid antagonist
    - Cyclosporine, angiotensin-converting enzyme (ACE) inhibitor, nonsteroidal anti-inflammatory drugs (NSAIDs), β-blockers
  - Urinary tract infections and obstructive uropathy
  - Rare: medullary necrosis and renal vein thrombosis

Diagnosis and Evaluation

- Hyponatremia, hyperkalemia, and metabolic acidosis with high renin and aldosterone levels
- High urine Na
- AR form has high sweat and salivary NaCl.
- Genetic testing is available.

Treatment

- Salt supplements may require up to 10 to 15 mEq/kg/d.
- K restriction, K binder (Kayexalate), or alkali (Bicitra or $NaHCO_3^-$) may be required, especially for AR form.

BARTTER SYNDROME

Overview

- Bartter syndrome results from autosomal recessive defects in Na, K, or Cl tubular transport proteins and is classified into five types (I–IVb) based on which transporter is defective.

Clinical Presentation

- Neonatal and infant forms present with FTT.
- Types I, II, and IV have severe polyhydramnios resulting in preterm delivery and continued significant polyuria.
- Type IV presents with deafness.
- Type III usually presents later in infancy.

Diagnosis and Evaluation

- All forms have hyponatremia, hypokalemia, hypochloremia, and metabolic alkalosis with high urine chloride.
- Type II will have an initial transient hyperkalemia before developing hypokalemia.
- Hypomagnesemia can be seen in types III and IV.
- Genetic testing is available.

Treatment

- Indomethacin is helpful except in type IV (for unknown reason).
- Na and water supplementation for all
- Potassium and magnesium supplements may be required.

RENAL TUBULAR ACIDOSIS

- All forms of renal tubular acidosis (RTA) are characterized by normal AG metabolic acidosis in the absence of gastrointestinal loss of $NaHCO_3^-$ or cysteine Cl supplementation in TPN.

- It results from either inadequate renal acidification or renal bicarbonate wasting.

PROXIMAL RENAL TUBULAR ACIDOSIS, TYPE II

Overview

- Impaired capacity to reabsorb HCO_3^- by the proximal tubule
- Reabsorption does not occur until serum HCO_3^- falls below the tubular threshold.
- Ability to secrete H^+ distally is intact so can maximally acidify urine when serum HCO_3^- is below the threshold.
- Isolated form is rare – usually part of generalized proximal tubular dysfunction (Fanconi syndrome).
- Genetic causes exist:
  - AR defect in $NaHCO_3^-$ cotransporter is associated with eye problems.
  - Rare AD form is without an identified gene thus far.

Clinical Presentation

- FTT, polyuria

Diagnosis and Evaluation

- Urine pH is variable.
  - If serum HCO_3^- is below the tubular threshold, urine pH will be maximally acidified (<5.5).
  - If treated to raise serum HCO_3^- above threshold, urine pH will be high.
- If present with Fanconi syndrome, will also have phosphate wasting, renal glucosuria, aminoaciduria, and tubular proteinuria

Treatment

- Administer alkali; typically requires 5 to 10 mEq/kg/d or more.
- Often requires K supplement.
- If part of a generalized proximal dysfunction, will need supplements of affected electrolytes

DISTAL RENAL TUBULAR ACIDOSIS, TYPE I

Overview

- Inability to properly acidify the urine
- In children, usually an isolated entity
- Genetic causes
  - AD or AR mutation in Cl^-/HCO_3^- exchanger (AE1)
  - AR mutation in B1 subunit of H^+-ATPase, which is associated with early-onset deafness
  - AR mutation in A4 subunit of H^+-ATPase, which is variably associated with later-onset deafness
- Drugs: classically amphotericin
- Congenital lesions cause tubular dysfunction, such as obstructive lesions.

Clinical Presentation

- FTT, lethargy, polyuria, vomiting, dehydration
- May have kidney stones or nephrocalcinosis

Diagnosis and Evaluation

- Urine pH < 5.5 rules it out.
- Urine pH > 6.5 with non AG metabolic acidosis is suggestive.
- Typically diagnosed by positive urine AG, but this is not reliable in neonates due to their high urine anions
- Can use urine PCO_2–blood PCO_2 gradient:
  - Administer alkali to raise serum HCO_3^- to slightly above normal.
  - Measure PCO_2 from urine and blood.
  - Difference should be >20 with normal function.
- Hypercalciuria, hypocitraturia, and hypokalemia are typical.

Treatment

- Alkali: amount required decreases with age; typically requires less than proximal RTA (2–3 mEq/kg/d)

HYPERKALEMIC DISTAL RENAL TUBULAR ACIDOSIS, TYPE IV

Overview

- Impaired potassium and hydrogen secretion in collecting duct
- Rare in children
- May be from drugs that impair release or action of aldosterone
- Also seen in genetic conditions that decrease production of or cause resistance to aldosterone (PHA type 1)

Clinical Presentation

- Acidosis is typically less severe than other forms: bicarbonate is in high teens.
- Hyperkalemia

Diagnosis and Evaluation

- Hyperkalemia
- High urine sodium
- Low urine potassium

Treatment

- If due to low aldosterone production, mineralocorticoid replacement
- Low potassium intake
- Potassium-binding resins
- Alkali

MIXED DISTAL RENAL TUBULAR ACIDOSIS, TYPE III

Overview

- Defect in both proximal and distal tubule
- Common in VLBW infants in first few weeks
- Genetic form results from defect in carbonic anhydrase II and presents with mixed RTA and osteopetrosis, growth restriction, mental retardation, and cerebral calcifications.

HORMONAL CONTROL OF RENAL FUNCTION

- The primary function of the renin–angiotensin system (RAS) is to protect ECW volume/blood pressure
  - Angiotensinogen is produced in liver.
  - Renin produced by the juxtaglomerular apparatus of afferent arterioles converts angiotensinogen to angiotensin I (Ang I).
  - ACE converts Ang I to angiotensin II (Ang II).
  - Ang II via its AT1 receptor subtype constricts efferent arteriole > afferent, resulting in increase in GFR.
  - Ang II also promotes Na, HCO_3^-, and water reabsorption along the nephron and aldosterone release.
  - Ang II via its AT2 receptor subtype is important in nephrogenesis.
  - Aldosterone increases K secretion and Na reabsorption in the distal tubule.
  - Pharmacologic RAS inhibition during pregnancy or mutation in genes involved in the RAS can result in hypotension, hypocalvaria, intrauterine growth restriction (IUGR), pulmonary hypoplasia, oligohydramnios, anuria, and fetal/neonatal death.
- Prostaglandins
  - Are synthesized in kidney via the cyclooxygenase pathway
  - Are important in maintaining the GFR when renal perfusion is low or vasoconstrictive state is activated.
  - Exposure to NSAIDs in utero results in a transient decrease in the GFR.
  - Use of indomethacin for PDA therapy is associated with a decrease in the GFR and AKI.
- Atrial natriuretic peptide (ANP)
  - Is released from atrial myocytes when stretched
  - Causes afferent arteriole vasodilation and efferent arteriole constriction with an increase in the GFR
  - Inhibits renin production; aldosterone release stimulates natriuresis
- Nitric oxide (NO) is a potent vasodilator synthesized by endothelial cells.
- Dopamine
  - Increases renal blood flow and the GFR
  - Inhibits Na reabsorption by inhibiting Na,K-ATPase
- Sympathetic nervous system
  - Low-level activation results in equal constriction of afferent and efferent arterioles, with a decrease in renal blood flow and no effect on the GFR.
  - Higher degree of activation results in constriction of mesangial cells and decreases the GFR.
  - It stimulates renin release, activating the RAS.

EVALUATION OF RENAL FUNCTION

- At 32 to 34 weeks' gestational age, the GFR is ~14 mL/min/1.73 m². At term, the GFR is 21 mL/min/1.73 m². This increases to ~50 mL/min/1.73 m² by 2 weeks, 77 mL/min/1.73 m² by 1 year, and 120 mL/min/1.73 m² by 2 years.
- Blood creatinine is most commonly used to assess renal function. It falls to 0.4 mg/dL by 2 weeks after term birth. Preterm infants may have a rise in creatinine over several days but then a slow fall to 0.4 mg/dL over the next month.

- Cystatin C has been proposed as an alternative estimate of GFR but is not as widely available as serum creatinine measurements.
- Urinalysis
  - Proteinuria is best assessed by spot urine protein/creatinine ratios. Preterm normal < 0.7 mg/mg, term < 0.5 mg/mg. High levels may be seen with acute tubular necrosis, fever, dehydration, heart failure, and nephrotic syndrome.
  - Hematuria > 5 RBC/HPF by microscopic exam may be seen with acute tubular necrosis, renal vein thrombosis, urine infection, or trauma from a catheter.
- $FENa = (U_{Na} \times S_{Cr})/(S_{Na} \times U_{Cr})$, where U_{Na} is urine sodium, S_{Cr} is serum creatinine, S_{Na} is serum sodium, and U_{Cr} is urine creatinine.
- Calculated serumos molality
$$= (2 \times S_{Na}[mmol/L]) + (glucose[mg/dL]/18) + (BUN[mg/dL]/2.8).$$

NEPHROTIC SYNDROME (NS)

Overview

- High-grade proteinuria, low serum albumin, edema
- Congenital NS presents in the first 3 months. Infantile NS presents at 3 to 12 months.
- Primary NS has a genetic cause. Most cases of congenital/infantile NS are from one of four genes:
  - *NPHS1* = nephrin (CNS of the Finnish type); most common AR form
  - *NPHS2* = podocin; second most common AR form, which presents later than nephrin mutation (4–12 months old)
  - *WT1* = Wilm's tumor suppressor gene, which can be isolated (diffuse mesangial sclerosis) or part of syndrome (WAGR, Fraser, or Denys-Drash syndromes)
  - *LAMB2* = laminin beta-2 chain
- Infectious causes include cytomegalovirus (CMV), syphilis, hepatitis B, toxoplasmosis, rubeola, and human immunodeficiency virus (HIV).

Treatment

- Does not respond to immunosuppression
- If infectious cause, treatment of infection may lead to cure of the NS.
- Symptomatic management until infant is big enough to undergo renal transplant; albumin infusions, diuretics, ACE-I, nephrectomy if recurrent complications
- Complications include infections, blood clots, FTT, and hypothyroidism.

Suggested Readings

Azhibekov T, Friedlich PS, Seri I. Regulation of acid-base balance in the fetus and neonate. In: Polin RA, Abman SH, Rowitch DH, Benitz WE, eds. *Fetal and Neonatal Physiology*. 6th ed. Philadelphia: Elsevier; 2022:1076–1081.

Baum M. Renal transport of sodium during development. In: Polin RA, Abman SH, Rowitch DH, Benitz WE, eds. *Fetal and Neonatal Physiology*. 6th ed. Philadelphia: Elsevier; 2022:1984–1992.

Bockenhauer D, Zieg J. Electrolyte disorders. *Clin Perinatol.* 2014;41(3): 575–590.

Dell KM. Fluid, electrolytes, and acid-base homeostasis. In: Martin RJ, Fanaroff AA, Walsh MC, eds. *Fanaroff and Martin's Neonatal-Perinatal Medicine.* 11th ed. Philadelphia: Elsevier; 2020:854–1870.

Segar JL. Renal adaptive changes and sodium handling in the fetal-to-newborn transition. *Semin Fetal Neonatal Med.* 2017;22(2):76–82.

Solhaug MJ, Jose PA. Development and regulation of renal blood flow in the neonate. In: Polin RA, Abman SH, Rowitch DH, Benitz WE, eds. *Fetal and Neonatal Physiology.* 6th ed. Philadelphia: Elsevier; 2022:965–974.

Wolf MT, Benchimol C, Satlin LM, Quigley R. Potassium homeostasis in the fetus and neonate. In: Polin RA, Abman SH, Rowitch DH, Benitz WE, eds. *Fetal and Neonatal Physiology.* 6th ed. Philadelphia: Elsevier; 2022:992–1005.

53 Abnormal Renal Development

ERIN RADEMACHER

Prenatal Ultrasound of Kidneys/Bladder

- The goal of fetal ultrasound (U/S) is to evaluate kidney size, shape, and echogenicity; amniotic fluid volume; and bladder size and shape.
  - See Box 53.1 for potential etiologies of different U/S findings.
- Fetal kidneys can be visualized at 9 to 12 weeks.
  - Average length is 1 cm at 12 weeks and 2.7 cm at 20 weeks.
  - Bladder can seen by the 15th week.
- Abnormal findings in the renal/urinary system account for 20% to 30% of anomalies detected on prenatal U/S.
- The risk of renal tract malformations is increased by maternal diabetes mellitus and certain drug exposures.
  - Cocaine and alcohol have also been reported to increase risk.

Prenatal Diagnosis: Hydronephrosis

- Hydronephrosis is defined as significant dilatation of upper tract involving dilatation of the calyces.
  - Pelviectasis or pyelectasis usually refers to dilatation of the renal pelvis only.
- Hydronephrosis or pelviectasis is seen in ~1% to 5% of pregnancies.
- The definition depends on which classification system used.
  - Measurement of the anterior–posterior diameter of the renal pelvis (APRPD) is most common.
    - >4 mm if < 33 weeks or >7 mm at > 33 weeks is predictive of postnatal problems.
    - >15 mm is highly predictive of ureteropelvic junction (UPJ) obstruction.
- Predictors of long-term renal impairment include oligohydramnios, lack of reniform shape of kidney, presence of cysts, and increased echogenicity.
- 50% to 70% of prenatally detected hydronephrosis cases are physiologic or idiopathic (no obstruction or reflux); most resolve over the first 2 years of life.
- Other causes of prenatal hydronephrosis:
  - UPJ obstruction (10–30%)
    - Most common cause of severe hydronephrosis
    - More common in males
    - May be part of syndrome

- Vesicoureteral reflux (VUR) (10–40%)
  - Caused by ectopic insertion of the ureter, resulting in shortened intravesicular segment
  - One-third have an affected first-degree relative.
- Ureterovesical junction (UVJ) obstruction (5–15%)
  - Usually isolated
  - Hydroureter also seen on U/S
- Multicystic dysplastic kidney (MCDK) (2–5%)
- Posterior urethral valve (PUV) (1–5%)
- Ureterocele (1–3%)
  - Usually from the upper pole ureter of the duplex collection system
- Eagle-Barrett syndrome, or "prune belly syndrome" (<1%)

POSTNATAL EVALUATION OF PRENATAL HYDRONEPHROSIS

- U/S in first 1 to 2 days of life is indicated for severe prenatal hydronephrosis, bilateral hydronephrosis, oligohydramnios, or concern of bladder obstruction.
- If initial early U/S is normal, follow up in 1 to 2 weeks when urine output is well established.
- Unilateral hydronephrosis: U/S at ~2 weeks of life
- Follow-up U/S is done at 4 to 6 weeks of life.
- If U/S at 1 to 2 weeks *and* at 4 to 6 weeks are both normal, then no further follow-up is needed.
- If severe hydronephrosis is present on a postnatal U/S, the infant should be placed on antibiotic prophylaxis and a voiding cystourethrogram (VCUG) obtained.

Prenatal Treatment of Suspected Bladder Outlet Obstruction With Oligohydramnios

- Controversial: Intervention has not been shown to reliably improve renal or pulmonary function.
- The most common intervention is a vesicoamniotic shunt placed in the second trimester in a fetus thought to have preserved renal function.
- Fetal renal function is assessed by fetal urine indices on serial bladder taps (need to empty the bladder to obtain fresh urine for analysis).
- Findings thought to predict good renal function:
  - Urine Na < 100 mEq/L
  - Urine Ca < 8 mg/dL
  - Urine osmolality < 200 mOsm/L
  - Urine β_2 microglobulin < 4 mg/L
  - Urine protein < 40 mg/dL

Box 53.1   Abnormal Findings of Urinary Tract Seen by Prenatal Ultrasound

Kidneys

- Dilated renal pelvis/hydronephrosis: physiologic, vesicoureteral reflux, obstruction
- Cystic kidney: MCDK, cystic dysplasia, ADPKD, severe obstruction
- Echogenic kidney: renal dysplasia, ARPKD
- Structural abnormalities: renal duplication fusion abnormalities (e.g., horseshoe, crossed fused ectopia), ectopic kidneys (pelvic, thoracic)
- Lack of visualization: renal agenesis, hypoplasia, ectopic
- Enlarged kidneys: ARPKD, obstruction, overgrowth syndromes (Simpson-Golabi-Behmel, Perlman, Beckwith-Wiedemann)
- Renal mass

Ureter

- Hydroureter

Bladder

- Dilation
- Ureterocele
- With thickened wall: posterior urethral valves
- Without thickened wall: megacystis–megaureter syndrome, neurogenic bladder, EBS
- Bladder exstrophy, cloacal exstrophy

- Lack of visualization: minimal or absent fetal urine production, obstructive uropathy

Ascites

- Urinary ascites (typically associated with thickened bladder wall and/or abnormal kidneys)

Hydrops Fetalis

- Most often due to non-renal causes; occasionally caused by bilateral renal cystic disease, urinary tract obstruction, or congenital nephrotic syndrome

Oligohydramnios

- Bilateral renal dysplasia, urinary tract obstruction, ARPKD
- Rupture of membranes, postmaturity, subacute fetal distress

Polyhydramnios

- Renal tubular disorder with urinary concentrating defect (NDI, Bartter syndrome)
- Multiple gestation: upper gastrointestinal tract obstruction, neurologic disorders, maternal diabetes, fetal hydrops

Placental Edema

- Congenital nephrotic syndrome

ADPKD, Autosomal dominant polycystic kidney disease; *ARPKD*, autosomal recessive polycystic kidney disease; *EBS*, Eagle Barrett syndrome; *MCDK*, multicystic dysplastic kidney; *NDI*, nephrogenic diabetes insipidus.
From Martin RJ. *Fanaroff and Martin's Neonatal-Perinatal Medicine*, 11th ed. Philadelphia: Elsevier/Saunders, 2020, p.1875, Box 93.1.

Oligohydramnios Sequence (Potter Syndrome)

- See Fig. 53.1.
- Syndrome is seen in babies with oligohydramnios or anhydramnios of any cause.
- Characteristic facies: wide-set eyes, depressed nasal bridge, beaked nose, receding chin, posteriorly rotated and low-set ears
- Other features include small chest, arthrogryposis, hip dislocation, and club feet.
- Respiratory failure is secondary to pulmonary hypoplasia.

Posterior Urethral Valves

- See Fig. 53.2.
- Occurs in 1/5000 to 1/8000 males
- U/S shows bilateral hydronephrosis/hydroureter and thickened, trabeculated bladder with "keyhole" sign (dilated posterior urethra).
- VCUG shows narrowing of urethra.
- Clinical exam: palpable bladder, poor urine stream
- Treatment: urethral catheter to relieve obstruction, followed by valve ablation (preferred) or vesicostomy if infant is too small to pass scope
- Prognosis: prone to dehydration due to poor concentrating ability, 12% to 15% progress to renal failure by adolescence (20–60% reach end-stage renal disease overall).

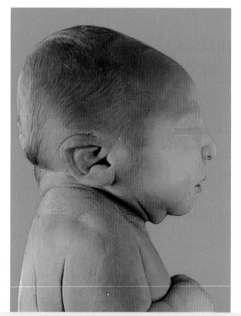

Fig. 53.1 Oligohydramnios sequence typical facial appearance. (From Gleason CA, Juul SE, eds. *Avery's Diseases of the Newborn*. 10th ed. Philadelphia: Elsevier; 2018:1252, Fig. 87.1.)

Eagle-Barrett Syndrome

- See Fig. 53.3.
- Full syndrome has triad of findings:
  - Poorly contractile, markedly enlarged bladder without urethral obstruction, megaureters, renal dysplasia

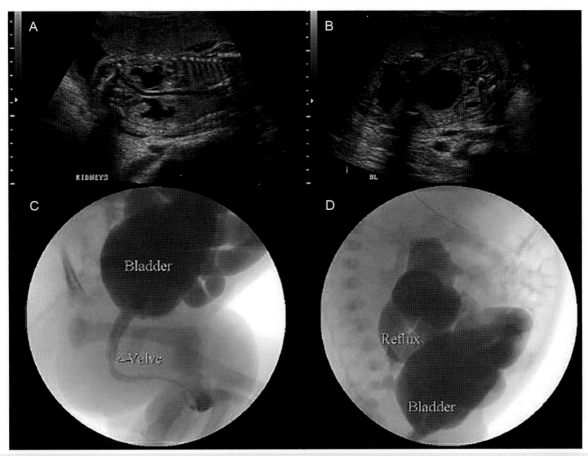

Fig. 53.2 Posterior urethral valve imaging. (A) Prenatal ultrasound (U/S) showing bilateral hydronephrosis. (B) Prenatal U/S showing dilated bladder. (C) Voiding cystourethrogram (VCUG) showing narrowing in posterior urethra. (D) VCUG showing reflux into dilated ureter. (From Clayton DB, Brock JW. Lower urinary tract obstruction in the fetus and neonate. *Clin Perinatol.* 2014;41:643–659.)

- Deficient abdominal wall musculature
- Cryptorchidism
- Can be incomplete and only display some of the features of the classic triad
- Occurs in 1/35,000 to 1/50,000, nearly all males (95%)
- May have abnormalities of other organs: cardiovascular, gastrointestinal, musculoskeletal
- Urinary tract infection prophylaxis is indicated due to poorly functioning bladder.
- About 50% develop chronic kidney disease, and 15% reach end-stage kidney disease.

Renal Agenesis

- Unilateral absence of kidney occurs in 1/500 to 1/3200 live births.
  - Expect compensatory hypertrophy of contralateral kidney (often seen in utero).
  - One-third have an abnormality in the contralateral kidney: VUR, UPJ, dysplasia, ureterocele.
  - Can be associated with defects in Müllerian duct structures; gastrointestinal, cardiac, and musculoskeletal anomalies are also seen.
  - Risk of chronic kidney disease in adulthood is increased due to hyperfiltration injury.

- Bilateral (1/4000–1/10,000), more common in males; will have oligohydramnios sequence
- May be associated with the vertebral, anorectal, cardiac, tracheal, esophageal, renal/genitourinary, and limb (VACTERL) syndrome, caudal regression syndrome, branchiootorenal syndrome, and chromosomal defects.

Renal Dysplasia

- Abnormal development of kidney resulting in disorganized structure and presence of cartilage
- Can be caused by genetic mutation, obstruction, or toxin/medication exposure
- Associations include VACTERL association; CHARGE (coloboma, heart defect, choanal atresia, retarded growth, genitourinary and ear anomalies) syndrome; Jeune syndrome; trisomies 13, 18, and 21; and more.
- Bilateral dysplasia usually results in chronic kidney disease.

Multicystic Dysplastic Kidney

- MCDK does not have any functional properties.
- Normal architecture is replaced by cysts, or "cluster of grapes" (see Fig. 53.4).

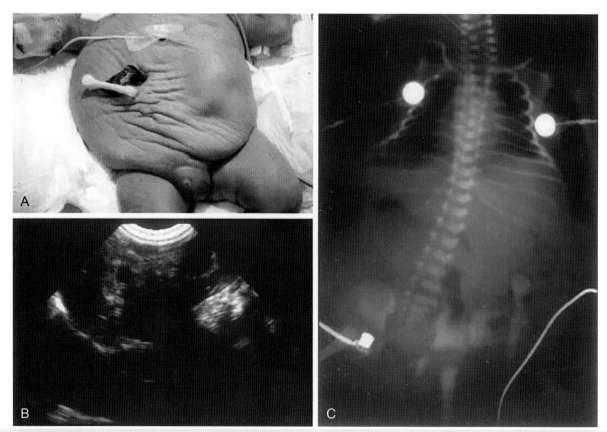

Fig. 53.3 Eagle-Barrett syndrome. (From Gleason CA, Juul SE, eds. *Avery's Diseases of the Newborn*. 10th ed. Philadelphia: Elsevier; 2018:1272, Fig. 88.9.)

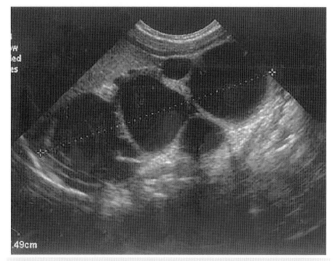

Fig. 53.4 Ultrasound appearance of multicystic dysplastic kidney. Note the "bunch of grapes" appearance of the multiple cysts, which do not communicate with each other. (From Gleason CA, Juul SE, eds. *Avery's Diseases of the Newborn*. 10th ed. Philadelphia: Elsevier; 2018:1263, Fig. 88.2.)

- Occurs in 1/4300 live births, more common in males
- Left-sided predominance
- Most involute over time.
- No increased risk of tumor or hypertension
- One-third have abnormal contralateral kidney (agenesis, dysplasia, VUR, ectopia).

- Should have VCUG if contralateral kidney or bladder has abnormal U/S appearance or if cryptorchidism is present.
- If opposite kidney is normal, should see compensatory hypertrophy.

Autosomal Recessive Polycystic Kidney

- Autosomal recessive polycystic kidney disease (ARPKD) is a polycystic kidney disease with congenital hepatic fibrosis.
- 1/20,000 incidence
- ARPKD is autosomal recessive, with a mutation in the *PKHD1* gene. Genetic testing is available but detects only 85% of cases. Expression is variable within a family.
- Prenatal U/S shows enlarged, echogenic kidneys; cysts are usually too small to be detected.
- May develop oligohydramnios in second trimester
- After birth, infant may have respiratory failure secondary to oligohydramnios and/or abdominal distention from large kidneys.
- May have severe hypertension
- Hyponatremia and polyuria are common.
- Nutrition may be compromised by large kidneys limiting feed volumes.
- 70% survive the neonatal period, and 80% of those individuals will survive to 10 years of age.
- 50% develop renal failure in the first decade.

Autosomal Dominant Polycystic Kidney Disease

- One in 1000 live births carry the mutation for autosomal dominant polycystic kidney disease (ADPKD), but it rarely manifests clinically until adulthood.
- May have visible cysts at birth
- Rarely has severe presentation similar to ARPKD
- Majority have a mutation in the *PKD1* or *PKD2* genes; 10% have a de novo mutation.

Renal Artery Thrombosis

- A major risk factor is the presence of an umbilical artery catheter (UAC).
- Presumed cause is endothelial injury after insertion of UAC.
- Other risk factors include shock, coagulopathy, and congestive heart failure.
- Incidence varies with the modality used to detect:
  - U/S with Doppler, 14–35%
  - Angiography, 64%
  - Autopsy, 9%–28%
- High UAC (T6–T10) and heparinized fluid are associated with *lower* incidence.
- Symptomatic in 1% to 3%
- Presents within first few days in term infant but is delayed in preterm ones (~8 days)
- Clinical presentation:
  - Minor clot—mildly decreased lower extremity perfusion, hypertension, hematuria
  - Moderate clot—decreased lower extremity perfusion, hypertension, oliguria, congestive heart failure
  - Major clot—multiorgan failure
  - Other features include thrombocytopenia, low fibrinogen, increased fibrin split products, variable prothrombin and thromboplastin times, conjugated hyperbilirubinemia, increased blood urea nitrogen (BUN) and creatinine, hematuria.
- Diagnostic imaging includes Doppler U/S or angiography.
- Treatment:
  - Asymptomatic/minor symptoms—removal of UAC and supportive care
  - More severe symptoms—systemic heparinization
  - Life-threatening—thrombolytic agents have been used, but few data are available regarding dosing, safety, or efficacy
- Prognosis
  - 9% to 20% mortality with clots involving both the aorta and renal artery.
  - Renovascular hypertension is the most common long-term complication but often resolves.
  - Chronic kidney disease not common but will always be present if the clot affected both renal arteries.

Renal Vein Thrombosis

- Renal vein thrombosis is the most common blood clot in infancy; the reported incidence varies from 2.2/100,000 live births (symptomatic clot) to 0.5/1000 neonatal intensive care unit (NICU) admissions.
- It is more common in males (67%).
- Left renal vein is more common (60%).
- It is unilateral in 70%.
- The inferior vena cava (IVC) is involved in 40%.
- Adrenal hemorrhage in 15%.
- Risk factors:
  - Prothrombotic factors play a significant role.
  - Maternal diabetes, hyperviscosity, hemoconcentration, traumatic delivery, prematurity, sepsis, birth asphyxia, cyanotic congenital cardiac disease, congenital renal vein defects
  - Most do *not* involve an umbilical venous catheter.
- Clinical presentation:
  - Classic triad: gross hematuria, decreased platelets, flank/abdominal mass (all three seen in <50% cases)
  - Decreased urine output
  - Associated signs: thrombocytopenia, hemolytic anemia, metabolic acidosis, increased BUN/Cr, variable prothrombin and partial thromboplastic times
- Diagnosis:
  - Renal ultrasound with Dopplers; appearance of U/S changes with time (see Box 53.2)
  - Clot in small intrarenal veins can cause increased resistance in the renal artery.
  - Angiography and magnetic resonance imaging are used in selected circumstances.
- Treatment:
  - Correct any fluid, electrolyte, or acid-base issues in all cases.
  - Avoid hypertonic solutions, nephrotoxins, hyperosmotic radiocontrast material, and diuretics.

Box 53.2 Ultrasound Changes in Kidney Affected by Renal Vein Thrombosis

Early (first week)

Globular enlargement of kidney

Increase in echogenicity

Loss of corticomedullary boundary

Echogenic streaks

Loss of normal sinus echoes

Intermediate (second week)

More prominent and diffuse renal enlargement

Diffuse "snowstorm" pattern of echogenicity

Loss of corticomedullary differentiation

May see coexisting hyperechoeic (hemorrhagic) areas and hypoechoeic (edema/resolving hemorrhagic) areas

May see thrombus extension in renal veins and inferior vena cava

Late (after second week)

May be normal in appearance

May become atrophic

May see calcifications in either or both kidneys and within the vascular system

From Brandão LR, Simpson EA, Lau KK. Neonatal renal vein thrombosis. *Semin Fetal Neonatal Med.* 2011;16:323–328, Box 1.

- It is unclear if heparinization leads to differences in long-term outcomes, but it usually is recommended in unilateral cases with IVC involvement.
- Fibrinolysis is only considered in bilateral cases.
- Prognosis:
  - Scarring and atrophy of the affected kidney are common.
  - 20% have hypertension.
  - Mortality is ~3% and is usually related to the underlying cause of the renal vein thrombosis.

Acute Kidney Injury

- Acute kidney injury (AKI) can be defined as sudden decline in glomerular filtration rate (GFR) or tubular function.
- The currently used definition of neonatal AKI divides AKI into stages based on rise in creatinine or drop in urine output (see Table 53.1).
  - Problems with creatinine-based definitions in neonates:
    - Creatinine does not change until 25% to 50% of GFR is lost.
    - Creatinine may rise in preterm infants over the first few days of life and then plateau for several days before falling.
    - Creatinine is secreted by tubules at a low GFR.
    - Most neonatal AKI does not involve oliguria.
- Rates of AKI in NICUs vary with the population studied:
  - Very low birth weight, 18% to 40%
  - Extracorporeal membrane oxygenation, as high as 70%

Table 53.1 Neonatal KDIGO AKI Definition

Stage	Serum Creatinine (SCr)	Urine Output Over 24 Hours
0	No change in serum creatinine or rise < 0.3 mg/dL	>1 mL/kg/h
1	SCr rise ≥ 0.3 mg/dL within 48 h or SCr rise ≥ 1.5–1.9 × reference SCr[a] within 7 days	>0.5 and ≤ 1 mL/kg/h
2	SCr rise ≥ 2–2.9 × reference SCr	>0.3 and ≤0.5 mL/kg/h
3	SCr rise ≥ 3 × reference SCr or SCr ≥ 2.5 mg/dL or receipt of dialysis	≤0.3 mL/kg/h

AKI, Acute kidney injury; KDIGO, Kidney Disease: Improving Global Outcomes.
[a]Reference SCr is the lowest prior SCr measurement.
From Nada A, Bonachea EM, Askenazi DJ. Acute kidney injury in the fetus and neonate. Semin Fetal Neonatal Med. 2017;22:90–97, Table 53.1.

- Perinatal asphyxia, 40%
- Cardiopulmonary bypass, 50% to 60%
- AKI is often divided into prerenal, intrinsic, and postrenal causes (see Table 53.2).
  - Prerenal AKI
    - Most common type in NICU
    - Results from short period of decreased perfusion of the kidneys
    - Typically reversible
    - If tubular function is intact, increased reabsorption of sodium and urea will be seen.
      - FENa < 1%
      - FEUrea < 35%
      - BUN/Cr ratio is increased.
    - Interpretation of the above tests can be difficult in preterm infants, salt-wasting states, or chronic kidney disease.
    - Treatment addresses the underlying cause of poor blood flow to kidneys and includes fluid boluses, blood products, and vasopressors as appropriate.
  - Intrinsic AKI
    - Prerenal AKI can progress to ischemic AKI if there is prolonged hypoperfusion to the kidneys resulting in cellular damage. Severity ranges from mild tubular dysfunction to acute tubular necrosis (ATN) to renal infarction to corticomedullary necrosis.
    - Nephrotoxic AKI results from drugs or endogenous substances: myoglobin, hemoglobin, uric acid (see Box 53.3).
  - Obstructive AKI
    - Results from congenital malformation (UPJ, UVJ, PUV), neurogenic bladder, extrinsic compression, fungal ball, or stone
- Evaluation and diagnosis of AKI:
  - History: maternal medical history/drug exposures, birth history, coexistent conditions (e.g., cardiac or liver issues, sepsis, necrotizing enterocolitis), intake, output, weights, blood pressure, drug exposures
  - Clinical presentation: assessment of fluid status, vital signs, fontanelle, skin turgor, mucus membranes, edema, crackles, murmurs/rubs, color, capillary refill
  - Labs: electrolytes, BUN, creatinine, albumin, complete urinalysis, urinary electrolytes
  - Radiology: renal/bladder U/S, chest x-ray
- Treatment of AKI
  - Remove inciting factors, if possible; restore perfusion via bolus, administer pressors if needed to support blood pressure, and remove nephrotoxic drugs.

Table 53.2 Causes of Acute Kidney Injury in Neonates

Prerenal	Intrinsic	Postrenal
Any cause of intravascular volume depletion (dehydration, bleeding, capillary leak)	Acute tubular necrosis	Congenital obstructions (posterior urethral valve, ureteropelvic junction obstruction, ureterocele)
Hypotension	Congenital: dysplasia, polycystic kidneys	
Sepsis	Pyelonephritis	Neurogenic bladder
Necrotizing enterocolitis	Renal tubule damage: uric acid nephropathy, hemoglobinuria, myoglobinuria	Kidney stones
Congestive heart failure	Drugs: aminoglycosides, amphotericin, acyclovir, radiocontrast dyes	Fungal balls
Drugs: angiotensin-converting enzyme, angiotensin receptor blocker, nonsteroidal anti-inflammatory drug	Renovascular	Extrinsic compression

Box 53.3 Nephrotoxic Medications

Drug	Mechanism
Acyclovir	Urinary precipitation, especially with low flow and hypovolemia, with renal tubular obstruction and damage and decreased GFR; may cause direct tubular toxicity (metabolites)
Angiotensin-converting enzyme inhibitors	Decreased angiotensin II production inhibiting compensatory constriction of the efferent arteriole to maintain GFR
Aminoglycosides	Toxic to the proximal tubules (transport in the tubule, accumulate in lysosome, intracellular rise in reactive oxygen species and phospholipidosis, cell death); intrarenal vasoconstriction and local glomerular/mesangial cell contraction
Amphotericin B	Distal tubular toxicity, vasoconstriction, and decreased GFR
Nonsteroidal anti-inflammatory drugs	Decreased afferent arteriole dilatation as a result of inhibiting prostaglandin production resulting in reduced GFR
Radiocontrast agents	Renal tubular toxicity secondary to increase in reactive oxygen species; intrarenal vasoconstriction may play a role
Vancomycin	Mechanism of AKI unclear; possible mechanism includes proximal tubular injury with generation of reactive oxygen species

AKI, Acute kidney injury; *GFR*, glomerular filtration rate.
From Gleason CA, Juul SE, eds. *Avery's Diseases of the Newborn*. 10th ed. Philadelphia: Elsevier; 2018:1285, Table 90.5.

- Specific therapy for AKI is limited:
  - Theophylline may have a protective effect, as it was shown to decrease AKI rates in asphyxiated infants in one small study.
  - "Renal dose dopamine" was not shown to decrease the rates of AKI in a meta-analysis.
- Manage the consequences of AKI (impaired homeostasis):
- Hyperkalemia (refer to Table 52.3 in Chapter 52):
  - Remove sources of potassium (TPN, feeds, medications such as potassium-sparing diuretic).
  - Correct hypovolemia, if present, with normal saline to deliver Na to distal nephrons to aid in potassium secretion.
  - Stabilize myocardium (calcium).
  - Shift potassium into cells (insulin, sodium bicarbonate, albuterol).
  - Remove potassium from the body using Lasix, binding resin (Kayexalate), or dialysis.

- Metabolic acidosis:
  - $NaHCO_3$ bolus, but note that repeated dosing may make infant hypernatremic
  - Use acetate in TPN/fluids.
- Hypocalcemia: Correct and replete.
- Hyperphosphatemia: Reduce phosphate intake by removing it from TPN, use low-phosphorus feeds (breast milk or Similac PM60/40) and phosphate binders with feeds.
- Hypermagnesemia: Limit intake.
- Fluid status:
  - Fluids should be tailored to individual patient needs.
  - In a fluid-overloaded patient, restrict intake to be less than output; careful use of diuretics may help with volume overload but will not hasten recovery from AKI. For severe overload, dialysis may be required for fluid removal.
  - Euvolemic: Intake = Output + Insensible losses

Table 53.3 Summary of Different Dialysis Modalities

	Peritoneal Dialysis (PD)	Hemodialysis (HD)	Continuous Renal Replacement Therapy (CRRT)
Access	PD catheter is tunneled through abdominal wall into peritoneal space. Non-PD catheters can be used (e.g., chest tube) but they are less ideal.	≥7Fr double-lumen HD catheter in internal jugular or femoral vein *or* two 5Fr single-lumen HD catheters	Same as HD access
Advantages	No anticoagulation is needed. Bedside nurses can do the therapy. If the patient requires chronic dialysis, PD can be done by families at home.	Rapid clearance of solute/toxin	Can be used in hemodynamically unstable patient Fluid removal goal is spread over much longer time (better tolerated than HD).
Disadvantages	Less efficient removal solutes Cannot program fluid loss Cannot be done in patient with abdominal wall defect	Requires specialized nursing Rapid volume shifts Anticoagulation usually needed Usually requires blood prime of circuit	Anticoagulation is needed. Depending on size of baby/machine used, may require blood primes
Complications	Peritonitis Fluid leaks/pleural effusion Loss of proteins into dialysate	Line sepsis Blood clots Air embolism Blood loss	Same as HD

- Hypovolemic: Use boluses or increased total daily fluids to restore normal blood volume.
- Post-obstructive AKI may have polyuria when the obstruction is relieved.

Dialysis

- See Table 53.3.
- Indications include metabolic derangements than cannot be managed medically, fluid overload, toxin/drug removal, and inborn errors of metabolism.
- Peritoneal dialysis is the instillation of dialysate through a catheter placed through the abdominal wall into the peritoneal space.
  - Cycle consists of fill, dwell, and drain; typically each cycle is about an hour in a neonate.
  - Clearance of solutes occurs mostly by diffusion across peritoneal membrane.
  - Ultrafiltration (fluid removal) occurs due to high dextrose concentration in dialysate fluid. Increasing dextrose and decreasing dwell times lead to more fluid removal.
  - Contraindications include abdominal wall defects (absolute), ventriculoperitoneal shunt, and previous significant bowel surgeries (relative).
- Hemodialysis (HD)
  - HD is typically a 3- to 4-hour treatment completed by a hemodialysis nurse.
  - Clearance of solutes occurs due to diffusion across the dialyzer.
  - Ultrafiltration volume can be programmed but is limited by the patient's hemodynamic tolerance.
- Continuous renal replacement therapy (CRRT) is the same principle as HD, but therapy is provided continuously.

Diuretics

- Loop diuretics (furosemide and bumetanide) are highly protein bound so they must be secreted into the tubular lumen, where they act on the thick ascending limb of the loop of Henle Na-K-2Cl transporter.
  - Half-life is much longer in preterm compared to term infants.

- With repeated doses, tolerance to its effect develops, likely due to a compensatory increase in Na reabsorption in other parts of the nephron.
- Adverse effects include hypokalemia, hypomagnesemia, hypocalcemia, hyponatremia, hypercalciuria, nephrocalcinosis, decreased bone density, and deafness.
- Thiazide diuretics (hydrochlorothiazide, chlorothiazide, metolozone) are secreted into the lumen and then bind to the Na-Cl cotransporter in the distal tubule.
  - Thiazide diuretics are less potent than loop diuretics but can be added to a loop diuretic.
  - They are particularly useful to increase the diuretic effect when tolerance to a loop diuretic has developed.
  - Adverse effects include hypokalemia and hyponatremia.
  - Unlike loop diuretics, thiazide diuretics lead to increased calcium reabsorption.
- Aldosterone receptor antagonist (spironolactone) is a weak diuretic.
  - It is primarily used in neonates as potassium-sparing agent in combination with thiazide.
- Other diuretics not commonly used in NICU
  - Mannitol, an osmotic diuretic
  - Carbonic anhydrase inhibitor (acetazolamide), a mild diuretic that acts on the proximal tubule; can be helpful in cases of metabolic alkalosis
  - Amiloride, a potassium-sparing diuretic that blocks the epithelial sodium channel in the collecting duct

Suggested Readings

Guignard JP, Iacobelli S. Use of diuretics in the neonatal period. *Pediatr Nephrol.* 2021;36(9):2687–2695.

Liu DB, Armstrong WR, Maizels M. Hydronephrosis prenatal and postnatal evaluation and management. *Clin Perinatol.* 2014;41(3):661–678.

Murugapoopathy V, Gupta IR. A primer on congenital anomalies of the kidneys and urinary tracts (CAKUT). *Clin J Am Soc Nephrol.* 2020;15(5):723–731.

Resontoc LPR, Yap HK. Renal vascular thrombosis in the newborn. *Pediatr Nephrol.* 2016;31:907–915.

Spector BL, Misurac JM. Renal replacement therapy in neonates. *NeoReviews.* 2019;20(12):e697–e710.

Starr MC, Charlton JR, Guillet R, et al. Advances in neonatal acute kidney injury. *Pediatrics.* 2021;148(5):e2021051220.

Vogt BA, Springel T. The kidney and urinary tract of the neonate. In: Martin RJ, Fanaroff AA, Walsh MC, eds. *Fanaroff and Martin's Neonatal-Perinatal Medicine.* 11th ed. Philadelphia: Elsevier; 2020:1871–1895.

Endocrine, Metabolic, Thermal

DAVID R. WEBER and ALISON FALCK

54 *Normal and Abnormal Sexual Differentiation*

DAVID R. WEBER

Normal Sexual Differentiation

- Sexual differentiation is a process by which the male or female phenotype develops. It begins early in fetal development (Fig. 54.1).
- Chromosomal sexual determination is the formation of XY (male) or XX (female) zygotes via fertilization between a spermatocyte (X or Y) and an oocyte (X).
- Gonadal differentiation is differentiation of the bipotential gonad into testes (male) or ovaries (female).
  - Migration of germ cells to genital ridge begins at week 6.
  - Testicular development is initiated by expression of the *SRY* gene and induces differentiation of Sertoli and Leydig cells.
  - Ovarian development includes differentiation of granulosa and theca cells and proceeds in the absence of *SRY* expression.
- Internal genital differentiation is differentiation of internal genital structures from Wolffian ducts (male) or Müllerian ducts (female)
  - Male:
    - Anti-Müllerian hormone (AMH) secretion by Sertoli cells causes regression of Müllerian ducts
    - It begins at 8 weeks.
    - Testosterone secretion by Leydig cells induces Wolffian ducts to differentiate into epididymis, vas deferens, and seminal vesicles.
  - Female:
    - Absence of AMH and testosterone results in persistence of Müllerian ducts and regression of Wolffian ducts.
    - Müllerian ducts differentiate into fallopian tubes, uterus, cervix, and upper vagina.
- Differentiation of external genital structures from the bipotential urethral folds, genital tubercle, and labioscrotal swellings
  - Males:
    - Virilization under the action of dihydrotestosterone (DHT)
    - Genital tubercle elongates into penis, urethral folds fuse into urethra, labioscrotal swellings fuse into scrotum, and urogenital sinus closes.
    - It begins at week 8, with virilization complete by weeks 12 to 14.
    - Testes begin descent into the scrotum at week 28.
  - Females:
    - External genitalia development proceeds in the absence of androgens.
    - Genital tubercle forms the clitoris and urethral folds.
    - Labioscrotal swellings form labia minora and majora.
    - Urogenital sinus forms the vagina.

Ambiguous Genitalia

OVERVIEW

- A difference in sexual development (DSD; formerly referred to as a "disorder of sexual development") is a discordance in chromosomal, gonadal, and/or genital sex that develops as a result of genetic mutation or environmental exposure.

CLINICAL PRESENTATION

- 46 XY DSD: undervirilized internal and/or external genitalia in a chromosomal male due to impaired androgen production/function
  - Gonadal dysgenesis is partial or complete, symmetric or asymmetric
    - mutation affects the early differentiation of bipotential gonad into testes.
      - Gonadal Yp deletion: mutations in *SRY*, *SOX9*, others
      - Denys-Drash syndrome: gonadal dysgenesis, nephropathy, Wilms tumor due to *WT1* mutation
    - Phenotype varies from complete sex reversal to mild undervirilization.
      - Internal structures and external genitalia can be undervirilized.
    - Low testosterone and AMH
  - Defective testicular hormone production
    - Defective Leydig cell differentiation
      - Mutations in the luteinizing hormone (LH)/human chorionic gonadotropin (hCG) receptor result in Leydig cell hypoplasia/aplasia.
      - Variable internal/external undervirilization is based on receptor activity.
      - AMH is not affected; regression of Müllerian ducts occurs.
      - Labs: elevated LH, low testosterone, no response to hCG stimulation
    - Testosterone biosynthetic defect: mutations affecting dehydrocholesterol reductase (DHCR), StAR, P450 side-chain cleavage, P450

Male development

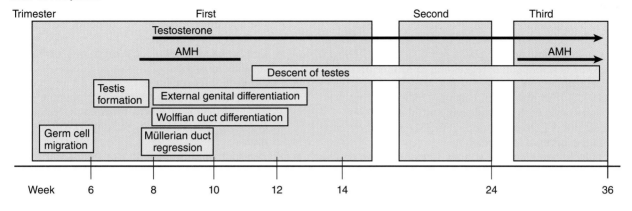

Female development

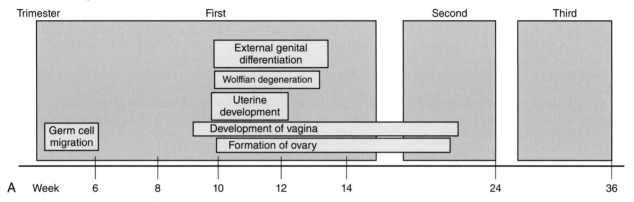

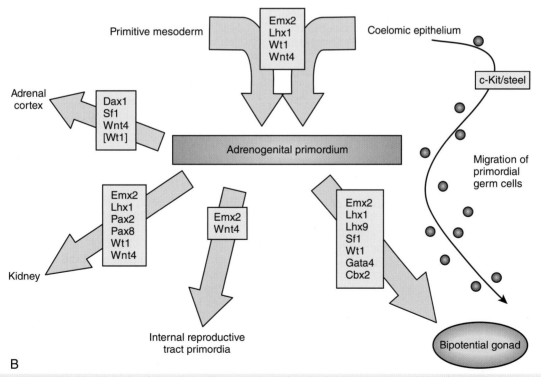

Fig. 54.1 Time line of sexual differentiation. (A) Timetable of gonadal and genital differentiation. (B) Genetic determinants of gonadal development. *AMH*, Anti-Müllerian hormone. (From Jameson JL, De Groot LJ, eds. *Endocrinology: Adult and Pediatric.* 7th ed. Philadelphia: Elsevier; 2016:2051–2085.)

oxidoreductase, 3-β-hydroxysteroid dehydrogenase (3β-HSD), 17α-hydroxylase/17,20-lyase deficiency, 17β-hydroxysteroid dehydrogenase (17β-HSD)
- Variable internal/external undervirilization based on enzymatic activity
- AMH is not affected; regression of Müllerian ducts occurs.
- *DHCR* mutation (Smith-Lemli-Opitz syndrome) is associated with multiple congenital anomalies.
- All but 17,20-lyase and 17β-HSD deficiency can cause adrenal insufficiency.
- Labs show elevated steroid hormone precursors upstream of defect.
- 5α-reductase deficiency: low/absent conversion of testosterone to DHT
  - AMH and testosterone are unaffected; internal structures are normal male.
  - External genitalia are undervirilized to a variable degree.
  - Virilization will occur at puberty as a result of increased testosterone.
  - Labs show an elevated testosterone-to-DHT ratio.
- Defective androgen receptor
  - Partial/complete androgen insensitivity (AIS): androgen receptor mutation
    - Variable undervirilization of external genitalia and internal structures
    - Complete AIS presents as primary amenorrhea in phenotypic female.
    - Labs during infancy may show normal or elevated testosterone.
- 46 XX DSD: virilized chromosomal female due to excess androgen production or phenotypically normal female with absent development of secondary sex characteristic due to impaired estrogen synthesis or action
  - Excessive androgen production due to congenital adrenal hyperplasia (CAH): mutations in p450 oxidoreductase, 3β-HSD, 11β-hydroxylase, 21-hydroxylase
    - Degree of virilization is determined by the magnitude of androgen production.
    - May be associated with adrenal insufficiency, salt wasting
    - See Chapter 55 for details.
  - Gonadal dysgenesis
    - Mutation affecting early differentiation of bipotential gonad into ovary
    - Normal female internal/external genitalia, present in adolescence with primary amenorrhea, absent breast development because of absent ovaries and estrogen

Other DSDs

- Sex chromosome DSD
  - Turner syndrome (45 X): atrophic gonads, normal female external genitalia
  - Klinefelter syndrome (47 XXY): normal male external genitalia at birth
  - Mixed gonadal dysgenesis (45 X/46 XY): phenotype varies from that of Turner syndrome to virilized female based on extent/timing of androgen production

- Ovitesticular DSD: presence of both ovarian and testicular tissue
  - Usually undervirilized XY, depends on the extent of androgen production
  - Can be XX with translocation of *SRY* or mosaicism of sex chromosomes
- Environmental exposures
  - Endocrine hormone disrupters: possible estrogenic/antiandrogenic effects of numerous chemicals
  - Potential contribution to undervirilization of XY males
- Placental aromatase deficiency: excess androgens cross placenta; virilization of XX female
- Maternal androgen/exposure: endogenous/exogenous androgens can cross placenta; virilization of XX female

DIAGNOSIS AND EVALUATION

- Requires early involvement of multidisciplinary team: neonatologist, endocrinologist, urologic/gynecologic surgeon, psychologist, others
- An algorithm for the workup of an infant with ambiguous genitalia is shown in Fig. 54.2.
- Initial workup must include clinical evaluation for signs of adrenal insufficiency and assessment of electrolytes/glucose.
  - Higher likelihood of adrenal insufficiency if infant has nonpalpable gonads
  - Karyotype should be obtained shortly after birth.
    - Chromosomal sex will guide differential diagnosis and further testing.
- Ultrasound, magnetic resonance imaging, and/or genitogram can identify presence of gonads and internal genital structures.
- Hormone studies may include gonadotropins, androgens, androgen precursors, and AMH.
  - Assessment of androgen levels after hCG stimulation may aid in diagnosis of Leydig cell hypoplasia, testosterone biosynthesis defect, and 5α-reductase deficiency.

TREATMENT

- Specific medical and surgical management depends on the disorder.
  - Hydrocortisone ± mineralocorticoid replacement is life sustaining in CAH with adrenal insufficiency (see Chapter 55).
  - Feminizing or virilizing genitoplasty as needed for ambiguous external genitalia
  - Gonadectomy in cases of atrophic/dysplastic gonads due to increased risk of malignancy
  - Sex hormone replacement may be needed at puberty to develop secondary sex characteristics concordant with gender.
- Gender assignment
  - Current practice is to assign gender as soon as possible (allowing for completion of diagnostic workup).
    - Values regarding the timing of this decision may vary based on personal or cultural perspectives.
  - Based on numerous factors, including:
    - Consideration of sex steroid exposure in utero and anticipated future sex steroid production

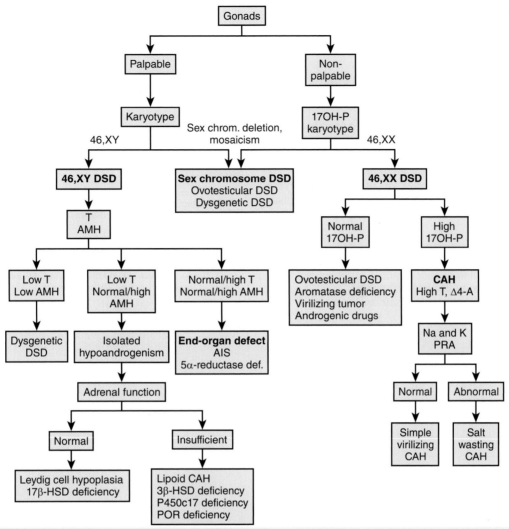

Fig. 54.2 Diagnostic workup of suspected disorder of sexual development. *AIS,* Androgen insensitivity syndrome); *AMH,* anti-Müllerian hormone; *CAH,* congenital adrenal hyperplasia; *DSD,* disorder of sexual development; *HSD,* hydroxysteroid dehydrogenase; *POR,* cytochrome P450 oxidoreductase; *PRA,* plasma renin activity. (From Jameson JL, De Groot LJ, eds. *Endocrinology: Adult and Pediatric.* 7th ed. Philadelphia: Elsevier; 2016:2086–2118.)

- Likelihood of adequate functional and cosmetic outcomes of virilizing versus feminizing surgery
- Potential for future fertility
- Individual cultural perspectives
- Female gender is typically assigned to
  - Virilized XX infants with CAH
  - Nonvirilized XX infants with gonadal dysgenesis
  - XY infants with complete AIS
- Male gender is typically assigned to
  - Undervirilized XY infants when virilizing genitoplasty is expected to be adequate
  - Cases in which significant virilization is expected during puberty (as in 5α-reductase deficiency)
- Incompletely virilized infants with XX or XY gonadal dysgenesis or sex chromosome mosaicism:
  - May be assigned male or female gender based on the degree of virilization of internal/external structures
    - In many instances, long-term data on patient satisfaction with gender assignment are incomplete or inadequate.

- Parents should be allowed to make the final decision regarding gender assignment.

Developmental Anomalies of the Penis, Urethra, and Testicles

CLINICAL PRESENTATION AND DIAGNOSIS

- Hypospadias: Urethral opening is located on the ventral shaft of the penis.
  - Locations: glanular, coronal, subcoronal, midpenile, penoscrotal, scrotal, perineal
- Epispadias: Urethral opening is on the dorsal shaft of the penis.
- Chordee: ventral curvature of penis
- Micropenis: Morphologically normal penis more than 2.5 SD below mean for size
  - Stretched penile length < 2 cm in term infants; cut-off depends on gestational age

- Can be the result of hypothalamic or pituitary dysfunction (growth hormone, gonadotropins); pituitary function should be tested
- Aphallia: congenital absence of penis
- Cryptorchidism: undescended testes
  - Relatively common: ~4% of term males and ~30% of preterm males
    - ~10% of cases are bilateral.
  - Location: abdominal, inguinal, gliding (can be pulled down), ectopic
  - Typically present at birth; may be seen in association with congenital syndromes with multiple midline defects
  - Bilateral nonpalpable testes or presence of severe hypospadias in association with cryptorchidism should be evaluated for DSDs as described above.

TREATMENT

- Hypospadias/epispadias
  - Avoid circumcision in newborn period.
  - Typical age of surgical repair is between 6 and 12 months.
- Micropenis
  - Recombinant human growth hormone if deficient
  - A short course of testosterone (25 mg intramuscular testosterone every 3–4 weeks over 3–4 months) can be given to increase penile size during infancy.
- Cryptorchidism
  - Spontaneous descent is unlikely after 4 months of age (corrected for gestational age).
  - Orchiopexy between 6 and 15 months of age
    - Orchiectomy if testis atrophic

Suggested Readings

Ahmed SF, Achermann J, Alderson J, et al. Society for Endocrinology UK Guidance on the initial evaluation of a suspected difference or disorder of sex development (Revised 2021). *Clin Endocrinol (Oxf)*. 2021;95(6):818–840.

Krishnan S, Wisniewski AB. Ambiguous genitalia in the newborn. In: De Groot LJ, Chrousos G, Dungan K, et al. eds. *Endotext [Internet]*. South Dartmouth, MA: MDText.com; 2017.

Lee PA, Houk CP, Ahmed SF, Hughes IA. Consensus statement on management of intersex disorders. *Pediatrics*. 2006;118:e488–e500.

55 *Adrenal Disorders*

DAVID R. WEBER

Adrenal Hormone Physiology

- Anatomy and histology (Fig. 55.1): Adrenal glands, located superior to kidneys, are composed of two distinct endocrine hormone–producing regions: adrenal medulla and adrenal cortex.
  - The adrenal medulla secretes catecholamine hormones (epinephrine, norepinephrine, dopamine), which are synthesized in chromaffin cells.
  - The fully developed adrenal cortex is organized into three different zones that synthesize and secrete steroid hormones:
    - Zona glomerulosa, which secretes mineralocorticoids (aldosterone)
    - Zona fasciculata, which secretes glucocorticoids (cortisol)
    - Zona reticularis, which secretes adrenal androgens (androstenedione and dehydroepiandrosterone [DHEA])
  - Fetal adrenal steroid hormone production occurs in a transient fetal zone.
- Embryology and fetal development: The hormone-secreting cells of the medulla are derived from the neuroectoderm; those of the cortex are derived from the mesoderm.
  - The adrenal gland is formed and begins to secrete steroid hormones by weeks 8 to 10.
  - The timing, location, and magnitude of steroid hormone synthesis after week 8 are regulated by the fetoplacental unit.
  - The mother provides cholesterol for steroid hormone synthesis and receives progesterone and estrogens at levels necessary to maintain pregnancy.
  - The placenta expresses enzymes (3β-hydroxysteroid dehydrogenase [3β-HSD], aromatase) necessary for the conversion of cholesterol into steroid hormone precursors and androgens into estrogens.
  - The fetus receives steroid hormone precursors for glucocorticoid and androgen hormone synthesis, provides androgens to the placenta, and receives estrogens necessary for organ/tissue development.
  - The fetal zone of the adrenal cortex involutes rapidly following birth and is largely undetectable by 6 to 12 months.
- In steroid hormone synthesis, steroid hormones are synthesized from cholesterol through a sequential series of enzymatic reactions (Fig. 55.2).
  - Steroid acute regulatory protein (StAR) is required for cholesterol transport to the inner mitochondrial membrane.
  - Conversion of cholesterol into pregnenolone is the rate-limiting step.

- Six enzymes expressed in the adrenal gland are responsible for steroidogenesis:
  - Five members of the cytochrome P450 family (CYP11A1, CYP17, CYP21, CYP11B1, and CYP11B2; see Fig. 55.2)
  - One additional steroid dehydrogenase: 3β-HSD
- The final steps of androgen conversion from DHEA and androstenedione into testosterone and estrogen occur only outside of the adrenal glands (gonads and some peripheral tissues).

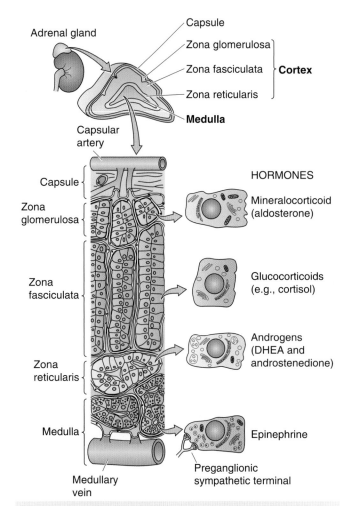

Fig. 55.1 The adrenal gland. Anatomy and organization of the adrenal gland. Catecholamine hormones are synthesized and secreted by the adrenal medulla; steroid hormones are synthesized and secreted by the adrenal cortex. *DHEA,* Dehydroepiandrosterone. (From Rhoades RA, Bell DR, eds. *Medical Physiology: Principles for Clinical Medicine.* 3rd ed. Philadelphia: Elsevier; 2016:1018–1034.)

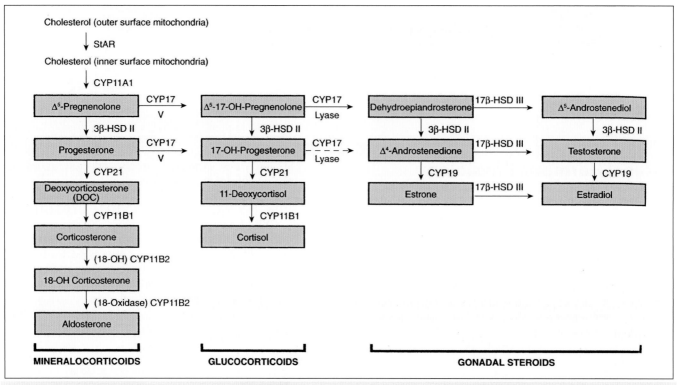

Fig. 55.2 Steroidogenesis. Diagram of the steroid synthesis pathway. Steroid hormones and precursors are shown in *boxes*; enzymes are shown next to *arrows*. *CYP11A1*, Cholesterol side-chain cleavage enzyme; *CYP11B1*, 11β-hydroxylase; *CYP11B2*, 18-hydroxylase and 18-oxidase, also known as aldosterone synthetase; *CYP17*, 17α-hydroxylase and 17,20-lyase; *CYP19*, aromatase; *CYP21*, 21-hydroxylase. (From Marcdante KJ, Kliegman RM. *Nelson Essentials of Pediatrics*. 7th ed. Philadelphia: Elsevier; 2015:607–611.)

- Pathophysiology: Steroid hormones exert their action through nuclear hormone receptors.
  - Aldosterone functions to promote sodium and water retention, raise blood pressure, and lower potassium.
    - The process is regulated by the renin–angiotensin system, potassium concentration, and the pituitary hormone adrenocorticotropic hormone (ACTH).
  - Cortisol regulates both resting physiology and the stress response.
    - The glucocorticoid receptor is expressed in most cells.
    - Glucocorticoids affect cellular action via regulation of gene transcription.
    - Key physiologic actions of glucocorticoids include regulation of glucose homeostasis, fat metabolism, cardiovascular reactivity and blood pressure, sodium and potassium balance, and mood and appetite.
    - At high levels, glucocorticoids cause immunosuppression and inhibit growth.
    - Cortisol secretion is under hypothalamic–pituitary control via the actions of corticotropin-releasing hormone (hypothalamus) and ACTH (pituitary)
  - Adrenal androgens (androstenedione and DHEA) are sex steroids essential to the function of the fetoplacental unit as above and contribute to the development of secondary sex characteristics in puberty.
    - The synthesis and secretion of adrenal androgens fall after birth and remain low until puberty.

  - Increased production at puberty contributes to physical signs of adrenarche (acne, body odor, pubic/axillary hair).
  - Sustained elevations of ACTH increase androgen production with physiologic consequences in congenital adrenal hyperplasia (CAH).

Congenital Adrenal Hyperplasia

OVERVIEW

- CAH is an inherited disease and is due to a defect in one of the enzymes necessary for steroidogenesis.
- All forms are autosomal recessive.
- Incidence is from 1 per 10,000 to 1 per 20,000 live births.
- Mutations in CYP21 (21-hydroxylase) account for ~95% of all cases of CAH.
  - 75% also have salt wasting due to aldosterone deficiency ("classic salt wasting").
  - The remainder have aldosterone synthesis preserved ("simple virilizing").
  - Non-classic 21-hydroxylase deficiency is a mild form with preserved cortisol and aldosterone synthesis; it typically presents later in life with androgen excess.
- Pathophysiology
  - Enzymatic defect results in decreased cortisol production.
  - ACTH levels increase in response to low cortisol.

Table 55.1 Identifying Features of Different Forms of Congenital Adrenal Hyperplasia Presenting in Infancy

CAH Form	Ambiguous Genitalia	Salt Wasting	Steroid Hormone Abnormalities	Other Notable Clinical Features
3β-HSD				
■ Classical	M ± F	Yes	↑ Δ5P, Δ517-OHP, DHEA	—
■ Nonclassical	F only	No	↑ PRA	
CYP11B1				
■ Classical	F only	Yes	↑ 11-DOC, 11-deoxycortisol, 17-OHP	■ Hypertension
■ Nonclassical	None	No	↓ PRA, aldosterone	■ Infantile gynecomastia
CYP17	M only	No	↑ 11-DOC, corticosterone, 18-hydroxycorticosterone	■ Low potassium hypertension
			↓ PRA, aldosterone	
CYP21				
■ Classical	F only	Yes	↑ 17-OHP, Δ5P, Δ517-OHP, DHEA, Δ5–A	■ Cause of >90% of all CAH
■ Simple virilizing	F only	No[a]	↑ PRA	
■ Nonclassical	None	No		
POR deficiency	M and F	No	↓ Levels of all CYP-dependent hormones	■ Skeletal and craniofacial anomalies
			↑ Progesterone, 17-OHP	■ Maternal virilization
StAR/CYP11A1 (congenital lipoid hyperplasia)	M only	Yes	↓ Undetectable levels of all steroids	■ Fatty infiltration adrenal glands
			↑ PRA, ACTH	■ Often fatal in infancy

3β-HSD, 3β-Hydroxysteroid dehydrogenase; *11-DOC*, 11-deoxycorticosterone; *17-OHP*, 17-hydroxyprogesterone; *Δ5P*, pregnenolone; *Δ5–A*, androstenedione; *17-Δ5P*, pregnenolone; *Δ517-OHP*, 17-hydrodxypregnenolone; *ACTH*, adrenocorticotropic hormone; *CAH*, congenital adrenal hyperplasia; *CYP*, cytochrome P450; *CYP11A1*, cholesterol side-chain cleavage enzyme; *CYP11B1*, 11β-hydroxylase; *CYP17*, 17α-hydroxylase and 17,20-lyase; *CYP21*, 21-hydroxylase; *DHEA*, dehydroepiandrosterone; *F*, female; *M*, male; *POR*, P450 oxidoreductase; *PRA*, plasmin renin activity; *StAR*, steroidogenic acute regulatory protein.
[a]An elevated PRA and some degree of salt wasting may be present in infancy.

- High ACTH leads to excess stimulation of adrenal cortex and increased production of steroid hormone precursors.
- Steroid hormone precursors are shunted into the androgen synthesis pathway, leading to increased production of sex steroids.
- Excess androgens/sex steroids result in virilization, rapid growth, early skeletal maturation, and precocious puberty.

CLINICAL PRESENTATION

- Clinical presentation in infancy varies based on sex, genotype, and residual enzymatic activity (Table 55.1).
  - Cortisol deficiency
    - Hypoglycemia
    - Hypotension
    - Hyponatremia/hyperkalemia
    - Poor feeding/vomiting
    - Poor weight gain
    - Typically manifests 7 to 10 days after birth
  - Aldosterone deficiency (if present)
    - Salt wasting with hyponatremia, hyperkalemia
    - In combination with cortisol deficiency can lead to hypovolemic shock
    - Typically manifests 7 to 10 days after birth
  - Androgen excess
    - Virilization manifested as ambiguous genitalia at birth in females
    - Hyperpigmentation and/or penile enlargement may be present in males.
    - Progressive androgen excess postnatally in males and females if untreated

- Androgen deficiency
  - Mutations blocking androgen synthesis (StAR, CYP11A1, 3β-HSD, CYP17) may manifest as ambiguous genitalia in males.

DIAGNOSIS AND EVALUATION

- Newborn screening for 21-hydroxylase CAH
  - Measurement of 17-hydroxyprogesterone (17-OHP) in capillary blood on day of life (DOL) 2
  - Levels drawn in the first 24 hours may be falsely elevated.
  - 17-OHP levels are higher in premature infants and must be interpreted against local lab reference ranges according to gestational age and/or weight.
  - Classic CAH is typically associated with 17-OHP levels > 10,000 ng/dL (300 nmol/L); unaffected individuals typically have values < 100 ng/dL (3 nmol/L).
  - Elevated or borderline levels should be repeated with a venous blood sample.
- Diagnosis can be confirmed with ACTH stimulation testing or CYP21 sequencing.
  - ACTH stimulation to measure serum 17-OHP at times 0 and 60 minutes after injection of 125 μg or 250 μg cosyntropin (Cortrosyn)
    - Stimulated 17-OHP > 10,000 ng/dL is consistent with classic CAH.
    - Stimulated 17-OHP <1000 ng/dL is normal.
    - Stimulated 17-OHP between 1000 and 10,000 ng/dL may represent nonclassic 21-hydroxylase CAH or another form of CAH (11β-hydroxylase).
  - Treatment should not be delayed while awaiting confirmation if there is clinical evidence of adrenal insufficiency or salt wasting.

- Diagnosis of salt wasting
  - Low sodium, high potassium
  - Elevated plasma renin activity (PRA)
  - Low aldosterone
  - Low aldosterone/PRA ratio
- Testing for other forms of CAH (non-21-hydroxylase disease)
  - Basal steroid profile: 17-OH pregnenolone, 17-OH progesterone, 11-deoxycorticosterone (DOC), 11-deoxycortisol, androstenedione, DHEA, cortisol
  - ACTH stimulation as described above, with additional steroids from above list added based on clinical suspicion (see Table 55.1)

TREATMENT

- Goal of treatment for all forms of CAH is physiologic glucocorticoid and mineralocorticoid (if necessary) replacement.
- Hydrocortisone 10 to 15 mg/m^2 of body surface area per day divided into three daily doses
  - Follow 17-OHP, androstenedione, testosterone, growth, and physical exam for signs of androgen excess to evaluate treatment.
  - ACTH is not a reliable marker of treatment adequacy.
  - 17-OHP levels in the normal range typically indicate overtreatment.
  - Overtreatment results in poor growth and obesity.
- Stress dosing with hydrocortisone 50 to 100 mg/m^2 of body surface area per day
  - Fever, acute illness
  - Surgery requiring general anesthesia
  - Trauma
- Treatment of salt wasting (if present)
  - Infants typically require higher doses of fludrocortisone and salt supplements then older children.

- Low sodium content of breast milk/formula
  - Immaturity of kidneys to reabsorb sodium
- Fludrocortisone 0.05 to 0.2 mg/d divided into one to two daily doses
- NaCl supplements 1 to 2 g/d mixed into two to three feedings per day
- Follow potassium, plasma renin activity, and blood pressure to evaluate treatment.
  - High potassium, PRA: increase fludrocortisone and/or NaCl dose
  - Suppressed PRA, hypertensive: decrease doses
- Prenatal treatment of affected fetuses remains experimental.
  - Goal of treatment is to suppress adrenal androgen production and minimize prenatal virilization of affected females.
  - Dexamethasone is used because it is not inactivated by placenta.
  - Treatment is instituted by 6 to 8 weeks in potentially affected fetuses.
    - Treatment would occur prior to the age when genetic confirmation and sex determination can be made.
    - Thus, seven out of eight fetuses would be exposed to therapy with no potential benefit.

Suggested Readings

Mallappa A, Merke DP. Management challenges and therapeutic advances in congenital adrenal hyperplasia. *Nat Rev Endocrinol.* 2022;18(6):337–352.

Merke DP, Auchus RJ. Congenital adrenal hyperplasia due to 21-hydroxylase deficiency. *N Engl J Med.* 2020;383(13):1248–1261.

Nimkam S, Gangishetti PK, Yau M, New MI. 21-Hydroxylase-deficient congenital adrenal hyperplasia. In: *GeneReviews [Internet].* Seattle, WA: University of Washington, Seattle; 2002.

Speiser PW, Wiebke A, Auchus RJ, et al. Congenital adrenal hyperplasia due to steroid 21-hydroxylase deficiency: an endocrine society clinical practice guideline. *J Clin Endocrinol Metab.* 2018;103(11):4043–4088.

56 *Thyroid Disorders*

DAVID R. WEBER

Thyroid Embryology and Physiology

- Embryology: The thyroid gland is derived from two distinct embryologic tissues.
  - Thyroid hormone-producing cells (follicular cells) are derived from endodermal cells lining the floor of the primitive pharynx (thyroid anlage).
    - Primordial thyroid is identifiable at 4 weeks.
    - It migrates downward through the tongue to its final location in the anterior neck.
    - It is connected to tongue via the thyroglossal duct.
    - The thyroglossal duct can persist as a thyroglossal duct cyst.
  - Calcitonin-producing cells (C-cells) are derived from neural crest cells in the fourth and fifth pharyngeal pouches (ultimobranchial bodies).
    - C-cells fuse with the thyroid anlage to form the definitive thyroid gland by 8 to 10 weeks.
- Physiology:
  - Thyroid hormone production occurs in the follicular cell.
    - Regulated by thyroid-stimulating hormone (TSH) secreted from the pituitary gland
    - Iodide is transported into cell via sodium iodide symporter.
    - Iodide is oxidized by thyroidal peroxidase and bound to tyrosine residues in thyroglobulin, forming monoiodotyrosine (MIT) and diiodotyrosine (DIT)
    - MIT and DIT molecules combine to form the thyroid hormones thyroxine (T4) and triiodothyronine (T3).
    - T4 and T3 are freed from thyroglobulin by enzymes and secreted in a ratio of ~5:1.
    - The majority of T4 and T3 circulates bound to thyroid-binding globulin (TBG).
  - Peripheral metabolism and regulation of thyroid hormones
    - T3 has three- to fourfold greater potency than T4.
    - T3 is generated from T4 peripherally via type I and II deiodinase (D1, D2).
    - T3 and T4 are inactivated into reverse T3 by type III deiodinase (D3).
  - Cellular action of thyroid hormones
    - Thyroid hormones enter peripheral cells via thyroid hormone transporters.
    - Signal via the thyroid hormone receptor (THR)
      - □ Expressed in nearly all tissues
      - □ Critical regulator of growth and metabolism (Fig. 56.1)

- Fetal thyroid physiology
  - Maternal T4 crosses the placenta and is essential for development until fetal thyroid hormone production begins.
    - Fetal thyroid hormone synthesis begins by 12 to 14 weeks.
    - Hypothalamic–pituitary–thyroid control is in place by 18 to 20 weeks.
  - T3 and TSH do not cross the placenta.
  - TSH receptor stimulating and blocking antibodies can cross the placenta.
- Thyroid physiology at transition
  - TSH surge at birth occurs in response to exposure to colder ex utero environment.
    - TSH peaks within 24 hours, then falls rapidly; there is a risk of false-positive TSH screens drawn in the first 24 hours.
    - T4 peaks on day of life (DOL) 2.
  - TSH and T4 peaks are lower in premature infants, although still present.

Congenital Hypothyroidism

OVERVIEW

- Epidemiology: incidence of congenital hypothyroidism is 1:2500–1:4000 live births.
- Etiology
  - Thyroid dysgenesis: defect in thyroid development (~80–90% of cases)
    - Ectopic thyroid (failure of thyroid gland to descend completely)
    - Hypoplasia (incomplete development of gland)
    - Athyreosis (complete absence of gland)
    - Genes implicated include *TTF1*, *TSHR*, *PAX8*, and others.
  - Thyroid dyshormonogenesis: defect in thyroid hormone synthesis (10–20% of cases)
    - Genetic defects in *NIS*, *TPO*, *TG*, *NIS*, *THOX-2*, and others
  - Central hypothyroidism: defect in hypothalamic/pituitary thyroid control (rare)
    - Genetic defects in *THRH*, *PROP*, *PIT-1*, and others
    - May be associated with other pituitary hormone defects
  - Peripheral forms of hypothyroidism (rare)
    - Defective thyroid hormone transport: monocarboxylate transporter 8 (MCT8) deficiency, others
    - Consumptive hypothyroidism

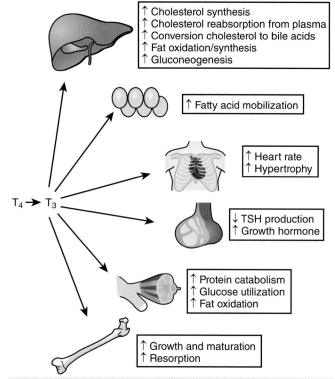

Fig. 56.1 Thyroid hormone action. Thyroid hormone acts in nearly all body tissues to promote growth and regulate metabolism. *TSH,* Thyroid-stimulating hormone. (From Jameson JL, De Groot LJ. *Endocrinology: Adult and Pediatric.* 7th ed. Philadelphia: Elsevier; 2016:1336–1349.)

□ Thyroid hormone deactivation because of D3 overexpression, most commonly in infantile hepatic hemangiomas
- Transient hypothyroidism
  - Exposure to maternal antithyroid medications in utero
  - Placental passage of maternal TSH receptor-blocking antibodies
  - Endemic iodide deficiency
  - Prenatal or postnatal iodide exposure
    □ Inhibits iodide organification (Wolff-Chaikoff effect)
- Transient hypothyroxinemia of prematurity (THOP)
  - Most common in premature infants less than 30 weeks' gestational age (WGA)
  - THOP may be associated with adverse neurodevelopmental outcomes, but there is insufficient evidence to determine if this relationship is cause or effect.

CLINICAL PRESENTATION

- Signs/symptoms are usually not present at birth, but if untreated the following may develop:
  - Jaundice
  - Lethargy/hypotonia
  - Poor feeding
  - Constipation
  - Hypothermia
  - Macroglossia

- Large/persistent anterior fontanelle
- Intrauterine growth restriction (IUGR)/failure to thrive
- Progressive developmental delay

DIAGNOSIS AND EVALUATION

- Newborn screening from capillary blood spot
  - Primary TSH screen with back-up T4 for elevated TSH
    - Cutoff selected to detect elevated TSH
    - False-positive result if drawn in first 24 to 48 hours (TSH surge)
    - False-negative result in newborns with central hypothyroidism
  - Primary T4 screen with back-up TSH for low T4
    - Cutoff set locally to detect low T4
    - False-positive result in newborns with TBG deficiency
      □ Most commonly because of X-linked mutation in *SERPINA7*
- Abnormal newborn screen
  - Confirm with venous TSH, T4 (or free T4) at DOL 2 or later.
  - Choice of T4, free T4, or T3 resin uptake test depends on local lab.
    - Free T4 should be checked if TBG deficiency is suspected, as the patient is euthyroid with normal free T4 and TSH but low T4.
  - Elevated TSH with low T4 (or free T4) is consistent with primary hypothyroidism.
    - Thyroid ultrasound or thyroid scan can be performed but is not required.
  - Low/normal TSH with low T4
    - Central hypothyroidism
      □ Testing of other pituitary hormones should be done
      □ Consider brain imaging
  - THOP (see earlier)
- Labs and clinical features in conditions of abnormal thyroid physiology are shown in Table 56.1.

TREATMENT

- Goal is to attain normal thyroid hormone levels as soon as possible.
  - Treatment should not be delayed if confirmatory labs are not readily available.
  - Normalize T4 within 2 weeks.
  - Normalize TSH within 4 weeks.
  - Follow labs every 1 to 3 months for the first 12 months.
- Levothyroxine (T4) should be initiated at 10 to 15 µg/kg/d.
  - Tablet and liquid preparations are approved for use in infants.
  - Local compounding of tablets into liquid solution is not advised due to questions about stability.
  - Intravenous dose of levothyroxine is 50% to 75% of the oral dose for patients who cannot take enteral medications.

Table 56.1 Laboratory Findings and Clinical Findings in Conditions of Abnormal Thyroid Hormone Physiology Affecting Neonates

Condition	TSH	T4	Free T4	T3	Free T3	Reverse T3	Notable Clinical Features
Congenital hypothyroidism–primary	↑	↓	↓	↓	↓	↓/nml	AGA/LGA
Congenital hypothyroidism–secondary/ tertiary	↓/nml/↑	↓	↓	↓	↓	↓/nml	▪ Jaundice ▪ Lethargy ▪ Hypotonia
Consumptive hypothyroidism	↑	↓	↓	↓	↓	↑	▪ Hemangioma
Neonatal hyperthyroidism	↓	↑	↑	↑	↑	↑/nml	▪ Tachycardia ▪ Hypertension ▪ IUGR ▪ FTT ▪ Exophthalmos
Transient hypothyroxinemia of prematurity	nml/↓	↓	↓	↓	↓	↓/nml	▪ <30 WGA ▪ Blunted TSH surge ▪ No abnormal clinical phenotype
TBG/other thyroid hormone carrier deficiency	nml	↓	nml	↓	nml	nml	▪ No abnormal clinical phenotype
MCT8/other thyroid hormone transport deficiency	nml/↑	nml/↓	nml/↓	↑	↑	↓	▪ Hypotonia ▪ Cognitive impairment ▪ Neurologic abnormalities

AGA, Appropriate for gestational age; *FTT*, failure to thrive; *IUGR*, intrauterine growth restriction; *LGA*, large for gestational age; *MCT8*, monocarboxylate transporter 8; *nml*, normal; *TBG*, thyroid binding globulin; *TSH*, thyroid stimulating hormone; *T3*, triiodothyronine; *T4*, thyroxine; *WGA*, weeks' gestational age.

- Thyroid function tests should be checked within ~2 weeks of changing from oral to intravenous formulations (or the reverse) to assess dose adequacy.
- Monitoring
  - Labs: Maintain T4 (or free T4) in the upper one-half of the normal range and TSH in the normal range for the first year of life.
  - Growth: Length should be checked regularly; growth rate should be normal.
  - Cognitive development should be assessed per routine developmental screening guidelines.
    - Infants with adequately treated hypothyroidism should meet developmental milestones.
- Follow-up
  - At 3 years of age, a trial off therapy can be considered to determine if hypothyroidism is permanent.
    - Initial TSH value of >50 mIU/L suggests permanent hypothyroidism.
    - Obtaining a thyroid ultrasound to confirm presence of thyroid gland can be considered prior to stopping therapy.
    - A rise in TSH or fall in T4 (or free T4) 30 to 45 days after stopping therapy indicates need for continued therapy.
- Transient hypothyroidism
  - Neonatal hypothyroidism because of maternal antithyroid treatment or blocking antibodies requires short-term levothyroxine therapy as above.
  - Transient hypothyroidism as a result of iodine deficiency is treated with levothyroxine and iodine supplementation (90 μg/d in term infants).
  - Current evidence does not support routine treatment of THOP.

Neonatal Hyperthyroidism

OVERVIEW

- Epidemiology: Neonatal hyperthyroidism is rare and is usually due to passage of TSH receptor-stimulating antibodies (TRAbs) in the setting of maternal Graves' disease.
  - Antibodies can persist in maternal circulation for years after definitive treatment with thyroidectomy or radioactive ablation.
  - 1% to 10% of neonates born to mothers with Graves' disease will develop thyrotoxicosis.
  - Rarely, maternal Hashimoto thyroiditis can cause passage of TRAbs.
  - Rare genetic diseases that cause neonatal hyperthyroidism include McCune-Albright syndrome (activating mutation in *GNAS*) or activating mutations in the TSH receptor.

CLINICAL PRESENTATION

- Neonatal Graves' disease typically presents within the first week but may be delayed up to 6 to 8 weeks.
  - Presentation is delayed in mothers treated with antithyroid med during pregnancy.
- Fetal tachycardia or goiter may be detected in utero in some but not all cases.
  - Increased risk of IUGR and premature delivery with fetal thyrotoxicosis
  - Microcephaly, craniosynostosis, or exophthalmos may be present at birth.
- Signs/symptoms of neonatal thyrotoxicosis

- Tachycardia/hypertension
- Jitters/poor sleep
- Spitting up/vomiting
- Failure to gain weight/weight loss

DIAGNOSIS AND EVALUATION

- All infants born to women with a history of Graves's disease should be monitored closely.
  - Maternal TRAb levels should be checked in the second and third trimesters.
  - Higher risk of neonatal Graves's disease in mothers with TRAb levels greater than three- to fivefold the upper limit.
- TSH, T4 (or free T4), and T3: TRAb levels should be assessed from cord blood or venous sample in high-risk infants (+ maternal TRAb; history of neonatal Graves's disease with previous pregnancy) at birth.
  - Suppressed TSH and elevated T4 are consistent with neonatal Graves's disease.
  - Initial lab values may be normal in mothers treated with antithyroid meds.
- Low-risk infants (low maternal TRAb levels) or normal TRAb levels at birth can be followed clinically.

TREATMENT

- Beta blocker to control symptoms of hyperthyroidism (propranolol 1–2 mg/kg/d divided every 8 hours)

- Antithyroid medication to reduce thyroid hormone production
  - Methimazole 0.25 to 1 mg/kg/d divided every 12 hours
  - Iodine (Lugol's solution 126 mg/mL) can be added at 1 drop (8 mg)/d for 1 to 2 weeks.
- Glucocorticoids can be considered in severely symptomatic infants
  - Decrease thyroid hormone production and decrease the conversion of T4 to T3
- Monitor labs every 1 to 2 weeks; the goal is normal TSH, T4 (or free T4), and T3 levels.
- Self-limited; typically resolves within 3 to 6 weeks but may persist 6 months or longer
- Neonatal thyrotoxicosis in the absence of maternal Graves' disease or that does not resolve within 6 months should be further evaluated for genetic etiology.

Suggested Readings

Brown RS. Congenital hypothyroidism. In: De Groot LJ, Chrousos G, Dungan K, et al., eds. *Endotext [Internet]*. South Dartmouth, MA: MDText.com; 2000–2015.

La Gamma EF, Korzeniewski SJ, Ballabh P, Paneth N. Transient hypothyroxinemia of prematurity. *Pediatrics*. 2016;17(7):e394–e402.

Rose SR, Wassner AJ, Wintergerst KA, et al. Congenital hypothyroidism: screening and management. *Pediatrics*. 2023;151(1):e2022060420.

Van der Kaay DCM, Wasserman JD, Palmert MR. Management of neonates born to mothers with Graves' disease. *Pediatrics*. 2016;137(4): e20151878.

57 *Glucose Metabolism*

DAVID R. WEBER

Physiology of Energy Metabolism

- Adenosine triphosphate (ATP) provides the energy for cellular metabolism.
- Three major fuel sources of ATP are carbohydrates, fat, and protein.
- Sufficient ATP availability for cellular function is achieved through a complex web of hormonal, neural, and enzymatic regulation termed intermediary metabolism.
- Carbohydrate metabolism
  - ATP is generated from glucose via glycolysis.
  - Plasma glucose is maintained in a tight range (70–100 mg/dL).
    - Hepatic glucose production (fasting/basal state)
      - Glycogenolysis (breakdown of glycogen to form glucose)
      - Gluconeogenesis (synthesis of glucose from substrates including lactate, glycerol, gluconeogenic amino acids); occurs mostly in liver, also in kidneys, brain, muscle, gut
    - Gastrointestinal absorption (fed state)
      - Regulated by rate of gastric emptying and controlled by incretins (glucagon-like peptide 1 [GLP-1], cholecystokinin [CCK], others) and vagal tone
      - Glucose is absorbed via sodium-dependent sodium–glucose cotransporter-1 (SGLT1) in the small intestine.
    - Glucose disposal
      - Transported into cells via glucose transporters (GLUTs)
        - GLUT-1 (red blood cell [RBC], blood–brain barrier) is glucose dependent.
        - GLUT-2 (pancreas, liver, kidney, gut) is the glucose sensor.
        - GLUT-3 (neurons, placenta)
        - GLUT-4 (liver, fat) is insulin dependent.
      - Insulin is released from pancreatic β cells.
        - Promotes glucose uptake
        - Promotes glycogenesis and blocks glycogenolysis
        - Promotes lipogenesis and blocks lipolysis
- Fat metabolism
  - Adipose tissue is the largest energy storage depot in the body.
    - Lipolysis is the catabolism of triglycerides into glycerol and free fatty acids.
      - Glycerol is used by liver for gluconeogenesis.
      - Free fatty acids (FFAs) generate ATP via β-oxidation and the tricarboxylic acid (TCA) cycle.
      - Can also be converted into ketone bodies by the liver
      - Ketones are used by the brain and peripheral tissue as an alternative fuel source for the TCA cycle and ATP generation.
- Protein metabolism
  - Catabolism of muscle during fasting releases amino acids into the circulation.
    - Gluconeogenic amino acids (alanine, others) are used for gluconeogenesis.
    - Ketogenic amino acids (leucine, lysine, others) are converted into ketone bodies.
- Counterregulatory hormones are secreted in response to falling blood sugar.
  - Glucagon (pancreas): plasma glucose < 65 to 70 mg/dL
    - ↑ Glycogenolysis and gluconeogenesis (liver)
  - Epinephrine (adrenal medulla): plasma glucose < 65 to 70 mg/dL
    - ↑ Glycogenolysis and gluconeogenesis (liver), antagonizes insulin
  - Cortisol/growth hormone (adrenal/pituitary): plasma glucose < 65 mg/dL
    - Antagonizes insulin, mobilizes fatty acids, mobilizes amino acids
- Fetal energy metabolism
  - Placental glucose accounts for the majority (~65%) of the fetal energy source.
    - Glucose provides a substrate for glycogen and adipose synthesis and deposition.
    - Fetus is capable of glycogenolysis, gluconeogenesis, and lipolysis.
    - It provides a protective mechanism in the setting of maternal starvation.
  - Lactate and ketone bodies also cross the placenta and provide an alternative fuel source.
- Energy metabolism during transition to postnatal life:
  - Acute loss in placental glucose transfer results in transient decline in plasma glucose.
    - Stimulate hormonal response to raise and stabilize glucose.
      - Increased secretion of counterregulatory hormones
      - Decreased secretion of insulin
    - Glycogen stores are depleted in hours, and the infant becomes dependent on gluconeogenesis from amino acids, lactate, and fatty acids, as well as oxidation of ketones from ketogenesis.
  - Plasma glucose levels rise to normal child/adult levels (70–100 mg/dL) by 48 hours.

Hypoglycemia

OVERVIEW

- Hypoglycemia is the glucose level at which brain function begins to be impaired.
  - By convention, glucose concentration is reported as plasma glucose; whole blood glucose concentration is 10% to 20% lower than plasma glucose.
  - Controversy exists regarding the numerical cutoff to define hypoglycemia in neonates.
  - Level varies by age and availability of alternate fuel availability (ketones, lactate).
    - Brain glucose utilization is impaired when plasma glucose < 55 to 65 mg/dL.
    - Conditions limiting the availability of ketones/lactate increase the risk of central nervous system damage and require maintenance of higher plasma glucose levels.
  - Generally, at <48 hours of life hypoglycemia is defined as plasma glucose < 47 mg/dL. Transient plasma glucose down to 30 mg/dL can be seen in healthy infants in the first 24 hours.
  - Generally, at ≥48 hours of life, hypoglycemia is defined as plasma glucose < 60 to 70 mg/dL, with only 2% of infants at >48 hours noted to have a plasma glucose < 50 mg/dL.
    - Above targets are individualized based on risk factors.
    - Glucose levels between 50 and 60 mg/dL may be tolerated beyond 48 hours in premature infants.
    - The presence of metabolic disease warrants maintaining glucose levels at >60 to 70 mg/dL in hyperinsulinism where ketogenesis is impaired.
    - The American Academy of Pediatrics and the Pediatric Endocrine Society periodically review new literature and reassess target serum glucose levels to maximize outcomes while minimizing overtreatment.

CLINICAL PRESENTATION

- Signs and symptoms
  - Often asymptomatic
  - Jitteriness, irritability, lethargy, seizures
  - Intrauterine growth restriction (IUGR), preterm, large for gestational age (LGA), and infant of diabetic mother (IDM) are associated with increased hypoglycemia risk.

DIAGNOSIS AND EVALUATION

- Confirm low plasma glucose on glucometer with venous sample.
- Full diagnostic workup is typically delayed until >48 hours.
- Critical sample ± glucagon stimulation test to establish diagnosis (Tables 57.1 and 57.2)
  - Follow-up testing may be required based on results.
- Transient forms of hypoglycemia
  - Infant of diabetic mother: hyperinsulinism

Table 57.1   Clinical Evaluation of Neonatal Hypoglycemia

Critical Sample (Obtained With Plasma Glucose < 50 mg/dL)

■ Basic metabolic panel	■ Growth hormone[a]
■ Insulin	■ Cortisol[a]
■ C-peptide	■ Ammonia
■ β-hydroxybutyrate	■ Lactate
■ Free fatty acids	■ Acylcarnitine profile
■ IGF-BP1	■ Free and total carnitine

Glucagon Stimulation Test

- Test is performed when blood glucose < 50 mg/dL.
- Administer 1 mg glucagon IM/IV.[b]
- Check blood glucose q10 minutes for 40 minutes.
- An increase of blood glucose > 30 mg/dL is consistent with hyperinsulinism.
- Test can be aborted if blood glucose has not risen by 20 mg/dL at 20 minutes.
- Provide dextrose bolus (D10 at 2 cc/kg or similar) to restore normoglycemia.

IGF-BP1, insulin like growth factor binding protein 1; *IM*, intramuscular; *IV*, intravenous.
[a]Low cortisol and/or growth hormone is not diagnostic of pituitary hormone deficiency. Appropriate follow-up provocative testing is required to make diagnosis.
[b]0.5 mg can be considered for premature or low birth weight infants.

- IUGR, small for gestational age, prematurity: limited glycogen stores
- LGA infants: etiology unclear
- Drug-induced
  - Surreptitious insulin, oral hypoglycemic agents
  - Ethanol, beta blocker, terbutaline
  - Suppressed C peptide with detectable insulin suggests exogenous exposure.
- Perinatal stress induced hyperinsulinism
  - May be severe, can last up to 12 months before resolving
- Late dumping
  - Relatively common in infants with G-tubes and Nissen fundoplication
  - Characterized by hypoglycemia 1 to 2 hours post-feed
- Congenital disorders of hypoglycemia
  - Hypopituitarism (growth hormone [GH] and/or cortisol deficiency)
    - Low GH/cortisol on critical sample must be confirmed with provocative test.
  - Congenital hyperinsulinism (HI)
    - Detectable insulin during hypoglycemia
    - Positive response to glucagon stimulation test
  - Beckwith-Wiedemann syndrome (BWS)
    - Hyperinsulinism
    - Often with macrosomia, hemihypertrophy
  - Glycogen storage disease (GSD)
    - Hepatomegaly (except GSD)
  - Disorders of fatty acid oxidation
    - Will have associated abnormalities on acylcarnitine profile
  - Congenital disorder of glycosylation

TREATMENT

- All hypoglycemia: enteral/parenteral dextrose to maintain plasma glucose above target
  - Age <48 hours, typical target plasma glucose is >50 mg/dL.

Table 57.2 Laboratory Findings on Critical Sample in Various Types of Neonatal Hypoglycemia

LABORATORY FINDINGS OBTAINED FROM CRITICAL SAMPLE (PLASMA GLUCOSE < 50 MG/DL)			
No Acidosis ↓ BOHB, ↓ FFA	**No Acidosis** ↓ BOHB, ↑ FFA	**+ Acidosis** ↑ Lactate	**+ Acidosis** ↑ BOHB
▪ Congenital HI[a] ▪ Stress HI[a] ▪ Beckwith-Wiedemann syndrome ▪ GH/cortisol deficiency[b] ▪ Congenital disorder of glycosylation ▪ Drug induced[c]	▪ Disorder of fatty acid oxidation	▪ GSD (types 0, 1) ▪ Fructose-1,6-bisphosphotase deficiency ▪ Pyruvate carboxylase deficiency	▪ GSD (types 3, 6, 9, 10) ▪ Ketotic hypoglycemia ▪ GH/cortisol[b] deficiency ▪ Delayed transition in prematurity

BOHB, Beta-hydroxybutyrate; *FFA*, free fatty acid; *GH*, growth hormone; *GSD*, glycogen-storage disease; *HI*, hyperinsulinism.
[a]Diagnosis of hyperinsulinism is confirmed with the glucagon stimulation test; consider genetic testing if there is suspicion of congenital HI.
[b]Low GH or cortisol on critical sample is not sufficient for diagnosis; provocative testing is required.
[c]Insulin, oral hypoglycemics, beta blockers, ethanol, and terbutaline.

▪ Age ≥48 hours, typical target plasma glucose is >60 mg/dL.
▪ Target glucose is >70 mg/dL for all patients with suspected hypoglycemia disorder.
  ▪ Suppressed ketogenesis and lipolysis limit the availability of alternative fuels.
▪ Hyperinsulinism
  ▪ Glucose infusion rates (GIRs) for congenital hyperinsulinism often exceed 20 to 30 mg/kg/min (normal is ~4–6 mg/kg/min); dextrose fluid concentrations > 12.5% require a central line.
  ▪ Medical management
    ▪ Glucagon infused intravenously (IV) at 1 mg/24 h (independent of weight)
      □ Can also be given PRN as subcutaneous (SC)/intramuscular (IM) injection
    ▪ Diazoxide
      □ Inhibits insulin secretion by opening the K_{ATP} channel
      □ Effective in stress-induced HI, some forms of congenital HI
      □ Effective dose ranges from 5 to 20 mg/kg/d divided bid.
      □ Potential side effects include edema/pulmonary hypertension, cytopenia, and hypertrichosis.
      □ Consider concomitant diuretics.
      □ Follow complete blood count (CBC) every 3 to 6 months.
    ▪ Octreotide
      ▪ Somatostatin analog that inhibits insulin secretion
      ▪ Given via intermittent SC injection or continuous IV (2–20 μg/kg/d)
        □ Tachyphylaxis is common.
      ▪ May be associated with risk of necrotizing enterocolitis in young infants
    ▪ Surgical management: Patients with congenital HI who fail medical management are surgical candidates.
      ▪ Transfer to specialized center is imperative.
      ▪ Genetics and imaging (positron emission tomography/computed tomography) can be used to determine focal versus diffuse HI.
        □ Focal resection versus near-total (95–98%) pancreatectomy

▪ Glycogen storage diseases
  ▪ Continuous glucose delivery with frequent daytime feeds and continuous feeds overnight
  ▪ Older children are transitioned to uncooked cornstarch administered multiple times per night.
▪ Disorders of fatty acid oxidation
  ▪ Continuous glucose delivery and dietary medication/supplementation are targeted to the defect.
▪ Late dumping
  ▪ Continuous feeds; slowing of bolus rate including tapering of rate
  ▪ Acarbose 12.5 to 75 mg/dose given with each bolus feed

Hyperglycemia

OVERVIEW

▪ Persistent hyperglycemia is uncommon in neonates.
▪ Controversy exists regarding the numerical cutoff to define hyperglycemia in neonates.
  ▪ Plasma glucose > 180 mg/dL is often used.

CLINICAL PRESENTATION

▪ Often asymptomatic initially
▪ Polyuria, polydipsia, polyphagia
▪ Failure to thrive or weight loss
▪ IUGR, very low birth weight (VLBW), and premature infants are at increased risk.

DIAGNOSIS AND EVALUATION

▪ Confirm elevated plasma glucose on glucometer with venous sample.
▪ Transient forms of hyperglycemia:
  ▪ Infection
  ▪ Exposure to high-dose enteral/parenteral glucocorticoids
  ▪ Delayed maturation of physiologic mechanisms for glucose disposal
    ▪ Exacerbated with exposure to high GIRs in total parenteral nutrition (TPN)

- Transient neonatal diabetes
  - Onset is in the first week of life, with a median duration of 12 weeks.
  - Most cases are a result of chromosome 6q24 mutations.
- Permanent forms of hyperglycemia
  - Permanent neonatal diabetes
    - Median onset is ~5 weeks; range is birth to 6 months.
    - Most cases are caused by mutations resulting in β-cell under secretion of insulin.
  - Type 1 diabetes
    - Exceedingly uncommon before 6 months of age
    - Autoimmune-mediated destruction of β cells
  - Congenital syndromes of insulin resistance
    - Insulin receptor mutations (Donohue and Rabson-Mendenhall syndromes)

TREATMENT

- Generally, the goal is to maintain plasma glucose between 80 and 180 mg/dL.

- Initial response
  - Reduce GIR
  - Hydration, especially if evidence of osmotic diuresis
- Persistent hyperglycemia requires treatment with insulin.
  - Initially, IV insulin infusion ranges from 0.03 to 0.1 units/kg/h to stabilize glucose.
  - Transition to SC insulin when clinically stable, with doses ranging from 0.2 to 2 units/kg/d.

Suggested Readings

Lemelman MB, Letourneau L, Greeley SAW. Neonatal diabetes mellitus: an update on diagnosis and management. *Clin Perinatol.* 2018;45(1):41–59.

Palladino AA, Bennett MJ, Stanley CA. Hyperinsulinism in infancy and childhood: when an insulin level is not always enough. *Clin Chem.* 2008;54(2):256–263.

Thornton PS, Stanley CA, De Leon DD, et al. Recommendations from the Pediatric Endocrine Society for evaluation and management of persistent hypoglycemia in neonates, infants, and children. *J Pediatr.* 2015;167:238–245.

58 Calcium, Phosphorus, and Magnesium Metabolism

DAVID R. WEBER

Bone Mineral Metabolism

- Skeletal composition
  - Cellular components include osteoblasts, osteoclasts, osteocytes, and organic matrix.
    - Osteoblasts build bone and secrete matrix; they are derived from mesenchymal stem cells.
    - Osteoclasts reabsorb bone and are derived from hematopoietic stem cells.
    - Osteocytes are osteoblasts that become trapped in the matrix; they form a mechanosensation network and secrete hormones.
    - Organic matrix is composed of collagen, proteoglycans, and stromal cells.
      - Provides flexibility to skeleton and a scaffold for mineral deposition
  - Bone mineral is primarily composed of hydroxyapatite, $Ca_{10}(PO_4)_6(OH)_2$.
    - Provides strength to skeleton, as well as a reservoir of calcium (Ca) and phosphorus (P)
    - Bone mineralization requires alkaline phosphatase (ALP).
      - ALP hydrolyzes pyrophosphate (inhibitor of mineralization), thereby allowing hydroxyapatite crystals to form.
- Skeletal development occurs via endochondral or intramembranous ossification.
  - Endochondral ossification (majority of skeleton)
    - Cartilaginous model of skeleton deposited by chondrocytes
      - Complete cartilage model by 9 weeks
    - Replacement of cartilage with bone through activity of osteoblasts
      - Ossification begins at 7 weeks.
  - Initiated at ossification centers
    - Primary ossification centers in diaphyses (center of bone)
    - Secondary ossification centers in epiphyses (growth plate)
  - Intramembranous ossification (flat bones such as skull, jaw, clavicle)
    - No cartilage intermediary
    - Osteoblasts differentiate directly from local mesenchymal stem cells.
    - Begins in the second trimester
- Bone modeling
  - Process by which the skeleton grows and takes on mature shape
  - Begins in utero and continues until skeletal maturation after puberty
- Bone remodeling
  - Lifelong process of skeletal maintenance where old bone is replaced
- Skeletal mineralization in utero
  - Majority of prenatal mineralization occurs in the third trimester.
    - Calcium accretion of 120 to 150 mg/kg/d
  - Fetal blood Ca levels are greater than postnatal/maternal levels to promote mineralization.
  - Maternal skeleton is an important source of mineral for fetal skeletal development.
  - Parathyroid hormone (PTH)
    - Secreted by fetal parathyroid glands
    - Maintains high blood fetal calcium levels
    - Promotes osteoblast-mediated bone formation
  - Parathyroid hormone–related protein (PTHrP)
    - Secreted mostly by placenta
    - Regulates calcium transport across placenta
    - Maintains high blood fetal calcium levels
    - Regulates ossification centers
- Physiologic changes at birth (Fig. 58.1)
  - Rapid decline in blood calcium
    - Loss of placental calcium supply and PTHrP
    - Calcitonin surge (decrease bone resorption)
    - Neonatal calcium accretion into bone ongoing at ~150 mg/kg/d
  - Compensatory increase in PTH secretion
    - ↑ Ca resorption (bone), reabsorption (kidney), absorption (gastrointestinal tract)
  - Normocalcemia is restored.
- Pathophysiology: regulation of bone–mineral homeostasis postnatally
  - Calcium, phosphorus, and magnesium sites of regulation
    - Gastrointestinal tract
      - Active/passive absorption versus excretion in stool
      - Predominantly small intestine
    - Renal tubules
      - Active/passive reabsorption versus excretion in urine

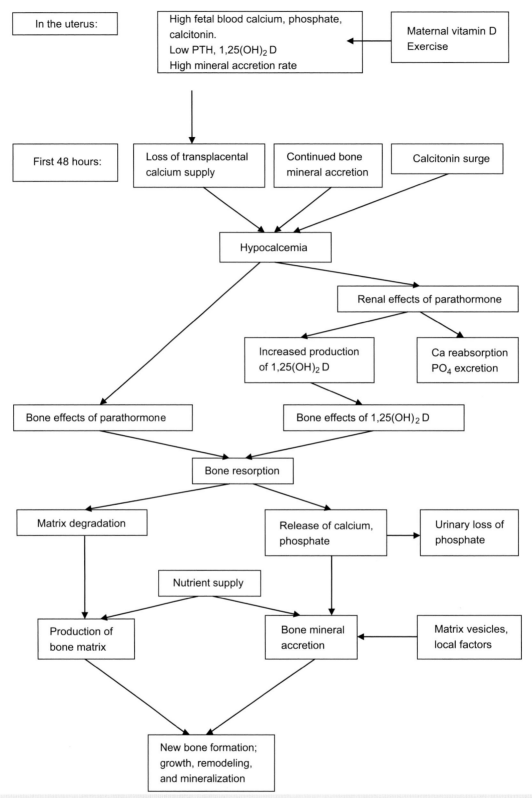

Fig. 58.1 Changes in calcium homeostasis at birth. Events influencing skeletal homeostasis around the time of birth in term infants. (From Glorieux FH, Pettifor JM, Jüppner H, eds. *Pediatric Bone*. 2nd ed. Amsterdam: Elsevier; 2012:655–677.)

- Bone
  - Deposition versus resorption
- Calcium and phosphorus hormonal regulators
  - PTH
    - All actions raise blood calcium levels.
    - PTH secretion requires normal magnesium.

- PTH is secreted from parathyroid glands in response to falling calcium, regulated by the calcium-sensing receptor (CaSR).
- Renal tubules
  - ↑ Calcium reabsorption
  - ↓ Phosphorus reabsorption

- Bone
  - ↑ Calcium and phosphorus resorption (via osteoclast activity)
- Gastrointestinal tract
  - ↑ Calcium and phosphorus absorption (indirect, via activation of vitamin D)
- Vitamin D
  - Hydroxylated from vitamin D_2 or D_3 into 25-hydroxyvitamin D (25-OHD) in liver via 25-hydroxylase (CYP2R1)
  - Activated to 1,25-OHD by 1-alpha-hydroxylase (CYP27B1) in kidney
  - ↑ Gastrointestinal absorption of calcium and phosphorus (primary impact)
  - ↑ Bone resorption and ↑ renal reabsorption of calcium (lesser impacts)
  - Inactivated by 24-hydroxylase (CYP24A1)
- Fibroblast growth factor 23 (FGF-23)
  - Secreted from osteocytes
  - ↓Phosphorus reabsorption
  - ↓ Activation of 1,25-OHD (inhibiting CYP27B1)
- Calcitonin
  - Secreted from C-cells in thyroid
  - ↓ Blood calcium due to decreased osteoclast activity

Neonatal Hypercalcemia

OVERVIEW

- Maternal factors (present shortly after birth)
  - Maternal hypoparathyroidism/hypocalcemia (hypertrophy of fetal parathyroid)
- Subcutaneous fat necrosis
  - Birth trauma
  - Local CYP27B1 activity increases 1,25-OHD production.
- Neonatal hyperparathyroidism
  - Neonatal severe hyperparathyroidism (NSHPT)/familial hypocalciuric hypercalcemia (FHH)
    - CaSR mutation (inactivating)
- Idiopathic infantile hypercalcemia
  - CYP24A1 (vitamin D 24-hydroxylase) mutation results in hypervitaminosis D.
- Williams syndrome (deletion on chromosome 7, unclear mechanism)
- Hypophosphatasia
  - Low calcium deposition in bone due to ALP mutation
- Nutritional factors
  - Excess calcium in total parenteral nutrition (TPN)/enteral feeds
  - Low phosphorus in TPN/enteral feeds
  - Hypervitaminosis D or A due to excess vitamin D or A supplementation
  - Congenital lactase deficiency
    - Presents with diarrhea in infancy
- Malignancy
  - PTH-, PTHrP-, or 1,25(OH)$_2$D-secreting sarcomas

CLINICAL PRESENTATION

- Lethargy, irritability
- Failure to thrive
- Polyuria/dehydration

DIAGNOSIS AND EVALUATION

- Biochemical assessment
  - Total calcium and/or ionized calcium
    - Calcium circulates bound to protein.
      - Corrected Ca = total Ca + 0.8 × 4-albumin
    - Binding altered by pH
      - Acidosis increases ionized calcium.
      - Source of lab error in improperly processed samples
  - Phosphorus
  - ALP
  - Intact PTH
  - 25-OHD (1,25-OHD if disorder of vitamin D metabolism is suspected)
  - Urine calcium (UCa), creatinine (UCr), phosphorus
    - Normal urinary calcium (UCa)/urinary creatinine (UCr) ratio in term infant is 1–1.2.
    - Altered by diuretics
  - Screen parents for total calcium and UCa/UCr ratio if NSHPT or FHH is suspected.
  - Genetics: Fluorescence in situ hybridization (FISH)/array for chromosome 7, gene sequencing as indicated
- Imaging
  - Renal US (nephrocalcinosis)

TREATMENT

- Targeted at etiology
- Acute therapy to decrease serum calcium
  - Hydration with normal saline at 1.5- to 2-times maintenance (natriuresis promotes calciuresis)
    - Lasix or loop diuretics should generally be avoided.
      - Minimally effective beyond fluids
      - Worsen dehydration, exacerbate renal tubular damage
- Calcitonin (4–16 units/kg/d in two or three doses)
  - May be effective in PTH, vitamin D–mediated etiologies (reduce bone resorption)
  - Limited long-term efficacy due to tachyphylaxis
  - May cause gastrointestinal symptoms in infants
- Bisphosphonates (doses vary based on agent)
  - May be effective in PTH, vitamin D–mediated etiologies (reduce bone resorption)
  - Contraindicated if renal insufficiency
  - May cause hypocalcemia, hypophosphatemia, fever, gastrointestinal symptoms with first dose
- Cinacalcet (dosing variable, 0.4–10 mg/kg/d reported)
  - Calcimimetic, lowers PTH secretion in NSHPT
- Corticosteroids (dose varies based on agent)
  - May be effective in reducing inflammation in subcutaneous fat necrosis
- Nutritional calcium restriction
  - Use of low-calcium formulas
- Dialysis
- Parathyroidectomy
  - If medical management of NSHPT fails

Neonatal Hypocalcemia

OVERVIEW

- Early neonatal hypocalcemia (onset prior to day of life [DOL] 4)

- Prematurity
  - Decreased skeletal stores
  - Inadequate intake (malabsorption, limitations of TPN)
  - Immature/inadequate PTH response to hypocalcemia
  - Renal resistance to PTH
  - Maternal factors
    - Diabetes
    - Hyperparathyroidism (suppresses fetal PTH)
    - Excessive calcium antacid use (suppresses fetal PTH)
    - Vitamin D deficiency
    - Anticonvulsant use
      - Cytochrome P450 inducers altering vitamin D metabolism
- Late neonatal hypocalcemia (onset after DOL 4)
  - High phosphorus load in cow's milk formulas
    - Renal immaturity results in decreased phosphorus excretion.
  - Malabsorption affects calcium, magnesium, and vitamin D absorption.
  - Transient or permanent hypoparathyroidism
    - Hypo- or hypermagnesemia
    - DiGeorge (22q.11.2 deletion) syndrome
    - Autosomal dominant hypoparathyroidism
      - Activating mutation in CaSR
      - Loss of function mutation in PTH
    - Other rare X-linked and recessive genetic diseases
  - PTH resistance
    - GNAS mutations resulting in pseudohypoparathyroidism
      - May be associated with Albright hereditary osteodystrophy (brachydactyly, heterotopic ossification)
  - Osteopetrosis (decreased bone resorption)

CLINICAL PRESENTATION

- Irritability, weakness
- Tetany (muscle spasm), myoclonic jerks
- Chvostek sign (facial twitch with tapping of facial nerve)
- Seizure
- Apnea/laryngospasm
- Heart failure

DIAGNOSIS AND EVALUATION

- Biochemical assessment for suspected hypocalcemia
  - Total calcium and/or ionized calcium
  - Magnesium
  - Phosphorus
  - ALP
  - Intact PTH
  - 25-OHD (1,25-OHD if disorder of vitamin D metabolism is suspected)
  - Urine calcium, creatinine, and phosphorus
- Electrocardiogram
  - Prolonged QTc interval
- Imaging (consider)
  - Chest x-ray (CXR) (absent thymic shadow in DiGeorge)
  - Anterior–posterior wrist (metaphyseal abnormalities in rickets)

- Genetics (consider)
  - FISH/array for 22q11.2 deletion, gene sequencing as indicated

TREATMENT

- Symptomatic hypocalcemia
  - Rapid correction of hypocalcemia with intravenous (IV) calcium gluconate
    - 100 to 200 mg/kg calcium gluconate over 5 to 10 minutes
    - Repeat PRN in 5 to 10 minutes.
    - Electrocardiogram (ECG) monitoring
    - Soft tissue necrosis with extravasation
  - Sustained IV calcium repletion may be necessary.
    - Continuous infusion is superior compared to intermittent dosing.
    - Doses vary from 25 to 100 mg/kg/d elemental calcium.
  - Correct underlying contributors.
    - Magnesium repletion
    - Vitamin D repletion
    - Acid–base status
  - Calcitriol can be added at 0.05 µg/kg/d divided into one or two doses if refractory.
- Asymptomatic hypocalcemia
  - Enteral replacement: 25 to 100 mg/kg/d of elemental calcium divided three or four times/day
  - Dose and duration of therapy will vary based on the underlying etiology.

Rickets

OVERVIEW

- Genetic and acquired disorders that result in impaired bone mineralization (Table 58.1)
  - Calcipenic rickets
    - Primary defect is diminished calcium availability.
  - Phosphopenic rickets
    - Primary defect is diminished phosphorus availability.
      - Gastrointestinal malabsorption: increased incidence with elemental formulas
      - Excess urinary wasting
  - Other defect in bone mineralization
    - Hypophosphatasia
    - Osteopenia of prematurity (metabolic bone disease of prematurity)

CLINICAL PRESENTATION

- Physical and clinical findings are variable and depend on the etiology, severity, and duration.
  - Bowing of long bones, craniotabes (soft skull)
  - Failure to thrive
  - Fracture
  - Signs/symptoms of hypocalcemia (including seizure)
- Radiographic findings
  - Global undermineralization
  - Frayed, cupped, or widened metaphases of long bones

Table 58.1 Biochemical Characteristics of Inherited and Acquired Forms of Rickets Affecting Neonates

Rickets Form	Ca	PO$_4$	25-OHD	1,25-OHD	PTH	ALP	UCa	UPO$_4$	Other
CALCIPENIC RICKETS									
Vitamin D deficiency	Nml/↓	↓	↓	Nml/↑	↑	↑	↓	↑	
1α-Hydroxylase rickets[a]	↓	↓	Nml	↓	↑	↑	↓	↑	
Vitamin D receptor rickets[b]	↓	↓	Nml	↑	↑	↑	↓	↑	Alopecia
25-Hydroxylase rickets	Nml/↓	Nml/↓	↓	Nml	↑	↑	↓	↑	
PHOSPHOPENIC RICKETS									
Nutritional PO$_4$ deficiency	Nml	↓	Nml	↑	Nml/↓	↑	Nml	↓	
X-linked hypophosphatemic rickets	Nml	↓	Nml	↓	Nml/↑	↑	Nml	↓	↑FGF23
Hereditary hypophosphatemic rickets with hypercalciuria	Nml	↓	Nml	↓	Nml/↓	↑	↑	↓	
OTHER MINERALIZATION DEFECTS									
Hypophosphatasia	↑	↑	Nml	Nml	↓	↓	↑	Nml/↑	Seizure
Osteopenia of prematurity	Nml/↓	Nml/↓	Nml/↓	Nml/↑	↑	↑	↑	Nml/↓	

[a]Vitamin D–dependent rickets type 1.
[b]Vitamin D–dependent rickets type 2.
25-OHD, 25-Hydroxy vitamin D; *1,25-OHD*, 1,25-hydroxy vitamin D; *ALP*, Alkaline phosphatase; *Ca*, calcium; *Nml*, normal; *PO$_4$*, phosphorus; *PTH*, parathyroid hormone; *UCa*, urine calcium; *UPO$_4$*, urine phosphorus.

- Widened costochondral junctions of ribs "rachitic rosary"
- Laboratory abnormalities
  - Variable based on etiology (see Table 58.1)
  - All patients on elemental formulas should have phosphorus and ALP levels checked regularly due to increased risk of malabsorptive hypophosphatemia.

TREATMENT AND MONITORING

- Vitamin D deficiency rickets
  - Ergocalciferol (D$_2$) or cholecalciferol (D$_3$) can be used for prevention and treatment.
  - Prevention
    - Vitamin D 400 IU daily (term), increase to 600 IU daily after 1 year of age
    - Vitamin D 200 to 400 IU daily (preterm)
  - Treatment
    - Vitamin D 2000 IU daily for at least 3 months
    - Elemental calcium 25 to 50 mg/kg/d
    - Vitamin D replacement in the absence of calcium can cause hypocalcemia
    - Calcitriol (0.05 μg/kg/d) can be added for severe hypocalcemia.
    - Continue treatment until normalization of labs and radiographic resolution.
- Hypophosphatemic rickets
  - Elemental phosphorus 20 to 40 mg/kg/d in three or four divided doses
  - Calcitriol 0.02 to 0.05 μg/kg/d to prevent secondary hyperparathyroidism

- Therapeutic goals are normal ALP, PTH, and urine Ca/Cr ratio.
- Repletion of phosphorus in malabsorptive hypophosphatemia can cause hypocalcemia.

Osteopenia of Prematurity (Metabolic Bone Disease of Prematurity)

OVERVIEW

- Form of rickets due to prematurity
  - Insufficient prenatal skeletal mineralization
  - Inadequate postnatal skeletal mineralization
    - Limitations of enteral/parenteral calcium and phosphorus provision

CLINICAL PRESENTATION

- Risk factors:
  - Birth weight <1500 g
  - Gestational age <28 weeks
  - TPN requirement >4 weeks
  - Delay in attaining full enteral feeds
  - Bone active medications
  - Loop diuretics
  - Corticosteroids
  - Anticonvulsants

- Often asymptomatic initially
- Need for routine biochemical screening
- At risk for fragility fractures
  - Often incidental finding on x-ray
  - Ribs, long bones typically affected

DIAGNOSIS AND EVALUATION

- Routine biochemical screening of at-risk infants has been proposed but is not standardized.
- Calcium, phosphorus, and ALP at 4 to 6 weeks' postgestational age
  - Abnormality in above triggers further testing with PTH, 25-OHD, and radiographs.
  - Screening should be repeated every 2 to 4 weeks in at-risk patients.

TREATMENT

- Maximize calcium, phosphorus, and vitamin D through enteral/parenteral nutrition.
  - Calcium 150 to 200 mg/kg/d elemental
  - Phosphorus 75 to 140 mg/kg/d elemental
  - Vitamin D 200 to 400 IU/d
- For TPN, target a calcium-to-phosphorus ratio of 1.7:1 (by weight).
- Consider supplementation with calcium, phosphorus, and vitamin D if nutritional targets are not met.
- Consider calcitriol 0.05 µg/kg/d to 0.2 µg/kg/d for persistently elevated PTH.
  - Suppresses PTH-mediated bone resorption and urinary phosphorus wasting
  - Can be given IV for patients on TPN
- Fractures
  - Splinting
  - Follow-up radiographs in 4 to 6 weeks to assess healing
- Consider physical therapy and passive exercise.
  - Mechanosensation promotes bone formation.

Hypo-/Hypermagnesemia

OVERVIEW

- Causes of hypomagnesemia
  - Insufficient stores
    - Placental insufficiency, intrauterine growth restriction (IUGR)
  - Intestinal malabsorption
    - Short gut, congenital or resection
  - Increased losses

- Chronic diarrhea
- Decrease renal reabsorption
  - Renal tubulopathies such as Bartter syndrome
- Causes of hypermagnesemia
  - Maternal treatment with magnesium sulfate
  - Excess enteral/TPN supplementation
  - Magnesium-containing antacids or enemas

CLINICAL PRESENTATION

- Hypomagnesemia
  - Signs and symptoms of hypocalcemia
  - Respiratory insufficiency or failure
  - Seizure
- Hypermagnesemia
  - Signs and symptoms of hypocalcemia
  - Respiratory depression, hypotonia, gastrointestinal hypomotility

DIAGNOSIS AND TREATMENT

- Biochemical assessment
  - Serum total and ionized magnesium
    - Magnesium circulates bound to protein; correct for albumin using the same equation as for calcium.
  - Urinalysis to look for other signs of tubulopathy
- Treatment
  - Hypomagnesemia
    - Magnesium repletion
      - Acute symptomatic: IV/IM $MgSO_4$ 2 to 5 mg/kg elemental magnesium, repeated PRN
      - Chronic: enteral magnesium supplementation (dose/duration vary)
      - Dose limited by diarrhea
  - Hypermagnesemia
    - Supportive
    - If severe or symptomatic, consider:
      - Fluids and loop diuretics to promote excretion
      - IV calcium gluconate to occupy magnesium receptors
      - Dialysis

Suggested Readings

Abrams SA. Calcium and vitamin D requirements of enterally fed preterm infants. *Pediatrics.* 2013;131(5):e1676–e1783.

Kovacs CS. Skeletal physiology: fetus and neonate. In: Favus J, ed. *Primer on Metabolic Bone Diseases and Disorders of Mineral Metabolism.* 6th ed. Washington, DC: American Society for Bone and Mineral Research; 2006:50–55.

Moreira A, Jacob R, Lavender L, Escarname E. Metabolic bone disease of prematurity. *NeoReviews.* 2015;16(11):e631–e641.

Rustico SE, Calabria AC, Garber SJ. Metabolic bone disease of prematurity. *J Clin Transl Endocrinol.* 2014;1:85–91.

59 *Thermoregulation*

ALISON FALCK and DAVID R. WEBER

Overview

- A neutral thermal environment offers a range of environmental temperatures in which an infant can maintain normal core temperature and that minimizes oxygen and energy consumption.
  - Normal core temperature range for infant is 97.7°F to 99.5°F (36.5°C–37.5°C).
  - Mild hypothermia is 36°C to 36.5°C; moderate hypothermia, 32°C to 36°C; and severe hypothermia, <32°C (metabolic processes begin to fail).
- Newborns are at risk of heat loss and hypothermia due to
  - High body surface area relative to body weight (up to 3 × that of adult)
  - Thin epidermis with increased evaporative losses, decreased subcutaneous fat, and increased body water also contribute.
  - Immature response to cold stress that is dependent on non-shivering thermogenesis as the primary mechanism for heat production
  - All three of the above are more pronounced with decreasing gestational age.
- Estimated heat loss after delivery
  - 0.18°F (0.1°C)/min of core body temperature
  - Cumulative loss of ~3.6°F to 5.4°F (2°C–3°C)
- Types of heat loss:
  - Conductive heat loss is due to direct contact with a cooler object.
  - Convective heat loss occurs from exposing warm skin to cooler air currents.
  - Evaporation leads to moisture loss from skin and respiratory tract.
    - Most common type at birth as amniotic fluid dries from skin
    - Markedly increased in preterm infants (up to 15 ×) due to premature skin
  - Radiant heat loss is due to heat radiating toward a cooler surface (e.g., cold window, wall, incubator wall); it is the most common type in late preterm or term infants.
- Physiologic response to cold stress:
  - Norepinephrine (NE) is key mediator of the following:
    - Peripheral vasoconstriction reduces conductive and convective heat losses.
    - Thermogenesis occurs via brown adipose tissue (non-shivering thermogenesis).
      - NE stimulates the release of thyroid hormones, thyroxine (T4) → triiodothyronine (T3)
      - T3 upregulates the expression of uncoupling protein 1 (UCP-1) in the mitochondria and uncouples oxidation from phosphorylation.
        - Adenosine triphosphate (ATP) synthesis is decreased; oxidation of free fatty acids → heat production.
  - In preterm, brown adipose tissue is present by 25 weeks but is inefficient; levels of UCP-1 and enzymes that convert T4 to T3 are low but increase by 32 weeks' gestation.

Hypothermia

CLINICAL PRESENTATION, DIAGNOSIS, AND EVALUATION

- Hypothermia is defined as a core temperature below normal range (<36.5°C).
  - Hypothermia occurs when body losses exceed body heat generation.
  - Temperature is measured via axillary, rectal, and skin probes.
  - Untreated consequences include metabolic acidosis, hypoxemia, hypoglycemia, and free water loss.
- Risk factors for development of hypothermia include:
  - Prematurity, birth weight < 1500 g
  - Small for gestational age (SGA), intrauterine growth restriction (IUGR)
  - Hypoxia
  - Acute illness
  - Abdominal wall or neural tube defects

TREATMENT

- After birth, infants should be dried immediately, removed from wet linens, and exposed to a heat source to reduce evaporative heat loss.
  - For term or late preterm, preheat radiant warmer and provide warm, dry blankets.
  - For preterm infants, the "golden hour" refers to achieving normothermia.
    - Delivery room temperature, 77°F to 79°F (25°C–26°C)
    - Radiant warmer turned on prior to delivery
    - Prewarmed blankets and hat
  - For infants <29 weeks gestation, a polyethylene bag and chemical mattress are recommended.
    - Transport from the delivery room in prewarmed incubator.
- Heat sources
  - Mother (skin-to-skin contact) is optimal in stable term or near-term newborn.
  - Radiant warmer is a temporary solution for infants needing resuscitation and acute care.

■ Incubator is used for premature or other at-risk newborns requiring ongoing management.
  ▫ Autonomous incubators provide a controlled heat, humidity, and oxygen environment and typically have automatic (servo) and manual control.
  ■ Provide warmed, humidified air for infants requiring oxygen and ventilatory support.
■ Thermoregulatory support is gradually weaned as the infant matures and begins to maintain appropriate core temperatures.

Hyperthermia

CLINICAL PRESENTATION, DIAGNOSIS, AND EVALUATION

■ Hyperthermia is defined as a core temperature above normal range (>37.5°C).
■ It occurs when body heat generation and absorption exceed dissipation.
■ Untreated consequences include increased metabolic demand and increased water and electrolyte losses; rarely, cardiac stress, central nervous system injury, and seizures.
■ Hyperthermia may be iatrogenic due to excessive clothing, inappropriate incubator settings, or failure of automatic control of autonomous incubators.
■ Persistent hyperthermia following correction of the thermal environment may be a sign of underlying infection or other metabolic derangement and should prompt a clinical evaluation.

TREATMENT

■ Treatment is directed at identifying and treating any environmental or infectious causes.
■ Acetaminophen and nonsteroidal anti-inflammatory drugs (NSAIDs) pharmacologically reduce body temperature through the inhibition of hypothalamic temperature control and blocking of pyrogenic cytokines, respectively.
  ▫ NSAIDS should be used with caution because there are no standard dosing recommendations in neonates, there is a lack of long-term data, and there are concerns over their potential toxicity.

Suggested Readings

Ashmeade TL, Haubner L, Collins S, Miladinovic B, Fugate K. Outcomes of a neonatal golden hour implementation project. *Am J Med Qual.* 2016;31(1):73–80.

Cannon B, Nedergaard J. Brown adipose tissue: function and physiologic significance. *Physiol Rev.* 2004;84(1):277–359.

Carlo WA. The newborn infant. In: Kliegman RM, Stanton BF, St. Geme JW, Schor N, eds. *Nelson Textbook of Pediatrics.* 20th ed. Philadelphia: Elsevier; 2015:794–802.

Ringer SA. Core concepts: thermoregulation in the newborn, part I: basic mechanisms. *NeoReviews.* 2013;14(4):e161–e167.

Ringer SA. Core concepts: thermoregulation in the newborn, part II: prevention of aberrant body temperature. *NeoReviews.* 2013;14(5):e221–e226.

Hematology and Oncology

LAURIE STEINER and JEFFREY R. ANDOLINA

60 Erythrocytes

LAURIE STEINER

Sites of Erythropoiesis in the Embryo, Fetus, and Neonate

- Sites of embryonic, fetal and neonatal erythropoiesis are shown in Fig. 60.1.
- Primitive red blood cells (RBCs) emerge from the yolk by 2 to 3 weeks after conception and support the growth of the embryo during the first trimester.
- Erythropoiesis shifts to the fetal liver during the late first trimester and continues to be a source of erythropoiesis through birth.
- By the end of the second trimester, the bone marrow is the primary site of erythropoiesis.

Developmental Biology of Hemoglobin

- Hemoglobin is a tetramer comprised of two α-type chains and two β-type chains. As erythropoiesis transitions from the yolk sac to the fetal liver and ultimately to the bone marrow, there are changes in the composition of the hemoglobin expressed. This is termed *hemoglobin switching* and is illustrated in Fig. 60.1.
- Embryonic hemoglobins (Hb Gower 1 [$\zeta_2\epsilon_2$], Hb Gower 2 [$\alpha_2\epsilon_2$], and Hb Portland [$\zeta_2\gamma_2$]) are expressed during the first trimester in primitive RBCs that come from yolk sac hematopoiesis.
- Fetal hemoglobin (HbF; $\alpha2\gamma2$) is the predominant hemoglobin of the fetus and newborn. Of note, there are two isoforms of γ globin, $^G\gamma$ and $^A\gamma$, which differ by only one amino acid and are functionally similar.
- Fetal hemoglobin does not efficiently bind 2,3-diphosphoglycerate and therefore has a higher affinity for oxygen than adult hemoglobin (Fig. 60.2).
- The major form of adult hemoglobin (HbA; $\alpha2\beta2$) increases in expression rapidly after birth. The minor form of adult hemoglobin (HbA$_2$; $\alpha2\delta2$) also increases in expression after birth.
- Adult hemoglobin has a lower oxygen affinity than either embryonic or fetal hemoglobin.
- By 6 months of age, the majority of infants express primarily adult globin and <1% of hemoglobin is HbF.

Red Cell Indices During Development

- The RBC count, hemoglobin, and hematocrit increase steadily throughout development (Table 60.1).

- Fetal and neonatal RBCs are larger than adult cells. The mean corpuscular volume (MCV) declines gradually with increasing gestational and postnatal age.
- Fetal and neonatal RBCs have a shorter life span than adult RBCs. RBCs from adults have a life span of 120 days. RBCs from term infants have a life span of 60 to 80 days with even lower RBC survival times in preterm infants.

Erythropoietin, Regulation of Erythropoiesis and Physiologic Anemia of Infancy

- Erythropoietin (EPO) is a glycoprotein hormone essential for the production of red blood cells.
- In the fetus, EPO is produced mainly in the liver, with production shifting to the kidney near the time of birth.
- EPO does not cross the placenta; therefore, erythropoiesis is primarily under the control of the fetus.
- Intrauterine conditions that result in fetal hypoxia, such as placental insufficiency or cigarette smoking, can result in increased EPO production by the fetus and subsequent polycythemia.
- EPO levels in cord blood are higher than EPO levels in adults, due to the relatively hypoxic intrauterine environment. EPO production declines rapidly after birth, contributing to the physiologic anemia of infancy.
- Physiologic anemia of infancy occurs in term infants at approximately 8 to 12 weeks of life, with an average hemoglobin nadir of 11 g/dL.

Anemia of Prematurity

OVERVIEW

- Anemia of prematurity (AOP) is an earlier and more dramatic physiologic anemia that occurs in preterm infants, often occurring by 6 weeks of age and reaching hemoglobin nadirs of 7 to 10 g/dL.
- AOP is a multifactorial disorder. Contributing factors include:
  - The shorter life span of preterm erythrocytes
  - Frequent blood sampling
  - Decreased EPO production in response to hypoxia compared to term infants, which may be due to developmental differences in the site of EPO production (liver vs. kidney)
  - Suppression of erythropoiesis due to systemic illness

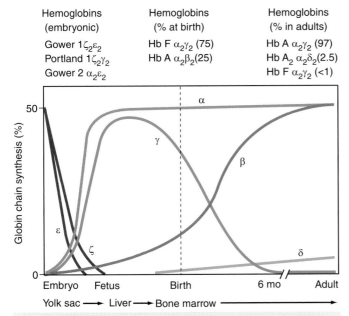

Fig. 60.1 Sites of erythropoiesis and pattern of hemoglobin expression during embryonic, fetal (F), and adult (A) development. (From Steinberg MH, et al. Pathobiology of the human erythrocyte and its hemoglobins. In: Hoffman R, Benz EJ, Shattil SJ, eds. *Hematology: Basic Principles and Practice*. 7th ed. Philadelphia: Elsevier; 2018:447–457, Fig. 33.8.)

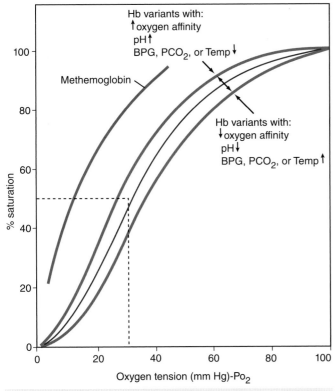

Fig. 60.2 The hemoglobin oxygen dissociation curve. Fetal hemoglobin shifts the P_{50} (the oxygen tension at which the hemoglobin is one-half saturated) to the left. *BPG*, Bisphosphoglycerate; *G6PD*, glucose-6-phosphate dehydrogenase; *PCO₂*, partial pressure of carbon dioxide; *PO₂*, partial pressure of oxygen. (From Steinberg M, et al. Pathobiology of the human erythrocyte. In: Hoffman R, Benz EJ, Shattil SJ, eds. *Hematology: Basic Principles and Practice*. Philadelphia: Elsevier; 2018: 447–457, Fig. 33.3.)

SYMPTOMS

- Some infants are asymptomatic, whereas others develop symptoms including tachypnea, pallor, poor feeding, and suboptimal weight gain that necessitate treatment with red cell transfusion.

TREATMENT

- Standard treatment for AOP is red cell transfusion.
- Careful attention to nutrition, particularly iron status, can aid in recovery from AOP.
- The use of EPO to treat anemia of prematurity is an area of active research and debate. EPO treatment can reduce, but not eliminate, the need for transfusions. In some studies, EPO treatment has been associated with an increased risk for retinopathy of prematurity.

Red Blood Cell Antigens

THE ABO BLOOD GROUP

- There are four major ABO blood groups that are distinguished by the type of oligosaccharide present on the red cell surface.
- The ABO blood groups are encoded by the ABO gene locus. The A and B alleles encode enzymes (glycosyltransferases) that catalyze the final step of the synthesis of the A and B antigen, respectively. The O allele encodes a catalytically inactive enzyme that does not place an antigen on the red cell surface.
- One allele from the ABO group is inherited from the mother and one is inherited from the father. The inheritance pattern for the ABO blood group is shown in Table 60.2.

THE RH LOCUS

- The Rh antigens are encoded by a linked group of two genes, *RHD* and *RHCE*. People are Rh positive or negative based on the presence or absence of the D antigen.

ABO Incompatibility

OVERVIEW

- ABO incompatibility refers to a mother with blood type O who has a fetus with blood type A, B, or AB. Hemolysis due to ABO incompatibility occurs when a woman with type O blood has antibodies that cross the placenta and interact with A or B antigens on the fetal erythrocytes.
- Maternal and fetal ABO incompatibility is common; however, hemolysis occurs in only a small fraction (~10%) of ABO incompatible pregnancies.
- The first pregnancy can be affected. Hemolysis does not worsen with subsequent pregnancies.

SYMPTOMS AND DIAGNOSIS

- Jaundice, often in the first 24 hours of life

Table 60.1 Normal Red Blood Cell Indices During Gestation

Weeks of Gestation	MEAN ± 1 SD			
	Erythrocytes (× 10^{12}/L)	Hemoglobin (g/dL)	Hematocrit (%)	Mean Corpuscular Volume (fL)
18–21	2.85 ± 0.36	11.7 ± 1.3	37.3 ± 4.3	131.11 ± 10.97
22–25	3.09 ± 0.34	12.2 ± 1.6	38.6 ± 3.9	125.1 ± 7.84
26–29	3.46 ± 0.41	12.9 ± 1.4	40.9 ± 4.4	118.5 ± 7.96
>36	4.7 ± 0.4	16.5 ± 1.5	51.0 ± 4.5	108 ± 5

From Dror Y, et al. Hematology. In: MacDonald MG, Seshia MMK, eds. *Avery & MacDonald's Neonatology: Pathophysiology and Management of the Newborn.* 7th ed. Philadelphia: Lippincott Williams & Wilkins; 2016:872–1199, Table 43.1.

Table 60.2 Inheritance Pattern of the ABO Blood Group

Paternal Allele	MATERNAL ALLELE		
	A	B	O
A	AA	AB	AO
B	AB	BB	BO
O	AO	BO	OO

- Positive direct Coombs test
- Evidence of neonatal hemolysis
  - Anemia with elevated reticulocyte count
  - Hyperbilirubinemia

TREATMENT

- Mainstay of treatment is preventing the severe hyperbilirubinemia that is associated with neurotoxicity through phototherapy.
- Severe cases may require exchange transfusion to control hyperbilirubinemia or packed red cell transfusion to treat anemia.

Rh Incompatibility and Alloimmune Hemolytic Disease of the Newborn

OVERVIEW

- Hemolytic disease of the newborn (HDN) is caused by the destruction of fetal/neonatal RBCs by maternal immunoglobulin (IgG).
- HDN is classically caused by antibodies targeting the D antigen of the Rh locus.
- HDN can also be caused by antibodies that target the C and E antigens of the Rh locus, as well as antibodies to other RBC antigens, such as anti-Kell and anti-Duffy. Maternal sensitization to these antigens is not prevented by RhoGAM (anti-D) administration.
- ABO incompatibility is *not* a common cause of HDN. ABO incompatibility causes anemia and hyperbilirubinemia after birth but rarely causes significant fetal anemia.
- HDN is typically mild with the first pregnancy and becomes more clinically significant with each subsequent pregnancy.

SYMPTOMS AND DIAGNOSIS

- Pregnant women are screened for antibodies to fetal red cell antigens.

- In women with high titers of anti-D or other antibodies targeting fetal RBC antigens, fetal anemia can be monitored noninvasively using middle cerebral arterial (MCA) Doppler studies. Elevated MCA Dopplers suggest fetal anemia, which can be verified using percutaneous umbilical cord blood sampling (PUBS).
- Symptoms in affected fetuses can range from mild anemia to hydrops fetalis due to severe anemia and high-output cardiac failure.
- Affected neonates can have significant jaundice, as well as ongoing hemolytic anemia, manifested by low hemoglobin and hematocrit, a high reticulocyte count, and a positive direct Coombs test.

PREVENTION AND TREATMENT

- RhoGAM (anti-D antibody) is given to Rh-negative mothers so that they clear Rh-positive fetal cells from their circulation before they generate anti-D antibodies.
- Severe fetal anemia is treated with in utero transfusion.
- The goal of neonatal therapy is to control hyperbilirubinemia with phototherapy or exchange transfusion, as appropriate. Anemia is treated with packed RBC transfusion, when necessary.
- Careful follow-up of the hematocrit after discharge is important. Infants with HDN can have an exaggerated physiologic nadir that may require packed red cell transfusion.

The Hemoglobinopathies

OVERVIEW

α-Thalassemia

- Humans have four copies of the α-globin gene, located on chromosome 16.
- Deletion of one, two, three, or four α-globin genes results in a silent carrier state, α-thalassemia trait, hemoglobin H disease (HbH; β4), and Hb Barts disease (γ4), respectively.
- α-Globin is the predominant α-type chain after the first trimester, therefore. severe α-thalassemia (HbH and Hb Barts disease) is often associated with *severe* fetal anemia that can result in hydrops fetalis and fetal demise.

β-THALASSEMIA

- Humans have two copies of the β-globin gene located on chromosome 11.

- The clinical phenotype of β-globin gene deletions is very heterogeneous and is strongly influenced by complex genetic interactions.
- There are four clinical classifications of β-thalassemia despite only having two β-globin genes: silent carrier, β-thalassemia trait, β-thalassemia intermedia, and β-thalassemia major.
- γ-Globin is the major β-type chain until after birth. The expression of γ-globin prevents infants with β-thalassemia from being symptomatic in the fetal and newborn period.

Sickle Cell Anemia and Other Sickle Cell Hemoglobinopathies

- Sickle hemoglobin (HbS) results from point mutation at position 6 in the β-chain that substitutes valine for glutamic acid. HbS is more common in patients of African and Mediterranean descent, and heterozygosity for HbS is thought to confer resistance to malaria.
- Patients homozygous for HbS have sickle cell anemia, characterized by sickling of red blood cells, moderate to severe anemia, painful crises, increased risk of stroke, and eventually end-organ damage to the kidneys and lungs.
- Patients with sickle cell trait (one copy of HbS and one copy of hemoglobin Beta [HbB]) are generally asymptomatic but can have difficulty tolerating extreme exertion, high altitude, or significant dehydration.
- Inheritance of HbSS with hereditary persistence of fetal hemoglobin results in a milder disease phenotype. Conversely, coinheritance of HbS with β-thalassemia can result in severe disease.
- HbS is a variant of the β-type chain. Symptoms of sickle cell anemia therefore do not present in the newborn period due to high levels of γ-globin expression.

Hemoglobin Variants

- Over 500 other hemoglobin variants have been described. Hemoglobin variants can impact hemoglobin stability, solubility, iron oxidation, and oxygen affinity.
- The clinical presentation of the hemoglobin variant depends on the specific mutation and hemoglobin chain affected.
- In general, only mutations in the α-, ^{G}γ-, and ^{A}γ-chains are symptomatic in the neonatal period.
- Anemia from mutations in either ^{G}γ or ^{A}γ resolves as hemoglobin switching occurs and the neonate begins to express significant amounts of β-globin.

DIAGNOSIS

- Diagnosis of hemoglobinopathies is generally made through hemoglobin electrophoresis.

SYMPTOMS AND TREATMENT

- Severe α-thalassemia (HbH and Hb Barts disease) is associated with severe fetal anemia and hydrops fetalis. Survival of these infants generally depends on in utero and postnatal transfusions, with phototherapy and exchange transfusion used to control hyperbilirubinemia. The α-thalassemia trait causes a mild anemia that is generally not symptomatic in the newborn period.

Table 60.3 Common Patterns of Hemoglobin Expression Identified on Newborn Screening

Hemoglobin Pattern	Interpretation
FA	Normal
A significantly greater than F	Transfusion prior to screening
FAS	Sickle cell trait
FSC	Hemoglobin sickle cell disease (HbSC)
FS	Sickle cell anemia or sickle-β^0-thalassemia
FAB	2–8% Hb Barts (γ4): α-thalassemia trait 25–50% Hb Barts: HbH disease

A, Adult hemoglobin; *B*, hemoglobin Barts; *C*, hemoglobin C; *F*, fetal hemoglobin; *S*, hemoglobin S.
Adapted from Diab Y, Luchtman-Jones. Hematologic and oncologic problems in the fetus and neonate. In: Martin RJ, Fanaroff AA, Walsh MC, eds. *Fanaroff and Martin's Neonatal-Perinatal Medicine.* 10th ed. Philadelphia: Elsevier; 2015:1294–1393, Box 88.5.

- The β-globinopathies, such as β-thalassemia and sickle cell anemia, are not symptomatic in the neonatal period due to the expression of fetal hemoglobin (HbF; α2γ2).
- Detection of a hemoglobinopathy, such as sickle cell anemia, by newborn screening requires referral to a pediatric hematologist for confirmation of the diagnosis and follow-up care.

Newborn Screening for Hemoglobinopathies

- All 50 states perform newborn screening for sickle cell anemia and other hemoglobinopathies, such as α- and β-thalassemia.
- The majority of newborn screening programs use a combination of isoelectric focusing and high-performance liquid chromatography for initial screening. Common patterns of hemoglobin expression detected by newborn screening are shown in Table 60.3. Abnormal test results are subjected to confirmatory testing, such as hemoglobin electrophoresis.
- Infants suspected of having a hemoglobinopathy based on newborn screening results should have testing repeated in 6 months under the supervision of a pediatric hematologist.
- Infants with sickle cell anemia are at risk of splenic dysfunction. Early identification of infants with sickle cell anemia allows for parent education, penicillin prophylaxis, and immunization against *Haemophilus influenzae* and *Streptococcus pneumoniae*. It also allows for earlier identification and treatment of life-threatening splenic sequestration syndrome.

Approach to the Anemic Infant

- Anemia is defined as a hemoglobin or hematocrit more than 2 standard deviations (SD) below the mean for gestational age.

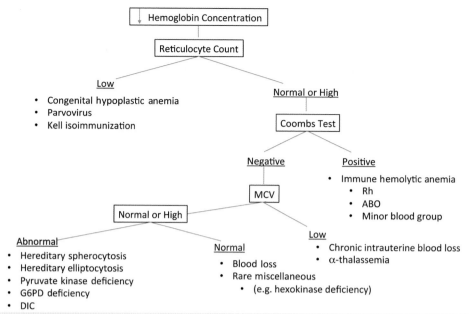

Fig. 60.3 Approach to the anemic infant. *DIC,* Disseminated intravascular coagulation; *MCV,* mean corpuscular volume. (Reprinted with permission from Elsevier *The Lancet,* 2007;370(9585):415–426.)

- The differential diagnosis for anemia presenting at birth is broad but can be divided into three main categories:
  - Blood loss (hemorrhage)
  - Destruction (hemolysis)
  - Hypoproduction
- An overview of the diagnostic approach to the anemic infant is provided in Fig. 60.3.

Blood Loss (Hemorrhage)

OVERVIEW

- Blood loss can be acute or chronic.
  - Chronic blood loss is generally better tolerated due to fetal compensation.
  - The hemoglobin and other red cell indices will be normal if sampled soon after an acute blood loss. Hemodilution will result in anemia by 3 to 4 hours after the event, with the true extent of the blood loss reflected in the hematocrit by 6 to 12 hours after the event.

Common Etiologies of Blood Loss

- Fetal: cephalohematoma, subgaleal hemorrhage, intraventricular hemorrhage, umbilical cord rupture, twin–twin transfusion syndrome
- Maternal/placental: placenta previa, abruptio placentae, vasa previa, fetal placental hemorrhage, fetal maternal hemorrhage (demonstrated by Kleihauer-Betke test, which is the presence of acid resistant fetal erythrocytes on maternal blood smear)
- Twin-to-twin transfusion syndrome primarily affects monochorionic diamniotic gestations and occurs due to an imbalance of blood flow through placental intravascular connections. The donor twin is at risk of anemia, hypovolemia, and oligohydramnios. The recipient twin is at risk of

polycythemia, hyperviscosity, polyhydramnios, and high-output cardiac failure. Severely affected pregnancies may be treated by reduction amniocentesis or laser ablation of abnormal vascular connections. Both twins are at risk for adverse neurologic and cardiac outcomes.

DIAGNOSIS AND TREATMENT

- The reticulocyte count is critical for distinguishing between chronic and acute blood loss, with a normal reticulocyte count suggesting acute blood loss and an elevated reticulocyte suggesting chronic blood loss.
- Acute blood loss can be treated with packed red blood cell transfusion.
- Chronic blood loss may require partial exchange transfusion to correct anemia without significantly increasing intravascular volume.

Blood Destruction (Hemolysis): Immune Mediated

- Please see earlier section on hemolytic disease of the newborn (HDN).

Hemolysis Due to Intrinsic Red Cell Defects (Nonimmune-Mediated Hemolysis)

RBC ENZYME DEFECTS

- Mature RBCs lack mitochondria and are therefore reliant on glycolysis (Embden-Meyerhof-Parnas pathway) and the hexose monophosphate shunt to generate energy (adenostine triphosphate [ATP]) and essential

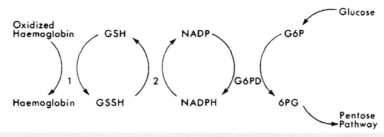

Fig. 60.4 Antioxidant defenses of the erythrocyte. *1*, Glutathione peroxidase; *2*, glutathione reductase; *G6PD*, glucose-6-phosphate dehydrogenase; *6PG*, 6-phosphogluconate; *G6P*, glucose-6-phosphate; *GSH*, reduced glutathione; *GSSH*, oxidized glutathione; *NADP*, nicotinamide adenine dinucleotide phosphate; *NADPH*, nicotinamide adenine dinucleotide phosphate, reduced. (From Dror Y, et al. Hematology. In: MacDonald MG, Seshia MMK, eds. *Avery & MacDonald's Neonatology: Pathophysiology and Management of the Newborn.* 7th ed. Philadelphia: Lippincott Williams & Wilkins; 2016:872–1199, Fig. 43.6.)

cofactors and antioxidants, most notably nicotinamide adenine dinucleotide phosphate (NADPH). Mutations of the enzymes in these metabolic pathways lead to hemolysis due to energy failure and/or inability to tolerate oxidative stress.

Glucose-6-Phosphate Dehydrogenase Deficiency

- Glucose-6-phosphate dehydrogenase (G6PD) deficiency is the most commonly inherited enzyme disorder of red blood cells. G6PD supplies NADPH and reduced glutathione to the red cell via the hexose monophosphate shunt (also referred to as the pentose phosphate pathway) (Fig. 60.4). Deficiency of this enzyme leads to hemolysis when challenged with oxidative stress. Over 100 variants of the G6PD enzyme have been described.
- Although G6PD deficiency can occur in people of all genetic backgrounds, G6PD deficiency is most common in people of African and Mediterranean descent, suggesting a selective advantage against malaria. In the United States, approximately 10% of African American males are affected.
- The G6PD variant common in African American populations (the A-variant) results in a mild reduction in enzymatic activity and enzyme stability. This variant is frequently associated with neonatal jaundice and can predispose to methemoglobinemia.
- The G6PD variant common in Mediterranean, Ashkenazi Jewish, and Asian populations is more severe and can result in fatal hemolytic anemia in the face of oxidative challenge.
- G6PD is X-linked recessive, although heterozygous females can be symptomatic if there is imbalanced X-inactivation.
- G6PD deficiency can be difficult to diagnose during a hemolytic episode. Reticulocytes and young RBCs have the highest levels of G6PD. Older RBCs, with lower levels of G6PD, are generally lost first during a hemolytic crisis, artificially elevating G6PD levels.

Other Enzyme Defects

- Pyruvate kinase (PK) deficiency is the next most common enzyme deficiency but is much less prevalent than G6PD deficiency, occurring in approximately one in 20,000 individuals. PK is the second enzyme in the ATP-producing glycolytic pathway, and PK deficiency results in hemolysis from energy deficiency. PK is most frequently autosomal recessive, although other modes of inheritance have been reported.

- Defects in other enzymes involved in glycolysis, the hexose monophosphate shunt, or nucleotide metabolism are much less common but can result in hemolytic anemia.

MEMBRANE PROTEIN DEFECTS

Overview

- Cytoskeletal proteins interact with the lipid bilayer of the red blood cell and provide the support and stability necessary for the red blood cell to successfully traverse the microvasculature. Mutations in cytoskeletal proteins result in defects in red blood cell shape and/or deformability resulting in removal of red blood cells from circulation by the reticuloendothelial system.

Hereditary Spherocytosis

- Hereditary spherocytosis (HS) is most commonly due to autosomal dominant defects in ankyrin but can also be due to mutations in spectrin, band 3, and protein 4.2 (Fig. 60.5).
- HS is characterized by a hemolytic anemia that can range from mild to severe and is accompanied by spherocytes on peripheral blood smear and increased sensitivity of red cells to osmotic (hypotonic) lysis.
- Affected infants can have splenomegaly and prolonged hyperbilirubinemia.
- HS occurs most commonly in infants of northern European ancestry but can occur in all ethnic backgrounds.

Other RBC Membrane Protein Defects

- Hereditary elliptocytosis (HE) is due to autosomal dominant mutations in α- or β-spectrin and is characterized by elliptical-shaped red blood cells (ovalocytes) and a hemolytic anemia, which is generally milder than in HS. HE tends to occur in infants of African and Mediterranean ancestry.
- Hereditary pyropoikilocytosis (HPP) is caused by homozygous or compound heterozygous mutations of α- or β-spectrin.

Defects in Hemoglobin Production or Stability

- Defects in hemoglobin quantity or quality can result in hemolytic anemia. For details, please see the earlier section on thalassemias and hemoglobinopathies.

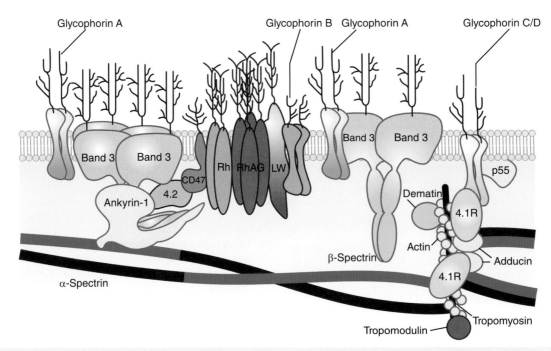

Fig. 60.5 A cross-section of the erythrocyte membrane. (From Gallagher PG. Red blood cell membrane disorders. In: Hoffman R, Benz Jr EJ, Silberstein LE, et al., eds. *Hematology: Basic Principles and Practice.* 7th ed. Elsevier; 2018:626–647, Fig. 45.1.)

RBC Hypoproduction

OVERVIEW

- Hypoproduction refers to anemia due to low production of RBCs and is typically characterized by a low reticulocyte count. Hypoproduction can be due to acquired disorders, most commonly parvovirus B19 infection, or it can be due to intrinsic bone marrow defects, such as Diamond-Blackfan anemia.

Parvovirus

- Parvovirus B19 binds to the P-antigen on the surface of red cell progenitors, disrupting erythroid maturation and resulting in a reticulocytopenic anemia.
- In utero infection with parvovirus can result in severe fetal anemia that may require in utero transfusions to prevent the development of hydrops fetalis.
- Parvovirus can also lead to aplastic crisis in patients with hemoglobinopathies or other inherited RBC disorders.

HDN Due to Anti-Kell Antibodies

- Although frequently discussed in the context of hemolytic disease of the newborn, maternal antibodies to the Kell antigen present on the surface of fetal red blood cells can cause hypoproduction in addition to hemolysis. The Kell antigen is expressed at highest levels on the surface of red blood cell precursors, resulting in the preferential destruction of those cells and a reticulocytopenic anemia.

Congenital Bone Marrow Failure Syndromes

- Diamond-Blackfan anemia (DBA) is a rare, autosomal dominant bone marrow syndrome characterized by macrocytic anemia and reticulocytopenia that are frequently accompanied by congenital abnormalities including short stature, abnormal facies, abnormal thumbs, and other skeletal abnormalities.
  - Patients with DBA frequently have mutations in genes that encode ribosomal subunits, with *RPS19* being the most commonly mutated gene in DBA.
- Fanconi anemia (FA) is a congenital bone marrow failure syndrome that can affect infants but is not typically diagnosed until late childhood.
  - FA can also be associated with thrombocytopenia and leukopenia. FA is due to a defect in DNA repair enzymes and is associated with an increased incidence of cancers later in life.
  - Diagnosis is typically made by DNA breakage analyses.
- Shwachman-Bodian-Diamond syndrome (SBDS) is a congenital bone marrow failure syndrome that is characterized by neutropenia and is often accompanied by anemia and/or thrombocytopenia, exocrine pancreatic insufficiency, and skeletal abnormalities.
  - SBDS is due to mutations in the SBDS gene on chromosome 7.
- Pearson syndrome is a rare mitochondrial disease characterized by anemia, exocrine pancreatic insufficiency, and renal and hepatic failure. Diagnosis is made by mitochondrial gene sequencing.

IRON HOMEOSTASIS

Overview

- The majority of the iron in the body (~75%) is bound to heme-containing proteins, including myoglobin and hemoglobin, with a small amount of iron contained in enzymes such as catalase or cytochromes. The remaining iron is contained in the storage proteins ferritin and hemosiderin.
- Hepcidin is a key hormone that regulates iron homeostasis. It inhibits intestinal iron absorption and release

of iron from macrophages. Hepcidin is also an acute-phase reactant and may contribute to anemia of chronic disease.

- Infants, especially preterm infants, require a higher percentage of daily iron intake than do adults to meet the demands of growth.
- The majority of iron is transferred to the fetus during the third trimester. Maternal anemia, diabetes, or hypertension with growth restriction can result in suboptimal iron transfer and low iron stores in the fetus.

IRON DEFICIENCY AND IRON DEFICIENCY ANEMIA

Overview

- Iron is an essential nutrient. Iron deficiency (ID) occurs when there is insufficient iron to maintain normal physiologic functions. Iron deficiency may precede the development of iron deficiency anemia (IDA).
- Iron is essential for normal neurologic development and function. Both ID and IDA have been associated with adverse neurologic outcome in numerous studies, although causality has not been definitively proven. Some studies have suggested that iron supplementation can improve cognitive function in children with ID.

Diagnosis

- IDA results in an increased RBC distribution width (RDW) and a microcytic, hypochromic anemia. The RBCs in IDA may have increased central pallor (hypochromia) and basophilic stippling.
- The most readily available measure of iron status is ferritin, with ferritin levels < 12 being diagnostic of iron deficiency. Ferritin is an acute-phase reactant, and measurement of ferritin during illness or inflammation may result in a false-negative result. Simultaneous measurement of C-reactive protein is often done to rule out elevation of ferritin due to inflammation.
- The reticulocyte Hb concentration and the serum transferrin receptor 1 are also recommended by the American Academy of Pediatrics to assess iron status. These tests are not affected by inflammation but are not widely available.
- Zinc protoporphyrin (ZPP) is formed when hemoglobin formation is disrupted by iron deficiency or lead toxicity. Elevated ZPP can therefore be an indirect indication of iron deficiency.

Prevention of Iron Deficiency Anemia

- Most full-term infants have sufficient iron stores for the first 4 to 6 months of life.
- Supplementation with 1 mg/kg of elemental iron is recommended beginning at 4 months of age and continued until iron-rich foods are added to the diet.
- Risk factors for IDA include severe maternal iron deficiency or diabetes, anemia at birth, frequent blood sampling or other ongoing blood loss, prematurity, and small for gestational age.
- Breast milk contains less iron than iron-supplemented formula; however, the iron in breast milk is highly bioavailable. Full-term infants who receive greater than half their feeds from breast milk require iron supplementation of 1 mg/kg beginning at 4 months of age. Term infant formulas are supplemented with sufficient iron (10–12 mg/L), and additional iron supplementation is not required unless clinically indicated.

- Preterm infants are at higher risk of IDA due to lower iron stores and more rapid rates of growth, although it is important to note that preterm infants who have had multiple blood transfusions may be at risk for elevated iron levels. In general, preterm infants should receive supplementation of 2 mg/kg elemental iron beginning at 1 month of age.
- Cow's milk should not be introduced before 1 year of age due to increased risk of IDA.

Polycythemia

OVERVIEW

- Polycythemia is defined as a Hgb or hematocrit (Hct) more than 2 SD above the mean.
- For a term infant, polycythemia is defined as an Hgb >22 g/dL or an Hct greater than 65%.
- Polycythemia often results from in utero hypoxia.
- It is associated with a number of conditions, including maternal hypertension, placental insufficiency, maternal use of vasoconstrictive drugs (such as tobacco or cocaine), maternal diabetes, genetic disorders (including trisomy 21 and Beckwith-Wiedemann syndrome), twin–twin transfusion syndrome, and delayed cord clamping.

SYMPTOMS AND TREATMENT

- Symptoms include jitteriness, hypoglycemia, and respiratory distress.
- Polycythemia is associated with persistent pulmonary hypertension of the newborn, as well as renal vein and cerebral sinovenous thrombosis.
- Treatment for symptomatic polycythemia is partial-exchange transfusion. Polycythemia has been associated with adverse neurologic outcomes; however, treatment with partial-exchange transfusion has not been shown to improve long-term neurologic outcomes.

Suggested Readings

Baker RD, Greer FR. Clinical report: diagnosis and prevention of iron deficiency and iron-deficiency anemia in infants and young children (0–3 years of age). *Pediatrics.* 2010;125:1040–1050.

Gallagher PG. The neonatal erythrocyte and its disorders. In: Orkin S, Fisher D, Ginsburg D, Thomas A, Lux S, Nathan D, eds. *Nathan and Oski's Hematology of Infancy and Childhood.* 7th ed. Philadelphia: Elsevier; 2015.

Kemper AR, Newman TB, Slaughter JL, et al. Clinical practice guideline revision: management of hyperbilirubinemia in the newborn infant 35 or more weeks of gestation. *Pediatrics.* 2022;150(3):e2022058859.

Juul S, Christensen R. Developmental hematology. In: Gleason C, Sawyer T, eds. *Avery's Diseases of the Newborn.* 11th ed. Philadelphia: Elsevier; 2024:957–964.

Widness JA. Pathophysiology of anemia during the neonatal period, including anemia of prematurity. *NeoReviews.* 2008;9(11):e520.

61 *White Blood Cells*

JEFFREY R. ANDOLINA

White blood cells (WBCs) are produced in the bone marrow and originally come from hematopoietic stem cells. The location of hematopoiesis transitions from primarily the liver and spleen in the fetus to the bone marrow after birth. Hematopoiesis is summarized in Fig. 61.1. Hematopoietic stem cells first differentiate into a common lymphoid progenitor and a common myeloid progenitor. The lymphoid progenitor will develop into all lymphocytes, including B lymphocytes, T lymphocytes, and natural killer (NK) cells. Conversely, the common myeloid progenitor will develop into all other blood cells, including red blood cells (erythrocytes), platelets, and all other white blood cells, including granulocytes, monocytes, and macrophages. Granulocytes include neutrophils, eosinophils, and basophils. Neutrophil developmental progression is summarized in Fig. 61.2. The development of WBCs is determined by the programmed expression of cell surface molecules, interactions by cytokines, and location. WBCs develop and mature in multiple locations, including the bone marrow, the thymus and lymphoid system, and the peripheral tissues. For further details on the development, components, and normal and abnormal function of WBCs, please refer to Section 4, Immunology and Infectious Diseases.

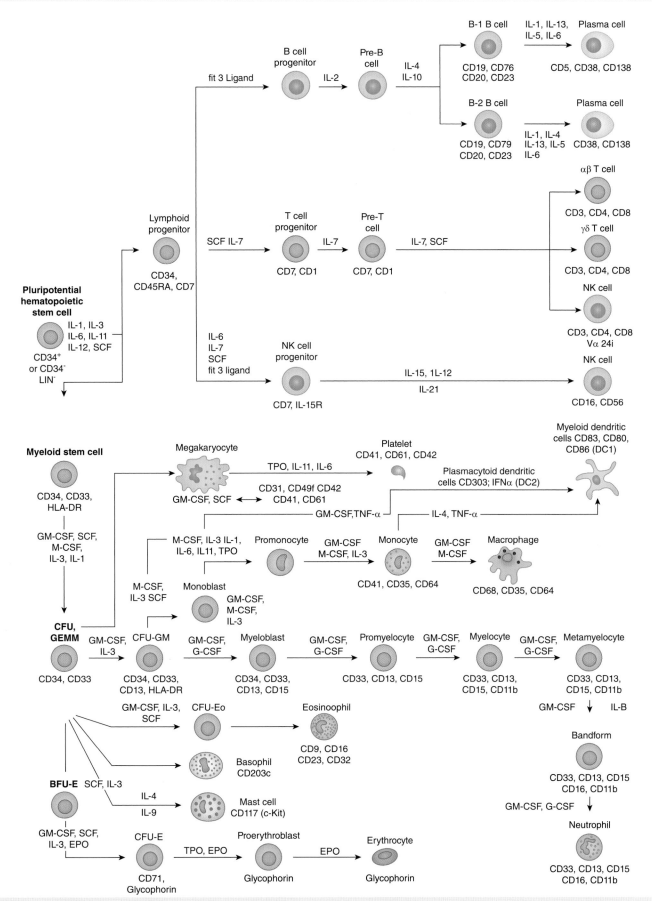

Fig. 61.1 Hematopoiesis. (From Lewis DE, Harriman GR, Blutt SE. Organization of the immune system. In: Rich RR, ed. *Clinical Immunology: Principles and Practice*. 4th ed. Philadelphia: Elsevier; 2013:16–34, Fig. 2.1.)

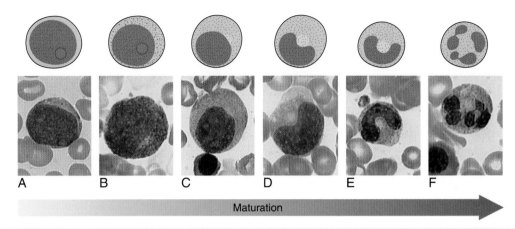

Fig. 61.2 Neutrophil maturation. (A) Myeloblast. (B) Promyelocyte. (C) Myelocyte. (D) Metamyelocyte. (E) Band. (F) Neutrophil. (Adapted from University of Virginia educational material (2019) and Medical-Labs.Net (2023). https://www.medical-labs.net/wp-content/uploads/2014/03/Neutrophil-Maturation-Diagram.jpg.)

62 *Platelets and Coagulation*

LAURIE STEINER

Platelet Production and Regulation of Platelet Levels

- Platelets are produced by specialized cells in bone marrow (megakaryocytes) in response to the hormone thrombopoietin (TPO).
- Maturing megakaryocyte progenitors replicate DNA without dividing, causing them to become polyploid (containing more than two copies of each chromosome, typically 4 to 18n). During this process, the cytoplasm of megakaryocyte progenitors matures and eventually produces platelets.
- The typical life span of a platelet in circulation is 7 to 10 days.
- The liver plays a central role in platelet homeostasis. TPO is produced constitutively by the liver. Platelets express TPO receptor and serve as a sink for circulating TPO. When platelet levels are low, circulating platelets do not adsorb TPO. TPO levels then rise, stimulating platelet production.
- Neonates have higher numbers of circulating megakaryocyte progenitors than older children and adults, but those progenitors are smaller and have lower ploidy. Thrombocytopenic neonates tend to have lower TPO levels than thrombocytopenic children or adults.

Thrombocytopenia

OVERVIEW

- Thrombocytopenia is generally defined as a platelet count less than 150×10^9/L; some otherwise healthy preterm and term neonates can have platelet counts in the range of 100 to 150×10^9/L.
- Thrombocytopenia is very common in sick neonates, affecting approximately 30% of neonatal intensive care unit (NICU) patients. Severe thrombocytopenia, defined as a platelet count less than 50×10^9/L, is less common but still affects roughly 5% to 10% of NICU patients.
- Thrombocytopenia can be due to maternal, placental, or fetal etiologies (each are detailed below); however, in many extremely low-birth-weight (ELBW) infants, no etiology for thrombocytopenia is found, despite a thorough diagnostic evaluation.

CLINICAL PRESENTATION

- Symptoms of thrombocytopenia include petechiae, bruising, and bleeding from sites such as the mucosa and heel sticks. Severe thrombocytopenia can also be associated with internal bleeding such as intraventricular hemorrhage.

TREATMENT

- Thrombocytopenia is treated by platelet transfusion.

Maternal Factors Associated With Neonatal Thrombocytopenia

- Neonatal thrombocytopenia can be associated with maternal illness including preeclampsia and HELLP (hemolysis, elevated liver enzymes, low platelets) syndrome.
  - Thrombocytopenia associated with preeclampsia typically nadirs at 2 to 4 days of life and resolves by 7 to 10 days.
- Maternal medications including heparin, thiazide diuretics, quinine, digoxin, hydralazine, and antiepileptics have been associated with fetal thrombocytopenia.
- Maternal infections, both bacterial and viral, can result in fetal or neonatal thrombocytopenia.
  - TORCH infections (*Toxoplasma gondii*, other agents, rubella, cytomegalovirus [CMV], and herpes simplex virus [HSV]), particularly CMV, are frequently associated with neonatal thrombocytopenia.
- Maternal antibodies to platelet antigens are relatively uncommon but can result in severe thrombocytopenia. There are two main classes of maternal platelet antibodies:
  - Alloimmune thrombocytopenia
  - Autoimmune thrombocytopenia

Neonatal Alloimmune Thrombocytopenia

OVERVIEW

- Neonatal alloimmune thrombocytopenia (NAIT) occurs when fetal platelets express a human platelet antigen (HPA) inherited from the father that the mother lacks. There are 16 different HPAs; however, HPA-1a accounts for approximately three-quarters of all cases of NAIT. In NAIT, the mother's platelet count is typically normal.

CLINICAL PRESENTATION

- NAIT can result in severe thrombocytopenia (platelet count < 50,000) in the first 72 hours of life that gradually improves over the first month of life as antiplatelet immunoglobulin G (IgG) levels decline.

- NAIT is associated with spontaneous mucocutaneous bleeding. Approximately 10% of affected infants will have intracranial bleeding, which can occur before or after delivery.

TREATMENT

- Platelet transfusion is the mainstay of therapy for severe thrombocytopenia.
  - Optimal treatment of severe thrombocytopenia due to NAIT is transfusion of HPA-1a–negative platelets. Maternal platelets, washed to remove antibody, may be used but HPA-1a–negative or washed maternal platelets are often not available.
  - Random pooled donor platelets can be quickly acquired and will rapidly increase platelet count. The survival of the random donor platelets in circulation may be short, but they are effective initial therapy, particularly in settings of severe thrombocytopenia or hemorrhage.
- Intravenous immunoglobulin (IVIG) is often effective as an adjunctive therapy and may reduce the number of platelet transfusions needed. Prednisone has been used in severe cases.
- Infants with NAIT and severe thrombocytopenia should have an ultrasound to screen for intracranial hemorrhage.
- The recurrence rate of NAIT is high (>75%). Women with known HPA antibodies may be treated with IVIG or glucocorticoids to decrease the risk of fetal/neonatal thrombocytopenia.

Neonatal Autoimmune Thrombocytopenia

OVERVIEW

- Neonatal autoimmune thrombocytopenia is caused by maternal antibodies that react with both maternal and fetal platelets. The mother is usually thrombocytopenic and often has an autoimmune disease such as immune thrombocytopenia purpura (ITP) or systemic lupus erythematosus (SLE).

CLINICAL PRESENTATION

- The platelet count of affected infants reaches nadir at 2 to 5 days of life. The thrombocytopenia may persist for weeks to months while maternal IgG persists in the infant's circulation.
- Persistent thrombocytopenia (>4 months) can be seen in breastfed infants due to antiplatelet IgA antibodies in the milk of affected mothers.

TREATMENT

- IVIG is effective at increasing the platelet count and should be given to infants with severe thrombocytopenia.

- Platelet transfusion can be used to transiently increase the platelet count in the case of severe thrombocytopenia (platelet count < 30,000) or bleeding.

Placental Factors Associated With Neonatal Thrombocytopenia

- Placental factors are a rare cause of fetal thrombocytopenia; however, placental abruption, thrombi, and vascular anomalies have been associated with fetal thrombocytopenia.

Neonatal Disorders Causing Thrombocytopenia

OVERVIEW

- The differential diagnosis of neonatal disorders causing thrombocytopenia can generally be divided into two categories:
  - Consumption and sequestration
  - Hypoproduction
- The approach to the diagnosis of the thrombocytopenic infant is shown in Fig. 62.1.

PLATELETS CONSUMPTION AND SEQUESTRATION

- Platelet consumption is one of the most common causes of neonatal thrombocytopenia. Common causes of platelet consumption include disseminated intravascular coagulation (DIC) and necrotizing enterocolitis (NEC).
- Thrombosis is also a common cause of thrombocytopenia.
  - Consider a deep vein thrombosis (DVT) investigation for infants for whom thrombocytopenia cannot be explained by another cause, particularly for infants with central venous catheters.
- Infections, particularly fungal infections, have also been associated with thrombocytopenia.
  - Thrombocytopenia associated with infection is likely due to increased consumption (DIC); however, damage to megakaryocytes may also play a role.
- Kasabach-Merritt phenomenon refers to thrombocytopenia and consumptive coagulopathy due to a vascular malformation, usually either a tufted angioma or a kaposiform hemangioendothelioma.
  - In Kasabach-Merritt, platelets are both sequestered in the vascular lesion and destroyed by the consumptive coagulopathy.
- Platelets may also be sequestered in an enlarged spleen.
  - Hypersplenism can be associated with hemolytic anemia, viral infections, and portal vein thrombosis.

HYPOPRODUCTION

- Perinatal hypoxic insult has been associated with mild thrombocytopenia that is attributed to decreased platelet production and does not usually require treatment.

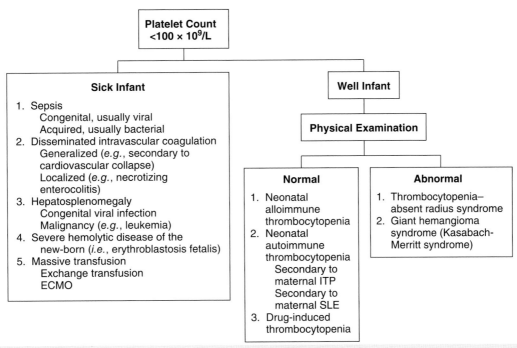

Fig. 62.1 Approach to the diagnosis of the thrombocytopenic newborn. *ECMO,* Extracorporeal membrane oxygenation; *ITP,* immune thrombocytopenic purpura; *SLE,* systemic lupus erythematosus. (Modified from Young G. Hemostatic disorders of the newborn. In: Gleason C, Devaskar S, eds. *Avery's Neonatology: Pathophysiology and Management of the Newborn.* 7th ed. Lippincott Williams & Wilkins; 2016:902, Fig 43.17.)

- Preeclampsia, placental insufficiency, and infections (particularly TORCH infections) can also be associated with neonatal thrombocytopenia due to decreased production.

Genetic Causes of Platelet Hypoproduction

- Chromosomal abnormalities (including trisomy 13, 18, and 21 and Turner syndrome) are associated with both fetal and neonatal thrombocytopenia.
- Thrombocytopenia-absent radius (TAR) syndrome is an autosomal recessive syndrome characterized by severe thrombocytopenia and bilateral absent radii.
    - Thumbs are present in TAR, helping distinguish it from Fanconi anemia.
    - Thrombocytopenia in TAR is due to a maturation defect in megakaryocyte progenitors and generally improves after the first year of life.
    - Infants with TAR are at high risk of intracranial hemorrhage due to severe thrombocytopenia.
- Fanconi anemia can be associated with thrombocytopenia, but it does not often present with thrombocytopenia in the neonatal period.
- Congenital amegakaryocytic thrombocytopenia results in severe thrombocytopenia due to mutations in the TPO receptor gene, which results in near absence of megakaryocytes in the bone marrow. Treatment is hematopoietic cell transplant.
- Wiskott-Aldrich syndrome is an autosomal recessive disorder characterized by thrombocytopenia with small platelets, eczema, and immunodeficiency.
- Bernard-Soulier syndrome is an autosomal recessive syndrome characterized by mild thrombocytopenia with large platelets with impaired function.

- May-Hegglin anomaly is an autosomal recessive condition characterized by mild to moderate thrombocytopenia with large platelets and often leukocyte inclusion bodies.

Thrombocytosis

- Thrombocytosis is generally defined as a platelet count > 450,000/μL; normative data based on chronological and gestational age are available. Thrombocytosis can be primary or secondary.
    - Primary thrombocytosis is rare and is due to mutations in the JAK2 protein.
    - Secondary, or reactive, thrombocytosis is much more common and can be associated with conditions including infection, inflammation, anemia, vitamin E deficiency, and iron deficiency.
- Thrombocytosis is generally well tolerated in neonates and does not require specific treatment to lower platelet levels.

The Coagulation System

- Coagulation factors are synthesized by the fetus and do not cross the placenta.
- There are well-described gestational-age-dependent differences in the quantity and function of hemostasis proteins.
- A comparison of neonatal and adult levels of coagulation factors is shown in Table 62.1.

Table 62.1 Differences in Coagulation Tests and Blood Factor Levels in Neonates Compared to Adults

Component		Neonatal Versus Adult Level
Primary hemostasis	↔	Platelet count
	↑	vWF
Coagulation factors	↓	FII, FVII, FIX, FX
	↓	FXI, FXII
	↓ to ↔	FV, FXIII
	↔	Fibrinogen
	↑	FVIII
Anticoagulant factors	↓	TFPI, AT, PC, PS
	↑	α_2M
Fibrinolysis	↓	Plasminogen
	↔ to ↑	PAI

α_2M, α_2-Macroglobulin; AT, antithrombin; F, factor; PAI, plasminogen activator inhibitor; PC, protein C; PS, protein S; TFPI, tissue factor pathway inhibitor; vWF, von Willebrand factor.

Used with permission from Guzzetta NA, Miller BE, Principles of hemostasis in children: models and maturation, Pediatric Anesthesia, John Wiley and Sons, 2010.

- Bleeding disorders can present with purpura, petechiae, ecchymosis, and mucosal bleeding, or as prolonged bleeding from heel stick or circumcision.
  - Bleeding in an otherwise well, term infant suggests an inherited bleeding disorder or immune-mediated thrombocytopenia.
  - Bleeding in an ill neonate is more likely due to an acquired hemostatic disorder.

Inherited Coagulation Disorders

HEMOPHILIA

Overview

- Hemophilia is the most common inherited bleeding disorder to present in the neonatal period. Hemophilia is due to a deficiency of factor VIII (hemophilia A) or factor IX (hemophilia B, also known as Christmas disease).
  - Both forms of hemophilia are X-linked recessive; however, 30% to 50% of mutations in factor VIII are due to de novo mutations.

Symptoms, Diagnosis, and Treatment

- Patients with hemophilia will have a prolonged activated partial thromboplastin time (aPTT) on routine coagulation testing. Definitive diagnosis requires measurement of factor levels.
  - Hemophilia A can be diagnosed at birth. Mild cases of hemophilia B can be difficult to diagnose in neonates, as factor IX levels are lower in neonates than older children and adults.
- Approximately one-third of infants with hemophilia will have clinically significant bleeding in the neonatal period and are at high risk for intracranial hemorrhage. Screening of affected infants for intracranial hemorrhage is recommended.
- Treatment of hemophilia is factor replacement.

Von Willebrand Disease

OVERVIEW

- von Willebrand disease (VWD) is a common inherited bleeding disorder; diagnosis is rarely made in the neonatal period because von Willebrand factor (VWF) levels are increased in the newborn (see Table 62.1).
  - VWD is generally inherited in an autosomal dominant manner, although recessive inheritance has been described for some subtypes.
  - Type 3 VWD is the rarest subtype but is the most likely subtype to present in the neonatal period and can be difficult to distinguish from severe hemophilia A.

Treatment

- Moderate to severe bleeding in the neonatal period can be treated using plasma-derived VWF-containing factor VIII concentrate. DDAVP (desmopressin) is sometimes used in older children to increase VWF levels but is contraindicated in neonates due to risk of hyponatremia.

Acquired Coagulation Disorders

VITAMIN K DEFICIENCY BLEEDING

- Vitamin K is an essential cofactor required for the carboxylation of factors II, VII, IX, and X.
- Neonates are at high risk for vitamin K deficiency bleeding (VKDB) because they have poor vitamin K stores at birth and the bacteria that produce vitamin K have not yet colonized the intestinal track.

SYMPTOMS

- Early VKDB presents in the first 24 hours of life and is usually associated with maternal medications such as warfarin, isoniazid, or antiepileptics. Early VKDB can result in skin and scalp hemorrhage, as well as severe intracranial, intra-abdominal, and intrathoracic hemorrhage.
- Classic VKDB presents from day of life (DOL) 2 to 7. It occurs more commonly in breastfed infants, although many cases are idiopathic. Classic VKDB generally presents as bruising and bleeding from the umbilical cord.
- Late VKDB occurs after 2 weeks of age and is frequently associated with intracranial hemorrhage. Infants at risk for late VKDB include exclusively breastfed babies who did not receive the vitamin K shot, infants with cholestatic liver dysfunction, and infants with chronic intestinal malabsorption.

DIAGNOSIS

- Prolongation of the prothrombin time (PT) is the earliest laboratory evidence of vitamin K deficiency. If the deficiency is not corrected, the aPTT eventually becomes prolonged.

TREATMENT

- A single intramuscular (IM) injection of vitamin K after birth is sufficient to prevent bleeding from vitamin K deficiency and is the standard of care in the United States. Oral vitamin K is not as efficacious as the IM preparation. Breastmilk is not a good source of vitamin K, and infants who are exclusively breastfed but do not receive IM vitamin K are at risk for VKDB.

Disseminated Intravascular Coagulation

OVERVIEW

- DIC is characterized by bleeding and microvascular thrombosis due to secondary activation of the coagulation cascade from tissue damage due to an underlying disease process.
- Neonates are more susceptible to DIC than older children and adults due to lower levels of antithrombin and protein C (see Table 62.1).
- DIC has been associated with numerous disease processes. Sepsis, NEC, and perinatal asphyxia are commonly associated with DIC in neonates.

DIAGNOSIS

- DIC results in the consumption of both platelets and coagulation factors. Although no single laboratory test is diagnostic for DIC, laboratory findings consistent with DIC include thrombocytopenia, prolonged PT and aPTT, positive D-dimers, fibrin degradation products, and low fibrinogen. When interpreting these laboratory values, it is important to use gestational age–appropriate normative values.

TREATMENT

- Successful treatment of DIC is dependent on identifying and treating the underlying cause. Supportive treatment includes transfusion of platelets, fresh frozen plasma, and cryoprecipitate. In patients with severe thrombosis, such as arterial or venous thromboembolism or purpura fulminans, cautious use of unfractionated heparin may be considered.

Neonatal Deep Vein Thrombosis

OVERVIEW

- The majority of cases of DVT in neonates are associated with central line use.
- Symptoms of DVT depend on its location and can include catheter dysfunction, limb or face swelling, effusion, and superior vena cava (SVC) syndrome.
- Persistent thrombocytopenia without another etiology is suggestive of DVT.

DIAGNOSIS

- DVT is typically diagnosed using Doppler ultrasonography.

TREATMENT

- Treatment of DVT is complex; many cases can be managed with supportive care.
- Clots that are large or occlusive or show evidence of extension may require anticoagulation therapy with low-molecular-weight heparin (LMWH), generally for 6 to 12 weeks.

Neonatal Renal Vein Thrombosis

OVERVIEW

- Renal vein thrombosis (RVT) is the most common non-catheter–related thrombotic event in neonates.
- Risk factors include gestational diabetes, prematurity, perinatal asphyxia, and congenital heart disease.

CLINICAL PRESENTATION

- The classic triad for diagnosis of RVT is thrombocytopenia, hematuria (macro- or microscopic), and a palpable flank mass. Acute renal injury and hypertension are also common.

DIAGNOSIS

- Definitive diagnosis is made by Doppler ultrasonography.

TREATMENT

- Treatment includes serial monitoring for extension of thrombosis. Anticoagulation is indicated for bilateral RVT or unilateral RVT that extends into the inferior vena cava (IVC).

Neonatal Arterial Thrombosis

OVERVIEW

- Arterial thrombosis is a rare, potentially life-threatening event that is most often associated with umbilical artery catheters.

CLINICAL PRESENTATION

- Affected infants may be asymptomatic or can have diminished pulses, catheter dysfunction, hypertension, renal dysfunction, and/or mesenteric ischemia.

DIAGNOSIS

- Diagnosis is made by Doppler ultrasound.

TREATMENT

- Treatment includes removal of line and anticoagulation therapy. For cases resulting in severe limb or organ ischemia, consider thrombolytic therapy or thrombectomy.

Neonatal Purpura Fulminans

OVERVIEW

- Neonatal purpura fulminans (PF) is a coagulation disorder characterized by cutaneous purpuric lesions and DIC.
- PF is due to inherited or acquired deficiency of protein C or protein S. Acquired PF is more common than inherited forms, is often secondary to sepsis, and has an association with group B *Streptococcus* (GBS) infection.
- PF can be associated with severe complications including cerebral thrombosis, renal vein thrombosis, vitreous hemorrhage retinal detachment, and necrosis resulting in loss of limb.

DIAGNOSIS

- Diagnosis is largely clinical. Infants with PF have a characteristic rash that begins as dark red lesions that progressively become dark purple or black and indurated. The lesions occur most commonly at sites of trauma, such as intravenous sticks.
- Inherited forms of PF are diagnosed by a combination of undetectable levels of protein C or protein S and genetic studies of either the parents or the affected child.

TREATMENT

- Treatment for PF includes replacement of proteins C and S with fresh frozen plasma or with protein C concentrate for patients with protein C deficiency.
- Infants with PF due to inherited deficiencies in protein C or S require anticoagulation.
- For acquired PF cases, it is imperative to treat the underlying cause.

Suggested Readings

Bussel J. Diagnosis and management of the fetus and neonate with alloimmune thrombocytopenia. *J Thromb Haemost.* 2009;7:253–257.

Cantor A. Hemostasis in the newborn and infant. In: Orkin S, Fisher D, Ginsburg D, Thomas A, Lux S, Nathan D, eds. *Nathan and Oski's Hematology of Infancy and Childhood.* 7th ed. Philadelphia: Saunders; 2015:128–157.

Fernández KS, Alarcón P. Neonatal thrombocytopenia. *NeoReviews.* 2013;14(2):e74–e82.

Monagle P, Chan A, Goldenberg N, et al. Antithrombotic therapy in neonates and children: Antithrombotic Therapy and Prevention of Thrombosis, 9th ed: American College of Chest Physicians Evidence-Based Clinical Practice Guidelines. *Chest.* 2012;141(2):e737S–e801S.

Saxonhouse M. Neonatal bleeding and thrombotic disorders. In: Gleason C, Juul S, eds. *Avery's Diseases of the Newborn.* 10th ed. Philadelphia: Elsevier; 2018:1121–1138.

63 *Transfusion Therapy in Neonates*

JEFFREY R. ANDOLINA

Transfusion Therapy in Neonates

- Transfusions of blood products are common in sick neonates in the neonatal intensive care unit (NICU).
- The majority of extremely low-birth-weight (ELBW) neonates will require at least one transfusion.
- Evidence-based data on transfusion indications are relatively scarce, so expert consensus often drives institutional protocols.
- Blood donors are the sole source of transfusion products.
- Whole blood is processed and divided into multiple separate blood products:
    - Packed red blood cells
    - Platelets
    - Fresh frozen plasma (FFP)
    - Cryoprecipitate
    - Granulocytes (used only very rarely)
- Complications may occur with any of the above blood products.
    - Critically ill neonates are more at risk of developing complications.

Packed Red Blood Cells

OVERVIEW

- Packed red blood cells (PRBCs) are commonly referred to as "blood" transfusions.
- PRBCs are stored refrigerated, with an anticoagulant/preservative such as citrate-phosphate-dextrose/citrate-phosphate-dextrose-adenine (CPD/CPDA-1).
- Donor PRBCs must be compatible with the patient by ABO group (O, A, B, or AB) as well as Rh type (positive or negative).
    - Type and screen will determine the patient's ABO and Rh type.
    - Type and cross or crossmatch consists of actual mixing of a tiny amount of donor and recipient PRBCs.
    - In emergent situations, O negative PRBC will always be compatible.
- PRBCs are most commonly given as "simple" transfusions.
    - PRBCs are dosed by volume, typically 10 to 15 mL/kg of PRBCs given over 4 hours.
- In rare instances, exchange transfusions can be performed, in which partial or complete volume of the patient's blood is removed at the same time that the transfused blood is given (e.g., for severe hyperbilirubinemia to avoid bilirubin encephalopathy, chronic in utero anemia to avoid volume overload/heart failure).
    - Extracorporeal membrane oxygenation (ECMO) is another setting in which large volumes of PRBCs are used.
- Neonates typically receive fresh PRBCs, meaning the most recently donated PRBC units.
    - Often this means the blood was collected from the donor less than ~14 days ago.
    - Data showing the efficacy of this approach are controversial.
- For neonates, PRBC units are leukocyte-reduced to reduce the risk of infection and reactions.
- For neonates, PRBC units are often irradiated, in addition to being leukocyte-reduced, to reduce the risk of transfusion-associated graft-versus-host disease.
    - If not irradiated, some centers may use cytomegalovirus (CMV)-negative PRBCs.
- Blood relatives are very strongly discouraged for neonatal patients, as blood from a relative holds no advantages and has multiple additional risks.
    - Neonates can make an immune response to similar antigens in blood products.
    - Risks of transfusion-associated graft-versus-host disease are higher.
        - Irradiation of blood products will completely remove the risk of transfusion-associated graft-versus-host disease.

CLINICAL INDICATIONS FOR PACKED RED BLOOD CELLS

- There is no exact laboratory value that would trigger a PRBC transfusion; the decision to transfuse should be based on the clinical status and symptoms of the patient.
- Studies have generally shown a lower hemoglobin trigger (7.0 g/dL) to be as safe and effective as a higher or more conservative value (8.0 or 9.0 g/dL).
    - Transfusing PRBC for hemoglobin < 7.0 g/dL would be reasonable.
    - For patients who have additional complications or surgeries, a higher threshold may be required.
- Symptoms and clinical indications that may trigger the need for PRBCs in an anemic patient include:
    - Acute blood loss
    - Anemia with anticipated blood loss during surgery
    - Significant tachycardia or tachypnea
    - Significant apnea or bradycardia
    - Hemodynamic instability

Platelets

OVERVIEW

- Platelets may be collected by two methods from blood donors:
  - Derived from whole blood units, referred to as random donor platelets
  - Collected through apheresis from a donor, referred to as apheresis donor platelets
    - Many centers prefer apheresis donor platelets, if available.
- Collected platelets are stored in plasma at room temperature and under agitation; thus, they only have a storage half-life of a few days.
- Platelets have to be ABO compatible between donor and patient.
- Platelets are dosed by volume; typically 10 mL/kg of platelets are given over 1 hour.

ETIOLOGY AND TREATMENT OF THROMBOCYTOPENIA

- Antibody-mediated thrombocytopenia is very common in neonates:
  - Neonatal alloimmune thrombocytopenia (NAIT) and maternal immune thrombocytopenic purpura (ITP) are both common causes of thrombocytopenia in this age group.
  - Platelet transfusions are used for these conditions; however, often the increase in platelet count is small or short-lived.
  - Intravenous immunoglobulin (IVIG) 1 g/kg for 1 to 3 days is a safe and effective therapy for antibody-mediated thrombocytopenia.
  - Steroids are no longer recommended, given the increased infectious risks.
  - For patients with severe NAIT, washed maternal platelets are considered the gold standard, when available.
- Thrombocytopenia may be from decreased production (e.g., bone marrow suppression from viral syndrome, maternal preeclampsia).
- Thrombocytopenia may also be from consumption from infection or disseminated intravascular coagulation (DIC).

CLINICAL INDICATIONS FOR PLATELETS

- The decision to transfuse should take into account the etiology of thrombocytopenia, clinical status, and symptoms of the patient.
- Active bleeding should trigger consideration of platelet transfusion if thrombocytopenic.
- Generally, neonates are kept at a higher platelet threshold than are older children or adults.
  - This is due to increased risk of major bleeding (e.g., intraventricular hemorrhage [IVH]) in very young and premature infants, particularly within the first week of life.
- Historically, neonates have often been transfused with platelets to maintain a platelet count > 50,000/µL. More recent data suggest that a higher target level is associated with a higher morbidity and mortality compared to a target of 25,000/µL.
- Patients may require a higher platelet threshold (e.g., >50,000/µL) if undergoing major surgery or ECMO, and they may tolerate a lower threshold if they are stable and clinically well (e.g., with antibody-mediated thrombocytopenia, a stable low platelet count, and no bleeding).

Fresh Frozen Plasma

OVERVIEW

- Fresh frozen plasma (FFP) is the liquid component of blood and consists of all of the clotting factors, including fibrinogen.
- Transfused FFP also should be ABO compatible between donor and patient.

CLINICAL INDICATIONS FOR FRESH FROZEN PLASMA

- The decision to transfuse FFP should take into account clinical status and symptoms.
- FFP is dosed by volume, typically 10 mL/kg.
- FFP is typically given to critically ill infants who have persistent bleeding secondary to DIC.
  - Patients with continued bleeding and oozing despite PRBCs and platelets may benefit from FFP infusion.
- There are no documented laboratory thresholds for FFP infusion; they vary by the risk or degree of bleeding, gestational age, and clinical status.
  - Most patients who receive FFP will have markedly abnormal coagulation studies (which vary with the gestational age of the neonate), with a very high prothrombin time (PT) or international normalized ratio (INR) and activated partial thromboplastin time (aPTT).

Rare Blood Products

- Cryoprecipitate consists of fibrinogen and only a few of the clotting factors.
- Cryoprecipitate is generally considered to be the blood product richest in fibrinogen.
  - Neonates with persistent, refractory hypofibrinogenemia may benefit from cryoprecipitate.

Complications From Transfusions

- The majority of neonates do well with transfusions.
- Although relatively uncommon, multiple risks and complications exist with the transfusion of any blood product.
- Hemolytic transfusion reactions
  - Hemolytic transfusion reactions occur when patients receive ABO-incompatible blood; most commonly, this occurs when patients with type O blood receive an incorrect A, B, or AB type blood.

- Hemolytic transfusion reactions are rare, and when they do occur, they are typically due to clerical errors.
- Massive hemolysis occurs, and symptoms include fever, hypotension, and hematuria.
- This is prevented by transfusing only ABO-compatible blood products and using a type and cross (cross-match) with every PRBC transfusion.
- Patients may also have a nonhemolytic transfusion reaction, which is thought to be antibody mediated.
- Infectious transmission from blood products
  - Despite significant donor screening and testing, infection transmission through blood products may rarely occur.
  - Historically, hepatitis B and C and human immunodeficiency virus (HIV) were the most common and most concerning.
    - Current risks of hepatitis or HIV transmission are now less than 1 in 500,000 (hepatitis) and less than 1 in 1 million (HIV).
    - Still, these tiny risks should be discussed with family prior to transfusion.
  - CMV transmission, which is rare, is a concern in the neonatal period.
    - Irradiation or CMV-negative blood products should eradicate the risk of CMV transmission.
  - Other very rare infectious transmissions remain theoretically possible.
  - Infections are prevented mainly by leukocyte depletion, which is done for all PRBC products in neonates.
  - Overall, blood products in the United States are extraordinarily safe, with absolute risk of infectious transmission of less than 1 in 100,000.
  - Very rarely, there can be bacterial contamination of a blood product, which can cause sepsis and may also present as new fever during or soon after transfusion.
- Transfusion-related acute lung injury (TRALI)
  - TRALI is now the most common cause of morbidity from transfusions.
  - TRALI is more common when high numbers of transfused blood products are given quickly.

- It is likely underrecognized and underreported in neonates.
- Symptoms of TRALI include the following:
  - Acute onset of symptoms, typically within 6 hours of transfusion
  - Respiratory distress/shortness of breath
  - Hypoxia
  - Pulmonary infiltrates/edema on chest x-ray
- TRALI is not due to a cardiac etiology.
- Its pathophysiology is thought to be due to antibody-mediated recipient neutrophil activation.
- Management of TRALI consists of discontinuing blood product (if still infusing) and good supportive care and respiratory support.
- Transfusion associated cardiac overload (TACO)
  - TACO may also cause significant morbidity after transfusions.
  - TACO is more common when high numbers of blood products are given quickly.
  - It is likely underrecognized and underreported in neonates.
  - Symptoms of TACO include the following:
    - Acute onset of symptoms, typically during transfusion
    - Respiratory distress/shortness of breath
    - Hypertension
    - Edema and fluid overload
    - Excessively positive fluid balance
  - Pathophysiology is thought to be due to fluid overload.
  - Management of TACO consists of diuretics, slowing down of blood transfusions (if able), and good supportive care and respiratory support.

Suggested Readings

Kelly AM, Williamson LM. Neonatal transfusion. *Early Hum Dev.* 2013;89(11):855–860.

New York State Council on Human Blood and Transfusion Services. *Guidelines for Transfusions of Pediatric Patients.* Albany, NY: New York State Department of Health; 2016. https://www.wadsworth.org/sites/default/files/WebDoc/ped_tx_guidelines_2.pdf.

Nickel RS, Josephson CD. Neonatal transfusion medicine: five major unanswered research questions for the twenty-first century. *Clin Perinatol.* 2015;42(3):499–513.

64 *Solid Tumors and Leukemias*

JEFFREY R. ANDOLINA

Overview

- Cancer in neonates and young infants is quite rare.
- The most common malignancies in neonates are teratomas and neuroblastoma.
- Diagnosis is often by prenatal ultrasound.
- Presumed most malignancies in this age group have a genetic basis, with causative events occurring in utero.
- Germline mutations and cancer predisposition genes and syndromes are also seen.
- Diagnosis is often confirmed by biopsy.
- Treatments include surgery and systemic chemotherapy.
- Therapies have significant toxicity, but the majority of patients can be successfully treated.
- See Table 64.1 for a summary of common neonatal tumors.

Congenital Leukemia

OVERVIEW

- Congenital leukemia is very rare and typically originates in utero.
- Acute myeloid leukemia (AML) is the most common congenital leukemia.
- Acute lymphoblastic leukemia (ALL) is the second most common.
  - Rarely, juvenile myelomonocytic leukemia (JMML) may occur.
- Down syndrome is a major risk factor, as it causes increased incidence of both AML and ALL.
- Transient abnormal myelopoiesis (TAM), formerly referred to as transient myeloproliferative disorder (TMD), is a form of transient leukemia only seen in neonates with Down syndrome.
  - TAM occurs in about 10% of neonates with Down syndrome.
  - TAM occurs in the first week of life, presents with leukemia cells in the blood, and may have other symptoms of leukemia.
  - Observation is recommended, as >80% of neonates with TAM will show spontaneous regression.
  - If a neonate with Down syndrome has TAM, that child will carry a 25% absolute risk of the development of AML by 4 years of age.

CLINICAL PRESENTATION

- Physical signs and symptoms
  - Hepatosplenomegaly is very common.
  - Skin nodules (consisting of leukemia cells, called leukemia cutis) are present in 60%, and this is unique in this age group.
  - Respiratory distress may occur from leukemia involvement in the lungs.
  - Central nervous systems (CNS) symptoms from stroke or bleed are also possible.
  - Classic symptoms of leukemia include fevers, petechiae, bruising, and lethargy.

DIAGNOSIS AND EVALUATION

- Laboratory evaluation including complete blood count (CBC) reveals the diagnosis.
  - Leukemia is characterized by an elevated white blood cell (WBC) count, blasts in the periphery, anemia, and thrombocytopenia.
  - Peripheral blood smear evaluation and consult with pediatric hematology/oncology are recommended.
  - Comprehensive chemistries, phosphorus, uric acid, and lactate dehydrogenase (LDH) should be obtained.
- Neonates typically have very high WBC counts and very often have hyperleukocytosis (WBC > 100×10^9 cells/L).
  - Leukemias tend to be very aggressive and rapidly growing.
- Diagnosis is confirmed by bone marrow aspiration.
  - Flow cytometry will classify the acute leukemia and cell of origin.
  - Cytogenetics will evaluate for any translocations or chromosomal abnormalities in the leukemia population.
- Infant ALL and AML are often characterized by a mixed lineage leukemia (MLL) genetic translocation; the MLL gene is on chromosome 11q23 and has multiple binding partners.

TREATMENT AND PROGNOSIS

- Congenital leukemia is very difficult to treat and generally carries a poor prognosis, with cure rates in the range of 20%.
- Chemotherapy may be given for therapy, and treatment regimens are very intense for the aggressive acute leukemias seen in this age group.
  - Neonates suffer much more toxicity from chemotherapy than do older children.
  - Lumbar puncture (LP) with intrathecal chemotherapy (for treatment and prophylaxis) is used as well.
  - Radiation is generally omitted given the severe late effects of this agent.
  - New, targeted agents are currently under investigation in clinical trials.

Table 64.1 Common Neonatal Tumors

Tumor	Benign or Malignant	Clinical Features	Lab and Imaging Characteristics	Treatment and Outcome
Congenital leukemia; AML > ALL	Malignant	Skin nodules; hepatosplenomegaly; bruising/bleeding	Elevated WBC count, anemia, thrombocytopenia; bone marrow and lumbar puncture	Chemotherapy; very poor prognosis
Transient abnormal myelopoiesis (TAM)	Malignant but transient	Symptoms similar to leukemia; only seen in Down syndrome	Elevated WBC count	Observation; most resolve with time; 25% future risk of AML
Langerhans cell histiocytosis (LCH)	Clonal; ± malignant	Scaly, eczematous rash; lytic bone lesions; multisystem involvement possible	Biopsy confirms histiocyte proliferation; cells stain positive for CD1a and CD207	Single-system disease has excellent prognosis; multisystem disease requires chemotherapy.
Teratoma	90% benign; 10% malignant	Large midline mass, typically in sacrococcygeal region	AFP and beta-hCG	Surgical resection; excellent outcomes
Hemangiomas	Benign	Varied and dependent on size and location; associations with syndromes and internal hemangiomas	If large size (>5 cm) or large number (>5), perform additional imaging	Natural history is proliferation in infancy followed by regression; propranolol is first-line treatment.
Neuroblastoma	Malignant	Adrenal mass; hepatomegaly; blue skin nodules; stage M-S (IV-S) common in neonates	Biopsy required; urine HVA/VMA; MIBG scan	Observation; excellent prognosis in neonates; spontaneous resolution
Cardiac rhabdomyomas	Benign	Cardiac mass(es); strong association with TS	Surgical resection if unstable; brain MRI and genetic testing for TS	Observation if able; regression; long-term care with TS
Wilms tumor	Malignant	Renal mass	Resection/nephrectomy	Excellent prognosis

AFP, Alpha-fetoprotein; *ALL*, acute lymphoblastic leukemia; *AML*, acute myeloid leukemia; *beta-hCG*, beta-human chorionic gonadotropin; *HVA*, homovanillic acid; *MIBG*, meta-iodobenzylguanidine; *MRI*, magnetic resonance imaging; *TS*, tuberous sclerosis; *VMA*, vanillylmandelic acid; *WBC*, white blood cell.

Langerhans Cell Histiocytosis

OVERVIEW

- Langerhans cell histiocytosis (LCH) is the preferred term for a group of disorders that includes histiocytosis X, eosinophilic granuloma, and other terms.
- LCH is a clonal disorder that results in proliferation of histiocytes.
- Classic pathology includes the "tennis racket"–shaped organelles referred to as Birbeck granules.
  - Cells stain positive for CD1a and/or CD207 (Langerin).
- LCH presentation is varied and can be a single-system or multisystem disorder.
  - Bone and skin are the most commonly affected organs.
  - Less commonly affected organs include the liver, spleen, lungs, bone marrow, and CNS.
  - Neonates and infants are more likely to have multisystem disease than older children.

CLINICAL PRESENTATION

- Physical signs and symptoms
  - Skin involvement and cutaneous lesions are very common presentations of LCH in neonates.
  - Rash is typically dry and scaly and not responsive to topical therapies.
  - Appearance is similar to severe "cradle cap."
  - LCH may also appear eczematous or include colored papules.
  - Additional signs can occur with other organ involvement, including bruising, hepatosplenomegaly, and respiratory distress.

DIAGNOSIS AND EVALUATION

- Diagnosis is confirmed by biopsy of the affected organ; biopsy is required.
  - Any severe, scaly rash not responding to topical therapy requires a skin biopsy.
  - LCH is confirmed by CD1a or CD207 (Langerin) positivity.
  - BRAF mutations may be seen in LCH, and BRAF inhibitors are a possible targeted therapy in refractory cases.
- Laboratory evaluation may reveal abnormalities depending on the organs affected.
  - CBC should be performed and may reveal cytopenias if bone marrow is affected.
  - Chemistries, liver function tests, and coagulation studies with fibrinogen are also recommended and may be abnormal if there is liver involvement.
  - Erythrocyte sedimentation rate (ESR), lactate dehydrogenase (LDH), and uric acid should also be performed.
  - Urinalysis for specific gravity and osmolality is recommended, as diabetes insipidus (DI) is a possible complication of CNS LCH.

- Bone marrow aspiration and biopsy should be considered if the CBC shows abnormalities.
  - Single-system LCH may have normal laboratory findings.
- Imaging is required to evaluate for bone and additional organ involvement.
  - Skeletal survey (x-ray of all bones) is required to evaluate for bone lesions.
  - LCH of bone typically presents as lytic lesions; associated granulomas may also occur.
  - Perform abdominal ultrasound to evaluate for liver and spleen involvement.
  - CNS imaging (brain magnetic resonance imaging [MRI]) if there are symptoms or signs of CNS involvement.
  - Additional imaging performed is related to signs and symptoms (e.g., positron emission tomography [PET] scan).

TREATMENT AND PROGNOSIS

- The management of LCH is varied and depends on disease location and disease spread.
- Single-system LCH in skin or bone may be managed with observation alone or surgical resection alone.
- LCH remains poorly understood, and mild cases may not require systemic therapies.
- Multisystem LCH (or multifocal bone LCH) will require systemic therapies.
- Systemic treatments consist of chemotherapy.
  - Steroids (prednisone) and vinblastine remain the mainstays of therapy.
  - Refractory patients may require more intensive chemotherapeutic agents.
  - BRAF inhibitor–targeted therapy may also be considered.
- Prognosis is excellent for single-system LCH.
- Multisystem LCH in the infant age group carries a more guarded prognosis and requires intensive chemotherapy for optimal management.
- DI may occur at presentation or as a late effect after LCH involving the CNS or "CNS-risk" bones.

Neonatal Teratoma

OVERVIEW

- Teratomas are the most common tumor seen in neonates.
- The vast majority (90%) of teratomas are benign, although about 10% will be malignant (and have the capacity to metastasize) in the neonatal age range.
- Teratomas arise from primitive germ cells.
  - Mature teratomas are benign.
  - "Immature" teratomas may have malignant features.
  - A small percentage of mature teratomas undergo malignant transformation over time.
- Malignant germ cell tumors may have elements of yolk sac tumor and/or choriocarcinoma.
  - These tumors secrete alpha-fetoprotein (AFP) and beta-human chorionic gonadotropin (beta-hCG).
- In neonates, teratomas occur in the midline.

- Most common location is the sacrococcygeal region; less common location is the mediastinum.
  - Sacrococcygeal teratomas are more common in girls.

CLINICAL PRESENTATION

- The majority of teratomas are now diagnosed before birth on prenatal ultrasound.
- Large sacrococcygeal tumors are an indication for cesarean section.

PHYSICAL SIGNS AND SYMPTOMS

- Physical exam reveals a mass or extruding tumor in the genitourinary or anal region.
- Sacrococcygeal teratomas present as a mass between the anus and coccyx.
  - Tumors will often have external extension and can be very large.
  - Teratomas may be very vascular, and significant bleeding can occur.
  - Significant neurologic symptoms are uncommon.
- Respiratory distress from teratoma as mediastinal mass is a less common presentation.

DIAGNOSIS AND EVALUATION

- Diagnosis is confirmed by pathology.
- Laboratory evaluation should include tumor markers (AFP and beta-hCG).
  - LDH is also obtained.
  - CBC should be considered if there is a concern for anemia from bleeding.
- Mature teratomas do *not* produce any AFP or beta-hCG; however, teratomas with immature or germ cell components will typically produce AFP ± beta-hCG.
- If teratoma produces these tumor markers, they can be helpful in monitoring for recurrence.
- Newborns have an average AFP level of 41,000 ng/mL, which decreases to the normal older child and normal adult range of 0 to 7 ng/mL by about 1 year of age.
- Imaging is extremely important to assess the extent of the tumor and for surgical planning.
- Ultrasound of the abdomen and pelvis is often done first line.
- Perform MRI to determine the extent of the mass and involvement in surrounding structures.
  - Computed tomography (CT) may also be used, although it is less desired due to the large amount of radiation exposure.
- If pathology shows completely mature (benign) teratoma, no additional imaging is needed.
- If malignant elements are identified on pathology, imaging of the chest is recommended to assess for metastases.

TREATMENT AND PROGNOSIS

- Surgical resection is the mainstay of therapy.
  - The majority of teratomas are able to be fully resected.
  - Achieving negative margins can be difficult or impossible in the sacrococcygeal region. The coccyx is always surgically removed.

- For the rare patient with metastatic disease, chemotherapy may be considered.
- Prognosis is excellent for teratomas in the neonatal period.
- Mature (benign) teratomas do not recur approximately 90% of the time.
  - If they do recur, they will only be local and are typically treated with repeat resection.
- Immature or malignant teratomas are also treated with surgery.
- These patients must be followed more closely, as there is a higher chance of recurrence.
- Surveillance imaging (ultrasound vs. MRI) and tumor marker (AFP ± beta-hCG) screening are recommended for approximately 5 years.

Hemangiomas

OVERVIEW

- Infantile hemangiomas are the most common vascular tumor in children, affecting approximately 4% to 5% of infants.
- Hemangiomas are benign.
- They typically occur on the skin, although they can occur anywhere, including mucous membranes, airway, and internal organs.
- Hemangiomas have a classic natural history.
  - They are typically small or subtle at birth.
  - They proliferate over the first year of life.
  - After about the age of 12 months, they slowly involute over the next few years.
- Hemangiomas are associated with numerous syndromes.
  - PHACES syndrome (posterior fossa malformations, hemangioma, arterial/aortic abnormalities, cardiac defects, eye abnormalities, sternal cleft/supraumbilical raphe syndrome)
- Numerous other vascular malformations may occur in neonates and infants, including malformations of capillaries and veins, arteriovenous malformations (AVMs), and lymphatic malformations.
  - Kaposi hemangioendothelioma

CLINICAL PRESENTATION

- Hemangiomas may occur on any region of the outer skin or internal organ.
- Thorough skin exam is required.
- Hemangiomas are typically red or pink and may be palpable.
  - Physical appearance is variable and heterogeneous.
  - Internal hemangiomas may be detected based on symptoms.
- Hemangiomas may be very faint, small, or undetectable at birth (as this is often prior to the proliferative phase).

DIAGNOSIS AND EVALUATION

- Hemangiomas are typically diagnosed on clinical grounds alone.
  - Biopsy typically is not required.
- Laboratory evaluation may be limited.
  - CBC is required to evaluate for thrombocytopenia or anemia.
  - Coagulation studies are typically performed to evaluate for DIC.
- In Kasabach-Merritt syndrome, very large hemangiomas may cause hematologic abnormalities, including thrombocytopenia and DIC.
- Imaging is not required for small and superficial hemangiomas.
- Very large or atypical lesions require imaging to evaluate for internal hemangiomas.
- MRI is typically the imaging modality of choice for internal hemangiomas.
  - Ultrasounds can also be considered.
  - Liver is a relatively common site for hemangiomas in infants.
- Single hemangiomas > 5 cm on the face or back require imaging to exclude syndromes.
- Cutaneous hemangiomas greater than 5 cm require imaging to assess for visceral involvement.

TREATMENT AND PROGNOSIS

- Observation is the treatment of choice, as the vast majority of hemangiomas will regress spontaneously and will not require system treatment.
- Generally, surgery is avoided whenever possible given that the surgical scar is typically significant and often worse than the hemangioma itself.
  - Biopsies are also often avoided given the bleeding risk with hemangiomas.
- Medical management is often required for very large hemangiomas or for those in critical areas (airway, brain).
- Corticosteroids are no longer commonly used due to side effects.
- Generally, a multidisciplinary approach is required for difficult hemangiomas, including dermatology, neonatology, interventional radiology, and pediatric hematology.
- Propranolol has developed into the first-line treatment for hemangiomas.
  - Intralesional steroids, vincristine, laser therapy, and embolization procedures have also been used.
- Sirolimus (also known as rapamycin) is a mammalian target of rapamycin (mTOR) inhibitor that has shown excellent response rates in massive hemangiomas and other vascular anomalies.

Neuroblastomas

OVERVIEW

- Congenital neuroblastoma is the most common malignancy of the newborn and the second most common tumor (second to teratoma, which is typically benign).
- Neuroblastoma arises from neural crest cells, and the most common site of primary tumor is the adrenal gland.
- Neuroblastoma is known for very unusual and unpredictable behavior, including spontaneous regression as well as rapid proliferation.

- Congenital and neonatal neuroblastoma is a very different disease than that of toddlers and older children.
  - Biologically, neonatal neuroblastoma is very likely to spontaneously regress or to differentiate into a benign tumor.
  - The incidence of neuroblastoma may be increased with additional surveillance (prenatal ultrasounds or urine screening).
  - It is assumed that the actual number of neuroblastoma cases is much higher than the number diagnosed, as many newborns have neuroblastoma that spontaneously regresses and is never detected.

CLINICAL PRESENTATION

- Many neuroblastoma cases are now diagnosed by prenatal ultrasound.
- Neuroblastoma presents as an adrenal mass or a mass along the sympathetic chain (may be in neck, chest, abdomen, or pelvis).
- Physical signs and symptoms are related to the site of primary tumor and any metastases.
  - Abdominal/retroperitoneal masses may or may not be palpable.
  - Hepatomegaly may indicate metastases to the liver.
  - Blue nodular lesions may reflect skin involvement of neuroblastoma.
  - Respiratory distress may result from a chest mass.
  - Additional masses in the chest, abdomen, pelvis, bones, or bone marrow may also be identified.
  - Neuroblastoma often has metastases at diagnosis.

DIAGNOSIS AND EVALUATION

- Tumor biopsy remains the gold standard to diagnose neuroblastoma.
  - Adrenal lesions that may be neuroblastoma typically require biopsy or resection.
- Tumor pathology is critical for staging and risk group determination for neonatal neuroblastoma.
  - Most neonates will have "favorable" histology.
  - Most neonates will not have the unfavorable n-MYC amplification.
- A complete laboratory evaluation is required for neuroblastoma.
  - CBC, chemistries, liver function tests, coagulation tests, LDH, ESR, uric acid
- Urine catecholamines can aid in the diagnosis.
  - Neuroblastoma produces urine homovanillic acid (HVA) and vanillylmandelic acid (VMA).
  - Urine HVA and VMA may or may not be elevated in neonatal neuroblastoma.
- Imaging is required in the workup of neuroblastoma.
  - CT or MRI of neck, chest, abdomen, and pelvis is required.
  - Meta-iodobenzylguanidine (MIBG) scan is a nuclear medicine scan specific to neuroblastoma that is required to evaluate for metastases.
- Neuroblastoma is staged based on extent of disease spread from localized disease (stages L1 and L2) to metastatic disease (stages M and M-S). This has replaced the prior staging system of I through IV, with stage I localized to the structure of origin and stage IV with distant metastases.
- There is a special stage for neuroblastoma, M-S (formerly IV-S), that is specific to infants.
  - Stage M-S (IV-S) includes patients age < 12 months, with metastatic disease to the liver, bone marrow, or skin.
    - The "S" stands for special and is associated with spontaneous regression.
  - The vast majority of stage M-S patients do not require any therapy and can be observed; the tumor regresses over the coming months.
  - These patients still require close observation.
  - Patients who become symptomatic (e.g., respiratory distress from hepatomegaly from liver involvement of neuroblastoma) may also require chemotherapy.

TREATMENT AND PROGNOSIS

- Treatment of neonatal neuroblastoma depends on disease stage and the resulting risk group.
- Neonatal age itself is a very favorable prognostic factor; the majority of newborns can be observed and do not require treatment.
  - Stage M-S (formerly known as IV-S) patients are typically observed (as noted earlier).
- For the unusual neonate with high-stage or high-risk disease, intensive systemic therapies are required to cure neuroblastoma.
  - Surgical resection of primary tumor
  - Very intensive chemotherapy
  - Additional therapies, including radiation therapy and antibody therapy
- Overall, the prognosis of neonates with neuroblastoma is excellent, with the vast majority being cured of their disease.

Rhabdomyomas

OVERVIEW

- Rhabdomyomas are benign tumors typically located in the heart.
- They arise from striated muscle and are typically cardiac in origin.
  - Rhabdomyomas are a separate entity from rhabdomyosarcomas (a malignant tumor occurring in children).
- Rhabdomyomas arise in utero.
- Most commonly they involve the myocardium of the ventricles or interventricular septum but can occasionally involve the atria.

CLINICAL PRESENTATION

- Rhabdomyomas may present with multiple cardiac symptoms.
- Symptoms may occur in utero or in the newborn period.

- Symptoms may include hydrops fetalis, fetal arrhythmias, respiratory distress, heart failure, or sudden death.
- Many rhabdomyomas occur as multiple; they are typically small but rarely can be very large.
  - The natural course of rhabdomyomas is spontaneous regression over time.
- Rhabdomyomas are very strongly associated with tuberous sclerosis (TS).
  - Approximately 80% of patients with rhabdomyomas will have TS.
  - Conversely, approximately 50% of TS patients will have rhabdomyomas.
- TS is an autosomal dominant genetic disorder causing numerous benign tumors in multiple organ systems, most notably in the brain.
  - Benign tumors, or "tubers," may grow in the brain and cause numerous problems including seizures.
  - TS also predisposes patient to numerous other tumors in the kidneys, liver, lungs, eyes, and skin, including astrocytoma and carcinomas.

DIAGNOSIS AND EVALUATION

- Many rhabdomyomas are diagnosed on prenatal ultrasound or fetal echocardiography.
- Echocardiogram or MRI will often confirm the suspected rhabdomyomas.
  - Electrocardiogram (ECG) is required to evaluate for arrhythmias.
- Biopsy is typically not done; surgery is reserved for very large rhabdomyomas in patients who require immediate intervention.
- If rhabdomyomas are suspected, full evaluation for TS is critical.
  - Perform MRI of the brain.
  - Consider genetic testing for TS of patient and parents.

TREATMENT AND PROGNOSIS

- Most rhabdomyomas are small and may not require any intervention.
  - Spontaneous regression over time is expected.
- Large rhabdomyomas or those causing significant symptoms may require cardiac surgery, although this is generally reserved for those infants with life-threatening tumors.
- Everolimus, an mTOR inhibitor, has been shown to have initial activity in cardiac rhabdomyomas.
- For those patients identified as having TS, lifelong multidisciplinary subspecialty care and screening for additional tumors are required.

Wilms Tumor

OVERVIEW

- Renal tumors are relatively uncommon in neonates.
- Congenital mesoblastic nephroma is benign and the most common kidney tumor in neonates.

- Wilms tumor is malignant and is the second most common primary kidney tumor in neonates (although the most common kidney tumor in children overall).
  - Wilms tumor is also known as nephroblastoma.
  - Wilms tumor is associated with numerous syndromes, including Beckwith-Wiedemann syndrome.
  - It has a low propensity to metastasize.

CLINICAL PRESENTATION

- Wilms tumor may present as an abdominal or flank mass on physical exam.
- Wilms tumor may also cause hematuria or hypertension.

DIAGNOSIS AND EVALUATION

- The majority of Wilms tumors in neonates are diagnosed by prenatal ultrasound.
- Laboratory evaluation may be normal but should include CBC, chemistries with blood urea nitrogen (BUN) and creatinine, liver function tests, and coagulation studies.
- Urinalysis should be performed to evaluate for hematuria.
- Imaging is required for the diagnosis of kidney tumors.
  - Ultrasound is often done first, as it is important to evaluate for local vascular spread.
  - CT scan of the abdomen/pelvis is most commonly used to evaluate kidney tumors; MRI is an acceptable alternative in neonates.
- Diagnosis is confirmed on pathology after nephrectomy.
- Wilms tumor pathology is "triphasic," as it includes blastemal, stromal, and tubular components.
  - Anaplasia is a sign of a more aggressive tumor.
- Wilms tumor, like all renal tumors, is staged I though V, with stage I being localized in an intact renal capsules, stage IV having distant metastasis, and stage V being bilateral.

TREATMENT AND PROGNOSIS

- Kidney tumors are managed with immediate nephrectomy, even in the neonatal period.
- Pediatric surgery consultation and surgical resection/nephrectomy are typically curative.
- Metastases are rare.
- Low-stage Wilms tumor patients may be treated with surgery alone.
- Higher-stage Wilms tumor patients may require adjuvant chemotherapy or radiation.
- Prognosis is excellent, and cure rates exceed 90% for all groups.

Suggested Readings

Askin DF. Neonatal cancer: a clinical perspective. *J Obstet Gynecol Neonatal Nurs.* 2000;29(4):423–431.

Lee KC, Bercovitch L. Update on infantile hemangiomas. *Semin Perinatol.* 2013;37(1):49–58.

Orbach D, Sarnacki S, Brisse HJ, et al. Neonatal cancer. *Lancet Oncol.* 2013;14(13):e609–e620.

Head (Ears, Eyes, Nose, Throat), Neck, and Skin

ANDREA AVILA, MATTHEW LLOYD HAYNIE, ASHLEY L. SOAPER, CATHERINE K. HART, JONATHAN LAI, NINA D'AMIANO and BERNARD A. COHEN

65 Eye Development, Retinopathy of Prematurity

ANDREA AVILA and MATTHEW LLOYD HAYNIE

Normal Development and Anatomy

- Development of the eye during the embryonic period occurs at 3 to 10 weeks' gestation.
  - It involves ectoderm, neural crest cells, and mesenchyme.
- Normal axial length is 17 mm in newborns (24 mm in adults).
- Corneal diameter is 10 mm in newborns (12 mm in adults).
- Retinal vasculature is mature in most full-term infants; see the Retinopathy of Prematurity (ROP) section.
- Central macula are underdeveloped at birth but become normal at 6 months.
- Visual function is about 20/400 at birth and becomes 20/20 by 6 months to 3 years depending on the measurement method.

Congenital Abnormalities

EYELIDS AND ORBIT

Overview

- Congenital ptosis
  - Abnormal drooping of the upper eyelid
  - Most common cause of childhood ptosis
  - Causes of congenital ptosis
    - Simple congenital (myopathic) ptosis
      - Most common cause of congenital ptosis
      - Due to developmental myopathy of the levator muscle
      - Ptosis is present at birth and remains stable throughout life.
      - Unilateral in 69%
      - Coexisting strabismus in 30%
    - Blepharophimosis syndrome
      - Severe bilateral ptosis with poor levator function
      - Palpebral fissures horizontally shortened (blepharophimosis)
      - Autosomal dominant inheritance
  - Marcus Gunn jaw-winking syndrome
    - Synkinetic (involuntary movement) ptosis
    - Predominantly unilateral
    - Sporadic, no inheritance pattern
    - Intermittent elevation of the ptotic eyelid occurs with contraction of the muscles of mastication, leading to a "winking" movement during eating or chewing.
- Acquired ptosis
  - Includes third nerve palsy, Horner syndrome, myasthenia gravis, mechanical ptosis (birth trauma, hemangioma, etc.)
- Orbital malformations
  - Typically in conjunction with craniofacial syndromes (Crouzon, Apert, etc.)

Clinical Presentation

- Drooping of upper eyelid in ptosis
- Orbital malformations can cause strabismus, proptosis, or optic nerve compression.

Diagnosis and Evaluation

- Check lid position with respect to pupil to determine if it is affecting vision.
- Check ocular rotations for strabismus.

Treatment

- Early surgical repair of ptosis if amblyogenic
- Topical or systemic beta blocker for large hemangiomas
- Possible craniofacial surgery for orbital malformations

CORNEAL OPACIFICATION

Overview

- Can lead to severe amblyopia if untreated

Clinical Presentation

- Localized or diffuse corneal clouding; may have microcystic edema or tears in Desçemet membrane

Diagnosis and Evaluation

- Forceps trauma: often with focal edema and vertical Desçemet tears
- Glaucoma: diffuse clouding with enlarged diameter and microcystic edema
- Metabolic diseases, including bilateral diffuse haze with thickened stroma
- Ocular disease: Peters anomaly, sclerocornea, dermoid, congenital hereditary endothelial dystrophy (CHED)

Treatment

- Lower intraocular pressure.
- Treat underlying metabolic disease.
- Perform corneal transplantation.

LEUKOCORIA

Overview

- White pupil due to decreased red reflex from the retina

Clinical Presentation

- Opacity of cornea or lens
- Vitreous opacity: vitritis, vitreous hemorrhage
- Retinal disease: detachment, retinoblastoma, coloboma, myelinated nerve fibers

Diagnosis and Evaluation

- Slit-lamp examination of cornea, iris, and lens
- Dilated fundus examination of vitreous, retina, and optic nerve
- Ultrasound to evaluate posterior segment

Treatment

- Cataract extraction
- Vitrectomy vitreous hemorrhage or retinal detachment
- Oncology evaluation for retinoblastoma

CONGENITAL CATARACT

Overview

- Can lead to severe deprivation amblyopia if left untreated
- Congenital cataracts: noted at birth
- Infantile cataracts: occur in first year of life

Clinical Presentation

- Abnormal or absent red reflex
- Decreased visual behavior or nystagmus
- Congenital cataracts associated with:
  - Trisomy 21
  - Trisomy 13
  - Trisomy 18
  - Cri du chat syndrome
  - Turner syndrome
  - Galactosemia
  - Fabry disease
  - Lowe syndrome
  - Alport syndrome
  - Congenital infections such as rubella
- Non-syndromic congenital cataract
  - One-third of all congenital cataracts are familial and not associated with other systemic disorders.
  - Bilateral cataracts tend to be inherited, whereas unilateral cataracts typically are not.

Diagnosis and Evaluation

- Slit-lamp examination to determine size and morphology
- Testing for syndromic, non-syndromic, and systemic disorders (as noted earlier)
- Genetics evaluation

Treatment

- If visually significant, lensectomy by 2 to 3 months old
- If small or faint, pharmacologic dilation
- Amblyopia management

CONGENITAL GLAUCOMA

Overview

- Increased intraocular pressure leading to corneal edema and optic nerve damage
- Congenital glaucoma can be autosomal recessive; two genes have been identified (*CYP1B1* and *LTBP2*).

Clinical Presentation

- Classic triad: photophobia, blepharospasm, and epiphora
- Associated with systemic disease: Sturge-Weber syndrome, neurofibromatosis type 1 (NF-1), Lowe syndrome
- Associated with ocular disease: Axenfeld-Rieger syndrome, aniridia, Peters anomaly, cataract

Diagnosis and Evaluation

- Corneal haze, increased corneal diameter (>11 mm in newborns)
- Increased intraocular pressure, optic disk cupping

Treatment

- Topical ocular hypotensive medication as a temporizing measure
- Surgical treatment to lower pressure (goniotomy, trabeculotomy)

OPTIC NERVE AND RETINA

Overview

- Optic nerve anomalies: hypoplasia, coloboma, morning glory disc anomaly
- Retinal disease: coloboma, Leber congenital amaurosis, rod–cone dystrophies

Clinical Presentation

- Decreased visual behavior, nystagmus
- Sluggish pupillary response, afferent pupillary defect

Diagnosis and Evaluation

- Dilated fundus examination
- Electroretinography for retinal disease
- Endocrine evaluation in septo-optic dysplasia

Treatment

- Management of associated systemic disorders
- Early intervention, low vision evaluation

Acquired Abnormalities

CONGENITAL INFECTIONS

Overview

- Due to transplacental or vaginal exposure to TORCH organisms (toxoplasmosis, other infections, rubella, cytomegalovirus [CMV], and herpes simplex virus [HSV])

Clinical Presentation

- Cataract: rubella, CMV
- Cornea (keratitis): HSV, syphilis
- Retinopathy: toxoplasmosis, rubella, CMV, syphilis

Diagnosis and Evaluation

- Titers and cultures for responsible agents

Treatment

- Targeted at the causative agent with consideration of systemic involvement

NASOLACRIMAL DUCT OBSTRUCTION

Overview

- Nasolacrimal duct obstruction occurs in 5% of newborns, due to failure of canalization of nasolacrimal duct.

Clinical Presentation

- Tearing with mucus buildup

Diagnosis and Evaluation

- Dye disappearance test
- Rule out congenital glaucoma.

Treatment

- Nasolacrimal probing and possible stent if not resolved by 6 to 12 months

OPHTHALMIA NEONATORUM

Overview

- Conjunctivitis within the first month of life
- At risk for systemic infection (*Neisseria*, *Chlamydia*, HSV)

Clinical Presentation

- Conjunctival injection, eyelid swelling, eyelid crusting, discharge (clear or mucopurulent)

Diagnosis and Evaluation

- Culture with gram stain.
- *Neisseria* gonorrhea: onset 3 days to 3 weeks, copious discharge
- *Chlamydia*: onset around 1 week, mild discharge
- HSV: onset in second week of life
- Chemical: onset within 24 hours of medicine administration, self-limited

Treatment

- Prophylaxis (erythromycin or tetracycline)
- Requires systemic treatment for *Neisseria* (ceftriaxone), *Chlamydia* (erythromycin), or HSV (acyclovir)
- May need topical antibiotic or antiviral as well

OCULAR TRAUMA

Overview

- Difficult deliveries and shaking injuries can cause damage to the retina and cornea.

Clinical Presentation

- Unilateral corneal opacity following forceps delivery
- Hemorrhages in the subconjunctival space or retina

Diagnosis and Evaluation

- Breaks in Descemet membrane are seen with forceps injury. There will be no other signs of glaucoma, ocular dysgenesis, or infection.
- Look for retinal hemorrhage on dilated funduscopic examination.
- Retinal hemorrhages from birth trauma are mild and resolve within 4 to 6 weeks.
- Retinal hemorrhages from nonaccidental trauma can be mild or severe and often involve multiple layers of the retina.
- Retinal detachment and retinoschisis may occur after shaking injury and are exceptionally rare in other forms of trauma.

Treatment

- Patching when at risk for amblyopia
- Vitrectomy for severe or nonclearing vitreous hemorrhage
- Evaluation for nonaccidental trauma when clinically suspected

RETINOBLASTOMA

Overview

- This is the most common malignant pediatric ocular tumor.
- Mutations in both alleles of the retinoblastoma gene (*RB1*) on chromosome 13 are found.
- 40% of cases result from the inheritance of one mutated allele:
  - A somatic mutation to the second allele is needed to develop retinoblastoma.
  - Most bilateral cases of retinoblastoma are inherited.
- 60% result from somatic nonhereditary mutations to both alleles.
- If a parent has bilateral retinoblastoma, each child has a 45% risk for the disease (90% penetrance).
- If a parent has unilateral retinoblastoma, each child has a 7% to 15% risk. If a child develops retinoblastoma, which indicates a heritable mutation, each subsequent child will carry a 45% risk.
- Chromosome 13q deletion may include the *RB1* gene and result in retinoblastoma.

Clinical Presentation

- Abnormal red reflex (leukocoria) and strabismus may be present.
- Poor vision in one or both eyes may be noted.
- Inherited and bilateral cases are typically diagnosed when the child is younger than 12 months of age.

Diagnosis and Evaluation

- Perform dilated fundus examination to look for a retinal mass.
- Ultrasound imaging may be helpful when a fundus examination is limited.
- Larger masses may have calcifications or vitreous seeding.
- Obtain magnetic resonance imaging (MRI) scans to rule out trilateral retinoblastoma (retinoblastoma with neuroectodermal tumor of the pineal gland).

- Children who have a parent or sibling with retinoblastoma need early and regular screening.

Treatment

- Systemic chemotherapy is the most common primary treatment.
- Local consolidation is needed after chemotherapy or as primary therapy in small tumors (typically photocoagulation or cryotherapy).
- Intraarterial or intravitreal chemotherapy may be used in select cases and may reduce the need for systemic chemotherapy.
- The survival rate is high (>95%), and most eyes are salvaged.
- Enucleation may be needed in advanced cases (especially unilateral).
- Heritable germinal mutations put a child at risk for secondary malignancies, including pinealoma, sarcoma, melanoma, and carcinomas (incidence rate, 1%/year of life).
- Lifetime monitoring is needed.

Vascular Development of the Retina

NORMAL DEVELOPMENT

- Retinal vasculature originates from the optic nerve at around 13 weeks' gestation.
- In the relatively hypoxic, in utero environment there are various proangiogenic growth factors, including vascular endothelial growth factor (VEGF), which develop and drive vessel growth from the vascular retina to avascular areas.
- Full vascularization is completed between 36 and 40 weeks' gestation.

ABNORMAL DEVELOPMENT IN PREMATURE INFANTS

- Infants born prematurely are exposed to a hyperoxic environment relative to the in utero environment.
- VEGF and other growth factors decrease, delaying vessel growth into the peripheral retina (phase 1 of retinopathy of prematurity [ROP]).
- Hypoxia develops in the peripheral avascular retina, accentuated by fluctuations in the supply of oxygen.
- An increase in proangiogenic factors causes abnormal vascular development at the border of the vascular and avascular retina (phase 2 of ROP).
- Most ROP will regress, but continued growth can lead to bleeding and retinal detachment.

RETINOPATHY OF PREMATURITY (ROP)

Overview

- Abnormal retinal vascular development in premature infants
- A leading cause of childhood blindness and visual impairment

Clinical Presentation

- Risk factors
  - Prematurity
  - Low birth weight
  - Prolonged duration of oxygen therapy
  - Poor weight gain
- No clinical signs are observed until advanced stage; it is identified on routine screening.

Diagnosis and Evaluation

- Dilated fundus examination should be performed by an ophthalmologist familiar with ROP.
- Screen if gestational age ≤ 30 weeks or birth weight ≤ 1500 g.
- Screen if 1500 to 2000 g or 30 to 32 weeks when the clinical course is unstable.
- Screening begins at 31 weeks corrected gestational age (CGA) or 4 weeks after birth (later of the two dates).
- ROP is graded based on zone and stage (Fig. 65.1).
  - Zones are geographic areas to which the vessels have extended:
    - Zone 1 is the most posterior and immature, a circle with a radius twice the distance from the optic nerve to the fovea centered on the optic nerve.
    - Zone 2 is an annulus around zone 1; the outer radius is the distance from the optic nerve to the nasal edge of the retina.
    - Zone 3 is the residual crescent of retina anterior to zone 2.
  - Stage refers to extent of anomalous vasculature. If more than stage 1 ROP is present in the same eye, it is classified by the most severe stage.
    - Stage 0: immature vasculature, no ROP (simply incomplete vascularization)
    - Stage 1: flat line of demarcation between vascular and avascular retina
    - Stage 2: elevated line or ridge
    - Stage 3: extraretinal neovascular proliferation extending from ridge into the vitreous
    - Stage 4: partial retinal detachment
      - Stage 4A: extrafoveal
      - Stage 4B: involves the fovea
    - Stage 5: total retinal detachment
  - Plus disease: dilation and tortuosity of the retinal blood vessels; determined from vessels within zone 1

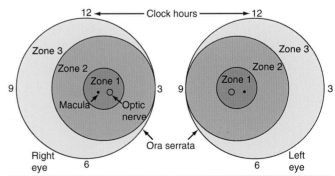

Fig. 65.1 Zones of the retina in retinopathy of prematurity. (From Anderson C, Kapoor S, Mark T, eds. *The Harriet Lane Handbook.* 23rd ed. Elsevier; 2024:503–528e1.)

- Aggressive retinopathy of prematurity was formerly termed "aggressive posterior ROP," or Rush disease. It features rapid development of pathologic neovascularization and severe plus disease without progression through the typical stages.
- Regression is spontaneous or after treatment and is considered either complete or incomplete.

Treatment

- Prevention—Provide prenatal care to limit risk for premature birth, avoid excessive oxygen, and limit extreme fluctuations in oxygenation.
- Treatment is indicated for type 1 ROP:
  - Zone I, any stage with plus disease
  - Zone I, stage 3 without plus disease
  - Zone II, stage 2 or 3 with plus disease
- Laser photocoagulation of the avascular retina is the current standard of care.

- Injection of VEGF inhibitors is better at treating posterior disease (zone 1) and is being used more often. Despite its widespread use, long-term systemic safety is still unclear.

Suggested Readings

Abramson DH, Shields CL, Munier FL, Chantada GL. Treatment of retinoblastoma in 2015: agreement and disagreement. *JAMA Ophthalmol.* 2015;133(11):1341–1347.

Chiang MF, Quinn GE, Fielder AR, et al. International Classification of Retinopathy of Prematurity, Third Edition. *Ophthalmology.* 2021;128(10):e51–e68.

Lee KA, Chandler DL, Repka MX. A comparison of treatment approaches for bilateral congenital nasolacrimal duct obstruction. *Am J Ophthalmol.* 2013;156(5):1045–1050.

Mintz-Hittner HA, Kennedy KA, Chuang AZ, et al. Efficacy of intravitreal bevacizumab for stage 3+ retinopathy of prematurity. *N Engl J Med.* 2011;364(7):603–615.

Plager DA, Lynn MJ, Buckley EG, et al. Complications in the first 5 years following cataract surgery in infants with and without intraocular lens implantation in the Infant Aphakia Treatment Study. *Am J Ophthalmol.* 2014;158(5):892–898.

Yanoff M, Duker JS. *Ophthalmology.* 4th ed. Philadelphia: Saunders; 2014.

66 *Ear Development and Anomalies*

ASHLEY L. SOAPER and CATHERINE K. HART

Outer Ear

NORMAL DEVELOPMENT

- Develops from the first and second branchial arches from six hillocks of His starting at 6 weeks' gestation
- Reaches adult shape by 20 weeks' gestation
- Position of ear
  - Average distance is 1.5 to 2 cm from helical rim to scalp.
  - Top of the external auditory canal (EAC) should be on a horizontal line drawn posteriorly from inferior orbital rim.

OUTER EAR PATHOLOGY

Congenital

- Pre-auricular tags are the most common ear anomalies.
  - Clinical presentation:
    - Due to extra hillocks of His
    - May be associated with branchiootorenal syndrome (especially if bilateral)
  - Diagnosis: clinical examination showing a preauricular tag, which may include cartilage
  - Treatment: elective surgical removal
- Pre-auricular pits
  - Clinical presentation:
    - Due to failure of fusion of the first and second arches of hillocks of His
    - May be associated with branchiootorenal syndrome (especially if bilateral)
  - Diagnosis: clinical examination demonstrating a pit at the helical root
  - Treatment:
    - Antibiotics if infected or draining (occasionally requires incision and drainage [I&D])
    - Surgical excision when not infected
- Prominauris (protruding ears)
  - Clinical presentation: underdevelopment of antihelix, deep conchal bowl
  - Diagnosis: larger than average distance from the helical rim to mastoid, usually bilateral
  - Treatment:
    - Ear molding: promising results if initiated before 3 weeks of age
    - Elective otoplasty (ear pinning) at 5 to 6 years of age
- Microtia: congenital abnormality in phenotype of the external ear
  - Outer ear develops early, so a malformed auricle implies malformation of the middle ear, mastoid, and facial nerve.
  - Clinical presentation:
    - Prevalence: one in 6000 to one in 12,000
    - Usually unilateral; more commonly affects males and the right side
    - 60% syndromic: Goldenhar syndrome, Treacher-Collins syndrome, CHARGE (coloboma, heart defect, choanal atresia, retarded growth, genitourinary and ear anomalies) syndrome
    - Often in conjunction with aural atresia
    - Most also have hearing loss (90%), usually conductive.
  - Diagnosis: Clinical assessment, including bone conduction auditory brainstem response (ABR) to assess hearing
  - Treatment:
    - Prosthesis (adhesive or bone anchored)
    - Surgical reconstruction around 6 years with Medpor (porous polyethylene) implant or costal cartilage graft
- Aural atresia, aural stenosis: congenital lack of or narrowing of the EAC due to failure of resorption of the meatal plug filling the bony portion of EAC by 28 weeks' gestation
  - Clinical presentation:
    - Prevalence: 1 in 10,000 to 1 in 20,000
    - Usually unilateral; more commonly affects males and right side
    - Normal auricle with canal atresia indicates abnormal development during the 28th week of gestation (after ossicle and middle ear development).
    - Associated syndromes: Goldenhar syndrome, Treacher Collins syndrome, Apert syndrome, Crouzon syndrome, Pfeiffer syndrome, Turner syndrome, trisomy 21, trisomy 18, and trisomy 13
  - Diagnosis:
    - Bone conduction ABR to assess hearing
    - Computed tomography (CT) scan of temporal bones
  - Treatment:
    - Hearing amplification
    - Bone-anchored hearing aid (BAHA) or surgical repair at 5 years

Middle and Inner Ear

NORMAL DEVELOPMENT

- Tympanic membrane
  - Two parts: pars flaccida and pars tensa
  - Three layers: epithelial (ectoderm), fibrous (mesoderm), and mucosal (endoderm)

- Middle ear space, mastoid air cells, inner layer of the tympanic membrane, and Eustachian tube arise from the endoderm of the first pharyngeal pouch.
  - Mastoid tip is poorly developed until 1 year of age, making the facial nerve more superficial and prone to injury (especially with surgery or birth trauma).
  - Eustachian tube measures 17 mm at birth and grows to 35 mm by adulthood, becoming less horizontal in orientation.
- Ossicles develop from the first and second branchial arches from 6 to 28 weeks' gestation.
- Inner ear (cochlea, vestibule, and internal auditory canal) malformations occur due to arrest of development from 3 to 10 weeks' gestation

INNER EAR PATHOLOGY

- Michel aplasia is complete agenesis of the petrous portion of the temporal bone due to disruption at or before 3 weeks' gestation.
  - Clinical presentation: normal outer and middle ear with no cochlear structures present and complete deafness
- Mondini dysplasia is a malformed cochlea with incomplete partitioning and reduced number of turns (1–1.5 turns rather than 2.5); it may be associated with an enlarged vestibular aqueduct due to disruption at 6 weeks' gestation.
  - Clinical presentation: range of normal to profound sensorineural hearing loss
  - Associated with Pendred syndrome, Waardenburg syndrome, Treacher Collins syndrome, Wildervanck syndrome, CHARGE syndrome, and cytomegalovirus (CMV) infection
- Scheibe dysplasia is pars inferior dysplasia or cochleosaccular dysplasia.
  - Clinical presentation:
    - Most common membranous inner ear malformation
    - Will have varying degree of sensorineural hearing loss (SNHL)
  - Associated with Usher syndrome, Refsum syndrome, Waardenburg syndrome, Jervell and Lange-Nielsen syndrome, and congenital rubella
- Alexander malformation is dysplasia of the basal turn of the cochlea; it is the least severe malformation.
  - Clinical presentation: high-frequency SNHL
- Enlarged vestibular aqueduct
  - Clinical presentation: variable, fluctuating SNHL that decreases in a stepwise fashion and worsens with head trauma or increased intracranial pressure (ICP)

CONGENITAL HEARING LOSS

- Hearing loss present at birth is 50% genetic and 50% acquired.
- Genetic hearing loss is 70% nonsyndromic and 30% syndromic.

Physical Examination and Testing

- Otoscopy: Evaluate external auditory canal and tympanic membrane.
- External ear: Evaluate auricle, pre-auricular pits and tags, and other facial anomalies.
- Conduct a hearing screen versus formal testing (ABR).
- Consider genetic testing.
- Consider CT of temporal bone.

General Management Concepts for Hearing Loss

- Early detection by 1 month of age, early intervention by 6 months of age
- If syndromic hearing loss is suspected, genetics consultation is appropriate.
- Hearing amplification should be offered early to facilitate development.

INFECTIOUS OR ACQUIRED CAUSES

- Acute otitis media
- Otitis media with effusion
- Fetal alcohol syndrome
- TORCH infections:
  - Toxoplasmosis (*Toxoplasma gondii*)
  - Other: syphilis (*Treponema pallidum*), varicella, parvovirus B19
  - Rubella
  - Cytomegalovirus
    - Most common infectious and nongenetic causes of hearing loss
  - Herpes simplex virus

GENETIC: NONSYNDROMIC AUTOSOMAL RECESSIVE CAUSES

- Connexin mutations are the most common cause of congenital deafness in developed countries.
  - DFNB-1 mutation: 80% due to a connexin 26 mutation (*GJB2* gene)
- Mitochondrial mutations are maternally inherited.
  - A1555G mutation causes increased susceptibility to aminoglycoside-related SNHL.

GENETIC: SYNDROMIC AUTOSOMAL RECESSIVE CAUSES

- Usher syndrome is the most common cause of deafness and blindness in the United States (50%).
  - Clinical presentation: SNHL and retinitis pigmentosa; may have balance issues
  - Degree of hearing loss depends on the designated syndrome type based on genetic mutation.
  - Type 1 is the most severe hearing loss at birth.
  - Diagnosis:
    - Type 1: mutations in at least six genes identified; most common *MYO7A* and *CDH23*
    - Type 2: mutations in at least three genes identified; most common *USH2A*
    - Type 3: most mutations in *CLRN1*
- Pendred syndrome
  - Clinical presentation: SNHL and euthyroid goiter

- Associated with enlarged vestibular aqueduct (85–100%)
- Diagnosis: Mutations of *SLC264A* gene or Pendrin gene on chromosome 7
- Jervell and Lange-Nielsen syndrome
  - Clinical presentation: SNHL and prolonged QTc interval (>500 ms)
  - Diagnosis: Mutations of *KCNQ1* (chromosome 11) and *KCNE1* (chromosome 21)

GENETIC: SYNDROMIC AUTOSOMAL DOMINANT (AD)

- Waardenburg syndrome
  - Waardenburg syndrome is the most common AD syndromic cause of hearing loss.
  - Prevalence is 1 in 10,000 to 1 in 20,000.
  - Associated features: orbital hypertelorism, pigment anomalies in hair ("white forelock"), skin (piebaldism, the absence of melanocytes in certain areas), eyes (pale blue eyes or heterochromia)
  - Clinical presentation:
    - Hearing loss is usually bilateral, profound, and stable over time.
    - Type I: dystopia canthorum (lateral displacement of inner canthi of eyes), white forelock, SNHL in 20%
    - Type II: absence of dystopia canthorum, SNHL in 50%
    - Type III: associated with unilateral ptosis and skeletal abnormalities
    - Type IV: associated with Hirschsprung disease
  - Diagnosis:
    - Mutations in *PAX3* gene (Waardenburg syndrome types I and III)
    - Mutations in *MITF* or *SNAI2* gene (Waardenburg syndrome type II)
    - Mutations in *SOX10*, *EDN3*, or *EDNRB* gene (Waardenburg type IV)
- Branchiootorenal (BOR) syndrome
  - BOR is the second most common AD syndromic cause of hearing loss.
  - Prevalence is 1 in 40,000.
  - Clinical presentation:
    - Ear abnormalities (preauricular pits or tags) with hearing impairment (90%)
    - Branchial cleft cysts, fistulas (25%), and renal anomalies (25%)
  - Diagnosis: Mutation in *EYA1* gene
- Craniofacial dysostosis (Apert syndrome and Crouzon syndrome)
  - Clinical presentation: conductive hearing loss and craniosynostosis
    - Apert: syndactyly of hands and feet of second through fourth digits and varying degrees of developmental; not seen in Crouzon
  - Diagnosis: *FGFR* gene mutation
- CHARGE syndrome
  - Clinical presentation: coloboma (eye), heart defects, atresia (choanal), retardation (growth), genitourinary anomalies, ear abnormalities
  - Diagnosis: *CHD7* gene mutation

- Treacher Collins syndrome (mandibulofacial dysostosis)
  - Clinical presentation:
    - Midface hypoplasia and micrognathia, down-slanting palpebral fissures
    - Auricular deformities and conductive hearing loss
  - Diagnosis: mutations in *TCOF1*, *POLR1D*, or *POLR1C* gene
- Stickler syndrome (hereditary arthro-ophthalmopathy)
  - Clinical presentation:
    - Pierre Robin sequence (micrognathia, glossoptosis, and possible cleft palate)
    - Hearing loss (80%)
    - Spondyloepiphyseal dysplasia
  - Diagnosis: *COL11A1* and *COL2A1* gene mutations
- Klippel-Feil syndrome
  - Clinical presentation: fusion of cervical vertebrae and hearing loss
  - Diagnosis: *GDF6*, *MEOX1*, and *GDF3* gene mutations on chromosomes 8q22, 17q21, and 12p13, respectively
- Other syndromes associated with hearing loss
  - Goldenhar syndrome
  - DiGeorge syndrome
  - Trisomy 13, 18, and 21
  - Turner syndrome
  - Congenital hypothyroidism

OTHER RISK FACTORS FOR HEARING LOSS

- Family history of permanent hearing loss in childhood
- Exposure to ototoxic medications: chemotherapy (carboplatin, cisplatin), loop diuretics (furosemide), aminoglycosides (gentamicin, tobramycin)
- Prematurity (<37 weeks) or birth weight < 1500 g
- Admission to neonatal intensive care unit (NICU) for >5 days
- Extracorporeal membrane oxygenation (ECMO)
- Prolonged mechanical ventilation (>10 days)
- Hyperbilirubinemia (>20 mg/100 mL serum or requiring exchange transfusion)
- Craniofacial anomalies or stigmata of a syndrome associated with hearing loss

NEWBORN HEARING SCREENING

- Universal newborn hearing screening (NBHS) has been instituted because as many as 50% of infants with hearing loss do not have identifiable risk factors.
- Types of NBHS
  - Otoacoustic emissions (OAEs) are acoustic emissions generated by the cochlear outer hair cells.
    - Evoked OAEs are generated in response to tone or click stimulus.
      - Most commonly used for NBHS
    - Benefits include that OAE screening is fast, efficient, and objective, providing frequency- and ear-specific data.
    - Limitations include that such screening is not a sufficient screening tool for infants at high risk or in the setting of middle ear disease.
    - Requirements include a calm, quiet subject and normal middle ear function.

- Auditory brainstem response (ABR) tests the cochlear nerve and brainstem by measuring electrical activity in response to click or tone burst stimuli.
  - It is not a true test of hearing but estimates hearing thresholds.
  - Automated ABR is used for screening.
  - Results are not affected by anesthetics or sedatives.
- Diagnostic ABR:
  - Not used for screening because it is time consuming and requires an audiologist to perform and interpret results
  - Allows determination of severity, nature (conductive or sensorineural), and frequency of hearing loss
  - Results are not affected by anesthetics or sedatives.
- Recommendations
  - All newborns should have hearing screening during the birth admission or by 1 month of life.
  - Automated ABR is recommended for all NICU infants or those admitted to the hospital for >5 days.
- If the infant does not pass the hearing screen, audiologic and otologic evaluations should be performed by 3 months of age.
- Rescreening should include both ears (not just ear that failed).
- At-risk newborns who pass the NBHS should be evaluated by an audiologist every 6 months for the first 3 years to identify changes in hearing.

Suggested Readings

Grindle CR. Pediatric hearing loss. *Pediatr Rev.* 2014;35:456–463.

Korver AM, Smith RJ, Van Camp G, et al. Congenital hearing loss. *Nat Rev Dis Primers.* 2017;3:16094.

Kraft CT, Malhotra S, Boerst A, Thorne MC. Risk indicators for congenital and delayed-onset hearing loss. *Otol Neurotol.* 2014;35:1839–1843.

Liming BJ, Carter J, Cheng A, et al. International Pediatric Otolaryngology (IPOG) consensus recommendations: hearing loss in the pediatric patient. *Intl J Pediatr Otorhinolaryngol.* 2016;90:251–258.

67 Nose, Mouth, and Throat Development and Anomalies

ASHLEY L. SOAPER and CATHERINE K. HART

Branchial (Pharyngeal) Arches

NORMAL DEVELOPMENT

- Most development occurs from 4 to 8 weeks' gestation.
- The five branchial arches (mesoderm) develop during week 4. See Table 67.1.
- Other pertinent structures:
  - Tongue
    - Anterior two-thirds derived from first branchial arch
    - Posterior third derived from third and fourth branchial arches
  - Thyroid gland
    - Thyroid diverticulum arises from endoderm at the foramen cecum (base of tongue) at 24 days' gestation.
    - Thyroid descends into the neck immediately anterior to the hyoid bone to reach its final position anterior to the trachea by week 7 of gestation.
  - Larynx, trachea, and proximal esophagus
    - The laryngotracheal groove develops in the ventral foregut at 3.5 weeks' gestation.
    - The tracheoesophageal septum forms to create two separate tubes:
      - Failure of recanalization results in laryngeal atresia and stenosis.
      - Failure of separation of the tubes results in tracheoesophageal fistula (TEF) and/or esophageal atresia (EA).

ANOMALIES OF DEVELOPMENT

Syndromes Associated With Branchial Apparatus

- Pierre Robin sequence (first branchial arch)
  - Clinical presentation:
    - Triad of micrognathia, glossoptosis, and cleft palate
    - Mandibular hypoplasia displaces the tongue, preventing fusion of the palatal shelves.
  - Diagnosis: clinical findings, assess for associated syndromes, polysomnography
  - Treatment:
    - Depends on degree of airway compromise
    - Interventions include prone positioning, nasopharyngeal airway, endotracheal intubation, lip–tongue adhesion, mandibular distraction, and tracheostomy.

- Other syndromes of first and second branchial arches: Goldenhar syndrome, hemifacial microsomia, Treacher Collins syndrome, and Nager syndrome
- DiGeorge syndrome (hypoplasia of first branchial arch, third and fourth branchial pouches)
  - Deletion of chromosome 22q11.2
  - Autosomal dominant (AD) if inherited, but usually sporadic
  - Clinical presentation ("CATCH-22"):
    - Cardiac and aortic malformations
    - Abnormal facies: micrognathia, ear anomalies, telecanthus, narrow palpebral fissures, high and broad nasal bridge, long face
    - Thymic aplasia, hypoplasia with associated immunodeficiency
    - Cleft palate (may be submucous cleft)
    - Hypocalcemia with tetany due to absence of parathyroid glands
  - Associated anomalies include glottic web, TEF, tracheomalacia, and hearing loss.
  - Diagnosis: cardiac echocardiography (echo), flow cytometry, calcium levels, parathyroid hormone (PTH) levels
  - Genetic testing: array comparative genomic hybridization (aCGH), fluorescent in situ hybridization (FISH), TBX1 gene analysis, karyotype
  - Treatment: amplification for hearing loss, cleft palate repair, manage immunodeficiency, calcium supplementation

NECK MASSES

- Branchial cleft anomalies (cysts, tracts, and fistulas)
  - Incidence unknown, but bilateral in 2% to 3%
    - If bilateral, check renal ultrasound for branchio-otorenal syndrome.
  - Cyst: no opening
  - Sinus: single opening to skin or internally
  - Fistula: opening to skin and internally
  - Diagnosis: clinical findings, imaging (computed tomography scan [CT] and/or magnetic resonance imaging [MRI])
  - Treatment: excision
- First branchial cleft anomalies
  - 1% of all branchial anomalies
  - Clinical presentation: pre-auricular cyst (type I) or in submandibular region (type II)

Table 67.1   Branchial Apparatus: Arches, Pouches, and Clefts[a]

Apparatus	Key Structures
ARCHES (MESODERM)	
First (mandibular) branchial arch	Ossicles, external ear, mandible, muscles of mastication
	Cranial nerve innervation: V (trigeminal)
Second (hyoid) branchial arch	Ossicles, hyoid, external ear, facial muscles
	Cranial nerve innervation: VII (facial)
Third branchial arch	Hyoid, muscles of pharynx
	Cranial nerve innervation: IX (glossopharyngeal)
Fourth branchial arch	Thyroid cartilage, cricothyroid muscle
	Cranial nerve innervation: X (superior laryngeal)
Sixth branchial arch	Cricoid cartilage, muscles of larynx
	Cranial nerve innervation: X (recurrent laryngeal)
POUCHES (ENDODERM)	
First branchial pouch	Auditory tubes, middle ear cavity
Second branchial pouch	Palatine tonsil
Third branchial pouch	Dorsal portion: inferior parathyroids
	Ventral portion: thymus
Fourth branchial pouch	Dorsal portion: superior parathyroids
	Ventral portion: ultimobranchial body, differentiates into parafollicular C cells of thyroid gland
Sixth branchial pouch	Ultimobranchial body
CLEFTS (ECTODERM)	
First branchial cleft	External auditory meatus
Second, third, fourth, and sixth branchial cleft	Usually obliterated (remnants may appear as cervical cysts or fistulas along the anterior border of the sternocleidomastoid muscle)

[a]Note: There is no fifth branchial apparatus.

- Second branchial cleft anomalies
  - Most common type of branchial cleft cyst (95%)
  - Clinical presentation: painless, fluctuant mass in anterior triangle of neck
- Third/fourth branchial cleft anomalies
  - Rare
  - Clinical presentation: mass in lower anterior neck
- Thyroglossal duct cyst
  - Most common congenital anomaly in the neck
  - Due to failure of obliteration of the thyroglossal duct tract (arises from foramen cecum)
  - Clinical presentation: painless midline neck mass in close proximity to the hyoid bone that elevates with swallowing or tongue protrusion
  - Diagnosis: ultrasound, CT (also need to confirm that there is normal thyroid tissue)
  - Treatment: surgical excision via Sistrunk operation (removal of duct cyst, middle part of hyoid bone, and surrounding tissue around the thyroglossal tract)
- Pseudotumor of infancy
  - Fibrotic lesion of the distal sternocleidomastoid muscle

- Clinical presentation:
  - Firm neck mass presents with torticollis in first weeks of life
  - Chin turned away and head tilted toward mass
  - Associated with breech presentation and forceps delivery
- Diagnosis: clinical examination, ultrasound
- Treatment: physical therapy
- Dermoid cysts
  - Mesoderm and ectoderm; may contain skin appendages
  - Clinical presentation: midline painless mass that does not elevate with tongue protrusion
  - Diagnosis: clinical examination and ultrasound
  - Treatment: excision
- Teratomas
  - Arise from misplaced embryologic germ cells containing all three germ layers
  - Clinical presentation:
    - Occur in 1 in 16,000 individuals
    - Larger midline or paramedian masses, present earlier in life, cause respiratory compromise.
    - 20% are associated with maternal polyhydramnios.
    - Termed *epignathus* when they arise from the palate
  - Diagnosis: ultrasound (often prenatal) as a mixed echogenicity lesion
  - Treatment:
    - Surgical excision
    - May require emergency airway management followed by excision at birth via ex utero intrapartum treatment (EXIT) procedure

Nose

NORMAL DEVELOPMENT

- Anterior neuropore represents the cranial aspect of the neural tube; it closes on the 24th day of gestation.
  - Failure of neuropore closure results in anencephaly.
- The skull base develops during the third week of gestation.
  - Faulty closure of the foramen cecum at the third week of development results in skull base defects, with the potential for midline nasal masses.

PATHOLOGY

- Midline nasal masses (glioma, encephalocele, dermoid)
  - Clinical presentation
  - Incidence is 1 in 20,000 to 1 in 40,000 live births (Table 67.2).
  - Diagnosis:
    - Clinical examination, CT scan, and MRI
    - Must determine if mass communicates with intracranial space (via MRI) and if there is a skull base defect (via CT)
  - Treatment:
    - Surgical excision with repair of skull base defect
    - Requires neurosurgery consultation if intracranial communication is present

Table 67.2 Midline Nasal Masses

Parameter	Glioma	Encephalocele	Dermoid
Pathophysiology	Sequestered glial tissue	Herniated meninges ± brain tissue	Dural tissue that does not obliterate
Connection to subarachnoid space?	No	Yes	Yes in 20–45%
Description	Firm, nonpulsatile mass	Soft, compressible mass that gets bigger with crying, straining (Furstenberg sign)	Firm, noncompressible with pit or fistula tract connecting to nasal dorsum
Transilluminates?	No	Yes	No
Location	Extranasal (60%) Intranasal (30%) Combined (10%)	Occipital (75%)	Nasal dorsum (most common), but anywhere along nose

- Left untreated, they can cause abscess formation, cerebrospinal (CSF) leak, meningitis, intracranial infection, and cosmetic deformity.

External Nose and Nasal Cavities

NORMAL DEVELOPMENT

- Nasal development occurs from 4 to 8 weeks' gestation.
- Frontonasal prominence develops into the nose.
  - Neural crest cells migrate into the frontonasal prominence at 4 weeks' gestation to form nasal placodes, oval-shaped thickenings of surface ectoderm.
  - Nasal placodes deepen into nasal pits at 6 weeks' gestation.
  - Nasobuccal membrane ruptures to create the primitive nasal cavity and choanae.
  - Medial and lateral nasal processes fuse with paired maxillary and mandibular processes to complete facial formation by 14 weeks' gestation.

PATHOLOGY

- Choanal atresia
  - Failure of resorption of the nasobuccal membrane at 5 weeks' gestation
  - Epidemiology:
    - Occurs in 1 in 5000 live births, with a 1:2 male-to-female ratio.
    - Unilateral (right > left) is twice as common as bilateral.
    - 50% have other congenital anomalies.
    - Associated with CHARGE (coloboma, heart defect, choanal atresia, retarded growth, genitourinary and ear anomalies) syndrome, Treacher Collins syndrome, Apert syndrome, and Crouzon syndrome
  - Clinical presentation:
    - Bilateral: cyanosis in infants relieved by crying
    - Unilateral: presents later with chronic, unilateral nasal drainage, obstruction
  - Diagnosis:
    - Inability to pass a suction catheter or absence of fogging of mirror under nose
    - Confirm with nasal endoscopy and CT scan.

- Treatment:
  - If bilateral, stabilize airway with oral airway, McGovern nipple, and endotracheal intubation followed by early surgical repair.
  - If unilateral, repair when symptomatic.

SYNDROMES ASSOCIATED WITH ABNORMAL NASAL DEVELOPMENT

See Table 67.3.

Table 67.3 Syndromes Associated With Abnormal Nasal Development

Low nasal bridge	Hurler syndrome
	Noonan syndrome
	Osteogenesis imperfecta
	Pfeiffer syndrome
	Valproic acid exposure in utero
	Growth hormone deficiency
	Congenital syphilis
Broad nasal ridge	Down syndrome
	Valproic acid exposure in utero
	Opitz G/BBB syndrome
	Otopalatodigital syndrome
	Cri du chat syndrome
Short, anteverted nostrils	Trisomy 18
	Valproic acid exposure in utero
	Opitz G/BBB syndrome
	Smith-Lemli-Opitz syndrome
	Lissencephaly
	Cornelia de Lange syndrome
	Cutis laxa
	Stickler syndrome
	Joubert syndrome
Abnormal philtrum	Fetal alcohol syndrome (smooth/flat)
	Perinatal HIV/AIDS (prominent, triangular shaped)
	Trisomy 13 (absent)
	Wolf-Hirschhorn syndrome (short)

AIDS, Acquired immunodeficiency syndrome; *HIV,* human immunodeficiency virus.

Mouth and Palate

NORMAL DEVELOPMENT

- Five facial primordia arising from first arch develop around stomodeum at 4 weeks' gestation:
  - Unpaired frontonasal prominence (superiorly)
  - Merging of medial nasal processes (5 weeks' gestation) that gives rise to the primary palate, philtrum of upper lip, and maxilla
  - Merging of paired maxillary prominences (6–7 weeks' gestation) to form upper lip, maxilla, and secondary palate
  - Secondary palate fuses with primary palate and nasal septum by 12 weeks' gestation.
  - Paired mandibular prominences (inferiorly) merge at 4 weeks' gestation to create mandible, lower lip, and lower part of face.

PATHOLOGY

- Cleft lip (CL) and cleft palate (CP)
  - Clinical presentation:
    - Most common congenital craniofacial malformations
    - Embryologic causes
      - CL ± CP: failure of fusion of the medial nasal processes with the maxillary prominences (4–6 weeks' gestation)
      - CP: failure of fusion of lateral palatine processes (8–12 weeks' gestation)
  - Epidemiology:
    - CL ± CP occur in 1 in 1000 live births.
    - More common in males
    - Up to 30% associated with syndromes
    - Isolated CP occurs in 1 in 2500 live births.
    - Risk for CL and CP in subsequent pregnancies if
      - Parents' normal, first child affected: 3% to 4%
      - One parent affected, first child affected: 10% to 15%
      - Both parents affected, first child affected: 45%
  - Diagnosis: physical examination findings at birth or prenatal ultrasound
  - Treatment:
    - Prior to surgical intervention
      - Manage feeding difficulties (Pigeon, McGovern, Haberman nipples)
      - Ensure adequate airway.
      - Audiologic evaluation
    - Surgical repair
      - CL repair: Remember the rule of 10s (10 weeks old, 10 pounds, hemoglobin of 10)
      - CP repair: Repair at 6 to 18 months of age.
      - 95% will have otitis media with effusion; most need ear tubes.

Neonatal Airway

SPECIAL CONSIDERATIONS FOR INTUBATION

- Anatomic differences

  - Larynx sits higher in the neck with a more acute angle from the oropharynx.
  - Cricoid cartilage is narrowest portion of the airway (compared to glottis in adults).
- Normal airway size for full-term neonate is a 3.5-mm endotracheal tube (ETT)
  - Adjust based on weight and gestational age.
  - ETT size is approximately 1/10th of gestational age (rounded down).
- Risks
  - Subglottic stenosis
    - Incidence has decreased over the past several decades: 8.3% in the 1970s compared to 0.63% in the 1990s.
    - Increased risk with prolonged, multiple or traumatic intubation, inappropriately sized tube, or high cuff pressures
  - Tracheal perforation
    - Contributing factors: difficult exposure, multiple intubation attempts, excessive force, improperly placed endotracheal tubes with stylets, airway anomalies
    - Clinical signs: subcutaneous emphysema, pneumothorax, pneumomediastinum

TRACHEOSTOMY

- Indications:
  - Prolonged ventilator dependence, such as with severe bronchopulmonary dysplasia
  - Upper airway obstruction
    - Craniofacial anomalies
    - Airway stenosis or trachea/bronchomalacia
    - Vocal fold paralysis
  - Neuromuscular or cardiac disease
- Complications:
  - Some complication is experienced in up to 80%.
  - Mortality rates as high as 42% have been reported, mostly due to comorbid conditions.
  - Tracheostomy-specific related deaths: 0.05% to 3.6%
  - Increased morbidity in children who are younger, low birth weight, have a history of heart or central nervous system (CNS) disease, or have had a tracheostomy at <100 days
  - Early complications (<7 days postoperatively): bleeding, subcutaneous emphysema, pneumothorax, pneumomediastinum, TEF
  - Late complications (>7 days postoperatively): peristomal granulation tissue, laryngeal or tracheal stenosis, tracheomalacia, TEF
  - Complications occurring in both time periods: accidental decannulation, mucus plugging, skin breakdown, infection, tracheoinnominate fistula, cardiopulmonary arrest, death

Necrotizing Tracheobronchitis

- Iatrogenic desquamation of the tracheobronchial mucosa, with formation of pseudomembranes of necrotic tissue
- Clinical presentation:

- Acute airway obstruction characterized by sudden unexplained increase in ventilatory requirements
- Mortality rate as high as 45%
- Seen in infants on mechanical ventilation, especially oscillator or jet ventilation
- Diagnosis and treatment:
  - Rigid bronchoscopy with removal of necrotic debris ± extracorporeal membrane oxygenation (ECMO)
  - Serial bronchoscopies due to risk of tracheal stenosis after resolution of the acute process
  - Culture and treatment of underlying infectious cause

EVALUATION OF STRIDOR

- Stridor: high-pitched sound created by turbulent airflow through a narrowed larynx or trachea
- History:
  - Onset (birth or several weeks after)
  - Progression (getting better or worse)
  - Chronicity (constant or intermittent)
  - Alleviating and aggravating factors (positioning, feeding, agitation, sleeping)
  - Prior intubation and/or congenital anomalies
  - Feeding difficulties
  - Quality (inspiratory, expiratory, biphasic)
- Physical examination: Assess work of breathing, retractions, and vital signs.
  - Determine the timing of stridor in the respiratory cycle.
    - Inspiratory stridor suggests supraglottic or glottic pathology.
    - Expiratory stridor suggests tracheal pathology.
    - Biphasic stridor suggests glottic or subglottic pathology.
- Evaluation and diagnosis:
  - Flexible awake laryngoscopy to evaluate dynamics of airway, levels of obstruction
  - Other studies: lateral, anteroposterior (AP) neck x-rays, chest x-ray, CT and MRI scans, barium swallow

PATHOLOGY

- Laryngomalacia is the most common congenital cause of stridor.
  - Clinical presentation:
    - Inspiratory stridor begins several weeks after birth and worsens with agitation, feeding, or supine positioning.
    - When severe, the infant may have apnea and/or cyanosis, difficulty feeding, or failure to thrive.
  - Diagnosis: Flexible laryngoscopy shows omega-shaped epiglottis that curls inward, shortened aryepiglottic folds, and arytenoids that prolapse on inspiration.
  - Treatment:
    - Most infants can be managed conservatively.
    - Approximately 10% will require surgical intervention.
    - Indications for surgery include apnea and/or cyanosis, increased work of breathing, failure to thrive, and cor pulmonale.

- Vocal cord paralysis is the second most common congenital cause of stridor.
  - It is typically idiopathic in neonates but can be iatrogenic.
  - Causes include cardiac surgery, CNS anomalies, Chiari malformation, intubation injury, infections, trauma, and some syndromes.
  - Clinical presentation:
    - Unilateral: may present with weak cry, feeding difficulties, and stridor
    - Bilateral: upper airway obstruction with biphasic stridor
  - Diagnosis:
    - Flexible laryngoscopy to evaluate vocal fold motion
    - If immobility is identified, brain MRI to rule out CNS lesions
  - Treatment:
    - May recover spontaneously over several years
    - Unilateral: rarely requires intervention
    - Bilateral: tracheostomy, anterior/posterior cricoid split
- Subglottic stenosis
  - Subglottic stenosis is the third most common cause of stridor in newborns.
    - Congenital (5%) is due to incomplete laryngeal lumen recanalization.
    - Acquired (95%) has a history of prolonged or traumatic intubation.
  - Clinical presentation: stridor, retractions, failure to extubate, feeding difficulties
  - Diagnosis: microlaryngoscopy and bronchoscopy with airway sizing
  - Treatment: balloon dilation, anterior/posterior cricoid split, tracheostomy, laryngotracheoplasty

OTHER CAUSES OF STRIDOR

- Laryngocele: enlarged laryngeal saccule with entrapment of air
- Saccular cyst: fluid-filled dilations of the laryngeal ventricle
- Subglottic hemangioma: subglottic mass, often with cutaneous hemangiomas; treat with propranolol depending on size/symptoms
- Recurrent respiratory papillomatosis: seen in neonates due to vertical transmission from affected mothers
- Laryngeal webs: due to incomplete recanalization of laryngeal lumen during embryogenesis
  - Typically glottic in location (75%), causing weak cry, biphasic stridor
  - Should prompt evaluation for 22q11 deletion
- Tracheal pathology
  - Congenital stenosis is often due to complete tracheal rings or sleeve trachea.
    - Associated with pulmonary artery slings
  - Acquired stenosis is usually due to intubation or tracheostomy.
  - Tracheomalacia is due to weak cartilage or extrinsic compression.

Tip: In general, MRI is better to assess soft tissue and CT is better to assess boney abnormalities.

Suggested Readings

Scott AR, Tibesar RJ, Sidman JD. Pierre Robin sequence: evaluation, management, indications for surgery and pitfalls. *Otolaryngol Clin North Am.* 2012;45(3):695–710.

Swibel Rosenthal LH, Caballero N, Drake AF. Otolaryngologic manifestations of craniofacial syndromes. *Otolaryngol Clin North Am.* 2012;45(3):557–577.

Yates PD. Stridor in children. In: Lalwani AK, ed. *CURRENT Diagnosis & Treatment in Otolaryngology: Head and Neck Surgery.* 3rd ed. New York: McGraw Hill; 2012:462–473.

68 Skin Development and Function

JONATHAN LAI, NINA D'AMIANO, and BERNARD A. COHEN

- Table 68.1 shows the embryology and development of skin.
- Differences between preterm and full-term skin (see Table 68.2):
  - Preterm babies have thinner skin, fewer keratinocyte attachments, more sun sensitivity, and less pigment, hair, sweat, and melanin.
  - Thinner skin increases transepidermal water loss (loss of water from inside the body to the surrounding environment through the epidermis via evaporation and diffusion) and increases the permeability of medications or toxic substances.
    - Avoid topical medications in newborns if systemic absorption would be harmful, particularly topical lidocaine, mydriatic agents, antiseptic agents, and biological agents.
  - Preterm and low-birth-weight infants may lack the vernix caseosa, a protective coating that increases hydration, lowers pH, and reduces heat loss.
  - Decreased epidermal and dermal thickness results in increased heat loss from radiation and conduction.
    - Minimize heat loss by swaddling the infant and increasing the ambient humidity and temperature, in addition to utilization of an incubator for controlled thermoregulation.
- Compared to older children and adults, preterm and term newborns
  - Are more likely to develop blisters or erosions in response to heat, chemical irritants, mechanical trauma, and inflammatory skin conditions
  - Avoid the application of monitors, adhesives, and harsh chemicals and cleansing agents, as they may compromise the skin barrier in neonates.
  - Have higher skin pH levels, leading to desquamation via serine protease activation and degradation of lipid-processing enzymes

Table 68.1 Neonatal Skin Embryology

Gestational Age (weeks)	Epidermal Development	Hair, Nail, and Gland Development
3–4	Single layer of ectoderm	
6	Outer periderm and inner germinal (basal) layer	Basal layer → epidermis
9–12	Epidermal stratification, appearance of anchoring filaments, hemidesmosomes, keratinization begins	Hair follicles and nail primordia seen
12–14	Fingerprints form	Eccrine and sebaceous glands develop
12–24	Melanin production (12–16 weeks) Melanosome transfer (20 weeks)	Hair follicle differentiation, mesenchymal cells associate with the epidermal bud, sebaceous glands apparent
24	Mature epidermis complete	Hair follicle elongation, all layers of epidermis keratinized

Adapted from Jain S, ed. *Dermatology: Illustrated Study Guide and Comprehensive Board Review*. Springer: New York; 2005:2.

Table 68.2 Structural and Functional Differences of Adult, Term Infant, and Preterm Infant Skin

Parameter	Adult	Term	Preterm (30 weeks)	Significance
Epidermal thickness	50 µm	50 µm	27.4 µm	Permeability to topical agents ↑ Transepidermal water loss[a]
Cell attachments (desmosome, hemidesmosome)	Normal	Normal	Fewer	↑ Tendency to blister
Dermis	Normal	↓ Collagen and elastic fibers	↓↓ Collagen and elastic fibers	↓ Elasticity ↑ Blistering
Melanosomes	Normal	Fewer; delayed activity for 1–7 days	1/3 of term infants	↑ Photosensitivity
Eccrine glands	Normal	↓ Neurologic control for 2–3 years	Total anhidrosis	↓ Response to thermal stress
Sebaceous glands	Normal	Normal	Normal	Barrier properties Lubricant Antibacterial
Hair	Normal	↓ Terminal hair	Persistent lanugo	Helpful in assessing gestational age

[a]Transepidermal water loss (*TEWL*) is the loss of water from inside the body to the surrounding environment through the epidermis via evaporation and diffusion. TEWL increases permeability to topical agents such as medications.
Adapted from Puttgen K, Cohen BA. Neonatal dermatology. In: Cohen BA, ed. *Cohen's Pediatric Dermatology*. 4th ed. Philadelphia: Saunders/Elsevier; 2013:14.

- Higher skin pH also leads to decreased defense against infection.
- Are not well equipped to handle thermal stress and sunlight due to underdeveloped eccrine glands
  - Avoid exposure to excess sun, and dress the infant in protective clothing when outdoors.
- Common skin injuries of neonates
  - Intravenous (IV) infiltration
    - Skin infiltration by IV fluids can cause blisters, inflammation, and subsequent necrosis.
    - Infiltration of hypertonic fluids, such as glucose and calcium, may result in full-thickness sloughing of the skin and later contractures.
    - Ensure proper placement of IV lines and watch for swelling or erythema near the IV site.
    - Discontinue IVs immediately if there is clinical suspicion.
    - Treatment includes elevation of the extremity and management with a temperature modality; may require splinting, physical therapy, and surgical repair, particularly if infiltration occurred over a joint.
  - Chemical burns
    - Topical agents, such as iodophors, cleaners, soaps, detergents, and solvents, may produce severe irritant reactions, particularly in premature infants.
    - Acids are associated with coagulative necrosis.
    - Alkalis are associated with liquefactive necrosis.
  - Treatment includes the application of a bland emollient; also consider a mild-potency topical steroid to suppress inflammation.
  - Thermal burns
    - Causes include heated water beds, radiant warmers, transcutaneous oxygen monitors, heated/humidified air, and, rarely, electrical discharge.
    - Prevention is key! Monitor the temperature of these devices.
    - Treatment includes antibiotic ointments, topical silver, and protective dressings.
  - Heel stick nodules
    - Often occur from repeated needlesticks
    - Clinically, they appear as tiny whitish papules or nodules resembling milia after several months and eventually calcify (termed heel-stick calcinosis cutis).
    - They appear between 4 and 12 months of age, then spontaneously resolve by age 18 to 30 months; no treatment is needed.

Suggested Readings

Jain S. Basic science and immunology. In: Jain S, ed. *Dermatology: Illustrated Study Guide and Comprehensive Board Review*. New York: Springer; 2005:1–28.

Hoath SB, Narendran V. The skin of the neonate. In: Martin RJ, Fanaroff AA, Walsh MC, eds. *Fanaroff and Martin's Neonatal-Perinatal Medicine*. 11th ed. Philadelphia: Elsevier; 2020:1898.

Puttgen K, Cohen BA. Neonatal dermatology. In: Cohen BA, ed. *Cohen's Pediatric Dermatology*. 4th ed. Philadelphia: Saunders; 2013:14–67.

69 *Neonatal Skin Lesions*

JONATHAN LAI, NINA D'AMIANO, and BERNARD A. COHEN

Newborn Dermatoses

See Table 69.1.

Table 69.1 Newborn Dermatoses

	Epidemiology	Clinical Features	Histology/ Pathology Findings	Prognosis and Treatment	Differential Diagnosis
Erythema toxicum neonatorum (see Fig. 69.1)	One-half of full-term newborns Less frequent in preterm More common in boys	Healthy infants, erythematous macules evolving into yellow–white pustules on trunk, appear between days 1 and 3 of life, "flea-bitten" appearance	Eosinophils in Wright-stained smear	Asymptomatic, resolves spontaneously in several days	Staphylococcal folliculitis, acne neonatorum, pyoderma, congenital candidiasis, Herpes simplex
Transient neonatal pustular melanosis (see Fig. 69.2)	5% of Black newborns, 1% of white infants	Small pustules that rupture leaving collarette of fine scale and significant postinflammatory hyperpigmentation Can involve palms and soles and may be present at birth	Neutrophils in Wright-stained smear, no organisms	Asymptomatic, pustules resolve within 48 hours, hyperpigmentation can last months	Transient neonatal pustular melanosis, miliaria, Infantile acropustulosis, eosinophilic pustular folliculitis
Congenital milia	Up to 40% of full-term infants If >2 mm and large number especially of face and scalp consider oral facial digital syndrome	1–2 mm white smooth papules usually on cheeks, forehead, chin. Epstein pearls occur on midline hard palate. Bohn nodules appear at gum margin. Sebaceous hyperplasia (smaller and more yellow)	Tiny epidermal inclusion cysts arising from vellus hair	Resolve over months without treatment	Sebaceous hyperplasia, comedonal acne, flat warts, milia-like idiopathic calcinosis cutis
Miliaria neonatorum	Healthy infants	Four clinical variants depending on depth of occlusion All resolve with cooling and avoidance of occlusive clothing. ▪ *Crystallina:* superficial, clear, noninflammatory vesicles within stratum corneum ▪ *Rubra:* erythematous grouped fine papules in skinfolds (see Fig. 69.3) ▪ *Pustulosa:* erythematous grouped pustules with possible bacterial infection ▪ *Profunda:* papular eruption within the deeper eccrine duct			Herpes simplex, varicella, congenital candidiasis, pityrosporum, staphylococcal folliculitis
Neonatal acne (see Fig. 69.4)	20% of healthy infants More common in boys	Comedones, inflammatory papules and pustules Neonatal acne appears at 1–2 weeks. Infantile acne appears at 3–6 months	Comedones	Infantile resolves by 3 months. Infantile can persist for years. 2.5% benzoyl peroxide daily. If severe, systemic erythromycin can be added.	Cephalic pustulosis with uniform 2–3 mm pustules is a variant in which *Malassezia* is implicated. No other disorders should feature comedones.
Diaper dermatitis	Occurs in about 50% of infants Peak incidence is around 9–12 months of age.	Redness and mild scaling of gluteal crease, buttocks, and pubic area May become erosive Caused by irritants including urine, feces, and cleansing materials	Spongiosis in the epidermis	Resolves with removing irritants, gentle skin care, zinc oxide paste as barrier ± mild potency topical steroid	Seborrheic dermatitis, allergic contact dermatitis, psoriasis (see Fig. 69.5), Langerhans cell histiocytosis, acrodermatitis enteropathica, *Candida*, *Staphylococcus* l, and streptococcal infections

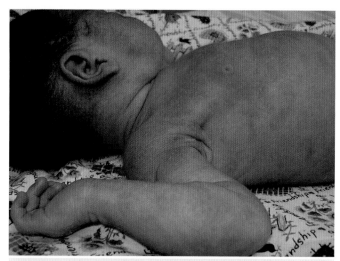

Fig. 69.1 Erythema toxicum neonatorum. Numerous yellow papules and pustules surrounded by large erythematous rings on the trunk. (Courtesy of Dr. Bernard Cohen. Dr. Cohen retains copyright of this figure.)

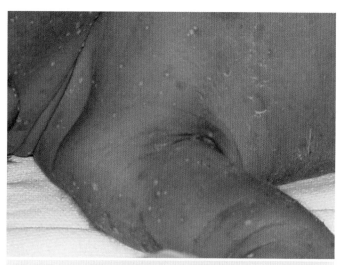

Fig. 69.2 Neonatal pustular melanosis. Numerous tiny pustules dot the trunk with healing pustules, leaving behind hyperpigmentation. (Courtesy of Dr. Bernard Cohen. Dr. Cohen retains copyright of this figure.)

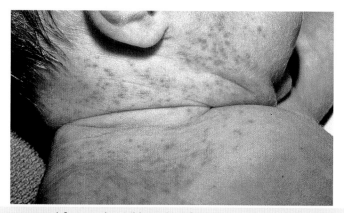

Fig. 69.3 Miliaria rubra. Erythematous, grouped, fine papules visible on this infant. (From Puttgen K, Cohen BA. Neonatal dermatology. In: Cohen BA, ed. *Pediatric Dermatology*. 4th ed. Philadelphia: Elsevier; 2013:21, Fig. 2.17.)

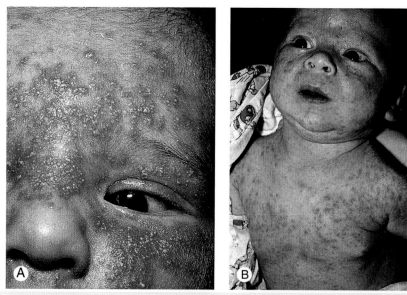

Fig. 69.4 Neonatal acne. Red papules mixed with pustules diffusely over face (A) and face and trunk (B) of infant. (From Puttgen K, Cohen BA. Neonatal dermatology. In: Cohen BA, ed. *Pediatric Dermatology*. 4th ed. Philadelphia: Elsevier; 2013:22, Fig. 2.19.)

Papulosquamous Disorders in Neonates

SEBORRHEIC DERMATITIS

- Clinical presentation
  - Occurs within the first 2 months of life
  - Greasy yellow scales on erythematous base on face, scalp, and/or diaper area
  - Transient hypopigmentation can develop and is more apparent in dark-skinned individuals.
- Diagnosis and treatment
  - Clinical diagnosis is based on lesion appearance and location.
  - Seborrheic dermatitis resolves spontaneously by the end of the first year of life. Most cases resolve spontaneously within weeks to a few months.
  - Treatments include ketoconazole, zinc pyrithione, selenium sulfide shampoos ± 1% hydrocortisone, low-potency topical corticosteroids, ketoconazole 2% shampoo or cream, zinc oxide and/or petrolatum, 1% hydrocortisone cream, selenium sulfide 2.5%, and salicylic acid.

ACRODERMATITIS ENTEROPATHICA

- Overview
  - Acrodermatitis enteropathica is caused by zinc deficiency that can be genetic or acquired.
  - Genetic: autosomal recessive (mutations in SLC394A gene) resulting in defects in intestinal absorption of zinc (zinc malabsorption)
    - Presents when breastfed infants are weaned off breast milk or earlier in infants who are formula fed.
  - Acquired: premature infants who carry the mutation and are exclusively formula fed
- Clinical presentation
  - Erosive periorificial, acral, and diaper rash with red, hemorrhagic crusted patches and plaques ± flaccid bullae (see Fig. 69.6)
  - Classical triad: alopecia, diarrhea, and a perioral and acral cutaneous rash

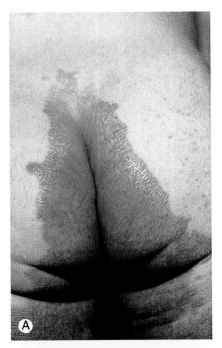

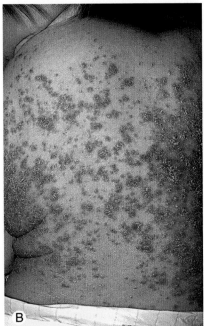

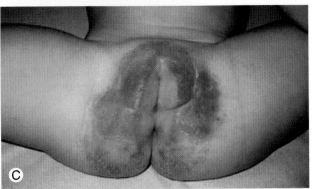

Fig. 69.5 Psoriasis. Beefy red diaper dermatitis involving skinfolds, which fails to respond to typical routine therapy. (A–C) Various presentations of psoriasis. (From Puttgen K, Cohen BA. Neonatal dermatology. In: Cohen BA, ed. *Pediatric Dermatology*. 4th ed. Philadelphia: Elsevier; 2013:33, Fig. 2.43.)

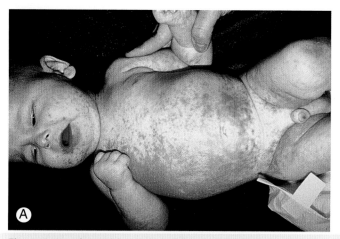
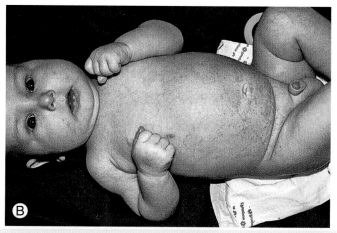

Fig. 69.6 Acrodermatitis enteropathica. (A) A bright red, scaling dermatitis that spreads to the intertriginous areas, face, and extremities of this 4-week-old infant. (B) After 4 days of zinc supplementation, many lesions were healing with desquamation. (From Puttgen K, Cohen BA. Neonatal dermatology. In: Cohen BA, ed. *Pediatric Dermatology*. 4th ed. Philadelphia: Elsevier; 2013:35, Fig. 2.39A.)

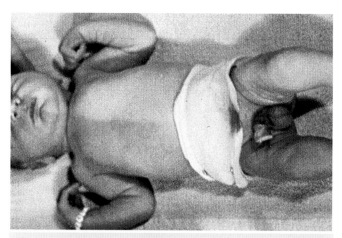

Fig. 69.7 Harlequin color change. (From Puttgen K, Cohen BA. Neonatal dermatology. In: Cohen BA, ed. *Pediatric Dermatology*. 4th ed. Philadelphia: Elsevier; 2013:19, Fig. 2.10.)

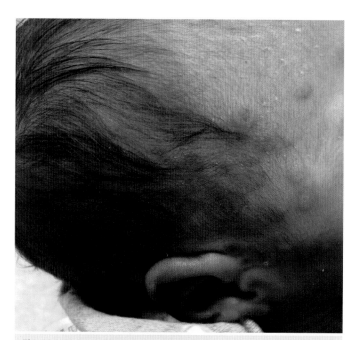

Fig. 69.8 Neonatal lupus. Characteristic erythematous, annular plaques on the lateral forehead and temple. (Courtesy of Dr. Bernard Cohen. Dr. Cohen retains copyright of this figure.)

- Diagnosis and treatment
  - Lab evaluation shows low serum zinc and alkaline phosphatase (which is zinc dependent). Also, measure serum albumin, which if low may indicate a falsely low serum zinc.
  - High-dose oral or intravenous (IV) zinc

NEONATAL LUPUS

- Clinical presentation
  - Atrophic, annular, reddish, hyperpigmented, subtly scarring plaques
  - Commonly located periocularly or on the forehead or scalp, but may be more widespread with prominent telangiectasias (see Figs. 69.7 and 69.8)
  - Associated with congenital heart block in up to 30% of patients, which may be detected before delivery
- Diagnosis and treatment
  - Associated with transplacental passage of anti-Ro/SSA, anti-La/SSb, and U1 RNP antibodies, so screen for antibodies starting at 16 weeks of gestation.
  - Obtain complete blood count (CBC; risk of thrombocytopenia), Liver Function Tests (risk of hepatobiliary disease), echocardiogram, and electrocardiogram (ECG).
  - Skin lesions often resolve with subtle scarring, dyspigmentation, and/or residual telangiectasias, so consider laser therapy or short course of topical steroids.
  - Heart block can be irreversible (mortality in 30% of cases) and requires a pacemaker.
  - Mother has 20% recurrence rate in subsequent pregnancies; consider oral hydroxychloroquine for the mother in subsequent pregnancies.

Congenital Infections of the Newborn

See Table 69.2.

Table 69.2 Congenital Infections of the Newborn

Infection	Epidemiology	Clinical Findings	Extracutaneous Findings	Diagnosis	Prognosis and Treatment	Differential Diagnoses
CMV	Presents at birth (transmitted from mother who contracted CMV during pregnancy)	Petechiae, purpura, blueberry muffin lesions	IUGR, deafness (most common infectious cause), chorioretinitis (common in HIV), microcephaly	CMV-IgM antibody, PCR for CMV DNA in plasma and tissue fluids	IV ganciclovir or oral valganciclovir Therapy should continue for a total duration of 6 months. Supportive care	Rubella, toxoplasmosis
HSV (see Fig. 69.9)	Neonates from mothers who acquired primary HSV2 are at greatest risk Presents at birth to 48 hours later	Grouped or diffuse vesicles, bullae, erosions, scarring	Prematurity, microcephaly, chorioretinitis, encephalitis (temporal lobes), seizures, multiorgan failure, lethargy, fever	Tzanck prep with multinucleate giant cells, HSVDFA from vesicle, viral dx	Aggressive treatment with high-dose IV acyclovir for 14–21 days depending on the severity of symptoms Supportive care	Epidermolysis bullosa, incontinentia pigmenti, varicella, bullous impetigo
Toxoplasmosis	Maternal infection in second or third trimester Later infection, lower risk	Blueberry muffin lesions on trunk	Chorioretinitis, hydrocephalus, blindness, deafness, DD, seizures, intracranial calcifications	IgM/IgG Toxoplasma *gondii*; *T. gondii* PCR; CT/ultrasound of brain with ring enhancing lesions	Combined pyrimethamine, sulfadiazine, and folinic acid	Disseminated CMV or HSV, rubella
Varicella	2% of neonates are from mothers infected with the virus before 20 weeks' gestation	Cutaneous scarring, limb hypoplasia If zoster, may see dermatomal lesions	Ocular abnormalities (e.g., chorioretinitis, cataracts), seizures, DD (can present without skin findings)	IgM/IgG VZV of mother or neonate, VZV PCR of fetal blood/amniotic fluid, lesions in dermatomal distribution	Supportive at birth Nonimmune pregnant women with recent contact should get PEP with varicellazoster IG	Toxoplasmosis, HSV, rubella
Syphilis, early	Infection with *Treponema pallidum* from mother Occurs before 2 years of age	Reddish-brown macules on face, buttocks, arms, legs ± diffuse acral scaling, condyloma lata	Snuffles, HSM, LAD, hemolytic anemia, thrombocytopenia, IUGR, periostitis	Nontreponemal serologic test (RPR or VDRL) performed on infant serum, clinical findings, positive darkfield test or PCR	IV penicillin G	Rubella, CMV
Rubella	Nonimmune mothers transmit virus to fetus. Severe defects within first 16 weeks' gestation	Blueberry muffin lesions, petechiae, Forchheimer sign in 20% (pinpoint petechia on palate)	Cataracts, deafness (50%), congenital heart disease, CNS effects (microcephaly, hydrocephaly)	Viral dx from oropharynx where viral particles are shed, echocardiogram	Once developed, cannot be treated Supportive care only	CMV, toxoplasmosis, HSV

CMV, Cytomegalovirus; *CNS*, central nervous system; *CT*, computed tomography; *DD*, developmental disability; *HIV*, human immunodeficiency virus; *HSM*, hepatosplenomegaly; *HSV*, herpes simplex virus; *HSVDFA*, herpes simplex virus direct fluorescent antibody; *IgG*, immunoglobulin G; *IgM*, immunoglobulin M; *IUGR*, intrauterine growth restriction; *IV*, intravenous; *LAD*, lymphadenopathy; *PCR*, polymerase chain reaction; *PEP*, post-exposure prophylaxis; *RPR*, rapid plasma reagin; *VDRL*, Venereal Disease Research Laboratory; *VZV*, varicella zoster virus.

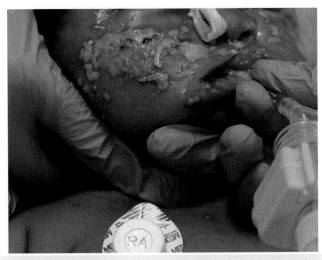

Fig. 69.9 Herpes simplex virus. Numerous clustered and coalescing vesicles with overlying serous exudate on the face of an intubated newborn. (Courtesy of Dr. Bernard Cohen. Dr. Cohen retains copyright of this figure.)

Vascular Anomalies (Vascular Tumors and Vascular Malformations)

See Table 69.3.

Table 69.3   Vascular Malformations

Vascular Malformation	Clinical Features	Diagnosis	Treatment	Extracutaneous Conditions	Other
Infantile hemangioma	4–5% of infants Red macules that rapidly grow into bright red soft tumors	Clinical Ultrasound or MRI if considering visceral involvement or extracutaneous syndromes	Regression expected Only treat if large or disfiguring or if function is impaired with propranolol, prednisone, timolol, surgical excision, or pulsed dye laser	May have visceral involvement If >5 hemangiomas, rule out liver involvement with ultrasound, UA, CBC, and stool guaiac	Large face/scalp IH → consider PHACE syndrome (posterior fossa brain malformations, hemangiomas, arterial anomalies, cardiac defects, and eye defects) Lumbosacral IH may have associated GU/spine, renal abnormalities (lumbar/sacral/pelvic syndromes).
Cavernous hemangiomas (venous malformation)	Bluish papules or nodules made of dilated vessels in the dermis/fat	Ultrasound/MRI may be helpful to delineate extent of lesion.	Sclerotherapy, Nd-YAG laser, or surgical excision	Can be associated with pain, swelling, or functional impairment of joints	—
Stork bite/salmon patches	Salmon patches: faint pink macules or patches usually located on the nape of neck (stork bite), glabella, forehead (angel kiss), upper eyelids, or sacrum	Clinical	Most regress with time	None	Darken with crying, breath holding, or exertion
Port wine stain	Well-demarcated red patch or plaque, typically unilateral Most common on head and neck, but any body part can be involved Does not regress	Clinical	Pulsed dye laser	If involving V1, obtain an MRI, which may show tram-track calcifications and delineate the extent of neurological involvement.	Sturge-Weber syndrome: port wine stain involving V1 distribution associated with an ipsilateral vascular malformation of the meninges, cortex, and eye (may develop HA, seizures, LD, or hemiparalysis).
Kasabach-Merritt syndrome	Large vascular or bulging nodules, plaques, or masses, purpura, with consumptive coagulopathy and low platelets	CBC, coagulation panel, and D-dimer Consider MRI. Biopsy may not be possible due to the risk of bleeding	Treatment is largely supportive. Control consumptive coagulopathy. Address the underlying tumor. Systemic steroids may be helpful.	Vascular tumors may be retroperitoneal.	Can be life threatening/fatal
Lymphatic malformation (cystic hygroma, cavernous lymphangiomas)	Skin-colored nodules made of dilated lymphatic vessels on the oral mucosa, head/neck, trunk, axillae, proximal extremities	Ultrasound/MRI may be helpful to delineate extent of lesion	Clinical	Can be deep on the head and neck, compressing important structures in the neck	—

CBC, Complete blood count; *GU*, genitourinary; *HA*, headache; *IH*, infantile hemangioma; *LD*, learning disabilities; *MRI*, magnetic resonance imaging; *UA*, urinalysis.

Aplasia Cutis Congenita

- Overview
  - Congenital absence of the skin
  - May be sporadic, autosomal dominant, or autosomal recessive
  - Association with limb abnormalities, central nervous system (CNS) dysraphism, vascular anomalies, and bony defects
  - Perinatal trauma from scalp electrodes or forceps may create similarly appearing lesions.
- Clinical presentation
  - One or several erosions/ulcerations are present on the vertex scalp with overlying crust or thin membrane; heals with a depressed, hairless scar over 3 to 6 months (see Fig. 69.10).
  - Bullous forms are seen.
  - Trunk or extremities may have similar findings.
  - Multiple, large, and nonvertex scalp lesions are more likely to be associated with extracutaneous lesions.
  - May be associated with a lipoma or vascular stain (which may be a sign of CNS involvement)

- Distinguish from hair collar sign: dark hairs noted circumferentially around a central papule or round plaque containing meningeal tissue; usually a solitary lesion, but may rarely be associated with neural tube defect
- Diagnosis and treatment
  - Rule out neonatal lupus and herpes simplex virus (HSV) if lesions are ulcerated.
  - Consider ultrasound and/or magnetic resonance imaging (MRI) for positive hair collar sign, lipoma, vascular patch, or large lesions to evaluate for connection to brain/bone.
  - Lesions should be cleansed daily, and topical antibacterial ointments can be applied for small lesions.
  - Surgical repair and/or skin grafting for larger lesions

Disorders of the Umbilical Cord

- Overview
  - Normally, the umbilical cord dries and separates from the umbilicus in 7 to 14 days with healing completed in 4 weeks.
  - Refer to Table 69.4 for disorders of the umbilical cord.

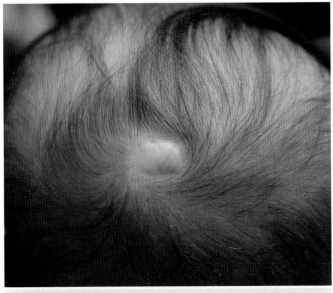

Fig. 69.10 Aplasia cutis congenita. This child and his father had similar hairless, atrophic plaques on the scalp. A thin, hemorrhagic membrane was noted at birth. (Courtesy of Dr. Bernard Cohen. Dr. Cohen retains copyright of this figure.)

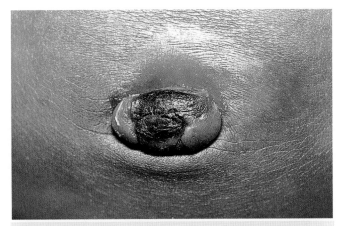

Fig. 69.11 Omphalitis. Omphalitis developed in this 10-day-old infant shortly after the cord separated from the umbilicus. The infection cleared after a 10-day course of parenteral antibiotics. (From Puttgen K, Cohen BA. Neonatal dermatology. In: Cohen BA, ed. *Pediatric Dermatology.* 4th ed. Philadelphia: Elsevier; 2013:25, Fig. 2.26.)

Table 69.4 Disorders of the Umbilical Cord

Disorder	Etiology	Clinical Presentation	Diagnosis/Treatment
Umbilical granuloma	Excessive moisture ± low-grade infection	Pink friable or firm papule on umbilicus	Silver nitrate cauterization; if persistent, excise
Umbilical polyp	Persistent vitelline duct (gastrointestinal mucosa) or patent urachus (urinary tract mucosa)	Firm, bright-red papule on umbilicus with chronic mucoid or watery discharge weeks to months after birth	Excision of patent urachus or persistent vitelline duct
Omphalitis (see Fig. 69.11)	Polymicrobial infection of umbilical stump Risk factors: instrumentation, low birth weight, premature rupture of membranes	Periumbilical erythema, tenderness, and/or foul-smelling purulent discharge from the umbilicus, which can lead to sepsis	Obtain culture/sensitivities and administer intravenous antibiotics.

Pigmented Lesions

See Table 69.5.

Table 69.5 Pigmented Lesions

Diagnosis	Etiology	Clinical Presentation	Differential Diagnoses	Associations
Café au lait macule	Increased number of melanocytes	Light to dark brown macule or patch May be solitary (10–20% neonates) or multiple	Transient neonatal pustulosis, lentigines	More than six spots: NF1/2, Legius syndrome, McCune-Albright syndrome, tuberous sclerosis, Fanconi anemia, others
Congenital smooth muscle hamartoma (hairy epidermal nevus)	Hamartomas made of smooth muscle and hair follicles (no nevus cells)	Typically single, tan/brown plaque in the lumbosacral area ± hair growth, approximately 1–5 cm in diameter	Becker hamartoma, congenital melanocytic nevus, piloleiomyoma, café au lait spots, and nevus pilosus	No risk of malignancy
Congenital nevi (see Fig. 69.12)	Onset at birth or first year of life (1–2% neonates) Nevus cells from neural crest produce melanin.	Pigmented macules or plaques, often with dense hair growth; may be tan initially and then darken Can be over 20 cm/10% BSA (giant congenital nevus)	Hairy epidermal nevus	Giant congenital nevi → 2–6% lifetime risk of melanoma If over scalp, neck, or back, consider MRI to evaluate for neurocutaneous melanosis.
Congenital dermal melanocytosis (Mongolian spot)	Dendritic melanocytes in the dermis; common in neonates with darker skin	Irregular, blue–gray macules or patches, usually over lumbosacral area or buttocks	Nevus of Ota (usually periorbital), nevus of Ito (usually on the neck, supraclavicular, and/or scapular regions)	May fade over time or persist

BSA, Body surface area; MRI, magnetic resonance imaging.

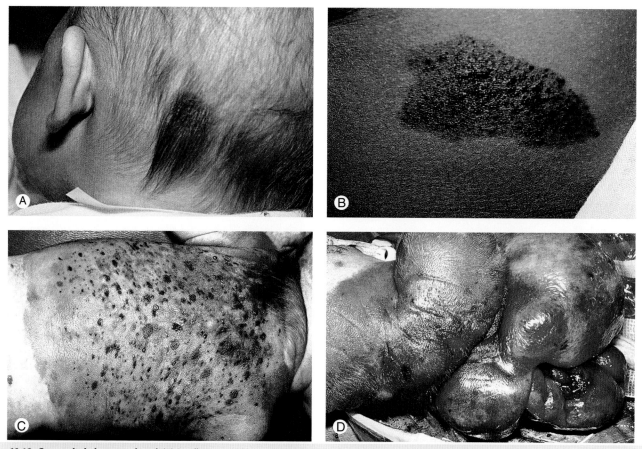

Fig. 69.12 Congenital pigmented nevi. (A) Small congenital nevi associated with tufts of dark hair. (B) An innocent medium-sized 5 cm by 3 cm nevus uniformly studded with numerous darkjly pigmented nodules. (C) A giant pigmented nevus with numerous darkly pigmented nodules. This child had neurocutaneous involvement and developed a malignant melanoma in the central nervous system. (D) A large tumor developed within a giant pigmented nevus which involved the diaper area of a newborn. The tumor contained structures that arose from various neuroectodermal elements. The tumor was excised in several stages. (From Puttgen K, Cohen BA. Neonatal dermatology. In: Cohen BA, ed. *Pediatric Dermatology*. 4th ed. Philadelphia: Elsevier; 2013:57, Fig. 2.85.)

Infectious Disease

STAPHYLOCOCCAL SCALDED SKIN SYNDROME (SSSS)

- Overview
  - Generalized, blistering eruption due to strains of *Staphylococcus aureus* that produce circulating epidermolytic exotoxin
- Clinical presentation
  - Abrupt onset of fever, irritability, and generalized skin redness with tender rash
  - Neonates will have facial swelling, and conjunctivitis, as well as crusting, exfoliating, erythematous lesions around the eyes, nose, and mouth.
  - Flaccid, delicate bullae often form followed by widespread desquamation of all skin within 2 to 3 days (see Fig. 69.13).
  - Must be distinguished from toxic epidermal necrolysis (TEN), which is typically triggered by a drug, causes full-thickness tissue necrosis, and involves mucosal surfaces.
- Diagnosis and treatment
  - Clinical suspicion
  - Bacterial cultures from common sites of primary infection (nasopharynx, umbilicus, conjunctiva) with sensitivities to help guide antibiotic choice
  - Blood cultures and cultures from skin lesions are often negative.
  - Gram stain from sites of common infection will be positive for gram-positive cocci in clusters.
  - IV penicillinase-resistant anti-staphylococcal antibiotics (nafcillin or methicillin)
  - Vancomycin if methicillin-resistant *Staphylococcus aureus* (MRSA) is suspected.
  - Supportive care: fluid and electrolyte replacement, bland emollient if needed

CANDIDA INFECTIONS

- Overview
  - *Candida albicans* is a pathogen of the female genitalia and is frequently noted in pregnancy.
  - *C. albicans* also colonizes the oral cavity and gastrointestinal tract of most newborns.

SYSTEMIC/DISSEMINATED CANDIDIASIS

- Overview
  - Systemic candidiasis (with blood, urine, or cerebrospinal fluid [CSF] involvement) affects low-birth-weight/premature infants more than full-term infants.
  - *C. albicans, C. parapsilosis,* and *C. tropiccalis* are implicated.
  - May be congenital (acquired in utero), due to untreated localized candidal infection, or from nosocomial spread
  - Risk factors: birth weight < 1500 g, indwelling catheters, broad-spectrum antibiotic use, systemic steroid

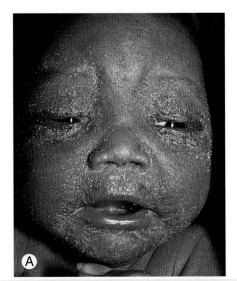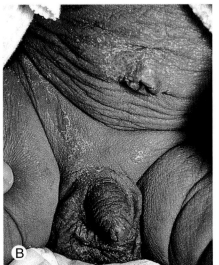

Fig. 69.13 Staphylococcal scalded skin syndrome. Staphylococcal scalded skin syndrome developed in this neonate a few days after his brother was diagnosed with impetigo. Erosive patches were most marked on the face (A) and diaper areas (B). (From Puttgen K, Cohen BA. Neonatal dermatology. In: Cohen BA, ed. *Pediatric Dermatology.* 4th ed. Philadelphia: Elsevier; 2013:38, Fig. 2.47.)

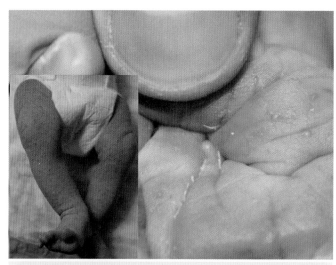

Fig. 69.14 Cutaneous candidiasis. Numerous inflammatory papules and pustules are scattered on the trunk and extremities, even the palms. (Courtesy of Dr. Bernard Cohen. Dr. Cohen retains copyright of this figure.)

use, history of instrumentation, premature (<27 weeks), intrauterine foreign bodies (e.g., intrauterine devices, cervical sutures), and total parenteral nutrition (TPN).
- Systemic involvement is secondary to hematogenous or lymphatic spread.
- Mortality is 40% to 94%; early recognition is paramount.
- Clinical presentation
  - Inflammatory papules or vesicopustules on a deeply erythematous base
  - May be sparse or diffuse on the body (see Fig. 69.14); the face and oral mucosa are usually spared
  - Progressive diaper dermatitis with papules, pustules, and abscesses
  - Systemic findings: Respiratory distress, bradycardia, temperature instability, hypotension, pneumonia, meningitis, and elevated white blood cells (WBCs) ± left shift all may suggest sepsis.
  - Umbilical cord exam shows clusters of small, round, whitish lesions.
- Diagnosis and treatment
  - Potassium hydroxide (KOH) prep from affected skin will demonstrate hyphae.
  - Skin biopsy for tissue culture

- Chest x-ray, blood culture, and cerebrospinal fluid culture may be helpful.
- IV antifungal therapy (e.g., amphotericin B) if clinical suspicion for disseminated disease given clinical findings and above stated risk factors
- Consider capsofungin for refractory cases.

HERPES SIMPLEX VIRUS (HSV)

- Overview
  - Often caused by vertical transmission via contact with mother's genital mucosa during delivery.
  - Two-thirds of cases are HSV-2 and one-third of cases are HSV-1.
  - Categorized by skin–eye–mucosa (SEM) disease (45%), CNS disease (30%), and disseminated disease (25%)
  - One-third of neonates have skin disease with vesicles at initial presentation.
  - Other presentations include sepsis, new-onset seizures, conjunctivitis, liver dysfunction, coagulopathy, and respiratory distress.
  - Disseminated disease has a 60% mortality rate and a 40% risk of neurologic impairment.
- Clinical presentation
  - Isolated or grouped vesicles on an erythematous base that evolve into pustules, crusts, or erosions
  - If infected in utero, the clinical presentation at birth is characterized by microcephaly, microphthalmia ± chorioretinitis, and skin lesions in the form of diffuse erosions, bullae, and/or scars.
- Diagnosis and treatment
  - Unroof a fresh vesicle to obtain viral culture, HSV polymerase chain reaction (PCR), or Tzanck smear, which will show multinucleated giant cells; can also swab other mucosal surfaces such as the mouth and nasopharynx.
  - Consider lumbar puncture for evaluation of CSF if disseminated disease is a concern.
  - Treat empirically with IV acyclovir for 14 days for SEM disease and 21 days for CNS or disseminated disease.
  - Delivery by cesarean section is indicated for mother with prodromal or active lesions at delivery and/or prophylactic antiviral therapy for mothers with known HSV history.
  - Low-dose prophylactic oral therapy for first 6 months of life reduces risk of cutaneous recurrence and improves neurodevelopmental scores in patients with CNS disease.

Genetic Neonatal Syndromes

See Table 69.6.

Table 69.6   Disorders of Hypopigmentation and Hyperpigmentation

	Cause	Clinical Findings	Diagnosis, Treatment, Prognosis
Oculocutaneous albinism	OCA1a	Near lack of pigment starting at birth, severely reduced visual acuity, high incidence of skin cancer	Genetic testing to distinguish subtypes Refer to ophthalmology because of risk of photophobia, nystagmus, and reduced visual acuity.
	OCA1b	No pigment at birth but develop pigment over time, better visual acuity	Refer to dermatology because of increased risk of basal cell and squamous cell carcinoma; OCA1 also has increased risk of melanoma.
	OCA2	Most common type, Africans, some pigment but variable, nevi and lentigines	
	OCA3	Reddish-bronze skin and red hair, very rare	
	OCA4	Variable, very rare, seen in Japan and Africa	
Chédiak-Higashi		Presents during infancy with decreased skin, eye, and hair pigment Silvery hair with pigment clumping in hair shaft Bleeding diatheses Increased bacterial infections of skin, gut, and lungs	Look for giant peroxidase-positive granules within cells. Death typically by age 10 from lymphoproliferative syndrome Severe neurologic degeneration
Phenylketonuria (PKU)	Deficiency of phenylalanine hydroxylase (autosomal recessive)	Diffuse pigmentation dilution Sweat with a musty odor Progressive developmental delay Eczema	Inborn error of metabolism Without treatment, accumulation of phenylalanine leads to profound mental retardation, seizures (rare because of screening). Refer to nutritionist.
Waardenburg syndrome	Mutations in *PAX3, MITF, EDNRB/EDN3/SOX10*	Skin: depigmented patch on the forehead with white forelock Eyes: heterochromic irises, synophrys, dystopia canthorum, square jaw	Referral to audiology/otolaryngology for congenital deafness. Normal life span
Piebaldism	c-Kit (autosomal dominant)	Associated with white forelock Congenital patches of spotty hypopigmentation (leukoderma) Heterochromic irises	Results in defective migration of melanoblasts Stable, permanent depigmentation but otherwise benign course
Incontinentia pigmenti (see Fig. 69.15)	NEMO (X-linked dominant)	Vesicular—birth to 1 month along lines of Blaschko Verrucous—warty papules from 8 weeks to 2 years Hyperpigmented curvilinear and whorled pattern—up to adolescence Hypopigmented and sometimes subtle atrophy—may persist through adulthood	Affected patient can have seizures, developmental delay, and blindness.
Tuberous sclerosis	*TSC1* (hamartia), *TSC2* (tuberis)	Major features: ≥3 angiofibromas, ≥3 ash-leaf macules, ≥2 ungual fibromas, shagreen patches, hamartomas in the central nervous system and skin, cortical dysplasia, giant cell astrocytoma, cardiac rhabdomyomas, lymphangioleiomyomatosis, ≥2 angiomyolipomas Minor features: confetti skin lesions (numerous scattered 1–3 mm hypopigmented macules), dental enamel pits, intraoral fibromas, renal cysts	At least one major or two minor criteria Definitive diagnosis with genetic testing Complications related to seizures and renal disease are the most common causes of mortality.
Peutz-Jeghers syndrome	SKT11 (autosomal dominant)	Dark blue, brown, or black macules on lips, buccal mucosa, and/or digits are seen by age 20. Mucocutaneous lentigines Hamartomatous polyps in jejunum and ileum may lead to intussusception, which is often the first presentation.	Number of melanocytic macules is not related to number of gastrointestinal polyps. Regular colonoscopy to assess polyposis Pigmented macules may fade with time. Increased risk of early-onset adenocarcinomas (most common gastrointestinal)
McCune-Albright syndrome	*GNAS1* (somatic mutation)	Triad: 1. Café au lait macules (large "coast of Maine–like") 2. Polyostotic fibrous dysplasia 3. Endocrine dysfunction (especially precocious puberty and hypophosphatemic rickets)	Clinical diagnosis, although genetic testing is available Pathologic fractures, gait abnormalities, and endocrine abnormalities need to be treated, but otherwise normal life span

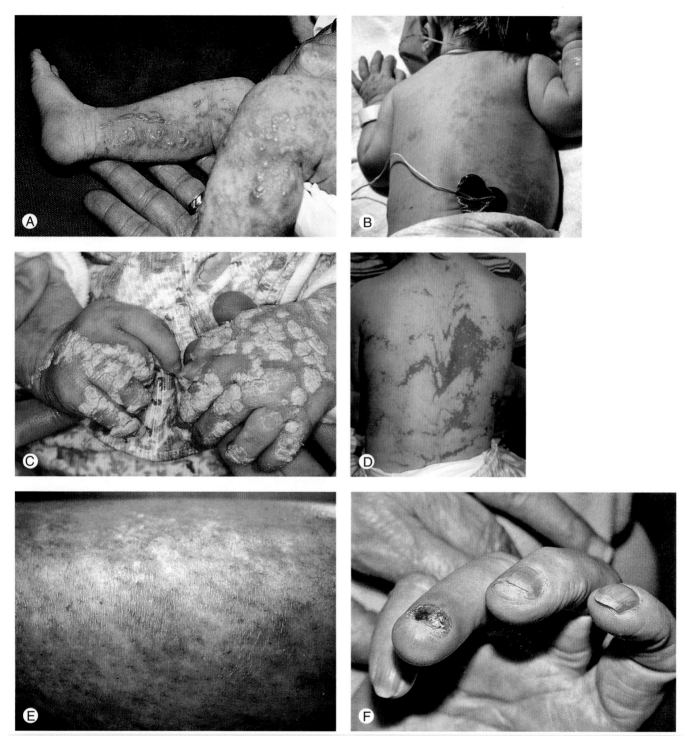

Fig. 69.15 Incontinentia pigmenti. (A, B) Vesicles along erythematous base following lines of Blaschko. (C) Progression to warty papules. (D) Resolving with hyperpigmentation. (E, F) Additional examples. (From Puttgen K, Cohen BA. Neonatal dermatology. In: Cohen BA, ed. *Pediatric Dermatology*. 4th ed. Philadelphia: Elsevier; 2013:47, Fig. 2.62.)

INHERITED ICHTHYOSES

- Overview
  - Spectrum of disorders linked by abnormal epidermal differentiation, epidermal hyperplasia, and excess stratum corneum formation
  - Treatment of all disorders is generally emollients and supportive care aimed at maintaining fluid balance and decreasing the risk of infections.
  - Progress is being made in the development of enzyme-replacement therapy, gene therapy, and biologics.

Harlequin Ichthyosis

- Clinical presentation
  - Most severe ichthyosis
  - Presents at birth with thick plates of scale with deep, erythematous fissures, extreme ectropion, eclabium, flattened nose, and dysplastic ears
- Diagnosis
  - Genetic testing with next-generation sequencing
  - Autosomal recessive: *ABCA12* gene mutation
- Prognosis
  - Often neonatal death from sepsis
  - Death usually occurs within first few days of life.
  - For the 55% of neonates who survive past the neonatal period, the average age ranges from 10 months to 25 years.

Congenital Ichthyosiform Erythroderma (CIE)

See Fig. 69.16.

- Clinical presentation
  - CIE is the number one cause of collodion membrane. After collodion membrane, infants have fine, white scale.
  - Collodion membrane is thickened parchment-like skin with distorting facial features such as ectropion and eclabium (see Fig. 69.17).
  - Temperature instability, defective barrier function, insensible water loss, and infection are common features.
- Diagnosis
  - Genetic testing, fetal skin biopsy similar to lamellar ichthyosis
  - Autosomal recessive: *ALOXE3*, *ALOX12B*, and others.

Lamellar Ichthyosis

- Clinical presentation: frequently collodion membrane and underlying erythroderma at birth, followed by thick, plate-like generalized brown scale
- Diagnosis
  - Genetic testing; in situ transglutaminase 1 (*TGM1*) expression
  - Autosomal recessive: *TGM1* is most frequently reported in 50% of patients, CYP4F22 in 5% patients.

Steroid Sulfatase Deficiency (X-Linked Ichthyosis)

- Clinical presentation
  - Presents in infancy with dark brown, adherent, polygonal scales that spare flexor surfaces
  - Associations: comma-shaped corneal opacities, cryptorchidism (which portends increased risk of testicular cancer), prolonged labor because of placental sulfatase deficiency, and impaired skin permeability
- Diagnosis
  - Genetic analysis
  - X-linked recessive: deletions or point mutations in steroid sulfatase gene

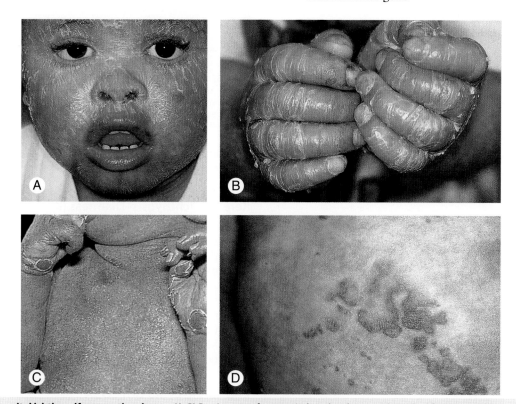

Fig. 69.16 Congenital ichthyosiform erythroderma. (A, B) Persistence of congenital erythroderma with marked fine white scale, especially on hands. (C, D) **Additional presentations.** (From Puttgen K, Cohen BA. Neonatal dermatology. In: Cohen BA, ed. *Pediatric Dermatology*. 4th ed. Philadelphia: Elsevier; 2013:28, Fig. 2.31.)

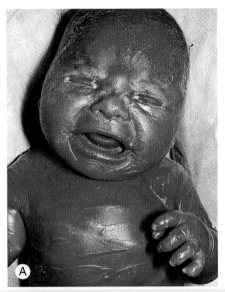
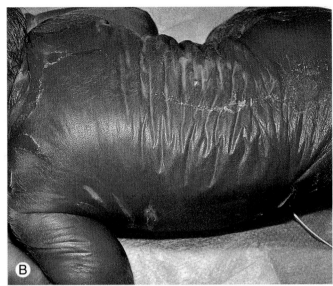

Fig. 69.17 Collodion membrane. Shiny transparent membrane covering baby at birth. Present in multiple conditions but most common in congenital ichthyosiform erythroderma. (A) Face, chest, and hand involvement. (B) Trunk involvement. (From Puttgen K, Cohen BA. Neonatal dermatology. In: Cohen BA, ed. *Pediatric Dermatology*. 4th ed. Philadelphia: Elsevier; 2013:26, Fig. 2.29.)

- Laboratory tests will show increased plasma cholesterol sulfate and/or decreased steroid sulfatase in leukocytes.
- Triple/quad screen will show decreased serum estriol.

Ichthyosis Vulgaris

- Clinical presentation
  - Most common and benign ichthyosis
  - Begins in later infancy with fine, white, adherent scale, mostly on the lower extremities; keratosis pilaris and hyperlinear palms
  - Associated with atopic dermatitis
- Diagnosis
  - Clinical diagnosis is sufficient, but genetic testing can be used.
  - Autosomal semidominant: defect in filaggrin (FLG), loss of function of *FLG*

Epidermolytic Hyperkeratosis

- Clinical presentation
  - Widespread blistering, skin denudation, and erythroderma at birth; later generalized hyperkeratosis with malodor and prominent flexural involvement.
- Diagnosis
  - Genetic testing
  - Autosomal dominant: keratin 1 (*KRT1*) and keratin 10 (*KRT10*).

OTHER ICHTHYOSIFORM SYNDROMES

Netherton Syndrome

- Clinical presentation
  - Erythema, collodion membrane, scale, and hypernatremia at birth
  - Later in infancy more atopic dermatitis-like with the addition of polycyclic erythematous scaling plaques (ichthyosis linearis circumflexa), trichorrhexis invaginata of hair (bamboo hair)

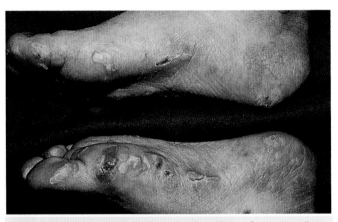

Fig. 69.18 Epidermolysis bullosa simplex. Blisters form primarily in areas of pressure such as hands and feet. (From Puttgen K, Cohen BA. Neonatal dermatology. In: Cohen BA, ed. *Pediatric Dermatology*. 4th ed. Philadelphia: Elsevier; 2013:41, Fig. 2.50.)

- Diagnosis
  - Genetic testing
  - Autosomal recessive: *SPINK5* gene.

Keratitis–Ichthyosis–Deafness (KID) Syndrome

- Clinical presentation
  - Mild hyperkeratosis, especially on face and extremities, palmoplantar keratoderma, recurrent bacterial and fungal infections, and alopecia
  - Associations: nonprogressive sensorineural deafness, vascularized keratitis, and erythrokeratoderma
- Diagnosis
  - Genetic testing
  - Mostly sporadic, some autosomal dominant: *GJB2* gene (connexin 26)

EPIDERMOLYSIS BULLOSA

- Clinical presentation

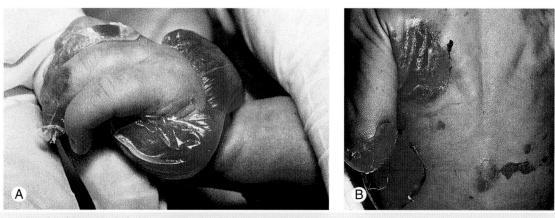

Fig. 69.19 Junctional epidermolysis bullosa. Widespread blisters at birth with erosions and denuded areas. (A) Hand involvement. (B) Trunk involvement. (From Puttgen K, Cohen BA. Neonatal dermatology. In: Cohen BA, ed. *Pediatric Dermatology.* 4th ed. Philadelphia: Elsevier; 2013:39, Fig. 2.51.)

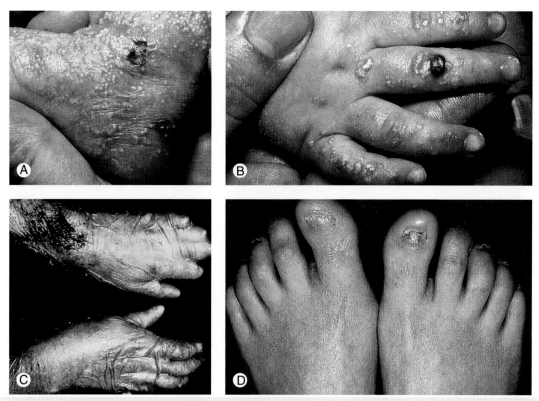

Fig. 69.20 Dystrophic epidermolysis bullosa. Blisters heal with hundreds of milia, especially on the hands and feet of this infant. (A–D) Various stages of healing. (From Puttgen K, Cohen BA. Neonatal dermatology. In: Cohen BA, ed. *Pediatric Dermatology.* 4th ed. Philadelphia: Elsevier; 2013:41, Fig. 2.52.)

- ▪ Heterogeneous group of inherited bullous disorders with very fragile skin and blistering that heals with atrophic scarring
- ▪ Often quite painful and deforming; nail and teeth dysplasia may be seen
- ▪ Often leads to early demise (see Figs. 69.18–20)
- ■ Diagnosis
  - ▪ Clinical and confirmed with biopsy
  - ▪ Definitive diagnosis can be done through genetic analysis.

Suggested Readings

Calonje E. *McKee's Pathology of the Skin: With Clinical Correlations.* 5th ed. Philadelphia: Elsevier; 2020:990–1014.

Cohen BA. *Cohen's Pediatric Dermatology.* 4th ed. Philadelphia: Elsevier; 2013.

Flint PW, Francis HW, Haughey BH, et al. *Cummings Otolaryngology: Head and Neck Surgery.* 7th ed. Philadelphia: Elsevier; 2021:2279–2292.

Gleason CA, et al. Congenital and hereditary disorders of the skin. In: Gleason CA, Juul SE, eds. *Avery's Diseases of the Newborn.* 10th ed. Philadelphia: Elsevier; 2018:1475–1494.

Kollmann TR, Mailman TL, Bortolussi R. Listeriosis. In: Wilson CB, Nizet V, Maldonado Y, Remington JS, Klein JO, eds. *Infectious Diseases of the Fetus and Newborn.* 8th ed. Philadelphia: Saunders; 2015:457–474.

Marcdante KJ, et al. Amino acid disorders. In: Marcdante KJ, Kliegman RM, Schuh AM, eds. *Nelson Essentials of Pediatrics.* 9th ed. Philadelphia: Elsevier; 2023:211–215.

Tenney-Soeiro R, et al. Hyperpigmented skin disorders. In: Tenney-Soeiro R, Devon EP, eds. *Netter's Pediatrics.* 2nd ed. Philadelphia: Elsevier; 2023:236–241.

Surgical and Complex NICU Patient Management

IGOR KHODAK, JONATHAN RYAN BURRIS, PATRICIA R. CHESS,

JONATHAN RYAN BURRIS, IGOR KHODAK and PATRICIA R. CHESS

General Pre- and Postoperative Management Tools/Checklist Tasks

OVERVIEW

Preoperative evaluation of any infant should include the infant's overall condition, any significant illness, and presence of any congenital anomalies or other abnormalities. Focus should be on the infant's cardiorespiratory status and requirements, serum chemistry derangements, and nutritional support.

ACCESS

- Consider central venous access based on extent of surgery and patient condition.
  - Umbilical venous access depends on age and surgery to be performed.
  - Central venous access location is based on the type of surgery.
- Determine the need for arterial access for blood pressure monitoring and frequent lab sampling.
- If central venous access is unobtainable, place two peripheral intravenous (IV) lines prior to surgery.

RESPIRATORY STATUS

- Establish and maintain a secure airway.
- If the infant is intubated, identify the tube size and review recent x-ray imaging to confirm appropriate tracheal tube position.
- Transition from high-frequency ventilation to conventional ventilation if feasible.
- Provide continuous saturation and an end-tidal CO_2 monitor or transcutaneous CO_2 monitor (TCOM) when muscle relaxed and if otherwise clinically indicated.

LAB EVALUATION

- Evaluate labs prior to surgical procedure to allow time for corrective actions.
- Obtain basic metabolic panel (BMP), complete blood count (CBC), blood gas, and/or coagulation factor.
  - Correct electrolyte derangements.
  - Correct coagulopathy; provide packed red blood cells (PRBCs) for anemia.
  - Correct respiratory, metabolic acidosis, and alkalosis.

FLUID SUPPORT

- Discontinue any enteral nutrition 2 to 6 hours prior to procedure (2 hours for clear liquids, 4 hours for breast milk, and 6 hours for formula).
- Transition off of parenteral nutrition within 1 to 2 hours prior to the procedure, and initiate crystalloid fluids.

TEMPERATURE REGULATION ON TRANSPORT

- Maintain normothermia throughout.
- Interhospital transport commonly leads to heat loss, so consider utilizing an incubator, bundling the infant, or the use of chemical warmer packs.

ANTIBIOTICS

- Antibiotics should be provided within 60 minutes before surgery (120 minutes prior for vancomycin). The following are suggestions for different types of surgery:
  - Prophylactic antibiotic regimen for neonates <72 hours of age: ampicillin + gentamicin
  - Prophylactic antibiotic regimen for neonates >72 hours of age
    - Cardiac surgery antibiotics
      - Primary: cefazolin
      - Alternative regimen: cefazolin + vancomycin (if methicillin-resistant *Staphylococcus aureus* [MRSA] is a concern)
      - If severe penicillin or cephalosporin allergy, use vancomycin + gentamicin
    - Gastrointestinal procedures (esophageal, gastroduodenal, hernia repair, gastrostomy tube placement)
      - Primary: cefazolin
      - Alternative regimen: cefazolin + vancomycin (if MRSA is known or likely)
      - If severe penicillin or known cephalosporin allergy, use vancomycin + gentamicin
    - Necrotizing enterocolitis
      - Broad-spectrum antibiotics covering gram-positive, gram-negative, and anaerobic bacteria, including
        - Commonly used regimen: ampicillin + gentamicin + metronidazole (or clindamycin, in place of metronidazole)
        - Piperacillin/tazobactam
    - Urogenital surgery
      - Primary: cefazolin
      - Alternative regimen: cefazolin + vancomycin (if MRSA is a concern)

ANESTHESIA

- Fentanyl
  - Synthetic opioid
  - Most commonly used anesthesia for premature infants
  - Fentanyl administration with a muscle relaxant is a standard for anesthesia in premature infants.
  - Useful in infants at risk or with pulmonary hypertension (e.g., congenital diaphragmatic hernia [CDH], persistent pulmonary hypertension of the newborn [PPHN])
  - Major adverse effect is respiratory depression.
- Morphine
  - Opium alkaloid
  - Less potent than fentanyl but with a longer duration of action
  - Commonly used for postoperative pain management
  - Causes significant histamine release, limiting its use as an anesthetic agent
  - Major adverse effect is respiratory depression
- Dexmedetomidine
  - An alpha-2 adrenergic agonist providing hypnotic, analgesic, and anxiolytic properties
  - Increased frequency of use with other anesthetics during surgical procedures
  - Benefits include little effect on respiratory function and reduced need for additional analgesics.
  - Adverse effects include bradycardia, hypotension, and paradoxical hypertension.
- Propofol
  - Approved for children <3 years old; infrequently used in premature infants
  - Used for induction and maintenance of anesthesia; little analgesic effect
  - Peripheral vasodilator; hypotension is a common adverse effect that limits its use in preterm infants
- Benzodiazepines (midazolam, lorazepam)
  - Produce sedation, anxiolysis, and amnesia but little analgesia
  - Midazolam is short acting; most commonly used when providing anesthesia; induces vasodilation, increasing the risk for hypotension, and may cause respiratory depression in high doses.
  - Lorazepam is longer acting.

NEUROMUSCULAR BLOCKING AGENTS

- Vecuronium
  - Nondepolarizing muscle relaxant (competitively inhibits acetylcholine at the neuromuscular junction)
  - Intermediate acting relaxant
  - Minimal effect on cardiac system; use with narcotics may cause bradycardia
- Rocuronium
  - Nondepolarizing muscle relaxant
  - Rapid onset of action; often used for rapid sequence intubation

POSTOPERATIVE CARE

- Recovery from anesthesia is usually prolonged due to immaturity of drug clearance; often these infants are not candidates for extubation directly after surgery.

- Neuromuscular blockade must be reversed.
- Monitor for hypothermia; as anesthesia can prolong neuromuscular blockage.

POSTOPERATIVE PAIN MANAGEMENT

- IV acetaminophen
- Opioids: morphine and/or fentanyl
- Epidural

Select Cardiac Surgical Intervention Considerations and Therapies

Congenital heart disease is grouped into cyanotic and acyanotic cardiac lesions. It is important to recognize whether the neonate is dealing with a ductal dependent lesion, right-to-left shunts affecting the infant's oxygenation, or left-to-right shunts typically resulting in volume overload.

GENERAL

Access: Central venous catheters and arterial monitoring lines prior to surgery are recommended.

- Single-ventricle patients who have umbilical venous catheters placed instead of femoral lines have lower rates of vascular thrombosis and occlusion.
- If non-umbilical access is required, use the smallest catheter necessary for medical management; a single lumen instead of a double lumen results in less vascular occlusion.
- Tunneling catheters is associated with less thrombosis and a decreased rate of central line–associated bloodstream infection (CLABSI).
- It is not recommended to place catheters in upper extremities or neck vessels in single-ventricle patients prior to the Fontan procedure.

RESPIRATORY STATUS

- Minimize pulmonary overcirculation.
  - Maintain pH in the normal range of 7.35 to 7.45 to avoid alkalosis.
  - Avoid hyperoxia.

MEDICAL MANAGEMENT

- Ductal-dependent congenital heart disease (CHD): Prostaglandin E1 (PGE1) should be initiated shortly after birth and can be provided through any vascular access site, including intraosseous route, until central access is obtained.
  - Monitor for potential side effects of PGE1, including apnea, fevers, hypotension, and bradycardia.
- Provide pre- and postoperative support of cardiac function with vasopressors as needed.

PATENT DUCTUS ARTERIOSUS (PDA) LIGATION

- Indications
  - Hemodynamically significant PDA resistant to closure with medical treatment

- Symptoms: respiratory failure, cardiac dysfunction including hypotension and signs of overt congestive heart failure, renal dysfunction
- Preoperative management
  - Optimize fluid status, cardiovascular status, ventilation, and oxygenation.
  - Assess for and treat possible infection based on symptoms and labwork.
  - Transition from high-frequency ventilation to conventional mechanical ventilation.
  - Consider stress dosing of hydrocortisone for infants already receiving steroids.
- Surgical approaches
  - Open thoracic approach (done at bedside or in the operating room)
  - Intravascular catheter approach with use of an occluding coil
- Postoperative complications
  - Postligation cardiac syndrome is defined as hypotension requiring inotropic support and failure of oxygenation and ventilation.
    - It can occur in the first 6 to 12 hours after surgery and is believed to be due to left ventricular systolic and diastolic dysfunction in the setting of an increased afterload postoperatively.
  - Pneumothorax, chylothorax, vocal cord paralysis, diaphragm paralysis, pulmonary artery hypertension
  - Catheter device closure specific complications include:
    - Device embolization
    - Fatal hemopericardium

BALLOON ATRIAL SEPTOSTOMY (BAS)

- Common indications:
  - d-Transposition of the great arteries with a restrictive atrial septum
  - Hypoplastic left heart syndrome
- Performed either in the catheterization lab or at the bedside
- Commonly performed through femoral venous access or an umbilical venous catheter
- BAS may be ineffective if the septum is thick or completely intact.
  - Completely intact atrial septum can be crossed using a radiofrequency wire, a radio-perforation transseptal needle, or standard transseptal needle.
  - Following opening of the atrial septum, multiple treatments can be performed, including static balloon septoplasty, blade atrial septostomy, and atrial septal stenting.
- Postprocedure complications
  - Rupture of the balloon with or without embolization of fragments
  - Inability to deflate the balloon
  - Rupture of atrial appendages, mitral valve damage, or vascular damage
  - Electrical rhythm abnormalities
  - Prolonged severe hypoxemia prior to and during the procedure may lead to pulmonary hypertension despite successful BAS.

Surgical Intervention Considerations and Therapies for Select Pulmonary Pathologies

CONGENITAL PULMONARY AIRWAY MALFORMATION (CPAM), PREVIOUSLY KNOWN AS CONGENITAL CYSTIC ADENOMATOID MALFORMATION (CCAM)

- Prenatal corrective surgery
  - Up to 15% of these lesions begin to resolve in the prenatal period, commonly beginning after 28 weeks' gestation.
  - Growth is unpredictable, requiring close follow-up.
  - Growth can be quite rapid, causing mediastinal shift, pulmonary hypoplasia, and obstructed venous return leading to fetal hydrops.
  - CPAM volume ratio (CVR) ≥ 1.6 predicts an increased risk for fetal hydrops.
  - Fetal surgery includes thoraco-amniotic shunting or cyst aspiration for macrocystic lesions.
  - Microcystic lesions necessitate open fetal surgery in the setting of hydrops.
  - Antenatal steroid use is a consideration for patients unsuitable for prenatal surgery.
  - The ex utero intrapartum treatment (EXIT) procedure can be considered for patients with substantial mediastinal shift causing a severely compromised airway and/or cardiac compression.
- Symptomatic lesions (respiratory distress/failure, failure to thrive): Early surgical excision is indicated (during initial hospitalization).
- Asymptomatic lesions: No consensus exists regarding observation versus elective surgical resection with low-risk characteristics. Majority opinion favors elective resection at 2 to 6 months of age.
  - Surgery may prevent future chest infection and sepsis and malignant transformation; early surgery may allow for compensatory lung growth.
- Perioperative ventilation strategies: There is potential need for one-lung ventilation due to extent of cyst and involved lung resection.
- Perioperative regional anesthesia: General anesthesia is preferred; thoracic epidural catheter placement may be considered as a supplement to help with intra- and postoperative pain relief.
- Postop complications: pneumothorax, pleural effusion, bronchopleural fistula, chylothorax, phrenic nerve palsy, prolonged air leak, bleeding, sepsis, pneumonia
- If feasible, attempt early extubation postoperatively to avoid ventilator-induced surgical site dehiscence.

BRONCHOPULMONARY SEQUESTRATION (BPS)

- Small cystic masses of nonfunctioning lung tissue, thought to develop from the primitive foregut
- Not usually connected to main airway, blood supply from systemic circulation
- Two forms: intralobar and extralobar
  - Intralobar masses develop before the pleura forms and are found within the normal lung.
  - Extralobar masses are primarily supradiaphragmatic with a small portion (<10%) infradiaphragmatic.

- They appear as solid echogenic masses on antenatal ultrasonography (USG). It is often difficult to differentiate between intralobar and extralobar unless they are surrounded by pleural effusion or are found beneath the diaphragm (extralobar).
- Intra-abdominal BPS can appear as a suprarenal solid mass; it is important to differentiate from other suprarenal masses (i.e., neuroblastoma).
- On chest x-ray (CXR), they appear as posterior thoracic masses, mostly on the left.
- Consider chest computed tomography (CT) or magnetic resonance imaging (MRI) to delineate systemic blood supply if unclear from previous Doppler ultrasound.
- Extralobar > intralobar masses can be associated with multiple congenital anomalies including CDH, congenital heart disease, and vertebral anomalies.
- BPS increases the risk for high-output cardiac failure due to redundant circulation.
- A large BPS can act as a space-occupying lesion presenting with respiratory distress from pulmonary hypoplasia or lung compression, prompting emergent surgical repair.
- There is a significant reduction in the size of most BPS as pregnancy progresses.
- BPS can also cause fetal hydrops secondary to mass effect, tension hydrothorax, or high-output cardiac failure.
- If asymptomatic in neonatal period, BPS can later present with recurrent pneumonia, atelectasis, bleeding, or high-output congestive heart failure.
- It is recommended that asymptomatic patients undergo elective resection to prevent infection and potential malignant transformation.
- Thorascopic surgical resection is the treatment of choice; embolization is an alternative approach.
- Presence of a systemic feeding artery increases the risk of perioperative hemorrhage.
- Postoperative complications include bronchopulmonary fistulas, secondary hemorrhage, need for reoperation, and increased risk for pulmonary hypertension.

BRONCHOGENIC CYST

- Single cyst made up of respiratory epithelium
- Develops due to abnormal budding of the ventral surface of the primitive foregut
- Largely found in the mediastinum near the carina, but does appear within the lung parenchyma, pleura, or diaphragm
- Most patients are asymptomatic during the neonatal period.
- Diagnosed commonly on prenatal ultrasound or fetal MRI
- Sometimes found incidentally on CXR during newborn period
  - When fluid filled, they appear radiopaque; however, they may be connected to the airway and can present with an air-fluid level.
- CT scan is the study of choice.
- Mass effect may cause symptoms related to obstruction of the airway, gastrointestinal tract, and/or cardiovascular system.
  - Smaller airway obstruction can lead to air trapping or overdistention, with an appearance similar to that of congenital lobar emphysema.

- Treatment is complete surgical excision.
- Cyst aspiration may be considered as a temporizing measure with complete resection following.
- Surgery can be delayed for asymptomatic newborns until they are several months of age.
- There are no long-term complications related to bronchogenic cyst resection.

Surgical Intervention Considerations and Therapies for Select Gastrointestinal Pathologies

GASTROSCHISIS SURGICAL MANAGEMENT OPTIONS: PRIMARY VERSUS STAGED (SILO) CLOSURE

- Delivery room management: Place lower body/abdomen/intestines in a sterile bag. Directly observe the bowel until surgery to ensure that the bowel is not kinked, which would obstruct blood flow. Manually reposition the intestines with sterile gloves to reestablish blood flow if kinking occurs. Place replogle as soon as possible.
- Timely closure or coverage of the abdominal wall defect is critical in helping prevent intestinal injury.
- NPO prior to closure; provide parenteral nutrition through a central venous catheter.
- Maintain bowel rest and gastric decompression with replogle until bowel function is demonstrated.
- Majority of gastroschisis cases can be corrected by primary closure.
  - If infant has pulmonary compromise, reintroduction of the bowel into the abdomen may lead to limited diaphragmatic expansion and worsening respiratory status.
  - Replacement of the bowel into the abdomen may compromise hepatic, mesenteric, and/or renal circulation.
- Staged closure with silo placement
  - Consider silo for repair when infant has respiratory problems or risk of elevated abdominal pressures prevents safe primary closure.
  - Silo use increases the risk of abdominal wall cellulitis in the setting of an open wound.
  - When reduction is complete, final closure is performed.
  - Provide broad-spectrum antibiotics until the silo is removed.
- Sutureless closure
  - When the bowel has been reintroduced into the abdomen, the umbilicus is placed over the defect with a dressing, allowing for the wound to heal without sutures.
  - It commonly results in an umbilical hernia, which often closes spontaneously.
- After primary closure or final closure after silo
  - If on mechanical ventilation, use a volume control mode to monitor changes in peak inspiratory pressures. Elevated peak inspiratory pressures may indicate an elevation to intra-abdominal pressures restricting diaphragmatic excursion.
  - Introduce enteral feeds slowly when the infant begins to show signs of ileus resolution, such as decreased

gastric replogle output, passage of meconium, and bowel sounds.

- If available, postoperative introduction of exclusive human milk enteral feeds has been shown to decrease the length of time to full enteral feeds and decrease time to discharge.
- Delayed enteral feeding and prolonged parenteral infusions raise the risk for hepatic cholestasis.
- Initiate small feedings early as tolerated, and reduce copper and manganese.
- Intestinal atresias can be found in 5% to 25% of patients with gastroschisis.
- If no intestinal patency is attained within 1 month of abdominal wall closure, obtain a water-soluble contrast enema to evaluate for atresia.
- Complex gastroschisis includes gastroschisis with atresia, necrosis, perforation, or volvulus.
  - Increases risk for sepsis, short bowel syndrome, and necrotizing enterocolitis
- Pain management immediately after surgery
  - IV acetaminophen; cautious administration of opioid analgesics (risk of slowed gut motility)

OMPHALOCELE

- Surgical closure options for omphaloceles are the same as those for gastroschisis.
- The difference is found in the preoperative management, as a thorough investigation must be performed to assess for associated genetic syndromes.

MIDGUT VOLVULUS

- Upper gastrointestinal (UGI) series is the gold standard for diagnosis. An abdominal radiograph is not sufficient for diagnosis; however, an acutely ill newborn with minimal or absent free air distal to the stomach and a presumed diagnosis of a volvulus can be sufficient to warrant emergent intervention.
- A volvulus commonly develops in the second or third portion of the duodenum, appearing as a bird's beak on an UGI series. Partial obstruction of the duodenum may appear as a spiral or corkscrew.
- Malrotation diagnosis on UGI: The duodenojejunal junction will present anterior, low, and often midline or to the right of midline. Normal positioning of the junction is at the level of the pylorus and posterior with duodenum making C sweep around the head of the pancreas.
- Patient is to be kept NPO on intravenous fluid (IVF). A peripherally inserted central venous catheter should be placed, time permitting. Broad-spectrum antibiotics are to be initiated.
- Time to surgery is critical in the setting of an acute malrotation with volvulus.
- Corrective surgical options include traditional Ladd's procedure (laparotomy/open) in emergent patients and laparoscopic Ladd's procedure for nonurgent malrotation patients.
- Postoperative complications include:
  - Intestinal dysmotility
  - Complications from intestinal ischemia post volvulus including reperfusion injury and hemodynamic instability and/or later onset stricture formation

- Bowel obstruction secondary to adhesions after a laparotomy
- Short gut syndrome

SPONTANEOUS PERFORATION

- Extremely low-birth-weight (ELBW) infants are at increased risk of perforation, especially in the first 1 to 2 weeks of life.
- Perforation occurs at the intestinal muscularis propria due to absence or thinning of this layer.
- Perforation presents with a distended abdomen secondary to perforation; it is not initially associated with significant intestinal inflammation or necrosis.
- ELBW infants are at additionally increased risk for spontaneous intestinal perforation (SIP) when prophylactic indomethacin is provided with postnatal steroid administration.
- Preoperative management: Make patient NPO, decompress the abdomen with replogle, provide supportive care with fluid resuscitation, provide vasopressors in the setting of hypotension, and initiate intravenous antibiotics.
- Surgical treatment options:
  - Bedside placement of a peritoneal drain may be performed initially and can potentially help avoid laparotomy.
  - The peritoneal drain is removed when there is resolution of meconium or intestinal drainage through the drain site.
  - Trial feeding can begin when there is evidence of bowel function or patency of the gastrointestinal tract has been confirmed with a contrast study.
- Laparotomy after peritoneal drain is indicated when air reaccumulates when the drain is removed or in the presence of persistent sepsis or fistula formation with meconium or intestinal drainage. Persistent bowel obstruction is often due to adhesions or a stricture at the perforation site.

NECROTIZING ENTEROCOLITIS (NEC)

- Preoperative management
  - Central venous and arterial access are important, as these infants require significant IV fluid resuscitation, are not fed for prolonged periods of time, and are at high risk for hypotension.
  - Close attention should be paid to electrolyte abnormalities and fluid balance, as these infants are at increased risk for third space fluid losses in the setting of intestinal edema.
  - Correct metabolic acidosis, severe anemia, thrombocytopenia, and/or coagulopathy.
  - Broad-spectrum antibiotics
- Surgical intervention indications: pneumoperitoneum, gangrenous bowel, persistent and severe hematological changes, failure of medical management
- Surgical approaches include exploratory laparotomy and primary peritoneal drainage (PPD) placement.
  - PPD placement is used primarily in infants who are deemed too ill to tolerate an exploratory laparotomy.
  - Surgery varies, usually involving resection of necrotic bowel and enterostomy creation.
  - A lethal intraoperative complication is liver hemorrhage.

- Consider surgery within the neonatal intensive care unit (NICU) for unstable critically ill infants requiring extensive supports.
- Postoperative gastrointestinal complications include intestinal strictures, short gut syndrome, and intestinal failure.
- Monitor enterostomy output, and consider replacement fluids if output is significant.
- If there is a persistent need for mechanical ventilation, volume control may have utility in helping identify abdominal compartment syndrome.
- Postoperative introduction of feeds should be resumed when bowel function has returned.

GASTROSTOMY TUBES

- Gastrostomy tubes can be placed endoscopically, surgically (laparoscopically or with an open approach), or radiologically (fluoroscopic or CT guided).
- Postoperative complications include dislodgement, excessive leakage around the gastrostomy tube site (mild drainage is expected), development of granulation tissue, surgical site cellulitis, and pressure necrosis.
- Postoperative pain management: IV or PO acetaminophen
- Feeds are typically initiated the day following placement; advance gradually.
- Routine care includes keeping the site clean and flushing the tube to prevent obstruction.

INGUINAL HERNIA

- Common in preterm infants
- The outcome is improved if the repair is delayed until 55 weeks' corrected gestational age (CGA) in preterm infants.
- If incarcerated hernia is unable to be reduced with sedation by an experienced provider, emergent surgery is indicated to avoid bowel necrosis regardless of age.

Surgical Intervention Considerations and Therapies for Select Neurologic Pathologies

NEURAL TUBE DEFECTS

- Open defects
  - Defect should be covered by a sterile dressing in the delivery room and maintained until surgical closure. Care should be taken to avoid pressure on the exposed neural tissue (e.g., if intubation is needed, position infant on side rather than back regardless of size of defect).
  - Prophylactic antibiotics are initiated ASAP.
  - Require urgent management and intervention, as neural tissue and cerebrospinal fluid are exposed, increasing the risk for infections such as meningitis.
  - Myelomeningoceles are most common and considered one of the most debilitating open defects, as they increase the risk for morbidities such as hydrocephalus, meningitis, and neurologic dysfunction (e.g., motor/somatosensory deficits, bladder and bowel impairment).
  - Corrective surgery involves closure of the defect and can be done prenatally or postnatally.

- Postnatal surgical repair should occur between 24 and 48 hours.
- Most common postoperative complication is hydrocephalus, requiring a shunt.
- Monitor with frequent head circumference measurements and head ultrasounds.
- Closed defects
  - Surgery may be delayed, as the defect is covered.
  - Urgent surgery is indicated with tethered cord syndrome presenting with neurologic deficits.
  - Surgical risks include neurologic deficits from a tethered cord or nerve injury during the procedure, poor wound healing, and infection/meningitis.

SACROCOCCYGEAL TERATOMA

- Rare germ cell tumor
- Prenatally, it can undergo rapid growth leading to complications such as high-output cardiac failure and hemorrhage, causing nonimmune fetal hydrops and fetal loss.
- A complicated and traumatic delivery can lead to tumor rupture and hemorrhage.
- There is no definitive set of prenatal surgical indications, but prenatal surgery is commonly considered in the setting of nonimmune hydrops or signs of eventual cardiac failure.
- Preoperative stabilization is focused on maintaining cardiovascular stability.
- Preoperative complications include tumor rupture and anorectal or urogenital obstruction.
- Initial surgery in the postnatal period is intended for stabilization in the setting of cardiovascular compromise. Surgery involves ablation, debulking, and devascularization to relieve cardiovascular strain.
- Complete resection is performed subsequently in the neonatal period.
  - Incomplete resection is the most common cause for recurrence.
- Postoperative complications include wound site infection, neuropathic bladder, diarrhea, bowel incontinence, and constipation.

Surgical Intervention Considerations and Therapies for Select Otolaryngology Pathologies

TRACHEOESOPHAGEAL FISTULA (TEF) AND ESOPHAGEAL ATRESIA (EA)

- Associated cardiac anomalies guide interventions and timing of surgery.
  - It is necessary to optimize infants in congestive heart failure prior to surgical intervention.
  - Infants with non-ductal–dependent cardiac lesions should not delay primary repair of TEF given the risk of aspiration through the TEF; EA repair may be delayed to optimize growth and a surgical approach to cardiac repair.
  - Infants with ductal-dependent lesions may need a palliative cardiac procedure prior to their TEF corrective surgery. If TEF repair is deemed necessary, infants should be taken to the operating room on PGE1.

- Position the endotracheal tube (ETT) tip distal to the fistula to avoid gastric overdistention.
- Postoperative management
  - Early extubation may be considered in nonpremature neonates who have mild or no respiratory impairment, appropriate lung compliance, and no tracheomalacia.
  - Lower-birth-weight neonates (<2 kg) typically require prolonged periods of ventilation postoperatively.
  - Reintubation may cause trauma to the corrected fistula site and potential stretching and shearing of the esophageal anastomosis.
  - Enteral feeding typically begins 48 hours after the surgical procedure and is administered through a nasogastric tube placed in the operating room.
  - Oral feeding may begin when a contrast swallow study rules out any esophageal leaks at the site of anastomosis, typically performed 5 to 7 days postoperatively.
  - Postoperative complications include respiratory distress due to tracheal edema (nebulized epinephrine and dexamethasone can be considered as therapies), anastomotic leaks, recurrent fistulas, esophageal motility dysfunction, and vocal cord dysfunction.

TRACHEOSTOMY

- Forty to sixty percent of pediatric tracheostomies are reported to beplaced in patients < 1 year of age.
- Ideally, a tracheostomy is performed when the patient weighs > 2500 g.
- Highest risk is the first week postoperatively when the tracheostomy tube can become dislodged and false track easily when replaced.
- Prenatal causes of airway obstruction include an obstructive neck mass, congenital high airway obstruction syndrome (CHAOS), micrognathia, and an obstructive chest mass.
  - These patients may require a tracheostomy as an EXIT procedure.

Surgical Intervention Considerations and Therapies for Select Urologic Pathologies

LOWER URINARY TRACT OBSTRUCTION: POSTERIOR URETHRAL VALVES (PUVs)

- Prenatal management
  - Prenatal findings include hydronephrosis, dilated ureters, thickened bladder, dilated proximal bladder, and oligohydramnios.
  - Indications for prenatal surgery include oligohydramnios.
  - Prenatal complications of oligohydramnios in the setting of lower urinary tract obstruction include pulmonary hypoplasia.
  - Prenatal surgical options
    - Insertion of a vesicoamniotic shunt (mixed outcome data)

- Festoscopic cystoscopy with posterior urethral valve ablation
- Open fetal vesicotomy
- Postnatal management
  - Ongoing monitoring of renal function and urine output, blood urea nitrogen (BUN)/creatinine (Cr) evaluation
  - Preoperative management
  - Correction of electrolyte derangements, metabolic acidosis, and uremia
  - Drainage of the bladder with urinary catheterization is critical.
  - Consideration of continuous antibiotic prophylaxis
  - Surgical management is performed at a later time with ablation of the valves.
  - Infants with continued obstruction may require vesicotomy.
- Long-term outcomes for these infants depend on the degree of associated renal dysplasia.
- Risk factors for progression to end-stage renal disease include serum Cr > 1 mg/dL, bladder dysfunction, and recurrent urinary tract infections.

BLADDER EXSTROPHY–EPISPADIAS COMPLEX

- Preoperative management
  - Cover the bladder to avoid abrasion.
  - Provide antibiotic prophylaxis.
- Surgical intervention
  - Modern staged repair (MSRE) of bladder exstrophy
  - Complete primary repair of exstrophy
  - Successful primary closure is most predictive of long-term bladder growth and voided continence.
  - Failure is usually due to wound dehiscence, bladder prolapse, bladder outlet obstruction, or vesicocutaneous fistula.
- Postoperative management
  - Initial pain management includes epidural infusions of local anesthesia (limited to first 2–3 days after surgery).
  - Immobilization of the pelvis and adequate pain control and sedation (acetaminophen, morphine, fentanyl) reduce the rates of postoperative complications and closure failure.
  - Keep the wound site clean and dry, without tension.
  - Continue antibiotic prophylaxis.

Suggested Readings

Abdelhalim A, Hafez AT. Antenatal and postnatal management of posterior urethral valves: where do we stand? *Afr J Urol.* 2021;27(1):140.

Bratzler DW, Dellinger EP, Olsen KM, et al. Clinical practice guidelines for antimicrobial prophylaxis in surgery. *Surg Infect (Larchmt).* 2013;14(1):73–156.

Kapralik J, Wayne C, Chan E, Nasr A. Surgical versus conservative management of congenital pulmonary airway malformation in children: a systematic review and meta-analysis. *J Pediatr Surg.* 2016;51(3):508–512.

Khen-Dunlop N, Farmakis K, Berteloot L, et al. Bronchopulmonary sequestrations in a paediatric centre: ongoing practices and debated management. *Eur J Cardiothorac Surg.* 2018;54(2):246–251.

Martin RJ, Fanaroff AA, Walsh MC, eds. *Fanaroff and Martin's Neonatal-Perinatal Medicine.* 11th ed. Philadelphia: Elsevier; 2020.

71 *Complex Neonatal Patient Management*

JONATHAN RYAN BURRIS, IGOR KHODAK, and PATRICIA R. CHESS

Overview

Neonates with complex conditions and multisystem organ involvement present challenges for management. Perinatal coordination of care occurs among neonatology, maternal–fetal medicine (MFM), and pediatric subspecialties to prognosticate and optimize chances for survival. Compassionate communication and counseling with the family are paramount skills for the neonatologist, as poor outcomes and life-threatening complications are more likely in these neonates.

Perinatal Counseling

- Periviable birth 22 to 24 weeks' gestation
  - Coordinate counseling with MFM and neonatology to discuss morbidity and mortality of both the mother and fetus.
  - The risk of mortality is higher in settings of sepsis (chorioamnionitis), premature rupture of membranes under 20 weeks' gestation (pulmonary hypoplasia), hydrops fetalis, complex congenital cardiac disease, and severe growth restriction (<1% percentile).
  - Assess parental understanding and cultural values.
  - Support emotional and spiritual needs.
  - Decision-making should not be based only on gestational age.
  - Provide objective, concise, and evidence-based national and regional data regarding survival, neurodevelopmental outcomes, delivery room interventions, respiratory morbidity, and risks for blindness and deafness.
  - Provide visual material regarding interventions and outcomes.
  - Discuss options and limitations for intervention when appropriate.
  - Offer option for comfort care in the delivery room and redirection of care in the neonatal intensive care unit (NICU) with family bonding when indicated.
  - Allow for questions and shared decision-making with respect to parental wishes.
  - Clearly document conversations with parents in the medical record.
- Complex fetal anomalies
  - Refer to tertiary/quaternary center with the needed pediatric subspecialty services.
  - Offer genetic counseling and testing (cell free DNA, amniocentesis) prior to delivery.
  - Coordinate more in-depth imaging (fetal magnetic resonance imaging [MRI], echocardiogram).
  - Ensure multidisciplinary service involvement for delivery room planning and coordination of care on admission.
  - Provide the family an opportunity for a second opinion, if requested.

Extreme Prematurity < 25 Weeks' Gestation

OVERVIEW

- Infants born less than 25 weeks' gestation have significant mortality and morbidity risk.
- When possible, delivery and management should be at a tertiary center.
- Following informed counseling, care should reflect the wishes of the parents.
- Birth leads to an abrupt ex utero transition of hypoxia to hyperoxia with resuscitation on developmentally immature organ systems.
- Risk of neurodevelopmental delay, cerebral palsy, blindness, deafness, and/or chronic lung disease is higher.

CLINICAL PRESENTATION

- *Lungs*: canalicular stage with respiratory bronchioles, primitive alveoli. Respiratory support and oxygen after birth can lead to derangements in alveolarization and arterialization with longer-term risks of bronchopulmonary dysplasia (BPD) and chronic pulmonary hypertension.
- *Heart*: disorganized sarcoplasmic reticulum, less mitochondria, less transverse tubules leading to impaired adaption of stroke volume with rapid changes in preload and afterload
- *Patent ductus arteriosus (PDA)*: modulates lower systemic perfusion in the fetus as oxygenated blood comes from the placenta. Postnatally, as pulmonary vascular resistance (PVR) drops, there is the potential for aortic to pulmonary shunting, increased pulmonary circulation/edema, and decreased organ perfusion (especially kidney and intestine).
- *Brain*: dysfunctional cerebral autoregulation. Neurons and glial cells arise from the germinal matrix and migrate outward to the cortex with fragile blood vessels. There is a high risk of ischemia–reperfusion injury, intraventricular hemorrhage, and white matter injury.
- *Retina*: interrupted normal vascular development, capillary constriction, neovascularization (vascular endothelial growth factor [VEGF]) with a risk for retinopathy of prematurity

- *Hearing*: intra-amniotic infection, including cytomegalovirus (CMV), TORCH infections (*Toxoplasma gondii*, other agents, rubella, CMV, and herpes simplex virus [HSV]), and bacterial infections; furosemide use; aminoglycoside use; and bilirubin toxicity are risk factors for sensorineural hearing loss.
- *Intestine*: spontaneous intestinal perforation (SIP) presents in the first week of life. Necrotizing enterocolitis (NEC) has the highest incidence between 28 and 33 weeks' corrected gestational age (CGA). Risk is higher in infants < 1000 g and earlier gestational age.
- *Nutrition*: calcium, phosphorus, and glycogen stores gained in last trimester. Risk is higher for protein deficits, growth restriction, hypoglycemia, and osteopenia of prematurity with high metabolic requirements, need for fluid restriction, therapeutic interventions for PDA and BPD.
- *Adrenal*: immature hypothalamic–pituitary–adrenal (HPA) axis. Cortisol production increases in the last trimester. Critical illnesses of very low-birth-weight (VLBW) and extreme prematurity lead to vasopressor-resistant hypotension, hyponatremia, and hypoglycemia.
- *Renal*: incomplete nephrogenesis and less glomeruli. Bicarbonate is lost, and risks are higher for renal injury with acidosis, hypotension, sepsis, antibiotics, and need for umbilical arterial catheters. Acute kidney injury raises the risk for mortality and increases the risks for chronic kidney disease, hypertension, and cardiovascular morbidity later in life.
- *Immune system*: reduced innate and adaptive immunity with deficits mucosal/epithelial barrier, lower production of cytokines, and less reserve of T-cell activation, monocytes, and neutrophils. Risk factors of intra-amniotic infection, need for invasive procedures (central lines, endotracheal tube, blood draws), and immature microbiome.
- *Hematologic*: anemia of prematurity is more pronounced than at term due to phlebotomy, reduced red blood cell (RBC) life span, and poor iron stores.
- *Skin*: stratum corneum is thin and underdeveloped. Rates of transepidermal water loss and transcutaneous heat loss are increased.

MANAGEMENT

- Antenatal steroids and magnesium are associated with improved survival and neuroprotection.
- Delay cord clamping for at least 30 seconds unless contraindicated (monochorionic multigestation, general anesthesia, acute blood loss, fetal bradycardia, apnea).
- Administer early surfactant within the first hour of life.
- Provide mechanical ventilation with early extubation to noninvasive nasal intermittent positive pressure ventilation (NIPPV) or continuous positive airway pressure (CPAP) to reduce ventilator-associated lung injury and pneumonia.
- Utilize high-frequency ventilation to reduce high mean airway pressure and peak inspiratory pressure (PIP).
- Target oxygen saturations of 90% to 95% to reduce reactive oxygen species (ROS) in lungs and retinopathy of prematurity (ROP).
- Use loop and thiazide diuretics intermittently to reduce oxygen requirements. Inhaled steroids may improve airway compliance.

- Provide maintenance caffeine for apnea of prematurity.
- Low-dose dexamethasone (DART protocol) for infants with ongoing invasive respiratory support > 28 days of life with high risk of BPD-associated mortality. A side effect of early dexamethasone use in the first 2 weeks of life is increased risk of cerebral palsy.
- Obtain echocardiographic screening for PDA within the first 5 days of life. Hemodynamically significant PDA may warrant closure medically or surgically. Findings are inconclusive with regard to whether PDA closure improves overall survival.
- Ensure effective thermoregulation, glucose, and blood pressure homeostasis to minimize fluid resuscitation and the risk for fluid overload, renal injury, pulmonary edema, and intraventricular hemorrhage (IVH).
- Consider hydrocortisone in infants with low cortisol and hypotension refractory to vasopressors. Use with caution if indomethacin has been given, due to increased risk of intestinal perforation.
- Anemia of prematurity presents a need for blood conservation, iron supplementation, and gestational age-based transfusion parameters.
- Prioritize maternal breast milk and donor breast milk, as both provide greater nutritional benefit and decreased risk of NEC compared to formula.
- Establish feeding protocols and optimize parenteral nutrition.
- Provide palivizumab prophylaxis against respiratory syncytial virus (RSV) in infants < 29 weeks' gestational age and younger than 12 months at the start of RSV season.
- Maintain immunization milestones based on corrected gestation age.
- Involve the services of occupational, physical, and speech therapy throughout the infant's NICU course.

PROGNOSIS

- Respiratory distress syndrome is the number-one cause of morbidity and mortality in extreme prematurity.
- Obtain echocardiographic screening for pulmonary hypertension in infants with chronic lung disease.
- Infants requiring chronic ventilation may need tracheostomy and an alternative enteral tube feeding regimen.
- Prolonged parenteral nutrition is associated with oral feeding delay and hepatic cholestasis.
- Grade III or IV periventricular cysts (PVLs) seen on head imaging carry a high risk of severe neurodevelopmental delay.
- Establish outpatient follow-up with a neurodevelopmental specialist.

Congenital Diaphragmatic Hernia (CDH)

OVERVIEW

- CDH is a diaphragmatic defect of the abdominal mesentery and viscera into the thorax.
- Herniated viscera compress lung tissue and impede normal micro- and macrostructural lung maturation, leading to varying degrees pulmonary hypoplasia, bronchovascular atresia, and pulmonary hypertension (PH).

- Intrapulmonary vasculature shows reduced arterial branching, resulting in increased muscularization of the pulmonary arterial tree and the inability to adapt to ex utero conditions with persistent PH.
- Incidence is one in 2000 to 3000.
- Defect locations: left-sided, 85%; posterolateral, 70%; anterior, 25% to 30%; central, 2% to 5%
- Associated anomalies occur in 40% to 60%.
- Antenatal ultrasound or fetal MRI can prognosticate survival with measurements of the ratio of observed to expected lung area to head (O/E LHR) or total lung volume (TLV).
- If O/E LHR < 15% or MRI fetal TLV < 20%, then survival is unlikely.
- If O/E LHR > 45% and liver down or MRI fetal TLV > 50%, then survival is >75%.
- With delivery at a tertiary center, anticipated overall survival ranges from 70% to 90%.

CLINICAL PRESENTATION

- Related to amount and timing of herniation. Small, late herniations may be asymptomatic.
- Symptomatology: scaphoid abdomen, absence of breath sounds on affected side of chest, often severe hypoxemic respiratory distress with failure to improve with ventilation
- Presence of bowel loops in chest with contralateral cardiomediastinal shift on chest radiograph

CLINICAL MANAGEMENT

- Target delivery at 39 to 41 weeks' gestation. If infant < 34 weeks' gestation, give antenatal steroids.
- Fetal therapies
  - Fetoscopic tracheal occlusion (FETO) in patients with severe pulmonary hypoplasia
- Delivery room
  - Immediately intubate and place orogastric tube for gastric decompression.
  - Provide gentle ventilation with PIPs of 20 to 22 with the goal of <25 and rates of 40 to 60 breaths per minute.
  - Resuscitate with 100% oxygen.
  - Give normal saline bolus for poor perfusion and delayed capillary refill.
- NICU
  - Start with conventional ventilation.
  - Target preductal oxygen saturations of 85%.
  - Accept permissive hypercapnia with pH >7.25 and partial pressure of carbon dioxide in arterial blood ($PaCO_2$) 45 to 65 to minimize barotrauma.
  - Place replogle tube to low intermittent wall suction to maintain intestinal decompression.
  - Support blood pressure to maintain adequate perfusion (dopamine, epinephrine, or dobutamine). High doses of vasopressors such as dopamine can induce pulmonary vasoconstriction and increase afterload. Consider a combination of multiple vasopressors to offset high-dose side effects of each medication and optimize cardiac output.
  - Use judicious fluid management to maintain appropriate renal output. Exercise caution regarding fluid overload, which increases the risk of mortality.
  - Place central venous lines. The right radial arterial line provides the most accurate blood pressure and gas monitoring.
  - Maintain adequate sedation with fentanyl or morphine, and consider dexmetomidine as a secondary agent to avoid heavy narcotic sedation.
  - Avoid neuromuscular blockage due to concerns about fluid overload and poor pulmonary clearance; outcomes are worse if the infant needs extracorporeal membrane oxygenation (ECMO).
  - Glucocorticoid support with scheduled hydrocortisone has shown benefit.

MONITORING

- Maintain close and continuous monitoring of oxygenation, blood pressure, urinary output, lactate, pH, and mean airway pressure.
- Obtain cardiac echocardiogram within the first 24 hours of life to assess ventricular function and persistent PH.

ADDITIONAL CONSIDERATIONS

- Use surfactant with caution, as it has been shown to be detrimental in term CDH babies.
- If there is evidence of poor lung compliance, low lung volumes, and poor gas exchange requiring higher conventional ventilation settings, then high-frequency ventilation may be utilized with slight benefit of jet ventilation (less cardiac compromise) over oscillatory. No true evidence has been obtained regarding the prophylactic benefit of starting over gentle conventional ventilation.
- Maintaining the patency of PDA should be considered in severe hypoxia and rising lactic acidosis as a bridge to improve cardiac output. There is unclear benefit for prophylactic PGE use without signs of right ventricular (RV) failure and PH.
- Administer milrinone for signs of severe PH and impending heart failure with ventricular dysfunction. Closely monitor for hypotensive side effects.
- Inhaled nitric oxide (iNO) improves oxygenation in the short term. Long-term concern for potential worsening of outcomes when used prior to repair is possibly related to delay of ECMO in severe cases.
- Left ventricular (LV) diastolic dysfunction in left-sided CDH leads to pulmonary venous hypertension. iNO can worsen pulmonary edema; consider it as a bridge to ECMO. Routine use is not recommended.

ECMO

- ECMO provides rescue therapy prior to repair with severe suprasystemic PH and RV dysfunction.
- Important to assess by clinical course (imaging, ECHO, arterial blood gases etc) before initiating ECMO if PH and degree of fixed PH indicate the ability to allow eventual decannulation.
- Surgical repair
  - Delay repair until improvement is seen in PH and overall stabilization of the patient.

- Consider primary closure versus synthetic patch for large defects.
  - Consider repair on ECMO in severe cases.
- Prognosis
  - Morbidity: failure to thrive, restrictive lung function pattern, neurodevelopmental delay secondary to hypoxemia, persistent PH
  - For persistent PH lasting > 6 weeks, consider cardiac catheterization and the phosphodiesterase inhibitor sildenafil.

Vein of Galen Aneurysmal Malformation (VGAM)

OVERVIEW

- VGAM is an arteriovenous malformation occurring between 6 and 11 weeks of gestation.
- Failure of the median porencephalic vein of Markowski to involute leads to high-flow and low-resistance arteriovenous shunting.
- Ischemic brain infarcts are due to parenchymal compression and vascular steal.
- Early presentation has 50% mortality; presentation at 5 months to 2 years has 90% survival.
- Mortality is due to high-output cardiac failure.

CLINICAL PRESENTATION

- Neonatal period: Arteriovenous shunting results in heart failure, pulmonary congestion, pulmonary hypertension, and multisystem organ failure.
- Hypotension, lactic acidosis, cyanosis, respiratory failure, seizures
- Hydrocephalus occurs if VGAM blocks CSF fluid drainage.
- Bruit over anterior fontanelle and orbits
- Cardiac exam: loud second heart sound, systolic ejection murmur

CLINICAL MANAGEMENT

- Diagnosis is confirmed with MRI or CT with angiography.
- Echocardiography shows right-sided dilation, PH, and diastolic runoff in ascending aorta.
- Treat heart failure to mitigate systolic dysfunction and PH.
- Severe pulmonary hypertension and ventricular systolic dysfunction: iNO and milrinone along with vasopressor support (epinephrine, dopamine, dobutamine)
- Monitor urine output with cautious use of loop diuretics based on fluid status and renal function.

PROCEDURAL INTERVENTION

- Endovascular embolization is the primary method to reduce atrioventricular (AV) shunting and heart failure.
- Neurosurgery is an option for embolization failure or evacuation of hematomas and management of hydrocephalus.

- In neonates with irreversible heart failure and brain atrophy at birth, discussion and counseling should weigh the benefit of treating the VGAM.

PROGNOSIS

- Infants treated in the newborn period with embolization have a 75% risk of neurodevelopmental delay.

Severe Anemia

OVERVIEW

- Neonatal anemia depends on hemoglobin (Hgb) concentration and ability to deliver oxygen to tissues.
- It results from blood loss, decreased RBC production, and/or RBC hemolysis.
- Chronic versus acute anemia dictates the body's circulatory adaption and pace at which blood should be repleted.
- Acute blood loss in the perinatal period with delayed intervention risk for ischemic brain injury, organ failure, and/or death.
- Acute blood loss surrounding delivery: fetal–maternal hemorrhage, placenta previa, vasa previa, placental abruption
- Internal blood loss in the neonate: subgaleal hemorrhage, pulmonary hemorrhage, intra-abdominal hemorrhage (adrenal), twin-to-twin transfusion syndrome (TTTS, with oligohydramnios of donor twin, polyhydramnios of recipient), and twin anemia polycythemia sequence (TAPS, with no amniotic fluid discordances in spite of large intertwin hemoglobin differences)

CLINICAL PRESENTATION

- Pale, tachycardic; >5 g/dL deoxygenated hemoglobin is needed to appear centrally cyanotic so often not cyanotic even though hypoxic.
- Low Hgb, jaundice secondary to hemolysis, or hydrops
- Acute blood loss: hypoxemia, hypotension, shock, disseminated intravascular coagulation (DIC)
- Chronic blood loss: well appearing, facing impending cardiac failure

MANAGEMENT

- Rapid transfusion is indicated in acute loss to replete intravascular volume and maintain cardiorespiratory status and oxygenation.
- Partial exchange or slow transfusion with chronic blood loss (e.g., TAPS, TTTS) or anemia from decreased RBC production minimizes increased preload on a failing heart.
- Support blood pressure and monitor for signs of coagulopathy.
- Obtain a Kleihauer Betke test for fetal maternal hemorrhage.
- Obtain a complete blood count with differential, reticulocyte count, fractionated bilirubin, and newborn investigation.
- Low reticulocyte count: parvovirus B19, viral suppression, Diamond-Blackfan anemia

- For an elevated reticulocyte count, obtain a direct antibody test (DAT).
- Negative DAT indicates RBC enzyme or membrane defect, ABO incompatibility, thalassemia, or chronic blood loss.
- Positive DAT indicates antibody-mediated hemolytic anemia.
- Hemolytic disease of the newborn with Rh disease: prophylactic anti-D is given prenatally if not previously sensitized. Consider fetal transfusion for severe anemia or hydrops when present. Postnatal therapies are aggressive phototherapy, hydration, and intravenous immunoglobulin. Partial or double volume exchanges are indicated in settings of severe anemia with or without hyperbilirubinemia.

Acute Kidney Injury (AKI) and Renal Failure

OVERVIEW

- AKI can evolve over hours to days and varies based on gestational age.
- 50% of infants 22 to 30 weeks' gestation experience AKI.
- Nephrogenesis begins at 5 weeks' gestation and continues until 32 to 36 weeks of gestation, with the majority during the third trimester.
- Premature birth may impede proper nephrogenesis, leading to chronic kidney disease.
- Functional renal capacity compared to an adult is not reached until 24 months of life.
- Renal hypoperfusion can occur via low intravascular volume and low cardiac output.
- AKI has negative effects on the lung relating to fluid balance, acid–base status, vascular tone, and erythropoietin production.

CLINICAL PRESENTATION

- AKI is defined by Kidney Disease: Improving Global Outcomes (KDIGO) guidelines as serum creatinine 0.3 mg/dL or >50% from previous Cr or drop in urine output (UOP) < 0.5 mL/kg/hr; relies entirely on serum creatinine and urinary output, which may be underdiagnosing kidney injury.
- Emerging evidence shows utility in urine biomarkers as early detectors of AKI, such as neutrophil gelatinase–associated lipocalin (NGAL).
- Prerenal: fluid losses (insensible, chest tubes, blood, gastrointestinal, diuretics), hypotension, infection, cardiac dysfunction
- Renal: acute tubular necrosis, renal dysplasia, polycystic kidney, renal vein thrombosis
- Postrenal: posterior urethral valves, bladder obstruction
- Risk factors include umbilical catheters, nonsteroidal anti-inflammatory drugs (NSAIDs), aminoglycosides, vancomycin, acyclovir, angiotensin-converting enzyme (ACE) inhibitors, and fluid shifts.
- High risk conditions: very low birth weight babies, extreme prematurity, perinatal asphyxia, complex cardiac disease.
- Symptomatology: oliguria, fluid overload, hypertension, electrolyte derangements (hyperkalemia, hypocalcemia, hyperphosphatemia), decreased medication clearance (sedation, antibiotics).

MANAGEMENT

- Correct underlying problem to restore adequate renal blood flow.
- Assess for volume depletion or overload (weight, urinary output).
- Obtain serum renal function panel and urine studies (analysis, culture, sodium, creatinine).
- Fractional excretion of sodium (FENa) greater than 3% is intrinsic AKI.
- Exclude prerenal by fluid challenge of 10 mL/kg normal saline over 1 to 2 hours.
- If hypotensive, support mean arterial pressure to provide adequate renal perfusion (dopamine).
- Exclude lower urinary tract obstruction with bladder scan/placement of urinary catheter.
- Adjust or discontinue renal toxic medications.
- Avoid potassium and phosphorus in intravenous fluids.
- For adequate fluid balance or fluid overload, restrict intake to insensible losses (30 mL/kg/d) + urine output.
- Avoid loop diuretics if the patient has anuria.
- Renal replacement therapy: peritoneal dialysis, continuous renal replacement therapy
- Monitor for comorbid effects of pulmonary edema, hypertension, compromised cardiac function, and anemia.
- A hemodynamically significant PDA may predispose a premature infant to AKI. It is inconclusive whether the timing and method of closure can prevent AKI.

PROCEDURAL INTERVENTION

- Continuous renal replacement therapy (CRRT) provides continuous renal replacement in infants 2.5 to 10 kg. Example: Cardio-Renal Pediatric Dialysis Emergency Machine™ (CARPEDIEM™). It is highly accurate and offers low blood and dialysis pump rates, precise scales, and requires low blood volumes.

PROGNOSIS

- The presence of AKI increases the mortality risk.
- Rates of chronic kidney disease and hypertension are higher in premature neonates.
- All infants with AKI warrant outpatient nephrology follow-up.

Hydrops Fetalis

OVERVIEW

- Hydrops fetalis is pathologic interstitial fluid accumulation in one or more body compartments (pleura, cardiac, abdomen, skin, or placenta).
- Immune mediated: RhD alloimmunization
- Nonimmune mediated: genetic causes, congenital heart disease (Ebstein's), arrythmia (supraventricular tachycardia [SVT] or complete heart block), viral infection (parvovirus), cardiomyopathy, TTTS, arteriovenous malformation (AVM), inborn error of metabolism, CDH, pulmonary mass (congenital pulmonary airway

malformation [CPAM]), airway obstruction (congenital high airway obstruction syndrome [CHAOS])

CLINICAL PRESENTATION

- Volume overload, anemia, heart failure, liver failure (hepatomegaly, ascites), lactic acidosis, hyponatremia (excess free water)
- Radiograph: cardiomegaly, pulmonary hypoplasia, pleural effusions

MANAGEMENT

- Immune-mediated prevention: RhoGAM for non-sensitized Rh-negative mothers
- Delivery room: establish ventilation, secure airway, consider surfactant for prematurity.
- Paracentesis or thoracentesis to allow lung expansion; send fluid for analysis.
- Obtain CBC with differential, serum electrolytes, albumin, and newborn investigation.
- Dysmorphic features: syndromic (chromosomal microarray), unclear (rapid genome)
- Place central venous and arterial umbilical access.
- Mechanical ventilation: consider high frequency if needing high PIP and mean airway pressure (MAP).
- Place chest tube for recurrent effusions.
- Administer octreotide for persistent chylothorax.
- Echocardiography and electrocardiogram (ECG) to assess cardiac function, arrythmia, and guide pericardiocentesis
- Provide vasopressor and ionotropic support (dopamine, epinephrine, dobutamine).
- Intractable hypotension (hydrocortisone)
- Judicious fluid monitoring with restriction is needed initially, as well as close monitoring of fluid losses with the potential use of albumin in parenteral nutrition.
- Careful use of furosemide depends on urinary output and renal function.
- Monitor for infection and give broad-spectrum antibiotics initially. There is a loss of immunoglobulins and white blood cells in pleural fluid.
- Obtain bacterial, viral cultures, and cell counts on fluid that is drained.

PROGNOSIS

- High risk of mortality is complicated by heart failure (approximately 50%).
- If diagnosed before 24 weeks' gestation, mortality > 95%.
- Autopsy and genetics can inform future pregnancies.

Congenital High Airway Obstruction Syndrome (CHAOS)

OVERVIEW

- CHAOS is complete or near complete laryngeal obstruction with atresia or stenosis.
- Larynx fails to recanalize around 10 weeks' gestation.

- Genetic testing is warranted (amniocentesis), as 50% of cases are associated with anomalies (skeletal) and genetic syndromes (Fraser, cri-du-chat, velocardiofacial).

CLINICAL PRESENTATION

- Prenatal ultrasounds by 16 to 20 weeks show hyperexpanded lungs, flat diaphragm, and dilated tracheobronchial tree.
- Pulmonary hyperexpansion causes decreased venous return and cardiac compression, leading to abdominal ascites, impaired cardiac output, and nonimmune hydrops.
- Compression of esophagus leads to polyhydramnios later in pregnancy.
- For an undiagnosed infant, look for severe cyanosis and apnea. Infant may appear large for gestational age (LGA) and edematous, with a firm abdomen. Breath sounds or chest rise with PPV cannot be heard, and it is not possible to pass an endotracheal tube (ETT).

MANAGEMENT

- Obtain fetal MRI to characterize airway and area of obstruction for delivery planning.
- Obtain fetal echocardiogram to evaluate for anomaly or compromised cardiac function.
- Obtain serial fetal ultrasounds to monitor for hydrops.
- Conduct needle centesis for pleural, abdominal, or pericardial effusions.

PROCEDURAL INTERVENTION

- Ex utero intrapartum treatment (EXIT) procedure: controlled cesarean-section delivery with a neonatologist and pediatric surgery or ENT present with MFM. Infant is delivered remaining attached to the placenta.
- High risk of uterine bleeding is due to the need for uterine atony to provide continued uteroplacental gas and nutrient exchange.
- Rigid bronchoscope is introduced into the airway to pass the ETT.
- If blockage is complete, a tracheostomy distal to the obstruction is performed.

PROGNOSIS

- It is a highly fatal condition even with intervention and is complicated by hydrops, heart failure, and genetic syndromes.

Complete Heart Block

OVERVIEW

- Complete AV block incidence is 1 in 10,000.
- Heart block is due to displacement of the AV node in congenital cardiac disease or by isoimmune damage by lupus antibodies (SSA).
- Fetal heart block develops around 16 to 24 weeks' gestation.
- Complete heart block is irreversible and associated with hydrops fetalis/congestive heart failure.

CLINICAL PRESENTATION

- Telemetry and ECG show QRS complexes conducted at their own rate independent of P waves.
- Symptoms include cyanosis, respiratory failure, and poor perfusion and oxygenation due to the inability of cardiac output to sustain systemic perfusion off placental circulation.
- Risks include AKI and renal failure, hypoxia and cerebral asphyxia, and lactic acidosis from poor end organ tissue perfusion.

MANAGEMENT

- Antenatal monitoring for ventricular rates, fetal growth, hydrops
- Mothers with positive lupus antibodies: fetal echocardiogram 18 to 20 weeks' gestation
- Coordinate delivery with MFM, cardiology, and neonatology. Specialized cardiac care following delivery is needed.
- Delivery room: in setting of bradycardia with poor perfusion and oxygenation despite appropriate airway resuscitation efforts, use cardiac pacing with automated external defibrillator (AED) and an intravenous infusion of isoproterenol.
- Be cautious about volume repletion in the delivery room, as it exacerbates cardiac failure and does not correct the underlying cause.
- Cardiac ventricular pacemaker can be placed externally or internally depending on the size of the infant.

PROGNOSIS

- Delivery that occurs at earlier gestations and is complicated by severe growth restriction, lung immaturity, or cardiac disease with hydrops has a high rate of mortality.
- Ventricular pacemakers pose a high risk of infection in the period following placement.

Transposition of the Great Arteries (TGA) With Intact Ventricular Septum (IVS)

OVERVIEW

- Ventricular arterial discordance
- Incidence is 5% of newborns with heart abnormalities.
- TGA is associated with ventricular septal defect (VSD), left ventricular outflow tract (LVOT), and coarctation of aorta.
- Intact ventricular and restrictive atrial (patent foramen ovale [PFO]) septum lead to parallel circulation with an inability to mix, resulting in severe hypoxemia, shock, and death.

CLINICAL PRESENTATION

- If fetal echocardiography shows cardiac outflow tract abnormality, prompt referral to a pediatric cardiac surgery center is necessary for delivery planning and postnatal care.
- Symptomatology at birth: severe cyanosis, poor perfusion, lactic acidosis
- Chest radiograph: cardiomegaly, increased pulmonary vascular markings
- ECG: right-axis deviation, right ventricular hypertrophy (RVH)

MANAGEMENT

- Immediately after birth, place IV and start prostaglandin (PGE1) to maintain ductal patency.
- Intubate and provide mechanical ventilation for persistent severe hypoxemia.
- Place ECG leads and upper/lower saturation monitoring.
- Maintain normal pH and CO_2, and judiciously raise the fraction of inspired oxygen (FiO_2) to facilitate a decrease in pulmonary vascular resistance as well as maintain systemic and cerebral oxygenation with goal saturation >80%.
- Obtain chest radiograph and echocardiogram.
- Echocardiography can determine if mixing between systemic and pulmonary circulation is adequate.
- Prompt placement of central access of umbilical venous and arterial lines is important.
- Support cardiac output with colloid and vasopressor (dopamine, epinephrine).
- Sedation and paralysis may be needed to decrease tissue O_2 consumption.

PROCEDURAL INTERVENTION

- Balloon atrial septostomy increases circulatory mixing and oxygenation.

SURGICAL REPAIR

- Timing of arterial switch depends on drop in pulmonary arterial resistance.

PROGNOSIS

- Persistent hypoxemia presents a risk for perinatal asphyxia, end organ failure (liver, renal, intestine), and coronary compromise with heart failure.
- TGA IVS presents a risk of persistent pulmonary hypertension with higher risk of mortality.

Suggested Readings

Baud O, Maury L, Lebail F, et al. Effect of early low-dose hydrocortisone on survival without bronchopulmonary dysplasia in extremely preterm infants (PREMILOC): a double-blind, placebo-controlled, multicentre, randomised trial. *Lancet.* 2016;387(10030):1827–1836.

Boardman JP, Groves AM, Ramasethu J, eds. *Avery and MacDonald's Neonatology: Pathophysiology and Management of the Newborn.* 8th ed. Philadelphia: Wolters Kluwer; 2021.

Chandrasekharan PK, Rawat M, Madappa R, Rothstein DH, Lakshminrusimha S. Congenital diaphragmatic hernia – a review. *Matern Health Neonatol Perinatol.* 2017;3:6.

Cummings J. Committee on Fetus and Newborn. Antenatal counseling regarding resuscitation and intensive care before 25 weeks of gestation. *Pediatrics.* 2015;136(3):588–595.

Jetton JG, Boohaker LJ, Sethi SK, et al. Incidence and outcomes of neonatal acute kidney injury (AWAKEN): a multicentre, multinational, observational cohort study. *Lancet Child Adolesc Health.* 2017;1(3):184–194.

Kirpalani H, Bell EF, Hintz SR, et al. Higher or lower hemoglobin transfusion thresholds for preterm infants. *N Engl J Med.* 2020;383(27):2639–2651.

Martin RJ, Fanaroff AA, Walsh MC, eds. *Fanaroff and Martin's Neonatal-Perinatal Medicine.* 11th ed. Philadelphia: Elsevier; 2020.

Polin RA, Abman SH, Rowitch DH, Benitz WE, Fox WW, eds. *Fetal and Neonatal Physiology.* 6th ed. Philadelphia: Elsevier; 2021.

SUPPORT Study Group of the Eunice Kennedy Shriver NICHD Neonatal Research Network, Carlo WA, Finer NN, et al. Target ranges of oxygen saturation in extremely preterm infants. *N Engl J Med.* 2010;362(21):1959–1969.

Basic Pharmacology Principles

TRACEY L. MCCOLLUM, GAL BARBUT and JONATHAN RYAN BURRIS

72 Drug Disposition and Pharmacokinetics

TRACEY L. MCCOLLUM and GAL BARBUT

Pharmaceutical therapy plays an integral role in the treatment of many conditions affecting the term and preterm neonate. Given the paucity of evidence-based dosing regimens, it is incumbent on the provider to use knowledge of developmental pharmacology to ensure that drug therapy is effective while minimizing the risk of toxicity. A thorough understanding of the maturational changes that affect drug disposition—absorption, distribution, metabolism, and elimination—as well as clinical pharmacokinetics will help guide this process.

Drug Disposition

ABSORPTION

- Absorption is the movement of a drug from the site of administration into the systemic circulation.
- Bioavailability (F) is the fraction of administered drug that reaches systemic circulation in its active form.
  - Intravascular administration = 100% bioavailability
- Extravascular absorption occurs by
  - Passive diffusion of unionized molecules across lipophilic membranes
  - Facilitated passive diffusion involving a carrier molecule
  - Active transport by a carrier that requires energy
- Absorption is influenced by
  - Route of administration
  - Biochemical properties and formulation of the drug
    - Lipid solubility—favors absorption
    - Degree of ionization (unionized molecules favored)
    - Molecular weight (smaller molecules favored)
  - Patient-specific factors
    - Gastric pH
    - Gastric emptying time
    - Intestinal transit time
    - Blood flow to the site of administration
    - Bacterial colonization
    - Bile acid production
- Bioavailability can be reduced by first-pass metabolism through the liver.
- Table 72.1 provides a summary of neonatal factors that affect drug absorption.

DISTRIBUTION

- Distribution is the movement of a drug from the bloodstream to the extravascular compartments, including fluids, organs, tissues, fat, and muscle.

- Distribution is influenced by
  - Size, composition, and pH of body compartments
  - Cardiac output (blood flow to tissues and organs)
  - Membrane permeability
  - Physiochemical properties of the drug
    - Lipid solubility, molecular weight, ionization constant, protein binding
- Volume of distribution (V_d) is the theoretic volume that would be necessary to contain the total administered dose of a drug at the same concentration observed in the plasma.
  - Lipophilic drugs generally have a larger V_d and longer half-life.
  - Hydrophilic and highly protein-bound drugs generally have a smaller V_d.
  - Drugs that have a larger V_d require a larger dose per unit of body measure to achieve the same serum concentration.
- Protein binding
  - Free drug is the fraction of drug not bound to protein, which can penetrate cell membranes and exert pharmacologic activity.
  - Binding proteins include albumin, lipoproteins, and alpha-1-acid glycoprotein.
    - Albumin has a greater affinity for acidic drugs.
    - Alpha-1-acid glycoprotein binds drugs that are bases.
  - Protein binding is a saturable, reversible process.
  - Serum drug concentration measurements reflect the total of free and bound drug. A greater percentage of free drug may result in an enhanced response for a given serum concentration.
- Characteristics of drugs that easily cross membranes, including the placenta and blood–brain barrier:
  - Highly lipophilic
  - Low degree of ionization (neutral)
  - Low degree of protein binding (protein-bound molecules generally incapable of crossing membranes)
  - Low molecular mass
- Table 72.2 provides a summary of neonatal factors that affect drug distribution.

METABOLISM

- Metabolism is the biotransformation of a drug to a more water-soluble compound to facilitate elimination.
- Metabolism primarily serves to weaken or inactivate a drug but sometimes may result in active metabolites or intermediates, or even transform an inactive prodrug into its active form.

Table 72.1 Summary of Neonatal Factors Affecting Drug Absorption

Route of Administration	Modifying Factor	Neonatal Function	Net Effect	Clinical Example(s)
Enteral, stomach	Gastric pH	Increased at birth; declines rapidly in term neonates but can remain elevated in preterm neonates (<32 weeks) for several weeks	Decreased absorption of weakly acidic drugs; weakly basic drugs readily absorbed	Phenobarbital, phenytoin, furosemide, amoxicillin, chlorothiazide, theophylline, penicillin, erythromycin, methadone, morphine, caffeine
	Gastric emptying	Delayed (up to 6–8 hours) in the preterm infant; variable in infancy up to 6–8 months of age; dependent on type of diet	Delayed absorption and reduced peak concentration	
Enteral, intestine (primary site of drug absorption)	Transit time	Generally delayed	Delayed peak serum drug concentration; reduced AUC	Ampicillin
	Presence of pancreatic enzymes and bile salts	Reduced	Decreased absorption of fat-soluble drugs	Vitamins A, D, E, and K; zinc; clindamycin
	Bacterial colonization	Reduced	Variable	Increased bioavailability of digoxin due to lack of digoxin-reducing bacteria
Intramuscular	Muscle mass and perfusion	Reduced muscle mass and blood flow	Reduced absorption; increased potential for injury	—
Percutaneous	Permeability and surface area	Increased in the preterm neonate due to immature stratum corneum and increased water content	Increased absorption; potential toxicity	Corticosteroids, alcohol-containing preparations
Rectal	Placement	Placement in lower rectum enhances absorption; placement in upper rectum subjects drugs to first-pass metabolism	Increased absorption; decreased bioavailability	Barbiturates, benzodiazepines acetaminophen

AUC, Area under the curve.

Table 72.2 Summary of Neonatal Factors Affecting Drug Distribution

Distribution Factor	Neonatal Function	Net Effect	Clinical Example(s)
Body composition	Greater percentage total body water[a]; ranges from 85% at 24 weeks to 75% at term	Increased volume of distribution of polar, water-soluble drugs	Aminoglycosides, vancomycin
	Lower percentage total body fat[a]; ranges from 1% or less at 24 weeks to 12% at term	Decreased volume of distribution of fat-soluble drugs	Propofol
Protein binding	Reduced concentrations of binding proteins	Increased fraction of free drug; increased volume of distribution	Digoxin, theophylline, phenobarbital
	Presence of fetal albumin	Decreased protein binding due to decreased affinity	—
	Presence of unconjugated bilirubin, free fatty acids	Decreased protein binding of drugs due to competition for binding sites	Ampicillin, penicillin, phenobarbital, phenytoin[b]

[a]Compared to values in older children and adults.
[b]Note that highly protein-bound drugs such as ceftriaxone and sulfonamides can displace bilirubin from binding sites.

- It occurs primarily in the liver, with contributions from the gastrointestinal tract, kidneys, lungs, plasma, skin, and other organs.
- Phase I (nonsynthetic) reactions
  - Commonly the first step in drug biotransformation, often preparing a drug for a phase II reaction
  - Include oxidation, reduction, hydrolysis, and hydroxylation
  - Cytochrome P-450 (CYP450) mixed-function oxidase system is responsible for 75% of phase I oxidative metabolism.

- Total CYP450 enzyme activity is about 30% of the adult level at birth.
- Enzymes mature at different rates, but most reach maturity by 1 year.
- This is important in drug interactions because many enzymes can be inhibited or induced by drug therapy, and drugs metabolized by the same pathway may compete for available enzymes.
- Other phase I enzymes include alcohol and aldehyde dehydrogenases, esterases, and monooxygenases.

- Phase II (synthetic) reactions
  - Involve conjugation of endogenous substances to the drug to create highly polar compounds and facilitate excretion
  - Include sulfation, acetylation, glucuronidation, and methylation
  - The capacity for sulfation and methylation is present at birth, whereas acetylation and glucuronidation develop over weeks to months (Fig. 72.1).
- Overall, the capacity for drug biotransformation is reduced in preterm and term neonates compared to adults.
  - Decreased hepatic blood flow and reduced cellular uptake limit delivery of the drug to the liver.
  - Activity of phase I and phase II enzymes is generally decreased, with variable rates of maturation.
  - Expression of hepatic enzymes is also associated with large interpatient variability, making it difficult to characterize the overall capacity for metabolism.
  - At various stages of development, a more developed metabolic pathway may compensate for one that is less developed.
- Modification of drug therapy in hepatic impairment
  - Reduce doses of drugs that are primarily hepatically metabolized as a result of:
    - Decreased metabolizing capacity of the hepatocytes
    - Increased bioavailability caused by a reduction in first-pass metabolism, as well as decreased protein binding
    - Impaired biliary elimination

ELIMINATION

- Elimination is removal of a drug or metabolite from the body, primarily via renal excretion.
- Minor routes of elimination include biliary, pulmonary, and fecal, as well as various body fluids.
- Renal clearance is the volume of plasma from which a drug is completely removed by the kidneys per unit of time; it is the sum of glomerular filtration, tubular secretion, and tubular reabsorption.
- Glomerular filtration rate (GFR)
  - Free drug, in solution, is filtered in the renal tubule.

- Highly protein-bound drugs will have a low rate of glomerular filtration.
- At birth, the GFR is ~30% of the adult value per unit surface area in term infants.
- The GFR increases rapidly in response to decreased renal vascular resistance, higher cardiac output, and increased renal blood flow, doubling by the end of the first month of life (see Fig. 72.1).
- The GFR in the preterm neonate is markedly reduced and may not reach adult values until 1 to 2 years of age.
- Tubular secretion and reabsorption
  - Drugs, particularly weak acids and bases, are secreted into the lumen of the renal tubule via active transporters in proximal tubule cells.
  - Secretion is not affected by protein binding.
  - Reabsorption of lipid-soluble drugs across the tubular epithelium occurs as the concentration of drug in the tubular fluid increases.
  - Tubular secretion is immature at birth, particularly in the preterm infant. It matures more slowly than the GFR, not reaching adult values until at least 6 months of age or later in preterm infants (see Fig. 72.1).
  - Drugs that require tubular secretion for elimination include penicillins, cephalosporins, furosemide, digoxin, and morphine. Neonates may have a reduced ability to clear these drugs.
- Renal elimination is largely dependent on cardiac output and renal blood flow. It is reduced in the setting of
  - Cardiovascular disease—heart failure, significant patent ductus arteriosus (PDA), left ventricular dysfunction
  - Hypotension—dehydration, sepsis, postsurgical
  - Renal disease or administration of nephrotoxic drugs
- Modification of drug therapy in renal impairment
  - Dose should be reduced for drugs that have a time-dependent profile (require maintenance of a minimum concentration) and/or exhibit toxicity at high concentrations (e.g., penicillins).
  - The administration interval should be extended for drugs that have a concentration-dependent profile (require achievement of a peak concentration for efficacy) and/or exhibit toxicity if not fully eliminated (e.g., aminoglycosides).

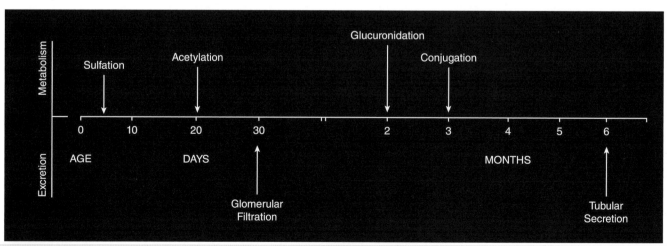

Fig. 72.1 Timeline of expected maturation of metabolic and renal pathways in the neonate to 6-month-old infant. (From Reed MD, Besunder JB. Developmental pharmacology: ontogenic basis of drug disposition. *Pediatr Clin North Am.* 1989;36:1064.)

Quantitative Pharmacokinetics

- Quantitative pharmacokinetics is the application of mathematical principles to predict changes in concentration of a drug in the body over time.
- Compartmental models (Fig. 72.2) are used to describe the distribution of a drug in the body:
  - A compartment represents a space (fluid or tissue) into which the drug can distribute.
    - The term *central compartment* generally refers to the blood (plasma) and highly perfused tissues (heart, lungs, liver, and kidneys).
    - Peripheral compartments include fat, muscle, and cerebrospinal fluid.
    - Compartments are not necessarily equivalent to physiologic or anatomic volumes.
  - The one-compartment model assumes the following:
    - All fluids and tissues belong to one compartment.
    - After administration, the drug distributes equally to all body areas instantaneously.
    - Changes to concentrations in plasma represent changes taking place in tissues.
    - A plot of the log drug concentration versus time will be linear (first-order elimination).
    - It is best used to describe polar drugs that are largely confined to the central compartment (e.g., aminoglycosides).
  - The multiple-compartment model assumes the following:
    - The drug is distributed between the central and peripheral compartments in such a way that maintains equilibrium.
      - After administration, the drug does not achieve instantaneous distribution and equilibration.
      - Rapid distribution to the central compartment occurs.
      - Distribution to the peripheral compartments is slow.
      - The model is best used to describe lipophilic drugs with extensive distribution (e.g., benzodiazepines).
- First-order, single-compartment elimination (linear pharmacokinetics)
  - The amount of drug eliminated over a given time is directly proportional to the amount or concentration in the body.
  - The fraction of drug in the body eliminated over a given time is constant.
  - First-order kinetics will demonstrate an exponential decay curve when plotted as plasma concentration versus time, but the curve will become linear when plotted as log plasma concentration versus time (Fig. 72.3).
  - First-order, one-compartment models can be used to describe the elimination of most drugs administered to neonates.
- First-order, multiple-compartment elimination
  - Rate of elimination is biphasic.
  - Drug concentration declines rapidly during the initial distribution phase, followed by a slower, steady elimination phase when equilibrium is achieved.
  - Because serum sampling is seldom done during the distribution phase, most pharmaceutical models assume first-order, single-compartment elimination.

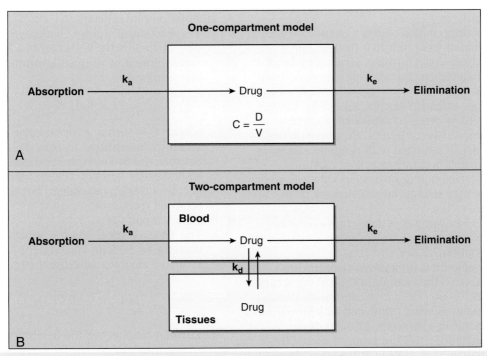

Fig. 72.2 One-compartment and two-compartment models of drug concentrations. (A) In the one-compartment model, the drug concentration (*C*) at any time is the amount of drug in the body at that time (*D*) divided by the volume of the compartment (*V*). Thus, *D* is a function of the dose administered and the rates of absorption and elimination represented by k_a and k_e, respectively. (B) In the two-compartment model, the drug concentration in the central compartment (the blood) is a function of the dose administered and the rates of drug absorption, distribution to the peripheral compartment (the tissues), and elimination from the central compartment. (From Brenner GM, Stevens CW. *Pharmacology.* 4th ed. Philadelphia: Elsevier; 2013:9–25.)

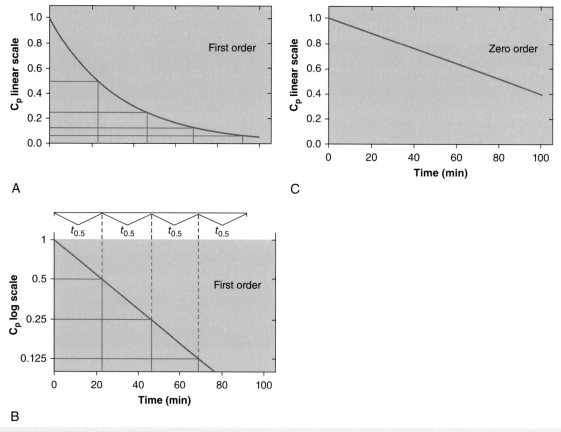

Fig. 72.3 Elimination of drugs. (A) First-order linear concentration scale. (B) First-order logarithmic scale. (C) Zero-order kinetics linear concentration scale. *Cp,* plasma concentration (drug). (From Dale MM, Hatlett DG. *Pharmacology Condensed.* 2nd ed. Philadelphia: Elsevier; 2009:24–25.)

- Zero-order elimination (nonlinear pharmacokinetics)
  - The amount of drug eliminated in a given amount of time is constant.
  - The fraction of drug eliminated over a given time varies.
  - Zero-order kinetics will produce a straight line when plotted as plasma concentration versus time and a curvilinear shape when plotted as log plasma concentration versus time.
  - Also known as *saturation kinetics,* zero-order kinetics can be displayed by drugs in situations of overdose or impaired clearance when enzymes or transport systems become completely saturated with drug, thus limiting the rate of metabolism or transport (Fig. 72.4).
  - When a drug is exhibiting saturation kinetics, small dose changes may lead to large increases in serum concentration.
  - See Table 72.3 for examples of drugs that exhibit zero-order kinetics.
- Volume of distribution
  - Dose (D) is the amount of drug administered (in mg/kg).
  - Concentration (C) is the amount of drug in the serum at a given time (in mg/L); C_0 is the serum concentration immediately following a dose and may have to be back-extrapolated in a two-compartment model.
  - Volume of distribution (V_d) is a proportionality factor that relates the amount of drug in the body (dose) to the serum concentration (in L/kg).
  - Thus:

$$V_d = D/C_0$$

- This equation can be rearranged to calculate a loading dose or dose increase.
- Elimination rate constant (k_e)
  - The fraction of a drug eliminated from the body per unit of time is the k_e. It can be calculated using the measurement of drug concentration at two different points in time:

$$k_e = \ln(C_1/C_2)/\Delta T$$

  where $C_1 =$ serum concentration at time T_1, $C_2 =$ serum concentration at time T_2, and $\Delta T =$ the time between the two measured concentrations.
  - In first-order kinetics, the amount of drug removed is concentration dependent, but the fraction of drug removed is constant.
- Elimination half-life ($t_{1/2}$)
  - The time required for the serum concentration to decrease by 50% (in hours) is the $t_{1/2}$.
  - It can be calculated from the elimination rate constant.

$$t_{1/2} = 0.693/k_e\,(\mathrm{hr}^{-1})$$

  - The elimination half-life determines the appropriate dosing interval.
- Clearance (Cl_s)
  - This is the volume of plasma from which a drug is cleared in a given time period.
  - It is the sum of clearances by various mechanisms.

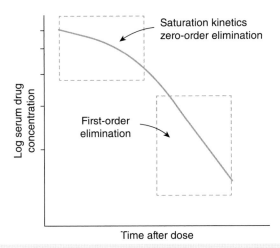

Fig. 72.4 Saturation kinetics, or zero-order and first-order pharmacokinetics. (From Allegaert K, Ward RM, Van Den Anker JN. Neonatal Pharmacology. In: Gleason CA, Juul SE, eds. *Avery's Diseases of the Newborn*. 10th ed. Philadelphia: Elsevier; 2018:419–431.)

- The rate of clearance is a constant, but the amount of drug cleared per unit of time is dependent on the serum concentration.
- It determines the steady-state concentration for a given dose:

$$Cl_s(\text{L/kg/hr}) = V_d(\text{L/kg}) \times k_e(\text{hr}^{-1})$$

Table 72.3   Kinetics of Drugs Commonly Used in Newborns

Zero-Order Kinetics	Saturation Kinetics[a]
Alcohol (as an excipient)	Caffeine
Heparin	Diazepam
Phenytoin	Furosemide
Theophylline	Indomethacin

[a]Even when administered at therapeutic doses.

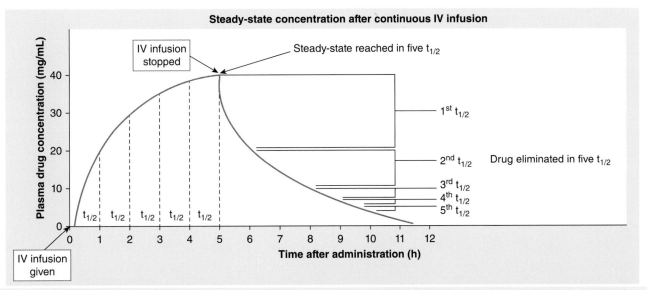

Fig. 72.5 Drug accumulation to the steady state. The time required to reach the steady state depends on the half-life ($t_{1/2}$); it does not depend on the dose or dosage interval. The steady-state drug concentration depends on the dose administered per unit of time and on the clearance or half-life of the drug. *IV*, Intravenous. (From Brenner GM, Stevens CW. *Pharmacology*. 5th ed. Philadelphia: Elsevier; 2018:11–26.)

- Steady-state concentration (C_{ss})
  - This refers to the point of therapy where the amount of drug being administered is equal to the amount of drug being cleared (in = out).
  - The length of time required to reach steady state is directly proportional to $t_{1/2}$, the half-life (~5 half-lives), and is independent of dose or dosing interval (Fig. 72.5):

  $$C_{ss} = (\text{dose}\,[D]/\text{dosing interval}\,[\tau])/Cl_s$$

- Basic calculations of dosages
  - The pharmacokinetic parameters described above, along with serum drug sampling, can be used to guide drug therapy.
  - This example uses gentamicin and assumes first-order kinetics at steady state:
    - A dose of 3 mg/kg administered every 12 hours results in a peak concentration of 5.2 µg/mL (note that µg/mL = mg/L) at a steady state.

- A trough level drawn 12 hours after the dose results in 2.6 µg/mL.
- These concentrations can be used to determine the V_d:

$$V_d(\text{L/kg}) = \frac{\text{Dose}\,(\text{mg/kg})}{\Delta C\,(\text{mg/L})}$$

$$= \frac{3\,\text{mg/kg}}{5.2 - 2.6\,\text{mg/L}} = 1.15\,\text{L/kg}$$

- As the serum level decreased by 50% (5.2 µg/mL to 2.6 µg/mL) over 12 hours, the $t_{1/2} = 12$ hours. After another 12 hours, the serum level would be expected to decrease to 1.3 µg/mL, within the desired range of 0.5 to 2 µg/mL, necessitating a 24- to 36-hour dosing interval (2–2.5 half-lives).

■ By rearranging the equation used to calculate V_d, one can determine the dose required to achieve a therapeutic peak level (6–10 µg/mL). Assume a desired peak of 7 µg/mL and dosing every 24 hours, as calculated above:

$$\text{Dose(mg/kg)} = V_d(\text{L/kg}) \times \Delta C(\text{mg/L})$$
$$= 1.15 \text{ L/kg} (7 \text{ mg/L} - 1.3 \text{ mg/L})$$
$$= 6.5 \text{ mg/kg every 24 hours}$$

Suggested Readings

Allegaert K, Ward RM, Van Den Anker JN. Neonatal pharmacology. In: Gleason CA, Sawyer T, eds. *Avery's Diseases of the Newborn*. 11th ed. Philadelphia: Elsevier; 2024:253–265.

Johnson PJ. Neonatal pharmacology–pharmacokinetics. *Neonatal Netw*. 2011;30(1):54–61.

Tayman C, Rayyan M, Allegaert K. Neonatal pharmacology: extensive interindividual variability despite limited size. *J Pediatr Pharmacol Ther*. 2011;16(3):170–184.

Ward RM, Lugo RA, Aranda JV. Drug therapy in the newborn. In: MacDonald MG, Seshia MMK, eds. *Avery's Neonatology: Pathophysiology and Management of the Newborn*. 7th ed. Philadelphia: Lippincott Williams and Wilkins; 2016:1093–1103.

73 *Clinical Toxicology*

TRACEY L. MCCOLLUM and JONATHAN RYAN BURRIS

Overview

The use of pharmaceuticals and other substances in pregnancy, childbirth, and lactation is common and often necessary. An understanding of the factors that determine fetal and infant exposure to these substances will assist the clinician in modifying risk while providing optimal care to both mother and baby.

Approach to Drug Categorization and Clinical Context

GENERAL CONSIDERATIONS

- US Food and Drug Administration (FDA) pregnancy risk categories (A–D and X) have been replaced by the Pregnancy and Lactation Labeling Rule.
- This Rule requires a drug label to include:
  - Pregnancy exposure registry
  - A risk summary detailing if the drug is contraindicated in pregnancy and supporting evidence that prioritizes human data, followed by animal data, then pharmacologic considerations
- The risk summary provides a description of adverse outcomes, including:
  - Structural abnormalities
  - Embryo, fetal, and infant mortality
  - Functional impairment
  - Alterations to growth
  - Information on the background population risk
  - A summary of established adverse outcome risk based on incidence, seriousness, reversibility, and relation to dose, duration, and gestational timing of exposure

Clinical Considerations and Guidance for Decision-Making in the Rule

- Risk of untreated disease to both mother and fetus
- Recommended dose adjustments for pregnancy
- Potential maternal or fetal adverse reactions
- Potential effects on labor and delivery
- All available human and animal data are available.

GUIDANCE FOR LABELING WITH REGARD TO LACTATION

- This guidance follows a similar format.
- The risk summary
  - Describes the extent to which the drug crosses into breast milk.
  - Includes effects of drug on milk production
  - Lists potential effects on the infant

Clinical Considerations

- The labeling guidance provides
  - Recommendations for dose adjustments, if required
  - Strategies to minimize infant exposure
  - Monitoring parameters for the infant
  - Data from all sources from which the information was gathered

DRUG USE DURING PREGNANCY AND LACTATION

- Drug use during pregnancy is guided by the principle that maternal benefits clearly outweigh risk to the fetus or infant.
- Principles regarding treatment should include the following:
  - Review treatment options to select drugs with significant safety data in pregnancy and lactation.
  - Consult multiple references to assess the most complete and up-to-date information.
  - Titrate maternal doses to the lowest effective dose, and use the shortest possible course.
  - Avoid the use of newer agents, because risks may not be identified for many years after marketing.

Drugs in Pregnancy

ADVERSE EFFECTS TO THE FETUS

- The risk of harm based on exposure to drugs in pregnancy is dependent on:
  - The teratogenic potential of the drug
  - The extent of fetal exposure
  - The developmental stage of the fetus at the time of exposure
- Fetal harm caused by drugs can be divided into two categories:
  - Teratogenic effects (Table 73.1)
    - Occur primarily during the embryonic period (2–8 weeks after fertilization)
    - Result in a disruption in tissue development or organ formation
    - Examples include neural tube defects, limb malformations, and craniofacial abnormalities.
  - Adverse fetal effects (Table 73.2)
    - Affect organs or systems that are already formed
    - Usually result in postnatal concerns

Table 73.1   Select Drugs With Known Teratogenic Effects in Pregnancy

Agent	Effects in Humans
ACEIs	In second and third trimesters: renal tubular dysgenesis, severe renal dysfunction with oligohydramnios, anuria, oliguria, hypotension, skull ossification defects (hypocalvaria), IUGR, fetal death
	In first trimester: congenital heart disease, CNS malformations
	Examples: captopril, enalapril, lisinopril
ARBs	In second and third trimesters: renal tubular dysgenesis, severe renal dysfunction with oligohydramnios, anuria, oliguria, hypotension, skull ossification defects (hypocalvaria), limb contractions, fetal death
	Early data do not demonstrate risk in first trimester.
	Examples: losartan, valsartan, candesartan
AEDs[a,b]	Carbamazepine—neural tube defects (especially meningomyelocele), IUGR, craniofacial defects, developmental delays
	Lamotrigine—facial cleft
	Phenytoin—FHS, with facial clefting, epicanthal folds, hypertelorism, short nose with broad nasal bridge, short neck, microcephaly, wide fontanel, low-set, abnormally formed ears, IUGR, digit and nail hypoplasia, mental deficiency (FHS features seen with other AEDs, as well)
	Topiramate—oral cleft, hypospadias
	Valproic acid—neural tube defects (especially meningomyelocele), cardiac defects; mental deficiency, FHS features as above
Antiretroviral drugs	Zidovudine—neuromitochondrial disease, congenital heart disease
	Efavirenz—neurologic defects
Cyclophosphamide	CNS malformations: facial and palate defects, absent fingers and toes, single coronary artery, imperforate anus, hernias, growth retardation, multiple eye defects, microcephaly, hypotonia, pancytopenia
Cocaine	Fetal loss, microcephaly, growth retardation, limb reduction, urinary tract malformations, cardiac abnormalities, placental abruption, poor neurodevelopmental outcomes
Ethanol	Fetal alcohol syndrome: IUGR, craniofacial abnormalities (short palpebral fissures, hypoplastic philtrum, maxillary hypoplasia, short nose, flat nasal bridge), microcephaly, growth retardation, developmental delay, behavioral abnormalities
Isotretinoin (retinoids)	Spontaneous abortion; multiple cardiac defects; craniofacial defects, including microtia, anotia, low-set ears, hypertelorism, hypoplastic maxilla and mandible, narrow sloping forehead, hydrocephalus; thymic hypoplasia
Lithium	Ebstein anomaly
Methotrexate	Neural tube defects; anencephaly; microcephaly; IUGR; craniofacial abnormalities, including synostosis of lambdoid, coronal sutures, and frontal bone, low-set ears, broad nasal bridge; syndactyly; tetralogy of Fallot
Misoprostol	Neural tube defects, limb defects, Möbius syndrome
Tetracyclines	Malformations of tooth enamel (including permanent discoloration) and bone
Thalidomide	Limb-shortening defects, hearing loss, abducens paralysis, facial paralysis, anotia, microtia, cardiovascular and gastrointestinal anomalies
Warfarin	Fetal warfarin syndrome: nasal hypoplasia, epiphyseal stippling, limb and digit hypoplasia, ophthalmic anomalies (e.g., optic atrophy, microphthalmia, blindness), low birth weight; CNS defects with exposure after first trimester, including agenesis of corpus callosum and Dandy-Walker syndrome

AEDs, Antiepileptic drugs; *ACEIs*, angiotensin-converting enzyme inhibitors; *ARBs*, angiotensin II receptor blockers; *CNS*, central nervous system; *FSH*, fetal hydantoin syndrome; *IUGR*, intrauterine growth retardation.
[a]Risk of defects increases with use of multiple agents and higher doses.
[b]Folic acid supplementation may reduce the risk of AED-induced teratogenic effects.

Table 73.2   Select Drugs Known to Cause Fetal or Neonatal Adverse Effects

Agent	Fetal or Neonatal Adverse Effects
Antipsychotic agents	Difficult adaption, breathing difficulties, jitteriness, irritability, poor feeding
Beta blockers	Neonatal hypoglycemia
Hypoglycemic agents	Neonatal hypoglycemia
Nicotine	Intrauterine growth retardation (IUGR), preterm delivery
Nonsteroidal anti-inflammatory drugs (NSAIDs)	Indomethacin, ibuprofen administered near term, at delivery
	Premature closure of the ductus arteriosus, necrotizing enterocolitis
Opioids, heroin	Neonatal abstinence syndrome
Selective serotonin reuptake inhibitors (SSRIs)	Preterm birth (low risk), persistent pulmonary hypertension, respiratory distress, difficult adaption, irritability, crying, poor feeding, sleep disturbances, increased tone, convulsions

Box 73.1   Drugs Contraindicated in Breastfeeding

Illicit drugs (unless mother actively in treatment program)
Radiopharmaceuticals
Antineoplastic chemotherapy agents

- Overall, the risk of fetal malformations due to drugs is very low when guided by appropriate clinical practice and decision-making.

Drugs in Lactation

CONSIDERATIONS FOR APPROACH TO BREASTFEEDING AND MOTHER'S MILK

- Very few drugs are truly contraindicated in breastfeeding (Box 73.1).

Relative Infant Dose

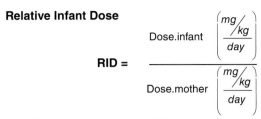

$$RID = \dfrac{Dose.infant\left(\dfrac{mg/kg}{day}\right)}{Dose.mother\left(\dfrac{mg/kg}{day}\right)}$$

Dose.infant = dose in infant/day

Dose.mother = dose in mother/day

Fig. 73.1 The relative infant dose (RID) expresses the infant's dose as a percentage of the mother's dose. (From Rowe H, Baker T, Hale TW. Maternal medication, drug use, and breastfeeding. *Pediatr Clin North Am.* 2013;60(1):274–294.)

- For other agents, consider the following:
  - Maternal need for the drug
  - Effects of the drug on milk production
  - Amount of drug excreted into breast milk (milk-to-plasma ratio)

- Extent of absorption by the infant
- Potential adverse effects to the infant
- Age and comorbid conditions of the infant
- The estimated infant drug exposure can be calculated.
  - The infant's daily dose (mg/kg/d) can be calculated by multiplying the average concentration in milk (mg/mL) × volume (mL) of milk ingested in 24 hours.
  - Calculate the relative infant dose (RID) using the equation shown in Fig. 73.1.
  - A RID of <10% is generally considered to be compatible with breastfeeding, although the toxicity of the drug should be considered.
  - The infant's daily dose (mg/kg/d) should fall well below the normal dosing range.
- See Table 73.3 for a listing of select drugs of concern in breastfeeding.

Suggested Readings

Djokanovic N, Boskovic R, Koren G. Maternal drug intake and the newborn. In: Yaffe SJ, ed. *Neonatal and Pediatric Pharmacology: Therapeutic Principles in Practice*. Philadelphia: Wolters Kluwer; 2010:158–168.

Greene MF. FDA drug labeling for pregnancy and lactation drug safety monitoring systems. *Semin Perinatol.* 2015;39(7):520–523.

Rowe H, Baker T, Hale TW. Maternal medication, drug use, and breastfeeding. *Pediatr Clin North Am.* 2013;60(1):274–294.

Sachs HC. Committee on Drugs. The transfer of drugs and therapeutics into human breast milk: an update on selected topics. *Pediatrics.* 2013;132(3):e796–e809.

Table 73.3 Select Drugs With Concerns in Breastfeeding

Agent	Infant Risk	Considerations
Alcohol	Psychomotor delay, drowsiness, decreased milk intake	Delay breastfeeding 2 hours for each drink consumed to allow for alcohol metabolism.
Amiodarone	Depressed thyroid function	Monitor infant cardiac and thyroid function.
Ergotamine	Vomiting, diarrhea, convulsions; may also decrease milk production	Use with caution; consider alternative agents.
Anticonvulsants, phenobarbital, primidone, ethosuximide	Sedation, levels approaching therapeutic, potential for seizures on withdrawal	Monitor serum levels, and reduce maternal dose if possible.
Cyclosporine	Immune suppression, renal toxicity	Monitor infant cyclosporine and serum creatinine levels.
Lithium	Changes to thyroid and/or renal function	Use only when alternatives are not suitable and only with healthy, full-term infants; monitor infant lithium, TSH, BUN, and creatinine levels frequently.

BUN, Blood urea nitrogen; *TSH*, thyroid-stimulating hormone.

74 Indications, Mechanisms, and Adverse Reactions for Common Drugs

TRACEY L. MCCOLLUM and JONATHAN RYAN BURRIS

Overview

Pharmaceutical therapy is a critical component in the care of the sick neonate. Babies in the neonatal intensive care unit receive dozens of medications a day, many of them unlicensed or off-label. This chapter examines the most commonly used medications and discusses the implications of unlicensed and off-label use.

Antibacterial Drugs

AMINOGLYCOSIDES (AMIKACIN, GENTAMICIN, TOBRAMYCIN)

- Indications: treatment of infections caused by aerobic gram-negative bacilli, including *Pseudomonas*; commonly used in combination with a β-lactam antibiotic for synergy in treating early-onset sepsis, meningitis, endocarditis
- Mechanism of action: Aminoglycosides inhibit protein synthesis in susceptible bacteria by binding to the 30S ribosomal subunit.
- Adverse effects include decreased creatinine clearance, renal tubular dysfunction resulting in electrolyte disturbances (e.g., hyponatremia, hypocalcemia, hypokalemia, hypomagnesemia), intrinsic neuromuscular blocking properties, potentiation of neuromuscular blockade in the presence of other neuromuscular blockers, and hypermagnesemia.
- Toxicity: renal toxicity with high trough levels, ototoxicity with high peak levels; toxicity is increased in combination with other ototoxic/nephrotoxic agents (e.g., vancomycin, furosemide)

PENICILLIN'S (β-LACTAM)—AMPICILLIN, PENICILLIN G, NAFCILLIN, OXACILLIN (PENICILLINASE-RESISTANT), PIPERACILLIN–TAZOBACTAM (ANTIPSEUDOMONAL)

- Indications: These broad-spectrum agents are useful in treating disorders such as sepsis, meningitis, pneumonia, urinary tract infections (UTIs); they are active against group B *Streptococcus*, *Listeria monocytogenes*, susceptible *Staphylococcus aureus* and enterococci, *Neisseria meningitidis*, and susceptible *Haemophilus influenzae* and *Escherichia coli* spp. Penicillin is also used to treat neonatal gonococcal and syphilis infections.

- Mechanism of action: β-Lactam antibiotics exert bactericidal action by binding to penicillin-binding proteins and inhibiting bacterial cell wall synthesis.
- Adverse effects include diarrhea; extended-spectrum agents can cause elevations in aspartate aminotransferase (AST) and alanine aminotransferase (ALT) levels.
- Toxicity: High doses can cause central nervous system (CNS) excitation, leading to seizures; piperacillin–tazobactam is nephrotoxic. These effects are increased in combination with other nephrotoxic agents, particularly vancomycin.

CEPHALOSPORINS (β-LACTAM)

See Table 74.1 for the classification and indications for cephalosporins.

- Mechanism of action: β-Lactam antibiotics exert bactericidal action by binding to penicillin-binding proteins and inhibiting bacterial cell wall synthesis.
- Adverse effects are rare but include rash, diarrhea, elevated hepatic transaminase levels, transient eosinophilia, and positive Coombs test.

VANCOMYCIN

- Indications: serious infections caused by methicillin-resistant staphylococci and penicillin-resistant pneumococci, including late-onset sepsis, meningitis, and pneumonia
- Mechanism of action: Vancomycin inhibits bacterial cell wall synthesis by inhibiting peptidoglycan synthesis; higher doses are required to be bactericidal.
- Adverse effects include rash and hypotension (red man syndrome), which can be relieved by extending the infusion time; also, phlebitis and neutropenia with prolonged therapy.
- Toxicity: ototoxicity with elevated peak levels and nephrotoxicity, which is increased when used with other nephrotoxic agents (piperacillin-tazobactam, aminoglycosides)

Antifungal Drugs

AMPHOTERICIN B (CONVENTIONAL, LIPID COMPLEX, OR LIPOSOMAL)

- Indications: treatment of systemic fungal infections; lipid complex or liposomal formulation indicated for patients with renal or hepatic impairment

Table 74.1 Classification of Cephalosporins Commonly Used in the Neonatal Intensive Care Unit

Generation	Antimicrobial Coverage	Indications
First generation (cefazolin, cephalexin)	Primarily gram-positive cocci[a] plus *Escherichia coli*, *Klebsiella*, and *Proteus*	Surgical prophylaxis, UTIs, skin and soft tissue infections
Second generation (cefoxitin)	Increased gram-negative coverage, including anaerobes (e.g., *Bacteroides fragilis*), Haemophilus *influenzae*, and *Neisseria gonorrhoeae*; reduced gram-positive coverage	Intra-abdominal, UTIs, skin and soft tissue infections
Third generation (cefotaxime, ceftriaxone,[b] ceftazidime)	Broad spectrum; effective against most gram-positive and gram-negative organisms; ceftazidime covers *Pseudomonas*	Sepsis, meningitis (excellent CNS penetration)
Fourth generation (cefepime)	Similar coverage to third generation but with increased resistance to β-lactamases	Sepsis, meningitis

CNS, Central nervous system; *UTIs*, urinary tract infections.
[a]None of the cephalosporins covers *Listeria* or *Enterococcus* spp.
[b]Ceftriaxone may displace bilirubin from albumin.

- Mechanism of action: Amphotericin B binds to ergosterol in the fungal cell wall, leading to alteration of cell membrane permeability; also causes leakage of cell components, with subsequent cell death.
- Adverse effects include decreased renal blood flow and glomerular filtration rate (increased hydration required with conventional form); renal losses of sodium, potassium, and magnesium; renal tubular acidosis; anemia; thrombocytopenia; fever and chills.
- Toxicity: nephrotoxic; caution advised in dosing because of 5- to 10-fold difference in dosing between conventional and lipid-based products

FLUCONAZOLE

- Indications: treatment of systemic infections caused by *Candida* and *Cryptococcus*, including meningitis, and superficial mycoses not relieved by topical treatment
- Mechanism of action: Fluconazole decreases ergosterol synthesis in the fungal cell membrane by interrupting fungal cytochrome P450 activity, thus inhibiting fungal cell membrane formation.
- Adverse effects include elevation of hepatic transaminase levels, hepatitis, jaundice, and rash.
- Toxicity: hepatic

Antiviral Drugs: Acyclovir

- Indications: treatment of infections caused by herpes simplex virus (HSV) or varicella zoster (VZV), including CNS and pulmonary infections
- Mechanism of action: Acyclovir triphosphate (a metabolite of acyclovir) acts as a specific inhibitor of herpesvirus DNA polymerase, thus inhibiting DNA synthesis and viral replication.
- Adverse effects include neutropenia, crystalluria (adequate hydration is required), and transient renal dysfunction.

Cardiovascular Drugs

ALPROSTADIL (PROSTAGLANDIN E1)

- Indications: maintenance of ductus arteriosus patency necessary for patients with congenital heart disease dependent on ductal shunting for oxygenation and perfusion.
- Mechanism of action: vasodilation of vascular and ductus arteriosus smooth muscle.
- Adverse effects: apnea, bradycardia, hypotension, fever, cutaneous flushing, leukocytosis; hypokalemia with long-term infusion.

VASOACTIVE DRUGS

See Table 74.2.

- *Indications*: Vasoactive drugs are used to increase perfusion due to hypotension, cardiac failure, and shock; agents affect cardiac contractility (inotropic effect), heart rate (chronotropic effect), and systemic vascular resistance (SVR).

IBUPROFEN AND INDOMETHACIN

- Indications: closure of patent ductus arteriosus (PDA); indomethacin is also used for prophylaxis of intraventricular hemorrhage
- Mechanism of action: nonsteroidal anti-inflammatory drugs that inhibit prostaglandin synthesis
- Adverse effects include decreased cerebral, renal, and gastrointestinal (GI) blood flow; oliguria; hypoglycemia; platelet dysfunction; and risk of gastrointestinal perforation (spontaneous intestinal perforation [SIP]) if used in conjunction with steroids.
- Toxicity: renal

SILDENAFIL

- Indications: treatment of persistent pulmonary hypertension
- Mechanism of action: Phosphodiesterase type-5 (PDE5) inhibitor limits the breakdown of cyclic guanosine monophosphate (cGMP), causing relaxation of the pulmonary vasculature.
- Adverse effects include systemic hypotension, exacerbation of dyspnea, visual disturbances, increased liver enzymes, and increased V/Q mismatch.
- Toxicity: possibly hepatic (case reports)

Table 74.2   Vasoactive Dugs

Agent	Contractility	HR	SVR	Adverse Effects[a] and Comments
Dobutamine	↑↑	↑	↓	Adverse effects: tachycardia, arrhythmias at high dose (ectopic beats), hypotension if volume depleted
				Synthetic catecholamine with primarily β1-adrenergic activity; useful for cardiogenic shock and myocardial dysfunction; no increase in afterload; no effect on renal blood flow
Dopamine	↑↑	↑↑	↑↑	Adverse effects: tachycardia/arrhythmias (ectopic beats), hypoxemia due to pulmonary vascular constriction, azotemia
				Catecholamine with α-adrenergic effects; effects vary with dosage; increases renal blood flow at low dose
Epinephrine	↑↑↑	↑↑↑	↑↑↑	Adverse effects: hypokalemia, arrhythmias (PVCs and VT), severe hypertension, renal vascular ischemia; stimulates alpha and beta receptors
Isoproterenol	↑↑↑	↑↑↑	↓↓↓	Adverse effects: tachycardia, arrhythmias, decreased coronary blood flow, hypoglycemia
				Stimulates beta-1 and beta-2 receptors; useful in bradycardia and to increase cardiac output; less helpful in shock due to decreased vascular resistance
Milrinone	↑↑		↑↑	↓↓	Adverse effects: hypotension if volume-depleted, thrombocytopenia, arrhythmias
				Phosphodiesterase inhibitor, decreases cAMP breakdown; decreases afterload

cAMP, Cyclic adenosine monophosphate; *HR*, heart rate; *PVCs*, premature ventricular contractions; *SVR*, systemic vascular resistance; *VT*, ventricular tachycardia.
[a]Note that all vasoactive agents can cause tissue ischemia and necrosis if extravasation occurs.

Central Nervous System Drugs

BENZODIAZEPINES (DIAZEPAM, LORAZEPAM, MIDAZOLAM)

- Indications: status epilepticus (refractory to standard anticonvulsants), maintenance of sedation, skeletal muscle spasticity
- Mechanism of action: Benzodiazepines enhance the effect of gamma-aminobutyric acid (GABA) at the GABAA receptor.
- Adverse effects include respiratory depression, hypotension, hypotonia, and seizure-like myoclonus in premature infants.
- Toxicity: Flumazenil is a reversal agent.

OPIOIDS (FENTANYL, MORPHINE, METHADONE)

- Indications: analgesia, sedation, anesthesia; methadone useful in narcotic weaning
- Mechanism of action: Opioids bind to opioid receptors in the CNS and inhibit ascending pain pathways.
- Adverse effects include respiratory depression (fentanyl < morphine), hypotension, bradycardia, urinary retention, ileus and delayed gastric emptying, pruritus, and seizures (especially with rapid weaning). Fentanyl has been associated with chest wall rigidity, especially with rapid administration. Tolerance with prolonged infusion (>5 days) requires slow weaning to avoid withdrawal.
- Toxicity: Naloxone is reversal agent.

PHENOBARBITAL

- Indications: seizures, sedation, narcotic withdrawal, hyperbilirubinemia
- Mechanism of action is largely unknown, but phenobarbital depresses the sensory cortex and limits the spread of seizure activity, possibly by increasing inhibitory neurotransmission.
- Adverse effects include CNS depression, sedation, respiratory depression at elevated serum concentrations, and apnea with rapid intravenous administration.
- Toxicity: reports of hepatic toxicity with prolonged use

US Food and Drug Administration Approval

- The US Food and Drug Administration (FDA) approves drugs based on adequate and well-controlled trials that provide substantial evidence of efficacy and safety.
- These trials rarely include neonatal or pediatric populations, so these populations are excluded from the approved labeling for many drugs.
- Off-label use refers to the use of a drug for an unapproved indication or an unapproved age group, dosage, or route of administration.
  - Lack of labeling does not imply that a drug is contraindicated or inappropriate for use in a disorder or population.
  - Off-label use is not illegal, nor is it considered investigational use.
- Professional standards for off-label use dictate that the drug is used:
  - In good faith
  - In the best interest of the patient
  - Without fraudulent intent
- Therapeutic decision-making should be guided by:
  - Benefit to the individual patient
  - Best available evidence, including:
    - Published literature
    - Expert opinion
    - American Academy of Pediatrics Practice Guidelines and Policy Statements
    - Handbooks and databases
- Practitioners have a duty to add to the body of knowledge by publishing or reporting notable experiences with off-label use.
- The Best Pharmaceuticals for Children Act (BPCA) and Pediatric Research Equity Act (PREA) have helped increase the number of drugs with pediatric labeling, but there is still a deficit in the neonatal and preterm populations.

Suggested Readings

American Academy of Pediatrics Committee on Drugs. Off-label use of drugs in children. *Pediatrics.* 2014;133(3):563–567.

Hsieh EM, Hornik CP, Clark RH, et al. Medication use in the neonatal intensive care unit. *Am J Perinatol.* 2014;31(9):811–821.

Takemoto CK, Hodding JH, Kraus DM. *Pediatric and Neonatal Dosage Handbook.* 23rd ed. Hudson, OH: Lexi-Comp; 2016.

Management of Neonatal Care Systems

MARLYSE F. HAWARD and ANNIE JANVIER

75 *Organization of Perinatal Care*

MARLYSE F. HAWARD and ANNIE JANVIER

Principles of Resource Organization, Utilization, and Management

- Overall goals are to decrease maternal and neonatal morbidity and mortality, as well as provide efficient and effective use of resources to promote value in health care.
- Perinatal/neonatal care includes:
  - Access to comprehensive perinatal health care services
  - Patient-centered, family-integrated care respectful of individual families' needs, preferences, and values
  - Clinically and linguistically competent care
  - Education
  - Accountability
- Health outcomes relevant to costs are expressed as *value*.
  - Value differs from *patient satisfaction* (how care is delivered) and *quality* (compliance).
- Assessments of system and care are evaluated by:
  - Evidence-based medicine (value = effectiveness)
  - Evidence-based economics (comparisons of incremental cost-effectiveness ratios (ICRs)
  - Quality improvement
    - Reflected in quality of life years (QALYs) and health-related QALYs (Hr-QALYs)
      - Quality improvement includes subjective (e.g., family perspective) and objective components.
      - Clinicians often underestimate QALYs for premature infants compared with parents.
- *Regionalization* refers to care delivered at larger centers as opposed to multiple smaller centers with less volume.
  - Regionalization leads to improved outcomes (small baby units), access to comprehensive perinatal health care services, system of referrals and consultations between institutions in a region, and early risk assessments matched to appropriate level of care.
  - It provides benefits for extremely low-birth-weight (ELBW) infants, extreme prematurity, extracorporeal membrane oxygenation (ECMO), and pediatric and cardiac surgery.
  - Challenges include financial competition and lack of governmental oversight.
- *Organization*:
  - The organization provides preconception care, prenatal care (basic, specialty, subspecialty, in-hospital care), and postnatal care (in-hospital care and outpatient follow-up).
  - Neonatal intensive care units (NICUs) can receive the designations of Level I, II, III, or IV (see Table 75.1).

Principles of Leadership

- *Leadership* involves future vision and improves outcomes, whereas *management* addresses current organizational issues.
  - Hospitals with physicians as leaders have better outcomes.
- Organizations involve *levels* of the workforce from the bedside (e.g., resident, nurse, physician) to the executive level (chief medical officer, dean, chair).
- *Core competencies* develop a vision, communicate that vision, inspire and empower others to share the vision, model expected behaviors, and develop future leaders.
- *Health care–specific competencies* target technical expertise in clinical areas, as well as industry expertise in operations, strategic thinking, finance, human resources, and information technology.
- Leadership *attributes* include emotional intelligence and self-awareness, self-management, social awareness, and relationship management.
- Leadership *behaviors* include assigning clear roles, goals, and responsibilities to team members; encouraging the inclusion of all individuals; providing psychological safety; encouraging self-reflection (e.g., "just culture"); and promoting health care virtues.
- Leadership *styles* include visionary, coaching, affiliative, democratic, pacesetting, and commanding.
- Strong leadership at multiple levels leads to decreased medical errors and delays, maximizes safety, increases job satisfaction, and reduces burnout.
- Clinical examples of leadership: (1) maintain an environmental awareness, (2) anticipate and plan, (3) assume a leadership role, (4) communicate effectively, (5) delegate workload, (6) allocate attention wisely, (7) use all available information, (8) use all available resources, (9) call for help when needed, and (10) maintain professionalism. (Refer to Weiner GM, Zaichkin J, eds. *Textbook of Neonatal Resuscitation*. 8th ed. American Academy of Pediatrics; 2021.)

Health Care Advocacy of the Mother–Fetal Dyad

- Advocating on behalf of the mother and fetus is a fine balance based on medical and ethical complexity and the psychosocial factors at play.
- *Medical complexity* exists due to the fetus being accessible only by going through a pregnant person; outcomes are linked and reliant on the pregnant person's well-being.

Table 75.1 Neonatal Intensive Care Units Level of Care

Level 1	Well-baby nursery with delivery room; 35–37 weeks to term
Level II	>32 weeks, >1500 g, mechanical ventilation < 24 hours
Level III	Level II plus ≤32 weeks, <1500 g, high-frequency ventilation, inhaled nitric oxide (iNO), medical and surgical subspecialties, advanced imaging
Level IV	Level III plus full range of surgical repairs including complex cardiac disease

- *Ethical complexity* stems from the fact that best interests of the fetus are balanced against maternal autonomy, legal rights of privacy, self-determination, informed consent, and protection from invasion of bodily integrity.
  - Societal debates exist in variety of circles; for example:
    - Are a pregnant person's moral obligations to an unborn fetus legal obligations?
    - When does a fetus gain rights and/or "personhood"?
  - Political, philosophical, legal, religious, and societal disagreements exist (e.g., abortion, frozen and discarded embryos, palliative care for very small preterm infants).
  - Implications of fetal rights legislation (Unborn Victims of Violence Act; Unborn Child Pain Awareness Act) have yet to be determined as abortion regulations shift.
  - There is no consensus on when personhood begins. Arguments range from conception to the acquisition of certain developmental milestones (e.g., pain sensation), viability, birth, human characteristics (smiling), or cognitive traits associated with personhood (e.g., capacity to communicate, self-consciousness).
  - Professional guidelines can favor respect for autonomy over fetal best interests.
  - *Mindset:* Preserve the patient–physician relationship so high-risk pregnant parents are not deterred from seeking care.
  - Few states prioritize fetal beneficence or prosecute pregnant persons with child endangerment who expose the fetus to harm (e.g., illegal drug use).
- Important case law and legislation
  - *In re A.C.*, 1987, Washington DC: terminal cancer patient at 26 weeks; parens patriae invoked; judge approved culture and sensitivity (C&S); overturned by DC Appellate Court; landmark ruling favoring autonomy
  - US Supreme Court: *Ferguson v. City of Charlestown*, 2001: women screened for drug use without consent; results to police: violation of Fourth Amendment; illegal search and seizure
  - Child Abuse Protection and Treatment Act (CAPTA) mandates that states have policies to address needs of drug-exposed infants; states differ as to whether illicit drug use is child endangerment.
  - *Muñoz v. John Peter Smith Hospital et al.*, 2017: 33-year-old woman, brain dead, 14 weeks pregnant; withdrawal of ventilator per patient's former wishes refused by hospital, alleging Texas Advance Directive Act prevents removal of "life-sustaining" treatment from pregnant women; district judge ruled in favor of

family based on brain death; no comment on constitutionality of the law
- Decision-making based on research and studies can be difficult when there is a lack of evidence to guide medical care and pregnant persons are under represented.
  - Fear of fetal harm from research overpowers fetal harm from lack of research.
  - Ensure justice for the pregnant person to benefit from research and respect for autonomy.
  - As stated by the American Congress of Obstetricians and Gynecologists (ACOG 2015) and endorsed by the American Academy of Pediatrics (AAP): Pregnant persons are "scientifically complex," not "vulnerable."
  - This statement led to a change of subpart B of the Common Rule, with removal of the consideration of pregnant persons as vulnerable.
  - Advocacy is important for equal representation of pregnant persons in research.
- Following birth, the mother–infant dyad is important beyond the hospital stay, and there are postdischarge supportive regulations regarding the family, parent, and infant. They are resource and state dependent and variable.
  - The Family Medical Leave Act protects a parent's job for 12 weeks, but the parent is unpaid (dependent on employer), and it is not universally available to all workers; it is state dependent.
  - Complex health care needs for an infant after NICU discharge are complicated by limited affordability for and access to appropriate medical care and daycare.
  - The AAP recommends team-based pediatric care and family-centered medical homes.
  - *Advocacy:* Neonatologists as individuals may join political groups advocating for universal health care, maternity leave, and disability support for children with complex medical care.

Health Equity and Health Disparities

- Health disparities exist for neonatal outcomes for minorities (Black, Hispanic, American Indian, and Puerto Ricans) compared to non-Hispanic white individuals.
  - Short-term outcome example: Black infants are more likely to be born premature.
  - Long-term outcomes examples: Elevated risks of morbidity, adverse neurodevelopmental outcomes, and behavioral deficits influence health and quality of life.
- Etiologies for disparities are multifactorial, and it is imperative to address deficits in access, care, resources, and social bias for those affected.
  - Access to the appropriate level of prenatal and postnatal care is important. Social biases can lead to unequal and worse care within the same functioning health care system.
  - Early programming life course theory: Exposures during the perinatal period (e.g., stress) can increase preterm birth.
  - Weathering hypothesis: Chronic stress leads to adverse health outcomes (e.g., preterm birth).

- Toxic stress can lead to epigenetic events, such as structural adaptations of chromosomal regions that result in mechanisms that manifest in utero and lead to chronic disease.
- Social determinants of health include environmental factors beyond individual genetics and biology that impact health, quality of life, and functioning as defined by the World Health Organization.
  - The five key areas that can help address disparities are economic stability, education, understanding social and community context, health care neighborhood, and built environment.
  - Racism is a social determinant of health that has a profound impact on the health status of children, adolescents, emerging adults, and their families.
  - Implicit bias is a subconscious attitude or stereotype of individual characteristics.

Transfer of Care and Transport Principles, Tools, and Communication Strategies

- Transport is an essential component in regionalization, and there are three types: maternal, neonatal, and return. Modes include ground or air (e.g., helicopter, plane).
- Antepartum transport is preferable if feasibly safe for both mother and fetus. It includes teams from the referring hospital, accepting hospital, or third hospital for transport only.
- Transport must adhere to federal and state law.
  - Emergency Medical Treatment and Labor Act: Emergency screening is required for Medicare patient.
- Components and process of a transport system:
  - Predetermined alliances and formal transfer plans between hospitals (ensures appropriate level of care for infant and mother)
  - Risk identification and anticipated benefits of transfer
  - Assessment of perinatal capabilities and conditions recommended for consultation and transfer
  - Safe, efficient, effective resource management
  - Financial and personnel support
  - Comprehensive and reliable communication systems
  - Clear responsibility of functions for transport team and receiving and referring institutions
- Transport team responsibilities:
  - Medical care: Referring hospital team retains responsibility until arrival at receiving hospital; receiving hospital team assumes responsibility on departure from referring hospital.
  - Procedures include proper identification of the newborn, medical records, and tests; providing a secure venous line; endotracheal tube (ETT) placement; STABLE protocol (sugar, temperature, airway, blood pressure, and emotional support); monitoring and performing patient care; and gaining appropriate consents.
  - Equipment should be checked regularly to ensure functionality.

- Staff responsibilities for developing and maintaining a transport system:
  - Appropriate level of training for transport team
  - Leadership director
  - Maintaining a database, protocols, and safety standards
  - Establishing alternative plans if transport is not possible
- Communication strategies, legal consent, and continued evaluation of system:
  - Policies and protocols in place for level of care, consultation, and transfer
  - Consent for transport and procedures, telephone consent for surgical procedures
  - Continued contact with supervising physician during transport
  - Continual quality evaluation and improvement procedures

Principles of Public and Population Health

- See Table 75.2.
- Morbidity and mortality:
  - Neonatal deaths (NDs) are more likely due to prematurity, congenital anomalies, and newborns affected by complications from pregnancy.
  - Postneonatal deaths (PNDs) are more likely due to infections, sudden infant death syndrome, and unintentional injuries.
  - Industrialized countries have higher NDs (2:1).
  - Underdeveloped countries have higher PNDs.
- Model State Vital Statistics Act and Regulations (Model Law)
  - Vital statistics reporting for infants born weighing more than 350 g at or more than 20 weeks' completed gestation are required.

Table 75.2 Perinatal, Neonatal, Postneonatal, and Infant Mortality

Term	Definitions
Perinatal death (PD) = Fetal death (FD) + Neonatal death (ND)	1. ND < 7 days + FD > 8 weeks
	2. ND < 28 days + FD > 20 weeks (most used)
	3. ND < 7 days + FD > 20 weeks
Perinatal mortality	Stillbirth + neonatal death
FD > 8 weeks; no live birth; any gestational age	Miscarriage: 8–20 weeks
	Stillbirth: >28 weeks
	Early: 20–27 weeks
	Late: 28–term
Infant death (ID) = Neonatal death (ND) + Postneonatal death (PND)	Any live birth resulting in death at < 365 days
Early neonatal death	<7 days
Late neonatal death	7–28 days
Postneonatal death	29–364 days
Live birth	Any gestational age completely out of uterus with umbilical pulsations, heartbeat, respirations, movement

States need to report on live births, fetal deaths, and infant deaths, but there is variability in reporting criteria among states, despite the Model Law.

Recognizing and Addressing Psychological Trauma

- *Moral distress* results from psychological disequilibrium in a health care provider who feels unable to take ethical action based on institutional or patient/family constraints; it includes feelings of anger, frustration, guilt, and powerlessness when caring for patients.
  - An example is providing aggressive, potentially painful intensive care in a situation assessed as futile.
  - Moral distress can lead to negative emotional consequences, burnout, and poor quality of care.
  - Moral distress is inevitable in the practice of neonatology due to the complexity and difficulties of patient care, and it impacts team members at all levels.
- *Burnout* refers to fatigue, detachment, and cynicism due to elevated levels of chronic stress.
- Parents of preterm and critically ill infants are at higher risk of acute stress disorders, anxiety, depression, and post-stress disorders including post-traumatic stress disorder.
- To address psychological trauma:
  - It is important to find strategies to harness into positive growth (e.g., advocacy, empathy) and provide access to resources for individuals to receive help.
  - Mental health (employee assisted behavioral therapy), social work, child life, and supportive/palliative care is recommended for those involved in the NICU.
  - Support of caregivers (parents) includes emotional support, screening, education, psychotherapy, and teleservices.
  - Health care team support should include education, emotional support, and debriefings.

Principles of Clinical Guideline Development and Evaluation

- Overall goal is to decrease variations in outcomes, minimize harm, be cost effective, improve outcomes, promote quality, eliminate race-based medicine, and deconstruct structural racism.
- The AAP is committed to eliminating race-based medicine:
  - Clinical practice guidelines (CPGs) are recommendations guiding practice that are evidence based; they include comprehensive literature reviews and data analyses.
  - Policy statements advocate, direct, or detail a public health position of concern.
  - Technical reports report reviews of the literature and data analyses.

- Clinical reports provide guidance on best practices and state-of-the-art medicine.
- The process of developing clinical guidelines involves determination of the quality of evidence (individual and aggregate assessments), assessment of the balance between benefits and harm, and assigning recommendations.
  - Systematic reviews are helpful (e.g., Cochrane Database).
  - Recommendations provided can be based on strong recommendations, recommendations, optional recommendations, or no recommendations.
- It is imperative to have a standardized approach. This consists of six criteria for assessing the quality of evidence and determining the strength of a recommendation, as developed by the Grading of Recommendations Assessment, Development and Evaluation (GRADE) working group.
- Based on standards for guideline development, methodology must meet the methodologic standards for the conduct of new Methodological Expectations of Cochrane Intervention Reviews (MECIR).

Suggested Readings

Value in Health Care

Ho T, Dukhovny D, Zupancic JA, Goldmann DA, Horbar JD, Pursley DM. Choosing wisely in newborn medicine: five opportunities to increase value. *Pediatrics*. 2015;136(2):e482–e489.

Perinatal Care Organization, Including Transport, Leadership, and Teams

Kilpatrick SJ, Papile L-A, eds. *Guidelines in Perinatal Care*. 8th ed. Elk Grove Village, IL: American Academy of Pediatrics; 2017.

Family-Centered Care

Davidson JE, Aslakson RA, Long AC, et al. Guidelines for family-centered care in the neonatal, pediatric, and adult ICU. *Crit Care Med*. 2017;45(1):103–128.

Leadership

Stoller JK. Leadership essentials for CHEST medicine professionals: models, attributes, and styles. *Chest*. 2021;159(3):1147–1154.

Maternal–Fetal Dyad and Research

Krubiner CB, Faden RR. Pregnant women should not be categorized as a 'vulnerable population' in biomedical research studies: ending a vicious cycle of 'vulnerability.' *J Med Ethics*. 2017;43(10):664–665.

Health Equity and Health Disparities

Sigurdson K, Mitchell B, Liu J, et al. Racial/ethnic disparities in neonatal intensive care: a systematic review. *Pediatrics*. 2019;144(2):e20183114.

Wright JL, Davis WS, Joseph MM, Ellison AM, Heard-Garris NJ, Johnson TL. Eliminating race-based medicine. *Pediatrics*. 2022;150(1):e2022057998.

Moral Distress

Prentice T, Janvier A, Gillam L, Davis PG. Moral distress within neonatal and paediatric intensive care units: a systematic review. *Arch Dis Child*. 2016;101(8):701–708.

Clinical Guidelines

American Academy of Pediatrics Steering Committee on Quality Improvement and Management. Classifying recommendations for clinical practice guidelines. Pediatrics. 2004;114(3):874–877.

76 Ethical and Legal Issues in Neonatology

MARLYSE F. HAWARD and ANNIE JANVIER

Ethical and Legal Principles (Limit of Viability, Futility, and Decision-Making)

- Controversies result from prognostic uncertainty, perceptions of sanctity of life and quality of life (QOL), beneficence and nonmaleficence, and inability to predict outcomes.
- Five factors influence prognosis at 22 to 25 weeks: birth weight, antenatal steroids, gender, multiple and singleton, and gestational age (see the National Institute of Child Health and Human Development calculator at https://www.nichd.nih.gov/research/supported/EPBO).
- Three categories of risk:
  - Early death likely, risk of severe morbidity high, intensive care not indicated
  - Survival likely, risk of severe morbidity low, intensive care indicated
  - Prognosis uncertain, survival associated with decreased QOL, parental discretion advised "gray zone"
- Shared decision-making is a two-way exchange of clinical information and parental values between physicians and parents to guide decision-making using infant's best interests.
- Personalized decision-making recognizes differences in decision-making (rational vs. intuitive), psychological makeup, life experiences, values, risk perceptions, and preferences.
- Personalized communication builds rapport and trust by addressing individualized information needs, values, emotions, and relationships; it includes frameworks such as the mnemonic SOBPIE (situation, opinion and options, basic politeness, perspectives, information, and emotions).
  - Support from relational autonomy (interdependency of infant and family interests and relationships) and feminist ethics (importance of relationships in making decisions)
- Historically, ethical debates have focused on nontreatment of children with disabling disorders.
- Current ethical debates focus on principles of justice and exposes biases:
  - Extremely premature infants are treated differently compared with other patient populations despite similar prognoses.
  - Predictions are pessimistic regarding the QOL for premature children surviving with disability compared with parents and the children themselves.
  - Parents of infants with trisomy 18 and 13 highlight alternative perspectives on QOL.
  - The data available reflect practices and self-fulfilling prophecies.
  - Practices vary; for example, survival is influenced by care practices for infants born 22 to 23 weeks' gestational age and other fragile children (T13–T18).
  - Other arguments about justice consider cost and resource allocation.
- Futility arises from definitions that are qualitative ("not worth it"), quantitative ("does not work"), or subjective versus objective. "Medically inappropriate care" has been suggested as an alternative terminology to replace "futility."
  - Futility may lead to moral distress.
  - Resolving conflict about "potentially inappropriate care" can follow a seven-step procedure based on a Society of Critical Care Medicine policy statement.
  - States have varied regulations regarding futility laws (e.g., California, Texas).
  - Regardless of gestational age, if survival is very unlikely and/or not in the interest of the child, interventions are not mandatory, and comfort care and palliative care are recommended.
- Parens patriae means that a state can intervene in protecting the best interests of a child; such intervention is reserved for extreme cases when parental decisions could cause direct, imminent, and irreversible harm (harm principle) or when decisions are clearly not in the best interests of the infant.
- Surrogate decision-making occurs when decisions are being made on behalf of individuals who lack capacity; parents are considered natural surrogate decision-makers, guided by the infant's best interests.
- Redirection of care toward comfort measures or noninitiation after thoughtful deliberation with parents is supported by the American Academy of Pediatrics (AAP) policy.
  - Withdrawal and noninitiation of care are ethically equivalent, with withdrawal of fluids and nutrition being ethically permissible under circumstances in which redirection is warranted.
- Research in the neonatal population is an important endeavor that has not been addressed until recent years.
  - Debates focus on informed consent procedures, research oversight, and "reasonable foreseeable risks" when evidence is absent, especially for emergency situations that occur at birth (e.g., intubation).
  - Parental participation can help determine research goals and outcome objectives; current outcome and disability categories may not align with parental experiences.

IMPORTANT FEDERAL REGULATIONS

- Rehabilitation Act of 1973, Section 504: Medical therapy cannot be withheld on the basis of disability.
- Baby Doe rules (US Department of Health and Human Services [DHHS])
  - Two sets (1982 and 1984); federal funds are jeopardized if Section 504 is violated, and the second rule addresses hotlines, posted announcements, and oversight committees
  - Prompted by the "Baby Doe" case (Bloomington, IN), Robinson case (surgery was refused for an infant with spina bifida, and the infant was placed for adoption), and a second Jane Doe case; rules were overturned and a Baby Doe Amendment was added to the Child Abuse Prevention and Treatment Act (CAPTA) which, if violated, would affect federal funding to hospitals
- 1983 President's Commission for the Study of Ethical Problems in Medicine and Biomedical and Behavioral Research: Deciding to Forgo Life-Sustaining Treatment: Section on Seriously Ill Newborns—parents are surrogate decision-makers
- CAPTA (1974)
- Baby Doe Amendment (1984): Hospitals could not withhold treatment based on QOL assessments unless the following criteria were met:
  - Infant is chronically and irreversibly comatose.
  - The provision of such treatment would merely prolong dying, would not be effective in ameliorating or correcting all of the infant's life-threatening conditions, or would be futile in terms of the infant's survival.
  - Treatment would be virtually futile or inhumane.
- Emergency Medical Treatment and Labor Act (EMTALA; 1986) included a provision to provide emergency care to those presenting to a hospital, regardless of ability to pay in an emergency medical situation.
- The Born Alive Infants Protection Act (BAIPA; 2002) defined "alive" as a product of conception outside of the uterus, regardless of means, with pulsation, heart rate, movement, or breathing.
- DHHS 2005 memo: Investigate claims of nonadherence under CAPTA and EMTALA; Neonatal Resuscitation Program (NRP) response: no impact on standard care

CASE LAW

- *Maine Medical Center v. Houle*, 1974: infant with multiple anomalies, parents refused repair, hospital petitioned, court ordered treatment
- *Baby Doe*, 1982: trisomy 21 with tracheoesophageal fistula (TEF) and esophageal atresia (EA); parents refused surgery due to mental disability; court-appointed guardian concurred; infant died of pneumonia; Indiana Supreme Court did not hear the case
- *Baby Jane Doe*: *Bowen v. American Hospital Association*; New York Supreme Court, 1983; US Supreme Court, 1986: meningomyelocele and hydrocephaly; parents opted against surgical repair; activist sued; New York Supreme Court upheld parents' decision; US Supreme Court concurred: state had no authority to give unsolicited advice
- *Miller v. HCA*, 2003: 23-week-old infant resuscitated, despite parental objections; Texas Supreme Court upheld actions, saying consent not necessary under emergent circumstances

- *Baby K*, 1994: anencephalopathic child had multiple visits to emergency room for resuscitation; hospital petitioned court to limit treatment; US Fourth Circuit of Appeals upheld EMTALA

Palliative Care Principles

- Know the components of bereavement counseling prior to, during, and after the death of a newborn infant, including palliative care.
- The AAP defines pediatric palliative care and pediatric hospice care goals that aim to:
  - Relieve suffering
  - Improve QOL (including family's adaptation)
  - Facilitate informed decision-making
  - Assist with care coordination
- Two models: integrative (prenatal, postnatal with life-threatening diagnoses, postnatal with worsening conditions) and consultative (primary team identifies patient and then consults palliative care expert)
- Goals are curative and palliative pain control and comfort but shift based on patient condition.
- Perinatal hospice: infants with conditions incompatible with life, as an alternative to termination
- Good parenting beliefs are paradigms parents utilize when coping with critical illness and can help with end-of-life decision-making.
  - Neonatal parents' processes involve more steps, including overcoming feelings of guilt, accepting their parenthood, and then feeling like good parents.
- Communication concepts:
  - Promote and help transition hopes, provide warning shots for bad news (what you are about to hear will be difficult), allow silence ("some very loving parents ... other very loving parents"), promote good parenting beliefs, reframe the decision so parents feel they are protecting their infants from pain and prolonged dying.
  - Provide a clear, consistent message about the infant's prognosis through a single spokesperson. Team collaboration and conflict resolution should occur prior to meeting with parents.
  - Frameworks: SOBPIE mnemonic
- Offer support regardless of care decision and recognize diversity.
  - Some parents find it helpful to witness resuscitation and codes.
  - Signatures for "do not resuscitate" or "do not intubate" orders are *not* mandatory and increase parental distress.
- Death and the grieving process:
  - Anticipatory guidance prior to death about dying process
  - Empathy and continued guidance during death
  - Private setting: limit distractions, encourage memories, allow privacy but be attentive and available
    - There is evidence of long-term psychological sequelae if parents do not have the opportunity to see their child during death, so in a culturally sensitive manner encourage parents to be with their infant.
  - Symptom management: Alleviate pain or other symptoms. Narcotics and sedatives do not shorten time to

death and should be given when needed; for example, if a neonate is dying and in pain, it is ethically permissible to provide morphine to relieve pain, even if this results in a decreased respiratory drive (doctrine of double effect).

- After death:
  - Offer pictures, hand/foot prints, etc. (can hold for later date if not ready for them).
  - Debrief with staff and follow up with parents regarding a memorial (family and hospital).
  - Phases of grief include shock and numbness, searching and yearning, disorientation, reorganization, and resolution.
  - Autopsy
    - An autopsy provides valuable information to facilitate closure for the family and generalizable knowledge for the scientific community, such as effects of treatment, iatrogenic complications, changing of presumed diagnoses, and cause of death, and it serves as quality control.
    - Declining autopsy rates have been suggested to be due to poor reimbursement, fear of litigation, lack of standards, parental concerns, or physicians not seeking consent.
    - Consent is obtained in an empathetic manner and is more likely to be obtained when death is sudden or unexplained. Parents often cite concerns for disfigurement as reasons for refusal, so limited autopsies can be considered.
  - Follow up with parents and primary consultant.

Genetic Testing and Gene Therapy

- Newborn genetic screening identifies individuals at risk in a population.
  - Selection of conditions: best interest standards and three Wilson and Junger criteria: natural history of the disorder, available interventions with cost-effective screening, and available confirmatory tests
  - Recommended Uniform Screening Panel (RUSP; federal guidance)
  - States retain authority on selection of disorders.
  - Parental refusal is permitted in all states but Nebraska; two states require active consent.
  - Ethical objections to parental refusal: States have interests in healthy children, benefits significantly outweigh risks, and consent leads to time-consuming refusals.
- Genetic testing is performed due to clinical suspicion, positive screens, family history, or other reasons to seek a definitive diagnosis. It includes karyotyping, microarray testing, testing for mutations, whole-exome sequencing (WES), and whole-genome sequencing (WGS).
  - WGS and WES should address concerns about incidental findings and disclosure procedures (e.g., who should be told and how to safeguard the information).
  - Genetic exceptionalism: Genetic information is unique and affects the entire family, with consequences on reproductive decisions.
  - Ethical debates: Carrier screening and testing for adult-onset disorders in minors challenge boundaries between infant and family interests. Protecting "open-future" is a primary concern of the AAP, which

recommends delayed testing unless treatment slows progression or parental anxiety is severe.
  - Research evolves faster than policies, and findings have uncertain significance, given variable penetrance.
- Legal considerations
  - The 10th Amendment states that states can implement programs for health and well-being of its citizens.
  - Common law: parens patriae
  - The 14th Amendment protects individuals' rights to refuse care and treatment (includes parental surrogate decision-making on behalf of the infant's best interests).
  - The Newborn Screening Saves Lives Act of 2008 (reauthorized 2014) provides national newborn screening guidelines and requires informed consent should blood spots be used in research.

Gene-Based Therapies and Treatments for Neonatal Conditions

- Gene therapy uses virus vectors and leads to potential risks such as immunologic responses or potentially higher rates of malignancy if they are inserted near proto-oncogenes.
  - Ethical concerns are related to justice and informed consent procedures (e.g., Wiskott-Aldrich syndrome, severe combined immunodeficiency, chronic granulomatous disease, ornithine transcarbamylase [OTC], adrenoleukodystrophy).
- Important historical case: Jesse Gelsinger, an 18-year-old with OTC deficiency, died during an institutional review board (IRB)-approved experimental gene therapy trial. The initial study was intended for infants who carried the lethal diagnosis of OTC, but the IRB thought that these patients were too vulnerable, potentially jeopardizing informed consent. Therefore, the study was performed with older, less severely affected OTC individuals who could provide active consent. The IRB balanced the potential for harm versus adequate consent. When Jesse died, a lawsuit followed.

Suggested Readings

Limits of Viability, Futility, and Decision-Making

Bosslet GT, Pope TM, Rubenfeld GD, et al. An Official ATS/AACN/ACCP/ESICM/SCCM Policy Statement: Responding to Requests for Potentially Inappropriate Treatments in Intensive Care Units. *Am J Respir Crit Care Med.* 2015;191(11):1318–1330.

Lantos JD. Ethical problems in decision making in the neonatal ICU. *N Engl J Med.* 2018;379(19):1851–1860.

Rysavy MA, Li L, Bell EF, et al. Between-hospital variation in treatment and outcomes in extremely preterm infants. *N Engl J Med.* 2015;372:1801–1811.

Palliative Care

Section on Hospice and Palliative Medicine and Committee on Hospital Care. Pediatric palliative care and hospice care commitments, guidelines, and recommendations. *Pediatrics.* 2013;132(5):966–972.

Weise KL, Okun AL, Carter BS, et al. Guidance on forgoing life-sustaining medical treatment. *Pediatrics.* 2017;140(3):e20171905.

Genetics

Kemper AR, Green NS, Calonge N, et al. Decision-making process for conditions nominated to the recommended uniform screening panel: statement of the US Department of Health and Human Services Secretary's Advisory Committee on Heritable Disorders in Newborns and Children. *Genet Med.* 2014;16(2):183–187.

Scholarly Activities and Quality Improvement

CARL T. D'ANGIO, COLBY L. DAY, RITA DADIZ and EMER FINAN

77 Biostatistics in Research

Carl T. D'ANGIO

Overview

- Statistics involves *inference*.
  - From a *sample* of the entire *population*, what can we understand about the whole population (Fig. 77.1)?
- Statistics attempt to measure the likelihood that an observed result reflects what is true in the population.
- A combination of *large differences* and a *large sample* makes a true difference more likely.

Understanding Variables

- Types of variables
  - *Continuous* variables can have any value on a scale (e.g., 1.0, 1.1, or 1.11).
    - Example: weight

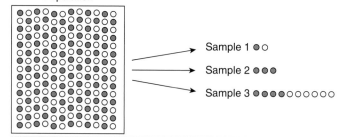

Population

Sample 1
Sample 2
Sample 3

Fig. 77.1 Sampling and inference. Statistics infers the nature of a population from a sample or samples drawn from the population. Larger samples provide more precise estimates of population characteristics.

- *Ordinal* variables are also ordered (e.g., 1, 2, 3), but
  - The variable cannot assume a value between those specified.
  - The distance between values is not necessarily constant.
  - Example: Apgar score
- *Categorical* or *nominal* variables describe categories without any implied order of the categories.
  - Examples (two categories): yes/no choices, RhD positive/negative
  - Example (>two categories): hair color
- Dependence
  - *Independent variables* are independent of other factors.
    - Example: age
  - *Dependent variables* are expected to be changed by other factors (e.g., disease or intervention).
    - They are typically the outcome variables in a study.
    - Example: In a study of vasodilators, pulmonary blood flow would be a dependent variable.

Distribution of Data

- *Normal distribution* implies that values are evenly distributed around a central value.
  - A *skewed distribution* is not evenly distributed around a central value (Fig. 77.2).
- Measures of *central tendency* (i.e., where is the middle of the data?)
  - Example: with the values (1, 1, 1, 2, 2, 3, 11),
    - *Mean* is the average.
    - *Median* is the middle value.
    - *Mode* is the most common value.

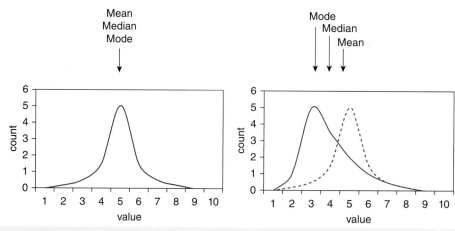

Fig. 77.2 Normal and skewed populations. The mean, median, and mode of a normally distributed population (left-hand panel) are the same. If the population is skewed (right-hand panel), the mode and median of the sample fall to one side of the mean value. The skew is toward the long "tail" of the data; in this case, to the right.

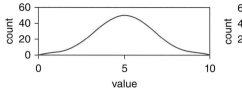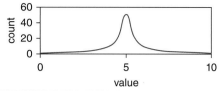

Fig. 77.3 Distribution widths. The data on the left have a wider standard deviation (and less certainty about the central value) than the data on the right.

- *Standard deviation* is a measure of the spread of the data (Fig. 77.3).
- *Standard error* is a measure of the precision of an estimate of the mean of a population.
    - The larger the population sampled, the smaller the standard error.
    - You are more likely to be sure that your estimate of the mean of 100 values is more accurate than if you only have 10 values.
- The *confidence interval* is the range within which a certain proportion of estimates of a value would fall.
    - For example, the 95% confidence interval (CI) is the range containing 95% of the estimates of a value.
        - If we made multiple estimates of the mean value of a measure using samples from the same population, 95% of them would fall within the 95% CI.
    - The CI is typically expressed as "1.5 (95% CI: 1.3, 1.7)" or "1.5 (95% CI, 1.3–1.7)."

Hypothesis Testing

- Statistical hypothesis testing starts with an assumption of no difference.
    - The *null hypothesis* (H_0) is that there is no difference between groups tested.
    - The *alternative hypothesis* (H_a) is that there is a difference between groups tested.
- The measure of statistical significance, usually the *p value*, is the likelihood that the observed differences within the *sample* reflect random chance rather than a true difference in the *population*.
    - Specifically, it is the likelihood that the observed results or results that are "more extreme" (larger difference) would be seen in the sample if the null hypothesis (no true difference in the population) were true.
        - A *high p* value (e.g., 0.80) reflects a *high* probability that any difference is due to chance.
        - A *low p* value (e.g., 0.01) reflects a *low* probability that the difference is due to chance; that is, the difference is likely to be due to a *true* population difference.
    - In the biomedical literature, a *p* value < 0.05 (<1 in 20 chance that the observed results or more extreme results are due to chance) is generally considered to be *statistically significant*, or there is a low enough likelihood of error to accept the result (Fig. 77.4).
- Types of error in statistical comparisons
    - A *type I* (or α) error is concluding that there is a true difference in the population when there is, in fact, no difference.
        - This error is minimized by choosing a restrictive (lower) *p* value cut-off to define significance.

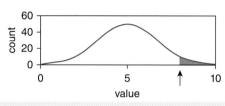

Fig. 77.4 Graphic representation of p value. Five percent of values in this distribution fall at or beyond the arrow, and a new observed value in the shaded range would have a 5% or lower likelihood of truly falling within this population.

- A *type II* (or β) error is concluding that there is no difference in the population when there is, in fact, a difference.
    - This error is minimized by using a large enough sample of the population (which increases the *power* of a study to find differences).
- Multiple comparisons
    - When multiple comparisons are made (e.g., among multiple groups of test subjects), the likelihood of an erroneous conclusion also rises.
        - For example, if 10 independent comparisons are made using a *p* value of 0.05 to define significance, the likelihood that none of the comparisons is due to chance is only 0.60 (0.95^{10}).
            - Technically, the likelihood that at least one result would be due to chance is $1 - (1 - 0.05)^{10}$, or 0.40.
        - The most common method for correcting for multiple comparisons (the *Bonferroni method*) is to divide the *p* value that will be used to determine statistical significance by the number of comparisons.
            - For 10 comparisons, a significant *p* value would be 0.05/10 = 0.005.

Statistical Tests

- Common statistical tests for varying data types
    - Tests that measure differences in central tendencies (e.g., means, medians) based on the central value and the spread of data are used for continuous or ordinal variables; in general,
        - A *t test* is used when the data are continuous.
        - The *t* test performs well when data are normally distributed.
        - Even if the data are not normally distributed, it still performs well if the number of observations is relatively large (over about 25).
        - The *t* test can be used only when two groups are being compared (not three or more groups; see analysis of variance [ANOVA], later).

- A *nonparametric* test (e.g., *Mann-Whitney U* test, also referred to as the *Wilcoxon rank-sum test*)
  - A nonparametric test is used when the data do not meet the "parameters" (e.g., normal distribution) for the *t* test.
  - It is also used when the data are ordinal.
- *Analysis of variance* (ANOVA) testing is used when three or more groups are being compared.
  - ANOVA tests whether the means are likely to be the same among all groups (null hypothesis).
  - If the null hypothesis is rejected, further testing is needed (with correction for multiple comparisons) to describe where differences exist.
- Tests that compare number of values in a category (e.g., number of males vs. number of females) are used with categorical variables.
  - *Chi square* (χ^2) test in most cases
  - *Fisher's exact* test with very small samples
- Test statistics
  - Statistical tests generate a *test statistic* (e.g., the *t* statistic or the χ^2 statistic) that can be translated into a *p* value.
  - Computerized statistics programs often report the test statistic but display the *p* value as well.
- Paired data
  - If the two continuous data points being compared are linked to one another (e.g., same patient before and after an intervention), a *paired t* test is used.
    - It compares the mean change in variable pairs, rather than change in means.
  - The *McNemar* test is used to compare paired categorical data.
- One- and two-tailed tests
  - A *one-tailed* test is used to evaluate if one mean varies from another in only one direction (greater or less).
    - It will detect smaller differences in the hypothesized direction but cannot be interpreted if the difference is in the opposite direction.
  - A *two-tailed* test evaluates differences in both directions.
    - Most clinical questions should be evaluated using a two-tailed test.
- *Bayesian* statistics
  - This branch of statistics, based on Bayes' theorem, uses both prior information and current data to estimate the probability of a specific result (see Chapter 79).
  - *Bayesian* statistics differs from traditional *frequentist* statistical tests (outlined in this chapter), which assess the likelihood that a given finding is due to chance.
  - Bayesian statistics are being used increasingly to describe biomedical results.

Assessing and Comparing Risks

- Measuring risk
  - The *risk* of an outcome is the number with the outcome divided by the total population.
    - If one person out of a population of four people has an outcome, the risk is $1/4 = 0.25$.
  - The *odds* of an outcome are the number with an outcome compared to the number without the outcome.

Relative Risk (RR) $\dfrac{[A/(A+C)]}{[B/(B+D)]}$

	Exposure	No exposure
Case	A	B
Non-Case ("Control")	C	D

Fig. 77.5 Relative risk. The relative risk (RR) of being a case with a particular exposure (as opposed to a case with no exposure) is the ratio of hatched blue/total blue (left column) to hatched green/total green (right column).

- If one person out of a population of four people has an outcome (i.e., one does and three do not), the odds are 1:3, also expressed as 1/3 or 0.33.
- With the exception of horse racing, clinicians usually think in terms of risk.
- Risk reduction
  - *Absolute risk reduction* is the *absolute* change in the risk of an event between one group and another.
    - If a certain treatment reduces the annual incidence of myocardial infarction in a population from 3/1000 to 2/1000, then the absolute risk reduction is 1/1000, or 0.1%.
  - *Relative risk reduction* is the *proportional* change in risk of an event between one group and another.
    - If a certain treatment reduces the annual incidence of myocardial infarction in a population from 3/1000 to 2/1000, then the relative risk reduction is $1/1000 \div 3/1000$, or 33%.
  - Note that these are two descriptions of the same result.
- Comparing risks
  - *Relative risk* or *risk ratio (RR)* is the ratio of the risk of an outcome in one group (typically a treated or comparison group) to the risk in another group (typically a control group) (Fig 77.5).
    - If a protective exposure decreases the risk of an outcome to 20% (2/10) from 30% (3/10), the relative risk of the outcome with exposure is $0.2/0.3 = 0.67$.
  - *Odds ratio (OR)* is the ratio of the odds of an outcome in one group to the odds in another group.
    - Using the same reduction as in the previous example, if a protective exposure therapy reduces an outcome to 20% (odds of 2:8) from 30% (odds of 3:7), the odds ratio with exposure is $0.25/0.43 = 0.58$.
- Relative risk versus odds ratio
  - When the prevalence of an outcome is rare, the odds ratio and relative risk are similar.
  - When the prevalence of an outcome is common, the odds ratio gives a bigger estimate of effect than does relative risk (as in the example above).
  - Why use an odds ratio?
    - Because of the characteristics of the math, odds ratios are not affected by the oversampling of disease that happens in *case–control* studies (see Chapter 78), making it possible to estimate the effect of an exposure on a disease from these

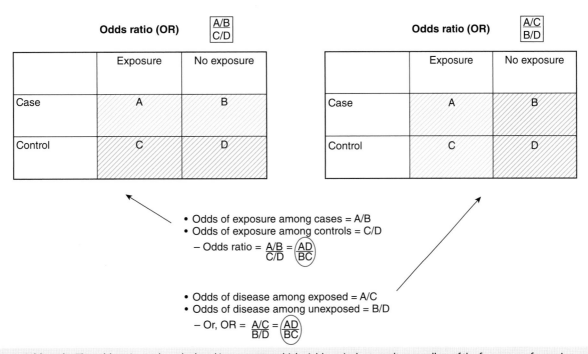

Fig. 77.6 Odds ratio. The odds ratio can be calculated in two ways, which yield equivalent results regardless of the frequency of cases in a sample.

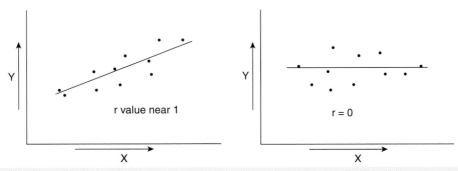

Fig. 77.7 Correlation coefficient (r value). A group of observations that closely approximate a linear relationship between X and Y (left) has r close to 1 (perfect correlation), whereas a group of observations in which one variable has no correlation to the other (right) has r = 0.

studies (despite the fact that they start by finding people with diseases rather than assessing exposure) (Fig. 77.6).

Measuring Correlation

- When comparing two continuous variables, we can measure the *correlation* between them.
  - The *correlation coefficient* (usually expressed as *Pearson product moment correlation*, or *r*) puts a number on this (Fig. 77.7).
    - A correlation coefficient of 1 ($r = 1$) indicates a perfect correlation; the variables line up on a straight line, and a change in one variable is directly correlated to a change in the other.
    - A correlation coefficient of 0 ($r = 0$) indicates no correlation between the two variables.
    - Correlations can be positive (slope of line is up) or negative (slope of line is down); the sign only indicates direction, not strength.

- Ordinal or skewed variables can be compared using *Spearman's rank-order correlation* (also known as *Spearman's rho*).
- Interpreting the *r* value
  - Definitions of levels of correlation are strictly descriptive
    - Above 0.70 to 0.75 = strong
    - Below 0.25 to 0.30 = weak
    - Everything in between is fair to moderate (sometimes split as below 0.50 = fair and above 0.50 = moderate).
  - Values of *p* can be assigned to correlations, but even weak correlations will be "statistically significant" if the number of observations is large.
    - The strength of the correlation is often a better indicator of correlation than a *p* value.
- The *coefficient of determination* describes how much of the variance in one variable is determined by the value of the other.
  - Calculated by the square of r (r^2)
  - For an *r* of 0.60 (a moderate correlation), 36% of the variance in one variable is described by the other ($r^2 = 0.60^2 = 0.36$).
    - 64% of the variance is described by something else.

Regression Analysis

- Regression analysis applies statistical testing to correlations.
- *Linear* regression is used to assess the effect of a continuous *independent* variable (or variables) on a continuous *dependent* variable.
    - The results are typically expressed as correlation coefficient (r), 95% CI, and p value.
- *Logistic* regression is used when the *dependent* variable is categorical.
    - The results are typically expressed as an odds ratio, 95% CI, and p value.
- Both linear and logistic regressions can incorporate multiple *independent* variables = *multiple regression*.
    - The analyses measure the effect of each independent variable on the outcome when the effect of all other independent variables is controlled.

Survival Analysis

- *Survival analysis* is used to compare the time to an event in two or more groups.
    - It is typically used to measure survival in patients following a therapy.
    - The *Kaplan-Meier* analysis (Fig. 77.8) is the most commonly used survival analysis and accounts for the fact that different patients may have been observed for differing periods of time since treatment, *censoring* a patient's data at the time that patient has been observed since treatment.
    - Survival curves may be compared using median time to an event or by calculating a *hazard ratio*: a specialized version of relative risk comparing outcome rates.

Diagnostic Tests

- Diagnostic tests are used to predict the presence of a disease and seldom do so perfectly.
    - When assessing the effectiveness of a diagnostic test, it should be compared to an independent *gold standard* known to correlate highly or definitely with disease.
        - Example: An imaging modality used to detect lymph nodes containing tumors might be compared to lymph node biopsy.
- Tests can result in four possible outcomes (Fig. 77.9):
    - Test positive and disease present = *true positive*
    - Test positive but disease absent = *false positive*
    - Test negative and disease absent = *true negative*
    - Test negative but disease present = *false negative*

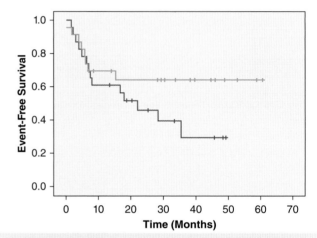

Fig. 77.8 Kaplan-Meier survival curve. Each step downward represents an event, and each tick mark represents a censored observation (subject has not yet had an event but has only been observed for that length of time). (Figure Courtesy of Craig Mullen.)

Bacterial infection present

Laboratory test result		Yes	No	
	Positive	True positives (a)	False positives (b)	***Positive predictive value*** (a)/(a+b)
	Negative	False negatives (c)	True negatives (d)	***Negative predictive value*** (d)/(c+d)
		Sensitivity (a)/(a+c)	***Specificity*** (d)/(b+d)	

Likelihood ratio, positive
Sensitivity/(1-specificity)

Likelihood ratio, negative
(1-sensitivity)/specificity

Prevalence
(a+c)/(a+b+c+d)

Fig. 77.9 Diagnostic test characteristics. Example uses the ability of a laboratory test to predict bacterial infection. Sensitivity, specificity, positive predictive value, and negative predictive value are commonly expressed as percentages or proportions; likelihood ratios represent fold increases or decreases in odds. Prevalence is not relevant in case–control studies (see Chapter 78). (From Weinberg GA, D'Angio CT. Laboratory aids for diagnosis of neonatal sepsis. In: Remington JS, Klein JO, Wilson CB, Nizet V, Maldonado YA, eds. *Infectious Diseases of the Fetus and Newborn Infant.* 8th ed. Philadelphia: Elsevier; 2015:1132–1146. Modified from Feinstein AR. Clinical biostatistics: XXXI. On the sensitivity, specificity, and discrimination of diagnostic tests. *Clin Pharmacol Ther.* 1975;17:104–116. Jaeschke R, Guyatt GH, Sackett DL. Users' guides to the medical literature. III. How to use an article about a diagnostic test. B. What are the results and will they help me in caring for my patients? *JAMA.* 1994;271:703–707. From Radetsky M. The laboratory evaluation of newborn sepsis, *Curr Opin Infect Dis.* 1995;8:191–199.)

Prevalence	Sensitivity	Specificity	PPV	NPV
25%	60%	92%	71%	87%
10%	60%	92%	45%	95%
5%	60%	92%	28%	98%

Fig. 77.10 Effect of changing prevalence of disease on positive and negative predictive values. In a test with constant sensitivity (disease producing positive test) and specificity (no disease producing negative test), as the prevalence of disease in a population increases, the positive predictive value (*PPV*; positive test implying disease) increases and the negative predictive value (*NPV*; negative test implying health) decreases.

- Test performance
  - *Sensitivity* is the ability of a test to detect those with disease (true positives/all patients with disease).
    - A highly sensitive test has few false negatives.
  - *Specificity* is the ability of a test to correctly identify patients without disease (true negatives/all patients without disease).
    - A highly specific test has a few false positives.
  - *Positive predictive value (PPV)* is the likelihood that a positive test means that a patient truly has disease.
    - A test with a high PPV has many true positives.
    - PPV is highly affected by disease prevalence in the population; if disease prevalence is very low, even the best test will have a lot of false positives (Fig 77.10).
  - *Negative predictive value (NPV)* is the likelihood that a negative test means that a patient truly does not have disease.
    - A test with a high NPV has many true negatives.
    - NPV is also highly affected by disease prevalence in the population; if disease prevalence is high, even the best test will miss disease (Fig. 77.10).

Assessing Diagnostic Tests

- *Likelihood ratios* are a measure of the change in likelihood of a disease based on results of a test.
  - Ratios vary with sensitivity and specificity of a test.
    - Likelihood ratio (positive, +) is the change in disease likelihood if a test is positive.
      - LR+ = sensitivity/(1 − specificity)
      - Example: A test with a sensitivity of 0.90 and a specificity of 0.80 would have a likelihood ratio (positive) of 0.9/0.2 = 4.5.
      - A highly predictive test has a likelihood ratio (positive) of about 10.
    - Likelihood ratio (negative, −) is the change in disease likelihood if a test is negative.
      - LR− = (1 − sensitivity)/specificity
      - Example: A test with a sensitivity of 0.90 and a specificity of 0.80 would have a likelihood ratio (negative) of 0.1/0.8 = 0.125.
      - A highly predictive test has a likelihood ratio (negative) of about 0.1.

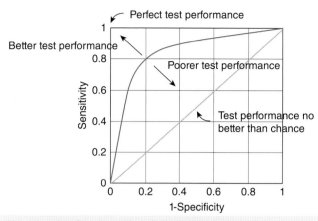

Fig. 77.11 Receiver operating characteristic (ROC) curve. This idealized curve shows a test with a sensitivity of 0.80 and specificity of 0.80 at the left "shoulder" of the curve. A perfect test would fill the entire graph (area under the curve [AUC] of 1.0), and a test without predictive value would describe a straight upward diagonal line (AUC of 0.50).

- The likelihood ratio tells you how much the odds (not risk) of an outcome are changed if a test is positive or negative (see Chapter 79).
- *Receiver operating characteristic (ROC) curves* compare the sensitivity and specificity of multiple cutoff values (to define a "positive" test) of a diagnostic test (Fig. 77.11).
  - The ROC curve plots 1 − specificity versus sensitivity.
    - Example: A test of fetal lung maturity would become more specific (include fewer false positives) but less sensitive (include more false negatives) as the surfactant cutoff value rose.
  - Curves with high "shoulders" (nearer to the left upper corner) imply better test performance.
  - Performance can also be described by the *area under the ROC curve (AUC)*.
    - An AUC of 1 describes a perfect test.
    - An AUC of 0.50 describes a test that performs no better than chance.

* Indicates required field

*Gestational Age (**Best estimate in completed weeks**)	Select ⌄
*Birth Weight (**from 401-1000 grams**)	⌄
* Infant Sex	○ Male ○ Female
* Singleton Birth	○ Yes ○ No
* Antenatal Steroids	○ Yes ○ No

Clear   Submit

Fig. 77.12 Clinical prediction rule applied to neonatal survival and morbidity. The Eunice Kennedy Shriver National Institutes of Child Health and Human Development Extremely Preterm Birth Outcomes Tool uses clinical factors combined in a multivariate regression derived from a large dataset to estimate survival and neurodevelopmental impairment. (From Eunice Kennedy Shriver National Institute of Child Health and Human Development, Extremely Preterm Birth Outcomes Tool, https://www.nichd.nih.gov/research/supported/EPBO/use.)

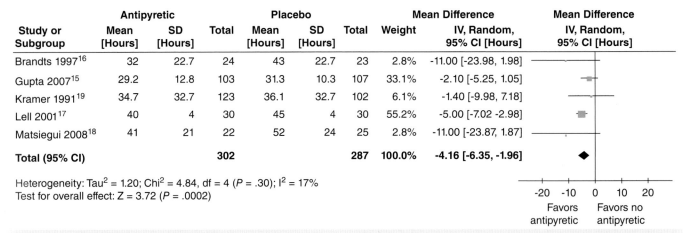

Study or Subgroup	Antipyretic			Placebo			Weight	Mean Difference IV, Random, 95% CI [Hours]	Mean Difference IV, Random, 95% CI [Hours]
	Mean [Hours]	SD [Hours]	Total	Mean [Hours]	SD [Hours]	Total			
Brandts 1997[16]	32	22.7	24	43	22.7	23	2.8%	-11.00 [-23.98, 1.98]	
Gupta 2007[15]	29.2	12.8	103	31.3	10.3	107	33.1%	-2.10 [-5.25, 1.05]	
Kramer 1991[19]	34.7	32.7	123	36.1	32.7	102	6.1%	-1.40 [-9.98, 7.18]	
Lell 2001[17]	40	4	30	45	4	30	55.2%	-5.00 [-7.02 -2.98]	
Matsiegui 2008[18]	41	21	22	52	24	25	2.8%	-11.00 [-23.87, 1.87]	
Total (95% CI)			**302**			**287**	**100.0%**	**-4.16 [-6.35, -1.96]**	

Heterogeneity: $Tau^2 = 1.20$; $Chi^2 = 4.84$, df = 4 ($P = .30$); $I^2 = 17\%$
Test for overall effect: Z = 3.72 ($P = .0002$)

-20 -10 0 10 20
Favors antipyretic   Favors no antipyretic

Fig. 77.13 Forest plot from a meta-analysis. Data are from studies showing effect of antipyretics on duration of febrile illness. Plot shows results from each individual study (green boxes and whiskers) and the weighted combination of studies (black diamond) and displays a mean difference in illness duration favoring antipyretics. (From Purssell E, While AE. Does the use of antipyretics in children who have acute infections prolong febrile illness? A systematic review and meta-analysis. *J Pediatr.* 2013;163(3):822–827.)

- *Clinical prediction rules* are methods that combine the results of a number of different parameters (e.g., patient characteristics, test results) to predict the likelihood of an outcome.
  - Examples: Score of Acute Neonatal Physiology (SNAP and its modifications) and the National Institute of Child Health and Human Development (NICHD) Neonatal Research Network outcome calculator (Fig. 77.12) use patient characteristics and/or physiologic parameters to predict neonatal morbidity and mortality.
  - Outcomes are usually listed as the percentages of patients in similar situations that will have a particular outcome; these percentages are seldom 0% or 100%.
    - Characteristics not measured by the rule will also affect outcomes, and the data used to generate the model may not apply to the specific patient (e.g., may be old or derived from a different population).
    - Application of results to an individual patient requires understanding of the patient's overall situation.

Systematic Reviews and Meta-Analysis

- *Systematic reviews* assess existing literature, taking advantage of electronic literature databases to identify all articles that meet reviewers' criteria and to avoid inclusion bias in articles reviewed.
  - Systematic reviews are limited by several factors, including search strategies used, publication bias that affects the articles available, and inherent subjective decisions regarding how to treat data.
- *Meta-analysis* is a statistical method of combining results of multiple trials to increase power of comparisons and to further decrease the bias in systematic reviews of therapies.
  - Studies to be included are sought systematically and must meet predetermined inclusion criteria.
  - Outcomes of individual studies and an overall weighted combination of the studies are expressed as a comparison between study groups (e.g., OR, RR, or mean difference) and 95% CIs, displayed as a *Forest plot* (Fig. 77.13).
    - Studies are typically weighted according to effect size.
    - 95% CIs that do not cross the line of identity (1 for OR and RR, 0 for mean difference) are statistically significant.
  - Meta-analyses are limited by search strategy and publication bias, as well as by undetected differences between studies that may make them inappropriate to combine.
  - Although potentially superior to small clinical trials (see Chapter 78), meta-analyses may not be as definitive of a large trial containing the same total number of patients included in the meta-analysis.

Suggested Readings

Adams ST, Leveson SH. Clinical prediction rules. *BMJ.* 2012;344:d8312.
Rindskopf D. Overview of Bayesian statistics. *Eval Rev.* 2020;44(4):225–237.
White S. *Basic & Clinical Biostatistics.* 5th ed. New York: McGraw-Hill; 2020.

78 *Epidemiology and Clinical Research Design*

CARL T. D'ANGIO

Study Types

- Based on timing of data collection
  - *Retrospective* studies collect data after study events have occurred.
    - They have the drawback of being unable to decide which data will be available.
    - They preclude being able to perturb the system; they are, by nature, *observational* rather than *experimental*.
  - *Prospective* studies collect data while study events are occurring
    - Data collection can be planned up front.
    - These studies can be either observational or experimental.
- Types of observational studies, which observe rather than cause outcomes (Fig. 78.1)
  - *Case reports* are descriptions of individual cases.
    - Advantage: useful for education and generating hypotheses
    - Disadvantage: may not be *generalizable* (one may not be able to draw conclusions about other cases from them)
  - *Case series* are a collection of cases, usually at least partially retrospective.
    - Advantage: potentially generalizable
    - Disadvantage: lack a *control* group of unaffected patients
  - *Cross-sectional* studies are evaluations of the state of a population at a particular point in time.
    - Advantage: can assess number of people with a disease or condition (*prevalence*), often in a large population
    - Disadvantage: provide no information about frequency of onset (*incidence*) or progression of disease
  - *Case-control* studies identify *cases* and compare them to *controls* without disease (Fig. 78.2).
    - These studies typically look retrospectively to evaluate previous exposures or conditions that may have preceded disease (and thus would be more common in cases).
    - Controls are often *matched* to cases (e.g., age or sex) to make the groups as similar as possible, other than the factors of interest.
    - Advantages
      - Allow for oversampling of cases, which is particularly useful with rare conditions
      - Example: Rather than following 1000 subjects to find 10 who develop a disease with an incidence of 1% over 10 years, one can find 100 cases and 100 healthy controls.
    - Disadvantages
      - Retrospective by nature
      - Regardless of matching, cases and controls are likely to differ in ways other than an exposure of interest, making conclusions difficult.
  - *Longitudinal studies* follow patients or test subjects over time.
    - Many, but not all, longitudinal studies are observational.
    - The simplest longitudinal studies follow a group of interest over time, an expanded version of a case series.
  - *Cohort studies* follow cohorts of subjects, typically at least one group with an exposure or condition of interest and a control group without that characteristic (Fig. 78.3).
    - Can be solely retrospective, identifying exposures in the past and assessing outcome in the present
      - Example: follow-up of a cohort with a known perinatal exposure and a control group without it
    - Can be prospective (identifying exposed and control cohorts now and following for outcomes)
    - Can also have *before–after* or *sequential* design (identifying cohorts before and after the addition or removal of an exposure)
      - Example: incidence of necrotizing enterocolitis before and after a change from formula to donor milk feedings
    - Advantages
      - All types of cohort studies are likely to yield more complete longitudinal data than case–control studies.
      - Prospective and before–after cohort studies are more likely to have complete information about exposure.
    - Disadvantages
      - It is difficult to study rare conditions.
      - Uncontrolled differences between cohorts beyond exposure of interest may cloud results.
    - Before–after studies may also be particularly affected by changes in other factors over time (known as *secular trends*).
- *Experimental* studies involve the investigator altering the conditions of study subjects—typically by administering a drug or an intervention (Fig. 78.4)
  - *Randomized controlled trials (RCTs)*, also referred to as *clinical trials*, are the classic experimental study.
    - Investigators assign participants *randomly* to an intervention or control (not receiving intervention) group and follow for outcomes of interest.
    - Control circumstance may be a *placebo* (inactive compound) or the best current therapy.

- These trials are often *blinded* (participants and/or investigators do not know which subjects are receiving which intervention), as well.
  - Advantages
    - Random assignment distributes unknown baseline differences evenly between groups.

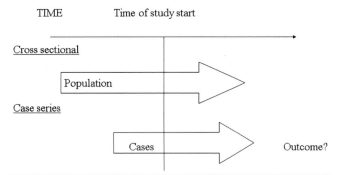

Fig. 78.1 Observational studies I. A case series reports accumulated cases of an illness. A cross-sectional study evaluates a condition in the population at one point in time (allowing estimates of *prevalence* (see text for discussion on prevalence and incidence).

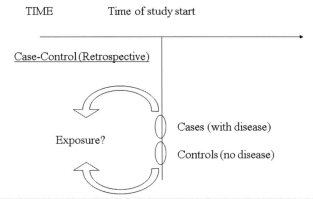

Fig. 78.2 Observational studies II: case–control study. A case–control study chooses cases (with disease) and controls (without disease) and looks retrospectively for exposures.

- They allow controlled investigation of a single factor on outcome with a concurrent control group.
  - Prospective nature allows investigators to collect research-quality data from outset of trial.
  - Disadvantages
    - Expensive
    - Lengthy
    - Investigators are manipulating conditions, potentially directly exposing participants to risks.
- In *crossover* studies, investigators assign subjects to a condition (e.g., intervention) and then cross them over to another condition (e.g., no intervention), observing the results of both conditions. They can also cross over two groups (Fig. 78.5).
  - Advantage: All participants experience both conditions.
  - Disadvantages
    - Sequence of conditions may *confound* (complicate interpretation of) results.
    - Secular trends over time may confound results.
- *Open-label* studies typically expose all subjects to an intervention.
  - Sometimes these studies are also referred to as a controlled, but nonblinded, trial.
  - Advantage: All subjects experience intervention.
  - Disadvantages
    - Lack of control group
    - When subjects know they are receiving an intervention, they may experience changes not truly due to the intervention (*placebo effect*).
- Experimental studies can also be described by the *phase* of investigation (Table 78.1)
- Additional analyses of planned trials
  - *Post hoc* analyses explore questions not initially planned for study.
    - Advantage: They allow investigators to adjust analyses based on findings.
    - Disadvantage: Findings may not be due to initial intervention.
  - *Subgroup* analyses explore outcomes in parts of the study groups.

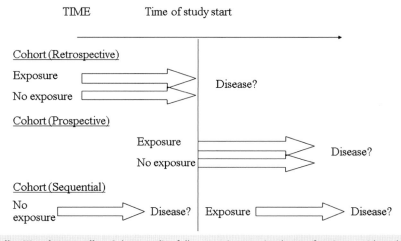

Fig. 78.3 Observational studies III: cohort studies. Cohort studies follow two (or more) cohorts of patients, with and without exposure, and assess the frequency of an outcome of interest. Cohort studies can be retrospective (cohorts chosen for known past exposure, which is relatively uncommon), prospective, or sequential (before–after).

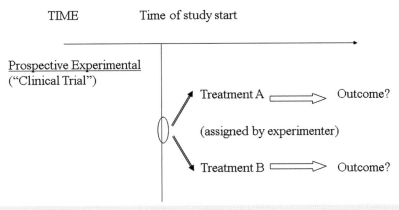

Fig. 78.4 Experimental study: randomized controlled trial. In an experimental trial, the investigator assigns participants to an intervention. Characteristics of randomized controlled trials can include random assignment to groups, control conditions (sometimes with a placebo), and double-blinding of investigators and participants as to who is exposed to the intervention condition (see Study Types section for description).

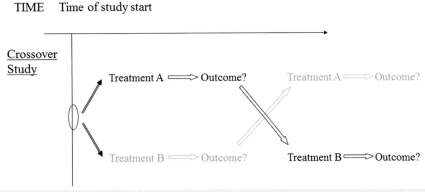

Fig. 78.5 Crossover study. Study participants are first exposed to one condition, followed by the other condition (e.g., control followed by intervention). Frequently, a second group (in gray) is exposed in the opposite order to control for the effect of sequence.

Table 78.1   Regulatory Terminology Describing Experimental (Particularly Drug) Studies

Phase I	Small safety trial, usually uncontrolled; does the drug do immediate harm?
Phase II	Larger, controlled safety and initial efficacy (effect in a research setting) trial
Phase III	Definitive, large, randomized controlled trial; studies drug efficacy
Phase IV	Postmarketing safety and effectiveness (effect in real world) surveillance

- Advantage: They allow investigators to explore effects in specific groups.
- Disadvantage: Lower numbers raise the risk of type II errors and multiple comparisons raise the risk of type I errors.
- Additional analyses are often best viewed as *hypothesis generating*, rather than *hypothesis testing*.

Sources of Error in Clinical Studies

- Random errors (e.g., type I or type II errors, random misclassification of subjects)
- *Bias* is a systematic, nonrandom error that leads to an erroneous conclusion about data.
  - Example: In a cohort study evaluating intensive monitoring to prevent preterm birth, women at risk for preterm birth are incidentally more likely to be included in an intensive monitoring arm, which leads to the incorrect conclusion that intensive monitoring increases preterm birth.
  - Bias can occur at any step in research process.
  - Bias can be minimized by strict enrollment criteria, randomization, matching, blinding, and clear outcome definitions.
- *Confounding* is the inappropriate attribution of effect to an independent variable, when, in fact, another variable, related both to the independent and dependent variables, is responsible.
  - Example: Paroxysmal atrial tachycardia among neonatologists is attributed to sleep deprivation, when, in fact, caffeine is the cause (Fig. 78.6).
  - Confounding can be minimized by
    - Distributing confounding variable equally between groups (e.g., randomization, *restriction* [choosing all subjects to have the confounding variable], or matching subjects on that variable, if it is suspected to be a confounder)
    - Using multivariate models (e.g., regressions) to identify effects of multiple independent variables
- *Effect modification* occurs when another variable modifies the effect of an independent variable.

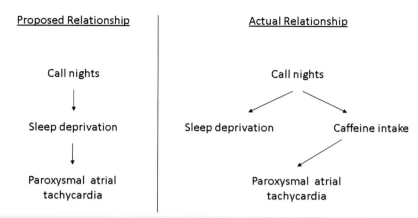

Fig. 78.6 Example of confounding. Although the initial hypothesis was that sleep deprivation during call nights caused paroxysmal atrial tachycardia, the actual causal pathway is through caffeine intake, which is related to sleep deprivation through call nights.

■ Example: Differing metabolism rates for a drug could modify drug toxicity in groups with differing enzyme alleles (slow metabolizers have more toxicity, regardless of dose, which is the independent variable being evaluated).

Causation Versus Association

■ One variable is *associated* with another variable if the two vary in tandem.
  ■ Association implies neither *causation* (A causes B) nor, if there is causation, the *direction* of causation (A causes B vs. B causes A).
■ *Causation* is best tested in experimental studies; if one adds an intervention and an outcome changes, causation is likely.
  ■ In observational studies, one can infer causation if certain things are true (e.g., temporal sequence, dose response, repetition in a different population, consistency with other studies, biologic plausibility), but it is more difficult to be certain (Box 78.1).

Incidence Versus Prevalence

■ *Incidence* is the rate of events over a certain period of time in a defined population.
  ■ Example: premature births per 1000 women per year
■ *Prevalence* is the number of cases in a population at a given time (i.e., a cross-sectional measure).
  ■ Example: former premature infants currently alive in the US population

Screening

■ In general, screening for a disease is most easily justified when the following are true (Box 78.2):
  ■ The combination of the test *accuracy* and disease prevalence will identify a suitable portion of people with the disease (*sensitivity*) with an acceptably low number of false positives (*positive predictive value*).
  ■ With low disease prevalence, even an excellent test will produce far more false positives than true positives.

Box 78.1   Factors Suggesting a Causative Relationship Between an Independent and a Dependent Variable

1. Shown in experimental studies
2. Temporal sequence
3. Dose response
4. Repetition in a different population
5. Consistency with other studies
6. Biologic plausibility

Box 78.2   World Health Organization Criteria for Optimal Usefulness of Screening

1. The condition should be an important health problem.
2. There should be a recognizable latent or early symptomatic stage.
3. The natural history of the condition, including development from latent to declared disease, should be adequately understood.
4. There should be an accepted treatment for patients with recognized disease.
5. There should be a suitable test or examination that has a high level of accuracy.
6. The test should be acceptable to the population.
7. There should be an agreed-upon policy on whom to treat as patients.
8. Facilities for diagnosis and treatment should be available.
9. The cost of screening (including diagnosis and treatment of patients diagnosed) should be economically balanced in relation to possible expenditure on medical care as a whole.
10. Screening should be a continuing process and not a "once and for all" project.

From Wilson JMG, Jungner G. *Principles and Practices of Screening for Disease.* Public Health Papers No. 34. Geneva, Switzerland: World Health Organization; 1968.

■ The burden caused by disease is high.
■ The burden of the testing is low.
■ There is a *presymptomatic* state during which the application of an intervention will prevent the onset of symptoms or ameliorate the disease process.
■ The screen can be performed for a reasonable *cost*.

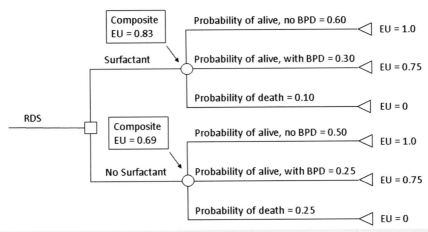

Fig. 78.7 Example of a decision tree for an imaginary population with respiratory distress syndrome (RDS). The tree attempts to quantify the values of outcomes when surfactant increases both survival and bronchopulmonary dysplasia (BPD). Based on the assumptions (which would be drawn from the literature and subjective judgments about value), the composite expected utility (EU) of surfactant use would be the sum of the probability of each outcome times the EU for each outcome, in this case $(0.60 \times 1.0) + (0.30 \times 0.75) + (0.10 \times 0) = 0.83$, whereas the composite EU of no surfactant would be $(0.50 \times 1.0) + (0.25 \times 0.75) + (0.25 \times 0) = 0.69$, implying that surfactant would be the preferred choice. See text for limitations of this analysis.

- These factors form a *risk–benefit* analysis for a proposed screen.
  - Example: As diagnostic accuracy of cystic fibrosis screening in the newborn improved with the addition of genetic techniques and evidence accumulated that screening improves nutritional outcomes, the risk–benefit balance improved (lower risk, more benefit).

Decision Analysis

- *Decision analysis* is a formalized method for evaluating the factors involved in clinical decision making.

  - Decision analysis attempts to identify the probability of each outcome, based on diagnostic or therapeutic decisions, and assign a value (*expected utility [EU]*) to that outcome.
    - Example: Assuming that life without disability would be the best outcome and death would be the worst, the EU (life without disability) would be 1.0 and the EU (death) would be 0 on a 0 to 1 scale.
  - By combining outcome probabilities and EUs, a best decision is suggested.
  - EU is most commonly depicted as *decision trees* with branch points for each decision (Fig. 78.7).
  - Advantage: EU quantifies and clarifies assumptions about probabilities and value of outcomes.
  - Disadvantages:
    - Decision trees tend to be complex, limiting clinical utility.
    - Even complex decision analysis uses only a limited number of variables, potentially omitting important factors.
  - If assumptions for analysis are inaccurate, analysis may yield misleading results.
  - Expected utilities are often subjective
    - Example: Is alive with disability = 0.75 or 0.5, and who decides?

Cost Analyses

- Cost analyses are a form of decision analysis, measuring outcomes in terms of monetary cost.
  - A *cost–benefit* analysis assigns a monetary value to each outcome and often seeks the outcome with the lowest cost-to-benefit ratio.
  - A *cost-effectiveness* analysis seeks to evaluate the cost to achieve an outcome.
- Outcomes that involve survival are often measured in years of life gained or in *quality-adjusted life years (QALYs)*, which assign a numerical estimate of quality of life (much like the EU, above)
- Costs can be estimated from multiple perspectives (e.g., patient, payors, society), and the conclusions may differ depending on perspective.

Sensitivity Analysis

- *Sensitivity analysis* measures the effect of alterations in assumptions on the outcome of an analysis; what if the data were different than the observed or projected values?
  - Example: in Fig. 78.7, a higher assigned EU of bronchopulmonary dysplasia (BPD) would increase the composite EU of surfactant use, whereas a smaller improvement in death would decrease the composite EU of surfactant use. Try varying the values to understand this.
- Like the initial data analysis itself, sensitivity analysis is limited by the validity of the assumptions (which may be entirely theoretical).

Qualities of Measurement

- Types of validity in measurement (i.e., does the test work?)
  - *Face* validity is a subjective impression of whether a tool is likely to measure what it is intended to measure.

- *Content* validity is the ability of a tool to measure all aspects of what it purports to measure.
- *Criterion* validity is the ability of a tool to predict other characteristics associated with the measured characteristic, either at the same time (concurrent validity) or in the future (predictive validity).
- *Construct* validity implies a high correlation with other measures of the same characteristic.
- *Internal* validity is the confidence that any proposed causal relationship is valid (a measure of experimental quality).
- *External* validity is the ability of the outcome of a study to be generalized to other similar populations.
- *Reliability* refers to the reproducibility of the data (i.e., can the test be applied?).
  - *Interobserver* or *interrater* reliability is the degree of agreement between observers measuring the same thing.
    - Interrater reliability is typically measured using the *kappa* (κ) statistic, which varies from 0 to 1; a high κ means high agreement between observers.
  - *Internal consistency* is the degree of relationship among items on a test that purport to measure the same thing (e.g., among three items measuring depression).
    - Internal consistency is typically measured by *Cronbach alpha* (α), which can vary from 0 to 1; a high α means high internal consistency.
  - *Test–retest* reliability is the ability of a tool to get the same result on a repeat measurement.
- *Accuracy* is the ability of a tool to measure the true value of a quantity.
- *Precision* is the ability of a tool to produce consistent results.
  - Accuracy and precision are separate characteristics (Fig. 78.8).

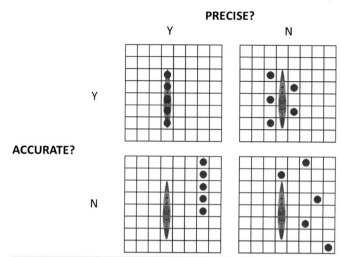

Fig. 78.8 Accuracy and precision. Accuracy is the ability of a measure (on average) to correctly reflect a true value. Precision is the reproducibility of the measure.

Suggested Readings

Dawson B, Trapp RG, eds. *Basic & Clinical Biostatistics*. 4th ed. New York: McGraw-Hill; 2004.

Moyer VA, Calonge N, Teutsch SM, Botkin JR. Expanding newborn screening: process, policy, and priorities. *Hastings Cent Rep*. 2008;38(3):32–39.

Paneth N. *Bias and Confounding, Part I*. Available at: http://www.umin.ac.jp/supercourse/lecture/lec18951/index.htm. Accessed November 23, 2022.

Paneth N. *Bias and Confounding, Part II*. Available at: http://www.umin.ac.jp/supercourse/lecture/lec18961/index.htm. Accessed November 23, 2022.

Pourhoseingholi MA, Baghestani AR, Vahedi M. How to control confounding effects by statistical analysis. *Gastroenterol Hepatol Bed Bench*. 2012;5(2):79–83.

79 Applying Research to Clinical Practice

CARL T. D'ANGIO

Assessment of Study Design, Performance, and Analysis

- Assessing the details of design, performance, and analysis allows a clinician to determine the *internal validity* of a study (see Chapter 78).
- Selecting control groups
  - Control groups for case–control studies (Fig. 79.1)
    - Think of cases and controls as belonging to the same cohort (i.e., similar in all ways other than the presence of the disease or condition of interest).
      - Criteria for choosing controls:
        - Representative of population from which cases are drawn
        - Should be sampled independent of exposure of interest (i.e., should not have any known factor that would make exposure more or less likely)
          - Example: In a study of risks for intraventricular hemorrhage, choosing a control group from another neonatal intensive care unit (NICU) with a differing rate of indomethacin prophylaxis would bias the exposure.
        - The same exposure information as used for cases should be available.
      - Methods to choose appropriate controls:
        - Drawing from the same database or population as cases
        - Matching on important, potentially biasing or confounding factors, without "overmatching" in a way that inadvertently equalizes exposures
          - Example: Matching on early respiratory support would equalize that exposure in a case–control study of bronchopulmonary dysplasia (BPD)
  - Control groups for cohort studies (Fig. 79.2)
    - Like controls in a case-control study, unexposed controls (also known as the *comparison group*) in a cohort study should be as similar to the exposed cohort as possible
      - Specifically, as similar as possible on possible confounding factors
      - Similar data about exposure and outcome should be available.
    - Sources of comparison groups
      - An *internal* comparison group is drawn from the same population, but differs in exposure.
        - Example: In a study of necrotizing enterocolitis (NEC), a group of premature infants from the same NICU differed only in exposure to human donor milk.

      - An *external* comparison group is drawn from another group that is similar, other than the exposure.
        - Example: In a study of NEC, a group of premature infants from another, similar NICU, differed only in the second NICU's use of human donor milk.
      - The general population
- Surrogate endpoints (Fig. 79.3)
  - A *surrogate endpoint* is a study outcome that stands in for another, more definitive endpoint.
    - Example: change in systolic blood pressure as a surrogate for lowering risk of stroke

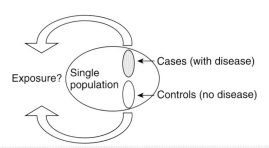

Fig. 79.1 Choosing controls in case–control studies. Controls drawn from the same population, differing only on presence of disease or condition of interest, are least likely to have other, confounding exposures. Matching also helps choose controls who are similar.

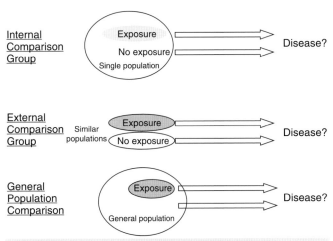

Fig. 79.2 Choosing controls for cohort studies. The control or "comparison" cohort should be as similar as possible to the exposed cohort and have the same information available. Internal (same population, differing only on exposure), external (similar population, differing only on exposure), and general population comparison groups are illustrated.

441

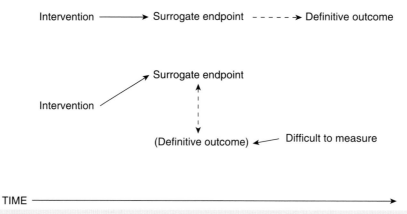

Fig. 79.3 Types of surrogate endpoints. An intermediate surrogate endpoint ("intermediate outcome") occurs before the definitive outcome and reliably (but nearly never perfectly) predicts the outcome (*top*). Surrogate endpoints can also be outcomes that are highly correlated to a definitive outcome, measured at the same time, when the definitive outcome is difficult to measure (*bottom*).

- *Biomarkers* (physical or other biological outcomes that are correlated with clinical outcomes) are a form of surrogate endpoints.
- Why use surrogate endpoints?
  - A definitive clinical endpoint may only occur a long time after the intervention, making the waiting period for a definitive outcome prohibitive.
  - The definitive clinical outcome may be prohibitively expensive.
  - The definitive outcome may not be possible to measure.
    - Example: In clinical studies aimed at improving intrapulmonary inflammation, it may not be safe to sample lung tissue.
- What are the characteristics of a good surrogate endpoint?
  - The relationship of the surrogate should be stronger than mere correlation.
    - A change in a good surrogate endpoint should predict a change in clinical outcome.
    - Surrogates shown in clinical trials to predict clinical outcomes are referred to as *validated surrogate outcomes* (Table 79.1).
  - Surrogate endpoints are ideally more timely, less expensive, and/or less risky than the definitive endpoint.
- Disadvantages:
  - The relationship between surrogates and definitive outcomes is seldom guaranteed.
  - Even some clinical endpoints usually considered definitive are actually surrogates for later outcomes, and may themselves be imperfect.
    - Examples: BPD does not always predict longer term pulmonary outcome; 5-year cancer survival does not always predict cure.
- *Intention-to-treat* analysis
  - In a randomized, controlled trial, some participants will not begin or complete treatment.
  - The temptation is to include those participants in the control group (if never treated) or exclude them.
    - However, participants who do not receive the full course of treatment are likely to differ systematically from fully treated participants (i.e., be biased) and will skew results if moved or eliminated.

Table 79.1   Examples of Surrogate Endpoints Allowed by the US Food and Drug Administration as Surrogate Markers of Efficacy in Drug Trials

Surrogate Endpoint	Correlated Clinical Outcome
Human immunodeficiency virus (HIV) viral load	Development of an acquired immunodeficiency syndrome (AIDS) diagnosis
Forced expiratory volume in 1 second (FEV_1)	Asthma
Estimated glomerular filtration rate or serum creatinine	Chronic kidney disease
Opsonophagocytosis assay titers	Invasive pneumococcal disease

Modified from https://www.fda.gov/drugs/development-resources/table-surrogate-endpoints-were-basis-drug-approval-or-licensure. Accessed November 23, 2022.

- Solution: Keep all participants in the treatment group in that group for analysis = intention-to-treat analysis.
  - Less likely to result in skewed results than any amount of attempting to control for incomplete treatment
- Sample size
  - The larger the sample size, the less likely a study is to have a type II error (i.e., the less likely it is to miss a true difference between conditions).
    - The likelihood of a type II error is known as the β *(beta) error*.
    - Resistance to type II error is the study *power*.
      - Study power is $1 - \beta$.
        - Example: In a typical study, where a β error of 0.20 would be tolerated, the power would be $1 - 0.20 = 0.80 = 80\%$.
      - Larger sample size = better power.
  - Power to detect adverse events also varies with sample size.
    - Because some adverse events may be rare, even a well-powered randomized controlled trial may miss them (i.e., type II error in detecting adverse events).
      - Extremely large, postmarketing, *phase IV* observational studies may be necessary to detect rare adverse events (see Chapter 78).

Table 79.2 Calculated Sample Size Given Differing Values for Difference, Standard Deviation, Type I Error, and Power

Difference					
Value Group 1	Value Group 2	Standard Deviation	Type I Error (α)	Power (1 – β)	Sample Size (Per Group)
20	30	15	0.05	0.80	36
20	*25*	15	0.05	0.80	142[a]
20	30	*30*	0.05	0.80	142[a]
20	30	15	*0.01*	0.80	53
20	30	15	0.05	*0.90*	48

The quantity varying in each row is shown in *italics*.
[a]Note that the effect size is the same for these two calculations (effect size = difference/standard deviation = 0.33).

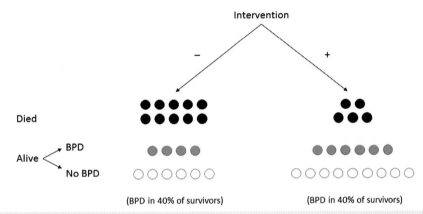

Fig. 79.4 Survival bias caused by competing outcomes. An imaginary intervention applied to extremely premature infants does not affect bronchopulmonary dysplasia (BPD) among survivors but results in a marked drop in early death (which precludes development of BPD), from 50% to 25%. Although the absolute incidence of BPD is higher in the intervention group (30% vs. 20%), the incidence of the composite outcome of death or BPD is lower (55% vs. 70%).

- Calculating sample size for a study
  - Four parameters drive sample size.
    - What difference would be *clinically meaningful?*
      - Choosing a small, meaningless difference (e.g., a 1% difference in respiratory distress syndrome [RDS] rates) inflates the sample size needlessly.
      - Choosing too large of a difference (e.g., a 50% difference in RDS rates) raises the likelihood of type II error and missing a clinically meaningful difference.
    - What is the spread of the data (variability in measurement)?
      - The wider the spread (e.g., standard deviation), the larger the sample size needed to detect the same difference.
      - The relationship of difference between the group means to the standard deviation is known as *effect size.*
        - Effect size = Difference/standard deviation.
          - If difference = standard deviation, effect size is 1.
          - If difference = one-half standard deviation, effect size is 0.5.
        - Smaller effect size requires a larger sample size.
    - What level of type I error is acceptable?
      - Type I or α error is typically set at 0.05.

- What level of type II error is acceptable?
  - Type II or β error typically is set at 0.10 to 0.20.
    - This gives a power of 80% to 90%.
- Sample size calculators use these parameters to calculate necessary sample size (Table 79.2).

Assessment of Generalizability

- Assessing the details of generalizability allows a clinician to determine the *external validity* of the study (see Chapter 78).
- Even a well-performed study, with excellent internal validity, may not reflect what is happening in the general population.
- Bias in enrollment or in who completes the study can imperil generalizability.
  - *Selection* or *enrollment bias* involves choosing enrollees or cases that do not actually reflect the general population.
  - *Survival bias* in who completes the study may result in outcomes that do not reflect the overall result of a therapy or condition.
    - *Competing outcomes* can cause survival bias; for example, early death would prevent evaluation of BPD at a later time (Fig. 79.4).
      - This is often handled with the *composite* outcome of "death or condition X."

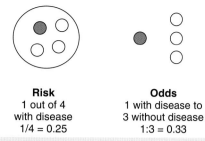

Risk
1 out of 4
with disease
1/4 = 0.25

Odds
1 with disease to
3 without disease
1:3 = 0.33

Fig. 79.5 Risk versus odds. Risk is the likelihood that a member of the population will have a condition = $(n_{condition})/(N_{population})$. Odds are the likelihood that a population member will have a condition versus the likelihood that he/she will not = $(n_{condition}):(N_{no\ condition})$. In both examples, one out of every four members of the population will have the condition.

- ▣ *Ascertainment* or *information bias*, with less information available about one group, may prevent accurate assessment of outcomes.
- ■ Clinical trials have a tension between being *standardized* enough for the population, intervention, and outcome to be interpretable but *practical* enough to represent the "real world" of clinical medicine, where these categories are not homogeneous.
  - ▣ Overstandardization can limit generalizability.
  - ▣ Practicality can limit interpretation.
- ■ The data source used to collect results can also influence external validity.
  - ▣ Example: Billing data (aimed at revenue) and a government database may yield differing estimates of disease prevalence.
  - ▣ Subjective measures such as diaries may be susceptible to the Hawthorne effect: the tendency of a group that knows it is being observed to act differently than if unobserved.

Application of Information for Patient Care

- ■ *Likelihood ratios*
  - ▣ Likelihood ratios are an application of Bayesian statistics, based on Bayes' theorem.
    - ▣ Rather than asking the question "What is the evidence that this difference is not due to chance?" of traditional *frequentist* statistics, Bayesian statistics ask how new information changes one's prior impression of the probability of an event.
  - ▣ To review, the likelihood ratio measures the change in the odds from pretest to posttest (see Chapter 77).
  - ▣ Clinicians usually think in terms of risk, not odds (Fig. 79.5).
    - ▣ Example: If the risk of a disease is 1/4 (0.25), then the odds of having the disease are 1 yes to 3 no, or 1:3 (0.33).
    - ▣ To convert:
      - ☐ Odds = $(numerator_{risk})/(denominator_{risk} - numerator_{risk})$.
        - ▣ If risk = 1/4, then odds = 1:(4−1) = 1:3 = 0.33.
      - ☐ Risk = $(numerator_{odds})/(denominator_{odds} + numerator_{odds})$.
        - ▣ If odds = 1:3, then risk = 1/(3 + 1) = 1/4 = 0.25.

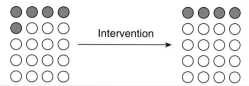

Fig. 79.6 Number needed to treat. In this example, if the intervention changes the likelihood of an outcome from 25% (5 out of 20) to 20% (4 out of 20), then 20 people must be treated to experience a different outcome.

- ▣ Likelihood ratios use odds because they are not bound by 1, whereas risk must be.
  - ▣ Odds of 99:1 are still a risk of 0.99 (99%); risk is never >1 (100%).
  - ▣ Conversely, if risk is low, say 1 in 100 (0.01), then the odds are similar (1:99 or 0.0101); neither ever falls below zero.
- ▣ Example of applying likelihood ratio:
  - ▣ If the pretest probability of a diagnosis is 20% (0.20) and the likelihood ratio of a positive test (LR[+]) is 8, then the posttest probability is
    - ☐ Pretest risk 0.20 → pretest odds 1:(5−1) = 1:4 = 0.25
    - ☐ Times LR(+) of 8 = 0.25 × 8 = posttest odds 2:1 →
    - ☐ Posttest risk 2/(1 + 2) = 2/3 = 0.67
    - ☐ Note: Posttest risk is not 0.20 × 8 = 1.6; that would be an impossibility.
  - ▣ Or, you can use a likelihood ratio nomogram that converts probabilities to odds and back again automatically, or use an online likelihood ratio calculator.
- ■ Risk reduction
  - ▣ To review, absolute risk reduction is the change in the raw numbers.
    - ▣ A drop from 3/1000 to 2/1000 is an absolute risk reduction of 1/1000.
  - ▣ Relative risk reduction is the percent change.
    - ▣ A drop from 3/1000 to 2/1000 is a relative risk reduction of 33%.
- ■ *Number needed to treat (NNT)*
  - ▣ NNT calculates the number of patients who would need to be treated with a therapy for one patient to experience a positive effect.
    - ▣ NNT = 1/(absolute risk reduction)
  - ▣ Example: If a therapy reduces death from 25% to 20%, an absolute risk reduction of 5% or 0.05, then NNT = 1/0.05 = 20 (Fig. 79.6).
  - ▣ If a therapy has risks, one can also calculate the "number needed to harm" using the same math.
- ■ Statistical significance versus *clinical importance*
  - ▣ If large numbers of subjects are treated, very small absolute risk reductions can be statistically significant but may not be of any clinical relevance (or importance).
    - ▣ For example, with about 1100 subjects per group, a study could expect to detect a drop in preeclampsia from 95% to 92% with a particular treatment, which is not likely to be very useful clinically.

Using the Medical Literature

- ■ Constructing a literature search
  - ▣ Specific, targeted questions will yield more specific and useful results.

- One approach is to construct a search question the way one constructs a research hypothesis, with the "PICOT" format:
  - **P**opulation (in this case, patients): In which patient group is the question being asked?
  - **I**ntervention: What is the therapy?
  - **C**omparator: Compared to what? (Another therapy? No treatment?)
  - **O**utcome: What is the outcome of interest?
  - **T**ime: Over what time?
    - Example: Among <u>infants born at 23 to 24 weeks' gestation</u>, does the use of <u>caffeine</u> in the first 14 days, compared to <u>no caffeine</u> therapy change the incidence of <u>death before discharge</u>?
- For a nontherapeutic question, a modified format using **P**atients, **P**rognostic factors, and **O**utcomes ("PPO") can be useful.
- A refined question also simplifies the sorting of articles that return from a search.
- Different literature databases cover different portions of the literature.
  - Most offer the ability to refine a search, but ease of use varies.
- Choosing a study type to answer specific sorts of questions
  - Accuracy of diagnostic tests
    - A cross-sectional study comparing a test to a gold standard

- Benefits or harms of an intervention
  - Randomized controlled trial is the preferred approach.
  - Observational cohort studies are another possibility but are more subject to bias.
  - For rare outcomes, a phase IV, postmarketing, extremely large registry study may be the best source of information.
- Prognosis of a condition
  - Longitudinal, long-term, observational study, either single group or traditional (with affected and comparison groups) cohort study
  - Administrative databases (insurance, state, or other large databases) may also provide long-term outcome data.

Suggested Readings

Boston University School of Public Health. *Case-Control Studies*. Available at: http://sphweb.bumc.bu.edu/otlt/mph-modules/ep/ep713_case-control/EP713_Case-Control-TOC.html. Accessed November 23, 2022.

Boston University School of Public Health. *Cohort Studies*. Available at: http://sphweb.bumc.bu.edu/otlt/MPH-Modules/EP/EP713_Cohort-Studies/EP713_CohortStudies_print.html. Accessed November 23, 2022.

Dawson B, Trapp RG, eds. *Basic & Clinical Biostatistics*. 4th ed. New York: McGraw-Hill; 2004.

Ecker ED, Skelly AC. Conducting a winning literature search. *Evid Based Spine Care J*. 2010;1(1):9–14.

Kukull WA, Ganguli M. Generalizability: the trees, the forest, and the low-hanging fruit. *Neurology*. 2012;78(23):1886–1891.

80 *Quality Improvement*

COLBY L. DAY

Concepts in Quality Improvement Science

OVERVIEW OF APPROACHES

Although there are several approaches to quality improvement (QI) science, it is important to understand the basics of the most common approaches in health care quality improvement science work.

- The Institute for Healthcare Improvement's Model for Improvement
  - The most common QI method used in health care
  - Following creation of a QI team, the following questions help guide the project:
    - What are we trying to accomplish?
    - How will we know that a change is an improvement?
    - What changes can we make that will result in improvement?
  - Based on these questions, the team develops a Specific, Measurable, Attainable, Relevant, Time-bound *(SMART) Aim, key driver diagram (KDD)*, measures, and a *plan–do–study–act (PDSA) cycle* strategy.
  - The team utilizes a *rapid cycle improvement model*.
    - Defined by the Agency for Healthcare Research and Quality (AHRQ) as a "practical and real-time approach that involves testing interventions on a small scale, permitting experimentation, and discarding unsuccessful tests. Numerous small cycles of change can successfully accumulate into large effects."
  - When interventions are deemed successful, there is also a focus on maintenance of improvement (aka sustainability).
- Lean
  - Toyota production system
    - Goal is to reduce waste and to improve value.
    - Focus is on streamlining processes and maximizing profit or value.
  - In business, the value is defined by the customer's wants.
  - In health care, the value is defined by the patient's wants.
  - The lean method is used primarily in business and manufacturing areas, but hospitals sometimes adopt this methodology in their quality improvement strategies.
  - The method uses *value stream mapping*, which involves visual process maps.
  - In a 5S organization, every work environment or process is reviewed using this systematic approach with the goal of reducing time waste:
    - Sort, Simplify, Standardize, Sweep/Shine, initiate Self-controls to maintain standardization.
- Six Sigma
  - Goal is to eliminate defects and waste in order to improve quality and efficiency.
  - The AHRQ defines a Six Sigma process as a "process where 99.99966% of production opportunities are expected to be free of defects."
  - It is the least utilized methodology in health care among the three methodologies mentioned, but it can add value in increasing reliability of processes.
  - It relies on heavy use of statistical tools.
  - It utilizes the *DMAIC methodology:* Define, Measure, Analyze, Improve, Control.

Summary of Approaches

Although the unique aspects of each of these approaches are detailed above, there are some similarities among the three:

- They utilize a systematic and structured methodology.
- The importance of a team with clear leadership is emphasized.
- They delineate the aims and goals for the quality improvement work, which are set at the initiation of the project.
- They utilize strategic planning of iterative changes or interventions.
- They rely on clear measures and robust analysis to determine whether improvement occurs.
- They emphasize the importance of communication within the team and with stakeholders.

Optimizing Healthcare Through Paired Goals

- *Crossing the Quality Chasm*, a publication by the Institute of Medicine (IOM), proposes that there are six dimensions that must be incorporated into quality improvement work in healthcare:
  - Safe
  - Effective
  - Patient-centered
  - Timely
  - Efficient
  - Equitable
- The 2008 article "Triple Aim: Care, Health, and Cost" suggests that, in order to improve the health care system, we must:

- Improve population health.
- Improve the experience of care.
- Reduce per capita cost.
- The 2014 article "From Triple to Quadruple Aim: Care of the Patient Requires Care of the Provider" incorporates the three components of the Triple Aim above to improve the health care system but adds recognition of physician and health care workforce burnout as an area for improvement focus.
- The 2022 article "The Quintuple Aim for Health Care Improvement: A New Imperative to Advance Health Equity" incorporates the four components of the Quadruple Aim above to improve the health care system but adds advancing health equity as an area for improvement.

Project Design

- The first step of a successful QI project is *identification of a team*. This team should:
  - Be multidisciplinary. All staff members and disciplines involved in the process being improved should have a role in the quality improvement team.
  - Have a clear leader responsible for organization, delegation of tasks, and accountability.
  - Include families. Most often these are families who no longer have an infant in the neonatal intensive care unit (NICU); many institutions have guidelines for which families may be appropriate to approach. Even in projects that may not have a clear family focus, such teams should involve family representatives, as they often have insight into processes that is unexpected.
  - Be diverse. Every effort should be made to be inclusive.
- The second step is creation of an *aim statement*. An aim statement has multiple purposes:
  - Provide direction.
  - Define the scope of project and keep project on task, avoiding waste.

Table 80.1   Goals for Developing a SMART Aim

S	Specific
M	Measurable
A	Attainable
R	Relevant
T	Time-bound

- Align multiple stakeholders and ensure buy-in from key participants.
- Aid in identifying appropriate measures.
- Serve as an elevator pitch for further support/resources.
- Specifically, you should create a *SMART* aim statement
  - You can utilize the six overarching goals of the IOM for health care improvement when developing your SMART aim statement (safe, effective, patient-centered, timely, efficient, equitable). See Table 80.1.
  - You can also consider the quintuple focuses when developing your SMART aim statement (improving population health, improving experience of care, reducing cost, improving workforce burnout, improving health equity).
- What does a "good" SMART aim statement look like? (See Table 80.2.)
  - It utilizes an iterative approach to defining goals, in addition to providing details.
- The next step is key for robust QI science: the *pre-implementation phase*. The following is not an exhaustive list but does include some of the most commonly used tools when planning QI work:
  - *Process mapping* is useful when a quality improvement problem involves workflow and processes involving multiple departments, staff, and locations.
  - *Fishbone diagram/Ishikawa diagram* is a cause-and-effect diagram that is useful to structure brainstorming, especially when determining primary drivers.
  - *Pareto chart* is useful when you need to delineate the most important factors among many.
  - *Bar charts* show individual values and a cumulative total line; they help identify the vital few factors on which the team should be focusing their efforts.
  - *Swimlane diagram* is a flowchart that specifically delineates who does what in a process.
- After you have created your team, defined your aim statement, and completed your pre-implementation work by describing the process or problem you hope to improve, it is time to create a *key driver diagram (KDD)*.
  - Purpose of a KDD is to graphically present the context of the problem, identifying potential key drivers that contribute to the desired project aim.
  - Key aspects of a KDD: It should be simple and visual, align change ideas to a bigger goal (the aim statement), keep the team on track, and provide a one-page synopsis of the project.

Table 80.2   Iterative Process to Develop SMART Aim

	Aim Statement Attempts	Lacking ...
First draft	We will decrease the number of unplanned extubations (UEs) in our neonatal intensive care unit (NICU).	Specific population, magnitude of change, time frame, details of "how," maintenance
Second draft	We will decrease the number of UEs in our very low birth weight (VLBW) infants.	Magnitude of change, time frame, details of "how," maintenance
Third draft	We will decrease the number of UEs by 20% in our VLBW infants by June 2022.	Details of "how," maintenance
Final draft	By multidisciplinary team strategies and a focus on respiratory practices, we will decrease the number of UEs by 20% in our VLBW infants by June 2022 and maintain this decrease through December 2022.	—

Note that this chapter uses the same sample project of UEs throughout examples when able.

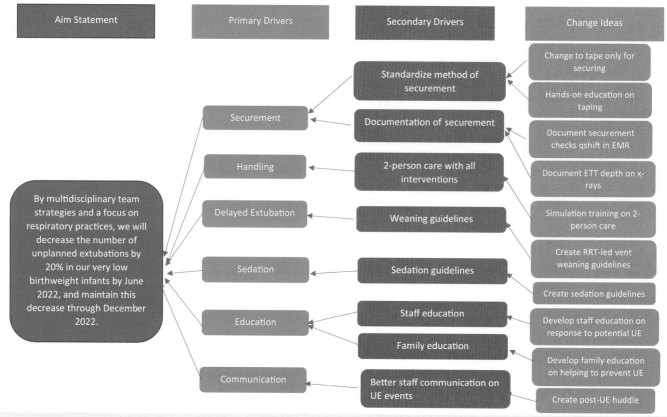

Fig. 80.1 Key driver diagram.

- Anatomy of a KDD (see Fig. 80.1):
  - Start with an aim statement (left in the figure).
  - In the figure, the next column shows *primary drivers*, which are overarching themes that are thought to be causative of the problem requiring improvement (or that will contribute to the desired aim). These can be broad categorizations.
    - Some KDDs further delineate *secondary drivers*, which impact the primary drivers.
  - The next column in the figure shows *change ideas*, which help drive small iterative interventions or PDSA cycles.
  - Some KDD include a column for process measures.
  - All arrows point left to demonstrate the ultimate goal is achieving the aim statement.
- Tips for KDD:
  - The KDD can change over time as your project progresses.
  - There may not always be secondary drivers.
  - Drivers can be co-dependent (i.e., more than one secondary driver can link to a primary driver).
  - If it is becoming too complicated, you may need multiple KDDs.
- In order to ascertain whether improvement is being achieved, you need to define measures to track over time.
- QI science requires that you analyze data over time, as opposed to pre- and post-intervention data, which is common practice in clinical research.
- Qualities of good measures are that they should be clinically important, evidence based, and well defined; it should be simple to obtain data, and timely data are available.

- *Outcome measures* represent what we want to achieve and may be clinical endpoints; every aim statement should describe an outcome measure.
  - Most important to patients and families, health care teams, administrators
  - May be slower to change
  - Examples: number of unplanned extubations per 100 ventilator days, percent of very low birth weight (VLBW) infants with necrotizing enterocolitis, neurodevelopmental outcome at 2 years of age, patient satisfaction, readmissions after NICU discharge
- *Process measures* represent how to obtain to the desired outcome; they are action metrics.
  - Process measures are often quicker to achieve so they can be tracked over time while waiting for outcome measure data.
  - Examples: If working on the ultimate outcome of reducing unplanned extubations (UEs), you may track process measures such as (1) percentage of endotracheal tubes (ETTs) properly taped, (2) percentage of rapid response teams (RRTs) receiving education on taping, (3) percentage of VLBW intubated patients with proper ETT securement documentation, (4) percentage of hands-on care for VLBW intubated infants utilizing two-person care, and (5) adherence to ventilator weaning guidelines, among others.
- *Balancing measures* represent the unintended effects of improving your process, the things that could go wrong.
  - Not every project will have balancing measures, but every project should be evaluated for balancing measures, and the majority should have them.

Examples: If you are working on reducing UEs, balancing measures could be (1) decreased kangaroo care in intubated patients, (2) increased reintubations (weaning too quickly), and (3) increase in other hospital-acquired conditions as you focus on UEs, among others.

Project Implementation

- When the team has been assembled, the aim defined, the KDD created, and measures discussed, it is time to plan the intervention, which includes small tests of change or PDSA cycles.
- Process measures may be developed further as you plan your PDSA cycles.
- PDSA cycles should:
  - Include small changes with a process that can be measured and tracked over time.
  - Implement only one change (or limited changes) at a time to determine what change leads to the desired outcome.
  - Be evaluated for their success in achieving the desired improvements, for costs, for workflow and social impacts, and for balancing measures and side effects.
- *Plan:* What questions are being answered? What is the predicted outcome of the test of change? (*Tip*: Keep it small.)
- *Do:* Carry out the test of change.
- *Study:* What worked? What didn't work? Was there anything unexpected or were any barriers encountered? Did the results match your prediction?
- *Act:* What changes should be made to the intervention? Can the change be scaled-up?
- Decide whether to abandon, adapt, or adopt the change.

Data Analysis

- When analyzing QI science data, we are looking for noise versus signal.
- *Noise* is statistically indistinguishable from other data and contains no new information. It is also known as *common cause variation.*
- *Signal* represents variation that is not part of the usual process and contains new information. It is also known as *special cause variation.*
- The most basic, minimum standard for analyzing data in quality improvement science is a *run chart*, which is a graphical display of data over time.
  - The purpose of a visual display of data is to make performance visible to staff and team members, to determine whether the changes resulted in improvement, and, if so, if they were sustained.
  - You *must* understand context when interpreting a run chart. In order to say a run chart shows improvement, you need to understand what may have caused the improvement.
  - Begin plotting your data in a run chart as soon as you have data, but you will need at least 10 data points to establish a baseline and apply rules for detecting special cause variation.
- Anatomy of a run chart (see Fig. 80.2):
  - The x-axis represents time order for data (often weeks, months, consecutive patients, etc.), and the y-axis is reflective of your measure.
  - In the line graph of data points:
    - The center line is the median, which was determined from the baseline data.
    - Annotations of when tests of change occurred are noted.
    - The goal line indicates the goal.

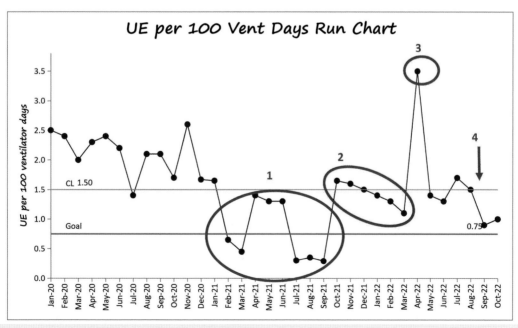

Fig. 80.2 Run chart of unplanned extubations per 100 ventilator days. (1) Shift; (2) trend; (3) astronomical point; (4) data crosses center line eight times, which means there are nine runs, too few for the number of total data points.

- After a baseline of at least 10 data points is achieved, you can apply rules to determine if special cause variation has occurred (see Fig. 80.2).
  - Rule 1. *Shift*: Six or more consecutive data points are either all above or all below the median; skip values that fall on the center line and continue counting.
  - Rule 2. *Trend*: Five points are all going up or all going down; if two or more consecutive points are the same value, only count one.
  - Rule 3. *Astronomical point*: Detects unusually large or small numbers in data/outliers.
    - This is the most subjective of the rules; it does not mean the highest or lowest data point.
  - Rule 4. *Number of runs*: A run is a series of points in a row on one side of the center line; to determine the number of runs, count the number of times the data line crosses the median/center line and add one.
    - You can have too few runs or too many runs; there are published tables to reference for the lower and upper limit of runs based on number of data points on the chart.
- *Control charts* (statistical process control [SPC] charts or Shewhart charts) are statistical tools used to distinguish between common cause variation and special cause variation.
  - Control charts differ from run charts in that:
    - The center line is often the mean, not the median.
    - Upper and lower control limits exist to reflect the extent of common cause variation; they represent three-sigma standard deviation.
    - Control charts are more sensitive and powerful to detect change.
  - In order to create the correct control chart, you must know what type of data you have
    - *Continuous/variable data* are quantitative numerical data.
      - X and MR chart: X plots individual value and MR plots the moving range of individual values.
      - X-bar and S chart: X-bar plots the sample average and S plots the standard deviation of sample.
    - Discrete/attribute data
      - *Classification*: presence or not of an attribute
      - *P chart*: percent observations with given attribute
      - *Count*: how many attributes occur in a sample
      - *U (unit) chart*: plot of the number of instances per opportunities to observe; for unequal or variable area of opportunity
      - *C (count) chart*: plot of raw numbers of instances; for equal or fixed area of opportunity

- Similar to run charts, control charts use rules to determine special cause variation; there are different combinations of rules used so, when using software to determine special cause variation, know which rule convention is being used. The following five rules are the designation suggested by Provost and Murray in 2011:
  - Rule 1 (variation of astronomical point but without the subjectivity): one point more than 3 standard deviations from the center line (outside upper or lower control limit)
  - Rule 2 (variation of astronomical point but without the subjectivity): two out of three points more than 2 standard deviations from center line
  - Rule 3 (variation of shift): eight points in a row on one side of center line
  - Rule 4 (variation of trend): six points in a row increasing or decreasing
  - Rule 5: 15 points in a row within 1 standard deviation of the center line

Publication

- As with all scholarly work, QI science projects should aim for publication in peer-reviewed journals.
- The *SQUIRE* guidelines (see Suggested Readings) exist to aid in putting together QI work for publication. These guidelines should be referenced from the start of a project onward to ensure that the project contains all of the necessary elements for eventual publication.

Suggested Readings

Agency for Healthcare Research and Quality (AHRQ). *The CAHPS Ambulatory Care Improvement Guide: Practical Strategies for Improving Patient Experience.* Available at: https://www.ahrq.gov/cahps/quality-improvement/improvement-guide/4-approach-qi-process/sect4part2.html. Accessed September 21, 2023.

Bodenheimer T, Sinsky C. From triple to quadruple aim: care of the patient requires care of the provider. *Ann Fam Med.* 2014;12(6):573–576.

Institute for Healthcare Improvement. *How to Improve.* Available at: https://www.ihi.org/resources/Pages/HowtoImprove/default.aspx. Accessed September 21, 2023.

Nundy S, Cooper LA, Mate KS. The quintuple aim for health care improvement: a new imperative to advance health equity. *JAMA.* 2022;327(6):521–522.

Perla RJ, Provost LP, Murray SK. The run chart: a simple analytical tool for learning from variation in healthcare processes. *BMJ Qual Saf.* 2011;20:46–51.

Provost L, Murray S. *The Health Care Data Guide: Learning from Data for Improvement.* 1st ed. Hoboken, NJ: Jossey-Bass; 2011.

SQUIRE. *Revised Standards for Quality Improvement Reporting Excellence: SQUIRE 2.0.* Available at: http://www.squire-statement.org/index.cfm?fuseaction=page.viewpage&pageid=471. Accessed September 21, 2023.

81 *Principles of Teaching and Learning*

RITA DADIZ and EMER FINAN

Educational Theory

Knowles' theory of "andragogy" (the science of adult learning) is based on certain assumptions regarding adult learners (Table 81.1). These characteristics have implications for the learning environment and the teaching methods that `educators incorporate.

SELF-DETERMINATION THEORY

- *Intrinsic motivation*: an internal drive to pursue learning
- *Extrinsic motivators*: external influences that impact the pursuit of learning (e.g., grades)
- Learners are self-directed and learn best when intrinsically motivated.
- Ryan and Deci (see Suggested Readings) noted three needs that drive intrinsic motivation:
  - *Competence*: the need to gain skill or expertise in an area
  - *Relatedness*: the need to connect and share experience with others
  - *Autonomy*: the need to take responsibility for one's own learning
- Extrinsic motivators may negatively impact intrinsic motivation by reducing learner autonomy.
- Strategies that educators may use to motivate learners include:
  - Make learning "problem centered" and relevant to learners' current or future roles.
  - Develop clear, focused objectives (learners often have many competing interests and may need help prioritizing their learning goals).
  - Engage learners in developing their own learning plans.
  - Create a "safe" learning environment where learners feel empowered to pose questions, discuss challenges, and share their experiences and insights.
- *Reflective practice* is the process of continual development and modification of practice through ongoing reflection on learning.
  - The "reflective practitioner," as originally described by Schön, reflects "in action" during an event to draw on past experiences and aid decision-making. After the event, the practitioner reflects "on action" to deconstruct and analyze management and to refine approaches to future scenarios.
  - Educators should model ongoing reflective practice and lifelong learning.
  - Educators have a role in fostering learners' critical and analytical thinking through reflection (e.g., case-based reflections and group activities such as debriefing). Such reflection helps learners identify future goals and learning needs and promotes longitudinal growth and development.
- *Effective learning environments* are comfortable physical spaces conducive to learning. In addition,
  - A safe environment is created with mutual respect between teachers and learners.
  - Learners must feel personally and professionally safe to ask questions and share opinions and ideas without negative consequences to promote deeper understanding of the educational content.
  - Learners' experiences and their contributions are valued and appreciated.
  - Learners are given autonomy and responsibility for their own learning.
  - Teaching is relevant and adapted to meet learning needs.
  - Educators engage learners through interactive approaches to learning that meet practical needs.
- *Hidden curriculum* is the unspoken institutional culture and views of educators that are learned through observed behaviors and actions. Although the formal curriculum is clearly outlined, the hidden curriculum may be experienced and modeled on a regular basis.
  - Medical educators and practitioners need to be aware of a hidden curriculum, as it may conflict with the formal curriculum (e.g., learners may be taught core elements of professionalism yet observe unprofessional team behaviors within the clinical environment).
  - Educators and learners should reflect on ways the hidden curriculum may be perpetuated within teaching and assessment and identify corrective strategies.

ASSESSMENTS

- Educators assess learners' knowledge and skills using different methods (Table 81.2). Assessment methods should align with learning goals. For example, knowledge acquisition may be measured using oral exams or short-answer questions, whereas performance of behavioral and technical skills may be measured using simulation or direct observation in the clinical environment.
- Assessments should be multimodal, reflect identified learning objectives, and appropriately target learners' level of training.
- Assessments *of* learning versus assessments *for* learning are used for different purposes:
  - Assessments *of* learning are assignments of a grade or the comparison of a learner's performance to others. These can be used *summatively* as a final evaluation

451

Table 81.1   Adult Learning Theory

Characteristics of Adult Learners	Implications for Educators
They are self-directed and goal-directed.	Educators need to engage learners in identifying their own needs and provide autonomy and responsibility.
Adults come with a vast array of previous experiences.	Educators and learners need to appreciate the experience that each learner brings to create a respectful learning environment.
	Educators and learners should recognize how opinions may be influenced by prior experiences.
	Diversity in past experiences creates a rich environment for learning, but educators may need to target teaching at different levels, depending on individual experiences and learning needs.
Readiness to learn is linked to "social roles."	Learning objectives need to be relevant to learners' needs, practical, and applicable to their current and future roles and responsibilities.
Knowledge acquired is generally applied more rapidly.	Adults often have a need for a problem-centered, goal-oriented approach to learning.
They have a motivation to learn.	Educators need to foster adults' internal motivation and provide learners with autonomy and responsibility for their learning.

that aims to measure how well learners have achieved a goal or predetermined endpoint for decision-making (e.g., end-of-rotation clinical evaluations, specialty board certification exams) or *formatively* to identify ongoing learning needs and develop individualized learning plans (e.g., in-training exams).

■ Assessments *for* learning are constructive appraisals of learner performance to provide feedback, promote reflective practice, and identify longitudinal learning goals. These are generally used *formatively* (e.g., direct observational assessments, periodic meetings between a learner and educator, a review of learner's reflective journals/portfolio).

FEEDBACK

■ Learner readiness to receive feedback reflects the learner's ability to receive feedback and fosters culture for personal growth (e.g., emotional readiness, quiet environment without distractions, psychological safety).

■ Characteristics of effective feedback
  ■ Timely: limits recall bias and helps learners make performance improvements in real time
  ■ Specific and based on observed behaviors: uses concrete examples directly observed in the learner's practice to provide context
  ■ Nonjudgmental: provides objective descriptions of learner behaviors to avoid the association of the educator's opinion with the learner's value or worth, which could demoralize and deactivate learning

Table 81.2   Types of Learner Assessments

What Is Being Assessed?	Assessment Methods	Strengths	Weaknesses
What is the learner's knowledge?	Multiple-choice exams	Represents foundational knowledge Assessments are not labor intensive	Do not assess integration and application of knowledge
Does the learner know how to use the knowledge?	Case presentations Short-answer questions Oral exams	Measure learners' ability to integrate and apply theoretical knowledge to patient care	Do not assess application of knowledge in the clinical environment
How well does the learner apply knowledge to perform requisite skills?	In the simulated environment: ■ Individual and team-based simulations ■ Objective structured clinical exams (OSCEs) In the clinical environment: ■ Hand offs ■ Direct observation of skills ■ Patient rounds	In the simulated environment: ■ Standardize experiences ■ Integrate a wide variety of uncommon and common cases In the clinical environment: ■ Performance reflects critical thinking and decision-making in the "real-world" environment. ■ Helps identify learning needs to promote reflective practice and identify longitudinal learning goals	Require equipment, personnel, and scheduled time as resources to prepare and perform assessments Performance in the simulated environment may not reflect what occurs in the clinical environment (e.g., degree of realism, learner engagement, Hawthorne effect of being observed) The reliability, validity, and feasibility of high-stakes assessment tools require testing Equipment, personnel, and scheduled time are required as resources to perform assessments In the clinical environment: ■ Requires time, engagement, and a balance with clinical responsibilities ■ May lack a diversity of clinical exposures ■ May require 360-degree evaluations to perform a comprehensive assessment

Adapted from Miller GE. The assessment of clinical skills/competence/performance. *Acad Med.* 1990;65(9):S63–S67.

Table 81.3 Strengths and Challenges of Teaching Methods

Teaching Method	Strengths	Challenges
Lecture	Can expose a large group of learners to the information, which can help standardize the delivery of content	Limited opportunity for interaction between educator and learner
	Efficient in the delivery of core theory/content, especially after learners are able to think through concepts beforehand	Unable to assess and cater to individual learner's needs
	Can provide over a virtual platform	Difficult to assess learners' understanding of content
		Unable to draw on learners' experiences
Small group discussion	Allows for interactive discussion and learner engagement	May require many facilitators and a higher teacher-to-learner ratio
	Can draw on learners' experiences	Learners may need to have an understanding of core concepts to optimize learning during group discussion.
	Allows for exploration of learners' critical thinking, application of knowledge	
	May enhance understanding of core concepts through group discussion	
	Can provide over a virtual platform	
Bedside teaching	Highly relevant, "problem-centered"	Need to balance clinical and educational responsibilities, requiring focused teaching methods due to time pressures (e.g., "one-minute preceptor")
	Allows for the opportunity to explore critical thinking and the application of knowledge, in addition to integrating basic science principles with diagnosis and clinical management	
	Promotes experiential learning (i.e., opportunity to learn through reflecting on practical experience)	Learners may feel vulnerable in the presence of families or other health care professionals.
	Can focus on clinical exam skills	
	Provides an opportunity for interprofessional team learning	
Simulation and debriefing	Promotes experiential learning	May be costly and require trained facilitators, instructors, technical operators
	Fosters an engaging and interactive learning environment	May require many facilitators and a higher teacher-to-learner ratio
	Provides opportunities to apply knowledge and practice behaviors, both individual and team-based	
	No patient safety concerns, as learners are encouraged to make errors in the simulation setting	
	Explicitly includes reflection on experience and behaviors to facilitate learning	
	Can control "clinical" exposure and learning environment	

- Focused on changeable behaviors or attainable goals: imparts constructive feedback on behaviors or goals that learners can target for improvement, rather than on the person
- Focused on positive consequences of change: balances positive and negative feedback to reinforce desirable behaviors and opportunities for change to target improvements in behavior

TEACHING METHODS

- A variety of teaching methods can be adopted by medical educators, depending on the teaching context and content to be covered (Table 81.3). All teaching sessions should incorporate:
  - Effective planning
  - Knowledge of learners and their needs
  - Clear, predetermined learning objectives
  - Content relevant for learners
  - Interactive learning
- Individuals have different learning goals and needs. Learners should be encouraged to reflect on their individual learning style and integrate complementary study aids to optimize learning.
- Educators should foster a learner-centered environment that promotes learner engagement and accommodates different approaches to learning.

Teaching Preparation and Planning

- Needs assessment is the process of determining core requirements along with gaps in learners' knowledge, skills, and attitudes. This process facilitates the formulation of individualized learning plans, curricula, and/or learning collaboratives.
- Methods include surveys, focus groups, exams, performance in clinical rotations, critical clinical incident reviews, etc.
- Goals can be specific short-, medium-, or long-term outcomes that learners work toward achieving in their continuing professional development.
- Learning objectives are concrete steps taken to achieve a goal.
  - Well-formulated learning objectives are *specific, measurable,* and *outcome-based,* stating what the learner should be able to do after a learning activity.
  - They serve as an educational guide for both learners and educators.
  - They help learners and educators choose the most appropriate educational methods to accomplish the learning objectives.
  - Learning objectives provide educators with a guide for evaluating the effectiveness of educational methods.

Table 81.4   Kirkpatrick's Model for Evaluating the Effectiveness of Training

What Is Being Evaluated?	Evaluation Methods	Strengths	Weaknesses
Reaction (level 1) How did learners react to the educational activity?	Surveys Verbal feedback Learner evaluations	Educators can use feedback to modify training so that learners are more motivated to participate again. It is generally quick and easy to obtain these data.	Activities that are reviewed unfavorably are not necessarily ineffective educational sessions. There may be reporting bias if evaluations are completed on a voluntary basis.
Learning (level 2) What knowledge and skills did learners learn from the educational activity?	Pre- and post-training tests Longitudinal retention tests	Measures knowledge acquisition and learners' theoretical approach to patient care	It is easier to measure knowledge than skill acquisition. Improved knowledge does not equate improved patient care. Knowledge attrition can occur over time; immediate assessment after an educational activity may not predict future knowledge retention.
Behavior (level 3) How did learners change their behaviors in the learning or clinical environment after the educational activity?	Simulated patient events Observed behaviors during patient care Peer and 360-degree evaluations Reflection journals or portfolios	Shows how new knowledge and skills are used in the work environment	Learners must be intrinsically motivated to apply new knowledge and skills in the learning or clinical environment. Outcomes depend on internal drivers and environmental conditions that must be conducive to change (e.g., motivation, collaboration from others).
Results (level 4) What are the patient care and/or organizational outcomes that resulted from the educational activity?	Quality assurance reviews Chart audits Patient satisfaction Staff retention	This is the "bottom line" outcome. Positive outcomes can foster organizational change.	Outcomes depend on environmental conditions that must be conducive to change. Improvements in patient care and at the organizational level are more difficult to measure. It may be difficult to directly link an educational activity to a specific change in outcome.

They use *measurable* verbs to convey the educational action item:

- ▪ Measurable verbs include identify, demonstrate, calculate, develop, assess, etc.
- ▪ Nonmeasurable verbs include know, understand, improve, appreciate, etc.

- ▪ Educators should acquire different types of information to evaluate the effectiveness and impact of their educational interventions and/or programs to identify opportunities for programmatic improvements (Table 81.4).

Suggested Readings

Amonoo HL, Longley RM, Robinson DM. Giving feedback. *Psychiatr Clin North Am.* 2021;44(2):237–247.

Brodsky D, Newman LR. A systematic approach to curriculum development. *NeoReviews.* 2011;12(1):e2–e7.

Knowles M. Andragogy: an emerging technology for adult learning. The assessment of clinical skills/competence/performance. *Acad Med.* 1990;65(9):S63–S67.

Ryan RM, Deci EL. Self-determination theory and the facilitation of intrinsic motivation, social development, and well-being. *Am Psychol.* 2000;55(1):68–78.

Schön DA. *The Reflective Practitioner: How Professionals Think in Action.* New York: Taylor and Francis Group; 1991.

Spencer J. Learning and teaching in the clinical environment. *BMJ.* 2003;326(7389):591–594.

Torralba KD, Jose D, Byrne J. Psychological safety, the hidden curriculum, and ambiguity in medicine. *Clin Rheumatol.* 2020;39(3):667–671.

82 Ethics in Research

CARL T. D'ANGIO

Overview

- Three landmarks:
  - The *Nuremberg Code* (Box 82.1) was promulgated in 1949 during the trial of Nazi physicians and scientists for war crimes committed against concentration camp prisoners.
    - It enunciated 10 components of ethical human subjects research.
  - *The Belmont Report* (Table 82.1) was issued in response to continued failings of the US research community in its obligation to protect research participants, including the *Tuskegee syphilis study*, which followed Black men with untreated syphilis long after treatment became available.
    - *The Belmont Report* laid out three ethical *principles* and their applications to research:
      - *Respect for persons*: an individual's autonomy to make decisions independently, applied in appropriate use of informed consent
      - *Beneficence* (and some add its twin, *nonmaleficence*): doing what is good for other people, applied through assessment of risks and benefits, minimizing risks
      - *Justice*: treating people in equal situations equally, applied by the equitable selection of subjects, avoiding having one group of people bear risks in finding information on or treatment for a disease that affects many groups
  - The *"Common Rule"* (45 CFR 46), issued by the US Department of Health and Human Services (DHHS) in 1991, governs human subjects research across nearly all federal agencies.
    - It has been updated several times since, with a recent major revision in 2018.
- Animal research is also governed by a wide variety of federal regulations.
  - The Department of Agriculture and other agencies enforce these regulations.
- Research misconduct is policed by several federal agencies, including the DHHS's Office of Research Integrity (ORI) and Office of Human Research Protection (OHRP).

Conflicts of Interest and Commitment

- *Conflicts of interest* can either consciously or subconsciously influence the way a researcher views, analyzes, and/or presents data.
  - As defined by the American Thoracic Society, a conflict of interest is "a divergence between an individual's private interests and his or her professional obligations" (Fig. 82.1)
  - They can be difficult to identify and depend heavily on individuals identifying and self-reporting them.
  - Some commonly identified conflicts of interest:
    - Financial conflict
    - Intellectual conflict
    - Personal/relationship conflict
    - Physician–researchers also have an inherent conflict of *fiduciary* (responsibility for the welfare of others) role between individuals as patients and research subjects.
  - Methods for managing conflicts of interest:
    - *Avoid* them.
    - *Disclosing* them allows reviewers, funders, and the scientific community to decide conflict.
    - *Manage* by
      - Reducing, modifying, or eliminating one's interest to decrease/remove conflict
      - Modifying one's role in research

Box 82.1 Ten Components of the Nuremberg Code, 1949

1. Voluntary consent
2. Fruitful results for good of society, not otherwise obtainable
3. Well designed
4. Avoid suffering and injury
5. No intended death
6. Benefit should outweigh risk
7. Proper preparation for ill effects
8. Conducted by scientists
9. Voluntary withdrawal
10. Ability of investigators to terminate for harm

National Institutes of Health. *Trials of War Criminals Before the Nuernberg Military Tribunals Under Control Council Law No. 10 Nuernberg, October 1946–April 1949*. Washington, D.C: US Government Printing Office; 1949:181–182.

Table 82.1 Components of *The Belmont Report*, 1979

Ethical Principle	Application to Research
Respect for persons (autonomy)	Informed consent
Beneficence	Assessment of risk and benefits
Justice	Selection of subjects

Summarized from National Commission for the Protection of Human Subjects of Biomedical and Behavioral Research. *The Belmont Report: Ethical Principles and Guidelines for the Protection of Human Subjects of Research*. Washington, DC: Department of Health, Education, and Welfare; 1979. Available at: https://www.hhs.gov/ohrp/regulations-and-policy/belmont-report/index.html.

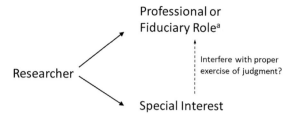

^a**Fiduciary role** = responsibility to promote another's interests (especially if the other person isn't able to do so themselves)

Fig. 82.1 Conflict of interest. A conflict of interest occurs when a personal or special interest interferes with the ability of a person to exercise a professional or fiduciary duty. As noted in the chapter text, special interests can be monetary or nonmonetary.

- ☐ Third-party oversight of the program to manage conflicting interests
- ☐ When in doubt, recusal from discussion or study performance
- *Conflict of commitment*
  - Researcher is dedicating time to personal or other activities (either for pay or not) that may detract from his or her primary responsibility to an institution or project.

Misconduct and Professionalism in Research

- According to the US ORI, "Research misconduct means fabrication, falsification, or plagiarism in proposing, performing, or reviewing research, or in reporting research results." (Definitions below have been modified from the ORI.)
  - *Fabrication* is manufacturing data or results that do not exist.
  - *Falsification* is the manipulation of materials, equipment, processes, or data to alter the representation of research results.
  - *Plagiarism* is representing another's words, images, or ideas as one's own, without giving appropriate credit.
- Research misconduct "does not include honest error or differences of opinion" (ORI).
- Authorship on scientific publications
  - The International Committee of Medical Journal Editors (ICMJE) suggested four criteria that all authors must meet to be listed on a publication.
    - Substantial contributions to the conception or design of the work or the acquisition, analysis, or interpretation of data for the work
    - Drafting the work or revising it critically for important intellectual content
    - Final approval of the version to be published
    - Agreement to be accountable for all aspects of the work

Definitions of Research With Human Subjects

- Under US federal research regulations, *research* is considered "a systematic investigation designed to develop or contribute to generalizable knowledge" (45 CFR 46.102).
- Human subjects research is research conducted on "a living individual about whom an investigator obtains (1) data through intervention or interaction with the individual, or (2) identifiable private information" (45 CFR 46.102).
- Humans taking part in research are interchangeably referred to as *subjects* or *participants*.

Role and Responsibilities of an Institutional Review Board

- An *institutional review board (IRB)* is a group established according to federal rules and regulations that is charged with reviewing and monitoring human subjects research.
  - The IRB can approve, require modifications of, or disapprove proposed research.
- Certain research activities are *exempt* from IRB review (i.e., do not have to be reviewed, but the decision of whether this is true still rests with the IRB):
  - Some educational, interview, and survey research
  - Use of existing records or specimens, provided that subjects are not identifiable
  - Some consumer preference testing
  - Scholarly (e.g., historical) research, oral history, public health surveillance, benign behavioral interventions, law enforcement/intelligence activities
  - Identifiable survey research and use of identifiable biospecimens allowed with "limited" IRB review
- Analysis of risks and benefits
  - IRBs are charged with evaluating risk and determining that:
    - Risks to subjects are minimized.
    - Risks are reasonable in relation to anticipated benefits to the subjects or society.
  - Risks can be thought of in terms of both *probability* and *magnitude.*
    - As an example, a 50% likelihood of experiencing transient flushing is of high probability but low magnitude, whereas a 1/10,000 likelihood of death is the opposite.
  - *Minimal risk* applies to a specific category of research involving research-specific risks that are "not greater than those ordinarily encountered in daily life" (45 CFR 46.102).

Further Application of Research Ethics to Human Subjects

- *Clinical equipoise* describes a state of uncertainty in the medical profession about the balance of benefits and harms of a proposed therapy.
- The *therapeutic misconception* or *therapeutic fallacy* is a belief on the part of a patient (and sometimes his/her provider) that an experimental intervention being applied as part of research is for the direct benefit of the patient.
- Ethical considerations in study design
  - Scientifically unsound research on human subjects is ipso facto unethical in that it may expose subjects to risks or inconvenience to no purpose (Council for International Organizations of Medical Sciences).
  - *Placebo* controls are often necessary to measure the *placebo effect* of a research subject knowing he/she is receiving an agent.
    - Placebos are generally not felt to be ethical if another, best current treatment for a condition is available; the appropriate control would be that treatment.

- *Deception* is sometimes permissible, usually in psychology research, when the value of the research is high, there are no alternatives, and subjects are debriefed (have the deception revealed) afterward.
- As is clear from the formative documents of research ethics, minimization of harms is a necessary prerequisite for ethical research.
- *Privacy* (right to be left alone) and *confidentiality* (right not to have your information shared) are protected by both federal research rules and the Health Insurance Portability and Accountability Act (HIPAA).
  - Privacy concerns generally prevent researchers without a bona fide relationship to a patient from contacting the patient directly for recruitment without the patient's consent.
  - Confidentiality concerns generally prevent the dissemination of identifiable data without a person's consent.
- *Data and safety monitoring boards* are independent groups of experts (usually in the condition being studied and in statistics and trial design) charged with monitoring the conduct of a study.
  - They monitor data integrity, safety, and accumulating efficacy information.
  - These boards often have access to group-specific data during the trial in blinded trials.
  - They can make recommendations to the study investigators or sponsor to alter, suspend, or terminate a study, based on their findings.

Consent, Assent, and Permission

- Definitions
  - *Consent* is an autonomous, voluntary decision made by someone with *decisional capacity* (i.e., possesses the understanding necessary to make a decision) to receive a treatment or participate in research.

- *Assent* is the agreement of a person without full decisional capacity (e.g., a child or an elder who has lost capacity) to a decision made by someone else to have the person receive a treatment or participate in research.
  - Infants and people with advanced dementia cannot assent.
- *Permission* is what someone with a legal responsibility for someone else (e.g., parent, guardian) gives for that person to receive a treatment or participate in research.
  - Permission has many characteristics of consent but is more limited than consent.
- Consent (and assent and permission) for research is expected to be *informed.*
  - Ethically, the person needs all the information necessary to make a decision.
  - Practically, the person needs to understand the purpose, procedures, risks and potential benefits, and context of the research.
  - Consent is a process, rather than merely a form, but regulations specify the information that should be present in a consent form (Box 82.2).
- The voluntary nature of consent can be undermined by inappropriate consent practices.
  - *Undue influence* or *undue inducement* is the application of positive enticements to participate in research.
  - *Coercion* is the actual or implied threat of harm if a potential subject does not participate.

Research in Vulnerable Populations

- Populations can be *vulnerable* due to lack of capacity (e.g., children, the mentally disabled, the elderly), lack of voluntariness (e.g., prisoners), risk of undue influence (e.g., economically or educational disadvantaged or desperately ill), or other factors (Fig. 82.2).

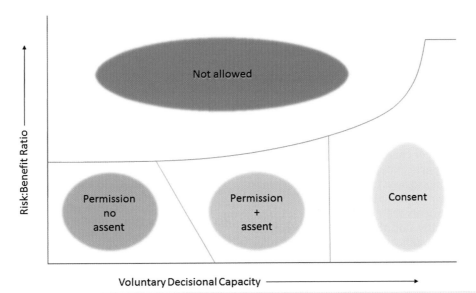

Fig. 82.2 Relationship among risk, benefit, and decisional capacity in research consent/permission. A person with full, voluntary, decisional capacity may consent to nearly any research (although note that research with very high risk and no benefit is not approvable). As the capacity to make voluntary, fully informed decisions diminishes (e.g., prisoners), some types of research are not allowed. People with limited or no decisional capacity (e.g., children or infants) depend on permission from others, with or without assent. Note that in some cases with a high chance of benefit to the individual (e.g., potentially lifesaving therapeutic trials), permission may override assent among persons who would otherwise be asked to assent.

Box 82.2 Required Components of Consent Forms

1. Identification as research
2. Purpose of study
3. Study procedures
4. Risks
5. Potential personal benefits
6. Alternatives to participation in research
7. Confidentiality
8. Compensation for injury
9. Contact information for investigators
10. Voluntary nature of participation

Summarized from 45 CFR 46.116, Federal Policy for the Protection of Human Subjects, US Department of Health and Human Services. 2018 changes to the Common Rule require more specific information in consent forms about reuse or dissemination of private information and biospecimens, and information about whether results will be shared with the research subject.

Table 82.2 Categories of Research in Children

Category	Description	Special Conditions
§46.404	Research not involving greater than minimal risk	None
§46.405	Research involving greater than minimal risk but presenting the prospect of direct benefit to the individual subjects	Risks no greater than alternative approaches
§46.406	Research involving greater than minimal risk and no prospect of direct benefit to individual subjects, but likely to yield generalizable knowledge about the subject's disorder or condition	Risk must be only a "minor increase over minimal risk" Two-parent permission is required
§46.407	Research not otherwise approvable which presents an opportunity to understand, prevent, or alleviate a serious problem affecting the health or welfare of children	Permission of Secretary of Health and Human Services is required

Descriptions are drawn verbatim from 45 CFR 46, Federal Policy for the Protection of Human Subjects, US Department of Health and Human Services, 2018.

- Federal regulations provide extra protections for vulnerable groups:
  - Pregnant women (not necessarily vulnerable themselves), fetuses, and nonviable newborns (45 CFR 46 Subpart B)
  - Prisoners (45 CFR 46 Subpart C)
  - Children (45 CFR 46 Subpart D); see next section

Research in Children

- Children are vulnerable due to their inability to provide informed consent for research.
  - As noted, parents instead provide permission—as in therapy, the overall criterion in deciding to provide permission is the *best interests* of the child, generally understood as minimizing risks and maximizing benefits.
  - When appropriate, children must give assent.
- Although *child* generally refers to someone below the age of majority (18 years old), specific definitions are dependent on the laws of the locality and specifics of proposed intervention.
- Allowable research in children (Table 82.2):
  - Children may generally participate in research that is of minimal risk (same definition as with adults) or has the prospect of direct benefit for the child, even if the risk is high (e.g., cancer chemotherapy trials).
  - Children may also participate in research that represents a "minor increase over minimal risk" and does not hold the prospect of direct benefit, but review and permission requirements are stricter.
  - Children are generally not allowed to participate in research that poses significant risks but does not offer a reasonable prospect of direct benefit to the child (see "best interests," above).

Suggested Readings

Code of Federal Regulations Title 45, Part 46 (45 CFR 46, "The Common Rule"), Protection of Human Subjects. Subpart D–Additional Protections for Children Involved as Subjects in Research. Available at: https://www.hhs.gov/ohrp/regulations-and-policy/regulations/45-cfr-46/index.html#subpartd. Accessed September 21, 2023.

CIOMS. *International Ethical Guidelines for Biomedical Research Involving Human Subjects.* Geneva, Switzerland: Council for International Organizations of Medical Sciences; 1993.

Emanuel EJ, Wendler D, Grady C. What makes clinical research ethical? *JAMA.* 2000;283(20):2701–2711.

Moreno JD, Schmidt U, Joffe S. The Nuremberg Code 70 years later. *JAMA.* 2017;318(9):795–796.

National Commission for the Protection of Human Subjects of Biomedical and Behavioral Research. *The Belmont Report: Ethical Principles and Guidelines for the Protection of Human Subjects of Research.* Washington, DC: Department of Health, Education, and Welfare; 1979. Available at: https://www.hhs.gov/ohrp/regulations-and-policy/belmont-report/index.html. Accessed September 21, 2023.

National Institutes of Health. *Trials of War Criminals Before the Nuernberg Military Tribunals Under Control Council Law No. 10 Nuernberg, October 1946–April 1949.* Washington, D.C: US Government Printing Office; 1949:181–182. Available at. https://history.nih.gov/research/downloads/nuremberg.pdf.

Schünemann HJ, Osborne M, Moss J, et al. An official American Thoracic Society Policy statement: managing conflict of interest in professional societies. *Am J Respir Crit Care Med.* 2009;180(6):564–580.

US Department of Health and Human Services, Office of Research Integrity. *Definition of Research Misconduct.* Available at: https://ori.hhs.gov/definition-misconduct. Accessed September 21, 2023.

Diagnostic Imaging

MITCHELL CHESS

83 *Neurologic Imaging*

MITCHELL CHESS

Germinal Matrix and Intraventricular Hemorrhage

- Ultrasound is the study of choice.
- Intraventricular hemorrhage (IVH) grading:
  - Grade I—Echogenicity is confined to caudothalamic groove (Fig. 83.1).
  - Grade II—Echogenicity extends into nondilated ventricles.
    - May have appearance similar to that of bulky choroid (Fig. 83.2A)
    - Echogenicity in occipital horns always hemorrhages (no choroid in this location) (see Fig. 83.2B).
    - May have secondary hydrocephalus from occlusion of brain foramena or aqueduct of Sylvius (Fig. 83.3).
  - Grade III—Ventricles are expanded by the accumulated blood (Fig. 83.4A).
    - Associated with venous infarction caused by deep terminal vein compression by pressure caused by blood (see Fig. 83.4B)
  - Grade IV—Bleeding extends into brain tissue around the ventricles (Fig. 83.5).
    - Cause is believed to be parenchymal hemorrhage into venous infarction.

Periventricular Leukomalacia (PVL)

- Ultrasound
  - Hyperechoic areas in the periventricular regions in mild and early cases (Fig. 83.6)
  - More severe—cysts revealed in these areas, cystic PVL (Fig. 83.7)
- Magnetic resonance imaging (MRI)
  - Early MRI—T1 hyperintensity/T2 hyperintensity (see Hypoxia and Ischemia section)
  - Subsequent periventricular cyst formation, develop after 2 to 6 weeks

Hypoxia and Ischemia

- MRI is the most sensitive and specific imaging study.
  - Findings indicating ischemia:
    - High T1 signal in the basal ganglia
    - Cortical laminar necrosis
      - T1—gray matter: hyperintense; white matter: hypointense (Fig. 83.8A)
      - T2—gray matter: variable; white matter: hyperintense (see Fig. 83.8B)
- MR spectroscopy with elevated lactate peaks (1.3 ppm; see Figs. 83.8C and 83.8D)

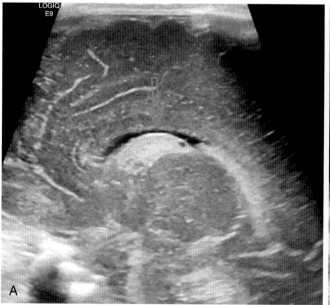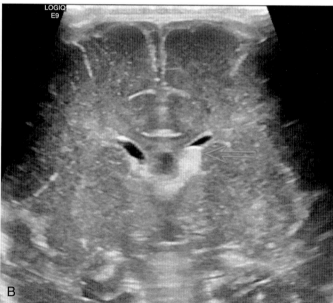

Fig. 83.1 Grade I germinal matrix and intraventricular hemorrhage (*arrows*). (A) Sagittal. (B) Coronal.

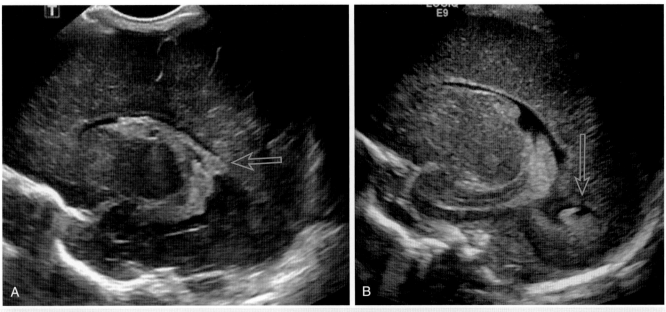

Fig. 83.2 (A, B) Grade II germinal matrix hemorrhage (*arrows*).

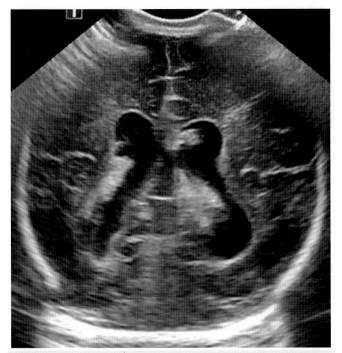

Fig. 83.3 Grade II germinal matrix and intraventricular hemorrhage with hydrocephalus.

- Diffusion-weighted imaging (DWI), apparent diffusion coefficient (ADC)—diffusion restriction, low signal (see Fig. 83.8E)
  - ADC normalizes at 7 to 10 days.
- Ultrasound findings indicating ischemia:
  - Increased echogenicity from edema in acute phase (see Fig 70.8F) frequently with mass effect

Mineralizing Vasculopathy

- Linear echogenicity in the basal ganglia (Fig. 83.9)
- Nonspecific causes include intrauterine TORCH infections (*Toxoplasma gondii*, other agents, rubella, cytomegalovirus [CMV], and herpes simplex virus [HSV]), chromosomal disorders, neonatal asphyxia, and maternal drug use.

Cavum Velum Interpositum

- Cystic space in the pineal region (Fig. 83.10)
  - Not to be mistaken for pineal or arachnoid cysts
  - Internal cerebral veins below the cystic space

Chiari II Malformation

- Posterior fossa (Fig. 83.11)
  - Inferiorly displaced cerebellar tonsils and vermis through foramen magnum
  - Low attachment of the tentorium, causing small posterior fossa

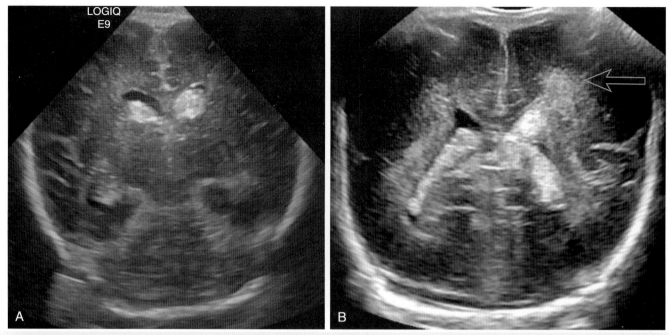

Fig. 83.4 (A, B) Grade III germinal matrix and intraventricular hemorrhage, with venous infarct (*arrow*).

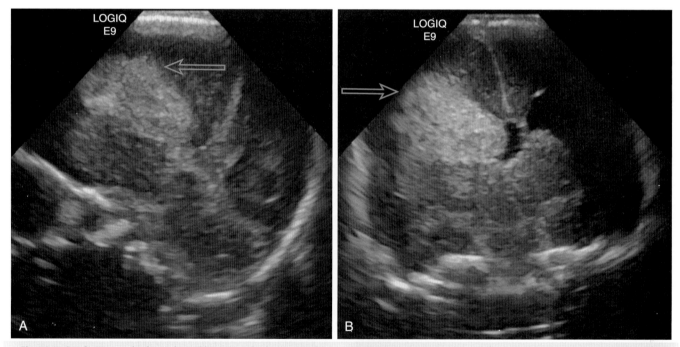

Fig. 83.5 Grade IV germinal matrix and intraventricular hemorrhage, with intraparenchymal hemorrhage (*arrows*). (A) Sagittal. (B) Coronal.

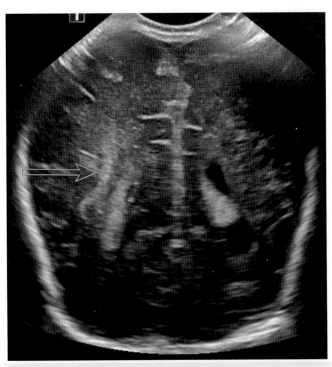

Fig. 83.6 Early periventricular leukomalacia (PVL)/ischemia (*arrow*).

- Flattened pons
- Elongated small fourth ventricle
- Tectal beaking, causing aqueductal stenosis and hydrocephalus

Holoprosencephaly

- Three general types:
  - Alobar holoprosencephaly
    - Single cortical structure without interhemispheric fissure
    - Fused thalami
    - Single large ventricle
    - Associated with facial abnormalities
  - Semilobar holoprosencephaly (Fig. 83.12)
    - Cerebral lobes present fused, most commonly anteriorly and at thalami
    - Absent septum pellucidum
    - Olfactory tracts and bulbs usually not present
    - Agenesis or hypoplasia of the corpus callosum
  - Lobar holoprosencephaly
    - Subtle midline fusion (cingulate gyrus and thalami)
    - Absent septum pellucidum
    - Olfactory tracts absent or hypoplastic
    - Hypoplasia or agenesis of corpus callosum

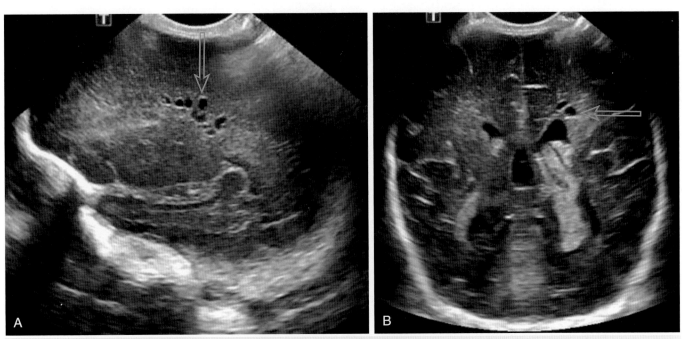

Fig. 83.7 Periventricular leukomalacia (PVL) (*arrows*). (A) Sagittal. (B) Coronal.

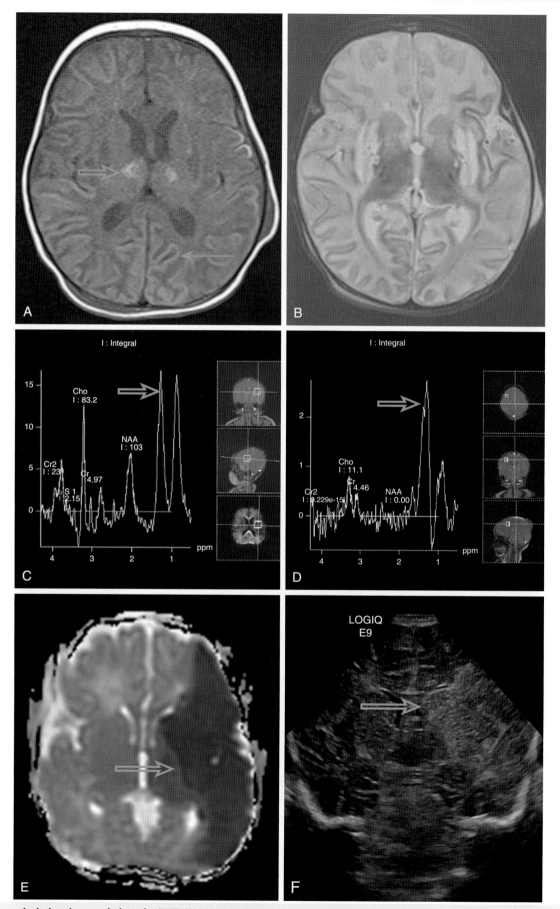

Fig. 83.8 Hypoxic–ischemic encephalopathy (HIE). (A) Magnetic resonance imaging (MRI) T1-weighted thalamic high signal (*open arrow*) and cortical necrosis (*closed arrow*). (B) MRI T2-weighted cortical necrosis (*closed arrow*). (C, D) MR spectroscopy lactate peak (*arrow*). (E) MRI diffusion weighted restricted diffusion (*arrow*). (F) Corresponding ultrasound with increased echogenicity (*arrow*).

Dandy-Walker Malformation (DWM) Spectrum

- Most common posterior fossa malformation (Fig. 83.13)
- Hypoplasia of the vermis and cephalad rotation of the vermian remnant
- Cystic dilation of the fourth ventricle posteriorly
- Enlarged posterior fossa with high tentorium

Syrinx

- Hydromyelia—dilation of the central canal of the spinal cord
- Syringomyelia—paracentral cavities lined by gliotic parenchyma due to disruption of the ependyma (Fig. 83.14)

Choanal Atresia

- Assessment with axial computed tomography (CT) (Fig. 83.15) may show the following:
    - Unilateral or bilateral posterior nasal narrowing, obstruction
    - Airway less than 3 mm at level of the pterygoid plates
    - Air-fluid level above obstruction
    - Thickening of vomer
    - Medial bowing of the posterior maxillary sinus

Suggested Reading

de Oliveira Schiavon JL, Grassi DC. *Neonatal and Infant Brain Imaging Evaluation.* Available at: http://reference.medscape.com/slideshow/neonatal-infant-brain-imaging-6009107. Accessed September 21, 2023.

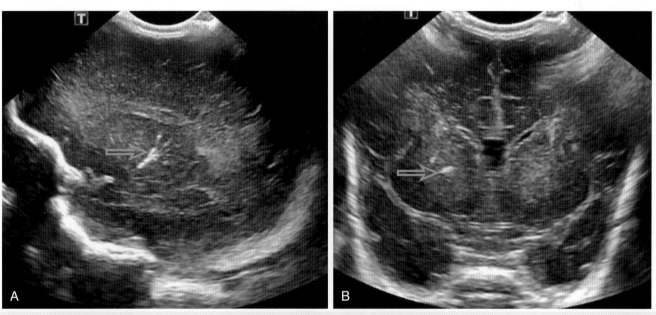

Fig. 83.9 Mineralizing vasculopathy (*arrows*). (A) Sagittal. (B) Coronal.

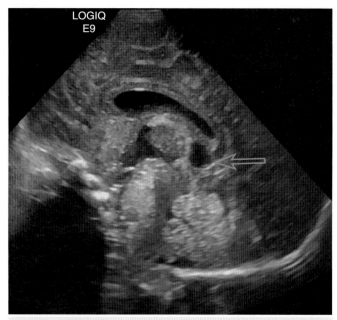

Fig. 83.10 Cavum velum interpositum (*arrow*).

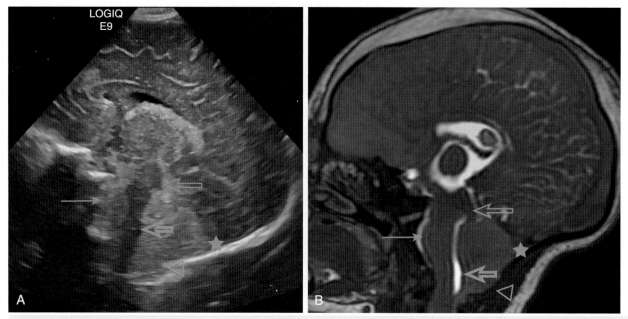

Fig. 83.11 Chiari II. Low cerebellar tonsils (*arrow head*), low tentorial attachment (*star*), flattened pons (*solid arrow*), elongated fourth ventricle (*short arrow*), tectal beaking (*long arrow*). (A) Ultrasound. (B) Magnetic resonance imaging (MRI).

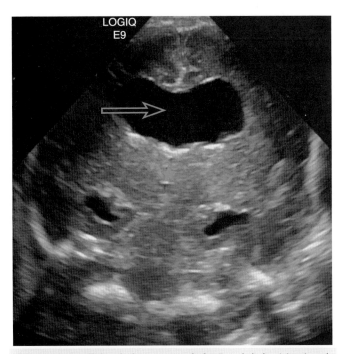

Fig. 83.12 Semilobar holoprosencephaly. Fused thalami (*star*) and absent septum pellucidum (*arrow*).

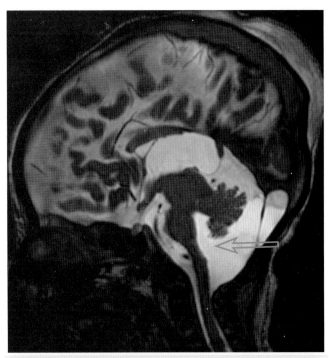

Fig. 83.13 Dandy-Walker malformation. Hypoplasia of vermis with retrocerebellar cyst (*arrow*).

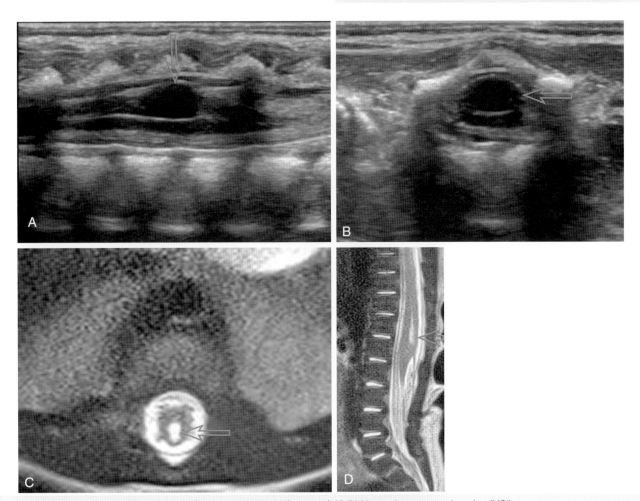

Fig. 83.14 Syrinx (*arrows*). (A, B) Ultrasound. (C, D) Magnetic resonance imaging (MRI).

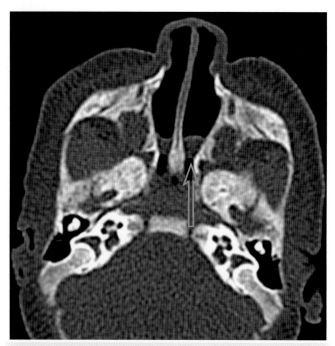

Fig. 83.15 Bilateral choanal atresia. Membranous obstruction (*arrow*) and thickened vomer (*star*).

84 *Chest Imaging*

MITCHELL CHESS

Surfactant Deficiency

- See Fig. 84.1.
- Diffuse ground-glass appearance, with fine granular pattern
- Bilateral and symmetric
- Air bronchograms
- Lung underexpansion
- Presents within hours of birth

Bronchopulmonary Dysplasia (BPD)

- See Fig. 84.2.
- Increased interstitial markings with areas of diffuse lucency
- Hyperinflated lungs
- Cardiomegaly may suggest pulmonary hypertension.

Pulmonary Interstitial Emphysema

- Cystic or linear lucencies extending from hilum
- May be focal (Fig. 84.3A) or generalized (see Fig. 84.3B)

- Hyperexpansion
- Associated with pneumothorax, pneumomediastinum, and pneumopericardium
- Increased pressure may lead to decreased venous return and smaller heart.

Pneumonia

- Variable appearance from hyperexpansion, alveolar densities, and interstitial disease
- Lung haziness may mimic surfactant deficiency but overexpansion rather than underexpansion.
- Alveolar pattern with bilateral air space disease and air bronchograms (Fig. 84.4A)
- Round pneumonia—well-defined, rounded opacities almost exclusively pediatric (see Fig. 84.4B)

Transient Tachypnea of the Newborn (TTN)

- See Fig. 84.5.
- Interstitial edema with normal heart size
- Present at birth, resolves within 48 hours postpartum

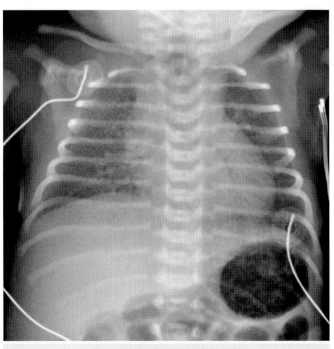

Fig. 84.1 Surfactant deficiency.

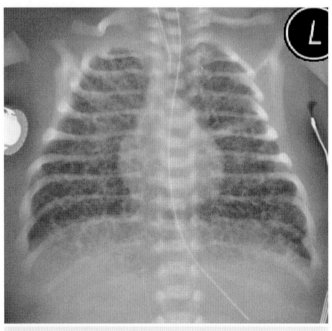

Fig. 84.2 Bronchopulmonary dysplasia (BPD).

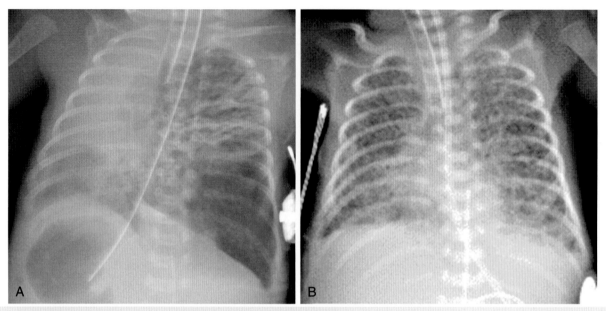

Fig. 84.3 Pulmonary interstitial emphysema. (A) Focal. (B) Generalized.

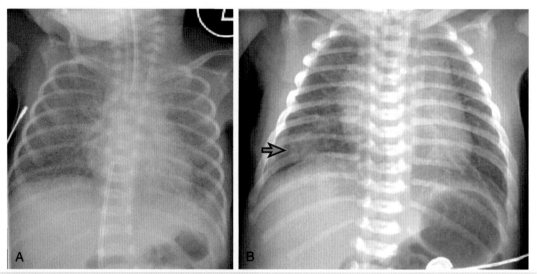

Fig. 84.4 Pneumonia. (A) Alveolar pattern. (B) Round pneumonia (*arrow*).

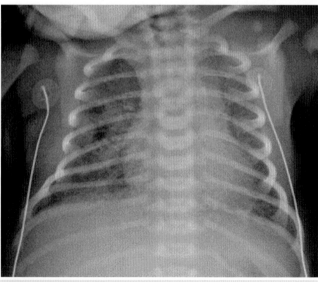

Fig. 84.5 Transient tachypnea of the newborn (TTN).

Meconium Aspiration

- See Fig. 84.6.
- Hyperexpansion due to small airway obstruction
- Asymmetric, patchy opacities
- May have pleural effusions
- Pneumothorax association

Congenital Diaphragmatic Hernia (CDH)

- Indistinct diaphragm (90% left-sided)

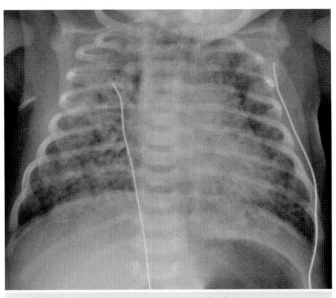

Fig. 84.6 Meconium aspiration.

- Preintubation or at intubation, bowel fluid-filled with opacification in hemithorax (Fig. 84.7A)
- Postintubation, bowel air with increased mass effect (see Fig. 84.7B)

Congenital Lobar Emphysema (CLE)

- Location
  - Left upper lobe: 40% to 45%
  - Right middle lobe: 30%
  - Right upper lobe: 20%
  - Much rarer in the lower lobe
- Immediate postpartum may appear opaque and homogeneous with fetal lung fluid (Fig. 84.8A).
- Later appears hyperlucent, with a paucity of vessels (see Fig. 84.8B)
- Mass effect (mediastinal shift, diaphragm depression)
- No change in lung volume on decubitus film

Congenital Pulmonary Airway Malformation (CPAM)

- This was previously known as a *congenital cystic adenomatoid malformation* (CCAM).
- CPAM is a multicystic (air-filled) lesion (Fig. 84.9A).
- It may cause mass effect (mediastinal shift, depression of diaphragm).
- Early neonatal cysts may be fluid-filled.
- Lesion may appear solid or with air–fluid levels (see Fig. 84.9B).

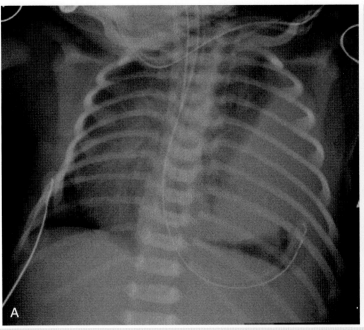
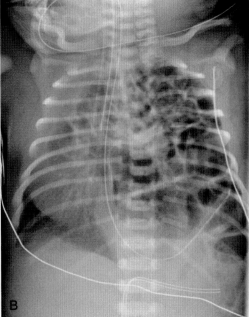

Fig. 84.7 **Congenital diaphragmatic hernia (CDH).** (A) Perinatal with bowel still fluid-filled causing opacification. (B) Bowel filling with air and increasing mass effect.

- Computed tomography (CT) more accurately delineates the location and extent (see Fig. 84.9C).
- CT angiography can identify the arterial supply (systemic vs. pulmonary).

Pleural Effusion

- Pleural effusion is most easily seen along the lateral chest wall or as a generalized hazy opacity (see Fig. 84.10) when supine because fluid layers dependently.

Pneumothorax

- Accumulates in a nondependent fashion
- Supine, pneumothorax is best seen as lateral chest, along the diaphragm, at a costophrenic angle as a deep sulcus

sign or as a generalized lucency of the lung as the air layers anteriorly (Fig. 84.11A).
- Decubitus pneumothorax is best seen on side that is up (see Fig. 84.11B).

Tension Pneumothorax

- See Fig. 84.12.
- Increased intercostal space
- Mediastinal shift
- Hemidiaphragm depression

Pneumomediastinum and Pneumopericardium

- See Fig. 84.13.

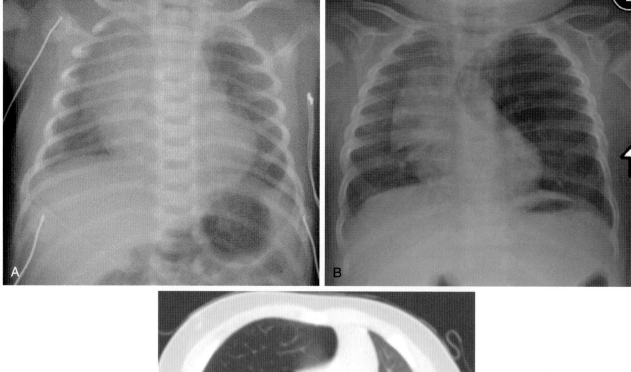

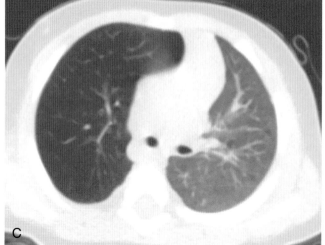

Fig. 84.8 Congenital lobar emphysema (CLE). (A, B) X-ray images of perinatal CLE with mild hyperexpansion (A) and increasing hyperexpansion over time (B). (C) Computed tomography (CT) scan.

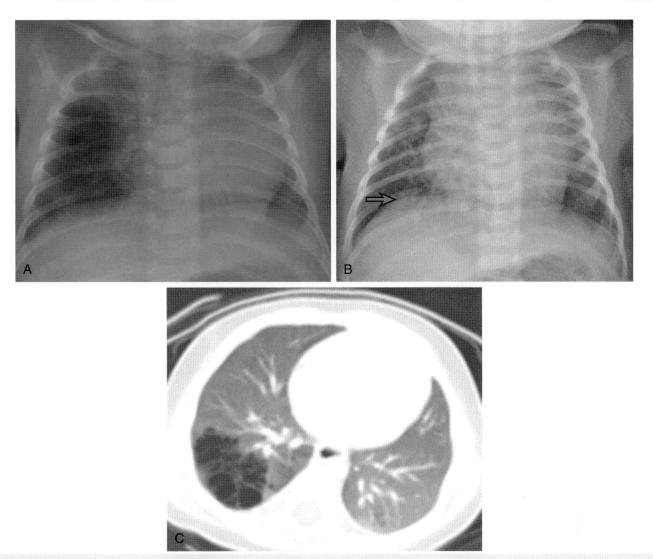

Fig. 84.9 Congenital pulmonary airway malformation. (A) X-ray of air-filled malformation. (B) X-ray of fluid-filled malformation (*arrow*). (C) Computed tomography (CT) scan.

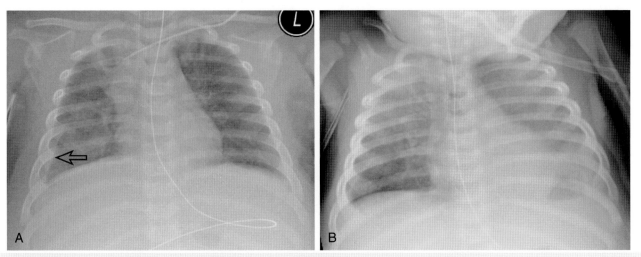

Fig. 84.10 Pleural effusion. (A) Along lateral chest wall (*arrow*). (B) Generalized opacity.

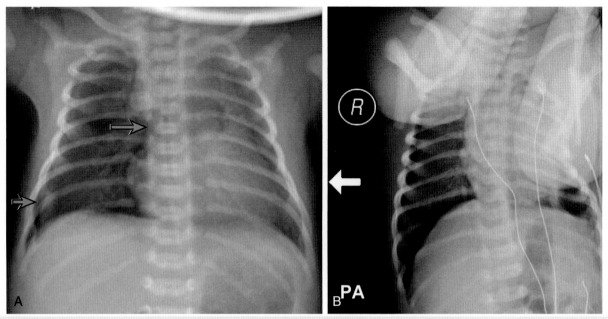

Fig. 84.11 **(A) Supine and (B) left lateral decubitus.** Lung margin (*arrows*).

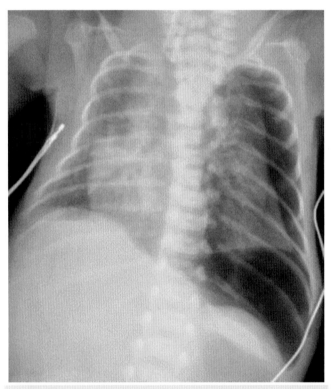

Fig. 84.12 **Tension pneumothorax.**

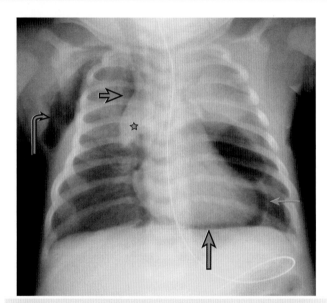

Fig. 84.13 **Pneumomediastinum and pneumopericardium.** Thymic wing sign (*star*), subcutaneous emphysema (*curved arrow*), mediastinal air (*short arrow*), pericardial air (*thin arrow*), continuous diaphragm sign (*long arrow*).

- *Pneumomediastinum:*
  - Elevated thymus, thymic wing sign
  - Lucency outlining mediastinal contour
  - Associated with subcutaneous emphysema
- *Pneumopericardium:*
  - Pericardium sharply outlined by air
  - Continuous diaphragm sign

Total Anomalous Pulmonary Venous Return (TAPVR)

- Right heart prominent due to increased flow volume
- Normal left atrium
- Cardiomegaly
- Type 1 (supracardiac) most common (Fig. 84.14)
  - Snowman appearance—Left vertical vein, brachiocephalic vein, and superior vena cava (SVC) form the head; enlarged right atrium forms the body.

Transposition of the Great Arteries (TGA)

- See Fig. 84.15.
- Cardiomegaly
- Egg-on-a-string sign—narrowed superior mediastinum with main pulmonary artery posterior to the aorta in d-transposition

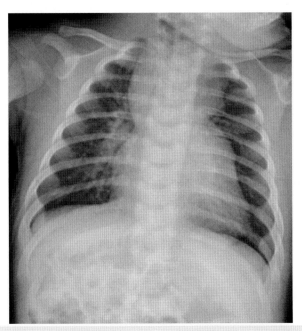

Fig. 84.14 Total anomalous pulmonary venous return (TAPVR).

Tetralogy of Fallot (TOF)

- See Fig. 84.16.
- Boot-shaped heart—upturned cardiac apex due to right ventricular hypertrophy and concave pulmonary artery
- Decreased pulmonary arterial flow related to pulmonary stenosis
- Right-sided aortic arch is seen in 25%.

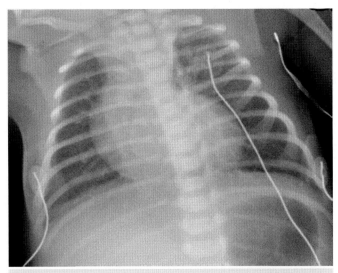

Fig. 84.15 Transposition of the great arteries (TGA).

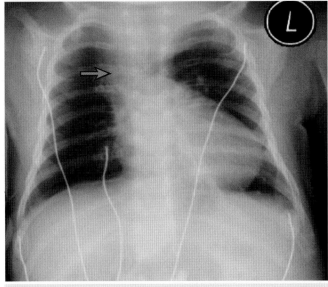

Fig. 84.16 Tetralogy of Fallot. Right sided aortic arch (*arrow*). Note lack of arch density to the left of the trachea.

Suggested Reading

Eklund MJ, Hill JG, Swift CC, et al. *Neonatal Imaging.* 1st ed. Chicago, IL: National Certification Corporation; 2017.

85 *Abdominal Imaging*

MITCHELL CHESS

Necrotizing Enterocolitis

- Bowel dilation, frequently with asymmetric distribution
- "Stacking" of bowel loops (Fig. 85.1A)
- Bowel wall thickening, with separation of bowel loops (see Fig. 85.1A) or thumbprinting
- Mottled appearance of colon (see Fig. 85.1A) and linear lucency (see Fig. 85.1A) representing pneumatosis intestinalis
- Portal venous gas (see Fig. 85.1A)
- Pneumoperitoneum indicating perforation, including Rigler sign (air on both sides of the bowel) and football sign (air outlining falciform ligament) (see Fig. 85.1B)
- May be diagnosed by ultrasound with bowel wall thickening, abnormal blood flow (hypervascular early and hypovascular late), and hyperechoic foci in the bowel wall representing air

Biliary Atresia

- Nuclear medicine hepatobiliary iminodiacetic acid (HIDA) scan—good hepatic uptake with no evidence of excretion into the bowel at 24 hours
- Pretreatment with phenobarbital can increase biliary secretion by stimulating hepatic enzymes; may minimize false-positive studies with patent biliary system but poor excretion.
- No small bowel tracer at 6 hours (Fig. 85.2A) or 24 hours (see Fig. 85.2B)

Hirschsprung Disease

- Contrast enema for diagnosis and assessing length of involvement; transition zone on enema not always accurate transition between aganglionic and ganglionic cells
- Affected segment—small caliber, with proximal dilation (Fig. 85.3)
- Early filling views—include rectum and sigmoid colon so rectosigmoid ratio may be determined

Microcolon

- See Fig. 85.4.
- Diagnosed with contrast enema
- Differential diagnoses include ileal atresia, meconium ileus, and total colonic Hirschsprung disease.

Esophageal Atresia With Fistula

- See Fig. 85.5.
- Dilated air-filled pharyngeal pouch with tube in pouch turning back to neck
- Air in the stomach in the presence of esophageal atresia implies fistula

Esophageal Atresia Without Fistula

- Dilated air-filled pharyngeal pouch and no air in the stomach imply esophageal atresia with no fistula (Fig. 85.6A).
- Contrast via gastrostomy tube demonstrates proximal, blind-ending, distal esophagus segment (see Fig. 85.6B).

Malrotation

- Upper gastrointestinal series is the examination of choice.
- Malrotation may be diagnosed with ultrasound with inversion of the superior mesenteric vessels (superior mesenteric artery [SMA] on the right and superior mesenteric vein [SMV] on the left).
- The duodenojejunal junction fails to cross the midline to the left of the vertebral body (Fig. 85.7A).
- The duodenojejunal junction lies inferior to the duodenal bulb (see Fig. 85.7B).

Duodenal Atresia

- See Fig. 85.8.
- Double-bubble sign with gas-filled distended stomach and duodenum with absence of distal gas

Hypertrophic Pyloric Stenosis

- See Fig. 85.9.
- The pylorus here is elongated and thick-walled.
- *Tip* to remember abnormal values: Remember that π (3.14) is abnormal.
  - Wall thickness > 3 mm is abnormal.
  - Length > 14 mm is abnormal.
- Stomach contents may pass through.

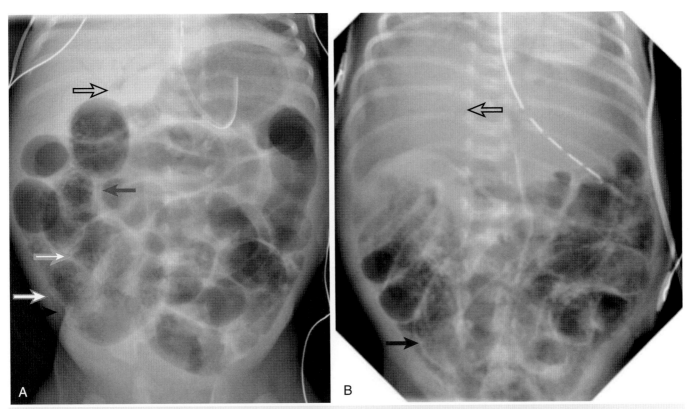

Fig. 85.1 Necrotizing enterocolitis. (A) Portal venous gas (*black arrow*), "stacking" of bowel loops (*green arrow*), separation of bowel loops (*red arrow*), mottled colon (*orange arrow*), and linear lucency (*blue arrow*) representing pneumatosis intestinalis. (B) Pneumoperitoneum (*black arrow*) and Rigler sign (*blue arrow*).

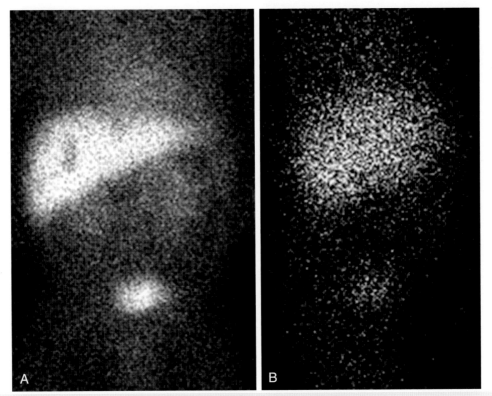

Fig. 85.2 Biliary atresia. (A) At 6 hours. (B) At 24 hours.

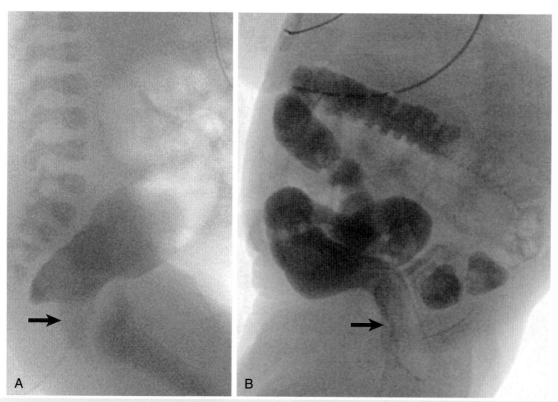

Fig. 85.3 (A, B) **Hirschsprung disease.** Narrowed aganglionic segment (*blue arrows*).

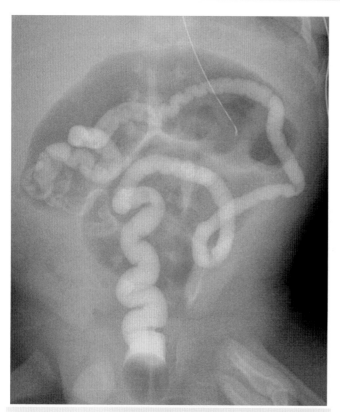

Fig. 85.4 Microcolon.

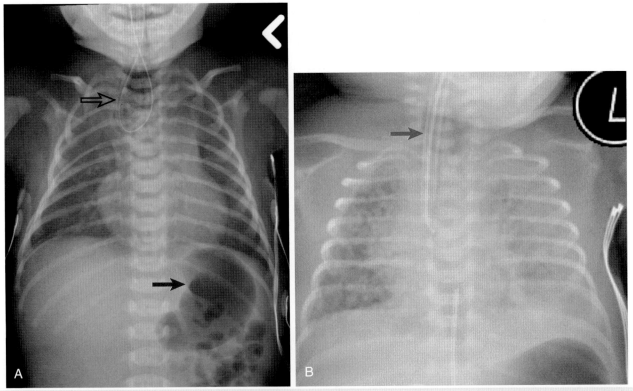

Fig. 85.5 (A, B) Esophageal atresia with fistula. Pharyngeal pouch (*red arrow*) with tube insertion in blind pouch (*black arrow*); air in the stomach (*blue arrow*).

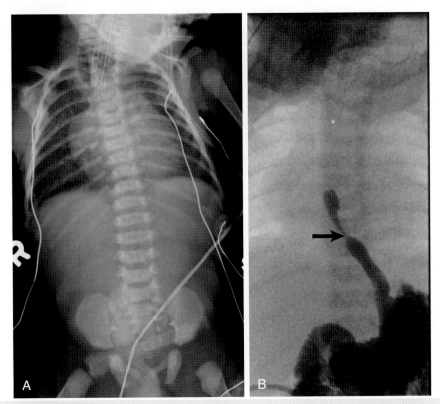

Fig. 85.6 Esophageal atresia without fistula. (A) X-ray. (B) Contrast via gastrostomy tube demonstrates distal esophagus (*arrow*).

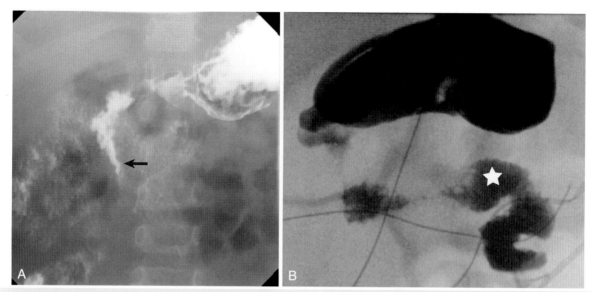

Fig. 85.7 Malrotation. (A) Duodenojejunal junction fails to cross the midline (*arrow*). (B) Duodenojejunal junction lies inferior to the duodenal bulb (*star*).

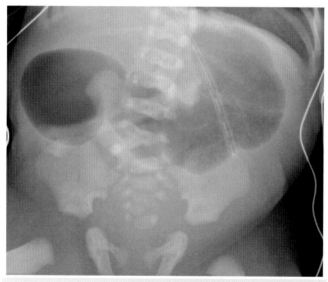

Fig. 85.8 Duodenal atresia.

Suggested Reading

Eklund MJ, Hill JG, Swift CC, et al. *Neonatal Imaging.* 1st ed. Chicago, IL: National Certification Corporation; 2017.

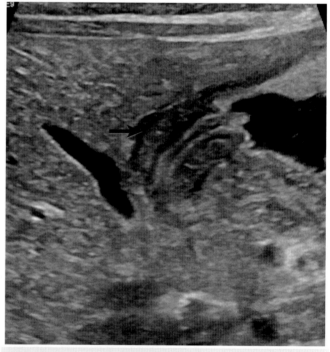

Fig. 85.9 Hypertrophic pyloric stenosis. Thickened, elongated pylorus (*arrow*).

86 *Miscellaneous Imaging*

MITCHELL CHESS

Normal Thymus/Clavicle Fracture

- See Fig. 86.1.
- Thymus is triangular and frequently toward the right of the mediastinum, without mass effect on the vascular structures or airway.
- Scalloped contour from anterior rib impressions
- Clavicular fractures are complete or incomplete, unilateral or bilateral.
- Incidence increases with increasing fetal weight.
- Frequently related to shoulder dystocia

Lines

- See Fig. 86.2.
- Umbilical vein (UV) courses anteriorly with a dip posteriorly in the liver through the ductus venosus; final position is above the diaphragm. Target position is the tip just above the diaphragm, not in the heart—ideally at the junction of the inferior vena cava and right atrium.
- Umbilical artery (UA) courses inferiorly to iliac artery before extending to the aorta. Target position is between T7 and T9, in the descending aorta above the origin of the celiac, mesenteric, and renal arteries.

Cystic Hygroma (Cystic or Nuchal Lymphangioma)

- See Fig. 86.3.
- Well circumscribed
- Fluid density
- Unilocular or multilocular
- Density variable; combination of fluid, soft tissue, and fat

Thanatophoric Deformity

- See Fig. 86.4.
- Limbs
  - Proximal limbs are short with rhizomelic appearance.
  - Long bones show "telephone handle" bowing and metaphyseal flaring.
- Iliac bones
  - Hypoplastic with squared iliac wings
  - May show a "trident" acetabular roof

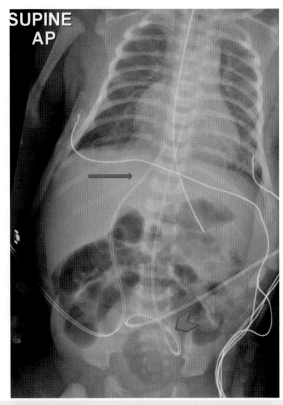

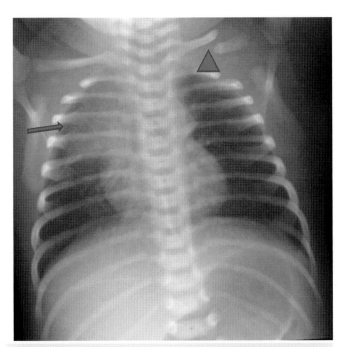

Fig. 86.1 Normal thymus (*arrow*) and clavicle fracture (*triangle*).

Fig. 86.2 The umbilical vein (*UV*) (*arrow*) courses anteriorly with dip posteriorly, and the umbilical artery (*UA*) (*arrow head*) courses inferiorly to iliac artery before extending to aorta.

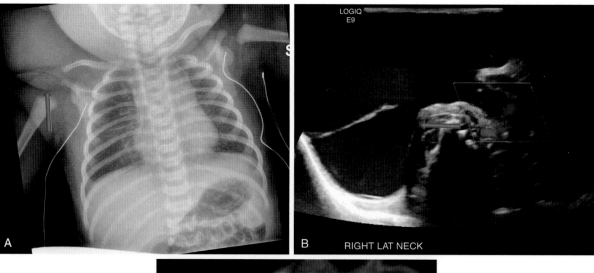

Fig. 86.3 Cystic hygroma (*arrows*). (A) X-ray. (B) Ultrasound. (C) Magnetic resonance imaging.

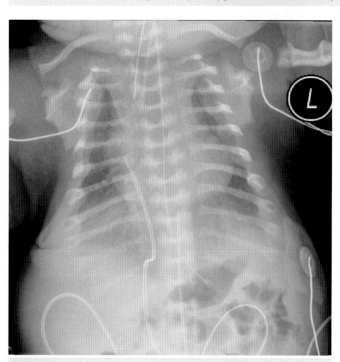

Fig. 86.4 Thanatophoric deformity.

- Chest
  - Narrow "bell-shaped" chest, short horizontal ribs, small scapulae
- Skull and face
  - Macrocephaly with frontal bossing, proptosis, and nasal bridge flattening
  - May have Kleeblattschaedel (cloverleaf skull from severe craniosynostosis of multiple sutures)
- Spine
  - Platyspondyly (flattened vertebral bodies)

Achondroplasia

- See Fig. 86.5.
- Chest
  - Anterior flaring of the ribs, with anteroposterior narrowing of the ribs
- Pelvis and hips
  - Decreased acetabular angle
  - Small squared iliac wings
  - Small trident pelvis

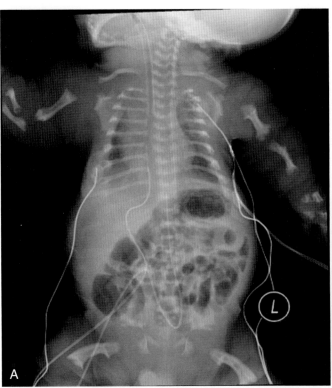

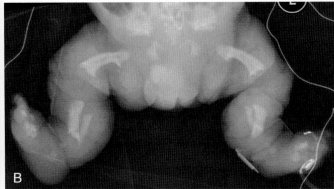

Fig. 86.5 (A, B) Achondroplasia.

- Champagne-glass type of pelvic inlet
- Short sacroiliac notches
- Limbs
  - Metaphyseal flaring
  - Femora and humeri most foreshortened (rhizomelic shortening)

Hydronephrosis

- See Fig. 86.6.
- Abnormal dilatation of the renal collecting system; see Suggested Reading for more complete classification of urinary tract dilatation
- Causes include ureteropelvic obstruction (most common), posterior urethral valves, vesicoureteral reflux, ureterocele, and other developmental anomalies of the genitourinary tract.

Urinary Tract Dilation—Posterior Urethral Valves (PUVs)

- Voiding cystourethrogram (VCUG) is the best imaging technique.
  - Dilation and elongation of posterior urethra (keyhole sign) (Fig. 86.7A)
  - Linear lucency corresponding to the valve (see Fig. 86.7A)
  - Vesicoureteral reflux is frequent.
  - Bladder trabecula and diverticula (see Fig. 86.7B)
- Ultrasound

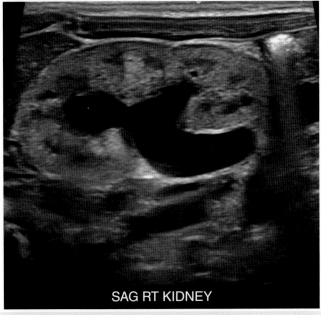

SAG RT KIDNEY

Fig. 86.6 Hydronephrosis.

- Bladder is thick-walled and trabeculated, with an elongated and dilated posterior urethra (see Fig. 86.7C).
- Hydronephrosis (up to 10% may appear normal)
- Valve may be seen as an echogenic line.
- Rupture of calyceal fornix may cause urinoma (anechoic fluid collections).

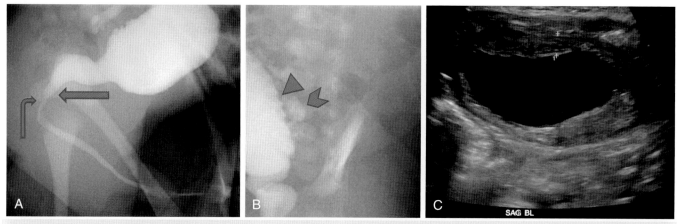

Fig. 86.7 Posterior urethral valves (PUVs). (A, B) Voiding cystourethrogram (*VCUG*) of keyhole sign (*arrow*), linear lucency corresponding to the valve (*curved arrow*), bladder trabecula (*triangle*), and diverticula (*chevron*). (C) Ultrasound of bladder shows that it is thick walled and trabeculated.

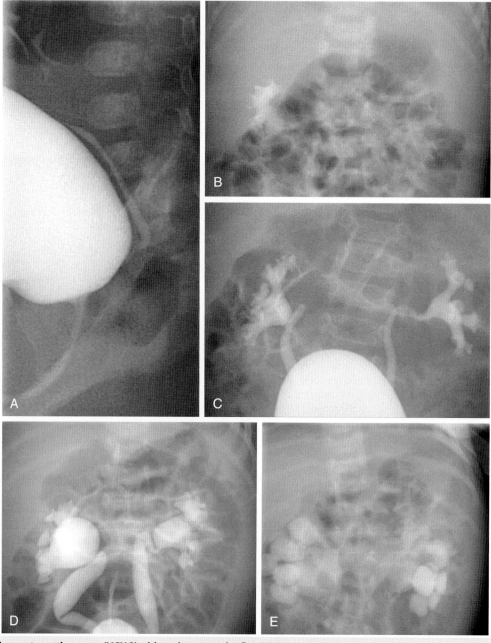

Fig. 86.8 Voiding cystourethrogram (VCUG) with vesicoureteral reflux (VUR). (A) Grade 1. (B) Grade 2. (C) Grade 3. (D) Grade 4. (E) Grade 5.

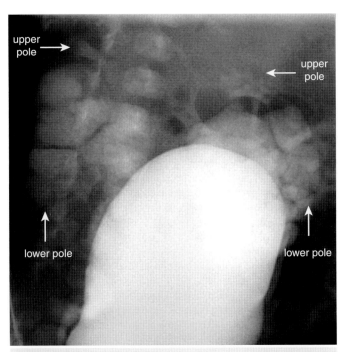

Fig. 86.9 Grade 2 vesicoureteral reflux (VUR), upper left; grade 3, upper right; grade 5, lower bilateral.

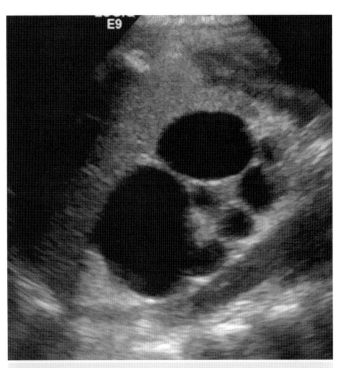

Fig. 86.10 Multicystic dysplastic kidney (MCDK) with non-communicating cysts.

Vesicoureteral Reflux (VUR)

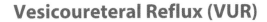

- Grade 1: reflux limited to the ureter (Fig. 86.8A)
- Grade 2: reflux up to the renal pelvis (see Fig. 86.8B)
- Grade 3: mild dilation of the urinary tract (see Fig. 86.8C)
- Grade 4: tortuous ureter with moderate dilation of renal collecting system, with preserved papillary impressions (see Fig. 86.8D)
- Grade 5: tortuous ureter with severe dilation of ureter and pelvicalyceal system, with loss of fornices and papillary impressions (see Fig. 86.8E)
- Reflux may not be symmetric bilaterally (Fig. 86.9).

Multicystic Dysplastic Kidney (MCDK)

- See Fig. 86.10.
- Lobulated renal contour with multiple cysts of varying sizes
- Absent or small hilar vessels
- Cysts typically cluster and are noncommunicating.

Suggested Reading

Chow JS, Darge K. Multidisciplinary consensus on the classification of antenatal and postnatal urinary tract dilation (UTD classification) system. *Pediatr Radiol.* 2015;45(6):787–789.

Questions Section

Chapter 1

1. An effective way to study for the boards is:
   a. Commit large blocks of time to cover more material at each sitting.
   b. Avoid 10-minute study periods because you are unlikely to learn anything relevant in this period of time.
   c. Develop detailed schematics because these are more likely to improve retention.
   d. Develop a study map incorporating topics and time to study each topic.

Chapter 2

1. Which of the following lung volumes cannot be measured using spirometry?
   a. Residual volume (RV)
   b. Total lung capacity
   c. Forced expiratory volume 1 second (FEV_1)
   d. Forced vital capacity (FVC)
   e. Tidal volume (TV)
2. A term infant is born with congenital diaphragmatic hernia and is in hypoxemic respiratory failure. The last postductal arterial blood gas has pH = 7.29, $PaCO_2$ = 52 mmHg, PaO_2 = 40 mmHg, HCO_3 = 20 mg/dL. The infant is on high-frequency oscillatory ventilation with MAP = 18 cmH_2O, frequency = 8 Hz, FIO_2 = 1.0. Atmospheric pressure is 760 mmHg; water pressure = 47 mmHg. Which of the following choices corresponds to the infant's A-a gradient and oxygenation index (OI)?
   a. A-a gradient = 621; OI = 45
   b. A-a gradient = 608; OI = 36
   c. A-a gradient = 648; OI = 36
   d. A-a gradient = 608; OI = 45
   e. A-a gradient = 648; OI = 18
3. Which of the following expected perturbations in oxygen parameters is TRUE?

	PaO_2	O_2 Saturation	O_2 Content
a. Severe anemia	Decreased	Unchanged	Decreased
b. Severe anemia	Decreased	Increased	Decreased
c. Severe V/Q mismatch	Decreased	Decreased	Decreased
d. Severe V/Q mismatch	Unchanged	Decreased	Decreased

4. Which of the following is true about dead space?
   a. Dead space is characterized by V/Q ratio >1.
   b. Dead space can be calculated using Fick's diffusion equation.
   c. Alveolar dead space is not affected by broncho-constriction.
   d. Physiologic dead space is always greater than anatomic dead space.
5. Which of the following is the most accurate statement about the neonatal versus adult respiratory system?
   a. The neonatal lung has a longer time constant than the adult lung.
   b. The neonatal lung has more anatomic dead space than the adult lung.
   c. The neonatal lung has lower residual volume compared to adults.
   d. Neonatal tidal volumes are lower than adult tidal volumes.
   e. Minute ventilation is similar between neonates and adults.
6. Answer "True" or "False" to each of the following statements:
   a. The ELBW infant born at 24 weeks' gestation is in the saccular stage of lung development.
   b. Aberrant development of the canalicular phase results in tracheo-esophageal fistula.
7. Several stages are involved in the development of the lung. At the end of which stage is the lung considered viable?
   a. Alveolar
   b. Saccular
   c. Pseudoglandular
   d. Canalicular
   e. Embryonic
8. The fluid that fills the fetal lung in utero is largely derived from the lung secretion rather than from amniotic fluid inhalation. The one major driving force responsible for the production of fetal lung liquid is the transepithelial secretion of:
   a. Bicarbonate
   b. Calcium
   c. Chloride
   d. Potassium
   e. Sodium
9. Sequence analysis of the relevant genes and an adjunct evaluation of lung tissues by histology (including electron microscopy) are ways to establish the diagnosis of an inherited disorder of surfactant metabolism. Which of the following is a typical lung histopathology finding of ABCA3 protein deficiency?
   a. Alveolar septal thinning
   b. Diffuse alveolar type II epithelial cell hypoplasia
   c. Interstitial protein deposition

d. Lamellar bodied with eccentric dense inclusions

e. Neutrophils in airspaces

10. Answer "True" or "False" to each of the following statements:

a. Laplace's law states that the pressure needed to expand a bubble is inversely proportional to the surface tension and directly proportional to the radius.

b. In the absence of surfactant, when two alveoli are connected through a common airway, gas from the larger one will flow into the smaller one until both of them are the same volume.

c. Surfactant is composed of phospholipids and three types of surfactant associated proteins.

d. Surfactant becomes more efficient as alveolar diameter decreases.

e. Atelectatic lungs are more compliant than normal volume lungs.

11. Which of the following is the most accurate equation for calculating resistance?

a. Change in flow divided by pressure

b. Change in volume divided by pressure

c. Change in volume divided by flow

d. Change in pressure divided by flow

e. Change in pressure divided by volume

12. Shorter time constants result in the collapse of lung units, and longer time constants result in overdistention. Which of the following is the most accurate equation for calculation of the time constant?

a. Resistance × elastance

b. Frequency × conductance

c. Resistance × compliance

d. Conductance × compliance

e. Conductance × elastance

13. Answer "True" or "False" to each of the following statements:

a. Static compliance is measured during gas flow.

b. Static compliance reflects elastic properties of the lung.

c. Dynamic compliance is measured during continuous breathing.

d. Elastic and resistive components of the lungs are not reflected by the dynamic compliance.

e. Compliance is a measure of distensibility of elastic tissue.

14. The apex of the upright human lung when compared to the base has:

a. Higher PO_2

b. Higher ventilation

c. Lower pH in end-capillary blood

d. Higher blood flow

e. Smaller alveoli

15. Answer "True" or "False" to each of the following statements:

a. Carbon dioxide elimination is determined by alveolar minute ventilation, surface area, and interstitium thickness.

b. Minute ventilation is a ratio of tidal volume and respiratory rate.

c. Increased physiological dead space will result in higher CO_2.

d. Infants with BPD have decreased physiologic dead space.

e. Pulmonary blood flow has no effect on CO_2 removal.

16. Oxygen delivery to the tissues depends on:

a. Cardiac output

b. Hemoglobin concentration

c. SpO_2

d. Patient's blood type

e. a, b, and c

17. Shifting of the oxyhemoglobin dissociation curve to the right due to increased CO_2 concentration in the blood is called:

a. Chloride shift

b. Donann equilibrium

c. Haldane effect

d. Bohr effect

e. Fick's principle

18. In which one of the following conditions does the oxygen dissociation curve shift to the right of a normal curve?

a. Decrease in pH

b. Decrease in $CO_2$2 concentration

c. Decrease in acidity

d. Decrease in temperature

e. Increased fetal hemoglobin

19. Answer "True" or "False" to each of the following statements:

a. Oxygen dissociation curve is shifted to the right at extreme altitude.

b. At moderate altitude, oxygen dissociation curve is shifted to the left.

c. Increased 2,3-DPG is responsible for the left shift of the oxygen dissociation curve at extreme high altitudes.

d. Increased 2,3-DPG is responsible for the left shift of the oxygen dissociation curve at moderately high altitudes.

e. Respiratory alkalosis is responsible for the left shift of the oxygen dissociation curve at extremely high altitudes.

20. Evaluate pH 7.50, $PaCO_2$ 16 mmHg, HCO_3 12 mEq/L.

21. Evaluate pH 7.27, $PaCO_2$ 29 mmHg, HCO_3 13 mEq/L.

22. Evaluate pH 7.32, $PaCO_2$ 24 mmHg, HCO_3 12 mEq/L.

23. Evaluate pH 7.35, $PaCO_2$ 65 mmHg, HCO_3 35 mEq/L.

24. A newborn female infant breathing in room air was admitted to the NICU in New York due to transient tachypnea of newborn with arterial PO_2 of 60, PCO_2 of 25, and respiratory quotient (RQ) of 0.8. What is her alveolar–arterial PO_2 gradient? Assume water vapor pressure is 47.

a. 40

b. 52

c. 59

d. 100

e. Unable to calculate given the above information

25. A 36 weeks' GA female infant was intubated at birth for respiratory failure with 4.0 mm ETT. Five minutes after extubation at 1 week of life, the infant developed severe respiratory stridor and required a reintubation. The vocal cord could only allow a placement of size 2.0 mm ETT (internal diameter). By what factor did the resistance of the ETT increase?

a. 2 ×

b. 4 ×

c. 8 ×

d. 16 ×

e. No change in resistance

26. A 2-day-old full-term infant on AC mechanical ventilator developed interval worsening of respiratory acidosis after surgery for gastroschisis. The respiratory acidosis resolved with $PaO_2 = 80$ when the respiratory support was switched to HFOV with MAP of 18, 0.8 FiO_2, and Hz of 10. What is the oxygenation index (OI)?
    a. 18
    b. 15
    c. 30
    d. 20
    e. 19

Chapter 3

1. Surfactant proteins B and C are essential components for surfactant replacement because they:
    a. Increase surfactant spreading at the air–liquid interface
    b. Coat bacteria and viruses to increase innate immunity
    c. Detoxify oxygen radicals and reduce injury to alveolar type II cells
    d. All of the above
2. Which of the following recommendations about postnatal glucocorticoid use in BPD are contained in the 2010 AAP policy statement?
    a. Therapy with high-dose dexamethasone cannot be recommended.
    b. There is insufficient evidence to make a recommendation regarding treatment with low-dose dexamethasone.
    c. Early hydrocortisone treatment may be beneficial in a specific population of patients; however, there is insufficient evidence to recommend its use for all infants at risk of BPD.
    d. All of the above
3. Which of the following treatments has been proven to prevent BPD?
    a. Antioxidants
    b. Surfactant
    c. Caffeine
    d. Vitamin E
    e. Inhaled glucocortioids

Chapter 4

1. A 41 weeks' gestation infant is born after induction of labor. There was thick particulate meconium at delivery. The neonatal resuscitation team that received the infant did initial resuscitation by stimulating the infant and, when there was no respiratory effort, initiated positive pressure ventilation (PPV). The infant eventually required endotracheal intubation and admission to the NICU. A chest x-ray revealed coarse bilateral opacities. Which of the following strategies is recommended in the further management of this infant?
    a. Lung lavage with dilute surfactant
    b. Exogenous surfactant at standard doses
    c. Respiratory alkalosis using high ventilator rates
    d. Routine use of muscle relaxants
2. A preterm infant born at 26 weeks' gestation is now 3 days old, and you are considering initiating trophic enteral feeds. The mother is known to be seropositive for cytomegalovirus (CMV), and she asks you about the risk of transmission of CMV through breast milk and the risk of pneumonia due to CMV. What is your response?
    a. CMV is eliminated by a freeze–thawing process.
    b. CMV only rarely causes pneumonia postnatally.
    c. CMV can cause interstitial pneumonia in preterm infants but can be eliminated by short-term pasteurization.
    d. Provide preterm formula, as the risk of pneumonia is very high.
3. A 5-hour-old infant delivered at term to a mother who was febrile and had rupture of membranes for 28 hours before delivery was noted to have decreased activity, poor feeding, increased work of breathing, and poor saturations. The infant is intubated, and supplemental oxygen has been provided. Which of the following is not indicated in this situation?
    a. Broad-spectrum antibiotics
    b. Maintenance of thermoneutral environment
    c. Assessment of upper and lower saturations
    d. Hyperventilation to achieve alkalosis, known to relax pulmonary vasculature

Chapter 5

1. A term infant has inspiratory stridor noticed in the normal nursery a few hours after birth. The stridor was most noticeable when the infant cried. There were mild retractions but no oxygen desaturation. The mother had gestational diabetes during pregnancy. The infant was born by spontaneous vaginal delivery at 39 weeks after forceps-assisted delivery with a birth weight of 4.3 kg. What is the most likely diagnosis?
    a. Unilateral vocal cord paralysis
    b. Subglottic stenosis
    c. Laryngomalacia
    d. Hemangioma
2. A newborn was born at 36 weeks following spontaneous labor. The mother had late onset of prenatal care, and the fetus was noted to have hydrops. At birth, the infant was noted to have poor respiratory effort and hydrops with skin edema and abdominal distention. Resuscitation included drainage of fluid from the chest and abdominal cavities, and the infant was admitted to the NICU. Examination in the NICU revealed dysmorphic features, down-sloping palpebral fissures, webbed neck, dysplastic pulmonary valve, and cryptorchidism. Analysis of the pleural fluid revealed serosanguinous fluid with lymphocyte predominant cell count. What is the likely diagnosis?
    a. Congenital empyema
    b. Immune hydrops
    c. Cardiac failure
    d. Chylothorax
3. A newborn with no prenatal care delivers shortly after the mother's arrival to the hospital. He is noted to have mild increased work of breathing, scaphoid abdomen, and decreased breath sounds on the left. Pulses and perfusion are normal for his age. All of the following initial steps are indicated to help this infant *except*:
    a. Provide supplemental oxygen to avoid severe hypoxia.
    b. Expedite CXR.
    c. Maintain normothermic temperature.
    d. Perform needle thoracostomy on the left.

Chapter 6

1. A 32-year-old pregnant mother at 28 weeks' gestation is referred to you for a neonatology prenatal consult. According to the obstetrician, the fetus has reduced fetal movements, thin bones, and polyhydramnios. The ultrasound also notes the near total absence of fetal breathing. How will you explain the significance of the lack of fetal breathing to the mother?
   a. Fetal breathing is not a significant indicator of fetal health.
   b. Lack of fetal breathing implies severe periodic breathing in neonate after birth.
   c. Regular fetal breathing at the rate of 30 to 40/min is essential for establishment of neonatal breathing.
   d. Fetal breathing is essential for lung development.
2. During teaching rounds with medical students, you point out periodic breathing in a 28-week preterm infant who is 2 weeks old. How would you best describe the response of this infant to hypoxia?
   a. Immediate and persistent hyperventilation
   b. Biphasic response, early ventilatory depression, and later hyperventilation
   c. Biphasic response, early hyperventilation, and later ventilatory depression
   d. No predictable response

Chapter 7

1. Which of the following are clinical situations for which ECMO is indicated?
   a. A neonate with transposition of the great arteries who has undergone a successful arterial switch palliation but is unable to maintain adequate blood pressure and oxygenation immediately postoperatively
   b. A 4-day-old with trisomy 21 and overwhelming sepsis and pneumonia on maximal ventilatory support, bilateral pneumothoraces, and an oxygenation index of 60 in spite of maximal medical therapy
   c. A 30-week-old, 1200-g infant with severe RDS unresponsive to multiple doses of surfactant on optimal ventilator support with an oxygenation index of 50
   d. A full-term infant with rupture of membranes at 18 weeks and persistent severe oligohydramnios whose parents chose to continue the pregnancy presents in the delivery room with severe increased work of breathing. The infant remains hypoxic with pO_2 of 20 mmHg and pCO_2 of 110 mmHg in spite of aggressive maximal cardiorespiratory support. A cardiac echocardiogram reveals normal anatomy, right ventricular dysfunction, and significant right to left shunting at the ductal and atrial level. CXR suggests pulmonary hypoplasia.
2. You are considering initiating iNO therapy for a 37-week-old infant of a diabetic mother with severe RDS. Which of the following is not indicated prior to initiation of iNO?
   a. Cardiac echocardiogram
   b. CXR
   c. Optimized lung expansion and ventilator support

   d. Surfactant replacement
   e. Steroid therapy
3. The only respiratory support that utilizes active inspiration and active expiration is:
   a. JET ventilation
   b. Volume targeted ventilation
   c. Pressure control ventilation
   d. Oscillatory ventilation
4. Which of the following regarding iNO is accurate?
   a. Starting dose is 40 ppm.
   b. It can be quickly weaned if started <2 hours earlier.
   c. iNO half-life is 15 to 20 seconds.
   d. iNO is FDA approved to treat left ventricular failure.
5. Effects of dexamethasone include all but which of the following?
   a. Improves compliance
   b. Decreases inflammation
   c. Increases risk of CP
   d. Increases risk of GI perforation when used in first 8 days
   e. Improves linear growth
6. Indications for JET ventilation include:
   a. Nonhomogeneous lung disease (e.g., aspiration pneumonitis)
   b. Air leak (pneumothorax, PIE)
   c. Pulmonary hypoplasia
   d. Cardiac compromise when high-frequency ventilation is indicated
   e. All of the above

Chapter 8

1. An infant was born with truncus arteriosus. What embryologic event led to this anomaly?
   a. Failure of the conotruncus to septate
   b. Failure of the second heart field cells to migrate
   c. Failure of the conotruncus to rotate
   d. Abnormal development of the 6th arch
2. The most common cyanotic congenital heart defect seen in infants of diabetic mothers is which of the following?
   a. d-Transposition of the great arteries
   b. Hypoplastic left heart syndrome
   c. Tricuspid atresia
   d. Tetralogy of Fallot

Chapter 9

1. Physiologic responses to asphyxia include which of the following?
   a. Tachycardia, decreased central venous pressure, vasoconstriction of the cerebral vessels
   b. Bradycardia, increased central venous pressure, vasoconstriction of the skeletal muscle vessels
   c. Bradycardia, decreased central venous pressure, vasodilation of the cerebral vessels
   d. Tachycardia, increased central venous pressure, vasoconstriction of the skeletal muscle vessels
2. Fetal stress is accompanied by which of the following cardiovascular changes?
   a. End-diastolic velocities increase in the umbilical artery

b. Development of a reverse S wave in the ductus venosus
c. Venous pulsations in the umbilical venous Doppler tracing
d. End-diastolic velocities increase in the cerebral arteries

Chapter 10

1. A 1-week-old infant with tetralogy of Fallot is undergoing a rule-out sepsis evaluation. The infant's baseline saturations are 98% with a 2/6 systolic ejection murmur along the left sternal border. During the blood draw, the infant's saturations drop to 60%, and the infant becomes visibly cyanotic. On auscultation, the lung sounds remain clear, but the murmur is no longer audible. What interventions should be performed?
   a. Intubation with 100% O_2
   b. STAT echocardiogram
   c. Arterial blood gas
   d. Morphine and phenylephrine administration
2. A newborn infant was found to have interrupted aortic arch type B with truncus arteriosus. What other features is the infant likely to have?
   a. Epicanthal folds with a single palmar crease
   b. Elfin facies
   c. Broad thumbs and toes
   d. Absent thymus on chest x-ray and hypocalcemia

Chapter 11

1. A term infant undergoes echocardiography after birth due to a murmur. Numerous small cardiac tumors are identified throughout the heart. Which genetic disease is likely?
   a. Down syndrome
   b. Williams syndrome
   c. Tuberous sclerosis
   d. Hunter syndrome
2. A 24 weeks' gestation infant (BW 500g) born in the setting of preterm labor without prolonged rupture of membranes is admitted to the NICU after delayed cord clamping. Apgar scores are 7 and 9, and no maternal risk factors have been identified. The infant is intubated in the delivery room due to ineffective respiratory drive given the prematurity. Soon after admission, the infant develops hypotension. What is the most likely pathophysiology?
   a. High afterload
   b. Low preload
   c. Left to right shunting across the PDA
   d. Low systemic vascular resistance

Chapter 12

1. An infant was born at full term to a 29-year-old woman with lupus by cesarean section due to persistent fetal bradycardia. The newborn appears vigorous, with normal capillary refill, blood pressure of 80/55 mmHg, and 2+ femoral pulses. The heart rate, however, is 65 beats/min, with a narrow QRS complex not associated with P waves. What is the best course of action?
   a. Begin isoproterenol.
   b. Begin cardiopulmonary resuscitation.
   c. Monitor closely on telemetry.
   d. Use transcutaneous pacing.
2. A 3-day-old infant suddenly develops tachycardia to 240 beats/min. Adenosine is administered, which slows the ventricular rate briefly to 140 beats/min, revealing a sawtooth-like pattern between the QRS complexes. Transesophageal pacing is used to terminate the tachycardia. Which drug is best to use as prophylaxis to prevent future tachycardia?
   a. Propranolol
   b. No prophylactic therapy is needed.
   c. Digoxin
   d. Amiodarone

Chapter 13

1. An infant with a large ventricular septal defect and congestive heart failure is being medically managed with digoxin, enalapril, and furosemide (Lasix). Spironolactone was added yesterday due to persistent hypokalemia. Overnight, the infant developed Mobitz II heart block. This is a toxicity of which medication?
   a. Spironolactone
   b. Digoxin
   c. Enalapril
   d. Lasix
2. A 10-day-old infant is being treated for sepsis with antibiotics and dopamine. The infant is requiring escalating doses of dopamine. All of the interventions below can increase the infant's response to the current dose of dopamine, except for one. Which intervention does not increase an infant's sensitivity to catecholamines?
   a. Beginning steroid administration
   b. Normalizing pH
   c. Normalizing serum calcium levels
   d. Normalizing potassium levels

Chapter 14

1. A 5-day-old infant presents with hypotonia. Which of the following findings would raise suspicion for a diagnosis of spinal muscular atrophy?
   a. Hypotonic facies
   b. Seizures found on EEG
   c. Absent deep tendon reflexes
   d. Poor feeding requiring NG
2. A 12-hour-old newborn is noted to have an asymmetric Moro with absent left-sided Moro. Where does this injury localize to?
   a. Right-sided MCA stroke
   b. Left-sided MCA stroke
   c. Left brachial plexus
   d. Right brachial plexus
3. A 2-day-old born at 26 weeks' GA has acute decrease in hematocrit and was found to have bilateral grade III IVH on cranial ultrasound. Patient is noted to have increased

number of apnea/bradycardia events clinically. Which of the following features on neurologic exam would support a diagnosis of acute increased intracranial pressure?
a. Tight at the popliteal angles
b. Absent dazzle reflex
c. Increased deep tendon reflexes
d. 4 beats of clonus unilaterally

Chapter 15

1. You are called to consult with a 25-year-old mother whose first child is wheelchair-bound due to a lumbar myelomeningocele. Her pregnancy history is significant for tobacco smoking and occasional cocaine use. She is now at 8 weeks' gestation, has started taking a prenatal vitamin this week, has stopped her acne medication this week, and is taking an antiemetic as needed. She is very worried about the risk of this baby being born with a myelomeningocele. Which of the following is true in regard to the recurrence risk?
a. She is reducing the risk of recurrence by starting a prenatal vitamin with folic acid in the first trimester.
b. Her cocaine use increases the risk of recurrence in this pregnancy.
c. Smoking cessation prior to pregnancy greatly reduces the incidence of myelomeningocele.
d. The recurrence risk is greater if this baby has the same father as her first child.
e. Acne medications do not affect the rate of myelomeningocele.

2. You are called to a term vaginal delivery due to fetal forebrain anomalies. Prenatal ultrasounds note no separation of cerebral hemispheres concerning for agenesis of the corpus callosum. Parents declined genetic testing during pregnancy. Parents have no known genetic anomalies. There are no notable infections or alcohol use in pregnancy. The infant born is male, well appearing with normal vital signs, and has no visible anomalies after birth. Parents would like to know what the next steps are after delivery and what the chances are of their baby not having anything wrong in their brain.
a. The infant should stay with her parents and have a head ultrasound prior to discharge; 75% chance the infant will not have agenesis of the corpus callosum.
b. The infant should be admitted to the NICU and an MRI of the brain should be performed urgently; 25% chance the infant will not have agenesis of the corpus callosum.
c. The infant should stay with her parents and undergo an MRI of the brain non-urgently; 25% chance the infant will have agenesis of the corpus callosum.
d. The infant should stay with her parents and have chromosomal analysis prior to discharge; 100% chance the infant will have agenesis of the corpus callosum, as this has already been noted prenatally.

3. A male infant born at 24 weeks, gestation is now 3 months old. He has a history of bronchopulmonary dysplasia and grade III intraventricular hemorrhage bilaterally. Over the past 3 weeks, his head circumference has been increasing rapidly, now crossing growth percentiles from the 25th to 50th percentile. The infant has been well until today when he started having episodes of apnea, with normal respiratory rate between these events and lethargy. The infant has stable vital signs. What would be your next step to care for this infant?
a. Page the neurosurgical team emergently to evaluate the patient.
b. Obtain an MRI emergently.
c. Intubate the infant to protect his airway.
d. Begin a sepsis evaluation and obtain a head ultrasound.

4. A 23-week preterm infant was born urgently without maternal steroids given. The infant receives indomethacin for neuroprotection. What is the appropriate mechanism of action on cerebral blood flow in this infant?
a. Decreases cerebral blood flow by prostaglandin inhibition
b. Decreases cerebral blood flow by antagonistic effects on adenosine
c. Increases cerebral blood flow by prostaglandin stimulation
d. Decreases cerebral blood flow by increased calcium levels

Chapter 16

1. You are admitting a newborn with suspected hypoxic–ischemic encephalopathy (HIE). Based on the physical exam, you are attempting to stage the infant based on Sarnat staging. On exam, you note that the infant is lethargic and floppy and exhibits an exaggerated grasp reflex and weak suck reflex. How would this infant be classified?
a. Mild HIE
b. Moderate HIE
c. Severe HIE
d. Normal infant
e. None of the above

2. You are clinically caring for a term infant that underwent therapeutic cooling following a cord prolapse prior to delivery with Sarnat staging consistent with moderate to severe HIE based on exam. The infant receives an MRI that reveals injury to deep gray matter or posterior limb of internal capsule. This is often associated with which of the following?
a. Adverse motor deficits
b. Mild speech deficits
c. Moderate memory deficits
d. No adverse deficits

Chapter 17

1. The appropriate time frame at which periventricular leukomalacia (cystic PVL) can first be identified is:
a. Just after birth (first 24 hours)
b. After 4 weeks of life
c. At 7 days after birth
d. After discharge home

2. Which neonate is at greatest risk of developing a significant intracranial hemorrhage?
a. Term infant after a vacuum-assisted delivery
b. A 32-week infant born after induction for maternal preeclampsia

c. A 26-week infant born after placental abruption who requires intubation and chest compressions at the time of birth
d. A 39-week IDM infant delivered after 5 minutes of shoulder dystocia

Chapter 18

1. A newborn presents to the ER after a home water birth and unknown breech presentation with subsequent head and left arm entrapment for 10 minutes. The infant was limp and had no respiratory effort and required resuscitation after birth. Significant traction and torsion were required to deliver the arm and head. The neonate is encephalopathic with some response to stimulation, few spontaneous movements, and poor tone. Given the history, in addition to HIE, which of the following birth injuries would be most likely to be identified in this patient?
   a. Cephalohematoma
   b. Skull fracture
   c. Brachial plexus injury
   d. High cervical spine injury
2. You are called to the well-baby nursery to evaluate a 2-hour-old term infant who was born after a prolonged second stage of labor and required forceps followed by vacuum application times three. The nursing staff is concerned that the baby appears pale and the head feels boggy. You assess the infant and agree that the baby is pale and poorly perfused with a fluctuant-feeling scalp that is diffuse around the head. You are most concerned about which of the following conditions depicted in Fig. 18.1?
   a. Caput
   b. Cephalohematoma
   c. Subgaleal hemorrhage
   d. Extradural hemorrhage
3. You are informed that the head circumference has increased by 2 cm over 1 hour. How much blood could this represent?
   a. 100 cc
   b. 20 cc
   c. 40 cc
   d. 80 cc
4. What is the next step in management of this patient?
   a. Continued monitoring of infant in mother's room with vital sign checks every 4 hours
   b. Close observation in well-baby nursery environment
   c. No follow-up needed
   d. Admission to NICU with placement of umbilical lines, volume resuscitation, and blood transfusion

Chapter 19

1. A term infant is born after an uncomplicated pregnancy and delivery. When the infant is 3 hours old, he begins to exhibit lethargy, poor feeding, and movements concerning for seizure. Upon admission to the neonatal intensive care unit, he requires intubation for apnea. Frequent seizures are confirmed on electroencephalography (EEG). The infant continues to have seizures despite treatment with three different antiepileptic medications. After administration of another substance, the infant's seizures cease. What is the most likely diagnosis?
   a. Maple syrup urine disease
   b. Hypoxic–ischemic encephalopathy
   c. Pyridoxine-dependent seizures
   d. Subdural hematoma
   e. Kernicterus
2. An infant is admitted to the NICU with seizures and associated finding of failed hearing screen. EKG is obtained and shows a prolonged long QT. Other workups and electrolytes are normal. Jervell and Lange-Nielsen syndrome is suspected as the underlying diagnosis leading to seizures. The parents ask what is the cause of the syndrome.
   a. Autosomal dominant mutation in sodium channels
   b. Autosomal recessive mutation in potassium channels
   c. Autosomal dominant mutation in potassium channels
   d. X-Linked recessive mutation in potassium channels

Chapter 20

1. Which is the most common pathogen isolated in meningitis in very low birth weight infants?
   a. Group B *Streptococcus* (GBS)
   b. *Escherichia coli*
   c. *Candida* spp.
   d. *Staphylococcus epidermidis*
2. Which of the following is incorrect regarding neonatal HSV infections?
   a. HSV-2 is responsible for the majority of cases.
   b. Almost all infections occur around the time of delivery.
   c. Skin lesions are typically the presenting feature of CNS HSV infections.
   d. Early and continued administration of acyclovir improves neurodevelopmental outcomes.
3. A 34-weeks' gestation neonate presented with temperature instability, irritability, and bulging fontanelle. CSF was obtained, and culture was positive for gram-negative bacteria. The baby was treated with appropriate antibiotics; however, 2 weeks later, the infant developed focal-motor seizures and fevers. What is the most appropriate step in determining etiology and treatment?
   a. Repeat CSF studies.
   b. Broaden antibiotic coverage.
   c. Add corticosteroids.
   d. Obtain neuroimaging.
4. Which of the following antibiotics is associated with ototoxicity and long-term hearing impairment?
   a. Vancomycin
   b. Ampicillin
   c. Cefotaxime
   d. Acyclovir
5. A 48-hour-old term baby, born at home, presents with poor feeding, irritability, hypothermia, and seizure-like activity. CSF is obtained, which shows pleocytosis (1800 WBCs), 11% neutrophils, 21% lymphocytes, and 68% monocytes with a protein of 205 and glucose of 22. What is the most likely pathogen?
   a. Group B *Streptococcus* (GBS)
   b. *Listeria monocytogenes*
   c. *Candida* spp.
   d. *Escherichia coli*

6. A 28-week-old, 1250-g neonate developed temperature instability, need for increased respiratory support, and vital sign instability. He is currently being treated for candidiasis, and you suspect systemic infection. Which of the following are you most likely to see on CSF studies?
   a. Elevated protein and normal glucose
   b. Normal protein and normal glucose
   c. Elevated protein and low glucose
   d. a, b, or c

Chapter 21

1. You are called to see a 50-hour-old term neonate for tremors, emesis, diarrhea, crying, and 12% weight loss. The maternal history is significant for maternal opiate dependence on buprenorphine 16 mg daily. Social history reveals cigarette smoking, half a pack per day. Prenatal course was otherwise uncomplicated with normal anatomic scan. Urine toxicology screens during pregnancy and on admission were all negative. Labor and delivery were unremarkable. Which of the following statements about this neonate is true?
   a. If the mother was treated with methadone instead of buprenorphine, the baby would likely have less significant withdrawal.
   b. The mother should be counseled against breastfeeding, given her dose of buprenorphine.
   c. Modified Finnegan abstinence scoring should be initiated to confirm the diagnosis of NAS.
   d. This patient will likely require increased caloric density and volume of feeds.
   e. The mother was noncompliant with her buprenorphine therapy before delivery.
2. You are counseling a birthing parent who is on prescription opioids for pain management about the effects and risks to the infant for the development of neonatal abstinence syndrome. Which of the following does not correlate to the overall severity of NAS symptoms in the neonate?
   a. Tobacco use
   b. Absolute dose of maternal opioid agonist medication
   c. Polysubstance exposures
   d. Duration of prescription opioids during pregnancy
3. Upon routine first-day examination of a full-term infant, you notice the infant has a smooth philtrum with a thin upper-lip vermillion border, short palpebral fissures, and hypoplastic nails. Which of the following is true about the underlying diagnosis?
   a. It is a diagnosis that has a dose-dependent spectrum of fetal and neonatal effects.
   b. Withdrawal symptoms do not occur.
   c. Behavior and IQ are unaffected.
   d. It is associated with fetal macrosomia.

Chapter 22

1. A 2-day-old infant born at 38 weeks requires intubation at birth secondary to poor respiratory effort. The pregnancy and delivery were otherwise uncomplicated. The following day, she fails an extubation trial. On your examination, you note an intubated baby who awakens easily to your examination but holds her mouth open around the endotracheal tube. She has bilateral talipes equinovarus. You note decreased spontaneous movements with a frog-leg position and significant head lag. You are unable to obtain deep tendon reflexes. Which of the following points in the history can lead to the final diagnosis?
   a. Maternal report of decreased fetal movements
   b. Maternal report of prior fetal losses
   c. Maternal report of hand weakness
   d. Maternal report of alcohol use during pregnancy
2. A 2-hour-old neonate born at 39 weeks, 6 days is examined for possible therapeutic hypothermia secondary to concern for hypoxic-ischemic encephalopathy. He was born to a 24-year-old G1 mother with gestational diabetes. The delivery was complicated by shoulder dystocia, with Apgar scores of 1, 1, and 2 at 1, 5, and 10 minutes of life. Initial blood gas pH in the baby is 6.9, with a base deficit of 13. On examination, the neonate is noted to be lying still with arms extended. On attempts to arouse him with stimulation, he is noted to make spontaneous movements; however, he returns to his initial state once you stop stimulation. On forced eye opening, you note small but reactive pupils. He is noted to have an incomplete Moro response and absent suck with gag reflex present. On tests of tone, you note a frog-leg position and excessive head lag. Deep tendon reflexes are brisk with spread to the adjacent joint. He is intubated but is noted to be breathing over the ventilator rate without difficulty. Which of the following best describes his level of encephalopathy based on his examination?
   a. Normal
   b. Mild encephalopathy
   c. Moderate encephalopathy
   d. Severe encephalopathy
3. A 1-day-old term neonate in the newborn nursery is noted to have a port-wine birthmark over the forehead bilaterally, extending to the frontonasal prominence. On exam, he is noted to be alert; he visually engages and fixates; and he has symmetric facies, normal tone, and brisk symmetric reflexes at 2, with intact palmar and plantar grasp as well as Moro. Which of the following is the best next step in his care?
   a. Cranial ultrasound prior to discharge home
   b. Referral to pediatric ophthalmology
   c. Referral for MRI with and without contrast
   d. Routine newborn follow-up/no additional evaluation
4. A prenatal echocardiogram raises concern for cardiac rhabdomyoma. Which of the following imaging findings may be seen postnatally?
   a. Intraventricular hemorrhage
   b. Perinatal arterial ischemic stroke
   c. Perisylvian polymicrogyria
   d. Subependymal nodules
5. A 14-day-old born at term is noted to have new onset of focal clonic movements confirmed as seizures on cEEG. Pregnancy was reported as unremarkable; Apgar scores at birth were 8/9. No reported feeding difficulties prior to delivery. On exam, patient is afebrile, breathing comfortably prior to treatment with antiseizure medications, and appears alert with normal tone. Skin is notable for

vesicular lesions over the chest, which the mother noted started on the day prior to admission. HSV PCR from the lesion is negative. Blood cultures are negative, and CBC is notable for eosinophilic predominance. CSF demonstrates 0 WBC, 10 RBCs, normal protein and glucose, and negative bacterial CSF cultures. HSV PCR is negative in the CSF. Which of the following disorders is most likely?
   a. Incontinentia pigmenti
   b. Pigmentary mosaicism
   c. Zellweger syndrome
   d. Tuberous sclerosis

6. Anatomy ultrasound at 22 weeks' gestation raises a concern for ventriculomegaly with potential mass present. At 35 weeks, there is ongoing enlargement of the ventricles, raising concern for hydrocephalus with macrocrania on ultrasound. Fetal MRI raises suspicion for a tumor arising from the third ventricle. Which of the following is indicated?
   a. Routine medical care with early consultation with oncology postnatally
   b. Consideration of delivery by C-section
   c. Neurosurgical consult for fetal biopsy
   d. cEEG for seizures postnatally

Chapter 23

1. An infant is born via stat cesarean section for cord prolapse prior to delivery and is assigned Apgar scores of 1, 3, and 5. The infant is intubated in the delivery room and spontaneously breathing at 8 minutes of life. Cord arterial gas is pH 6.90 with base excess of −18. The infant's neurological exam at 1 hour of life shows lethargy, decreased spontaneous activity, distal flexion, hypotonia, weak suck and incomplete Moro, and normal heart rate; the infant is periodically breathing above the ventilator. Based on your assessment, how would you classify the degree of encephalopathy and qualification for therapeutic cooling?
   a. Mild encephalopathy; do not initiate therapeutic cooling.
   b. Mild encephalopathy; initiate therapeutic cooling.
   c. Moderate encephalopathy; initiate therapeutic cooling.
   d. Severe encephalopathy; initiate therapeutic cooling.

2. In neonates born extremely prematurely at less than 25 weeks' gestation, all of the following are protective or mitigating factors at reducing neurodevelopmental impairment *except*:
   a. Betamethasone prior to delivery
   b. Dexamethasone use in the first week of life
   c. Antenatal magnesium sulfate
   d. Systematic resuscitation with early surfactant delivery

3. In neonates who have experienced fetal growth restriction, the morphologic structure and functionality of their brains exhibit:
   a. Increased total cerebral volume and total number of brain cells
   b. Thicker cortical thickness and abnormal gyration
   c. Acceleration in myelination
   d. Reduced structural complexity of gray and white matter

Chapter 24

1. A male infant born at 23 weeks' gestation, 500 g, is now 2 weeks old and remains mechanically ventilated with difficulty weaning on ventilator. The infant is placed in the prone position for all of the following associated physiologic effects *except*:
   a. Increased respiratory rate
   b. Improved chest wall synchrony
   c. Increased rate of gastric emptying
   d. Improved gas exchange

2. A former 24 weeks' gestation infant born at 650 g is now 2 months old with a clinical course complicated by necrotizing enterocolitis and subsequent bowel resection of terminal ileum and proximal colon. There is a risk of malabsorption and deficiency of which of the following nutrients?
   a. Vitamin B_{12}
   b. Copper
   c. Zinc
   d. Iron

3. Socioeconomic status and access to care and resources contribute to the multifactorial causes contributing to health disparities amongst families and their neonates. One important factor contributing to health disparities is the mother–infant dyad. Those with poor attachment and bonding have the following outcome:
   a. Lower rates of child abuse as it pertains to negligence
   b. Lower rates of breastfeeding but higher rates of feeding by pumped breast milk
   c. Higher rates of failure to thrive
   d. Developmental delay primarily related to vision and memory

4. Which of the following nutrient deficiencies in pregnancy is appropriately associated with its fetal/neonate outcome?
   a. Zinc—blindness
   b. Folate—spina bifida
   c. Vitamin D—deafness
   d. Iodine—hyperthyroidism

Chapter 25

1. A mother brings her now 18-month-old infant for developmental follow-up at your clinic. The infant was born at 25 weeks' gestation and had an uneventful NICU course after initial low Apgar scores with intubation. The infant extubated to CPAP on day of life 2 and weaned to room air by 32 weeks of life with left-sided grade I IVH followed through the NICU course. The mother asks what the Bayley assessment will determine. You explain:
   a. The infant's intelligence quotient (IQ) will be determined with a score of 100 as the mean and a 15-point standard deviation.
   b. The scoring system is devised to control for effects of environmental exposure the infant has had since discharge.
   c. The scoring system will not be affected by visual, hearing, attention, or behavioral issues.

d. The purpose of the system is to detect developmental delay to direct early intervention services.

e. The system will determine developmental functioning of infants and young children from birth to 42 months of age.

2. A mother used assisted reproductive technologies to become pregnant, which resulted in a twin gestation. The di-di female infants are born at 31 weeks + 3 days gestational age weighing 1505 g and 1570 g after the mother goes into preterm labor and is found to have chorioamnionitis. The mother is otherwise well on prenatal vitamins and levothyroxine for hypothyroidism. Which factors in this pregnancy are not risk factors for developing cerebral palsy in the infants?

a. Female gender of the infants

b. The use of assisted reproductive technologies

c. The development of chorioamnionitis in the mother

d. The history of hypothyroidism

e. The twin gestation

3. Which of the following neonates will have the highest chance of developing neurodevelopmental impairments during their lives?

a. 28-week infant born with inadequate maternal steroid administration

b. 23-week infant born after preterm labor

c. 30-week infant who developed necrotizing enterocolitis at 34 weeks

d. 27-week infant who developed BPD

e. 39-week infant with meconium aspiration who developed pulmonary hypertension

Chapter 26

1. An infant is successfully resuscitated following vaginal delivery at 23 0/7 weeks due to intrauterine infection. You are concerned that this patient could quickly develop overwhelming sepsis due to her extreme prematurity and exposure to infection. Which of the following immune-related factors does not contribute to this patient's increased susceptibility to infection?

a. An underdeveloped stratum corneum increases the permeability of skin to pathogens.

b. Definitive hematopoiesis (bone marrow–derived) begins at 28 weeks' gestation, so extremely premature infants rely on primitive hematopoietic immune lineages for protection.

c. There is impaired interferon-γ production by T cells and monocytes in neonates.

d. Preterm infants and full-term neonates have decreased lectin-mediated complement activation.

Chapter 27

1. In accordance with guidelines, a newborn screen was carried out prior to the first blood transfusion in an infant born at 23 0/7 weeks' gestational age. The screening test is positive for severe combined immunodeficiency (SCID), showing low, but not absent, T cell receptor excision circles (TRECs). The most appropriate next step for this patient is which of the following?

a. Urgent hematology and oncology consult to assess for bone marrow transplantation candidacy

b. Newborn screen repeated until patient reaches term-equivalent gestational age

c. Antimicrobial prophylaxis started with sulfamethoxazole-trimethoprim (Bactrim)

d. Blood specimen sent to laboratory for measurement of lymphocyte subsets by flow cytometry

2. Vaccines against *Haemophilus influenzae* type b and *Pneumococcus* infections are highly successful in reducing the incidence of invasive disease. The vaccine platform against these pathogens is well tailored for the neonatal immune system in that:

a. The polysaccharide antigen is T independent, and the protein toxin enables T cell help in inducing B cell memory differentiation and antibody class switching.

b. They contain monophosphoryl lipid A adjuvant, which boosts a newborn's naïve adaptive response.

c. The antigens are recombinant proteins, which more specifically target antigen-specific naïve T cells and therefore generate more effective memory.

d. The polysaccharide antigen is conjugated to a DNA fragment, which provides costimulation of antigen-specific T cells through Toll-like receptors.

3. A term newborn's antibody concentration at birth is which of the following?

a. Higher in IgG compared to maternal circulation due to active transport across the placenta

b. High in IgA due to mucosal immune responses

c. High in maternal IgM in the setting of maternal infection with *Toxoplasmosis*

d. Similar in IgE due to passive transport across the placenta

Chapter 28

1. You are asked to evaluate a term infant born 4 hours ago by scheduled cesarean section for persistent central cyanosis. The infant is male, appropriate weight for gestational age, and appears in no distress. Vital signs are within normal limits with the exception of oxygen saturation, which measures 81% preductal and postductal. Your examination reveals a hyperdynamic precordium with a single S2 and a regurgitant murmur. You obtain an x-ray, which shows dextroposition of the heart and a midline liver and stomach. You determine that, when stable, this infant may ultimately require antimicrobial prophylaxis with which of the following?

a. Bactrim due to high risk for *Pneumocystis* pneumonia

b. IVIG due to low antibody levels

c. Amoxicillin due to high risk for infection with encapsulated bacteria

d. FFP to restore complement levels

2. A term infant is admitted to the NICU for evaluation and management of her prenatally diagnosed pulmonary stenosis. On examination, she is found to have hypertelorism, hooded lids, a short philtrum, and micrognathia. Her oral examination reveals a bifid uvula. Her postnatal

echocardiogram shows anatomy consistent with tetralogy of Fallot, and there is adequate flow through the outflow tract without prostaglandins. Her vital signs remain stable on the monitors. Electrolytes remain within normal limits with the exception of a low ionized calcium level detected on day of life 4. The tests most likely to reveal a contraindication to live vaccine administration in this patient include which of the following?

   a. Lymphocyte subsets by flow cytometry
   b. Complement levels
   c. Complete blood count with differential
   d. Immunoglobulin levels

3. A term infant presents to the special care nursery with a 24-hour total serum bilirubin of 13 (11.9 indirect, 1.1 direct). The mother's blood type is O, Rh+. The infant's blood type is B, Rh+, and her hematocrit and reticulocyte counts are 38 and 9.2%, respectively. In this setting, the likely mechanism of the therapeutic effect of intravenous immunoglobulin is which of the following?

   a. IVIG inhibits NK cell activation.
   b. IVIG saturates B-antigen sites on the erythrocytes, thereby blocking maternal antibodies from attaching.
   c. IVIG binds to Fc portion of anti-B maternal antibodies, rendering bound erythrocytes "invisible" to the infant's immune system.
   d. IVIG saturates Fc receptor on infant's phagocytes, thereby blocking recognition and destruction of antibody-bound erythrocytes.

4. A healthy-appearing term infant presents with a newborn screen that is positive for severe combined immunodeficiency (SCID). The laboratory report details that the T cell receptor excision circle content is "absent." Lymphocyte subsets by flow cytometry reveal a T-negative, B-positive, NK-positive SCID phenotype. The most likely genetic defect explaining this patient's T cell deficiency is which of the following?

   a. Absent IL-7 α-receptor expression, leading to T cell maturation defects
   b. RAG1 deficiency (Omenn syndrome), causing defective T cell receptor production
   c. Low CD40L expression, causing T cell cycle arrest
   d. Low adenosine deaminase (ADA) expression, leading to accelerated apoptosis of T cells

5. A 26-week-old infant presents at birth in shock from *Escherichia coli* sepsis and is found to have an absolute neutrophil count of 500/mL, which falls to 200/mL on a subsequent CBC. Which of the following is most accurate regarding medical therapy for sepsis-induced neutropenia?

   a. Dexamethasone increases the absolute neutrophil count by stimulating bone marrow production.
   b. IVIG improves sepsis outcomes by blocking complement-induced cytolysis and neutrophil consumption.
   c. Granulocyte-colony stimulating factor (G-CSF) increases bone marrow monocyte and neutrophil production.
   d. G-CSF will improve neutrophil count by stimulating bone marrow neutrophil production.

6. A term infant is admitted to the NICU for tachypnea and increased work of breathing after delivery complicated by preeclampsia. On physical examination, he is found to have a narrow chest but otherwise appears normal. A chest radiograph reveals a narrow chest, increased vascular markings, and fluid in the minor fissure. Some long bones also have metaphyseal sclerosis. A CBC with differential shows an absolute neutrophil count of 500 cells/mL, absolute lymphocyte count of 700/mL, hemoglobin of 9.4 g/dL, and platelets of 110×10^3/mL. His blood cultures remain negative, the absolute neutrophil count (ANC) improves to >1500 cells/mL, his respiratory symptoms resolve, and he is discharged to home. He is seen repeatedly at the pediatrician for foul-smelling, oily stools; recurrent respiratory infections; and persistent growth failure. His CBC again shows anemia (Hgb, 7.6 g/dL) and neutropenia (400 cells/mL). This patient's most likely diagnosis is which of the following?

   a. Cystic fibrosis
   b. Asphyxiating thoracic dystrophy
   c. Shwachman-Diamond syndrome
   d. Hemophagocytic lymphohistiocytosis

Chapter 29

1. What are the major causes of neonatal early-onset sepsis?
   a. Group B beta-hemolytic streptococci, *Escherichia coli*, and *Listeria monocytogenes*
   b. *Candida albicans*, coagulase-negative staphylococci, and *Staphylococcus aureus*
   c. Enteroviruses and herpes simplex viruses

2. What are the major causes of neonatal late-onset sepsis?
   a. Group B beta-hemolytic streptococci
   b. *Escherichia coli* and *Listeria monocytogenes*
   c. Coagulase-negative staphylococci and group D enterococci
   d. All of the above

3. A 2-day-old preterm neonate is found to have increasing apnea, tachycardia, and tachypnea. What are the optimal diagnostic tests to diagnose sepsis and meningitis?
   a. Complete blood count and differential (CBC/diff), CRP, and procalcitonin
   b. CBC/diff, CRP, head ultrasound, chest radiograph, and blood culture
   c. CBC/diff, blood culture, and lumbar puncture for CSF analysis and culture
   d. CBC/diff, CRP, and blood culture

Chapter 30

1. Which of the following statements is true concerning neonatal group B beta-hemolytic streptococcal meningitis (GBS meningitis)?
   a. Early-onset GBS disease (0–7 days of chronologic age) is more likely to include meningitis than is disease that occurs later.
   b. Late-onset GBS disease (7–90 days of chronologic age) is more likely to include meningitis than is disease that occurs earlier.
   c. GBS meningitis occurs at equal incidence rates throughout the first 3 months of chronologic age.

2. When is syphilis most commonly transmitted to the fetus?
   a. Transmission decreases as pregnancy continues toward term.
   b. Transmission increases as pregnancy continues toward term.
   c. Transmission occurs more often in mothers with advanced syphilis (latent infection more often than primary or secondary infection).
   d. Transmission occurs more often in mothers with early syphilis (primary or secondary infection more often than latent infection).
   e. a and c above.
   f. b and d above.
3. What is the leading non genetic cause of congenital sensorineural hearing loss?
   a. Congenital syphilis
   b. Congenital rubella
   c. Neonatal group B beta-hemolytic streptococcal meningitis
   d. Congenital cytomegalovirus infection
   e. Congenital toxoplasmosis

Chapter 31

1. Intrapartum antibiotic prophylaxis has significantly reduced the incidence of which of the following infections in the United States?
   a. Late-onset sepsis from group B streptococci (GBS)
   b. Both early-onset and late-onset sepsis from GBS
   c. Early-onset sepsis from GBS
   d. Syphilis
2. A baby is born to an HIV-infected mother who is in excellent virologic control with undetectable plasma HIV viral load. What is the appropriate schedule for HIV virologic testing to best exclude infection in the neonate?
   a. Weekly for the first 6 months of life (6 tests in all)
   b. At 2 to 3 weeks, 4 to 8 weeks, and 4 to 6 months of age (three tests in all)
   c. No testing is indicated, as transmission is unlikely enough so as not to be needed
   d. At birth and at 12 months of age (two tests in all)
3. A pregnant woman was exposed to varicella 3 days ago; she is currently in labor. Which of the following additional scenarios would be an indication to give VariZIG varicella immune globulin therapy to her neonate when it is delivered?
   a. The pregnant woman is in labor at 27 weeks, gestation.
   b. The pregnant woman is in labor at term and has a history of varicella immunization before pregnancy.
   c. The pregnant woman had varicella infection (chickenpox) 3 weeks before her labor began at term.
   d. Upon further information, you find out that actually the pregnant woman has shingles right now, and she is at 35 weeks' gestation.
   e. All of the above

Chapter 32

1. During the third trimester of fetal growth, the largest fractional increase in body composition is the result of:
   a. Water
   b. Fat

c. Brain
d. Lean body mass
2. Essential amino acids are
   a. Used for oxidation
   b. Used for protein synthesis
   c. Used for growth of the brain
   d. Required as part of nutrient supplies
   e. All of the above
3. Which of the following is false?
   a. Basal energy requirements are about 50 kcal/kg/d for most preterm infants.
   b. Growth requires an additional 15 kcal/kg/d for lean mass growth and 20 to 30 kcal/kg/d for fat mass growth (in the third trimester).
   c. Physical activity requires a large increase in energy supply to prevent growth faltering.
   d. Stool energy losses and heat losses to the environment are small.
4. Which of the following regarding neonatal nutrition is false?
   a. Rates of protein synthesis and the requirements for amino acid and protein supply to meet them are the same in preterm infants as in normally growing fetuses of the same gestational age.
   b. The critical amount of amino acid or protein nitrogen for preventing growth faltering in very preterm infants <30 to 32 weeks is less than 1.5 g/kg/d.
   c. There is no advantage to protein metabolism or growth (body weight or composition) with more than 3.5 to 4.0 g/kg/d parenterally or 4.0 to 4.5 g/kg/d enterally in very preterm infants.
   d. Excess amino acid or protein intake almost always produces higher blood urea and ammonia concentrations, but these seldom are in toxic ranges.
5. Which of the following are true?
   a. Preterm infants cannot synthesize the two primary LC-PUFAs, linoleic acid and α-linolenic acid.
   b. Clinical cases of essential fatty acid deficiency are relatively rare, even in very preterm infants, because of IV lipid emulsion and enteral milk/formula feeding.
   c. The primary end-product LC-PUFAs (DHA and ARA) are produced from α-linolenic acid and linoleic acid, respectively.
   d. Both DHA and ARA are important for neuronal development in the fetal and preterm infant brain.
6. Which of the following is false?
   a. Energy intake above 90 to 110 kcal/kg/d will promote more net protein balance.
   b. Energy intake from 90 to 110 kcal/kg/d will reduce amino acid oxidation and support protein synthesis.
   c. Energy above 90 to 110 kcal/kg/d will produce more body fat.
   d. Energy intake from 90 to 110 kcal/kg/d is necessary to support basal metabolic rate and energy production and provide sufficient fatty acids for brain growth and development.
7. Preterm infants often grow more slowly than normal healthy fetuses of the same gestational age because (choose the one *incorrect* answer):
   a. They are often not provided enough nutrition support to grow.

b. They often experience stressful, catabolic clinical conditions.

c. Preterm birth prevents the capacity for growth.

d. Treatments, such as steroids, catecholamines, diuretics, and ventilation, are catabolic.

Chapter 33

1. Which of the following is *true* about calcium and phosphorus supplements for preterm infants?
    a. Calcium and phosphorus are readily absorbed from the preterm infant GI tract and do not need to be supplemented.
    b. Calcium and phosphorus are easily soluble in IV nutrition solutions.
    c. Recommended intravenous intakes of calcium are higher than enteral requirements, ranging from 150 to 220 mg/kg/d for calcium.
    d. Risk factors in preterm infants for calcium and phosphorus deficiency and subsequent rickets include gestational age <27 weeks or birth weight <1000 g, long-term parenteral nutrition (>4–5 weeks), severe BPD requiring diuretics and fluid restriction, long-term steroid treatment, a history of necrotizing enterocolitis (NEC), and intolerance to enteral formula or human milk.

2. Which of the following statements about potential manganese (Mn) toxicity is true?
    a. There is a potential for nephrotoxicity.
    b. Mn supplementation should be stopped with any signs of hepatic dysfunction cholestasis.
    c. The contaminant levels of Mn in parenteral nutrient solutions are too low to meet requirements without additional supplementation.
    d. Parenteral calcium gluconate to prevent osteopenia does not contribute to Mn contamination and potential toxicity.

3. The infant of a 29-year-old G2P1 with severe pre-eclampsia at 36 weeks presents with respiratory distress and low tone at birth. Infant demonstrates poor suck that continues at 36 hours. What vitamin/mineral abnormality is the most likely cause?
    a. Hypercalcemia
    b. Hypocalcemia
    c. Hypermagnesemia
    d. Hypomagnesemia

4. An outborn 28-week infant was admitted to the NICU. What vitamin/mineral medication therapy should be confirmed as received at the outside hospital in a timely manner?
    a. Parenteral nutrition trace elements
    b. Oral multivitamin
    c. Vitamin B_{12} injection
    d. Oral folate
    e. Intramuscular vitamin K

5. Which of the following statements is *false* regarding iron supplementation?
    a. The iron content of human milk fortifiers varies among products.
    b. Recommended intake for term and preterm infants is 6 mg/kg/d.

c. Iron toxicity can lead to decreased growth, impaired neurodevelopment, and increased infection risk.

d. Formula-fed infants should receive only iron-fortified formula.

6. The patient is a preterm infant with poor tolerance of human milk fortifier and has been on unfortified donor human milk feeds for 1 week. The nurse reports continued watery stools and a scaly rash in the diaper area. What deficiency should be on the differential?
    a. Vitamin A
    b. Vitamin E
    c. Thiamine
    d. Zinc

Chapter 34

1. Which of the following is a *true* statement regarding human milk being the ideal enteral diet for human neonates?
    a. It provides sufficient energy, protein, fat, carbohydrate, micronutrients, and water for normal metabolism, growth, and development in term infants.
    b. It does not require supplements of protein and certain minerals.
    c. It is enriched in nutrients when it comes from a milk bank as mature donor milk.
    d. It is associated with delayed neurodevelopmental outcomes compared with term formulas.

2. Which of the following statements about a mother's own milk produced at home or in the NICU and stored is *true*?
    a. Varying degrees of nutrient loss may occur with long-term storage, particularly in frozen conditions.
    b. Vitamin C loss does not occur, even during the process of feeding freshly expressed human milk by bottle.
    c. For multiple human milk components, significant degradation generally occurs with even very short-term storage and multiple freeze–thaw cycles.
    d. Donated human breast milk does not contain pathogenic microorganisms that could be transferred to the infants who consume it.

3. Which of the following statements about heat treatment (pasteurization) of human milk are *false*?
    a. Heat treatment (pasteurization) of human milk may reduce the concentration and functional capacity of many bioactive components.
    b. Holder pasteurization does not adversely affect the protein content of donor milk (average value of about −4%).
    c. Total lipid generally is increased (as much as by 60%), but free fatty acids are reduced, which might increase their nutritive potential.
    d. No significant reductions in lactose have been noted, both as free molecules and as part of biologically active compounds such as oligosaccharides.

4. Which of the following is not a contraindication to the use of maternal milk?
    a. Active herpes virus lesions on the breast
    b. Receiving chemotherapy
    c. Positive test for narcotics
    d. Enrolled in a drug treatment program
    e. Human immunodeficiency virus (HIV) infection on antiretroviral therapy

5. The mother of a 2-day-old, former 30-week preterm infant expresses concern about the small amount of milk she has produced, 8 mL per pumping session. What responses would be appropriate?
   a. Acknowledge her concern about the low volumes and offer lactation support to help get the volumes up to a normal level for this stage of lactation.
   b. Inquire about the type of pump she has access to and whether she is comfortable using it.
   c. Provide positive feedback for her efforts to provide milk for her baby and discuss additional ways she will be caring for her infant while in the NICU.
   d. b and c
   e. All of the above

6. Which of the following is *false* regarding how preterm infant formulas differ from term infant formulas?
   a. Higher in calcium and phosphorus for bone mineralization
   b. Higher in protein and whey predominate to support increased protein turnover
   c. Higher in lactose to meet increased energy needs
   d. Fat blends include 20% to 50% MCTs to compensate for lower bile salts and lipases

Chapter 35

1. Which of the following statements regarding TPN and enteral neonatal nutrition is *false*?
   a. Normal fetal metabolic and growth rates and nutritional requirements stop with birth, precluding routine use of IV nutrition.
   b. The smaller, more preterm, and less developed the infant, the less body stores (protein, fat, glycogen) are available to provide nutrients for metabolic needs.
   c. The metabolic and thus nutrient requirements of the newborn are equal to or greater than those of the fetus of the same gestational age.
   d. First-week protein and energy intakes are associated with improved 18-month developmental outcomes in preterm infants.

2. Which of the following statements regarding TPN is *false*?
   a. The amino acid composition of current neonatal parenteral amino acid solutions is based on providing plasma concentrations similar to those of term, fully breastfed infants, which is appropriate for preterm infants who are growing at much faster rates than term infants.
   b. A standard parenteral infusion of 3 g/kg/d amino acids, 10% dextrose, and 3 g/kg/d lipid at 100 mL/kg/d would provide 82 kcal/kg/d, according to the following calculations: 3 g amino acids × 4 kcal/g = 12 kcal; 10 g of dextrose × 4 kcal/g = 40 kcal; 3 g/kg/d of lipid would add 30 kcal/kg/d.
   c. Cholestasis or parenteral nutrition associated liver disease (PNALD) is more common in infants (extremely preterm infants, and those with short gut syndromes such as gastroschisis or those with severe enteral feeding intolerance) who receive parenteral nutrition exclusively and for prolonged periods (weeks vs. days).
   d. The principal metabolic complication of parenteral nutrition is hyperglycemia.

3. Which of the following is not a common contaminant of parenteral nutrition components?
   a. Chromium
   b. Lead
   c. Aluminum
   d. Manganese

4. An 8-day old former 24-week infant is 800 g and has had feeding interruptions due to hemodynamic instability. The infant is currently on small trophic feeds. Current TPN contains 2.2 g amino acids/kg, 6% dextrose, and 1.6 g/kg of fish oil-containing fat emulsion at 4.5 mL/hour via a umbilical venous catheter. What complication of parenteral nutrition is of lowest concern?
   a. Line infection
   b. Inadequate caloric intake
   c. Intestinal failure associated liver disease
   d. Essential fatty acid deficiency

5. Essential amino acids include:
   a. Valine, tryptophan, and isoleucine
   b. Linoleic acid and alpha-linolenic acid
   c. Aspartic acid, glutamic acid, and alanine
   d. Arginine and tyrosine

6. Parenteral nutrition components should be photoprotected due to concerns for:
   a. Phytosterols
   b. Refeeding syndrome
   c. Sepsis risk
   d. Peroxide formation

Chapter 36

1. Nutritive sucking is evident at what gestational age?
   a. 20 weeks
   b. 28 weeks
   c. 32 weeks
   d. 36 weeks

2. Failure of the primitive gut tube to recanalize results in which of the following?
   a. Intestinal atresia
   b. Intestinal malrotation
   c. Intestinal duplication
   d. Gastroschisis

3. Which disaccharidase enzyme activity is reduced by 75% in preterm infants compared to term infants at birth?
   a. Sucrase
   b. Alpha-glucosidases
   c. Dipeptidases
   d. Lactase

4. Peyer patches found in the small intestine contribute to which of the following?
   a. IgA production
   b. Intestinal motility
   c. Bile acid reabsorption
   d. T and B cell activity

5. At what gestational age do the ductal systems of the two buds of the pancreas fuse?
   a. 6 weeks
   b. 8 weeks
   c. 12 weeks
   d. 16 weeks

6. Preterm infants are at increased risk to develop cholestasis due to which of the following?
   a. Sepsis
   b. Decreased bile acid pool
   c. Increased bile acid production
   d. a and b

7. The intrahepatic biliary tree is formed by which gestational week?
   a. 4
   b. 6
   c. 8
   d. 10

8. Omphalocele is the result of which of the following?
   a. Failure of recanalization of the primitive gut tube
   b. Failure of midgut loop to return to the abdominal cavity
   c. Partial rotation of the midgut loop around the superior mesenteric artery (SMA)
   d. Herniation of midgut loop through the abdominal ring

9. Incomplete fusion of the lateral grooves of the primitive foregut results in which of the following?
   a. Tracheoesophageal fistula (TEF)
   b. Duplication cyst
   c. Pancreatic divisum
   d. Biliary atresia

Chapter 37

1. Epstein pearls:
   a. Typically require surgical excision
   b. Can lead to respiratory and/or feeding difficulties
   c. Disappear within one month
   d. Involve the soft palate

2. Which one of the following is not a cause of bilious vomiting?
   a. Intestinal obstruction
   b. GERD
   c. Pyloric stenosis
   d. Intussusception

3. Which is not a cause of delayed passage of meconium?
   a. CF
   b. Small left colon syndrome
   c. Hirschsprung disease
   d. Milk protein intolerance

4. In infants with TEF, coexisting congenital anomalies occur in:
   a. 5%
   b. 30%
   c. 70%
   d. 90%

5. Which is the most common form of TEF?
   a. Esophageal atresia with distal TEF
   b. Esophageal atresia with no TEF
   c. H-type TEF
   d. Esophageal atresia with proximal TEF

6. What causes reflux in infants?
   a. Low resting pressure of the upper esophageal sphincter
   b. Immature esophageal peristalsis
   c. Increased gastric acidity
   d. Transient relaxation of the lower esophageal sphincter

7. Which is most consistent with pyloric stenosis?
   a. Hypochloremic alkalosis
   b. Hyperchloremic acidosis
   c. Hypochloremic acidosis
   d. Hyperchloremic alkalosis

8. With what syndrome would you most commonly see double bubble?
   a. Trisomy 21
   b. Beckwith-Wiedemann syndrome
   c. Smith-Lemli-Opitz syndrome
   d. Trisomy 18

9. A 3-day-old infant has not yet stooled. What is the next step in management?
   a. UGI with SBFT
   b. Abdominal ultrasound
   c. Rectal suction biopsy
   d. Barium enema

10. Poor motility is a long-term consequence of which condition?
    a. Gastroschisis
    b. Omphalocele
    c. Intestinal atresia
    d. Pyloric stenosis

Chapter 38

1. Which is true of sucrose-isomaltase deficiency?
   a. It presents after the introduction of standard infant formula.
   b. It presents with bloody diarrhea.
   c. It presents when secondary foods are introduced.
   d. Treatment is use of an amino acid–based formula.

2. Which is true of congenital lactase deficiency?
   a. It presents after introduction of standard infant formula.
   b. It presents with bloody diarrhea.
   c. It presents when secondary foods are introduced.
   d. Treatment is use of amino acid–based formula.

3. A 2-week-old female infant presents with severe watery diarrhea, acidosis, and lethargy. The workup reveals that stools are positive for reducing substances, intestinal biopsies are normal, and diarrhea resolves when the infant is made NPO. This disorder is due to which of the following?
   a. Defect found on chromosome 3
   b. Defect in sodium–glucose linked transporter (SGLT) protein
   c. Autosomal recessive disorder of lipoprotein assembly
   d. Defect in sodium–hydrogen exchanger in jejunal brush border

4. Treatment of hypobetalipoproteinemia involves which of the following?
   a. Low-fat diet
   b. High-fat diet
   c. Supplementation with docosahexaenoic acid (DHA)
   d. Supplementation with zinc

5. A 6-hour-old infant is admitted to the NICU with severe watery diarrhea that persists when the infant is made NPO. The infant is found to have hyponatremia,

hypochloremia, and metabolic alkalosis. The likely diagnosis is which of the following?
a. Microvillous inclusion disease
b. Tufting enteropathy
c. Congenital sodium diarrhea
d. Congenital chloride diarrhea

6. Which one of the following is not a risk factor for necrotizing enterocolitis (NEC)?
a. Bowel ischemia
b. Immaturity of the immune system
c. Enteral feeding
d. Exposure to antibiotics

7. Which is not a complication of short bowel syndrome?
a. Gastric hypersecretion
b. Small bowel intestinal overgrowth
c. Enterocolitis
d. Stricture

8. Appropriate management of small bowel syndrome consists of all but which of the following?
a. Acid suppression
b. Chronic antibiotic use to treat for bacterial over-growth
c. Total parenteral nutrition (TPN)
d. Enteral feeds with medium chain triglycerides (MCTs)

9. A 3-week-old breastfed infant presents with irritability and bright red blood in the stool. The complete blood count (CBC) reveals a white blood cell count (WBC) of 7000/μL, hematocrit (Hct) of 13%, and platelets (Plts) of 300,000/μL. Electrolytes are within normal limits. Weight gain has been stable, but mother reports recent feeding refusal. The most likely diagnosis is which of the following?
a. NEC
b. Gastroesophageal reflux disease (GERD)
c. Infection
d. Milk protein allergy

10. Which of the following is true regarding cases of neonatal intussusception?
a. Most involve the small bowel
b. Most involve large bowel
c. Very common
d. Always require surgical intervention

Chapter 39

1. A 5-week-old infant is found to have direct hyperbilirubinemia, heart murmur, and triangular facies. This syndrome is:
a. More common in females
b. Inherited in an autosomal recessive fashion
c. Due to mutation in *FIC1* gene
d. Due to mutation in *JAG1* gene

2. Symptoms concerning for biliary atresia include all of the following *except*:
a. Acholic stools
b. Triangular facies
c. Hepatosplenomegaly
d. Prolonged jaundice

3. Treatment of chylous ascites in the neonate typically includes:
a. Surgical decompression
b. Dietary restriction of protein
c. Dietary restriction of long chain triglycerides
d. Biliary drainage

4. With extrahepatic biliary atresia, the goal is to perform the Kasai procedure:
a. Before 60 days old
b. Before 90 days old
c. Before direct bilirubin reaches 8 mg/dL
d. Before direct bilirubin reaches 10 mg/dL

5. The distinguishing laboratory finding of progressive familial intrahepatic cholestasis type 2 (PFIC2) as opposed to PFIC1 or PFIC3 is:
a. Elevated gamma-glutamyltransferase (GGT)
b. Low GGT
c. Elevated aspartate aminotransferase (AST)
d. Elevated alanine aminotransferase (ALT)

6. Which of the following is not a presentation seen with Alagille syndrome?
a. Triangular facies
b. Butterfly vertebrae
c. Cardiac defects
d. Low GGT

7. Which of the following laboratory values are you most likely to find with biliary ascites?
a. High triglyceride count
b. Bilirubin >4 g/dL
c. Low sodium level
d. Elevated urea level

8. Which of the following can occur if a choledochal cyst goes without treatment?
a. Biliary atresia
b. Pancreatitis
c. Cirrhosis
d. b and c

9. All of the following are mechanisms for pathogenesis of biliary atresia *except*:
a. Defect in morphogenesis of biliary tract
b. Regurgitation of pancreatic secretions in to the biliary tree
c. Viral infection
d. Defect in fetal or prenatal circulation

10. Which of the following is most likely to be present in a neonate with alpha-1 antitrypsin deficiency?
a. High levels of alpha-1 antitrypsin
b. MM phenotype
c. High GGT levels
d. Normal ALT and AST levels

Chapter 40

1. All of the following are true statements about bilirubin metabolism *except*:
a. Bilirubin is formed from biliverdin catalyzed by biliverdin reductase.
b. Carbon monoxide is produced during the conversion of bilirubin to biliverdin.
c. Bilirubin is converted back to biliverdin by reactive oxygen species.
d. Iron eliminated from heme oxidation catalyzed by heme oxygenase is recycled.

2. Which of the following substances is lipophilic and crosses the placenta from the fetus?
   a. Conjugated bilirubin
   b. Unconjugated bilirubin
   c. Lumirubin
   d. Biliverdin

3. All of the following are measures of bilirubin *except*:
   a. Serum bilirubin
   b. Transcutaneous bilirubin
   c. ETCO
   d. Reticulocyte count

4. All of the following are risk factors for hyperbilirubinemia *except*:
   a. Formula feeding
   b. Ethnicity
   c. Gestational age
   d. Bruising

5. Which of the following enzymes are involved in bilirubin conjugation?
   a. Heme oxygenase
   b. Beta-glucuronidase
   c. UDP-glucuronyltransferase
   d. All of the above
   e. a and b
   f. b and c

6. All of the following contribute to an increased propensity for hyperbilirubinemia in neonates compared with adults *except*:
   a. Increased RBC turnover
   b. Immature conjugating enzymes
   c. Decreased enterohepatic circulation
   d. Relatively high bacterial flora

7. Factors affecting albumin to bilirubin binding include:
   a. Low serum albumin level
   b. Acidosis
   c. Medications such as ceftriaxone
   d. All of the above

8. The rate-limiting step in bilirubin metabolism in a preterm infant is:
   a. Heme oxygenase activity
   b. UDP-glucuronyltransferase activity
   c. Beta-glucuronidase activity
   d. All of the above
   e. None of the above

9. Bilirubin is transported from the bilirubin-albumin complex into hepatocytes by which of the following?
   a. Ligandin
   b. Glucuronyl *S*-transferase
   c. All of the above
   d. None of the above

10. Which of the following methods is most commonly used to measure the serum bilirubin levels?
    a. Spectrophotometry
    b. Fluorimetry
    c. High-pressure liquid chromatography
    d. All of the above
    e. None of the above

11. All of the following influence the binding of bilirubin to albumin *except*:
    a. Postnatal age
    b. Ampicillin use
    c. Ceftriaxone use
    d. Free fatty acid level
    e. Calcium level

Chapter 41

1. All of the following parts of the brain are typically affected in bilirubin toxicity *except* the:
   a. Hippocampus
   b. Cranial nerve nuclei
   c. Cerebral cortex
   d. Basal ganglia

2. Which of the following are features of acute bilirubin encephalopathy?
   a. Severely elevated serum bilirubin
   b. Abnormal brainstem auditory evoked response
   c. Abnormal otoacoustic emission test
   d. Abnormal MRI
   e. All of the above
   f. a, b, and d

3. Which of the following are mechanisms contributing to bilirubin toxicity?
   a. Increased bilirubin production
   b. Alteration of the blood-brain barrier
   c. Decreased serum albumin
   d. Increased in situ bilirubin production
   e. All of the above
   f. None of the above

4. Extraneural injuries due to bilirubin include:
   a. Intestinal necrosis
   b. Renal tubular necrosis
   c. Pancreatic necrosis
   d. None of the above
   e. All of the above

5. Long-term sequelae of kernicterus include:
   a. Cerebral palsy
   b. Abnormal gaze
   c. Dental dysplasias
   d. Normal intellect
   e. All of the above
   f. None of the above

6. Efficacy of phototherapy depends on:
   a. Wavelength
   b. Irradiance
   c. Distance from surface
   d. Surface area of exposure
   e. All of the above
   f. None of the above

7. Of the following diagnoses, which is the most common complication of exchange transfusion?
   a. Hypocalcemia
   b. Stroke
   c. Renal failure
   d. Intraventricular hemorrhage (IVH)

8. Which of the following is not a known side effect of phototherapy?
   a. Rash
   b. Acute intermittent porphyria
   c. Bronze baby syndrome
   d. Hypocalcemia

9. Which of the following sequelae of bilirubin toxicity is reversible?
   a. Lethargy
   b. Seizures
   c. Choreoathetoid movements
   d. Opisthotonus
   e. Dental dysplasia
10. Assessment of the cause of kernicterus includes:
    a. Liver function tests
    b. Peripheral smear
    c. Osmotic fragility
    d. Glucose-6-phosphate dehydrogenase
    e. All of the above
    f. None of the above

Chapter 42

1. A 6-day-old term infant presents to the emergency room with a history of exclusive breastfeeding, clinical jaundice, and decreased urination. The physical examination reveals a quiet but easily arousable clinically jaundiced infant with dry mucous membranes and poor skin turgor. Vital signs show a heart rate of 160 beats/min, temperature normal, and blood pressure of 55/32 mmHg. The serum bilirubin drawn in the emergency room is 24 mg/dL. The first step in the management of this infant is:
   a. Draw complete blood count with a reticulocyte count.
   b. Start an IV, and give a normal saline bolus.
   c. Start intensive phototherapy.
   d. Prepare for an exchange transfusion.
2. A 10-day-old exclusively breastfed infant presents to the clinic for a well child visit. The mother reports frequent breastfeeding with six to eight wet diapers per day and one or two stools per day. The physical examination reveals normal vital signs, a jaundiced infant, and no palpable hepatosplenomegaly. Fractionated serum bilirubin drawn in clinic = total 21, direct 0.7 mg/dL. The baby demonstrates no signs of anemia, and there is no evidence of hemolysis. The next step of management of this infant is:
   a. Suspension of breastfeeding and supplementation with formula
   b. IV fluid hydration
   c. Intensive phototherapy
   d. Reassurance and close follow-up
3. Factors contributing to breast milk jaundice include the following:
   a. Presence of high concentrations of beta-glucuronidase in maternal milk
   b. Factors in breast milk such as metal ions, steroids, and nucleotides, which could control uridine diphosphatase glucuronyl transferase
   c. Serum elevation of bile acids or taurine–glycine conjugates, which may be related to the cause
   d. All of the above
   e. None of the above
4. Breast milk jaundice peaks at:
   a. 1 to 3 days
   b. 7 to 14 days
   c. 14 to 21 days
   d. 2 to 6 days

5. All of the following are factors contribute to breast-feeding jaundice *except*:
   a. Cleft lip
   b. Engorgement
   c. Cracked nipples
   d. Maternal age
6. Evaluation of hyperbilirubinemia may include:
   a. Fractionated serum bilirubin
   b. Complete blood count with reticulocyte count
   c. Serum electrolytes
   d. All of the above
   e. None of the above
7. Factors influencing the severity of physiologic jaundice include:
   a. Polycythemia
   b. Maternal medications such as diazepam
   c. Gestational age
   d. Delayed feeding
   e. All of the above
   f. None of the above
8. The goal of assessment and treatment of hyperbilirubinemia is to:
   a. Prevent neurotoxicity
   b. Reduce readmission
   c. Reduce length of stay
   d. Decrease the risk of late onset sepsis
9. Risk factors for developing significant hyperbilirubinemia include all of the following *except*:
   a. Lower gestational age
   b. Jaundice in first 24 hours
   c. Phototherapy before discharge
   d. Blood transfusions

Chapter 43

1. Which of the following is true regarding maternal adaptation to pregnancy and the impact on chronic disease?
   a. Serial echocardiography should be done in mothers with cardiac disease because pregnancy-induced cardiovascular changes may worsen cardiac dysfunction.
   b. Peak flow monitoring cannot be used for asthma management because peak expiratory flow and FEV1 are altered by pregnancy.
   c. Increased doses of antihypertensives are required in pregnancy because of the increase in systemic vascular resistance.
   d. Pregestational diabetics require less insulin during pregnancy because of lower renal clearance of insulin.
   e. Free T4 levels cannot be used to monitor thyroid disease because these values are increased in pregnancy.
2. An Ashkenazi Jewish couple with a child affected by Tay-Sachs disease presents for preconception counseling. Their child's genetic analysis has identified a causative mutation that is detectable on routine screening panels. Neither partner has had prior genetic testing. The wife has chronic hypertension treated with lisinopril. All of the following are recommended *except*:
   a. Folic acid supplementation prior to conception
   b. Discontinuing lisinopril and transitioning to labetalol before conception

c. Expanded carrier screening for Eastern and Central European Jewish descent

d. An interpregnancy interval of less than 18 months

e. Gamete donation from a known Tay-Sachs negative donor to conceive the next pregnancy

3. A 30-year-old G3P1011 woman presents at 12 weeks with known Kell sensitization (red blood cell alloimmunization). She had an uncomplicated pregnancy 4 years ago and a 24-week fetal demise that occurred last year. After a motor vehicle accident 5 years ago, she required multiple blood transfusions. She is wondering if Kell sensitization caused the fetal demise. How would you answer her question?

a. It definitely caused the fetal demise.

b. It cannot cause fetal demise unless there was bleeding in the pregnancy.

c. It did not cause the fetal demise because her first pregnancy was uncomplicated.

d. It may have caused the demise; paternal antigen testing is required to determine if other pregnancies are at risk.

4. Which of the following is not routinely recommended in the management of pregestational diabetes in pregnancy?

a. Nutrition consult to review dietary and lifestyle modifications

b. Fetal echocardiography at 20 weeks due to increased risk of congenital heart defects

c. Frequent blood glucose checks and insulin or oral hypoglycemics as needed

d. Cesarean delivery if the EFW ≥ 4500 g, given the high risk of shoulder dystocia

e. All patients delivered at 37 weeks due to an increased risk of stillbirth

5. A 27-year-old G1P0 at 29 weeks is admitted with new severe-range hypertension. Antihypertensives and a steroid course are ordered. Laboratory evaluation shows 1400 mg/d proteinuria, creatinine of 1.0 mg/dL, AST of 106 mg/dL, platelet count of 95,000/μL, and hematocrit of 28%. Other laboratory tests are normal. An NST is reactive, and fetal growth is normal. The patient has no symptoms. What is the diagnosis, and what is the most appropriate next step in management?

a. Gestational hypertension; discharge from the hospital with close outpatient follow-up

b. Preeclampsia without severe features; expectant management until 37 weeks

c. HELLP syndrome; delivery after completion of steroid course

d. Preeclampsia with severe features; delivery after confirmation of fetal lung maturity

e. Preeclampsia with severe features; expectant management until 34 weeks of gestation if controlled hypertension, stable laboratory results, and reassuring fetal status

6. A patient has a normal fetal anatomy survey at 18 weeks. She decides to have quad screening for aneuploidy, which shows an elevated risk of trisomy 21. Which of the following is true?

a. The anatomy survey must have overlooked features of trisomy 21 because the false-positive rate of the quad screen is low.

b. The quad screen must be a false-positive because no sonographic features of trisomy 21 were detected.

c. Diagnostic testing for trisomy 21 should be offered.

d. The fetus has trisomy 21.

Chapter 44

1. A patient at 32 weeks is having fetal growth surveillance for renal disease. The EFW is at the seventh percentile with a normal amniotic fluid volume. The umbilical artery S/D ratio is elevated. Twice-weekly NSTs and weekly assessments of amniotic fluid volume are started for surveillance. Which of the following findings require delivery?

a. Fetal EFW <10th percentile on the next growth assessment

b. Biophysical profile of 8/10

c. Umbilical artery velocimetry showing reversed end-diastolic flow

d. Intermittent variable decelerations noted on reactive NST

2. A woman with diabetes is having a biophysical profile assessment at 34 weeks. Fetal NST shows four accelerations in the fetal heart rate of 10 beats/min above the baseline. Fetal breathing was seen. The single deepest vertical pocket (SDP) of amniotic fluid exceeds 2 cm. Many fetal body movements are seen, including at least one kick, with return to flexion. What is the BPP score, and what additional testing do you recommend?

a. 6; no further testing required at this time

b. 6; continuous electronic fetal monitoring

c. 8; no further testing required at this time

d. 8; consider a repeat biophysical profile within 24 hours

e. 10; no further testing required at this time

3. A patient with preeclampsia with severe features is undergoing fetal surveillance. She is having a biophysical profile assessment at 33 weeks. An NST shows no accelerations in heart rate and displays intermittent late decelerations. Baseline fetal heart rate is 120 beats/min with minimal-to-moderate variability. Fetal breathing was seen for 15 seconds. The single deepest vertical pocket (SDP) of amniotic fluid is 1 cm. Gross fetal body movements are seen, but no episodes of extension with return to flexion were noted. What is the BPP score, and what additional steps do you recommend?

a. 4; continuous electronic fetal monitoring

b. 2; urgent delivery

c. 2; consider delivery at 34 weeks for preeclampsia

d. 0; consider a repeat biophysical profile within 24 hours

e. 0; immediate delivery

4. A 36-year-old pregnant patient presents for routine prenatal care. She experienced a lot of anxiety in her last pregnancy secondary to a false-positive aneuploidy screening result, but she is interested in aneuploidy risk assessment. She asks you to recommend a testing strategy that has the lowest possibility of false-positive results while maximizing aneuploidy detection. What do you advise?

a. Detailed anatomy survey to look for anomalies and aneuploidy markers

b. First trimester screen

c. Cell-free DNA screening

d. Diagnostic CVS

e. Diagnostic amniocentesis

5. Which of the following patients are appropriate for diagnostic genetic testing, assuming they have no contraindications and are accepting of the small procedural risks?

a. 41-year-old multipara; multiple anatomic defects noted on anatomy survey

b. 41-year-old multipara; non-anomalous fetus

c. 21-year-old primipara; multiple anatomic defects noted on anatomy survey

d. 21-year-old primipara; non-anomalous fetus

e. a, b, and c

f. All of the above

6. A 25-year-old primigravid African American patient is attending her first prenatal visit with a spontaneously conceived pregnancy. She has no significant past medical history. There is no family history of structural birth defects, genetic disease, or intellectual disability. She has not had any preconception genetic testing. Which genetic screening tests do you recommend?

a. Aneuploidy screening

b. Aneuploidy screening, cystic fibrosis carrier testing, SMA carrier testing, hemoglobin electrophoresis

c. Aneuploidy screening, cystic fibrosis carrier testing, SMA carrier testing, hemoglobin electrophoresis, expanded carrier screening

d. Aneuploidy screening, cystic fibrosis carrier testing, SMA carrier testing, hemoglobin electrophoresis, expanded carrier screening, fragile X premutation testing

Chapter 45

1. For which of these clinical situations would you recommend a prompt, planned cesarean delivery?

a. 30-year-old G3P2002 at 39 weeks; one previous cesarean delivery (for breech)

b. 20-year-old G1P0 at 39 weeks; fetal gastroschisis

c. 24-year-old G2P1001 at 39 weeks; fetal hypoplastic left heart, unrestrictive atrial septum

d. 23-year-old G1P0 at 36 weeks; fetal sacrococcygeal teratoma with signs of fetal hydrops

e. 35-year-old G4P1112 at 39 weeks with maternal dilated cardiomyopathy who has a left ventricular ejection fraction (LVEF) of 40%

2. A 31-year-old G4P3003 presents at 35 weeks with heavy vaginal bleeding and a known placenta previa. She previously received a steroid course for an episode of vaginal bleeding. She had two prior vaginal deliveries. Fetal heart rate tracing shows tachycardia, moderate variability, and intermittent variable decelerations that have persisted in spite of maternal repositioning and IV fluid administration. Maternal vital signs are within normal limits. There is no purulent vaginal discharge or fundal tenderness. Lab evaluation is notable for mild maternal anemia with normal WBC count. The most appropriate next step in management is:

a. Prompt cesarean section for presumed chorioamnionitis

b. Prompt labor induction due to non-reassuring fetal status in the setting of vaginal bleeding

c. Prompt cesarean section for non-reassuring fetal status in the setting of vaginal bleeding

d. Repeat steroid course followed by cesarean delivery

e. Expectant management until term

3. A 34-year-old G7P5015 patient presents in active spontaneous labor, 10 cm dilated, with contractions having started 2 hours ago. Pregnancy is complicated by pregestational diabetes, grand multiparity, chronic hypertension, history of macrosomia, and prior precipitous delivery. An estimated fetal weight is 4500 g. Which of the following is not a risk factor for shoulder dystocia in her current pregnancy?

a. Pregestational diabetes

b. Grand multiparity

c. Chronic hypertension

d. Current macrosomic infant

e. Prior precipitous delivery with rapid labor course

4. During the initial evaluation of the patient in question #3, fetal bradycardia of uncertain duration is noted. She has a strong urge to push, and the fetal head is now crowning. She has a history of successful vaginal delivery of a similarly sized infant. The most appropriate next step is:

a. Coached maternal pushing efforts

b. Immediate episiotomy to facilitate delivery of the fetal head

c. Immediate operative vaginal delivery

d. Immediate cesarean delivery

5. A 22-year-old G1P0 at 38 weeks is undergoing labor induction for preeclampsia without severe features. Current maternal blood pressure is 145/96. The fetal heart rate tracing shows a baseline rate of 130 beats/min, moderate variability, no accelerations, and persistent early decelerations. The cervix is 4 cm dilated with the fetal head well applied. What is the most appropriate intervention?

a. Urgent cesarean delivery due to recurrent decelerations

b. Antihypertensives to control maternal blood pressure

c. IV fluid bolus and maternal repositioning

d. Amnioinfusion

e. No intervention needed

6. The patient in question #5 is now 7 cm dilated with bloody show and recently received an epidural for pain management. Bloody show has been noted since the patient had spontaneous rupture of membranes 30 minutes ago. The fetal heart rate tracing shows new-onset changes with a baseline of 160 beats/min, recurrent and deep variable decelerations, and some late decelerations. Maternal blood pressure is 82/43 mmHg. What is the most appropriate intervention?

a. Urgent cesarean delivery due to recurrent decelerations

b. Phenylephrine administration

c. IV fluid bolus and maternal repositioning

d. Amnioinfusion

e. b, c, and d

f. All of the above

Chapter 46

1. You are called to the delivery of a 39-week infant with no known maternal complications of pregnancy. Meconium was noted at the time of delivery. You arrive in the delivery room ~1 minute after birth and find the infant

is on a warmer, is apneic, and is being vigorously stimulated by the nursing staff. The HR is noted to be less than 100 beats/min. Of the following, which is the most appropriate next step to improve the patient's heart rate?
   a. Continue vigorous stimulation of the patient.
   b. Deep suction the posterior pharynx.
   c. Provide positive-pressure ventilation via bag-mask ventilation.
   d. Intubate the patient.
   e. Obtain umbilical access and administer intravenous epinephrine.

2. Based on current evidence and practice guidelines, which of the following describes an infant who would most benefit from therapeutic whole-body cooling?
   a. 33-week infant born due to maternal preeclampsia; required intubation at birth; Apgar scores of 1 at 1 minute, 3 at 5 minutes, and 8 at 10 minutes
   b. 37-week infant born after prolonged shoulder dystocia; Apgar scores of 1 at 1 minute, 3 at 5 minutes, and 8 at 10 minutes; arterial cord gas of pH 6.98; CO_2 of 88 mmHg; PaO_2 of 24 mmHg; bicarbonate of 20 mmol/L; base excess of −17; who at 1 hour of age appears hyperalert, with mildly increased tone, a weak suck, HR of 190 beats/min, and respiratory rate (RR) of 75 breaths/min
   c. 39-week infant born after uterine rupture; Apgar scores of 1 at 1 minute, 3 at 5 minutes, 8 at 10 minutes; arterial cord gas of pH 6.98; CO_2 of 88 mmHg; PaO_2 of 24 mmHg; bicarbonate of 20 mmol/L; base excess of −17; who at 1 hour of age appears comatose, remains intubated, is lethargic with decreased activity, hypotonia, incomplete Moro reflex and suck, and intermittent spontaneous respirations on the ventilator
   d. 37-week infant, now 12 hours old, found in mother's room to be unresponsive and received CPR with two doses of epinephrine before spontaneous return of circulation

3. Which of the following is the preferred dose of epinephrine to be given during a neonatal resuscitation?
   a. 0.2-mg/kg/dose of a 1:10,000 solution IV
   b. 0.5-mL/kg/dose of a 1:1000 solution via ETT
   c. 0.02-mg/kg/dose of a 0.1-mg/mL solution (1:10,000) IV
   d. 1-mL/kg/dose of a 1:10,000 solution via ETT

4. Which of the following is an advantage of a self-inflating bag over a T-piece resuscitator?
   a. It can administer PPV without a source of compressed air or oxygen.
   b. It can provide PEEP when applied continuously to the face.
   c. It provides consistent PIP and PEEP with each breath, with minimal variation between breaths.
   d. It can be used to deliver oxygen concentrations >FiO_2 21%.

5. The hypercapnia, hypoxemia, and acidosis that result from asphyxia will initially cause a redistribution of blood flow to which organs?
   a. Heart, kidneys, and adrenal glands
   b. Heart, intestines, and brain
   c. Heart, brain, and adrenal glands
   d. Brain, intestines, and kidneys
   e. Brain, kidneys, and heart

6. Which of the following is a feature of primary energy failure from hypoxic brain injury?
   a. Occurs 6 to 48 hours after hypoxic injury
   b. Necrotic cell death
   c. Apoptosis
   d. Decreased glutamate reuptake by damaged cells
   e. Increases in cerebral ATP stores

7. All of the following are symptoms or consequences of IUGR due to in utero hypoxia *except*:
   a. Polycythemia
   b. Necrotizing enterocolitis
   c. Hypoglycemia
   d. Decreased risk of adult-onset cardiovascular disease
   e. Increased risk of neurodevelopmental delays

Chapter 47

1. A male infant has hypotonia, poor feeding, and cryptorchidism. You suspect Prader-Willi syndrome (PWS). Evaluation of the 15q11-13 region does not reveal any deletions. You should next evaluate for:
   a. Point mutations in the PWS critical region
   b. Duplication of the 15q11-13 region
   c. Uniparental disomy of the 15q11-13 region
   d. Other causes of neonatal hypotonia

2. Diseases with this mode of inheritance are almost exclusively transmitted from the mother.
   a. Imprinted
   b. Autosomal recessive
   c. Trinucleotide repeats
   d. Mitochondrial

3. You are asked to evaluate an infant for hypotonia. You note that the infant has significant hypotonia and feeding difficulties. The mother is well appearing but has difficulty releasing your handshake. Both the mother and infant are subsequently diagnosed with myotonic dystrophy. The phenomenon described here, where the infant is more severely affected than the mother, is known as:
   a. Anticipation
   b. Imprinting
   c. Mitochondrial inheritance
   d. Uniparental disomy

4. You are called to evaluate an infant with tetralogy of Fallot, cleft palate, and hypocalcemia. After your initial evaluation, you suspect the child may have DiGeorge syndrome. What is the most appropriate initial test to order?
   a. Karyotype
   b. Fluorescence in situ hybridization (FISH)
   c. Whole exome sequencing (WES)
   d. Sequencing of the *TBX1* gene

5. Which of the following is a limitation of newborn screening?
   a. Preterm or critically ill neonates often have false-positive results.
   b. Current screening techniques can only evaluate for a few metabolites on each sample.
   c. Cystic fibrosis is not reliably detected by most newborn screening programs.
   d. Many states do not screen for sickle cell disease.

Chapter 48

1. A 38-weeks' gestation newborn infant at birth is noted to be small for gestational age with microcephaly, cleft lip and palate, and narrow hyperconvex fingernails; the infant developed central apnea shortly after birth, and an echocardiogram showed ventricular septal defect (VSD). This infant most likely has:
   a. Trisomy 21
   b. Fetal alcohol syndrome
   c. Trisomy 13
   d. Trisomy 18
   e. Prader-Willi syndrome
2. A full-term, appropriate for gestational age (AGA) male infant has persistent hypoglycemia despite adequate calorie feeds orally. He is also noted on physical examination to have a large tongue and exophthalmos. What is the mode of inheritance of this infant's condition?
   a. Autosomal dominant
   b. Uniparental disomy
   c. Autosomal recessive
   d. X-linked recessive
   e. X-linked dominant
3. All of the following statements are true about trisomy 21 *except*:
   a. Most are a result of meiotic nondisjunction.
   b. There is an increased rate of hip dysplasia compared to the general population.
   c. It is the most common chromosomal abnormality.
   d. Females are always infertile.

Chapter 49

1. The diagnosis of partial fetal alcohol syndrome requires:
   a. Short palpebral fissures
   b. Smooth philtrum
   c. Thin upper lip
   d. Central nervous system abnormalities
   e. Evidence of prenatal alcohol exposure
2. An infant is born with profound hypotonia and poor feeding. Genetic evaluation reveals Prader-Willi syndrome. Which of the following would be a more likely finding on the mother's history?
   a. Maternal phenylketonuria
   b. Maternal seizures
   c. Conception by ART
   d. Bicornuate uterus
   e. Late prenatal care
3. Structural heart defects are more likely to be caused by teratogen exposure during what phase of pregnancy?
   a. First trimester
   b. Second trimester
   c. Third trimester
   d. Any time in the pregnancy
   e. No association is known

Chapter 50

1. Several studies have shown that there is a small but definite increase in congenital malformations in neonates following artificial reproductive technology (ART) conception. In which type of ART is an increased incidence of urogenital abnormalities, specifically hypospadias, likely to occur?
   a. In vitro fertilization (IVF)
   b. Gamete intrafallopian tube transfer (GIFT)
   c. Intracytoplasmic sperm injection (ICSI)
   d. Embryo cryopreservation
   e. Blastocyst culture
2. Amniotic band sequence is caused by:
   a. Deformation
   b. Disruption
   c. Malformation
   d. Syndrome
   e. Association
3. Deformations most commonly occur during:
   a. The zygote period
   b. The blastula period
   c. The embryo period
   d. The fetal period
   e. The birth process
4. Arthrogryposis (congenital joint contractures) can be described as a:
   a. Dysplasia
   b. Syndrome
   c. Disruption
   d. Deformation
   e. None of the above

Chapter 51

1. A 3-day-old girl began feeding poorly on day 2 of life. She now has depressed mental status, clonus, and respiratory alkalosis. Which test should be sent for emergently?
   a. Very long-chain fatty acids
   b. 7-Dehydrocholesterol
   c. Ammonia
   d. Lysosomal enzymes
   e. Cholesterol
2. A newborn male has profound hypotonia and features suggestive of trisomy 21. He is found to have hepatomegaly, hyperbilirubinemia, and synthetic liver dysfunction. Which diagnosis should be considered?
   a. Zellweger syndrome
   b. Mucopolysaccharidosis
   c. Smith-Lemli-Opitz syndrome
   d. Pyruvate carboxylase deficiency
   e. Krabbe disease
3. A breast-fed newborn girl has high anion-gap acidosis, hypoglycemia, and altered mental status. Urinalysis reveals 4+ ketones. The ketosis is suggestive of:
   a. Normal response to hypoglycemia
   b. Fatty acid oxidation defect
   c. Peroxisomal defect
   d. Organic acidemia
   e. Lysosomal storage disease
4. Poorly treated maternal phenylketonuria puts a fetus at risk for having:
   a. PKU
   b. Cataracts
   c. Intracranial calcifications

d. Limb defects

e. Microcephaly

Chapter 52

1. A 24-week, 600-g infant is admitted to the NICU. The baby is intubated and sedated. Due to being quite unstable and requiring frequent hands-on care, she is under a radiant warmer. You estimate her baseline insensible fluid loss as 100 mL/kg/d. Based on the above information, what will you write her total fluids for the next 24 hours?
   a. 75 mL/kg/d
   b. 110 mL/kg/d
   c. 140 mL/kg/d
   d. 175 mL/kg/d
   e. 200 mL/kg/d

2. A full-term infant is being cared for in your NICU following a difficult delivery. He was initially prescribed D5W at 70 mL/kg/d for DOL 0 to 2. On DOL 3, he is noted to have a sodium of 130, a potassium of 4.8, and a creatinine of 0.7. His weight has been stable since birth. He appears euvolemic on exam. Urine lytes show a sodium of 40 mEq/L. What is the most likely etiology of the hyponatremia?
   a. AKI
   b. Bartters syndrome
   c. Inadequate intake of sodium
   d. SIADH
   e. Pseudohypoaldosteronism

3. An ex-25-week-old infant is now 11 days old. Her serum sodium has trended down from 137 to 126. Her creatinine is 0.8. Her TFs are written as 130 mL/kg/d. Her TPN has 3 mEq/kg/d of sodium with an additional 1 mEq/kg/d provided in her carrier fluids. You obtain urine lytes that show a sodium of 80 and a creatinine of 10. What is her FENa, and how does it explain her serum sodium?
   a. 12.6%, tubular wasting from immature tubule
   b. 7.9%, tubular wasting from acute tubular necrosis
   c. 5%, tubular wasting from prematurity
   d. 2.5%, prerenal AKI
   e. 0.05%, inadequate Na intake

4. The lab calls with a critical potassium value of 7.2 in a 4-day-old, ex-26-week infant. His weight is 15% below birth weight. The rest of the chemistry panel shows a Na of 151 and a bicarbonate of 10. Which of the following mechanisms would not perpetuate hyperkalemia?
   a. Avid sodium reabsorption by the proximal tubule secondary to volume depletion
   b. Lack of Maxi-K channels in neonates
   c. Inhibition of ROMK channels by acidosis
   d. Neonate's blunted response to aldosterone
   e. Acidosis stimulating Na,K-ATPase, which increases the intracellular to urine gradient

5. A 33-week cGA infant has been on thiazides for about 6 weeks for CLD. She develops acute vomiting. A chemistry panel shows a bicarbonate of 32 with potassium of 3.0 and creatinine 1.1. A blood gas confirms metabolic alkalosis. What mechanism is not involved in stimulating or maintaining the alkalosis?
   a. Vomiting leads to loss of protons.
   b. Vomiting leads to decrease in intravascular volume, which results in a decrease in GFR.
   c. Hypokalemia limits the shift of H^+ out of cells.
   d. Intravascular depletion stimulates proximal Na reabsorption, which leads to increase distal H^+ secretion.
   e. Intravascular depletion stimulates RAS, driving further potassium loss.

6. A 1-week-old, ex-37-week infant is admitted with the following chemistry: Na 127, K 7.3, bicarbonate 15. His mother reports he is not very interested in feeding but has been making a normal amount of wet diapers. His weight is 12% below his birth weight. His father reports that he has been told he was often admitted to the hospital as a baby, but he doesn't know any details. He is currently well and not on any medications. What advice could be given to the family about what to expect as their child grows up?
   a. Resolution of symptoms by age 2
   b. A chronic cough
   c. Persistent rashes
   d. Growth failure
   e. A need for salt supplementation throughout life

7. A 950-g infant is noted to have a 6% loss of weight from birth weight. His UOP has increased from DOL 1 to 2. His electrolytes and creatinine are normal for age. So far, he has been on 90 mL/kg/d TF without any Na or K in the TPN. Which statement below regarding his fluid/electrolytes management is correct?
   a. Increase TF to 130 mL/kg/d because he is losing too much weight.
   b. He is at a decreased risk of a PDA based on the numbers above.
   c. His risk of NEC is higher than that of an infant of similar BW who did not lose weight.
   d. Adding 1 mEq/kg/d potassium to the TPN would be dangerous.
   e. Your management has increased his risk of chronic lung disease.

8. A FT infant with bilateral pneumothoraces develops respiratory acidosis. Regarding neonatal respiratory acidosis, which statement is true?
   a. Preterm infants can respond to respiratory acidosis by increasing their tidal volume.
   b. Providing a dose of bicarbonate using the following formula is helpful: base deficit × BW × 0.3.
   c. Renal compensation is as efficient as in older children.
   d. Intubation may be needed.
   e. Administered bicarbonate stimulates hyperventilation.

9. A 1-month-old, ex-33-week infant has been having difficulty gaining weight. Her feeds have been fortified to 28 kcal/oz. but she still gains <5 g/d. Her mother reports her son had a similar issue with weight gain. You obtain a chemistry panel, which shows Na 137, K 4.1, bicarbonate 12, BUN 14, creatinine 0.3, glucose 85, Ca 9.4, and phosphorus 6.0. A urine sample has a specific gravity of 1.010 and pH 5.4 and is negative for blood, protein, LE, or nitrates. What is the baby's diagnosis?
   a. Distal RTA
   b. Type IV RTA
   c. Hemolyzed blood sample

d. Proximal RTA

e. Pseudohypoaldosteronism

10. You are treating an ex-27-week infant for a moderate sized PDA. The baby has developed worsening pulmonary edema despite restricting fluids. You start indomethacin. After the second dose, the baby's urine output is noted to drop from 1 to 0.6 mL/kg/hr. Which statement explains the drop in UOP?

a. Release of ANP has caused dilatation of the efferent arteriole.

b. Indomethacin has disrupted the intrarenal production of prostaglandins.

c. Ang II is constricting the afferent arteriole only.

d. The indomethacin has closed the PDA, resulting in shunting of blood away from the kidneys.

e. Dopamine is stimulating NA,K-ATPase.

Chapter 53

1. You are asked to consult on a woman at 21 weeks of her pregnancy for an abnormal prenatal ultrasound at 20 weeks. The ultrasound showed kidneys measuring 3.4 cm each with increased echogenicity. The bladder could not be seen. There is no family history of kidney disease. What is the likely etiology of these findings?

a. ADPKD

b. MCDK

c. Renal dysplasia

d. ARPKD

e. Beckwith-Wiedemann

2. You are asked to do another prenatal consult on a woman who was noted at her 20 week ultrasound to be carrying a fetus with abnormal kidneys. The left kidney is of normal length but has multiple cysts of similar size. The right kidney is of normal echogenicity and shape with good corticomedullary differentiation and no cysts. It measures 3 cm. No hydronephrosis or hydroureter is seen. The amniotic fluid volume is normal. Family history is negative for renal disease. What is the most likely diagnosis?

a. MCDK

b. ADPKD

c. Left sided UPJ

d. Left UVJ obstruction

e. ARPKD

3. A couple is considering prenatal intervention for their baby suspected to have a posterior urethral valve. Which of these statements regarding prenatal intervention for suspected bladder obstruction is *false*?

a. The most common intervention performed is a vesicoamniotic shunt.

b. Urine Na <100 mEq/L on serial taps suggests a good renal prognosis.

c. Intervention has been shown to improve both renal and lung function long term.

d. Serial bladder taps are preferred when assessing fetal renal function.

e. Urine Osm <200 mOsm/L predicts good renal function.

4. A 6-day-old, ex-24-week infant is noted by his bedside nurse to have decreased pulses in his lower extremities.

His blood pressure is also noted to be trending up. His urine has a pink tinge. Urine output is normal. His respiratory status is unchanged. He has a UAC in place. Ultrasound shows a small unilateral renal artery clot. What is the most likely long-term outcome?

a. End-stage renal disease as an infant

b. Necrosis of toes bilaterally

c. Persistent hematuria

d. Hypertension

e. Small bowel necrosis

5. A 4-week-old, ex-30-week infant undergoes a renal ultrasound for workup of UTI. The ultrasound shows a small left kidney with some echogenic spots. His past medical history includes treatment for culture negative sepsis with ampicillin and gentamycin for which he had a UVC in place. He was noted to have a transient drop in platelets shortly before his antibiotics finished. What is the most likely etiology of the ultrasound findings?

a. Kidney stones

b. Dysplasia

c. ARPKD

d. Old renal vein thrombosis

e. Nephrocalcinosis

6. A full-term baby with congestive heart failure is noted to have a rise in creatinine from a baseline of 0.7 to 1.6 by DOL 3. Urine output remains more than 1 mL/kg/hr. What stage of AKI is the baby in using the KDIGO system?

a. Stage 0

b. Stage 1

c. Stage 2

d. Stage 3

7. A 5-day-old FT infant is admitted to the NICU after seeing her PCP for a weight check. She was noted in the office to have a 15% decrease in weight since birth. On exam, she has dry mucus membranes, a sunken fontanelle, and capillary refill of 3 seconds. Her creatinine is 1.6. She receives fluid resuscitation with significant clinical improvement. Over the next 2 days, her creatinine falls to 1.2. Her vitals are normal for age. She appears euvolemic on exam. Her renal ultrasound is normal. Her urine output is 1.1 mL/kg/hr. What should be your next step in management?

a. NS bolus

b. Start renal dose dopamine

c. Kidney biopsy

d. Insert a bladder catheter

e. Observation

8. A cGA 30-week infant weighing 1900 g develops stage 3 AKI using the neonatal KDIGO definition. His daily fluid intake has been severely restricted due to oliguria, and thus he is receiving next to no nutrition. His potassium is 6.2, bicarbonate 15, BUN 42, and phosphorus 8. Which statement is *incorrect* regarding dialysis options for this baby?

a. PD can be performed by his NICU nurses.

b. PD does not require any anticoagulation.

c. PD removes immunoglobulins.

d. HD involves rapid volume shifts that may not be tolerated.

e. CRRT fluid goals are set on the machine once every 24 hours and cannot be adjusted in between.

9. A 28-week-old infant is receiving daily Lasix for fluid overload. His response to the Lasix dose seems to be decreasing despite increasing from 1 to 2 mg/kg/d. What strategy can be used next to optimize diuresis?
   a. Increase the frequency to q8 dosing.
   b. Add spironolactone.
   c. Increase the dose to 3 mg/kg.
   d. Add a thiazide diuretic.
   e. Space dosing to q48 hours.
10. The parents of a 10-week-old, ex-24-week infant are nervous about his medications causing long-term damage. They ask what the side-effects of his diuretics may be. Which of these is a true statement?
   a. Long-term use of thiazides is linked to bone fractures.
   b. Lasix has not been associated with hearing loss.
   c. Loop diuretics can lead to nephrocalcinosis.
   d. Thiazides are associated with increased numbers of kidney stones.
   e. Spironolactone causes hypokalemia.

Chapter 54

1. A term infant is noted to have bilateral (BL) undescended testes palpable in the inguinal canal. Penis is morphologically normal with stretched penile length of 3.2 cm. Which of the following is true about the management of this condition?
   a. Immediate surgical consultation is necessary because this infant is at increased risk of germ cell malignancy.
   b. Immediate endocrinologist evaluation is necessary because this infant likely has a disorder of sexual development.
   c. Spontaneous descent is likely; surgery should be delayed until after mini-puberty of infancy.
   d. Spontaneous descent is likely; surgery should be delayed until after onset of puberty.
2. A term infant born with cleft palate and large atrial septal defect has a morphologically normal penis with stretched penile length of 1.5 cm. Which of the following hormone defects is the most likely cause of his micropenis?
   a. Hypothyroidism due to impaired synthesis of thyroid-stimulating hormone
   b. Growth hormone deficiency
   c. Testosterone deficiency due to 17β-hydroxysteroid deficiency
   d. Dihydrotestosterone deficiency due to 5α-reductase deficiency
3. Which of the following conditions is typically associated with significant clinical virilization at the time of puberty?
   a. XY with 5α-reductase deficiency
   b. XY with complete androgen insensitivity
   c. XX with 21-hydroxylase CAH
   d. XY with 17β-HSD CAH
4. Who should make the final decision regarding gender assignment for an infant with ambiguous genitalia?
   a. The surgeon, who can best discuss functional and cosmetic outcomes of genitoplasty

b. The endocrinologist, who can best discuss past and future hormone exposure and will be guiding any sex-hormone replacement at the time of puberty
   c. The neonatologist, after reviewing the consults from the surgeon, endocrinologist, geneticist, and psychologist
   d. The family, after hearing recommendations of the full multidisciplinary team
5. Which of the following statements regarding hormones and their actions in sexual differentiation is not correct?
   a. The production of estrogen by granulosa cells in an XX female causes regression of the primordial male internal genitalia structures.
   b. The production of anti-Müllerian hormone by Sertoli cells in an XY male causes regression of the primordial female internal genitalia structures.
   c. The production of testosterone by Leydig cells in an XY male results in differentiation of internal structures into the epididymis, vas deferens, and seminal vesicle.
   d. The conversion of testosterone into dihydrotestosterone results in the virilization of external genitalia in an XY male.
6. Which of the following clinical presentations of ambiguous genitalia is associated with high risk of adrenal insufficiency?
   a. Testes palpable in a normally formed scrotum BL, microphallus with stretched penile length of 1 cm
   b. Testes palpable in a bifid scrotum BL, urethral opening at the ventral penile-scrotum junction
   c. Partially fused scrotum, phallic structure 1.5 cm in length, no palpable gonads
   d. Testis palpable on one side of scrotum, stretched penile length of 2.7 cm
7. A term infant is noted to have ambiguous genitalia. Karyotype was found to be XY; labs drawn on DOL 2 showed undetectable testosterone, normal AMH, and normal androgen precursors, including androstenedione and dehydroepiandrosterone (DHEA). HCG stimulation test showed no increase in testosterone levels. What is the most likely diagnosis?
   a. 17β-HSD deficiency
   b. Androgen insensitivity syndrome
   c. Leydig cell hypoplasia
   d. 5α-reductase deficiency
8. A term infant is found to have ambiguous genitalia. Rapid karyotype is XX; repeated androgen precursor hormones including 17-hydroxyprogesterone are normal. All of the following are appropriate next steps in the evaluation, except:
   a. Questioning of mother to determine if any performance enhancing drugs were used during early phases of pregnancy
   b. Questioning/examination of mother for new-onset hirsutism
   c. Genetic testing for presence of SRY
   d. Whole exome sequencing
9. Which of the following statements is true regarding gonadal dysgenesis?
   a. A karyotype showing XY sex chromosomes rules out gonadal dysgenesis.
   b. Patients with gonadal dysgenesis are at increased risk of gonadoblastoma.

c. All patients with XY gonadal dysgenesis should be assigned male gender at birth.

d. Wolffian duct differentiation is unaffected in patients with XY gonadal dysgenesis.

10. An infant with ambiguous genitalia has been found to have an XY karyotype. At which of the following time points will a serum testosterone level be informative?

a. 1 day of life

b. 1 week of life

c. 2 months of age

d. 6 months of age

e. 16 years of age

f. a, b, and c

g. a, c, and e

h. All of the above

Chapter 55

1. Which of the following hormones is not produced in the adrenal cortex?

a. Cortisol

b. Dopamine

c. Aldosterone

d. Dehydroepiandrosterone

e. All of the above are produced in the adrenal cortex

2. Which of the following statements is true regarding fetal adrenal steroid hormone production?

a. The adrenal glands develop and begin secreting hormones at 12 weeks.

b. The histopathologic organization of the adrenal gland in the fetus is identical to that of an adult.

c. The fetal adrenal gland does not express 3β-hydroxysteroid dehydrogenase and is therefore dependent on the placenta in order to synthesize cortisol.

d. The cells of the adrenal cortex are derived from neuroectodermal precursors.

3. Which of the following genes (enzymes) is not expressed in the adrenal gland?

a. CYP19 (aromatase)

b. CYP21 (21-hydroxylase)

c. CYP11B1 (11β-hydroxylase)

d. CYP11B2 (11β-hydroxylase)

e. All of the above enzymes are expressed and active in the adrenal gland

4. A patient is born with ambiguous genitalia and is found to have a genetic defect leading to loss of function of CYP11A1 (cholesterol side-chain cleavage enzyme). Which of the following is likely true about the patient's karyotype?

a. The karyotype is most likely XX, and the patient is overvirilized because of excess ACTH production.

b. The karyotype is most likely XY, and the patient is undervirilized because of elevated 5α-reductase activity.

c. The karyotype is mostly likely XX, and the patient is overvirilized because of decreased aromatase activity.

d. The karyotype is most likely XY, and the patient is undervirilized because of insufficient substrate for androgen hormone biosynthesis.

5. You are alerted that one of your patients admitted for transient tachypnea of the newborn had an abnormal newborn screen for CAH. The patient is now a 5-day-old infant, born 40 weeks, gestational age (WGA) via scheduled cesarean delivery, and has normal appearing male genitalia. Patient is clinically improving with decreasing oxygen requirement and normal blood pressure and is tolerating feeds. The newborn screen specimen was drawn at 36 hours of age, and electrolytes drawn on DOL 1 showed normal sodium and potassium. What is the most appropriate next step?

a. Immediately start hydrocortisone only at a dose of 15 mg/m²/d.

b. Immediately start hydrocortisone at a dose of 15 mg/m²/d and fludrocortisone at a dose of 0.1 mg/d.

c. Obtain a venous blood sample for measurement of 17-hydroxyprogesterone.

d. Obtain a venous blood sample for measurement of 17-hydroxyprogesterone and electrolytes.

6. You are caring for a 1-week-old, former 27 WGA infant with birth weight of 1000 g transferred to your NICU from a community hospital on DOL 1. Patient is phenotypically male and intubated and has required multiple fluid boluses, inotropes, and vasopressor support to maintain adequate perfusion. You receive a copy of the newborn screen report sent from the community hospital reporting a 17-hydroxyprogesterone value of 15,000 ng/dL. What is the appropriate next step?

a. Do nothing; the abnormal newborn screen result is likely the result of prematurity.

b. Obtain a venous blood sample for measurement of 17-hydroxyprogesterone; wait until results are back to start hydrocortisone.

c. Obtain a venous blood sample for measurement of 17-hydroxyprogesterone, and start hydrocortisone 100 mg/m²/d.

d. Obtain a venous blood sample for measurement of 17-hydroxyprogesterone, and start hydrocortisone 15 mg/m²/d.

7. A newborn is found to have ambiguous genitalia including partial fusion of the labioscrotal folds and clitoromegaly. No testes are palpable on exam. Which of the following scenarios is *not* likely to be responsible for the clinical presentation in this case?

a. 21-hydroxylase deficiency with karyotype XX

b. 3β-hydroxysteroid dehydrogenase with karyotype XX

c. 17-hydroxylase deficiency with karyotype XX

d. 11β-hydroxylase deficiency with karyotype XX

8. An 11-month-old infant male in your unit is found to be hypertensive. Review of his medical records shows that blood pressures have been gradually increasing over the past several weeks to months. Which of the following is true regarding hypertension in congenital adrenal hyperplasia?

a. Hypertension in 21-hydroxylase deficiency CAH is a sign that the Florinef dose needs to be increased.

b. Serum aldosterone levels are typically low.

c. The patient cannot have 17-hydroxlase deficiency because he has normal appearing genitalia.

d. The majority of patients who will develop hypertension due to 11β-hydroxylase deficiency are identified on the CAH newborn screen.

9. Which of the following assessments is *not* standardly used to assess adequacy of medical treatment in a patient with classic 21-hydroxylase CAH?
   a. Linear growth
   b. Radiograph of left hand for bone age
   c. Androstenedione
   d. ACTH
   e. Plasma renin activity
10. You are asked to provide prenatal counseling to a mother who previously gave birth to a virilized female with 21-hydroxylase CAH. Which of the following statements should you provide to the mother?
   a. The incidence of CAH is the same in males and females.
   b. She has a one in four chance of having another virilized female with CAH.
   c. There is a decreased incidence of virilization in female infants with CAH born to mothers who take maintenance doses of hydrocortisone during pregnancy.
   d. Fetal sexual differentiation does not occur until the third trimester, so she would only have to take dexamethasone for the last few weeks of her pregnancy to reduce the risk of virilization for an affected female.

Chapter 56

1. Which of the following statements is true regarding the potential effects of maternal Graves' disease on the fetus/neonate?
   a. Maternal T_3 is inactivated by the placenta; therefore, there is no risk of fetal hyperthyroidism.
   b. The fetus/neonate will be at an increased risk of hypothyroidism.
   c. There is no risk to the fetus/neonate in mothers who had definitive therapy for Graves' disease with thyroidectomy prior to conception.
   d. Maternal antithyroid therapy with methimazole or propylthiouracil (PTU) should be discontinued during pregnancy because of the risk of birth defects.
2. A full-term, newborn male is found to have an abnormal thyroid screen with elevated TSH of 500 mIU/mL and low T_4 of 2 μg/dL. Which of the following is not a possible cause of this child's hypothyroidism?
   a. Activating mutation in the TSH receptor
   b. Overexpression of deiodinase 3
   c. Inactivating mutation in the *NIS* gene
   d. Presence of a lingual thyroid gland
3. A 36 weeks' gestational age infant born to a 16-year-old first-time mother has a hypoglycemic seizure on DOL 4. Brain imaging reveals absence of corpus callosum and hypoplasia of optic nerves. Which pattern of thyroid hormone tests is most likely to be present?
   a. Elevated TSH, low T_4, low free T_4
   b. Normal TSH, low T_4, normal free T_4
   c. Normal TSH, low T_4, low free T_4
   d. Low TSH, elevated T_4, elevated free T_4
4. All of the following statements are true regarding fetal goiter *except*:
   a. A finding of fetal goiter on prenatal ultrasound is pathognomonic for the presence of thyroid dyshormonogenesis in the fetus.

   b. It is associated with increased risk of fetal upper airway obstruction at delivery.
   c. There is increased incidence of fetal goiter in areas where iodine deficiency is endemic.
   d. Fetal thyroid testing can be performed via percutaneous umbilical vein sampling after 20 weeks if fetal thyroid status is uncertain.
5. An otherwise healthy, appropriate-for-gestational-age (AGA) 34-week male is found to have an abnormal thyroid newborn screen on a blood spot obtained on DOL 2. You live in a state with a primary T_4 screening strategy. Follow-up venous blood sample on DOL 4 showed a normal TSH for age, low T_3, low T_4, normal free T_4, and normal free T_3. Which of the following statements is true about the most common form of his condition?
   a. He will be at risk for cognitive impairment if not started on levothyroxine immediately.
   b. His lab abnormalities are due to the fact that he was born prematurely.
   c. Evaluation of maternal serum would reveal elevated TRAb.
   d. He will be able to pass on his condition to a daughter, but not to a son.
6. An infant with which of the following conditions would be most likely to have elevated reverse T_3 levels?
   a. Congenital hypothyroidism due to athyreosis
   b. Consumptive hypothyroidism
   c. TBG deficiency due to *SERPIN7A* mutation
   d. Transient hypothyroxinemia of prematurity
7. Which of the following statements is true regarding the treatment of neonatal Graves' disease?
   a. All infants born to mothers with Graves' disease should be started on prophylactic antithyroid therapy with methimazole at birth.
   b. Prednisone dosed at 1 mg/kg/d is the first-line therapy for neonatal thyrotoxicosis.
   c. Infants with suppressed TSH and elevated T_4 levels at birth will require lifelong therapy.
   d. Treatment with Lugol solution is limited to 1 to 2 weeks because of "escape" from the Wolff-Chaikoff effect.
8. A term infant male with neonatal seizures is found to have abnormal thyroid studies, including elevated T_3 and free T_3 but low-normal T_4 and free T_4 levels. Which of the following statements is true regarding this condition?
   a. High-dose levothyroxine (T_4) treatment should be instituted.
   b. High-dose cytomel (T_3) treatment should be instituted.
   c. The clinical manifestations of this condition result from low intracellular concentrations of T_3 in neurons.
   d. It is inherited in an autosomal recessive manner.

Chapter 57

1. A term infant is readmitted to the NICU at 3 weeks of age in shock with cardiorespiratory failure and oliguric renal failure. Labs at presentation showed plasma glucose of 25 mg/dL and metabolic acidosis with elevated lactate.

Hepatomegaly is noted on physical exam. Parents state that the infant had not been feeding well for the past 3 days and slept through the night last night without waking to feed. What is the most likely diagnosis?

a. Congenital hyperinsulinism due to K_{ATP} channel mutation
b. Glycogen synthase deficiency
c. Glucose 6-phosphatase deficiency
d. Disorder of fatty acid oxidation

2. Laboratory results of a critical sample show venous glucose of 45 mg/dL, cortisol 2 µ/dL (normal stressed value, >18 µg/dL), growth hormone 12 ng/mL, free fatty acids 0.1 mmol/L (normal, <1 mmol/L), and β-hydroxybutyrate 0.2 mmol/L (normal, <1.5 mmol/L). Plasma glucose increased to 80 mg/dL 30 minutes after administration of 1 mg glucagon. Which of the following is an appropriate next step?

a. Start hydrocortisone 15 mg/m² BSA per day.
b. Perform an arginine/clonidine growth hormone stimulation test.
c. Resume intravenous dextrose infusion to maintain plasma glucose >60 mg/dL.
d. Trial diazoxide at dose of 15 mg/kg/d.

3. Which of the following is true regarding the use of diazoxide in neonates?

a. All infants with congenital hyperinsulinism will respond to diazoxide.
b. Diazoxide should be used with caution in patients with congenital heart disease.
c. Diazoxide causes hair loss.
d. Neonates on diazoxide need to have regular monitoring of CBCs for development of polycythemia.

4. Which of the following conditions of neonatal glucose disturbance is not associated with increased risk of diabetes as an adult?

a. Transient neonatal diabetes due to chromosome 6q24 mutation
b. Permanent neonatal diabetes due to activating mutation in K_{ATP} channel
c. Diffuse hyperinsulinism due to inactivating mutation in K_{ATP} channel
d. Neonatal panhypopituitarism

5. Which of the following statements is not true regarding energy utilization by the brain?

a. Glucose is the main source of ATP used by the brain.
b. Glucose is transported into brain cells via GLUT 3.
c. Fatty acids cross the blood-brain barrier and can be utilized as a source of ATP.
d. Ketone bodies cross the blood-brain barrier and can be utilized as a source of ATP.

6. A 3-week-old, AGA term male has persistent pre-fed plasma glucose levels between 45 and 60 mg/dL. Other notable clinical findings include partial cleft lip and palate and absent corpus callosum. Critical sample shows plasma glucose 47 mg/dL, cortisol of <1 µg/dL, growth hormone <1 ng/dL, β-hydroxybutyrate <0.1 mmol/L, and free-fatty acids <0.1 mmol/L. Which of the following statements is not consistent with these laboratory findings?

a. The patient will likely need lifelong hydrocortisone replacement.
b. Thyroid function with total or free T_4 should be checked ASAP.

c. Growth hormone therapy should be started immediately once diagnosis is confirmed.
d. Uncooked cornstarch can be used to help manage his hypoglycemia.

7. A 10-month-old, former 24 weeks' gestational age (WGA) male infant has recently developed intermittent episodes of hypoglycemia with plasma glucose levels as low as 30 mg/dL. He was receiving continuous feeds via a G-tube; recently, you have been working to condense his feeds, and he is now receiving daytime bolus feeds every 4 hours. Which of the following is true about his condition?

a. Critical sample is likely to show inappropriately normal insulin and suppressed β-hydroxybutyrate.
b. This condition is characterized by fasting hypoglycemia.
c. The patient will have lifelong hypoglycemia.
d. Hepatomegaly is an associated clinical finding.

8. Which of the following hormones is not involved in intermediary metabolism?

a. Glucagon
b. Insulin
c. Thyroid hormone
d. Growth hormone

9. Which of the following tests is most helpful in determining if the source of hyperinsulinism is endogenous (i.e., congenital hyperinsulinism) or exogenous (i.e., surreptitious in Munchausen by proxy)?

a. Insulin level
b. β-hydroxybutyrate level
c. Glucose response to glucagon administration
d. C peptide level

Chapter 58

1. Which statement is true regarding skeletal development?

a. The femurs are formed via intramembranous ossification.
b. A genetic defect resulting in impaired chondrocyte maturation would be expected to cause early onset arthritis but would not negatively affect the skeleton.
c. A genetic defect resulting in reduced alkaline phosphatase activity would negatively affect bone mineral density during infancy.
d. PTHrP is the primary regulator of osteoblast-mediated bone formation in neonates.

2. Neonatal magnesium status affects calcium metabolism in which way?

a. Hypermagnesemia results in hypercalcemia due to excessive secretion of PTH.
b. Hypermagnesemia results in hypocalcemia by binding calcium in the GI tract and thereby decreasing calcium availability for GI absorption.
c. Hypomagnesemia results in hypocalcemia via decreased PTH secretion.
d. Hypomagnesemia leads to hypercalcemia because magnesium is required for renal calcium excretion.

3. What is the mechanism of hypocalcemia in DiGeorge (22q11.2 deletion) syndrome?

a. Inactivating mutation in CYP27B1
b. Hypoplasia/aplasia of parathyroid glands

c. Renal resistance to parathyroid hormone
d. Activating mutation in PHEX with associated hyperphosphatemia

4. All of the following are signs/symptoms of hypocalcemia *except*:
   a. Shortened QTc interval
   b. Laryngospasm
   c. Involuntary muscle contraction
   d. Seizure

5. A 5.1-kg, 39 weeks' gestational age (WGA) infant suffers a hypocalcemic seizure on DOL 2. What is the most likely etiology?
   a. Hyperparathyroidism due to inactivation mutation in CaSR
   b. Transient hypoparathyroidism due to hypomagnesemia
   c. Familial hypocalciuric hypercalcemia
   d. Permanent hypoparathyroidism due to 22q11.2 deletion

6. A 32 WGA infant develops respiratory failure shortly after birth. Radiographs show marked undermineralization of bones and multiple rib fractures. Labs are notable for a serum calcium of 12.5 mg/dL, serum phosphorus of 8.5 mg/dL, and ratio of urine calcium to creatinine of 2.5. Which of the following tests will be most helpful in confirming the diagnosis?
   a. Urine phosphorus
   b. 25-OHD
   c. Alkaline phosphatase
   d. Intact PTH

7. Which of the following is not a risk factor for osteopenia of prematurity?
   a. Postnatal furosemide exposure for CHD
   b. Large for gestational age due to maternal diabetes
   c. History of necrotizing enterocolitis
   d. Birth weight of 1250 g

8. Which of the following is true regarding the clinical management of osteopenia of prematurity?
   a. Duration of TPN should be extended because this provides more phosphorus for bone mineralization compared to enteral feeds.
   b. DXA scans should be obtained every 4 weeks to screen for osteopenia in infants born <26 WGA.
   c. The goal calcium intake from enteral feeds in infants at risk of osteopenia of prematurity should be 150 to 200 mg/kg/d.
   d. All infants with birth weights <1500 g should be supplemented with 1000 IU of vitamin D daily.

9. A 2-week-old, term male infant is readmitted to the NICU with weight loss and dehydration. Labs are notable for serum calcium of 13.5, undetectable PTH, 25-OHD of 32 ng/mL, and 1,25-OHD of 175 pg/mL (normal range, 31–87). He has been breastfed and is receiving 400 IU of vitamin D_3 daily. Which of the following statements about the patient's underlying condition is false?
   a. He will be at increased risk of kidney stones in young adulthood.
   b. Initial therapy should include administration of normal saline at 1.5- to 2-times maintenance.
   c. His condition is iatrogenic due to excess vitamin D supplementation.

d. A low calcium formula may be needed to manage his condition during infancy.

10. A 12-month-old, former 26 WGA female infant with short gut maintained on elemental formula for the past 6 months is found on AM rounds to have acute-onset swelling and decreased movement of the left femur. Radiograph confirms a mid-shaft femur fracture and cupping and fraying of the distal femoral and proximal tibia metaphysis. Which of the following is true regarding the patient's underlying diagnosis?
    a. Urine labs will show elevated phosphorus.
    b. Hypocalcemia is a potential side effect of the treatment for her condition.
    c. Her condition is expected to be lifelong.
    d. Alkaline phosphatase will be low.

Chapter 59

1. Which of the following hormones is the primary driver of the acute physiologic response to cold stress?
   a. Cortisol
   b. Thyroid hormone
   c. Norepinephrine
   d. Growth hormone

2. Which of the following statements is true regarding brown adipose tissue?
   a. Fatty acids are the substrates for thermogenesis.
   b. Thermogenesis occurs in the nucleus of brown adipose tissue.
   c. It results in heat generation as a result of shivering.
   d. Infants have less brown adipose tissue, in proportion to body size, compared to adults.

3. Which of the following is not a mechanism of heat loss in premature infants?
   a. Convective heat loss due to cooler air environment in delivery room compared to womb
   b. Evaporative heat loss due to thin epidermis
   c. Excessive nonshivering thermogenesis
   d. Conductive heat loss to resuscitation bed because of decreased subcutaneous fat

4. Which of the following exposures is not a potential source of heat loss to a neonate?
   a. Mother's skin
   b. Inspired air via nasal cannula
   c. North-facing window in the NICU
   d. Blanket

Chapter 60

1. What is the primary site of erythropoietin production for the fetus?
   a. The kidney
   b. The liver
   c. The bone marrow
   d. The mother

2. Anemia of prematurity (AOP) is a multifactorial disease. Which of the following does NOT contribute to the development of AOP?
   a. Frequent blood sampling of premature neonates
   b. Suppression of erythropoiesis due to systemic illness

c. Inability of EPO to stimulate erythropoiesis in premature infants

d. Shorter life span of erythrocytes in preterm infants

3. ABO incompatibility is a common cause of neonatal hemolysis and jaundice. Which of the following statements about ABO incompatibility is true?

   a. The majority of pregnancies with ABO incompatibility will result in hemolysis and jaundice.

   b. ABO incompatibility worsens with each pregnancy.

   c. ABO incompatibility often results in fetal anemia that can lead to hydrops fetalis.

   d. Only infants with an A or B blood group whose mother has the O blood type are at risk of hemolysis due to ABO incapability.

4. What is the main hemoglobin produced by the fetus during the second trimester?

   a. HbF ($\alpha_2\gamma_2$)

   b. Hb Gower 1 ($\zeta_2\varepsilon_2$)

   c. Hb Gower 2 ($\alpha_2\varepsilon_2$)

   d. Hb Portland ($\zeta_2\gamma_2$)

5. Which of these diseases is symptomatic in the neonatal period?

   a. α-thalassemia major

   b. β-thalassemia

   c. Sickle cell anemia

6. Your patient, who has never been transfused, has a newborn screen that demonstrates a predominance of HbF with small amounts of HbS and HbA detected. What is the correct interpretation of the screening results?

   a. Sickle cell anemia

   b. Sickle cell trait

   c. Normal

7. The inheritance pattern of G-6-PD deficiency is

   a. Autosomal dominant

   b. Autosomal recessive

   c. X-linked recessive

   d. X-linked dominant

8. When is the majority of iron transferred from the fetus to the mother?

   a. First trimester

   b. Second trimester

   c. Third trimester

9. Iron supplementation should be considered for breast-fed term infants at what age?

   a. 1 month

   b. 4 months

   c. 1 year

   d. Never; it is not necessary

10. What is *not* an appropriate clinical reason to consider a partial exchange transfusion (PET) for polycythemia?

    a. To prevent neurodevelopmental delays

    b. For an extremely elevated central hematocrit (>70)

    c. For an elevated central hematocrit (>65) with persistent symptoms of polycythemia such as jitteriness or hypoglycemia

Chapter 61

1. What best describes the primary location of hematopoiesis in the fetus and in the full-term newborn?

   a. Fetus: thymus; newborn: bone marrow

   b. Fetus: liver and spleen; newborn: bone marrow

   c. Fetus: bone marrow; newborn: liver and spleen

   d. Fetus: liver and spleen; newborn: thymus

2. In the normal development of all blood cells from a hematopoietic stem cell, what is the first branch point of differentiation after an undifferentiated hematopoietic stem cell?

   a. White blood cells versus red blood cells and platelets

   b. Lymphocytes versus myeloid white blood cells, red blood cells, and platelets

   c. Red blood cells versus white blood cells and platelets

   d. Myeloid white blood cells versus red blood cells and platelets

3. A 2-day-old, ex-30-week premature neonate develops fevers and suspected sepsis. His white blood cell count is elevated at 23 (K/μL), and the differential includes white cell forms not normally seen including bands (14%), metamyelocytes (3%), myelocytes (2%), promyelocytes (1%), and blasts (1%). The hemoglobin and platelet counts are normal. What is the best explanation for the immature white blood cell forms seen in the peripheral blood?

   a. The white blood cells seen are immature forms representing the so-called "left-shift" and are likely due to bone marrow activation secondary to sepsis.

   b. The abnormal forms are worrisome and suggestive of infant leukemia.

   c. The white blood cell forms seen are immature cells and are likely due to the patient's prematurity.

   d. The abnormal forms are worrisome and suggest bone marrow dysfunction and a genetic syndrome.

Chapter 62

1. Neonatal thrombocytopenia associated with pre-eclampsia typically:

   a. Requires platelet transfusion

   b. Lasts 2 to 4 months

   c. Reaches a nadir within 2 to 4 days

   d. Is often associated with significant bleeding

2. Which of the following are true about neonatal alloimmune thrombocytopenia (NAIT)?

   a. It is associated with maternal thrombocytopenia.

   b. It is due to maternal antibodies against fetal platelet antigens.

   c. It does not cause severe thrombocytopenia.

   d. Random donor platelets are not an effective treatment.

3. Neonatal autoimmune thrombocytopenia is:

   a. Associated with maternal thrombocytopenia

   b. Due to maternal antibodies against the fetal platelet antigen HPA1a

   c. Not associated with severe thrombocytopenia

   d. Not effectively treated with random donor platelets

4. DIC is more common in neonates than older children and adults because:

   a. Neonates have lower von Willebrand levels than adults.

   b. Coagulation factors pass from the mother to the fetus.

c. Neonates have lower platelet levels than adults.

d. Neonates have lower levels of antithrombin and protein C.

5. Early-onset vitamin K deficient bleeding (VKDB) is associated with:
   a. Oral vitamin K
   b. Breastfeeding
   c. Maternal medications
   d. Malabsorption

6. Late-onset vitamin K deficient bleeding (VKDB) is associated with:
   a. Intracranial hemorrhage
   b. Mucosal bleeding
   c. Umbilical cord bleeding
   d. Excessive bleeding from circumcision

7. The classic triad of renal vein thrombosis is:
   a. Thrombocytopenia, hematuria, and a palpable flank mass
   b. Thrombocytopenia, high blood pressure, and hematuria
   c. High blood pressure, hematuria, and a palpable flank mass
   d. Hematuria, anemia, and thrombocytopenia

8. Unexplained thrombocytopenia in an infant with a central line should prompt an evaluation for:
   a. Fanconi anemia
   b. DVT
   c. Wiskott-Aldrich syndrome
   d. NAIT

9. Infants with thrombocytopenia absent radii (TAR):
   a. Often have anemia and immune deficiency
   b. Have improvement in platelet levels over the first year of life
   c. Lack thumbs
   d. Have mild thrombocytopenia

10. Neonatal purpura fulminans (PF) is due to all of the following *except*:
    a. Inherited deficiency of protein C
    b. Inherited deficiency of protein S
    c. Group B *Streptococcus*–associated sepsis
    d. Central line placement

Chapter 63

1. A 7-day-old, ex-28-week premature neonate has multiple medical problems and is found to be severely anemic with hemoglobin of 6 g/dL. There is no evidence of hemolysis, and the reticulocyte count is 1%. Your team plans a packed red blood cell transfusion for this patient. Which of the following red blood cell processing interventions by the blood bank would *not* be required for this patient?
   a. Type and cross to ensure ABO compatible blood
   b. Leukocyte-depleted PRBC to prevent viral infection transmission
   c. Irradiation to prevent CMV transmission
   d. Washing of the PRBC to prevent allergic reaction

2. A 4-day-old neonate with immunodeficiency has had significant blood loss after a major surgery. She now requires multiple transfusions of packed red blood cells. Her blood type is O positive. She has multiple family members offering to personally donate blood to her. Which of the following would be the most preferred donor?
   a. Random donor, blood type O positive
   b. Random donor, blood type A positive
   c. Patient's uncle, blood type O positive
   d. Patient's mother, blood type O positive

3. A 4-week-old neonate remains critically ill with multiple medical problems and is currently on oxygen by nasal cannula. After finishing a platelet transfusion, he suddenly develops multiple new symptoms, including hypoxia and increasing oxygen requirement, and low-grade fever. Chest x-ray shows new, widespread pulmonary edema. Cardiac silhouette is normal in size. What is the most likely etiology of this patient's reaction?
   a. Hemolytic transfusion reaction from ABO incompatible platelets
   b. CMV transmission from the platelet transfusion
   c. Transfusion related acute lung injury (TRALI)
   d. Transfusion associated circulatory overload (TACO)
   e. Sepsis from contaminated platelets

4. A 2-day-old full-term neonate is found to have bruising. The neonate has no bleeding and is otherwise well. Exam is unremarkable, although multiple bruises are noted. Complete blood count shows isolated thrombocytopenia with platelet count 15 ($\times 10^9$/μL). White blood cell count, hemoglobin, and white blood cell differential are normal. Maternal platelet count is normal. You suspect neonatal alloimmune thrombocytopenia (NAIT). In addition to giving IVIG, what would you recommend regarding transfusion therapy?
   a. Do not transfuse platelets, as the neonate is not bleeding currently.
   b. Obtain washed platelets from the father, and transfuse them to the neonate.
   c. Transfuse random donor platelets to the neonate.
   d. Transfuse fresh frozen plasma to the neonate.

5. A 2-day-old, ex-26-week neonate is extremely ill with sepsis and is found to have abnormal coagulation studies, including a very low level of fibrinogen. She is actively bleeding from her IV sites. What would be the best blood product to efficiently replace fibrinogen?
   a. Red blood cells
   b. Platelets
   c. Fresh frozen plasma (FFP)
   d. Cryoprecipitate

6. A 7-day-old, ex-30-week neonate is found to have an abnormal newborn screen with a severe decrease in TRECs (T cell receptor excision circles). Given this, you suspect a diagnosis of severe combined immunodeficiency (SCID). In addition to repeat and confirmatory blood testing and consulting the pediatric immunology and stem cell transplantation teams, what would you suggest regarding blood products for this patient?
   a. Avoid all packed red blood cell transfusions given the risks of allergic reaction.
   b. Avoid all platelet transfusions given the risks of bacterial infections with platelet transfusions.
   c. Ensure that all blood products are from a family member given the increased risk of infections with blood products.

d. Ensure that all blood products are radiated and CMV-negative given the risks of CMV infection in this neonate.

Chapter 64

1. A 1-day-old neonate in the newborn nursery develops respiratory distress. On exam, he is noted to have significant increased work of breathing as well as hepatosplenomegaly. Skin exam is notable for both significant bruising as well as numerous erythematous nodules. What is the most likely diagnosis?
   a. Acute myeloid leukemia
   b. Leukemoid reaction
   c. Neuroblastoma
   d. Cardiac rhabdomyomas
   e. Langerhans cell histiocytosis (LCH)

2. A 4-day-old neonate is suspected to have Down syndrome. Vital signs are stable, and she has no concerning symptoms or physical abnormalities other than stigmata of trisomy 21. Screening complete blood count (CBC) shows that the patient has a white blood cell count of 60×10^9 cells/L, and the white blood cell differential consists of 65% myeloblasts. She also has mild anemia and moderate thrombocytopenia. Which of the following is the most likely diagnosis?
   a. Acute myeloid leukemia (AML)
   b. Acute lymphoblastic leukemia (ALL)
   c. Leukemoid reaction
   d. Transient abnormal myelopoiesis (TAM)
   e. Neuroblastoma

3. For the neonate described in the previous question, short-term and long-term management would consist of which of the following?
   a. Observation and no long-term follow-up
   b. Observation followed by screening history, physical, and laboratory tests every 3 months for at least 4 years
   c. Chemotherapy for AML followed by screening history, physical, and laboratory tests every 3 months for at least 4 years
   d. Chemotherapy for AML followed by bone marrow transplant

4. A 2-month-old infant presents with persistent eczematous rash over his scalp and behind his ears. Eventually, skin biopsy is performed and shows abnormal histiocyte proliferation with immunostains positive for CD1a and CD207. The pathologist strongly suspects Langerhans cell histiocytosis. What would your next step be in the management of this patient?
   a. CT scan of the chest, abdomen, and pelvis to evaluate for additional tumors
   b. Bone marrow aspiration and biopsy
   c. Skeletal survey
   d. Repeat skin biopsy to confirm the diagnosis
   e. BRAF genetic testing

5. On prenatal ultrasound, a newborn was identified to have a large mass extruding from her body near her anus. The mass is quite large though there is no bleeding. The newborn was born via cesarean section and was stable at birth. You suspect a sacrococcygeal teratoma and consult the pediatric surgery team. What would your recommendations be for laboratory workup?
   a. No laboratory tests are required for this patient
   b. Alpha-fetoprotein (AFP) and beta-human chorionic gonadotropin (beta-hCG), although these tests are actually normal in the majority of teratomas
   c. Alpha-fetoprotein (AFP) and beta-human chorionic gonadotropin (beta-hCG); the majority of teratomas will produce AFP, and thus AFP will be elevated
   d. Alpha-fetoprotein (AFP) and beta-human chorionic gonadotropin (beta-hCG); the majority of teratomas will produce beta-hCG, and thus beta-hCG will be elevated

6. A 2-week-old neonate is found to have a large (5-cm) raised erythematous lesion over her right forehead, which seems consistent with a hemangioma. Which would be the most appropriate next step in her evaluation?
   a. Complete skin exam by dermatology
   b. Ultrasound of the abdomen looking for internal hemangiomas
   c. MRI of brain
   d. Laboratory evaluation looking for thrombocytopenia and DIC

7. The 2-week-old neonate in the prior question is also found to have a large hemangioma that is compressing her airway. Surgical management and embolization are not thought to be feasible for her. Which would be the first-line medical management for her hemangioma?
   a. Prednisone
   b. Propranolol
   c. Vincristine
   d. Sirolimus

8. A newborn was identified to have what appears to be a mass in his right adrenal gland on prenatal ultrasound. Further imaging on the child shows a massively enlarged right adrenal gland with lesions in the liver. Exam reveals hepatomegaly as well as blue nodular lesions on his skin. You suspect congenital neuroblastoma. Your next step in management would be:
   a. Pediatric surgery consultation for adrenal resection or biopsy
   b. Observation alone, as you are confident that the diagnosis is neuroblastoma and that it should regress with time
   c. MIBG (metaiodobenzylguanidine) scan
   d. Induction multi-agent chemotherapy
   e. Chemotherapy followed by tandem autologous stem cell transplant

9. A 1-week-old female is found to have multiple, small lesions in her heart, which seem to be in the lining of the ventricles as confirmed on echocardiography and MRI. She is stable and does not require immediate surgery. You suspect that she has cardiac rhabdomyomas. Which of the following conditions is very closely associated with rhabdomyomas and must be tested for immediately?
   a. Sturge-Weber syndrome
   b. Beckwith-Wiedemann syndrome
   c. Down syndrome
   d. Rhabdomyosarcoma
   e. Tuberous sclerosis

10. A 1-day-old neonate is found to have a palpable abdominal mass. Further imaging confirms a large retroperitoneal mass arising from the middle of the left kidney. The mass is relatively large, although the kidney capsule appears intact on CT scan. The child is otherwise healthy and has no symptoms. Which of the following would be the next step in management?
    a. Pediatric surgery consultation for immediate nephrectomy
    b. Genetic testing for familial cancer syndromes
    c. MIBG (metaiodobenzylguanidine) scan and urine HVA/VMA
    d. 24-hour urine collection for evaluation of hematuria
    e. Full-body MRI to evaluate for metastases

Chapter 65

1. A 1-month-old girl is brought to your office because her mother thinks the right eye "looks funny." She has tearing and photophobia when examining the right eye, which shows diffuse corneal edema with a corneal diameter of 12 mm. Her left eye appears normal. The most appropriate next step is:
    a. Corneal scraping for culture and institution of moxifloxacin eye drops four times a day
    b. Check intraocular pressure and refer to ophthalmology for glaucoma surgery
    c. Metabolic workup and referral to geneticist
    d. Corneal biopsy and referral for corneal transplant
2. A 10-day-old boy is brought to see you with a 2-day history of bilateral copious drainage and marked conjunctival injection. The most appropriate initial treatment is:
    a. Intramuscular ceftriaxone
    b. Oral erythromycin
    c. IM ceftriaxone and PO erythromycin
    d. Topical sulfacetamide
3. During a 1-month well-child check, the patient's mother reports a "strange glint" in her daughter's left eye. She was full term and is otherwise developing normally. You find a normal red reflex in the right eye but find a white pupillary reflex in the left eye. The most likely diagnosis is:
    a. Retinoblastoma
    b. Retinopathy of prematurity
    c. Strabismus
    d. Congenital rubella
4. A 2-day-old, full-term, otherwise healthy baby is noted to have drooping of the left upper eyelid. The right eye and eyelids appear normal. When you lift the lid, the pupil appears reactive and symmetric to the other eye, and the eyes appear well aligned. You tell the parents that this condition is most likely due to:
    a. Birth trauma in the setting of shoulder dystocia
    b. Damage to the third cranial nerve due to an intracranial lesion
    c. Poor development of the muscle in the upper eyelid
    d. Abnormal growth of blood vessels weighing down the upper eyelid
5. A baby boy is born to a healthy mother at 29 weeks and weighs 1700 g. Should this baby be seen for ROP screening, and, if so, when?

a. Yes. This patient should be seen 4 weeks after birth for ROP screening.
b. Yes. This patient should be seen at 30 weeks' GA for ROP screening.
c. No. Because of a birth weight of >1500 g, this baby does not need ROP screening.
d. No. Because this baby was born at >28 weeks, no ROP screening is needed.

6. A 1 week-old girl, born full term at home, presents to you for her first medical visit. The mother, who is 38 years old and has had four other children, reports that her husband delivered the baby at home without any complications and no medical care was needed. She reports that the child has been doing well. On exam, you note flattened facial features, upward slanting palpebral fissures, and a protruding tongue. What ophthalmic problem is this child at higher risk for?
    a. Congenital hereditary corneal dystrophy
    b. Congenital cataract
    c. Retinopathy of prematurity
    d. Marcus Gunn jaw-winking syndrome

Chapter 66

1. Genetic congenital hearing loss is most commonly which of the following combinations?
    a. Syndromic and autosomal recessive
    b. Syndromic and autosomal dominant
    c. Non-syndromic and autosomal recessive
    d. Non-syndromic and autosomal dominant
2. Which of the following statements is *false* regarding newborn hearing screening?
    a. Otoacoustic emissions and automated brainstem responses can be used for newborn hearing screening.
    b. Newborn hearing screening should be performed during the birth admission.
    c. If screening cannot be done during the birth admission, it should be done by 1 month of age.
    d. The goal of newborn hearing screening is to identify children with hearing loss prior to 12 months of age.
    e. At-risk newborns should undergo automated ABR screening.
3. Which of the following is considered a risk factor for hearing loss?
    a. Family history of permanent hearing loss in childhood
    b. Treatment with gentamicin
    c. Admission to the NICU >5 days
    d. Hyperbilirubinemia
    e. Prolonged mechanical ventilation
    f. All of the above are risk factors for neonatal hearing loss
4. Which of the following is the most common infectious cause of congenital hearing loss?
    a. Toxoplasmosis
    b. Syphilis
    c. Rubella
    d. Cytomegalovirus (CMV)
    e. Herpes
5. A 2-day-old infant is noted to have bilateral preauricular pits without evidence of drainage or infection. The child

does not pass their newborn hearing screen performed prior to discharge. Which of the following is the most appropriate next step?
   a. Surgical excision of the pre-auricular pits
   b. CT scan of the face
   c. Renal ultrasound
   d. Genetic testing
   e. Ophthalmology evaluation
6. A former 27-week premature infant with a birth weight of 1400 g passed her newborn hearing screen. Which of the following is appropriate follow-up after discharge from the NICU?
   a. Otolaryngology evaluation in 3 months
   b. Repeat audiometric evaluation in 6 months
   c. Repeat audiometric evaluation at 3 years of age
   d. Repeat audiometric evaluation only if hearing concerns develop
   e. Otolaryngology evaluation only if hearing concerns develop

Chapter 67

1. Which of the following is *not* a commonly described feature of the Pierre Robin sequence?
   a. U-shaped cleft palate
   b. Unilateral cleft lip
   c. Micrognathia
   d. Glossoptosis
   e. All of the above are associated with Pierre Robin sequence
2. A newborn is noted to have abnormal facies, including micrognathia, microtia, and telecanthus, as well as tetralogy of Fallot. You suspect DiGeorge syndrome. Which of the following would *not* help support your diagnosis?
   a. Genetic testing showing a 22q11 deletion
   b. Presence of a submucous cleft palate
   c. Anterior glottic web on laryngoscopy
   d. Serum calcium level of 11 mg/dL
   e. Absence of a thymus on ultrasound
3. A 3-month-old child was noted to have a small draining pit in his neck at the anterior aspect of the sternocleidomastoid muscle. The area intermittently gets swollen and drains. You suspect he has a branchial cleft cyst. Where would the fistula tract for this lesion most likely terminate?
   a. External auditory canal
   b. Parotid gland
   c. Tonsillar fossa
   d. Pyriform sinus
4. Which of the following is the narrowest portion of the airway in a child and adult, respectively?
   a. True vocal folds in both
   b. True vocal folds, cricoid cartilage
   c. Cricoid cartilage, true vocal folds
   d. Cricoid cartilage in both
5. A 3-week-old child born at 34 weeks' gestational age begins having inspiratory stridor worsened by agitation while feeding and when lying supine. There is no oxygen requirement and no apneic or cyanotic events. The child continues to gain weight appropriately and has a normal

cry. Which of the following is *not* appropriate in the initial management of this patient?
   a. Prone positioning
   b. Anti-reflux therapy
   c. Bedside flexible laryngoscopy
   d. Supraglottoplasty
   e. All of the above are appropriate interventions at this point
6. An 8-week-old child born at 30 weeks' gestational age begins having soft biphasic stridor that is progressively worsening over several days. The child's history is notable for several cutaneous hemangiomas, including one covering the right side of his cheek and chin. He was on CPAP after birth but did not require intubation and has been on room air. A bedside scope performed by ENT showed no evidence of laryngomalacia, and the vocal folds are mobile. You are suspicious for a subglottic hemangioma, which is confirmed on rigid bronchoscopy and shows 25% narrowing of the airway. What is the most appropriate intervention at this point?
   a. Tracheostomy
   b. Start propranolol therapy
   c. Biopsy the lesion to confirm the diagnosis
   d. Start steroid therapy
   e. Supplemental oxygen and racemic epinephrine

Chapter 68

1. At what gestational age has the epidermis fully matured?
   a. 6 weeks
   b. 12 weeks
   c. 16 weeks
   d. 20 weeks
   e. 24 weeks
2. Compared to the skin of full-term babies, the skin of preterm babies has:
   a. More keratinocyte attachments
   b. More pigment
   c. More hair
   d. More sweat
   e. More sun sensitivity
3. Underdevelopment of which skin structure predisposes neonates to increased thermal sensitivity?
   a. Sebaceous glands
   b. Collagen
   c. Melanosomes
   d. Eccrine glands
   e. Hemidesmosomes
4. You are seeing a neonate in the pediatric clinic with an irritant contact dermatitis sparing the skin folds. The rash is localized to the diaper region. Underdevelopment of which structure in the neonatal skin predisposes your patient to this condition?
   a. Stratum granulosum
   b. Stratum lucidum
   c. Stratum corneum
   d. Dermis
   e. Hair follicle
5. A 4-year-old patient presents to the pediatric clinic with multiple white nodules in the heels that have been

present since he was 5 months old. Although initially asymptomatic, these lesions have become painful. What is the most appropriate curative treatment?
a. Topical emollients
b. Watchful waiting
c. Topical steroids
d. Surgical excision
e. Rituximab

Chapter 69

1. Which congenital infection of the newborn presents at delivery with prominent scarring on the body?
   a. Cytomegalovirus
   b. Toxoplasmosis
   c. Varicella
   d. Rubella
   e. Syphilis
2. Which syndrome describes a vascular tumor with associated ophthalmologic defects, posterior fossa brain malformations, and arterial/cardiac defects?
   a. PHACES syndrome
   b. SACRAL syndrome
   c. LUMBAR syndrome
   d. PELVIS syndrome
   e. LAMB syndrome
3. You are working in the newborn nursery when you are called to see a neonate with diffuse redness; crusting around the eyes and mouth; and desquamation of the neck, axilla, antecubital fossa, and inguinal folds. You suspect staphylococcal scalded skin syndrome. To further help evaluate this neonate, where should you obtain bacterial cultures from?
   a. Conjunctiva
   b. Umbilical stump
   c. Circumcision wound
   d. Nasopharynx
   e. All of the above
4. You are seeing a neonate in clinic who was born with a giant congenital nevus. You counsel the patient's parents that there is an approximately _____ chance of malignant transformation of the nevus.
   a. 1%–3%
   b. 2%–6%
   c. 10%–15%
   d. 15%–20%
   e. 20%–25%
5. You are seeing a neonate in pediatric clinic who has a stubborn diaper rash with red, hemorrhagic plaques and some flaccid bullae, along with a red rash around the mouth, hands, and feet. What is the most likely diagnosis?
   a. Langerhans cell histiocytosis
   b. Irritant dermatitis
   c. Psoriasis
   d. Acrodermatitis enteropathica
   e. None of the above
6. Which of the following is *false* regarding the difference between neonatal pustular melanosis and erythema toxicum neonatorum?
   a. Erythema toxicum neonatorum presents in up to half of all full-term newborns.
   b. Transient neonatal pustular melanosis appears more commonly in Blacks.
   c. Erythema toxicum neonatorum usually is not present at birth.
   d. Transient neonatal pustular melanosis is characterized by eosinophils on Wright-stained smear.
   e. Transient neonatal pustular melanosis resolves with hyperpigmentation.
7. What is the most sensitive marker of neonatal lupus?
   a. Anti-dsDNA
   b. Anti-Ro/SSA
   c. Anti-La/SSB
   d. U1-RNP
   e. ANA
8. Which of the following is the most likely cause of collodion membrane at birth?
   a. Netherton syndrome
   b. Ichthyosis vulgaris
   c. Epidermolysis bullosa simplex
   d. Lamellar ichthyosis
   e. Congenital ichthyosis erythroderma
9. What mutation causes the mitten deformity seen in dystrophic epidermolysis bullosa?
   a. Missense mutation in Collagen VII
   b. Mutation in keratin 5
   c. Mutation in keratin 14
   d. Mutation in pectin
   e. Mutation in laminin 332
10. Which congenital ichthyosis is associated with prolonged labor?
    a. Ichthyosis vulgaris
    b. Lamellar ichthyosis
    c. Steroid sulfatase deficiency
    d. Epidermolytic hyperkeratosis
    e. Sjögren-Larson syndrome

Chapter 70

1. A preterm infant born at 29 weeks, gestational age, delivered via induced vaginal delivery in the setting of known severe IUGR, is currently 3 weeks old and has developed necrotizing enterocolitis. The infant is undergoing treatment with medical management. Which of the following are indications for surgical intervention in the setting of NEC?
   a. Pneumoperitoneum
   b. Portal venous gas
   c. Pneumatosis on abdominal imaging
   d. Significant cardiorespiratory compromise despite maximal escalation of medical support
   e. Fixed distended bowel loops on abdominal imaging
   f. a, b, c
   g. a, b, e
   h. a, d
   i. All of the above
2. Which of the following is not true regarding CPAM?
   a. Up to 15% of these lesions begin to resolve after 28 weeks' gestation.
   b. Rapid growth can lead to hydrops.
   c. CPAM volume ratio (CVR) <1.6 predicts an increased risk for fetal hydrops.

d. Ex utero intrapartum treatment (EXIT) procedure can be considered for severe cases.

3. Which of the following is true regarding gastroschesis?
   a. Intestinal torsion in utero or ex utero can result in bowel necrosis.
   b. Syndromes or chromosomal anomalies are often identified in these patients.
   c. Surgery is ideally performed at 24 to 48 hours to allow the infant's pulmonary pressures to fall.
   d. Once repaired, feeding can be quickly established.

Chapter 71

1. You are notified by the obstetrics team of a G1P0 mother who presented to triage at 23 weeks 0 days gestation with advanced cervical rupture of membranes 1 hour prior to arrival to the hospital, and she is intermittently contracting with signs of preterm labor. The fetus had a normal anatomic scan at 21 weeks' gestation, and the pregnancy has otherwise been uncomplicated. You are asked to provide counseling to the mother regarding resuscitation should the mother deliver under 25 weeks of gestation. You should incorporate all of the of the following in your discussion *except*:
   a. Assess parental understanding of the situation.
   b. Provide objective, concise, and evidence-based data surrounding neurodevelopmental outcomes.
   c. Provide counseling regarding survival primarily based on gestational age.
   d. Discuss limitations to interventions and care based on information available.
   e. Offer option for comfort care in the delivery room and redirection of care in the NICU with family bonding.

2. You are called to the delivery room of a term neonate born via vaginal delivery with signs of increased work of breathing, hypoxia, and poor perfusion. On exam, you find that the infant is macrocephalic with splayed suture lines. You additionally auscultate a loud systolic murmur over the LSB and astutely appreciate a bruit over the anterior fontanelle and orbits. You stabilize the infant and, on arrival to NICU, perform head imaging that demonstrates an intracranial arteriovenous vascular malformation. The likelihood of mortality is highest due to:
   a. Brain herniation
   b. Encephalopathy
   c. Seizure
   d. High output cardiac failure

3. You are at a prenatal diagnostic committee conference with your maternal fetal medicine colleagues and discuss the anatomic ultrasound findings of a fetus at 20 weeks' gestation. The imaging demonstrates hyperexpanded lungs, flat diaphragm, and dilated tracheobronchial tree. The findings are concerning for a syndrome with all of the following features *except*:
   a. Failure of the larynx to recanalize
   b. High association with other anomalies
   c. Pulmonary hyper-expansion leading to immune-mediated hydrops
   d. Carries a high mortality risk

4. You attend a delivery of a neonate with suspected transposition of the great arteries and intact ventricular septum and restrictive mixing based on a fetal echocardiogram. Following delivery, in the first hour of life, the infant experiences respiratory failure with profound hypoxemia, shock, and acidosis. Which of the following is the best intervention to relieve the hypoxemia acutely in the hour following delivery?
   a. Prostaglandin infusion for patency of the ductus arteriosus
   b. Balloon atrial septostomy
   c. Arterial switch operation
   d. Blalock-Taussig shunt

Chapter 72

1. A newborn 3-kg infant is admitted to your NICU and found to be hypotensive. You administer a single normal saline bolus with slight improvement in the blood pressure and then decide to initiate a pressor at an initial rate of 15 µg/min. You know the drug is cleared by first-order kinetics and are interested in determining how long it will take to reach steady state of the drug. Which variable will allow you to determine how long this will take?
   a. Elimination half life
   b. Dosage rate (mcg/min)
   c. Bioavailability
   d. Volume of distribution
   e. Saturation kinetics of the drug

2. Which of the following factors does not affect the transplacental passage of drugs from the maternal circulation to that of the fetus?
   a. The molecular weight of the drug
   b. pKa (pH at which the drug is 50% ionized) of the drug
   c. The extent of drug binding to the plasma protein
   d. Concentration gradient across the placenta
   e. The bioavailability of the drug

3. Phase II reactions occur after phase I reactions and facilitate the elimination of a drug from the circulation. Which of the following is true of phase II reactions?
   a. They include oxidation, reduction, hydrolysis, and hydroxylation.
   b. They are also referred to as "nonsynthetic reactions."
   c. They involve the cytochrome P-450 system.
   d. They include sulfation, acetylation, glucuronidation, and methylation.
   e. Alcohol dehydrogenases, esterases, and monoxygenases may be involved.

Chapter 73

1. A 29-year-old woman with a history of seizures has been well controlled on her maintenance medication and desires to be pregnant. She approaches her obstetrician and neurologist about an alternative antiepileptic. She read that her current medication can result in the fetus and infant having fetal growth restriction, cleft palate, midface hypoplasia with short nose, nail hypoplasia, and mental deficits. These characteristics are described by the use of:
   a. Carbamazepine
   b. Phenytoin

c. Valproic acid

d. Levetiracetam

2. A neonate born at 31 weeks' gestation in the setting of severe oligohydramnios is found to have bone ossification defects. The infant experiences severe renal failure with anuria following birth and dies by DOL 2. Autopsy and histology of the kidneys confirm severe renal tubular dysgenesis. The fetus was likely exposed to the following medication during pregnancy:

a. Enalapril

b. Cyclophosphamide

c. Zidovudine

d. Thalidomide

3. The Pregnancy and Lactation Labeling Rule requires a drug label to include all of the following *except*:

a. Pregnancy exposure registry

b. Description of adverse outcomes limited to structural abnormalities

c. A risk summary detailing if drug is contraindicated in pregnancy and supporting evidence

d. Information on background population risk

4. A mother is being managed on amiodarone and wishes to breastfeed her infant. The infant is at risk for which condition?

a. Adrenal insufficiency

b. Growth hormone suppression

c. Pancreatic insufficiency

d. Thyroid dysfunction

Chapter 74

1. Milrinone serves as an effective medication for heart failure with ventricular dysfunction through which of the following mechanisms?

a. Inotropy and lusitropy

b. Inotropy and chronotropy

c. Chronotropy and lusitropy

d. Chronotropy and dromotropy

2. A former 25-weeks' gestation infant is now 40 weeks corrected gestational age and noted to have new onset apnea and movements concerning for seizure. Past medical history is complicated by history of septicemia and BPD. A workup for sepsis including evaluation for meningitis is conducted. The cerebrospinal fluid (CSF) studies show concern for invasive bacterial meningitis. Which of the following cephalosporins has the lowest ability to penetrate the CSF?

a. Cefepime

b. Cefotaxime

c. Cefazolin

d. Ceftriaxone

3. Administration of amphotericin can result in which of the following serum abnormalities?

a. Hypokalemia, hypernatremia, hypermagnesemia, hypocalcemia

b. Hyperkalemia, hypernatremia, hypermagnesemia, hypercalcemia

c. Hypokalemia, hyponatremia, hypermagnesemia, hypercalcemia

d. Hypokalemia, hyponatremia, hypomagnesemia, hypocalcemia

4. Sildenafil can be an effective therapy in the treatment of persistent pulmonary hypertension. The following describe its mechanism of action *except*:

a. Phosphodiesterase-5 inhibitor

b. Enhances the effect of nitric oxide

c. Facilitates the breakdown of cGMP to GMP

d. Relaxes pulmonary vasculature

Chapter 75

1. The following factors impact outcomes for premature infants:

a. Transportation

b. Poverty

c. Exposure to crime

d. All of the above

e. b and c

2. Which of the following is consistent with value in health care?

a. Whether patients are satisfied with the delivery of care

b. Whether guidelines are followed in delivery of care

c. Whether outcomes are improved at lower cost

d. Whether care is delivered close to home

3. The following can measure value in health care:

a. Evidence-based medicine

b. Patient satisfaction

c. Professional guidelines

d. None of the above

4. Moral distress:

a. Can lead to poor quality of care

b. Is inevitable in the practice of neonatology

c. Can lead to greater empathy

d. a and b

e. All of the above

5. A 1000-g infant on BCPAP at 21% should be cared for in a:

a. Level 1 NICU

b. Level 2 NICU

c. Level 3 NICU

d. Level 4 NICU

e. Small baby unit

Chapter 76

1. Newborn screens are important in diagnosing conditions. The following are true statements *except*:

a. Federal guidelines dictate conditions to be screened.

b. Parents must sign consent for newborn screen in some states.

c. Conditions on a screen must meet three Wilson Junger criteria.

d. Blood spots are routinely used for research and do not require parental consent.

2. The following are ethically permissible:

a. Parents delegate clinicians to make decisions on their behalf after being given an opportunity to hear information and participate in decision making.

b. Clinicians feel that parents are too anxious and that delivering bad news would be too burdensome, so they avoid discussions about end-of-life care.

c. Morphine is provided for symptom relief in an infant who is dying knowing that an unintentional side effect is respiratory depression.
d. All of the above are ethically permissible
e. Both a and c are ethically permissible.

Chapter 77

1. Investigators are studying two methods ("new" and "old") of preventing intraventricular hemorrhage (IVH). The new method reduces the proportion of infants with IVH compared to the old method. The p value on a χ^2 test is 0.04. The clearest interpretation of the results would be:
   a. There is a 4% chance that the groups are different.
   b. The probability of finding a difference of this magnitude or more extreme, if there were truly no difference between groups, is 4%.
   c. There is a 4% chance that the old method works.
   d. There is a 96% chance that the new method works.
2. A nonparametric test (e.g., Mann-Whitney U test) might be the most appropriate statistical test to compare two groups of numerical values with each of the following characteristics *except*:
   a. Five observations per group
   b. Skewed distribution
   c. Normal distribution
   d. Ordinal data
3. The following groups of infants with hypoxic respiratory failure are treated with a selective pulmonary vasodilator: (1) infants with meconium aspiration syndrome, (2) infants with idiopathic pulmonary hypertension, (3) infants with congenital pneumonia, and (4) infants with congenital diaphragmatic hernia. Mean changes in right ventricular pressure are measured and compared using analysis of variance (ANOVA), which generates a p value of 0.01. The most appropriate interpretation of the result is:
   a. The null hypothesis of no difference among groups can be rejected.
   b. Each of the groups differs from each of the others.
   c. No statistically significant differences among groups are present.
   d. One of the first two groups differs from one of the second two groups.
4. In a preclinical test of a new surgical dressing, 7 out of 10 dressings in one group and 3 out of 10 dressings in the other fail after 30 minutes of water exposure, with a p value of 0.07 by χ^2. The investigators are concerned about a type II error. The most appropriate response would be to:
   a. Repeat the analysis using a more stringent p value.
   b. Repeat the experiment using a larger N.
   c. Repeat the analysis using a Fisher's exact test.
   d. Repeat the experiment using different surgical dressings.
5. An echocardiographic study compares two measures of left ventricular end diastolic volume. The two measures are compared in eFig. 77.15. The correlation coefficient (r) is 0.90. We can conclude that:
   a. 90% of the variance in one measure is described by the other measure.

b. The two measures are strongly correlated.
c. 95% of the variance in one measure is described by the other measure.
d. Measure 1 is a better reflection of left ventricular end diastolic volume than Measure 2.

6. Investigators are testing a new serum cytokine panel to predict the development of necrotizing enterocolitis (NEC) among infants with feeding intolerance. The performance of the test in predicting Bell stage II or above NEC is shown in eFig 77.16. The sensitivity of the test is:
   a. 75%
   b. 60%
   c. 80%
   d. 89%
7. The specificity of the test in eFig 77.16 is:
   a. 75%
   b. 60%
   c. 80%
   d. 89%
8. The positive predictive value (PPV) of the test in eFig 77.16 is:
   a. 75%
   b. 60%
   c. 80%
   d. 89%
9. The negative predictive value (NPV) of the test in eFig 77.16 is:
   a. 75%
   b. 60%
   c. 80%
   d. 89%
10. A proposed diagnostic test to predict the occurrence of a positive blood culture among infants with clinical signs consistent with sepsis is evaluated using a receiver operating characteristic (ROC) curve. The area under the ROC curve (AUC) is 0.60. We can conclude that:
    a. Infants with a positive test have a 60% chance of having a positive blood culture.
    b. At a cutoff for positive that provides a sensitivity of 100%, the test specificity will be 60%.
    c. This is not likely to be a very useful test.
    d. At a cutoff for positive that provides a specificity of 100%, the test sensitivity will be 60%.

Chapter 78

1. An advantage of case–control over cohort studies is that they:
   a. Can more accurately predict causation
   b. Are more likely to yield accurate exposure data
   c. Can oversample for rare outcomes
   d. Allow better assessment of relative risk
2. Investigators are considering a study to assess the effect of diuretic administration on the development of bronchopulmonary dysplasia. Compared to a case–control study, a randomized controlled trial would:
   a. More strongly infer causation of any observed effect
   b. Be less resource intensive
   c. Involve fewer additional risks to subjects
   d. Be completed more quickly

3. Investigators studying the effect of a new, oral angiogenesis inhibitor on diabetic retinopathy in a randomized controlled trial are concerned about bias in participant-reported side effects. Methods to avoid this might include:
   a. Developing a table of side-effect severity
   b. Concealing treatment allocation from study participants and investigators
   c. Using no treatment, rather than placebo, in the control group
   d. Asking about side effects weekly rather than monthly

4. Investigators are concerned about confounding factors in a study of the effect of a new breast milk fortifier on feeding intolerance. They could best minimize the chances of missing confounding by:
   a. Avoiding matching of control to case subjects
   b. Performing multivariate outcome analysis
   c. Performing an observational study
   d. Minimizing data collection about feeding-intolerance–related factors

5. Factors that make it more likely that an association between variables A and B in an observational study reflects A causing B include all of the following, *except*:
   a. Patients with higher exposure to A are more likely to develop B.
   b. A affects an enzyme pathway known to produce B.
   c. B always precedes A.
   d. Several previous studies in different populations have shown an association between A and B.

6. The most appropriate way to report the incidence of postneonatal sepsis in a pediatric population would be:
   a. 0.05%
   b. Five cases per 10,000 children
   c. Five cases per year
   d. Five cases per 10,000 children per year

7. A factor that improves the suitability of a screening test includes:
   a. Low sensitivity of the test
   b. Presence of a presymptomatic period
   c. Low prevalence of disease
   d. Lack of effective treatment

8. Factors that increase the advisability of a course of action in decision analysis include:
   a. Low likelihood of desired outcome
   b. Unclear data about probability of outcome
   c. High expected utility of the likely outcome
   d. Low agreement on value of expected utility of outcome

9. A neuroimaging scoring system to predict later neurodevelopmental impairment has been shown in previous studies to have good sensitivity and specificity but is complicated to derive from the images. A second neuroradiologist is being added to the study team. An appropriate approach to ensuring that the data that will be generated would be reliable would be to:
   a. Assess the face validity of the scoring system.
   b. Assess the internal consistency (Cronbach α) of the scoring system.
   c. Assess the interrater reliability (κ) of the scoring system.
   d. Assess the predictive validity of the scoring system.

10. Which of the following tests is accurate but not precise?
    a. Pulmonary arterial pressure is 50 mmHg, and echocardiographic estimates yield 48, 50, and 52 mm Hg.
    b. Pulmonary arterial pressure is 50 mmHg, and echocardiographic estimates yield 58, 60, and 62 mmHg.
    c. Pulmonary arterial pressure is 50 mmHg, and echocardiographic estimates yield 23, 42, and 58 mmHg.
    d. Pulmonary arterial pressure is 50 mmHg, and echocardiographic estimates yield 42, 51, and 56 mmHg.

Chapter 79

1. Neonatologists are interested in evaluating the effect of a new therapy on the development of hearing loss among infants with congenital cytomegalovirus (CMV). Which of the following would be the most appropriate surrogate endpoint for the effect of therapy on hearing loss diagnosed by behavioral audiometry at age 3 years?
   a. Brainstem auditory evoked response at birth
   b. Brainstem auditory evoked response at 6 months of age
   c. Death from CMV
   d. Cholestatic jaundice

2. Which of the following would allow a smaller sample size but maintain the power of a study?
   a. Larger expected difference between groups
   b. Smaller acceptable alpha (α) error
   c. Larger variability within groups
   d. Smaller acceptable beta (β) error

3. Which of the following regarding using surrogate endpoints in clinical research is false:
   a. The relationship between the surrogate and the actual endpoint should be stronger than a correlation.
   b. Surrogate endpoints should be less risky than definitive endpoints.
   c. The relationship between surrogate endpoints and definitive endpoints should be guaranteed.
   d. Surrogate endpoints ideally occur before definitive endpoints.

4. A new preventive therapy for bronchopulmonary dysplasia (BPD) among high-risk infants reduces the need for supplemental oxygen at 36 weeks postmenstrual age from 70% to 50%. The relative risk reduction in this study is closest to:
   a. 20%
   b. 29%
   c. 1.4
   d. 0.7

5. A new intervention to prevent retinopathy of prematurity reduces the likelihood of disease from 40% to 33% in a group of infants. Which value is closest to the number needed to treat?
   a. 14
   b. 7
   c. 7%
   d. 3

6. A therapy for upper respiratory infection is tested in a large trial. It shortens the duration of cough in upper respiratory infection from (mean ± standard deviation) 48 ± 12 hours to 46 ± 15 hours, with $p = 0.02$. The result is:
   a. Clinically important and statistically significant
   b. Not clinically important and not statistically significant
   c. Clinically important, but not statistically significant
   d. Not clinically important, but statistically significant

7. A cross-sectional study with comparison to a gold standard would be most appropriate for a study of the:
   a. Association of a rare disease with an earlier exposure
   b. Benefits and harms of an intervention
   c. Accuracy of a diagnostic test
   d. Prognosis of a condition

8. A case-control study would be most appropriate for a study of the:
   a. Association of a rare disease with an earlier exposure
   b. Benefits and harms of an intervention
   c. Accuracy of a diagnostic test
   d. Prognosis of a condition

9. A longitudinal cohort observational study, either with or without a comparison group, would be most appropriate for the study of the:
   a. Association of a rare disease with an earlier exposure
   b. Benefits and harms of an intervention
   c. Accuracy of a diagnostic test
   d. Prognosis of a condition

10. A randomized controlled trial would be most appropriate for a study of the:
    a. Association of a rare disease with an earlier exposure
    b. Benefits and harms of an intervention
    c. Accuracy of a diagnostic test
    d. Prognosis of a condition

Chapter 80

1. A multidisciplinary team decides to focus their next quality improvement effort on reducing hypothermia on admission to the NICU as they note that their percentage of infants with an admission temperature less than 36.5°C has increased threefold over the last 6 months. As a first step, they decide to meet to brainstorm potential cause-and-effects for the increase in hypothermia. Which diagram would likely help to organize their brainstorming session the best?
   a. A swimlane diagram
   b. An Ishikawa or fishbone diagram
   c. A pareto chart
   d. A run chart

2. Which of the following is *not* a requirement for a run chart?
   a. A line graph of time-series data
   b. A center line that is the median
   c. A p-value analyzing the trend line of the data
   d. An indication of your goal or desired direction

e. Annotations to describe what is happening during the timeline of your project

3. A fellow in your program is designing a quality improvement project focused on increasing the rates of skin-to-skin care in the NICU. She is deciding on a group of measures to track as she implements her change ideas. Which of the following is an example of a balancing measure?
   a. Percentage of infants receiving skin-to-skin care prior to discharge home
   b. Number of unplanned extubations occurring per month
   c. Staff completion of standing transfer simulation education
   d. Compliance with guidelines to have an additional provider at bedside for every transfer

4. You are tracking compliance with a new feeding guideline developed in your unit for extremely low birth weight infants. What type of control chart should be used to display your percent compliance data?
   a. P chart
   b. X and MR chart
   c. U chart
   d. X-bar and S chart

Chapter 81

1. You have been supervising a medical student in the newborn nursery and observed him speaking to the parents about their daughter's jaundice. After the encounter, you decide to provide him with formative feedback. Which of the following statements are consistent with the principles of providing effective feedback?
   a. "You did a great job talking to the parents about jaundice. They didn't have any questions afterwards."
   b. "When the parents asked how long their daughter will need to stay in the hospital, you estimated 1 to 2 days. I also suggest letting them know what their baby should accomplish before going home so that they understand the discharge criteria, just in case their baby does not respond to phototherapy as anticipated."
   c. "Let's say you have another baby with jaundice, but this child needs phototherapy. How would you explain phototherapy to the parents?"
   d. b and c only
   e. All of the above

2. You are preparing a workshop on developing a quality improvement project for a small group of pediatric residents. As you think about what you would like the residents to learn, you remember that learning objectives should include which of the following characteristics:
   a. Be specific in content, such as, "To list three ways statistical process control charts may be used in quality improvement initiatives."
   b. Detail how learning would be measured, such as, "To describe the pros and cons of using different quality improvement models such as PDSA, Six Sigma, and CQI."
   c. Identify the goals of learning, such as, "To understand the principles of quality improvement."
   d. a and b
   e. All of the above

3. You are developing the plan for a new workshop. You remember there are some key concepts in creating an effective learning environment for adults. An effective learning environment would include which of the following?
   a. A very bright room so that learners stay alert and engaged
   b. An interactive environment where learner input is encouraged
   c. Educational sessions that strictly follow learning objectives obtained from the chapter outline of a well-known textbook
   d. Educational sessions with large slide presentations that comprehensively cover core physiology topics
   e. Teaching that focuses on what learners need to know to pass the subspecialty board exam

4. As a neonatal fellow, you are responsible for teaching residents in a number of settings from lectures to simulation-based training. One of the pediatric residents is interested in learning more about various teaching strategies and asks about the benefits and challenges of each method. Which of the following is a true statement?
   a. Bedside teaching enables the facilitator to explore the application of learners' knowledge.
   b. Lectures allow the delivery of large amounts of teaching material in an individualized manner.
   c. It is challenging to standardize learner exposure using simulation-based training.
   d. Small group discussions are effective for learning when a dominant facilitator steers discussions to achieve the desired learning objectives.
   e. Virtual learning requires a higher facilitator-to-learner ratio than small group discussions.

5. You are the pediatric training program director, and you are looking at the current assessment methods within your program to ensure an integrative approach to trainee assessment both formatively and summatively. Which of the following statements is true?
   a. Multiple-choice exams are an efficient way to assess a breadth and depth of knowledge and conceptual understanding.
   b. An OSCE exam is the best tool to assess knowledge and the application of knowledge.

c. Formative assessments are used to make high-stakes decisions (e.g., certification examinations).
   d. Direct observation assessments in the clinical environment may help to identify learning needs and longitudinal goals.
   e. Short-answer questions do not assess the application of knowledge.

Chapter 82

1. *The Belmont Report* outlined three principles that are applied to clinical research. Each of the following represents an application *except*:
   a. Informed consent
   b. Subject selection
   c. Data analysis
   d. Assessment of risks and benefits

2. An investigator is the inventor of a drug delivery system and the owner of the company that makes the system. The investigator wishes to conduct a clinical study using the system as a step toward marketing it. What would be the most appropriate resolution of the investigator's conflict of interest?
   a. Choosing an independent investigator to perform the trial
   b. Performing the trial while turning day-to-day management of the company over to a colleague while maintaining stock ownership
   c. Choosing a subordinate at the company to conduct the clinical study
   d. Conflict of interest? What conflict of interest?

3. You are reviewing a manuscript detailing the development of a new drug treatment. You notice the figures depicted in Fig. 82.3 and mention the similarities between them in your review. The author returns the manuscript with no changes to the figures and no comment. This is a case of:
   a. Falsification
   b. Fabrication
   c. Plagiarism
   d. Honest difference of opinion

4. You have been an investigator on a project since its inception. You were instrumental in designing and

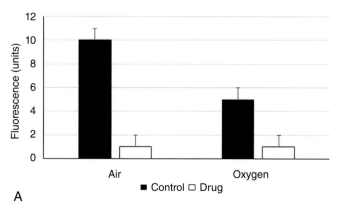

A

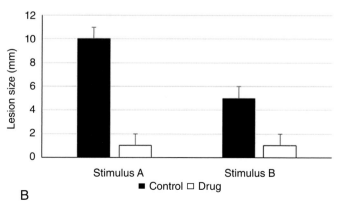

B

Fig. 82.3 Figures from an imaginary manuscript. (See question section.)

analyzing one of the assays in the manuscript. You drafted that portion of the manuscript and provided comments on the remainder of the manuscript. You have reviewed and understand the other components of the manuscript. You receive an email notifying you that the manuscript has been submitted. You open the attached file and notice that your discussion of your assays has been altered in a manner that changes the interpretation of the results. Which requirement for authorship do you not meet?

a. Approving the manuscript in its final form
b. Performing all assays
c. Drafting the entire manuscript
d. Reviewing the primary data from all assays

5. Investigators plan to study a new drug to reduce the risk of preeclampsia in pregnant women in a large randomized trial. They propose to screen women for preeclampsia risk but not share the results of the screen with the women. All women will be started on the drug or placebo. High-risk women will be randomized to the drug or placebo. Low-risk women will all be treated with placebo. Because the safety of the drug in pregnancy is incompletely studied, all women will be followed for adverse pregnancy outcomes, with the low-risk group serving as a concurrent comparison group to establish the baseline rate of complications in the population. Which of the following is most likely true of this study?

a. Risks have not been minimized, and potential benefits have not been maximized.
b. Risks have been minimized, but potential benefits have not been maximized.
c. Risks have not been minimized, but potential benefits have been maximized.
d. Risks have been minimized, and potential benefits have been maximized.

6. A clinical practice group is considering participating in a large randomized trial of an already available drug now being tested for amelioration of osteopenia of prematurity. One large observational trial suggested the drug might be effective and did not report new side effects. Small uncontrolled trials have yielded mixed results. One small controlled trial suggested efficacy but did not reach statistical significance. A meta-analysis concluded that there were insufficient data to combine to measure efficacy. In the practice group, some members routinely use the drug, whereas others avoid it. Which statement best describes the situation?

a. The data suggest efficacy; the group should not join the trial.
b. There is clinical equipoise; it would be reasonable to join the trial.
c. Because members of the group disagree, there is no clinical equipoise.
d. In the absence of firm evidence of efficacy, the group should not join the trial.

7. A newborn with severe sepsis and shock is eligible for a phase I, first-in-human trial of a new biological agent that decreases systemic inflammatory response in animal studies. The parents are eager to enroll their infant in the trial, stating that they are sure that the new treatment recommended by the doctors will help their baby. This is an example of which of the following?

a. Appropriate informed consent
b. Need for assent
c. Deception in research
d. The therapeutic misconception

8. A 12-year-old with leukemia is eligible for a study involving several additional blood draws and assays on 1-mL additional marrow samples at the time of clinical bone marrow aspirates. The aim of the study is improved understanding of tumor biology. Which best describes the consent process for this study?

a. The child can provide informed consent.
b. Due to the serious nature of the illness, parental permission without assent from the child is most appropriate.
c. Due to the risks, this research is not approvable.
d. Parental permission with assent from the child is most appropriate.

9. Given the existence of special protections of pregnant women and fetuses, which of the following would you expect is *not* likely to be approvable under federal regulations?

a. Research with the prospect of direct benefit to the mother and fetus and risk of significant harm to the fetus
b. Research with the prospect of direct benefit to the mother and risk of significant harm to the fetus
c. Research with no prospect of direct benefit to the mother or fetus and with the risk of significant harm to the fetus
d. Research with the prospect of direct benefit to the fetus and risk of significant harm to the fetus

10. Investigators wish to learn more about modifier gene effects on osteogenesis imperfecta (OI) phenotypes. They propose to perform open bone biopsies on unaffected school-age siblings of children with OI. Which of the following is true?

a. This would be considered minimal risk research.
b. This would be considered greater than minimal risk research with the prospect of direct benefit.
c. This would be considered research with a minor increase over minimal risk.
d. This research would not be considered approvable without permission of the Secretary of Health and Human Services.

Chapter 83

1. What is the study of choice to evaluate neonatal intracranial hemorrhage?
a. CT
b. US
c. MRI

2. Grade III intraventricular hemorrhage is associated with:
a. Cerebral palsy
b. Anatomic congenital anomalies of the brain
c. Venous infarct
d. a and c
e. All of the above

3. Evidence of hypoxic ischemic injury includes:
   a. MRI high T1 signal in the basal ganglia
   b. MRI low T1 signal in the cortex
   c. Increased echogenicity on ultrasound
   d. a and c
   e. b and c
4. Absent cerebellar vermis is a feature of:
   a. Chiari II malformation
   b. Holoprosencephaly
   c. Dandy-Walker
   d. Agenesis of the corpus callosum.

Chapter 84

1. What is the earliest sign of tension pneumothorax?
   a. Mediastinal shift
   b. Increased rib separation
   c. Hemidiaphragm depression
   d. Subcutaneous emphysema
2. Signs of bronchopulmonary dysplasia include:
   a. Coarse interstitial pattern, hypoexpanded lungs, pleural effusion
   b. Ground glass appearance, hyperexpanded lungs, rounded lucent areas
   c. Coarse interstitial pattern, hyperexpanded lungs, rounded lucent areas
   d. Pleural effusion, ground glass appearance, hyperexpanded lungs
   e. Coarse interstitial pattern, ground glass appearance, rounded lucent areas
3. Meconium aspiration may exhibit all but:
   a. Hypoexpansion
   b. Pneumothorax
   c. Asymmetric, patchy opacities
   d. Increased interstitial markings
   e. Pleural effusion
4. Match the congenital cardiac findings and associated x-ray findings:
   a. Transposition of the great vessels
   b. Tetralogy of Fallot
   c. Supracardiac total anomalous pulmonary venous return: snowman
   1. Boot-shaped heart
   2. Snowman
   3. Egg-on-a-string

Chapter 85

1. What finding suggests esophageal atresia without fistula?
   a. Dilated air-filled pharyngeal pouch
   b. No air in the stomach
   c. Distended small bowel
   d. Pneumothorax

2. Microcolon is associated with all of the following *except*:
   a. Malrotation
   b. Ileal atresia
   c. Total colonic Hirschsprung disease
   d. Infant of diabetic mother
   e. Meconium ileus
3. Necrotizing enterocolitis may exhibit all but:
   a. Bowel dilatation
   b. Bowel wall thickening
   c. Biliary air
   d. Pneumoperitoneum
   e. Pneumatosis
4. Malrotation is a condition:
   a. That may be diagnosed with ultrasound
   b. In which the duodenojejunal junction fails to cross the midline
   c. That is usually diagnosed by upper GI
   d. In which the duodenojejunal junction projects below the duodenal bulb
   e. All of the above

Chapter 86

1. Posterior urethral valves exhibit all *except*:
   a. Keyhole sign
   b. Vesicoureteral reflux frequent
   c. Hydronephrosis
   d. Distended small bowel
   e. Bladder trabecula and diverticula
2. All of the following are true for umbilical artery catheters *except*:
   a. Optimal position of tip between T7 and T9
   b. Dips posteriorly
   c. Extends toward groin from umbilical region
   d. Normally toward the left of the spine
3. All of the following are true for umbilical vein catheters *except*:
   a. The optimal position of tip is just above the diaphragm.
   b. They extend toward the chest from the umbilical region.
   c. They extend toward the groin from the umbilical region.
   d. They dip posteriorly.
4. Findings of achondroplasia include all of the following *except*:
   a. Anterior flaring of the ribs
   b. Small trident pelvis
   c. Metaphyseal flaring
   d. Platyspondyly

Answers Section

Chapter 1

1. **d.** *Explanation:* It is better to develop a detailed study map including topics to cover and time for each spread over a longer period of time. Short study periods, as short as 10 minutes, demonstrate improved retention compared to studying for hours at a stretch. If studying for >1 hour, incorporate a 10-minute break per hour. There is much work to cover. Don't worry about creating fancy schematics or charts. Focus on core content when developing study material, adding to this as time allows.

Chapter 2

1. **a.** *Explanation:* The residual volume cannot be measured because it is impossible to completely breathe out.
2. **d.**
3. **c.**
4. **d.**
5. **d.**
6. **a.** **False** (canalicular stage).
   b. **False** (embryonic).
7. **d.** *Explanation:* The canalicular stage is completed by approximately 26 weeks' gestation.
8. **c.**
9. **d.**
10. **a.** **False.** *Explanation:* It is directly proportional to surface tension and inversely proportional to radius.
    b. **False.** *Explanation:* Gas will flow into the larger one, as air flows in the part of least resistance.
    c. **False.** *Explanation:* There are four proteins.
    d. **True.**
    e. **False.**
11. **d.**
12. **c.**
13. **a.** **False.** *Explanation:* Measured with no air flow.
    b. **True.** *Explanation:* Static compliance reflects the elastic properties of the respiratory system, including lungs and chest wall, at rest.
    c. **True.**
    d. **False.** *Explanation:* Dynamic compliance reflects both elastic and resistive components.
    e. **True.**
14. **b.**
15. **a.** **True.**
    b. **False.** *Explanation:* Product of tidal volume and respiratory rate.
    c. **True.**

    d. **False.** *Explanation:* Physiologic dead space is increased in BPD.
    e. **False.** *Explanation:* CO_2 removal is dependent on pulmonary blood flow.
16. **e.**
17. **c.**
18. **a.**
19. **a.** **False.** *Explanation:* Shifted to the left at extreme altitude due to hypoxia.
    b. **False.** *Explanation:* Oxygen dissociation curve is shifted to the right at moderate altitude due to increased 2,3-DPG.
    c. **False.**
    d. **False.**
    e. **False.**
20. **Partially compensated respiratory alkalosis.** *Explanation:* pH and $PaCO_2$ levels are alkalotic, so the primary mechanism is respiratory alkalosis. The metabolic acidosis is compensation for the $PaCO_2$, but pH is not within normal limits, so it is only partially effective.
21. **Partially compensated metabolic acidosis.** *Explanation:* pH and HCO_3 levels are acidotic, so the primary mechanism is metabolic acidosis. The respiratory alkalosis is compensation for the HCO_3, but pH is not within normal limits, so it is only partially effective.
22. **Partially compensated metabolic acidosis.** *Explanation:* pH and HCO_3 levels are acidotic, so the primary mechanism is metabolic acidosis. The respiratory alkalosis is compensation for the HCO_3, but pH is not within normal limits, so it is only partially effective.
23. **Fully compensated respiratory acidosis.** *Explanation:* pH is at low end of normal (toward the acidotic side), but the HCO_3 and $PaCO_2$ indicate that something abnormal is happening. The acidotic factor is the primary culprit. Here, there is respiratory acidosis, and the normal pH means that it has been fully compensated by a metabolic alkalosis.
24. **c.** *Explanation:* The A-a gradient uses knowledge of alveolar gas equation: $PAO_2 = FiO_2(PB - PH_2O) - PaCO_2/RQ$, where PAO_2 is alveolar PO_2, FiO_2 (fraction of oxygen in inspired gas) = 0.21, PB = barometric pressure (760 mmHg at sea level), PH_2O (humidification of inspired air) = 47, $PaCO_2$ is the partial pressure of CO_2 in arterial blood, and RQ (respiratory quotient) = 0.8. $PAO_2 = 0.21(760 - 47) - 25/0.8 = 119$ (approximately). The A-a gradient = $PAO_2 - PO_2 = 119 - 60 = 59$.
25. **d.** *Explanation:* Calculate using Poiseuille's equation for laminar flow: $R = 8\eta l/\pi r4$. The resistance R changes by changes in the radius to the power of 4: $R = \frac{1}{2} \times \frac{1}{2} \times \frac{1}{2} \times \frac{1}{2} = 16 \times$.

26. **a.** *Explanation:* Oxygenation index (OI) = MAP × FiO_2 × 100/PaO_2; OI = 18 × 0.8 × 100/80 = 18.

Chapter 3

1. **a.** *Explanation:* Surfactant proteins are categorized as either hydrophobic (SP-B and SP-C) or hydrophilic (SP-A and SP-D). The hydrophobic proteins are secreted with surfactant in lamellar bodies and are required for production of lamellar bodies and for the normal spreading of surfactant phospholipids into a monolayer at the alveolar air-liquid interface. SP-B and SP-C are developmentally regulated. SP-A and SP-D are collectins that bind to carbohydrates on the surfaces of bacteria, fungi, and viruses. They are developmentally regulated and are important components of the lung host defense system.

2. **d.** *Explanation:* The 2010 AAP policy statement on the use of glucocorticoids to mitigate BPD does not recommend high-dose dexamethasone because of the potential for an adverse neurologic outcome. No subsequent policy has been issued. Both low-dose dexamethasone and the use of low-dose hydrocortisone require more randomized controlled trials, particularly focusing on neurodevelopmental outcome, before they can be recommended. Short courses of low-dose glucocorticoids are commonly used to treat BPD in ventilator-dependent patients. Their use should balance the potential benefits of these agents with potential harm they may cause. The decision to use these drugs should be individualized for selected patients.

3. **c.** *Explanation:* Caffeine therapy has been shown to prevent BPD in randomized controlled trials. Surfactant prevents RDS but does not prevent BPD. Antioxidants, vitamin E, and inhaled glucocorticoids do not have enough evidence to routinely recommend their use. Vitamin A therapy, however, does improve BPD rates.

Chapter 4

1. **b.** *Explanation:* Lung lavage with dilute surfactant does not have clear evidence to support its routine use. MAS is associated with inactivation of surfactant, and use of surfactant has been associated with less use of ECMO. Use of high ventilator rates can increase air trapping and increase the risk for pneumothorax. Further, hypocarbia can be detrimental to cerebral circulation. Muscle relaxants may be useful to improve oxygenation in severe MAS with PPHN, but routine use of muscle relaxants is not recommended.

2. **c.** *Explanation:* CMV transmission and disease are rare in term infants, as the mother will likely have transferred passive immunity to the infant during pregnancy. In preterm infants, passive transmission of immunity is incomplete and cannot be relied upon. In a prospective cohort study of very low birth weight infants born to CMV-seropositive mothers, the cumulative incidence of CMV infection at 12 weeks was 6.9%. About 17% of the infected infants developed the disease. Sepsis-like syndrome, interstitial pneumonia, hepatitis, and necrotizing enterocolitis are important clinical presentation of CMV disease in preterm infants. Holder pasteurization (62.5°C [144.5°F] for 30 minutes) and short-term pasteurization (72°C [161.6°F] for 5 seconds) of expressed breast milk can inactivate CMV. It is likely the short-term pasteurization will preserve more nutrients than the Holder method. Freezing of expressed milk does not reliably eliminate CMV.

3. **d.** *Explanation:* This baby is likely to have sepsis/ pneumonia. ABX will help treat an underlying bacterial infection. Avoiding hypothermia helps minimize pulmonary vasoconstriction. Assessing upper and lower saturations helps assess for reactive pulmonary hypertension. Although hyperventilation-induced alkalosis can result in short-term increase in PaO_2, it is not associated with change in long-term survival and has known long-term negative side effects.

Chapter 5

1. **a.** *Explanation:* Unilateral vocal cord paralysis is the second leading cause of stridor in infants. This is more common on the left side following damage to the recurrent laryngeal nerve. Surgery in the neck or the chest is the most common cause of the palsy, but trauma around birth, especially with the use of forceps, is also an important cause. Subglottic stenosis is usually acquired and is not present at birth, but laryngomalacia tends to present after the first few days of life, with the symptoms peaking at around 4 to 6 weeks of age. Similarly, hemangioma also presents after the first few weeks when the tumor enters the proliferative phase.

2. **d.** *Explanation:* Infant likely has Noonan syndrome with chylothorax. Noonan syndrome is associated with lymphatic abnormalities and is a common cause of congenital chylothorax. Fluid in congenital chylothorax is serosanguinous prior to initiation of feeds and may turn milky with onset of feeding. Diagnosis of chyle includes demonstration of lymphocyte preponderance (contributes to milky color), chylomicrons in the fluid, fluid triglycerides >110 mg/dL, and pleural fluid/serum cholesterol <1. Cardiac failure associated with anemia (immune and nonimmune) and cardiomyopathy can also present with fetal hydrops and serosanguinous fluid but usually do not have a lymphocyte preponderance of cell counts. Empyema has a high neutrophil count and protein in the fluid and can be caused by intra-amniotic shunt placements.

3. **d.** *Explanation:* This baby has a clinical diagnosis of congenital diaphragmatic hernia. Most infants are now diagnosed with CDH on prenatal ultrasound. It is important to expedite a CXR to confirm the diagnosis and rule out pneumothorax. Intubation based on the clinical diagnosis of CDH and current symptoms and gastric decompression to avoid air in the GI track can be considered prior to the CXR while being ready to address a tension pneumothorax should symptoms progress. Avoiding severe hypoxia and maintaining normothermia help minimize pulmonary hypertension seen in CDH babies. The reassuring pulses and perfusion

do not support a tension pneumothorax warranting an emergent thoracostomy at this time in the setting of probably CDH.

Chapter 6

1. **d.** *Explanation:* Fetal breathing is essential for lung development. Fetal breathing movements begin in the first trimester and are initially "tonic," with irregular tonic contraction of diaphragm and prolonged periods of apnea. The breathing becomes phasic in the third trimester but is still associated with apneic periods. Lack of fetal breathing due to neuromuscular diseases or ineffective fetal breathing movements (e.g., when the anterior chest wall is experimentally replaced with a silicone membrane) are associated with pulmonary hypoplasia. The fetus in this question is likely to have significant pulmonary hypoplasia, which will complicate the postnatal ventilatory management and may not be compatible with prolonged life.

2. **c.** *Explanation:* Biphasic response to hypoxia is characteristically noted in preterm infants, especially in those with apnea of prematurity. Adults normally respond to hypoxia with a sustained increase in rate and depth of breathing. In preterm infants, there is an initial increase in the rate of breathing, which is thought to be the result of peripheral chemoreceptor stimulation. After 1 to 2 minutes, though, a period of respiratory depression follows. This is primarily due to reduced rate rather than reduced tidal volume and is thought to be due to hypoxia-mediated central ventilatory depression. The mediators for such ventilatory depression include adenosine, GABA, and endorphins. Such inhibition of ventilation is noticed in the fetus too, leading to the hypothesis that the purpose of the inhibition is to reduce the metabolic rate, which, in a fetus dependent on placental oxygen delivery, will lead to reduced oxygen demand.

Chapter 7

1. **a** and **b.** *Explanation:* ECMO is used for reversible conditions unresponsive to less invasive treatment options. Given the need to anticoagulate and the technical limitations related to cannulation, it is not standard of care to attempt ECMO in infants <34 weeks and <1800 to 2000 g. It is also important to assess if a condition is reversible before initiating ECMO. Case (d) describes an infant with pulmonary hypertension related to severe pulmonary hypoplasia, which developed as a result of prolonged anhydramnios during an important stage of pulmonary development early in pregnancy. The pulmonary hypertension is related to structural maldevelopment of the pulmonary capillary bed, resulting in a poor prognosis.

2. **a.** *Explanation:* Infants of diabetic mothers can have delayed maturation of the surfactant, resulting in increased incidence of RDS at an older gestational age. Cardiac echocardiogram is indicated to rule out cardiac defect and confirm diagnosis of pulmonary hypertension. CXR assesses lung expansion and possible presence

of pneumothorax. Surfactant replacement is indicated before iNO when treating RDS. Steroid therapy has not been shown to benefit infants with RDS, with or without pulmonary hypertension.

3. **d.**

4. **c.** *Explanation:* NO (and therefore iNO) has a very short half-life of 15 to 20 seconds. It is given as an inhaled gas to avoid systemic hypotension from venous administration. While higher doses were used for early studies, there was little benefit and significantly increased risk of toxic metabolites, so recommended maximum and starting dose is 20 ppm. It can be weaned quickly if no response within an hour. After that, a slow wean is indicated due to downregulation of endogenous NO. iNO can lead to pulmonary edema in the setting of left ventricular failure and should be avoided.

5. **e.** *Explanation:* Dexamethasone has been shown to hinder linear growth.

6. **e.** *Explanation:* Jet attenuates pressure, allowing healing in air leak conditions and gentle ventilation with pulmonary hypoplasia. It is associated with less impeding of venous return to the heart at comparable pressures to other types of high frequency. The spiral expiratory air flow dynamic can aide in clearance of aspirated material and secretions.

Chapter 8

1. **a.** *Explanation:* Truncus arteriosus results from failure of the conotruncus to separate.

2. **a.**

Chapter 9

1. **b.**

2. **d.**

Chapter 10

1. **d.** *Explanation:* The infant is this scenario is having a hypercyanotic spell caused by an acute decrease in PBF. These are commonly triggered by medical procedures such as blood draws. Morphine and phenylephrine are first-line agents to counteract the hypercyanotic spell.

2. **d.** *Explanation:* Both type B interrupted arch and truncus arteriosus are associated with 22q11 deletion syndrome. Infants with 22q11 deletion syndrome frequently have hypocalcemia and an absent thymus.

Chapter 11

1. **c.** *Explanation:* Numerous cardiac tumors found in a neonate are almost always rhabdomyomas, which are strongly associated with tuberous sclerosis.

2. **a.** *Explanation:* Very preterm infants frequently develop hypotension because the immature left ventricle is

unable to mount the dramatic increase in output needed to adapt to the sudden increase in systemic vascular resistance with the removal of the low-resistance placental circuit.

Chapter 12

1. **c.** *Explanation:* This baby has complete heart block related to transplacental transfer of SSA and/or SSB antibodies from maternal lupus. Although the heart rate is low, the infant has adequate cardiac output, as evidenced by good capillary refill and blood pressure. Monitoring is all that is required at this time.
2. **b.** *Explanation:* This infant had an episode of atrial flutter, which is very unlikely to recur and does not warrant prophylaxis.

Chapter 13

1. **b.** *Explanation:* Atrioventricular block is a well-described result of digoxin toxicity. Digoxin toxicity is more likely to occur in the setting of hypokalemia.
2. **d.**

Chapter 14

1. **c.** *Explanation:* Spinal muscular atrophy (SMA) can present in the newborn and is now present on the newborn screen in 48 of 50 states in the United States. Spinal muscular atrophy is a disorder of the anterior horn cell and will present with absent deep tendon reflexes and tongue fasciculations. Seizures and brain malformation are not typically present, although nonspecific brain findings have been reported in the most severe form of SMA, SMA type 0. Hypotonic facies and poor feeding are commonly seen in various causes of neonatal hypotonia and are not specific to SMA. Typically, the face is spared in SMA, with the exception of tongue fasciculations.
2. **c.** *Explanation:* The Moro reflex arises at well formed by 37 weeks' gestational age and remains until approximately 4 to 6 months of age. An asymmetric Moro reflex should raise concern for a brachial plexus injury on the ipsilateral side of the asymmetry. Patients with perinatal stroke do not have an asymmetric Moro reflex. Newborns with encephalopathy will often have depression or complete absence of developmental reflexes such as the suck or Moro reflex.
3. **a.** *Explanation:* Signs of increased intracranial pressure in the preterm can include splayed sutures, bulging fontanelle, skew deviation of the eyes in primary gaze, and increased tone in the popliteal angles. Skew deviation can occur, as sixth cranial nerve palsy can occur with increased intracranial pressure. Increased tone or "tightness" at the popliteal angle can occur due to stretching of the motor fibers caused by acute changes in intracranial pressure. This can be tested by assessing the range of motion at the knee.

Chapter 15

1. **d.** *Explanation:* The greatest risk for recurrent myelomeningocele for a mother is having a prior affected child with the same father. This pattern indicates a yet unidentified genetic factor for neural tube defects. Folic acid supplementation starting now, at 8 weeks' gestation, will not affect the risk of myelomeningocele. Open neural tube defects are a result of neurulation errors occurring at 3 to 4 weeks' gestation. Folic acid supplementation initiation is recommended pregestation with 400 µg daily for most women and 4000 µg daily for women with a prior affected child. Vitamin B_{12} deficiency is also a risk factor for neural tube defects and should be considered in women on vegan diets and in women with pernicious anemia. Cocaine use and smoking are not documented risk factors for the development of neural tube defects. Alcohol is weakly associated with increased rates. Her acne medication may be isotretinoin, which is a known teratogen and does increase the development of neural tube defects. Other classic medication risks include valproate and carbamazepine. The maternal metabolic environment also elevates the risk of neural tube defects including maternal obesity, maternal pregestational diabetes, and first-trimester maternal hyperthermia.
2. **c.** *Explanation:* MRI is the standard of care for determining if an infant has agenesis of the corpus callosum, and with phenotypically normal parents, this is likely an autosomal recessive inheritance pattern with 25% risk of the infant being affected. The infant does not need to be admitted to the NICU. The infant is well appearing, with stable vitals and no abnormalities in phenotypic appearance that would be concerning for immediate evaluation and treatment. Though this infant most likely has agenesis of the corpus callosum with notable findings on the fetal ultrasound, it can be difficult for parents to see a well appearing infant and their infant still has a notable neurological finding. Agenesis of the corpus callosum can have a wide range of outcomes, from a normal life to global developmental delay, seizures, and other anomalies. Many with agenesis of the corpus callosum have an associated genetic/metabolic defect that may not have a phenotypical appearance at birth. Despite etiology, affected infants are at increased risk for seizures later in life. With a well appearing infant, despite prenatal findings, you should first confirm the infant has agenesis of the corpus callosum by MRI of the brain before further workup. MRI of the brain, not head ultrasound, is the standard of care to diagnose this finding. If confirmed, chromosomal analysis should be considered for both the infant and parents. With phenotypically normal parents and no history of infections or alcohol use with a well appearing male infant, the most likely cause of this infant having agenesis of the corpus callosum is an autosomal recessive inheritance pattern. In X-linked dominant inheritance, there is a 50% risk of inheritance of the affected X-chromosome. Female infants have a milder presentation, and male infants present with more severe findings. It would be unlikely that a male infant with X-linked dominant inheritance would be well appearing and phenotypically normal at birth.

3. **d.** *Explanation:* Although this infant likely has post hemorrhagic hydrocephalous resulting in the macrocephaly and acute neurological clinical signs observed, you must also consider a sepsis evaluation. Although this infant is having apnea episodes, he has a normal respiratory rate and stable vital signs between the episodes. This would not indicate the infant needs intubation, emergent neurologic subspeciality consultation, or an emergent MRI. Anytime an infant has apneic events and becomes lethargic, despite all information suggesting hydrocephalous, you must consider a sepsis evaluation and broad-spectrum antibiotics alongside any neurological workup. A head ultrasound is noninvasive, can be performed at bedside, and will allow initial diagnosis of hydrocephalus in an infant with an open fontanelle.

4. **a.** *Explanation:* Indomethacin is neuroprotective and decreases the risk of intraventricular hemorrhage in preterm neonates through a decrease in cerebral blood flow by prostaglandin inhibition. Cerebral blood flow can be regulated by local chemical factors that affect vascular resistance. Cerebral blood flow vasodilators increase arterial blood pressure and include hypoxia, acidosis (or high H+), hypercarbia, hyperkalemia, hypocalcemia, adenosine, prostaglandin, nitric oxide, and hyperosmolarity. Cerebral blood flow vasoconstrictors increase venous blood pressure (increase right atrial pressures, intraventricular hemorrhage) and include hyperoxia, hypocarbia, hypokalemia, hypercalcemia, antagonist to adenosine (caffeine), and prostaglandin inhibition (indomethacin). Prophylactic indomethacin has been shown to be an effective intervention in reduction of morbidity and mortality of preterm infants in both cardiopulmonary and neurodevelopmental outcomes. Particularly, the decrease in cerebral blood flow is neuroprotective and reduces the risk of intraventricular hemorrhage. With hypercarbia, hypotension, and hyperoxia that may occur in preterm infants, particularly in very low birth weight infants without maternal steroids, there are hyperemic responses that increase permeability through the blood–brain barrier. Indomethacin is an inhibitor in the cyclooxygenase pathway and reduces these hyperemic responses, thus reducing the cerebral perfusion induced ischemia risk to preterm brains.

Chapter 16

1. **b.** *Explanation:* Moderate HIE. Lethargy, hypotonia, exaggerated grasp reflex, and weak suck are present in Sarnat stage 2 (moderate encephalopathy).

2. **a.** *Explanation:* MRI findings with injury to deep gray matter or posterior limb of internal capsule is associated with adverse motor deficits and outcomes.

Chapter 17

1. **b.** *Explanation:* Periventricular leukomalacia represents injury and maldevelopment of the periventricular white matter that may be cystic or non-cystic and is best identified on ultrasound at about 4 weeks after birth. Although injurious processes may be occurring in the time period just after birth, the development of white matter abnormalities that are visible on an ultrasound takes time and thus will not be apparent at 24 hours after birth and is unusual to see at just 7 days after birth.

2. **c.** *Explanation:* Significant intracranial hemorrhages are not usually associated with the routine uncomplicated use of a vacuum to assist in the delivery of a term infant. A 32-week infant who does not require significant resuscitation at the time of birth is also unlikely to develop a significant intracranial hemorrhage. Neonates born at 26 weeks in the setting of a placental abruption that require significant resuscitation after birth are at high risk of developing significant intracranial hemorrhages in the form of intraventricular hemorrhage.

Chapter 18

1. **c and d.** *Explanation:* Risk of these is increased from traction and torsion of the head. These movements would not increase the risk of cephalohematoma and skull fracture.

2. **c.** *Explanation:* Subgaleal hemorrhage: pale baby, boggy head, fluctuant scalp

3. **d.** *Explanation:* For every increase in head circumference of 1 cm, estimated blood loss is 30 to 40 cc.

4. **d.** *Explanation:* Large subgaleal hematoma is a life-threatening complication that carries a high mortality if not treated with replacement of blood products and monitoring for disseminated intravascular coagulopathy.

Chapter 19

1. **c.** *Explanation:* Neonatal seizures that present early (in the first hours after birth) and are resistant to multiple antiepileptic medications, in the context of an uncomplicated pregnancy and delivery, are unlikely to be hypoxic–ischemic encephalopathy. These will rapidly improve with administration of pyridoxine. Other causes listed are unlikely to present this early and should have additional history (jaundice in the case of kernicterus, perinatal risk factors/events in case of hypoxic–ischemic encephalopathy).

2. **b.** *Explanation:* Jervell and Lange-Nielson syndrome is an autosomal recessive mutation in the genes *KCNE1* and *KCNQ1*, coding for potassium channels that affect the cardiac conduction system, leading to long QT syndrome as well as affecting the auditory system, leading to congenital sensorineural hearing loss. Patients with cardiac arrhythmias may experience seizures, and ECG is a useful diagnostic tool.

Chapter 20

1. **b.** *Explanation:* Although group B *Streptococcus* (GBS) is the most common cause of neonatal meningitis overall, *Escherichia coli* has become the most commonly isolated organism in very low birth weight infants. Other major

pathogens causing early onset meningitis in neonates include *Listeria* and *Streptococcus pneumoniae.* Other pathogens causing late-onset meningitis include coagulase-negative *Staphylococcus, Staphylococcus aureus, Klebsiella, Enterococcus, Enterobacter,* and *Pseudomonas.*

2. **c.** *Explanation:* HSV-2 is responsible for 70% of neonatal HSV infections, and almost all infections occur at the time of delivery. Although there have been a few case reports of congenitally acquired HSV, it is extremely rare. Early administration and continued therapy for 6 months have been shown to improve long-term neurodevelopmental outcomes. Skin lesions may or may not be associated with CNS disease, but they often do not present until well into the course of the disease.

3. **d.** *Explanation:* This patient likely has a brain abscess. These are more common in the gram-negative species including *Citrobacter, Proteus,* and *Pseudomonas.* Repeating CSF studies may not yield information, especially if the patient is on appropriate antibiotics. Although antibiotics may treat brain abscesses, they may require surgical drainage. Imaging to identify the size, location, and presence of a brain abscess is the next step in management. Corticosteroids have not been shown to improve outcomes.

4. **a.** *Explanation:* Aminoglycosides are well known for causing ototoxicity, and gentamicin has been shown to lead to long-term hearing impairment. However, vancomycin and meropenem have also been shown to have ototoxic side effects. Amphotericin B is also associated with ototoxicity.

5. **b.** *Explanation:* Although the most common cause of neonatal meningitis is group B *Streptococcus* (GBS), the percentage of monocytes seen in this patient's CSF make it more likely to be *Listeria.* Although slightly elevated protein is not uncommon in both term and preterm neonates, this patient's CSF suggests clear infection and elevated CSF protein beyond the expected range.

6. **d.** *Explanation:* CSF studies for suspected CNS involvement of *Candida* spp. are inconclusive and can sometimes be normal. There are no consistent CSF profiles associated with CNS *Candida* infection. *Candida* often forms abscesses that can make lumbar puncture results appear normal. Treatment of CNS disease should be initiated if infection is suspected regardless of CSF results.

Chapter 21

1. **d.** *Explanation:* This neonate has classic symptoms of neonatal opioid withdrawal syndrome from opiate withdrawal. The timing of symptom onset depends on both the medication and timing of last dose prior to delivery. In utero clearance occurs much more rapidly than neonatal opiate clearance. Withdrawal symptoms from chronic maternal short-acting opiate use may peak in the first 1 to 2 days; long-acting opiate withdrawal (methadone/buprenorphine) peaks at days 3 to 4 and may extend for weeks to months. Maternal buprenorphine does not cross the placenta as readily as methadone. This is likely the physiology behind the association between buprenorphine therapy and less frequent/severe withdrawal in neonates when compared with

methadone. The modified Finnegan scoring has been the scoring system recommended by the AAP. It is used for serial evaluation of neonatal withdrawal from opiates and is not diagnostic of opiate withdrawal. Many neonatal states can result in increased scores. Optimizing nonpharmacological interventions combined with functional assessment tools evaluating feeding, sleeping, and the infant's ability to console (eat, sleep, console) are being increasingly used in clinical treatment and evaluation of symptoms of withdrawal. Routine urine toxicology screens do not include buprenorphine and methadone. These synthetic opiates do not result in a positive opiate result on routine screen. This mother's negative urine screen does not indicate buprenorphine noncompliance. Breastfeeding is recommended in this setting and is associated with reduced withdrawal. The effects are not attributed to medication exposure in breast milk, as buprenorphine and methadone only cross into the breast milk in small amounts. Breastfed babies benefit from increased frequency feeds. Formula-fed neonates often require increased volume and caloric density feeds.

2. **b.** *Explanation:* Tobacco is a common substance used in combination with opioids and can adversely affect the total amount of opioid used to treat NAS symptoms as well as the length of treatment. In addition, polysubstance exposure is a strong predictor of the severity of the NAS. This includes exposure to cocaine, SSRIs, and benzodiazepines. Exposure to two or more psychotropic drugs increases the risk for NAS twofold for infants exposed prenatally to opioids. Shorter duration of opioid use during pregnancy has a lower risk of NAS as compared to longer use (>30 days). However, the absolute maternal dose of opioid agonist medication has not significantly or consistently been found to correlate to the severity of NAS symptoms.

3. **a.** *Explanation:* This infant has clinical findings characteristic of exposure to alcohol in utero. This is a dose-dependent disease that ranges from having effects of alcohol to fetal alcohol syndrome. Infants can have withdrawal from alcohol, and it is thought to be underrecognized. Alcohol exposure in utero has been associated with differences in long-term outcomes, specifically behavioral changes and a reduction in IQ. Fetal growth is adversely affected by alcohol, and the fetus typically has poor growth and is more likely to be SGA and microcephalic.

Chapter 22

1. **c.** *Explanation:* Congenital myotonic dystrophy is an autosomal dominant disorder typically inherited from the mother. In the congenital form, neonates are hypotonic at birth, often demonstrating poor respiratory effort. Classic examination findings include facial hypotonia, with decreased nasolabial folds bilaterally, with a carp-like appearance to the mouth and severe hypotonia on examination. Deep tendon reflexes are absent, and talipes equinovarus is frequent. Many require respiratory support initially with ventilator or positive pressure ventilation, such as bilevel positive airway pressure (BiPAP) or continuous positive airway pressure (CPAP).

The disorder demonstrates anticipation, with each generation affected more significantly than the prior, which is caused by a CTG repeat in the 3'UTR of the *DMPK* gene on chromosome 19. Unaffected individuals have between 5 and 27 repeats, but affected neonates present with greater than 1000 repeats. The number of repeats correlates with disease severity, and affected mothers have between 50 and 1000 repeats. Frequently, the mother may not be diagnosed with a neuromuscular condition but, on discussion, has a history of hand weakness or cramping. Examination of the mother reveals facial hypotonia, myotonic response of the hand muscles, and frontal balding. Although decreased fetal movements or prior fetal losses may be present in congenital myotonic dystrophy and may support the diagnosis, these are features present in numerous neuromuscular and genetic conditions. Fetal alcohol syndrome does not present with neuromuscular weakness.

2. **c.** *Explanation:* This examination is most consistent with a moderate encephalopathy. The description of the mental status is equivalent to lethargy, given the necessity for persistent stimulation to arouse the neonate. This is supported by the absence of some primitive reflexes and the hypotonic examination. Severely encephalopathic neonates do not arouse to stimulation but may show posturing on stimulation. Primitive reflexes such as plantar grasp, Moro reflex, and suck are absent, and deep tendon reflexes may be hyperreflexic or completely absent.

3. **b.** *Explanation:* Port-wine birthmarks involving the bilateral forehead with extension to the frontonasal prominence are considered high risk for Sturge-Weber syndrome. However, the patient described is noted to have a normal neurologic exam with no events raising suspicion for seizures. Based on this, imaging is not currently indicated. However, given the high-risk location of the port-wine birthmark, referral to pediatric ophthalmology is warranted for baseline neurologic examination.

4. **d.** *Explanation:* Cardiac rhabdomyomas are associated with tuberous sclerosis complex (TSC). Patients with tuberous sclerosis may develop cortical tubers and epilepsy, but they are also at risk for subependymal nodules and subependymal giant cell astrocytomas. Genetic testing for TSC should be considered, alongside genetic counseling. Cranial ultrasound should be considered for patients known to have cardiac rhabdomyomas. The remaining findings are not associated with TSC.

5. **a.** *Explanation:* Incontinentia pigmenti (IP) is a neurocutaneous disorder that can present in the neonatal period, initially with vesicular lesions that follow the lines of Blaschko. HSV should be ruled out in the patient; however, clinical suspicion for IP should increase if negative HSV PCR, vesicular lesions that follow the lines of Blaschko, and eosinophilic predominance are present.

6. **b.** *Explanation:* The fetus described raises concern for a congenital cerebral neoplasm resulting in obstructive hydrocephalus with subsequent macrocrania. Given this, considerations regarding the safest mode of delivery are necessary, such that a cesarean-section is highly likely. Although neurosurgery consultation is indicated prenatally for postnatal planning, fetal biopsy is risky and not currently recommended. Oncology and

neurology support is indicated postnatally, but cEEG is not necessarily indicated.

Chapter 23

1. **c.** *Explanation:* The infant exhibits moderate encephalopathy based on Sarnat staging criteria, with moderate category for level of consciousness, spontaneous activity, posture, tone, suck reflex, and respirations. The infant meets biochemical and neurologic criteria with a history of an acute perinatal event (cord prolapse) that warrants therapeutic cooling. Note: Therapeutic cooling is not recommended for infants with mild encephalopathy due to lack of demonstrated benefit and potential for harm.

2. **b.** *Explanation:* Early dexamethasone use within the first week of life is associated with worse neurodevelopmental outcomes and higher rates of cerebral palsy.

3. **d.** *Explanation:* Infants with fetal growth restriction have decreased total cerebral volume and total number of brain cells, thinner cortical thickness, abnormal gyration, delayed myelination, and reduced structural complexity of gray and white matter.

Chapter 24

1. **a.** *Explanation:* Prone position in VLBW premature infants has shown better physiologic stability with improved gas exchange (increased PaO_2, decreasing PCO_2), decreased respiratory rate, improved chest wall synchrony, increased overall sleep state, decreased energy expenditure, more rapid gastric emptying, and less reflux.

2. **a.** *Explanation:* Vitamin B_{12} binds to intrinsic factor and is mostly absorbed in the terminal ileum. Dietary iron is mostly absorbed in the duodenum and proximal jejunum. Zinc absorption primarily occurs in the jejunum. Copper absorption mainly occurs in the stomach and duodenum.

3. **c.** *Explanation:* Failure of bonding and poor attachment between mothers and their infants result in higher rates of failure to thrive, higher rates of child abuse/negligence/abandonment, developmental delays (various categories), and lower rates of feeding via breastfeeding and breast milk.

4. **b.** *Explanation:* Folate deficiency is associated with spina bifida and anencephaly. Iodine deficiency is associated with hypothyroidism. Zinc modulates neurogenesis and neuronal apoptosis and can lead to neural impairment and poor growth. Vitamin D deficiency is associated with lower cognitive and language development with no direct association to deafness.

Chapter 25

1. **d.** *Explanation:* The Bayley scoring system does not determine the IQ but rather a DQ (developmental quotient); however, scoring of the DQ does have a mean of 100 and a 15-point standard deviation. Differences in

educational exposures as well as environmental exposures may affect how a child scores in the Bayley Scales. Cognitive testing systems may be affected by perceptive (visual, hearing) or attention/behavioral issues. The system will determine developmental function of infants and young children starting from 16 days of age (not immediately at birth) up until 42 months of age. The correct answer choice is d because the Bayley Scales are used to identify infants and children with developmental delay in order to direct early intervention services.

2. **a.** *Explanation:* The female gender is not a risk factor for cerebral palsy (CP); males are at a higher risk of CP than females. The use of assisted reproductive technology does pose a higher risk of CP in the children born from these pregnancies, mostly explained by preterm delivery and/or multiple births. Infections during pregnancy due to cytokines and fevers in the mother lead to increased CP risk. These include chickenpox, rubella, cytomegalovirus, and bacterial infections. Mothers with thyroid problems, intellectual disability, or seizures also have a slight increase in risk of their infants having CP. Finally, multiple births, especially if a twin or triplet dies before or shortly after birth, add an increased risk of CP. Notably, the highest risk factors remain premature birth, especially <28 weeks' gestation, and lower birth weights, especially <1500 g.

3. **b.** *Explanation:* Although all of the above infants described are at risk of developing neurodevelopmental impairments, the strongest predictor is prematurity, with the 23-week infant born in preterm labor being at the highest risk. The 28-week infant is at risk due to both prematurity and inadequate maternal steroid administration but is likely at lower risk than a 23-week infant. The development of necrotizing enterocolitis (NEC) has been shown to lead to an increased risk of neurodevelopmental impairments, as well, compared to age-matched infants who did not develop NEC. Infants who develop bronchopulmonary dysplasia and chronic lung disease are at higher risk of developmental impairment, as are infants who develop pulmonary hypertension. Another notable subset of infants at increased risk are those with congenital heart defects.

Chapter 26

1. **b.** *Explanation:* Extremely low-gestational-age infants are highly susceptible to infection for multiple reasons. Many natural defenses, including skin barriers, ciliary clearance, and gastric pH, are naturally underdeveloped and also decreased due to medical interventions such as percutaneous catheters. Interferon-γ, a cytokine central to initiating and propagating many protective (and inflammatory) immune mechanisms, is suppressed in neonatal innate and adaptive immune cells. There are three pathways to complement activation, including the classic (antibody-activated), lectin (lectin and IgA activated), and alternative (spontaneous hydrolysis). Generally speaking, all three pathways have diminished activity in neonates compared to adults, and the classic and lectin pathways, due to lower maternal antibody

transfer, are more affected in preterm infants born prior to 28 weeks' gestation. Primitive hematopoiesis, which takes place in the fetal yolk sac, transitions to definitive hematopoiesis by 5 to 8 weeks' gestation.

Chapter 27

1. **b.** *Explanation:* Testing for SCID is currently included in the Recommended Uniform Screening Panel of Core Conditions, compiled by the Secretary of the Department of Health and Human Services. The SCID screen is considered positive when the TREC content falls below a threshold value that varies by laboratory. T cell receptor excision circles are circular episomal DNA fragments present in recent thymic emigrants that are formed during T cell receptor rearrangement. Cell TREC content is normally diluted through cell division, but overall content in the blood is kept relatively steady in the healthy term newborn by her or his high rate of new T cell release. Preterm infants have a lower TREC content developmentally, but, due to the many comorbid conditions that can blunt their thymic function, there are no published standards to account for gestational age when measuring TRECs. The false-positive rate for SCID, therefore, is much higher in preterm infants. Furthermore, there are no agreed standards for lymphocyte subsets measured by flow cytometry in the preterm infant, which makes confirmatory testing by flow problematic. In this case, the infant had measurable but low TRECs. In the absence of a family history or obvious stigmata for SCID, the recommended practice is to repeat the screen until the patient reaches term-corrected gestational age.

2. **a.** *Explanation:* Conjugate vaccines contain a linked polysaccharide–protein antigen and are tailored to improve the B cell response to polysaccharide (encapsulated bacteria) antigens. A major source of protection against encapsulated bacteria is antibody generated by B cells in a T-independent fashion. T-independent responses bypass normal antigen processing and presentation by antigen-presenting cells (APCs) and interact directly with B cell receptors. Splenic marginal zone B cells (MZBs) are highly active against T-independent antigens, but neonates are deficient in MZBs. Linked polysaccharide–protein antigens in conjugate vaccines simultaneously activate B and T cells, providing necessary secondary cytokine signals from T cells that can then stimulate B cell and antibody maturation. Aluminum adjuvant, not monophosphoryl lipid A, is used in both Hib and pneumococcal vaccines. Hepatitis B is the only recombinant protein vaccine given to children. Recombinant protein vaccines generally stimulate a weaker immune response and require adjuvant. There are no current DNA vaccines administered to newborns in the United States.

3. **a.** *Explanation:* IgG is actively transported from the mother to the fetus via IgG-specific receptors that are expressed on the placenta during the late second trimester. By term gestation, the neonate's IgG concentration is higher than the mother's. IgA is produced mainly at mucosal surfaces following exposure to commensal

microbes, which does not occur to a substantial degree until after delivery. IgM forms pentamers, which cannot cross the placenta, and there are no IgM-specific receptors to facilitate transport. IgE also does not cross the placenta but may be similar between mother and fetus due to a genetic predisposition to allergy.

Chapter 28

1. **c.** *Explanation:* This patient presents with heterotaxy syndrome, including inappropriate cardiac and abdominal situs. The midline liver and stomach suggest that there is a right-sided isomerism, which is associated with asplenia or hyposplenia. Splenic anatomy can be evaluated by ultrasound, and diminished function can be assessed by detection of Howell-Jolly bodies or pitted erythrocytes or by nuclear imaging modalities. Patients with asplenia are at high risk for infection with encapsulated bacteria, such as *Klebsiella pneumonia*, *Haemophilus influenzae* type b, and *Streptococcus pneumoniae.* The spleen is enriched with marginal zone B cells, which rapidly produce neutralizing IgM antibodies against polysaccharides. The spleen also plays a central role in generating memory B cells against T-independent antigens, such as polysaccharides and haptens.

2. **a.** *Explanation:* This infant's presentation (conotruncal cardiac anomaly, craniofacial findings, and hypocalcemia) is most consistent with 22q11 deletion syndrome (22q11DS), which affects pharyngeal pouch-derived structures. Patients with complete 22q11DS syndrome may suffer from athymia. The thymus is essential for common lymphoid progenitors to differentiate into naïve T cells, and athymic newborns will have low or absent naïve T cells in their circulation. Live vaccines, therefore, are contraindicated in athymic individuals who have not received immune replacement therapy. Enumeration of naïve T cell subsets is best accomplished by flow cytometry. A complete blood count with differential quantifies lymphocytes, combining T cells, B cells, and NK cells. T cells may be diminished, even when the absolute lymphocyte count falls within the normal range. Furthermore, maternal memory T cell engraftment can occur in the absence of an endogenous T cell population in the newborn and will falsely elevate the neonate's absolute lymphocyte count on a CBC. Flow cytometry can be used to differentiate memory and naïve T cell subsets and can therefore distinguish maternal from fetal T cells. Older athymic patients often have diminished immunoglobulin levels, but immunoglobulin in a term neonate is largely derived by placental transfer and is likely to be normal at birth. Complement levels are typically normal in patients with 22q11DS.

3. **d.** *Explanation:* IVIG is pooled donor, concentrated human immunoglobulin. IVIG contains mostly IgG, but some IgA and IgM are present. IVIG modulates immune system activity through multiple mechanisms, including inhibitory complement activation, inhibition of cytotoxic T cells, and inhibition of phagocytosis. The antibody structure includes a variable portion, which binds to its specific antigen. Once bound, the constant portion (Fc) is available to bind to Fc receptors on phagocytes, such as splenic macrophages, and it signals internalization and destruction of bound erythrocytes. IVIG neutralizes macrophage activity by saturating their Fc receptors, which then leaves antibody-bound erythrocytes free to circulate.

4. **a.** *Explanation:* The lymphocytes affected (T, B, NK) for a given SCID syndrome are dependent on the differential effects that molecular pathways have on the development of each lymphocyte subset. IL-7 signaling is critical during thymic T cell development, and, in its absence, T cells fail to mature. IL-7 is not an essential cytokine for either NK or B cell development; therefore, B and NK cells are unaffected in IL-7rα deficiency. The RAG complex is necessary for V(D)J recombination, which occurs in both T and B cells, and a deficiency therefore leads to failed T and B cell development. T cell CD40L binds to CD40 on B cells and signals antibody class switching and affinity maturation. Absent expression causes X-linked hyper IgM, or failure to produce mature, high-affinity antibodies. T, B, and NK cell numbers are intact in CD40L deficiency. ADA is involved in purine salvage, and intracellular accumulation of purines in ADA SCID causes apoptosis of T, B, and NK cells.

5. **d.** *Explanation:* G-CSF is a growth factor that selectively stimulates neutrophil production in the bone marrow and improves survival in preterm infants with sepsis-induced neutropenia. Granulocyte-macrophage colony-stimulating factor (GM-CSF) is a growth factor for multiple hematopoietic cell lineages, including both neutrophils and macrophages. Dexamethasone inhibits the adhesion and margination of neutrophils, which increases the number of measured circulating neutrophils in a blood sample without increasing the total body number. IVIG can dampen complement-induced inflammatory pathways, but it does not directly improve neutrophil number. IVIG has not been shown to improve survival in neonatal bacterial sepsis.

6. **c.** *Explanation:* This patient presents with pancytopenia, a pronounced neutropenia, skeletal abnormalities, and signs of pancreatic insufficiency, consistent with a diagnosis of Shwachman-Diamond syndrome (SDS). The bone marrow failure of SDS places patient at risk for life-threatening infections and blood cell dyscrasias and may require bone marrow transplantation for treatment. Cystic fibrosis is the most common cause of pancreatic insufficiency in children but does not typically present with skeletal abnormalities. Asphyxiating thoracic dystrophy presents with respiratory failure due to poor development of the thoracic ribs, but it does not include pancreatic insufficiency or cytopenias. Hemophagocytic lymphohistiocytosis (HLH) can also present with cytopenias but is usually associated with immune system activation, including hepatomegaly, lymphadenopathy, rash, and fever. HLH is not associated with skeletal anomalies.

Chapter 29

1. **a.**
2. **d.**
3. **c.**

Chapter 30

1. **b.**
2. **f.**
3. **d.**

Chapter 31

1. **c.**
2. **b.**
3. **a.**

Chapter 32

1. **d.** *Explanation:* Lean body mass, including structural components of cells that have been proliferating, muscle, and bone, accounts for the largest fractional increase in body weight, indicating the large nutritional requirements for protein during this period of growth.
2. **e.**
3. **c.** *Explanation:* Physical activity accounts for only 0% to 5% of total energy expenditure.
4. **b.** *Explanation:* The critical amount of amino acid or protein for preventing growth faltering in very preterm infants <30 to 32 weeks is at least 1.5 g/kg/d.
5. **All are true.**
6. **a.** *Explanation:* Energy intake above 90 to 110 kcal/kg/d only adds more calories for fat production, whereas protein intake is the primary contributor to net protein balance at any energy intake.
7. **c.** *Explanation:* Preterm infants who were not growth restricted in utero grow normally when sufficient nutrition is provided and stressful clinical conditions and their treatments resolve.

Chapter 33

1. **d.** *Explanation:* Risk factors in preterm infants for calcium and phosphorus deficiency and subsequent rickets include gestational age <27 weeks or birth weight <1000 g, long-term parenteral nutrition (<4–5 weeks), severe BPD requiring diuretics and fluid restriction, long-term steroid treatment, a history of necrotizing enterocolitis (NEC), and intolerance to enteral formula or human milk. All of these are true and self-explanatory. Calcium and phosphorus nutrition of very preterm infants is deficient for all of these reasons.
2. **b.** *Explanation:* Mn supplementation should be stopped with any signs of hepatic dysfunction or cholestasis. This is true, as excess Mn damages the liver.
3. **c.** *Explanation:* Magnesium sulfate is a common treatment for maternal preeclampsia and can result in hypermagnesemia in the newborn. Symptoms include low tone and respiratory depression. Treatment may include monitoring levels and withholding magnesium supplementation.
4. **e.** *Explanation:* A one-time intramuscular shot of vitamin K within 6 hours of birth is recommended to protect against vitamin K deficiency bleeding; vitamin K is essential to multiple clotting factors. Answers (a) and (b) are standard ongoing care dependent on gestational age but are nonurgent. Vitamin B_{12} injection may be required in the setting of diagnosed deficiency, most often seen with a strict and unsupplemented vegan or vegetarian maternal diet. Oral folate is added to maternal prenatal vitamins to reduce rates of neural tube defects.
5. **b.** *Explanation:* 6 mg/kg/d is the recommended intake during erythropoietin therapy. General recommendation is 2 to 3 mg/kg/d. Changes in type, fortification, and brand of feeding should be followed by reassessment of total Fe delivery. The iron content of products varies considerably. There are risks associated with both under- and over-supplementation of Fe; the risks for toxicity are listed here.
6. **d.** *Explanation:* Zinc. The patient has risk factors for low zinc intake (unfortified feeds of mature donor human milk and diarrhea) as well as symptoms of Zn deficiency (diarrhea and scaly rash). Vitamin A deficiency symptoms/signs include photophobia, conjunctivitis, failure to thrive, vitamin E hemolytic anemia, reticulocytosis, thrombocytosis, and acanthocytosis. Thiamine deficiency (beriberi) is seen with pyruvate dehydrogenase complex deficiency and maple-syrup urine disease and presents with neurological and cardiac symptoms.

Chapter 34

1. **a.** *Explanation:* True for term infants. Human milk provides sufficient energy, protein, fat, carbohydrates, micronutrients, and water for normal metabolism, growth, and development in term infants. Human milk has been the result of several million years of evolutionary development to produce the optimal nutrition for human newborn infants.
2. **a.** *Explanation:* Varying degrees of nutrient loss may occur with long-term storage, particularly in frozen conditions. This is true, especially when there are multiple freeze–thaw cycles, and is one reason why fresh mother's milk is superior.
3. **c.** *Explanation:* Total lipid generally is increased (as much as by 60%), but free fatty acids are reduced, which might increase their nutritive potential. This is false. Total lipids are generally reduced by up to 60%, but free fatty acids (FFAs) will increase.
4. **c.** *Explanation:* With mothers who test positive and are enrolled in drug reduction programs, the advantages of mother's own milk (MOM) generally outweigh the risks.
5. **d.** *Explanation:* Access to a quality pump is essential for establishing supply after a premature delivery. Encouragement from providers and being able to contribute to the care of their baby in other ways have been shown to reduce maternal stress and anxiety, both of which negatively affect milk production. Lactation support is key; however, 8 mL per session is a normal volume for 48 hours after birth (lactogenesis I).
6. **c.** *Explanation:* Lactose is reduced due to concern for early lactase deficiency. Preterm formulas are available in 20-, 24-, and 30-kcal/oz preparations with similar osmolalities and renal solute loads to help meet higher energy needs.

Chapter 35

1. **a.** *Explanation:* There is no reduction in metabolism or potential for growth with birth, thus the infant will require the same amount of nutrients. If the infant is very small, there will be insufficient nutrient stores to maintain normal metabolism or growth, requiring early IV nutrition and early and continued enteral nutrition.
2. **a.** *Explanation:* Term infants do not have as high a fractional protein synthetic rate or growth rate as the earlier gestation fetus does. Fetal amino acid concentrations are generally higher than those of term infants who are fed mature mother's milk, an indication of the premature infant's need for more amino acid and protein intake to meet their greater requirements.
3. **b.**
4. **c.** *Explanation:* TPN has been provided for 8 days, >14 days is considered prolonged, and the infant is receiving trophic amounts of feeding. Checking direct (conjugated) bilirubin concentrations in about 1 week would be appropriate if the patient remains on predominately TPN. Prolonged UVC line (>5–7 days) increases the risk of invasive bacterial infection and systemic sepsis. Current TPN provides 52 kcal/kg/d, which is below the amount needed to promote both protein accretion and fat deposition. Multicomponent IV lipid emulsions should be infused at ≥2 g/kg/d to prevent essential fatty acid deficiency.
5. **a.** *Explanation:* Valine, tryptophan, and isoleucine are included in the nine essential amino acids. Linoleic acid and alpha-linolenic acid are essential fatty acids. Aspartic acid, glutamic acid, and alanine are nonessential amino acids. Arginine and tyrosine are conditionally essential amino acids.
6. **d.** *Explanation:* Peroxide formation occurs when lipids, amino acids, vitamins, and trace elements are exposed to ambient light and phototherapy at any point and contributes to oxidative stress. Phytosterols found in lipid emulsions may contribute to cholestasis. Refeeding syndrome usually presents as hypophosphatemia in very low birth weight and growth-restricted infants. Sepsis risk is not affected by photo-protection.

Chapter 36

1. **c.** *Explanation:* Swallowing is first seen as early as week 16, nonnutritive sucking can be seen as early as gestation week 20, and nutritive sucking does not appear until weeks 32 to 34.
2. **a.** *Explanation:* Primitive gut tube forms by week 4, when a portion of the yolk sac incorporates into the embryo during craniofacial and lateral folding. The lumen is occluded as third epithelial lining rapidly proliferates and then later recanalizes. Failure to recanalize results in intestinal atresia or stenosis.
3. **d.** *Explanation:* At gestation week 24, lactase activity is <25% of that found in term infants. Increase in lactase activity occurs during weeks 32 to 34.
4. **d.** *Explanation:* Peyer patches are lymphoid follicles that are the sites of T and B cell activity.

5. **b.** *Explanation:* The duodenum rotates, resulting in movement of the ventral pancreatic bud, which becomes located poster and inferior to the dorsal pancreatic bud. The ductal systems of the two buds join during week 8.
6. **d.** *Explanation:* The bile acid pool size in preterm infants is one-third of that seen in term infants. Sepsis is another contributing factor in preterm infants for the development of cholestasis.
7. **a.** *Explanation:* By week 4 of gestation, the intrahepatic biliary tree is formed.
8. **b.** *Explanation:* At week 11, the midgut loop rotates counterclockwise around the superior mesenteric artery as it returns to the abdominal cavity. Failure of this loop to return to the abdomen results in omphalocele.
9. **a.** *Explanation:* Incomplete fusion of the lateral grooves results in failure of separation of the dorsal and ventral tubes, leading to a tracheoesophageal fistula (TEF).

Chapter 37

1. **c.** *Explanation:* Epstein pearls are small cystic lesions on the hard palate. They typically disappear within one month of life.
2. **b.** *Explanation:* Symptoms of GERD include poor weight gain, irritability, feeding aversion, apnea, cyanosis, and bradycardia. Bilious emesis is indicative of intestinal obstruction and is not seen with GERD.
3. **d.** *Explanation:* Cystic fibrosis, small left colon syndrome, and Hirschsprung disease are all associated with delayed passage of meconium. Milk protein intolerance can present with blood in the stool and irritability.
4. **c.** *Explanation:* In infants with TEF, coexisting congenital anomalies can occur in up to 70%. Up to 7% of infants have a chromosomal abnormality.
5. **a.** *Explanation:* Esophageal atresia with distal TEF accounts for 85% of cases.
6. **d.** *Explanation:* GER is a normal physiologic condition in neonates. Most cases are related to transient relaxation of the lower esophageal sphincter.
7. **a.** *Explanation:* Pyloric stenosis presents between 3 and 6 months of age with progressive projectile emesis. Hypochloremic hypokalemic alkalosis is seen.
8. **a.** *Explanation:* This abdominal radiograph illustrates the "double bubble" sign. It is associated with duodenal atresia, which is more common in infants with trisomy 21.
9. **d.** *Explanation:* This presentation is concerning for Hirschsprung disease. A barium enema would be the next step in management. Contrast enema would demonstrate a different caliber of the smaller aganglionic segment and proximal dilated segment of bowel.
10. **a.** *Explanation:* Long-term consequences of gastroschisis include poor motility, feeding intolerance, and need for prolonged parenteral nutrition.

Chapter 38

1. **c.** *Explanation:* Congenital sucrose–isomaltase deficiency is the most common congenital enzyme deficiency. This

commonly presents around age 3 to 6 months when a baby is introduced to foods containing sucrose.

2. **a.** *Explanation:* It typically presents with the introduction of lactose into the diet in the form of either breast milk or a lactose-based formula.

3. **b.** *Explanation:* This infant is suffering from glucose–galactose malabsorption. This is an autosomal recessive disorder that leads to a defect in sodium–glucose linked transporter protein.

4. **a.** *Explanation:* Hypobetalipoprotenemia is due to low or absent plasma concentrations of apolipoprotein B lipoproteins and low-density lipoprotein cholesterol. Treatment is a low-fat diet and fat-soluble vitamin supplementation.

5. **d.** *Explanation:* Congenital chloride diarrhea is the most common cause of congenital secretory diarrhea. Patients have severe watery diarrhea beginning immediately after birth. This persists when NPO.

6. **d.** *Explanation:* Risk factors associated with NEC are intrauterine growth restriction, small size for gestational age, birth asphyxia, congenital heart disease, gastroschisis, polycythemia, hypoglycemia, sepsis, and exchange transfusion.

7. **d.** *Explanation:* Complications of short bowel syndrome include malabsorption of nutrients, gastric hypersecretion, small bowel bacterial overgrowth, intestinal adaptation difficulties, cholestatic liver disease typically from chronic use of parenteral nutrition, catheter-related complications, and enterocolitis.

8. **b.** *Explanation:* Intermittent treatment with antibiotics for bacterial overgrowth is used in the management of short bowel syndrome. Chronic antibiotic use may predispose patients to antibiotic resistance.

9. **d.** *Explanation:* In an otherwise thriving infant with stable blood work, the most common cause of blood in the stool is milk protein allergy. Diagnosis is based on clinical improvement with a milk-free diet or recurrence of symptoms with the reintroduction of milk.

10. **a.** *Explanation:* Neonatal intussusception presents as abdominal distention, feeding intolerance, vomiting, and bloody stools. Most cases involve small bowel.

Chapter 39

1. **d.** *Explanation:* This infant is presenting with Alagille syndrome. This is due to mutations in the *JAG1* and *NOTCH2* genes.

2. **b.** *Explanation:* Infants with biliary atresia do not typically have characteristic or abnormal facies. Infants with Alagille syndrome are seen to have triangular facies.

3. **c.** *Explanation:* Chylous ascites is most commonly due to the congenital failure of lymphatic channels to communicate. Treatment can include paracentesis and formula containing medium-chain triglycerides.

4. **a.** *Explanation:* The Kasai procedure is a Roux-en-Y jejunostomy that allows for biliary drainage. Infants have a better prognosis if this is done before 60 days of age.

5. **b.** *Explanation:* PFIC presents as severe cholestasis, intractable pruritis, and possible coagulopathy. GGT is

decreased or normal in types 1 and 2 and is increased in type 3.

6. **d.** *Explanation:* Infants with Alagille syndrome present with very high GGT, which may be up to 20 times the normal value.

7. **b.** *Explanation:* In biliary ascites, the bilirubin is typically found to be >4 g/dL.

8. **d.** *Explanation:* If a choledochal cyst goes untreated, it can result in obstructive symptoms such as cholangitis, pancreatitis, hepatitis, cirrhosis, and/or portal hypertension.

9. **b.** *Explanation:* The pathogenesis of extrahepatic biliary atresia is not clearly elucidated at this time. Proposed mechanisms for the pathogenesis include a defect in morphogenesis of the biliary tract, a defect in fetal or prenatal circulation, environmental toxin exposure, and viral infections.

10. **c.** *Explanation:* A1AT deficiency presents with neonatal jaundice. GGT is often high, and A1AT level is low. A1AT abnormal phenotypes include ZZ, SZ, and MZ.

Chapter 40

1. **b.** *Explanation:* The iron eliminated from heme oxidation is recycled. Bilirubin is formed from biliverdin catalyzed by biliverdin reductase. Carbon monoxide is produced as a byproduct during the production of biliverdin, not bilirubin.

2. **b.** *Explanation:* Unconjugated bilirubin is lipophilic and crosses the placenta easily. Conjugated bilirubin and its derivatives are lipophobic and do not cross the placenta. Lumirubin is a photoisomer of bilirubin created by phototherapy.

3. **d.** *Explanation:* Serum bilirubin is measured by blood sampling using spectrophotometric measurement of a chemical reaction between bilirubin or its derivatives with a diazo agent, which yields a yellow pigment. Transcutaneous bilirubin is a noninvasive method of measurement using optical technology. End-tidal carbon monoxide (ETCO) is an indirect measurement of carboxyhemoglobin generated as a byproduct of bilirubin metabolism and is excreted via the lung. The reticulocyte count, on the other hand, is a measure of red blood cell production from the bone marrow and does not reflect bilirubin levels.

4. **a.** *Explanation:* Ethnicity (Asian), gestational age (inversely proportional), and bruising (directly proportional) are all risk factors for hyperbilirubinemia. Formula-fed infants are at lower risk for hyperbilirubinemia compared to breastfed infants.

5. **f.** *Explanation:* Beta-glucuronidase is involved in the uptake of the bilirubin-albumin complex by hepatocytes. UDP-glucuronyltransferase catalyzes the binding of bilirubin to glucuronic acid, converting it to a water-soluble form that can be excreted in bile. Heme oxygenase is an enzyme that breaks down hemoglobin to produce biliverdin. This step initiates bilirubin metabolism but is not part of bilirubin conjugation.

6. **d.** *Explanation:* The RBC life span in a newborn is shorter than adults (90 vs. 120 days), conjugating enzymes are immature in a newborn, and bacterial flora are

typically lower, reducing enterohepatic circulation and increasing the likelihood of hyperbilirubinemia.

7. **d.** *Explanation:* A low serum albumin level and acidosis, as seen in sick infants, reduce the binding capacity of free bilirubin. Medications such as ceftriaxone competitively bind with bilirubin, reducing albumin to bilirubin binding.

8. **b.** *Explanation:* UDP-glucuronyltransferase, an enzyme involved in conjugation, is developmentally regulated and increases after 30 weeks' gestation. At term, this enzyme is present at 1% of adult values.

9. **a.** *Explanation:* Ligandin is a carrier protein that helps transport the bilirubin-albumin complex into the hepatocyte for conjugation. Glucuronyl *S*-transferase is a conjugating enzyme.

10. **a.** *Explanation:* Spectrophotometry is the most commonly used technique to measure serum bilirubin. The other choices can measure serum bilirubin but are less commonly used.

11. **e.** *Explanation:* Bilirubin–albumin binding is proportionate to postnatal age. Use of ampicillin and ceftriaxone and free fatty acids negatively influence bilirubin binding with albumin by competitive inhibition.

Chapter 41

1. **c.** *Explanation:* Bilirubin toxicity affects the neurons in the subthalamic nuclei, hippocampus, and basal ganglia. These areas are typically seen as stained yellow on pathology. The cerebral cortex is usually spared.

2. **f.** *Explanation:* Acute bilirubin encephalopathy is associated with a severely elevated serum bilirubin level, abnormal auditory brainstem response, and an abnormal MRI. Because cochlear function is spared, the otoacoustic emission (OAE) test is usually normal.

3. **e.** *Explanation:* Increased bilirubin production and in situ production and/or decreased serum albumin reduce albumin–bilirubin binding and increase free bilirubin, which is then able to cross the blood–brain barrier. Alteration of the blood–brain barrier in situations such as infection increase its permeability, thereby increasing the possibility of bilirubin crossing the barrier.

4. **e.** *Explanation:* Extraneural injuries due to bilirubin toxicity include intestinal and pancreatic necrosis, renal tubular necrosis, and accumulation of bilirubin crystals.

5. **e.** *Explanation:* Long-term sequelae of kernicterus may include choreoathetoid cerebral palsy, abnormal upward gaze, dental dysplasias, and sensorineural hearing loss. The intellect is typically normal.

6. **e.** *Explanation:* Photoisomerization that occurs with phototherapy is influenced by wavelength of light (420–490 μm, blue range), irradiance, distance to the baby (closer more effective), and surface area of exposure (directly proportional to the surface area of exposure).

7. **a.** *Explanation:* Hypocalcemia is a known risk from exchange transfusions. Other potential complications include necrotizing enterocolitis, graft-versus-host disease, thrombosis, and thrombocytopenia. Stroke, IVH,

and renal failure are not known to be associated with exchange transfusions.

8. **d.** *Explanation:* Hypocalcemia is a known complication of exchange transfusions, not phototherapy. Rash, dehydration, gonadal and retinal injury, bronze baby syndrome, and acute intermittent porphyria are known side effects of phototherapy.

9. **a.** *Explanation:* Lethargy is an early sign of bilirubin toxicity and can be reversed by appropriate, timely therapy such as exchange transfusions.

10. **e.** *Explanation:* Along with the listed assessment modalities, thyroid panel and blood cultures are recommended for assessment of cause of kernicterus.

Chapter 42

1. **c.** *Explanation:* The clinical history of this infant is consistent with breastfeeding jaundice. Symptoms include a history of exclusive breastfeeding and decreased urine output, as well as signs of dehydration on physical exam with reassuring vital signs. Initiating intensive phototherapy immediately in the emergency room minimizes the risk of neurological sequelae from bilirubin toxicity. The team can assess what additional laboratory tests are needed and if rehydration can be done orally with enteral supplementation or via IVF based on factors such as percent weight loss (with >10% weight loss being concerning), exam findings, and vital signs.

2. **d.** *Explanation:* The infant described in this clinical vignette is experiencing breast milk jaundice. Because signs and symptoms suggest adequate hydration status and there is no evidence of anemia or hemolysis, reassurance and close follow-up are appropriate. Suspension of breastfeeding and supplementation with formula would help aid the diagnosis and treatment but are not the mainstay of therapy. Intensive phototherapy is not indicated acutely unless close follow-up cannot be ensured.

3. **d.** *Explanation:* The presence of beta-glucuronidase in maternal milk, metal ions, steroids that affect the conjugation enzymes, and elevation of serum bile acids have all been known to increase the potential for breast milk jaundice.

4. **b.** *Explanation:* Although breast milk jaundice typically occurs after 7 days of life, it may range anywhere from 5 to 15 days of life and last for up to 3 months. Breastfeeding jaundice is known to occur at 2 to 6 days of life, and pathologic jaundice due to other causes such as blood group incompatibility presents at 1 to 3 days of life. Jaundice before 24 hours is pathologic and requires immediate assessment to identify an etiology and establish an appropriate treatment plan.

5. **d.** *Explanation:* Any process that interrupts an infant's ability to latch, suck, and swallow contributes to breastfeeding jaundice. Cleft lip, engorgement, or cracked nipples are examples of such scenarios. Maternal age does not increase the risk of breastfeeding jaundice.

6. **e.** *Explanation:* Evaluation of hyperbilirubinemia should be directed at an evaluation of severity and identification of the cause. Fractionated serum bilirubin levels help determine the severity and whether bilirubin is direct

or indirect, guiding further workup and therapy. A complete blood count and reticulocyte count help identify ongoing hemolysis. When combined with a thorough exam and history, it can aid in detection of infection. Serum electrolyte level determination can reveal dehydration. All of these tests help determine the diagnosis and direct further evaluation and treatment of the underlying cause.

7. **e.** *Explanation:* All of the listed factors increase the severity of physiologic jaundice. Polycythemia and subsequent normalization of hematocrit by breakdown of extra RBC results in bilirubin precursors. Maternal diazepam crosses the placenta and binds competitively to albumin, increasing free bilirubin in the fetal blood. Conjugating enzymes are developmentally regulated, and this increases the likelihood of unconjugated hyperbilirubinemia in preterm infants. Delayed feeding reduces enterohepatic circulation, thereby increasing the risk of hyperbilirubinemia.

8. **a.** *Explanation:* The goal of assessment and treatment of hyperbilirubinemia is to prevent neurotoxicity.

9. **d.**

Chapter 43

1. **a.** *Explanation:* Increased cardiovascular demand may cause or worsen cardiac dysfunction in women with cardiac diseases. Echocardiography is recommended in each trimester or with new cardiac symptoms. Peak flow monitoring should be used because expiratory respiratory indices are unchanged in pregnancy. Systemic vascular resistance decreases in pregnancy; thus, antihypertensive doses often can be lowered or eliminated. Insulin dose increases are common because of progressive insulin resistance in pregnancy. Although total T_4 and T_3 increase in pregnancy, steroid-binding globulin also increases, so free levels are unchanged.

2. **d.** *Explanation:* An interpregnancy interval of at least 18 months is advised. Folic acid supplementation is recommended for all women to prevent neural tube defects. Lisinopril use is contraindicated in pregnancy; transition to a preferred medication should be carried out. Gamete donation can prevent genetic disease in the offspring if parents are known carriers. Expanded carrier screening is offered to all patients of Eastern and Central European Jewish descent. Although this couple may be presumed to be Tay-Sachs carriers, mutation analysis will confirm recurrence risk and screen for other at-risk conditions.

3. **d.** *Explanation:* Alloimmunization may have caused demise if the fetus was Kell positive. Absence of bleeding does not rule out Kell sensitization; anemia develops from transplacental passage of maternal antibodies. Sensitized patients may have uncomplicated pregnancies if a fetus is antigen negative. Paternal antigen testing will show if a pregnancy is at risk—there is no fetal risk if the father is Kell negative but possibly so if the father is Kell positive (may be heterozygous or homozygous).

4. **e.** *Explanation:* Stillbirth risk is increased with DM; fetal surveillance is recommended from 32 weeks. If glycemic control is poor, then 37- to 38-week delivery is considered. Delivery is delayed until 39 weeks in well-controlled

patients to allow time for fetal maturity. Nutrition consultation is recommended in all diabetic pregnancies. Fetal echocardiography is advised due to the increased risk of anomalies. Frequent blood glucose checks are necessary to guide dosing of medications. Metformin, glyburide, and insulin may all be used to achieve glycemic control.

5. **c.** *Explanation:* This patient has HELLP syndrome. If maternal and fetal statuses are reassuring, delivery should take place after completion of a steroid course. Severe features of preeclampsia syndrome (HELLP syndrome and severe hypertension) are present; thus, (a) and (b) are incorrect. If the only severe feature is controllable hypertension, then expectant management detailed in (e) is appropriate. Fetal lung maturity testing is not advised because delivery is indicated regardless of fetal maturity.

6. **c.** *Explanation:* Many, but not all, fetuses with trisomy 21 have structural anomalies or soft marker ultrasound findings. The lack of anomalies or markers does not rule out a trisomy 21 diagnosis. Maternal serum quad testing is a screening test for aneuploidy; a positive screening result should not be considered diagnostic. Although the detection rate of the serum quad test is high ($\sim$80%), the false-positive rate is also high.

Chapter 44

1. **c.** *Explanation:* Umbilical artery Doppler velocimetry defines a group of fetuses at high risk for adverse perinatal outcomes. Reversed end-diastolic flow should prompt delivery after 32 weeks. An EFW < 10th percentile defines growth restriction, but fetal tests of well-being are used to make delivery decisions. A biophysical profile score of 8/10 is reassuring, as this reliably excludes fetal asphyxia. Intermittent variable decelerations on a reactive NST do not portend imminent compromise.

2. **c.** *Explanation:* This fetus receives 2 points each for amniotic fluid volume, movement, tone, and breathing (total of 8 points). No points are received for the NST because the fetus is not reactive (15 beat accelerations are required at 34 weeks). A BPP score of 8 or 10 is predictive of normal fetal oxygenation, and no further testing is required. A BPP score of 6 is an equivocal test and requires follow-up testing (BPP at 8 and 24 hours) to determine if delivery is required.

3. **b.** *Explanation:* This fetus receives 2 points only for movement. No points are received for the NST because the fetus is not reactive (15 beat accelerations are required at 34 weeks). A BPP score of 2 is highly indicative of fetal hypoxemia and in this setting should prompt urgent delivery. A repeat BPP in 24 hours is typically used to reevaluate a preterm fetus with a BPP of 6/10. Although it is preferable to defer delivery until 34 weeks to improve fetal maturity in the setting of preeclampsia with severe features, expectant management is only appropriate when maternal/fetal status is stable.

4. **e.** *Explanation:* Although fetuses with aneuploidy may have structural anomalies or visible sonographic markers, ultrasound alone has a low detection rate for aneuploidy. First trimester screening has an improved

detection rate for trisomy 21 over sonography alone, but up to 20% of aneuploid fetuses will be missed. Cell-free DNA screening offers a significantly improved detection rate but also a 1% to 8% risk for indeterminate results. Both diagnostic CVS and amniocentesis offer excellent detection rates for aneuploidy and would be good options for this patient; amniocentesis is preferred, as it eliminates the risk of confined placental mosaicism.

5. **f.** *Explanation:* The risk for aneuploidy is highest in patients of advanced maternal age, and many fetuses with chromosomal abnormalities or genetic syndromes will display structural anatomic defects. However, all genetic screening tests have imperfect sensitivity and carry a risk of false-positive or false-negative results. Although many patients prefer to avoid procedural risks of diagnostic testing, any patient who desires diagnostic testing regardless of age, parity, or fetal anomaly status should be offered the procedure.

6. **b.** *Explanation:* All pregnant patients should be offered aneuploidy screening; CF and SMA carrier testing should be offered if not previously completed. Those with African American heritage should also be offered hemoglobin electrophoresis to screen for hemoglobinopathies. Expanded carrier testing can be considered but is not currently recommended for all patients. Fragile X premutation testing is only recommended for those with family history suggestive of fragile X.

Chapter 45

1. **d.** *Explanation:* Large fetal masses are at risk of rupture or dystocia during attempted vaginal delivery; thus, cesarean delivery is recommended. Hydrops is an indication for delivery near term. Women with two or one low-transverse cesareans may consider a trial of labor. Cesarean delivery is not required for fetal gastroschisis. Labor and vaginal delivery are well tolerated by fetuses with congenital heart disease; cesarean delivery is considered only in extreme cases. Most women with cardiac disease can have safe vaginal deliveries.

2. **c.** *Explanation:* History and exam features are suggestive of significant vaginal bleeding, which could put maternal health at risk. In addition, FHR tracing is notable for non-reassuring features (persistent tachycardia and variable decelerations). Prompt cesarean delivery is warranted. Although fetal tachycardia may be present with chorioamnionitis, there are no other clinical findings suggestive of this; thus, (a) is incorrect. Placenta previa is a contraindication to labor and vaginal delivery, so (b) is incorrect. Repeat steroid courses are not given after 34 weeks of gestation; thus, (d) is incorrect. Answer (e) is incorrect because expectant management is not appropriate in a setting of active hemorrhage and fetal distress.

3. **c.** *Explanation:* Chronic hypertension is not a known risk factor for shoulder dystocia. Pregestational diabetes, fetal macrosomia, and history of prior shoulder dystocia have the greatest association with risk for shoulder dystocia. Precipitous delivery and grand multiparity (a risk factor for recurrent precipitous delivery) increase the probability that a fetus will not descend in the birth canal in an optimum position for vaginal delivery, thus increasing the risk of shoulder dystocia.

4. **a.** *Explanation:* Although prompt delivery is recommended due to fetal bradycardia, the most expeditious method to affect delivery is likely coached maternal pushing efforts as the fetal head is crowning. Episiotomy may shorten the time to successful vaginal delivery of the fetus but is only recommended if it appears that delivery will not be achieved though maternal expulsive efforts alone or if additional room is needed to perform shoulder dystocia maneuvers (which has not yet been encountered). Operative vaginal delivery is not typically performed when the fetal head is crowning. Cesarean delivery is likely to take longer to achieve and poses increased risk to a fetus that is deeply engaged in the birth canal.

5. **e.** *Explanation:* Early decelerations occur due to compression on the fetal head, which leads to a vagally mediated heart rate deceleration. These often occur between 4 and 7 cm dilation in labor and are not associated with fetal compromise. Antihypertensives are warranted for severe hypertension (systolic blood pressure ≥160 mmHg or diastolic ≥110 mmHg). Intrauterine resuscitation with IV fluid bolus and repositioning are recommended for late or variable decelerations. Amnioinfusion is used for recurrent variable decelerations.

6. **e.** *Explanation:* The clinical picture is most consistent with fetal distress secondary to maternal hypotension following recent epidural analgesia. Though cesarean delivery may be warranted if the changes are refractory to resuscitative measures, it is most reasonable to first attempt interventions that may restore uteroplacental perfusion and ameliorate any umbilical cord compression. Ephedrine will raise maternal blood pressure. IV fluid bolus, used judiciously, will increase preload and maternal venous return. Maternal repositioning may relieve umbilical cord and aortocaval compression. Amnioinfusion will restore intrauterine fluid volume and may alleviate umbilical cord compression.

Chapter 46

1. **c.** *Explanation:* This patient is likely in secondary apnea. The appropriate next step is to provide effective positive-pressure ventilation. Continuous stimulation is unlikely to induce spontaneous respirations and improvement in heart rate in this infant. Deep suctioning may further exacerbate bradycardia by inducing a vagal nerve stimulatory response. If the patient does not respond to effective bag-mask ventilation, obtaining a more secure airway and administration of epinephrine may become necessary, but not before a period of effective positive-pressure ventilation and chest compressions has been attempted.

2. **c.** *Explanation:* The infant in choice (c) presents with signs of moderate encephalopathy after a known perinatal hypoxic event and is most likely to have a neurologic benefit from whole-body cooling. The infant in (b) has also experienced a significant hypoxic event at birth but shows signs of only mild encephalopathy on examination and therefore does not meet the criteria for

whole-body cooling. The infant in (a) is preterm; cooling in this population has not yet been established to be beneficial. The infant in (d) had an unwitnessed hypoxic event 12 hours after birth; whole-body cooling for neonates who experience this type of arrest is not the standard of care.

3. **c.** *Explanation:* This is the preferred dosage and route of administration for epinephrine during a neonatal resuscitation.

4. **a.** *Explanation:* Of the most commonly used devices used in neonatal resuscitation, the self-inflating bag is the only device that can deliver positive-pressure breaths without being attached to a source of compressed air or flow. A self-inflating bag cannot deliver PEEP unless additional valves or mechanisms are attached to the device, whereas a T-piece resuscitator can. Additionally, the benefit of a T-piece resuscitator is that it will deliver consistent PIP and PEEP to the patient, provided that a good seal is made between the mask and the patient's face and/or the ETT remains in place. Both devices can deliver PPV with an increased FiO_2 concentration if attached to an oxygen source.

5. **c.** *Explanation:* The hypercapnia, hypoxemia, and acidosis that result from asphyxia will initially cause a redistribution of blood flow to the most vital organs, the heart, brain, and adrenal glands.

6. **b.** *Explanation:* Necrotic cell death occurs after primary energy failure due to depletion of cerebral ATP stores and inactivation of the Na/K membrane pumps. Secondary energy failure occurs 6 to 48 hours after the initial hypoxic injury and results in decreased glutamate reuptake, which leads to the induction of apoptosis.

7. **d.** *Explanation:* Infants born after intrauterine growth restriction have an increased risk of adult onset cardiovascular disease and metabolic syndrome. This may be due to epigenetic effects during fetal development.

Chapter 47

1. **c.** *Explanation:* PWS is caused by lack of the paternally inherited genes in the 15q11-13 region. PWS can occur secondary to deletion of the 15q11-13 region on the paternally inherited chromosome. Alternatively, PWS can be due to inheritance of both copies of 15q11-13 from the mother (uniparental disomy).

2. **d.** *Explanation:* Mitochondria are organelles that have their own chromosome that encodes several genes essential for mitochondrial function. Mitochondrial DNA is inherited almost exclusively from the mother.

3. **a.** *Explanation:* Anticipation occurs in trinucleotide repeat diseases. Trinucleotide repeats tend to be unstable, with their size increasing with each subsequent generation, resulting in a more severe phenotype.

4. **b.** *Explanation:* Of the choices listed, FISH for 22q11 is the most appropriate test to evaluate for suspected DiGeorge syndrome. Although not listed, aCGH would also have been an appropriate choice. A karyotype does not have sufficient resolution to reliably detect the 22q11 microdeletion. A small fraction (<5%) of patients with DiGeorge syndrome will have normal cytogenetic studies. In those patients, targeted evaluation of DiGeorge

locus genes, such as *TBX1*, may be indicated. WES is not indicated in the evaluation for DiGeorge syndrome.

5. **a.** *Explanation:* Preterm or critically ill term infants are more likely to have false-positive newborn screening results. Most newborn screening programs utilize tandem mass spectrometry, which can analyze multiple metabolites, simultaneously enabling screening for many disorders with a single blood sample. Newborn screening panels do vary from state to state, but all states screen for sickle cell disease and cystic fibrosis.

Chapter 48

1. **c.** *Explanation:* Trisomy 13 (Patau syndrome) incidence is one in 5000 to 10,000 live births, with 95% of trisomy 13 conceptions resulting in spontaneous abortion; of those born live, 90% die within the first year of life. Abnormalities include cleft lip and palate, polydactyly, narrow hyperconvex fingernails, colobomas, umbilical or inguinal hernia, cryptorchidism, microcephaly, holoprosencephaly, seizures, cardiac defects (VSDs), and apnea.

2. **b.** *Explanation:* 20% of cases of Beckwith-Wiedemann syndrome are caused by paternal uniparental disomy (UPD).

3. **d.** *Explanation:* Although individuals with T21 typically have primary gonadal failure resulting in infertility, there are rare cases of female fertility.

Chapter 49

1. **e.** *Explanation:* Diagnosis of partial fetal alcohol syndrome (PFAS) requires evidence of prenatal alcohol exposure.

2. **c.** *Explanation:* Some studies have reported an increased risk of imprinting defects after conception using intracytoplasmic sperm injection, a form of assisted reproductive technology.

3. **a.** *Explanation:* The period of greatest vulnerability for cardiac development is within the first 7 weeks of pregnancy.

Chapter 50

1. **c.** *Explanation:* Current evidence suggests an association between ART and a small but definite (more than 1.3 times than in spontaneous conception) incidence of congenital malformations. This includes congenital heart defects, neural tube defects, facial cleft, gastrointestinal malformations, genitourinary malformations, and imprinting disorders. The rates of congenital malformations are similar for each type of ART, except for increased urogenital abnormalities with ICSI. The cause for the increase in malformations with ART has yet to be determined.

2. **b.** *Explanation:* Amniotic band sequence is an example of disruption. Disruption defects are due to destruction or interruption of a normal developmental process. It usually affects a body part rather than a specific organ.

3. **d.** *Explanation:* Deformations are defects caused by abnormal mechanical forces on morphologically normal tissue in utero. They are associated with multiple gestations, uterine malformations, and oligohydramnios.

TYPES OF CONGENITAL ANOMALIES			
Malformations	**Disruptions**	**Deformations**	**Dysplasias**
Morphologic defects resulting from intrinsically abnormal developmental processes	Breakdown of, or interference with, an originally normal developmental process	Abnormalities of form or position of a part of the body caused by nondisruptive mechanical forces	Abnormal structure because the tissues from which individual structures are formed are abnormal
Occur early in embryogenesis	May occur at any time during gestation	Usually develop during the second half of pregnancy	Often due to single abnormal genes

Adapted from Moh W, Graham Jr JM, Wadhawan I, Sanchez-Lara PA. Extrinsic factors influencing fetal deformations and intrauterine growth restriction. *J Pregnancy.* 2012;2012:750485.

4. **d.** *Explanation:* Deformations result when normal tissue is exposed to abnormal mechanical forces in utero.

Chapter 51

1. **c.** *Explanation:* Infants with urea cycle defects usually become symptomatic in the first days to months of life. Clinical presentation includes lethargy, hypothermia, poor feeding, tachypnea, irritability, vomiting, and coma. Differential diagnosis includes sepsis or an organic acidemia. Hyperventilation due to cerebral edema causes respiratory alkalosis.
2. **a.** *Explanation:* Zellweger spectrum disorder (ZSD) is a disorder of peroxisomal biogenesis caused by a defect in the *PEX* gene. A newborn with ZSD presents with dysmorphic features which include flattened face, epicanthal folds, upslanting palpebral fissures, broad nasal bridge, and hypoplastic supraorbital ridges with severe hypotonia and hepatic dysfunction.
3. **d.**
4. **e.** *Explanation:* Uncontrolled maternal phenylketonuria leads to complications in the offspring. These complications include microcephaly, intellectual disabilities, congenital heart disease, and intrauterine growth restriction. Dietary management prior to conception and during pregnancy is important to decrease complication risks in the offspring.

Chapter 52

1. **c.** *Explanation:* The baby is intubated and receiving 100% humidified air, which will reduce their insensible losses (15%–30%) from respiration. Sedation also decreases the insensible fluid loss by an additional 5% to 25%. Being under a radiant warmer, however, will increase insensible loss by 50% to 100%. Combining these factors will lead to a net increase of 15% to 45% above the baseline value ($-15 + -5 + 50 = 25$ to

$-30 + -25 + 100 = 45$). Therefore, total fluids would be 115 to 145 mL/kg/d as a rough estimate. Because this is only an estimate, electrolytes (particularly sodium), ins/outs, and weights should be followed closely.

2. **d.** *Explanation:* SIADH can be triggered by birth asphyxia. To make this diagnosis, renal, thyroid, and adrenal function tests must be normal. Confirmation of the diagnosis is made by the finding of urine osmolality higher than serum osmolality, and urine sodium should be greater than 20. A finding of urine sodium less than 20 would be suspicious for intravascular volume depletion leading to an increase in urine sodium reabsorption. In such cases, ADH release is appropriate to preserve volume, even at the expense of plasma osmolality. A creatinine of 0.7 in a 3-day-old infant would be in the normal range, making AKI unlikely to be the cause of the hyponatremia. Bartter syndrome is a tubular disorder leading to salt wasting, polyuria, and dehydration. Infants typically do not need sodium supplementation until day of life 3. Pseudohypoaldosteronism presents with low sodium and high potassium levels.

3. **c.** *Explanation:* The baby's FENa is calculated as $[(U_{Na} \times S_{Cr})/(U_{Cr} \times S_{Na})] \times 100 = (80 \times 0.8)/(10 \times 126) = 0.05 \times 100 = 5\%$. While term babies conserve sodium well with FENa <1 and often closer to 0.5%, preterm infants' immature tubules lead to sodium wasting and high FENa. A creatinine of 0.8 in an 11-day-old, ex-25 week infant would fall in the normal range, so AKI is unlikely.

4. **e.** *Explanation:* Alkalosis stimulates the Na,K-ATPase on the basolateral membrane. This will increase intracellular potassium levels and stimulate potassium exit to the urine space. Alkalosis also increases the amount of time the luminal potassium channels are open, further encouraging urine potassium secretion and leading to hypokalemia. Avid sodium reabsorption in the proximal tubules as seen in volume-depleted states leads to less sodium delivery to the distal tubule. The reabsorption of sodium by ENaC in this segment leaves the lumen electronegative, which allows for secretion of potassium. Neonates do initially lack the potassium maxi-K channels (although these are stimulated by high urine flow, which would not be present in the baby in the scenario). The potassium channel ROMK is inhibited by acidosis, which would lead to less potassium secretion to the urine. Although aldosterone levels are high in infants, they exhibit less of a response to it.

5. **d.** *Explanation:* In a state of volume depletion, alkalosis will persist by the following three mechanisms: (1) a decrease in GFR leads to less filtered bicarbonate; (2) the proximal tubule avidly reabsorbs Na, which leads to increased bicarbonate reabsorption; and (3) the volume depletion stimulates RAS, which leads to an increase in aldosterone. The aldosterone leads to increased activity of the epithelial Na channel (ENaC), making the lumen more electronegative. This favors both H^+ and K^+ secretion. Typically in alkalosis, H^+ would shift out of the cell in exchange for K^+. Hypokalemia inhibits this process.

6. **a.** *Explanation:* The baby has pseudohypoaldosteronism type 1, autosomal dominant type. PHA type 1 presents with vomiting, FTT, hyponatremia, hyperkalemia, and

acidosis with high urine sodium. Renin and aldosterone levels are high. It can be inherited as an autosomal recessive or dominant trait. The dominant form is clinically outgrown usually by age 2. It is limited to renal findings. In contrast, the recessive form is a lifelong, systemic illness involving the skin, lungs, and kidney predominantly.

7. **b.** *Explanation:* A weight loss of up to 15% is normal in premature infants. Studies have shown that not allowing this weight loss to occur is associated with increased rates of PDA, NEC, and CLD. Potassium should be withheld from the TPN until urine output is established. The baby in the above scenario is urinating normally and has a normal creatinine, so standard of care would be to add potassium to his TPN. His TF should be increased to allow more nutrition, not because of the expected and normal weight loss.

8. **d.** *Explanation:* Term infants increase both respiratory rate and tidal volume, but preterm infants increase only their respiratory rate. Bicarbonate is not helpful to treat respiratory acidosis because it decreases respiratory rate. Preterm infants have a decreased ability to reabsorb filtered bicarbonate.

9. **d.** *Explanation:* Proximal RTA is most commonly seen in children as part of the renal Fanconi syndrome with wasting of glucose, amino acids, phosphorus. However, rare genetic causes have been reported. With proximal RTA the defect lies in the reabsorption of the filtered bicarbonate. The distal acidification mechanism is intact. When the serum bicarbonate is low, the distal acidification results in a low urine pH. When alkali therapy is started, the filtered bicarbonate load increases, which raises the urine pH. Therapy of proximal RTA requires large amounts of alkali, often 10 to 15 mEq/kg/d. Distal RTA is due to an acidification defect. It is suggested by a normal AG acidosis with urine pH > 6.5. Hypercalciuria is often present. Type IV RTA presents with mild acidosis (bicarbonate levels in high teens) and hyperkalemia. Technical difficulties obtaining blood samples can lead to factitiously low bicarbonate levels, but hyperkalemia and hyperphosphatemia should also be seen in that case. Pseudohypoaldosteronism can have a mild metabolic acidosis, but hyperkalemia and hyponatremia are major features of the disease.

10. **b.** *Explanation:* Renal prostaglandins play a crucial role in maintaining GFR when the kidney is not receiving normal blood flow due to volume depletion, hemorrhage, etc., or when angiotensin II levels are high. NSAIDs disrupt the production of prostaglandins and can lead to AKI. ANP is released by stretch of the atrium. It acts on the kidney to increase GFR by dilating the afferent arteriole and constricting the efferent arteriole. Ang II constricts both the afferent and efferent arterioles. If the PDA closed, blood would stop shunting away from the kidneys. Dopamine is natriuretic by decreasing the activity of Na,K-ATPase, which provides the driving force for Na reabsorption.

Chapter 53

1. **d.** *Explanation:* The normal size of fetal kidneys at 20 weeks is 2.7 cm. The bladder can be seen by 15 weeks.

The combination of large, bright kidneys with presumably no urine (cannot visualize the bladder because it is empty) is very suggestive of ARPKD. ADPKD can present in neonates, but a severe presentation such as this with anuria is very rare. More often, just large kidneys or cysts are seen with normal renal function. The lack of family history argues more for ARPKD than ADPKD, although 10% of people affected by ADPKD have new mutations. Bilateral MCDK would be associated with anuria, but large cysts should be seen in the kidneys. Dysplastic kidneys are usually (but not always) small. The kidneys in Beckwith-Wiedemann can be large, but severe impairment of function in utero would be atypical.

2. **a.** *Explanation:* The characteristic MCDK ultrasound picture is of multiple cysts of similar size giving an appearance of a cluster of grapes. A MCDK has no function. Often, the contralateral kidney will show compensatory hypertrophy in utero. With the normal kidney on the right, you would expect normal amniotic fluid levels. ADPKD is possible but rarely presents in neonates with ultrasound findings. ARPKD rarely presents with visible cysts and affects both kidneys. A UPJ obstruction leads to hydronephrosis, whereas a UVJ obstruction would lead to hydroureter.

3. **c.** *Explanation:* Intervention of suspected fetal bladder outlet obstruction has not definitely been shown to improve long-term function of lungs or kidneys. When an intervention is done, the vesicoamniotic shunt is the most common procedure. Serial bladder taps are preferred to obtain fresh urine to analyze the urine electrolytes. Urine Na <100 and urine osm >200 are predictive of preserved renal function. Other tests predictive of good renal function are urine Ca <8 mg/dL, urine protein <40 mg/dL, and urine beta-2 microglobulin <4 mg/L.

4. **d.** *Explanation:* The baby likely has a renal artery clot due to the UAC. Clots are thought to form due to disruption of the endothelium during line placement. A low-lying UAC is more likely to have a renal artery clot as compared to a high-lying UAC. The findings of decreased LE perfusion, hypertension, and hematuria without oliguria, congestive heart failure, or multi-organ failure suggest a "minor" clot. The treatment would be removal of the catheter and symptomatic therapy. Hypertension is common following a renal artery clot. The hypertension should resolve, but this may take months or years. ESRD is seen with bilateral renal artery clots. Loss of toes or bowel ischemia would be expected with a more severe clot involving the Aorta.

5. **d.** *Explanation:* The baby has several risk factors for renal vein thrombosis: sepsis, prematurity, and presence of UVC. The classic clinical findings suggestive of RVT are flank mass, low platelets, and hypertension. The presence of all three findings is actually rare. Although preterm kidneys are more likely to have stones or nephrocalcinosis, the affected kidney would not be small. Dysplastic kidneys are often small but should not have calcifications. Kidneys affected by ARPKD are large and diffusely echogenic.

6. **c.** *Explanation:* A rise in serum creatinine between 2 and 2.9 times the lowest creatinine obtained in the

prior 7 days or UOP >0.3 and ≤0.5 mL/kg/hr defines stage 2 AKI by the KDIGO definition.

7. **e.** *Explanation:* You have assessed him as euvolemic, so further fluid boluses are unlikely to help. If his hydration was in question, though, a NS bolus could be trialed. Renal dose dopamine has not been shown to hasten renal recovery. Because there is no hydrone-phrosis or abnormal bladder on ultrasound, placement of a bladder catheter would not improve his renal function. Kidney biopsies are rarely required in neonates to make a diagnosis of AKI. The baby likely has ATN from prolonged renal hypoperfusion. There is no spe-cific treatment for this other than ensuring good hydra-tion, avoiding further renal insults, and managing any electrolytes issues or hypertension. ATN should resolve over days to weeks, depending on its severity.

8. **e.** *Explanation:* PD has several advantages in the NICU, including that it is comparatively technically simple compared to HD or CRRT. It is performed with manual exchanges of fluid done by NICU nurses. The baby is not anticoagulated with PD. It may be easier to get a PD catheter inserted than obtain reliable vascular access for HD or CRRT. The disadvantages of PD include the removal of beneficial proteins such as immunoglobu-lins, slow efficiency at solute and fluid removal, and risk of peritonitis. It is contraindicated in babies with abdominal wall defects. HD can quickly remove solutes, but rapid fluid removal is usually not tolerated well. One of the principal advantages of CRRT is that slow, hourly removal of fluid that can be adjusted each hour.

9. **d.** *Explanation:* Preterm infants have slower metabo-lism of furosemide so should not be dosed multiple times per day. Spironolactone is a weak diuretic used mostly as a potassium-sparing agent in the NICU. The baby is likely not responding as well to the Lasix because the tubule segments past the loop of Henle are avidly reabsorbing the sodium due to a state of volume depletion. The Na-Cl cotransporter can be blocked by a thiazide diuretic, which should increase diuresis. Care must be taken, though, not to induce AKI from intra-vascular depletion. Close attention to electrolytes is also necessary.

10. **c.** *Explanation:* Thiazides can cause increased reabsorp-tion of calcium from the urine. In contrast, loop diuret-ics are associated with hypercalciuria, kidney stones, and nephrocalcinosis. They are also associated with an increased risk of bone fractures and with hearing loss. Spironolactone is a potassium-sparing diuretic used most often in the NICU in conjunction with a thiazide to mitigate potassium loss in the urine.

Chapter 54

1. **c.** *Explanation:* The majority of palpable undescended testes will descend spontaneously after the testosterone surge that accompanies the mini-puberty of infancy, which occurs within the first few months of age. Spon-taneous descent is unlikely after 4 months of age. There is an increased risk of germ cell malignancy in undescended testes, but malignancy is uncommon in patients who had orchiopexy prior to 2 years of age.

Endocrine evaluation for DSD should be performed in patients with BL nonpalpable testes or those with undescended testes and hypospadias or micropenis.

2. **b.** *Explanation:* There is a high suspicion that micrope-nis in a patient with multiple congenital midline anom-alies is due to deficient pituitary secretion of LH (leading to testosterone deficiency) or growth hormone. Central hypothyroidism is also possible but does not cause micropenis. Most infants with 17β-hydroxysteroid deficiency or 5α-reductase deficiency will have a more severe phenotype with ambiguous external genitalia or external genitalia that appear female. Neither condi-tion is commonly associated with other midline defects.

3. **a.** *Explanation:* XY males with 5α-reductase may have severe undervirilization at birth due to a lack of 5-DHT production, the androgen responsible for the majority of external genitalia in the male virilization fetus. At puberty, testosterone levels increase dramatically and, because the androgen receptor is present, will cause virilization. There is no function androgen receptor in complete androgen insensitivity, so increased testoster-one has no effect. Individuals with partial AI will likely undergo some virilization at puberty. Virilization in an XX female is due to excess androgen production in set-ting of cortisol deficiency and will not be appreciably affected by female puberty. XY males with 17β-HSD CAH lack an enzyme necessary to produce testosterone so will not have significant virilization at puberty.

4. **d.** *Explanation:* Gender assignment remains complex, and there usually is not a "right" or "wrong" decision. It is essential that families be involved in the discus-sion and make the ultimate decision. Some people with DSDs have argued that gender assignment and surgi-cal intervention should be put off until the patient is old enough to decide and provide consent. This is cur-rently not standard practice due to the perceived diffi-culty in raising a child with an indeterminate gender and because in some cases, surgical outcomes may be better when performed earlier. Given the changing cul-tural perceptions on gender, however, it is likely that counseling will evolve to allow for delaying gender assignment as a reasonable possibility.

5. **a.** *Explanation:* Estrogen plays no known role in fetal sexual differentiation; the Wolffian ducts (primordial male internal structures) regress spontaneously in the absence of testosterone. Normal male virilization requires the coordinated production of several differ-ent hormones, as described in answers (b) to (d).

6. **c.** *Explanation:* Adrenal insufficiency should be sus-pected and urgently evaluated in any case of ambiguous genitalia with nonpalpable gonads. This presentation is commonly seen in patients with mutations in adrenal hormone biosynthesis resulting in congenital adrenal hyperplasia. In XX females with CAH causing adrenal insufficiency and ambiguous genitalia, there will be no testes; virilization is due to excessive androgen produc-tion. In XY males with CAH causing adrenal insuffi-ciency and ambiguous genitalia, undervirilization will be due to absent/impaired testosterone production, and testes will have not descended. Micropenis (a) and hypospadias (b) in the setting of descended testes are most likely due to structural developmental defects,

although the former can be the result of growth hormone deficiency, and the infant should be monitored for hypoglycemia. Unilateral cryptorchidism (d) with otherwise normal genitalia is relatively common and unlikely to be associated with CAH.

7. **c.** *Explanation:* Laboratory workup confirms isolated testosterone deficiency (normal AMH shows that testes/Sertoli cells are present), and the absence of elevated androgen hormone precursors rules out CAH. 17β-HSD deficiency (a) would show elevated androstenedione and DHEA; AIS (b) and 5AR (d) would show normal/elevated testosterone levels. Patients with Leydig cell hypoplasia can be treated with a short course of testosterone in infancy for penile enlargement and will develop normal secondary sexual characteristics with testosterone hormone replacement starting at the time of puberty.

8. **d.** *Explanation:* Presence of virilization in an XX female with absence of laboratory findings of CAH suggests possibility of exposure to maternal endogenous/exogenous androgens or presence of an ovotesticular DSD. Maternal use of androgens as athletically performance-enhancing drugs early in pregnancy (in some cases, before pregnancy was recognized) can cause virilization. Development of maternal hirsutism during pregnancy suggests the possibility of placental aromatase deficiency resulting in accumulation of excess androgens in both maternal and fetal circulation. Ovotesticular DSD is a condition associated with both ovarian and testicular tissue; degree of virilization depends upon amount of testicular tissue and testosterone production. In many cases, these patients are mosaics for chromosomes (possessing both XX and XY), which can be missed on initial karyotype but will be detected with DNA testing for *SRY*. In the absence of *SRY*, pursuit of other genetic abnormalities (such as *RSPO-1*) with tests such as WES can be considered, but that would not be the next step in the case here due to the expense and delay in results.

9. **b.** *Explanation:* Patients with dysgenetic gonads, including XY gonadal dysgenesis, are at increased risk of gonadoblastoma and germ cell malignancy; therefore, dysgenetic gonads should be identified and removed. Presence of XY karyotype does not rule out gonadal dysgenesis; mutations of *SRY* and other genes involved in early sexual differentiation can be responsible for the clinical phenotype. There is wide clinical phenotype in XY gonadal dysgenesis ranging from completely feminized internal and external genitalia (complete gonadal dysgenesis) to a range of undervirilization of internal (i.e., Wolffian ducts) and/or external genitalia depending on the extent of androgen production (partial gonadal dysgenesis).

10. **g.** *Explanation:* Testosterone production is present at birth and then rapidly declines in the first several days until rising again at 20 to 30 days of life ("mini-puberty of infancy"). Testosterone production in infancy peaks between 2 and 3 months of age before falling to non-detectable levels by 6 months of age. Testosterone production again rises at the onset of puberty (range, 9–14 years of age). Assessment of unstimulated testosterone outside of these times will not provide any useful clinical information; however, an hCG stimulation test can be performed to assess for the capability of testosterone production.

Chapter 55

1. **b.** *Explanation:* Dopamine is a catecholamine synthesized in the adrenal medulla.

2. **c.** *Explanation:* The fetal zone of the adrenal cortex produces pregnenolone, 17-hydroxypregnenolone, and DHEA, which then must be converted into progesterone, 17-hydroxyprogesterone, and androstenedione by the placenta, which expresses 3β-HSD in abundance.

3. **a.** *Explanation:* Aromatase, because the conversion of androgens into estrogens is expressed primarily in gonads but is also found in other tissues such as adipose, liver, skin, and brain.

4. **d.** *Explanation:* CYP11A1 mutation blocks the ability of cholesterol to be transported to the inner mitochondrial membrane; therefore, synthesis of all steroid hormones will be diminished and will typically result in an undervirilized male.

5. **d.** *Explanation:* In a well-appearing infant without clinical signs of adrenal insufficiency or salt wasting, it is appropriate to assess a venous blood sample for 17-hydroxyporogesterone and electrolytes as the next step. Perinatal stress is one possible source of a false-positive newborn screen for CAH. Because clinical signs and electrolyte abnormalities of salt wasting may not manifest in the first few days of life, it is also prudent to repeat electrolytes at this time.

6. **c.** *Explanation:* Based on the clinical picture and the finding of a 17-hydroxyprogesterone level greater than 10,000 ng/dL, this patient most likely has 21-hydroxylase deficiency CAH. Prematurity and timing of sample before 48 hours of age increase the possibility of a false-positive newborn screen result, although typically not to levels >10,000 ng/dL. A venous 17-hydroxyprogesterone sample should be obtained, but treatment should not be delayed, as the clinical picture is concerning for adrenal crisis. During times of crisis, stress doses of hydrocortisone at 50 to 100 mg/m²/d should be used.

7. **c.** *Explanation:* 17-Hydroxylase deficiency may cause ambiguous genitalia in XY males due to undervirilization as a result of decreased androgen synthesis. All other listed enzymatic defects can lead to ambiguous genitalia in XX females due to overvirilization as a result of excess androgen production.

8. **b.** *Explanation:* Forms of CAH associated with early-onset hypertension include 11β-hydroxylase CAH and 17-hydroxylase CAH. Both conditions are marked by dramatically elevated serum levels of 11-deoxycorticosterone. 11-Deoxycortisone has mineralocorticoid activity; when present at high levels, it leads to volume expansion with resultant suppression of renin and aldosterone. Hypertension is a sign of overtreatment with Florinef in 21-hydroxylase CAH, the dose of which typically needs to be weaned after infancy. The clinical presentation of all forms of CAH are variable; therefore, normal virilization does not rule out

17-hydroxylase CAH in an XY male. Some patients with severe 11β-hydroxylase deficiency may have 17-hydroxyprogesterone levels high enough to trigger an abnormal newborn screen result, although the majority will be diagnosed later. An elevated 11-deoxycorticosone level on ACTH stimulation is the gold-standard diagnostic technique.

9. **d.** *Explanation:* ACTH is not a reliable marker for the adequacy of hydrocortisone dose. Linear growth should be monitored for signs of undertreatment (increased growth velocity) and overtreatment (suppressed growth velocity). Bone age is checked every 1 to 2 years for evidence of androgen-induced skeletal maturation. Androstenedione should be followed and maintained in the normal range for age. Plasma renin activity is used to assess adequacy of mineralocorticoid replacement.

10. **a.** *Explanation:* 21-Hydroxylase is an autosomal recessive disorder that affects males and females equally. Statistically, assuming that both mother and father are carriers, there is a one in four chance of giving birth to an affected child with each pregnancy, so the risk of having another affected female is one in eight. Prenatal treatment with dexamethasone to reduce virilization of affected females is controversial; existing protocols suggest starting treatment at 6 to 8 weeks' gestational age, around the time that external sexual differentiation occurs. Hydrocortisone is not effective because it is metabolized by the placenta.

Chapter 56

1. **b.** *Explanation:* Graves' disease is associated with a mix of both TSH receptor stimulating and blocking antibodies; therefore, the fetus/neonate is at risk of both hyper- and hypothyroidism. T3 is inactivated; however, TSH antibodies do cross the placenta. Antibodies can persist even after definitive therapy, so the fetus/neonate is at risk even if the mother has had surgery/ablation. Untreated maternal hyperthyroidism results in increased risk of miscarriage, premature labor, intrauterine growth restriction, and hyper- and hypothyroidism. PTU is generally considered first-line treatment for Graves' disease in the United States, although methimazole is used in other countries, and it is unclear whether the risk of birth defects is actually higher in PTU versus methimazole. Either way, the goal of therapy is to maintain maternal free T4 levels in the upper end of the normal range on the lowest possible antithyroid dose.

2. **a.** *Explanation:* An activating mutation in the TSH receptor gene leads to hyperthyroidism and is a rare form of neonatal thyrotoxicosis. Consumptive hypothyroidism is due to overexpression of deiodinase 3, typically hepatic hemangiomas, that leads to excessive inactivation of thyroid hormones. Inactivating mutations in the sodium–iodine symporter prevent iodine from entering the follicular cell and are a form of thyroid hormone dyshormonogenesis. Ectopically located thyroid glands are a common cause of congenital hypothyroidism; often they are located near the base of the tongue.

3. **c.** *Explanation:* The infant likely has septo-optic dysplasia with clinical evidence of pituitary hormone deficiency (hypoglycemic seizure) and is therefore at risk for having central hypothyroidism. Central hypothyroidism is marked by low thyroid hormone levels; TSH can be low, normal, or even slightly elevated. As such, states that employ a TSH-only newborn screen may miss infants with central hypothyroidism. An elevated TSH with low thyroid hormone levels is diagnostic of primary hypothyroidism. A low T$_4$ with normal TSH and free T$_4$ is consistent with TBG deficiency. A pattern of low TSH with elevated thyroid hormone levels is seen in hyperthyroidism.

4. **a.** *Explanation:* A finding of fetal goiter can be a sign of either fetal hypo- or hyperthyroidism. Large goiters can cause airway obstruction and subsequent respiratory failure at birth. Fetal goiters due to hyperthyroidism that result from placental passage of TSH receptor stimulating antibodies can be treated with maternal antithyroid medication (methimazole or PTU) administration; therefore, fetal blood sampling may be indicated if there is a significant goiter and the thyroid status of the fetus is not apparent. Fetal blood sampling is associated with a 1% to 2% risk of miscarriage, so risks and benefits must be weighed on a case-by-case basis.

5. **d.** *Explanation:* Labs are most consistent with TBG deficiency, a benign condition characterized by low TBG. Treatment with levothyroxine is not indicated, as free thyroid hormone levels are normal. The inherited form of this condition is due to mutations in *SERPIN7A*. This gene is located on the X-chromosome; therefore, a father can only pass an abnormal copy to a daughter. TBG deficiency due to *SERPIN7A* can be partial (with one abnormal copy in a female) or complete (with no normal copies in either a male or female). Acquired forms of TBG deficiency are also possible in the setting of protein-losing conditions. THOP is characterized by low levels of all thyroid hormones; elevated TRAb levels can be seen in mothers with Graves' disease.

6. **b.** *Explanation:* Consumptive hypothyroidism will result in elevated reverse T$_3$ levels due to overexpression of deiodinase 3. Reverse T$_3$ levels are most likely to be low in congenital hypothyroidism and normal in TBG deficiency and THOP. The etiology of hypothyroxinemia in premature infants is not well understood; defective TSH surge and diminished iodide stores have been suggested as possible contributors, but definitive data are lacking.

7. **d.** *Explanation:* Only 1% to 10% of infants born to mothers with Graves' disease are affected; therefore, treatment is initiated only with clinical and biochemical evidence of hyperthyroidism. Therapy includes management of symptoms of hyperthyroidism with a beta-blocker and reduction in thyroid hormone production with an antithyroid medication (typically methimazole). High-dose iodine (as provided in Lugol solution) transiently inhibits thyroid hormone production by blocking iodide organification (Wolff-Chaikoff effect). The thyroid gland escapes this effect in 7 to 10 days, possibly due to decreased transport of iodine across the sodium–iodine symporter. Neonatal Graves' disease is transient and usually resolves by 6 months of age or sooner.

8. **c.** *Explanation:* This patient most likely has defective thyroid hormone transport due to a mutation in *MCT8* (also known as *SLC16A2*). This transporter is required for the transport of T_3 into neurons; in its absence, low intracellular T_3 levels result in abnormal neurologic findings, including seizure, hypotonia, and developmental delay. Other body cells are able to transport T_4 across the cell membrane with intracellular conversion into T_3. Therefore, treatment with either T_4 or T_3 can result in a hypermetabolic state in conjunction with hyperthyroidism. *MCT8* deficiency is inherited in an X-linked recessive pattern.

Chapter 57

1. **c.** *Explanation:* The patient most likely has glycogen storage disease 1 (GSD-1) due to glucose 6-phosphatase deficiency. This mutation blocks gluconeogenesis from glycogenolysis during fasting and presents with severe lactic acidosis. It often presents at a few months of age when infants begin to decrease feeding frequency and sleep through the night. Glycogen synthase deficiency (GSD-0) leads to inability to synthesize glycogen and therefore does not present with hepatomegaly. Neither congenital hyperinsulinism nor fatty acid oxidation disorder presents with severe acidosis.

2. **d.** *Explanation:* The labs are most c/w hyperinsulinism. Neither adrenal nor growth hormone deficiency can be diagnosed based on a critical sample alone. An ACTH or CRH stimulation test to confirm normal hypothalamic–pituitary–adrenal axis would be appropriate in this case. GH was normal, so growth hormone stimulation testing is not needed. If clinically appropriate, the next step in the management of hyperinsulinism would be try diazoxide. It can take up to 5 days to see the full effect of treatment; infants will continue to need intravenous or continuous enteral dextrose support, targeting BG >70 mg/dL.

3. **b.** *Explanation:* Diazoxide can cause fluid retention and may be associated with development of pulmonary hypertension; therefore, it must be used with caution in patients with congenital heart disease with frequent monitoring of cardiac status. Most infants with stress-induced HI will respond to diazoxide, whereas only some forms of congenital HI (GCK-HI, SCHAD-HI, GDH-AD AD-HI) are responsive; patients with mutations in the K_{ATP} channel will need surgery. Diazoxide causes hypertrichosis (reversible when discontinued) and can cause cytopenia.

4. **d.** *Explanation:* Patients with transient neonatal diabetes typically have a remission period during childhood where insulin is not needed but permanent insulin requirement is likely to return in adulthood. The diffuse HI d/t K_{ATP} channel will require near-total pancreatectomy; there is an increased risk of diabetes and insulin requirement after this surgery. Hypopituitarism is not associated with an increased risk of diabetes.

5. **c.** *Explanation:* Glucose is the main source of energy for the brain. During times of prolonged fasting, ketone bodies and lactate can be used as alternative fuel sources. Free fatty acids do not cross the blood–brain barrier so are unable to be utilized directly by the brain for energy.

6. **d.** *Explanation:* Labs and clinical findings are strongly suggestive of neonatal hypopituitarism; however, GH and ACTH or CRH stimulation tests should be done to confirm the diagnosis. The patient will most likely require lifelong hormone replacement. He is also at risk of central hypothyroidism, which could have been missed on a newborn screen in states that use a primary TSH screening program. Uncooked cornstarch is used to manage patients with glycogen storage disease and has no role here.

7. **a.** *Explanation:* The patient most likely has late-dumping syndrome. This condition is characterized by postprandial hypoglycemia, most commonly in patients with gastrostomy and history of Nissen fundoplication. The etiology is not entirely understood but appears to be a condition of excessive insulin secretion as a result of rapid glucose absorption and altered incretin hormone signaling. These patients do not have fasting hypoglycemia, and hypoglycemia will not persist when oral feeds have been established. In some cases, hypoglycemia can be prevented by lowering the rate of bolus feeds and tapering the rate over the last 30 minutes; acarbose given with each bolus feed is also effective.

8. **c.** *Explanation:* The secretion and action of a number of hormones contribute to intermediary metabolism. As plasma glucose levels fall below 70 mg/dL, insulin secretion decreases, and secretion of glucagon increases. Further declines in glucose levels induce secretion of epinephrine, growth hormone, and cortisol. Thyroid hormone is not known to play a role in intermediary metabolism.

9. **d.** *Explanation:* Distinguishing between endogenous and exogenous hyperinsulinism can be difficult. Biochemically, laboratory results at the time of the critical sample and a glucagon stimulation test will be identical, with the exception of C-peptide, which is expected to be elevated or inappropriately elevated with endogenous insulin oversecretion but suppressed in the setting of exogenous administration.

Chapter 58

1. **c.** *Explanation:* Mutations in the alkaline phosphatase gene cause hypophosphatasia, a type of early onset osteoporosis characterized by absent/diminished skeletal mineralization. The femurs, like all long bones, are formed by endochondral ossification. Defects in chondrocyte function lead to a number of skeletal dysplasias because of impaired endochondral ossification. PTHrP is an important regulator of calcium status and osteoblast function prenatally but has a limited role after birth.

2. **c.** *Explanation:* Normal magnesium levels are required for PTH. Both high and low magnesium levels inhibit PTH secretion; the mechanism is not fully understood. Both calcium and magnesium form divalent cations, so magnesium would not be expected to bind to calcium and decrease availability for absorption (as is seen with phosphate anions).

3. **c.** *Explanation:* DiGeorge syndrome results in hypocalcemia because of defective parathyroid gland

development. In many cases, the hypoparathyroidism is transient, although it can be exacerbated by illness and acute stress. Mutations in CPY27B1 cause vitamin D–dependent rickets type 1A and can result in hypocalcemia due to decreased synthesis of active vitamin D. PTH resistance as seen in pseudohypoparathyroidism is due to mutations in GNAS. Inactivating mutations in PHEX cause hypophosphatemia in X-linked hypophosphatemic rickets.

4. **a.** *Explanation:* Severe hypocalcemia can result in a prolonged QTc interval and resultant cardiac dysfunction.

5. **b.** *Explanation:* Large for gestational age is suggestive of an infant of a diabetic mother, which is a risk factor for early neonatal hypocalcemia related to low magnesium levels and impaired parathyroid hormone release. Inactivating mutations in the CaSR causing NSHPT and FHH cause hypercalcemia and typically do not present with seizure. Infants born with DiGeorge (22q11.2 deletion) syndrome are typically small in size.

6. **b.** *Explanation:* This child most likely has congenital rickets due to hypophosphatasia. This condition is caused by mutations in the ALP gene and results in markedly low serum alkaline phosphatase levels. Urine phosphorus is most helpful in differentiating malabsorptive from renal hypophosphatemic rickets, which is not present based on the elevated serum phosphorus. 25-OHD would be the test of choice if vitamin D deficiency rickets is suspected, which would not typically present with this severity and would be associated with low/normal serum calcium and phosphorus. An elevated intact PTH would, in the setting of hypercalcemia, confirm diagnosis of hyperparathyroidism, which would not present with rickets as described here.

7. **b.** *Explanation:* Large for gestational age and/or infant of a diabetic mother are not risk factors for osteopenia of prematurity, although they may be associated with other disorders of bone mineral homeostasis such as early postnatal hypocalcemia.

8. **c.** *Explanation:* The amount of calcium/phosphorus that can be provided in TPN is limited; transition to full enteral feeds should be encouraged as soon as feasible. DXA scans are capable of assessing bone mineral density, but there are only limited data in neonates, so these scans are not currently a recommended procedure in the monitoring of osteopenia of prematurity. Premature infants should be supplemented with 200 to 400 IU of vitamin D, increasing as needed for confirmed vitamin D deficiency.

9. **b.** *Explanation:* Based on a finding of elevated calcium and 1,25-OHD with appropriately suppressed PTH, the patient most likely has infantile hypercalcemia due to 24-hydroxylase mutation. This condition is associated with hypercalciuria and a risk of nephrocalcinosis and kidney stones in late childhood/early adulthood. Vitamin D intoxication would be associated with elevated 25-OHD (typically above 70–100 ng/mL). Low calcium formulas can be helpful in managing this condition; he should also avoid vitamin D supplementation and sun exposure.

10. **b.** *Explanation:* The patient most likely has nutritional hypophosphatemic rickets related to exposure to elemental formula. Labs will show low serum phosphorus,

undetectable urine phosphorus, and elevated alkaline phosphatase. Treatment includes oral phosphate supplementation and requires close laboratory monitoring for the development of hypocalcemia as a result of exuberant gastrointestinal phosphorus absorption. This condition is self-limited and will resolve with appropriate phosphorus supplements.

Chapter 59

1. **c.** *Explanation:* Norepinephrine is the key counter-regulatory hormone released in response to acute cold stress. Actions include peripheral vasoconstriction to reduce heat loss and stimulation of brown adipose tissue for thermogenesis. Thyroid hormone secretion ± cortisol secretion play a role in the long-term adaption to cold but are not thought to play a crucial role in the acute response to cold stress. Growth hormone is not known to have a regulatory role in the response to short- or long-term cold exposure.

2. **a.** *Explanation:* Free fatty acids, released via lipolysis, form the substrate for thermogenesis by brown adipose tissue. Thermogenesis occurs in the mitochondria of the brown adipocyte and is "nonshivering" as heat is generated in the absence of muscle contraction. Brown adipose tissue is more prominent in newborns than adults and was once thought to be an embryonic remnant, but it is now recognized as being present throughout the life span.

3. **c.** *Explanation:* Neonates can lose heat through conduct convective, conductive, radiant, and evaporative heat loss. Premature infants are at greater risk for convective, conductive, and radiant loss as a result of diminished subcutaneous fat that acts as an insulator, and they are at greater risk of evaporative heat loss because of thinner skin. Nonshivering thermogenesis is a primary physiologic response to generate heat in response to cold stress.

4. **a.** *Explanation:* Skin-to-skin contact with the mother is the optimal heat source for stable infants immediately following delivery. Air and oxygen used for respiratory support can be a source of both convective and evaporative heat loss; therefore, warmed or humidified air is recommended, if available. Windows or other cool objects can be a source of radiant heat loss. Nonwarmed blankets can be a source of conductive heat loss.

Chapter 60

1. **b.** *Explanation:* Erythropoietin is produced primarily in the fetal liver and does not shift to the kidney until near the time of birth. Erythropoietin does not cross the placenta. Bone marrow erythropoiesis requires erythropoietin, but the bone marrow is not a primary site of erythropoietin production.

2. **c.** *Explanation:* Frequent blood sampling, the shorter life span of preterm erythrocytes compared to the erythrocytes of term infants, and suppression of erythropoiesis due to systemic illness are major contributors to AOP. Preterm infants are capable of increasing

erythropoiesis in response to EPO treatment; however, they have lower EPO production in response to hypoxia than term infants. The use of EPO to treat AOP is controversial.

3. **d.** *Explanation:* ABO blood group incompatibilities between mother and fetus are common; however, only ~10% of such pregnancies result in an infant affected by hemolysis and jaundice. In contrast to Rh disease, ABO incompatibility does not worsen with each pregnancy and is not a common cause of fetal anemia.

4. **a.** *Explanation:* The other choices are embryonic globins present in the primitive erythroblasts produced by the yolk sac in the first trimester.

5. **a.** *Explanation:* Severe forms of α-thalassemia, including hemoglobin H and hemoglobin Barts (due to deletion or disruption of three or four of the four α-globin genes), can lead to severe fetal anemia and hydrops fetalis. Milder forms of α -thalassemia (silent carrier state and α-thalassemia trait) may not be diagnosed until later in childhood. β-Thalassemia and sickle cell anemia are due to mutations in the β-chain and do not manifest until after fetal hemoglobin levels decline, generally around 6 months of age.

6. **b.** *Explanation:* Following birth, it is appropriate for HbF (fetal hemoglobin) to predominate. The presence of both HbS and HbA indicates that the patient has one normal β-chain and one β-chain with the sickle cell mutation (HbS). A newborn screen suggestive of sickle cell anemia would show HbF with HbS and no HbA. A normal newborn screen would show only HbF and HbA.

7. **c.** *Explanation:* Due to this inheritance pattern, the majority of affected individuals are male; however, females can be affected if they are homozygous for the mutated G6PD allele or in the setting of unbalanced X-inactivation.

8. **c.** *Explanation:* During the third trimester.

9. **b.** *Explanation:* Iron supplementation is important, as iron deficiency has been associated with neurologic deficits and anemia. Term neonates have sufficient iron stores for 4 to 6 months, and iron supplementation is recommended starting at 4 months for term infants who receive more than half their feeds from breast milk. Breast milk has lower levels of iron than formula, but the iron in breast milk is highly bioavailable. Iron supplementation should be considered for preterm infants beginning at 1 month of age. Preterm infants have higher iron requirements due to more rapid rates of postnatal growth.

10. **a.** *Explanation:* Polycythemia has been associated with neurodevelopmental delays; however, PET has not been shown to improve neurologic outcomes.

Chapter 61

1. **b.** *Explanation:* Hematopoiesis, or the production of blood cells, occurs primarily in the liver and spleen in the fetus and occurs primarily in the bone marrow in full-term neonates, children, and adults.

2. **b.** *Explanation:* In the normal development of blood cells, the first branch point from a hematopoietic stem cell is lymphoid versus myeloid. Lymphoid precursors develop into lymphocytes; myeloid precursors develop into all other blood cells, including all other white blood cells (except lymphocytes), red blood cells, and platelets.

3. **a.** *Explanation:* This neonate clearly has multiple immature white blood cells present in the peripheral blood. Each of these forms (bands, metamyelocytes, myelocytes, promyelocytes, and blasts) represents normal maturation stages of a neutrophil, and each of these forms is normally present in the bone marrow. In conditions of extreme stress such as sepsis or severe illness, the bone marrow responds by trying to produce more neutrophils quickly, and this is the likely reason why these forms are seen in the blood. This is also known as the so-called "left shift." A tiny percentage of blasts is not likely to be leukemia in this setting, especially with other immature forms seen and with a normal hemoglobin and platelet count.

Chapter 62

1. **c.** *Explanation:* Neonatal thrombocytopenia is associated with preeclampsia and is typically a self-limited mild thrombocytopenia that nadirs by 2 to 4 days and resolves at around one week of life.

2. **b.** *Explanation:* NAIT is due to maternal antibodies against fetal platelet antigens. Maternal thrombocytopenia is suggestive of autoimmune thrombocytopenia. NAIT can cause severe thrombocytopenia. Random donor platelets will increase the platelet count and are more readily available than type-matched platelets, although the response may be transient.

3. **a.** *Explanation:* Neonatal autoimmune thrombocytopenia is frequently associated with maternal thrombocytopenia and maternal ITP or SLE.

4. **d.** *Explanation:* Neonates have lower levels of antithrombin and protein C. Coagulation factors do not pass from the mother to the fetus. Neonates have higher von Willebrand factor levels than adults. Normative platelet values are similar for neonates and adults.

5. **c.** *Explanation:* Early-onset VKDB occurs in the first 24 hours of life and can result in severe bleeding. It is associated with maternal medications including warfarin, isoniazid, or antiepileptics. The other factors are associated with late onset VKDB.

6. **a.** *Explanation:* Intracranial hemorrhage. Late-onset VKDB occurs after 2 weeks of age and is frequently associated with intracranial hemorrhage. Infants at risk for late VKDB include exclusively breastfed babies who did not receive the vitamin K shot, infants with cholestatic liver dysfunction, and infants with chronic intestinal malabsorption.

7. **a.** *Explanation:* The classic triad of renal vein thrombosis is thrombocytopenia, hematuria, and a palpable flank mass.

8. **b.** *Explanation:* DVTs are frequently associated with central lines and often result in thrombocytopenia.

9. **b.** *Explanation:* Infants with TAR have severe thrombocytopenia at birth that improves over the first year of life. The presence of thumbs helps to distinguish infants with TAR from infants with Fanconi anemia.

10. **d.** *Explanation:* PF can be due to an inherited deficiency in protein C or protein S, or PF can be secondary to

infection. Central lines are associated with DVTs, which cause thrombocytopenia, but generally not PE.

Chapter 63

1. **d.** *Explanation:* Of the choices listed, the first three are thought to be critically important for a safe PRBC transfusion in a neonate. All patients of all ages will require a type and cross to ensure ABO matching and no reaction. All patients, but especially neonates, should have PRBC products leukocyte reduced to decrease viral infectious transmission. Irradiation (or CMV negative units) would be strongly preferred for neonates. In addition, giving fresh PRBC (ideally <14 days old) would also be preferred by most centers. Washing, which is done to reduce the risk of allergic reaction, is typically only done if a patient has had a previous allergic reaction; it would not be necessary for all neonates.

2. **a.** *Explanation:* Random donor PRBC are almost always preferred to related family member donors. There are multiple reasons for this. First, in neonates, and also in patients with any immune system dysfunction, related donor blood products pose additional risks, including the risk of alloimmunization and the risk of transfusion-associated graft-versus-host disease. Second, many family members are first-time donors and present a statistically higher risk of having an infection. Random donor units need to be ABO compatible, and type O patients require type O blood, as they have naturally occurring anti-A and anti-B antibodies.

3. **c.** *Explanation:* Transfusion-related acute lung injury (TRALI) is now the most common cause of morbidity and mortality during blood product transfusions. However, it remains relatively rare in neonates and children. Management consists of stopping the infusion (if still running), considering diuresis, and providing good supportive care and respiratory support. TRALI is thought to occur through immunologic mechanisms including recipient neutrophil activation by donor antigens. Hemolytic transfusion reaction is unlikely unless there is a clerical error. CMV transmission would not present as acute symptoms and signs. Transfusion-associated circulatory overload (TACO) is relatively excluded by the normal cardiac size. Sepsis is also much less likely than TRALI.

4. **c.** *Explanation:* The management of severe thrombocytopenia in the neonatal period includes platelet transfusions. Neonates are thought to have a much higher risk of bleeding with thrombocytopenia in comparison to older infants, children, and adults. Consequently, the platelet count is typically maintained >30 ($\times 10^9/\mu$L) in the first week of life. Neonates with this level of thrombocytopenia should also be monitored closely for bleeding, and head ultrasound should be performed to exclude intracranial hemorrhage. NAIT is managed with IVIG, as well as intermittent random donor platelet transfusions. In NAIT, there is a finite number of anti-platelet antibodies (IgG anti-platelet antibodies); thus, platelet transfusions are helpful to reduce the antibody load and help the neonate to recover his or her platelet count more quickly. This patient would be managed with random donor platelets, as those are the most readily available platelet source. Washed maternal (not paternal) platelets would be the gold standard therapy for severe NAIT.

5. **d.** *Explanation:* Critically ill neonates will often require multiple blood product transfusions including all of the blood products listed. However, cryoprecipitate is a blood product that includes high levels of fibrinogen (as well as factor 8, factor 13, von Willebrand factor, and fibronectin) and is the most efficient and low-volume product to replete fibrinogen.

6. **d.** *Explanation:* Patients with severe combined immunodeficiency (SCID) have a severe absence or decrease in T lymphocyte infections and are thus at risk of life-threatening infections at a very early age. Most patients require a stem cell transplant (or gene therapy) within the first few months of life. SCID is now tested for in many states as part of the newborn screen. SCID patients are also susceptible to CMV infection, and all blood products must be irradiated and/or from CMV-negative donors to avoid any risk of primary CMV infection. (This is also the rare indication where a mother should consider not breastfeeding her baby if the mother is CMV positive.)

Chapter 64

1. **a.** *Explanation:* Respiratory distress, hepatosplenomegaly, significant bruising, and palpable nodules may all be symptoms of congenital leukemia. The most common subtype of congenital leukemia is acute myeloid leukemia (AML), and the prognosis is very poor. Leukemia cutis is the term for leukemia nodules, which may be seen. This should be differentiated from bluish nodules, which may be seen in neuroblastoma, as well as the dry, scaly rashes consistent with Langerhans cell histiocytosis (LCH). For the patient in this vignette, the next steps would include complete blood work, bone marrow aspiration/biopsy, lumbar puncture, and pediatric hematology/oncology consultation. Unfortunately, the prognosis for congenital leukemia is poor.

2. **d.** *Explanation:* Children with Down syndrome have a markedly increased risk of multiple hematologic abnormalities, including AML, ALL, TAM, and thrombocytopenia. However, the most common and most likely diagnosis in the first week of life is transient abnormal myelopoiesis (TAM, formerly referred to as transient myeloproliferative disorder [TMD]). TAM is truly a transient leukemia and is specific to neonates (age <7 days) with Down syndrome, occurring in about 10% of neonates with Down syndrome. Neonates with TAM develop proliferation of a leukemia clone, the cells are indistinguishable from AML cells, and the presentation is otherwise identical to AML. However, for reasons that are unclear, TAM typically resolves spontaneously and does not require therapy.

3. **b.** *Explanation:* As the majority of neonates with Down syndrome will have the TAM resolve, observation is typically recommended. A small number of neonates may require some chemotherapy if significantly symptomatic, but this is not the norm. However, neonates with TAM do have a very high absolute risk of 25% for

the development of true AML within the first 4 years of life. For this reason, very close follow-up, including screening CBCs, is recommended.

4. **c.** *Explanation:* Langerhans cell histiocytosis may affect any organ, although it most commonly affects bone and skin. A skeletal survey would be the only test above required for all patients with LCH. Additional diagnostic workup would be considered if the patient had localizing symptoms or signs. Ultrasound rather than CT is typically used to evaluate for hepatic and splenic involvement, if indicated. Complete laboratory screening, including CBC, chemistries, kidney and liver function testing, and coagulation studies, is also required in all patients. The treatment and prognosis of LCH are dependent upon disease extent and organ involvement. Infants with disease limited to skin or bone do extremely well, whereas those with multiple-organ involvement will typically need chemotherapy for cure. Vinblastine and prednisone are the most commonly recommended agents for LCH.

5. **b.** *Explanation:* Neonatal teratoma is the most common tumor in newborns, when benign and malignant tumors are taken together. The vast majority of teratomas are "mature" or benign; thus, they do not have any malignant potential, and they do not produce AFP or beta-hCG. About 10% of teratomas will have malignant elements and may be labeled "immature" or have germ cell tumor components. Immature or germ cell tumors do often produce AFP or beta-hCG, and these tumor markers can be used to follow patients. Surgical resection is the mainstay of therapy and is recommended up front.

6. **c.** *Explanation:* Large facial hemangiomas raise concern for PHACES syndrome (posterior fossa malformations, hemangioma, arterial/aortic abnormalities, cardiac defects, eye abnormalities, sternal cleft/supraumbilical raphe syndrome). An MRI of the brain is required to evaluate for brain abnormalities, typically in the posterior fossa. In general, large hemangiomas (>5 cm) or multiple hemangiomas (>five cutaneous lesions) will require additional workup and often imaging for internal abnormalities. Kasabach-Merritt syndrome is the association of thrombocytopenia and DIC, which may be associated with giant hemangiomas or vascular anomalies.

7. **b.** *Explanation:* Historically, corticosteroids (prednisone) were the mainstay of treatment; however, steroid side effects are significant and have led to decreased use. Currently, propranolol is a very well tolerated, safe, and effective medical treatment for hemangiomas, and it should be considered first-line. Additional or second-line therapies may include laser therapy, embolization procedures, and sirolimus.

8. **a.** *Explanation:* This patient very likely does have congenital neuroblastoma; however, biopsy and pathology confirmation is absolutely required to make the diagnosis. Especially in a neonate with multiple systems affected, biopsy or adrenal resection is critical to gain additional histologic information about the neuroblastoma, including evaluating for favorable histology and n-MYC amplification. This patient likely has stage M-S (IV-S) neuroblastoma, which often may be safely observed, as neonates with this presentation of neuroblastoma are very likely to have spontaneous resolution of their disease. However, one would not observe without first confirming the diagnosis. MIBG scan as well as urine HVA/VMA would also be supportive of the diagnosis, although they would not supersede tissue biopsy. Most neonates will not require intensive chemotherapy or stem cell transplants for cure. The prognosis for neonates with neuroblastoma is excellent.

9. **e.** *Explanation:* There is a very strong association between rhabdomyomas and tuberous sclerosis (TS). In fact, about 80% of patients with rhabdomyomas will be diagnosed with TS; half of TS patients will have rhabdomyomas. Workup for TS would include brain MRI as well as consideration of genetic testing. Sturge-Weber syndrome is a neurological disorder associated with a port-wine stain on the face, as well as intracranial abnormalities. Beckwith-Wiedemann is a syndrome including large tongue, hemihypertrophy, and risk of pediatric tumors including Wilms tumor and hepatoblastoma. Down syndrome has no association with solid tumors. Rhabdomyomas are benign and have no association with malignant rhabdomyosarcomas.

10. **a.** *Explanation:* Renal masses are relatively uncommon in neonates, although they may occur. The most common renal mass is congenital mesoblastic nephroma, whereas the most common malignant renal mass is Wilms tumor. However, without biopsy and pathology, it can be impossible to determine the tumor type. For that reason, immediate pediatric surgical consultation and nephrectomy are advised. Genetic testing for familial syndromes could be considered if there is a family history of pediatric cancer, although this would not be urgent. MIBG and urine HVA/VMA would be helpful in the diagnosis of neuroblastoma, which is an adrenal tumor. Hematuria may present with Wilms tumor, and a simple urinalysis is adequate for evaluation.

Chapter 65

1. **b.** *Explanation:* The presence of unilateral corneal edema, enlarged corneal diameter, tearing, and photophobia is most consistent with unilateral congenital glaucoma. The intraocular pressure would be expected to be high, and treatment is usually surgical. Microbial keratitis usually presents as a localized infiltrate in the cornea and would not cause an increased corneal diameter. Storage diseases can cause diffuse corneal clouding but would be bilateral with normal corneal diameter in most cases. There is no role for corneal biopsy in congenital glaucoma, and corneal transplant is not indicated for the primary treatment of glaucoma.

2. **c.** *Explanation:* Common causes of ophthalmia neonatorum include *Neisseria*, *Chlamydia*, herpes virus, and chemical. While awaiting results of Gram stain and culture, it is appropriate to cover both *Neisseria* and *Chlamydia* with systemic ceftriaxone and erythromycin.

3. **a.** *Explanation:* The most concerning diagnosis in this scenario is unilateral retinoblastoma, which requires prompt diagnosis and treatment. Retinopathy of prematurity is not likely to develop in a full-term infant.

Strabismus may cause a bright red reflex when viewing both eyes simultaneously, but it would not cause leukocoria. Congenital rubella syndrome can cause an abnormal red reflex due to cataract, but would be expected to be a bilateral disease.

4. **c.** *Explanation:* This case appears most consistent with simple congenital/myopathic ptosis, in which there is poor development of the levator muscle of the upper eyelid. This is often unilateral, remains stable throughout life, and may affect vision and lead to amblyopia. It will likely require surgery at a later time, but it can often be delayed several years. With an otherwise normal exam, including pupils and eye movements, there is low suspicion for Horner's syndrome (associated with shoulder dystocia) or CN III palsy. A hemangioma of the eyelid could cause a mechanical ptosis, but this would be obvious on exam.

5. **a.** *Explanation:* ROP screening is required for babies born at ≤30 weeks *or* birth weight of ≤1500 g. They do not need to meet both criteria. Additionally, screening can occur for babies 1500 to 2000g or >30 weeks if the clinical course is unstable. The timing of screening is 31 weeks or 4 weeks after birth, whichever comes later.

6. **b.** *Explanation:* The description of this child, born to a mother of advanced maternal age, makes a diagnosis of trisomy 21 likely. Trisomy 21 is associated with congenital cataracts, as noted above, in addition to a higher incidence of strabismus, keratoconus, refractive error (need for glasses), nasolacrimal duct obstruction, and several other ophthalmic conditions. There is not a significant association between trisomy 21 and CHED or Marcus Gunn jaw-winking. This child's gestational age leaves us with no concern for ROP.

Chapter 66

1. **c.** *Explanation:* Genetic congenital hearing loss is 70% non-syndromic and approximately 80% autosomal recessive.

2. **d.** *Explanation:* The goal of newborn hearing screening is to identify hearing loss by 1 month of age and institute early intervention by 6 months of age.

3. **f.**

4. **d.** *Explanation:* CMV accounts for up to 20% of hearing loss at birth in the United States.

5. **c.** Bilateral pre-auricular pits should raise concern for branchiootorenal (BOR) syndrome, so a renal ultrasound should be performed. Genetic testing may be appropriate if the renal ultrasound raises further concern for BOR. Surgical excision would be premature at this point because the lesions are asymptomatic. CT of the face and ophthalmology evaluation are not indicated at this time.

6. **b.** At-risk newborns who pass the NBHS should be evaluated by an audiologist every 6 months for the first 3 years of life to identify any changes in hearing.

Chapter 67

1. **b.** The triad of findings in Pierre Robin sequence is cleft palate, micrognathia, and glossoptosis. A cleft lip is not commonly seen.

2. **d.** Patients with DiGeorge syndrome are at risk for hypocalcemia.

3. **c.** This scenario describes a type 2 branchial cleft anomaly, which will commonly have a tract that opens internally in the tonsillar fossa.

4. **c.**

5. **d.** The child in this scenario has laryngomalacia, but, given the lack of significant respiratory symptoms or failure to thrive, no surgical intervention is indicated.

6. **b.** *Explanation:* In the absence of significant airway symptoms, propranolol should be initiated. A tracheostomy is not necessary, given that the airway obstruction is mild and the child does not have significant respiratory symptoms.

Chapter 68

1. **e.**
2. **e.**
3. **d.**
4. **c.**
5. **d.**

Chapter 69

1. **c.**
2. **a.**
3. **e.**
4. **b.**
5. **d.**
6. **d.**
7. **b.**
8. **e.**
9. **a.**
10. **c.**

Chapter 70

1. **c.** The goal of surgical intervention with NEC is to limit and regulate enteric leakage and remove any frankly necrotic intestine to maximize the length of viable intestine. Pneumoperitoneum is the only absolute criteria for surgical intervention. Continued clinical deterioration despite maximal medical intervention is considered a relative indication. Although the presence of pneumatosis and fixed distended bowel loops are commonly seen in settings of NEC, they are not considered indications for surgical intervention.

2. **c.** CVR is a ratio of CPAM size to head circumference. If the CPAM is large and the head circumference, which is unaffected by the CPAM, is normal for age, a larger CVR occurs. A CVR >1.6 has a higher risk of hydrops and worse prognosis.

3. **a.** Gastroschesis is thought to be due to a vascular accident and is not associated with other anomalies. Surgery should be performed as soon as possible after birth to minimize further damage to the exposed intestines. It may take weeks to months to establish full feed due to prolonged ileus in infants with gastroschesis.

Chapter 71

1. **c.** *Explanation:* Counseling should take into consideration a variety of factors, including gestational age, weight, rupture or intact membranes, single/multiple gestation, antenatal steroids, sex, infection, and congenital abnormalities. An example that can be utilized to aid in counseling and data for <25 weeks' gestation is the NICHD calculator or extremely preterm birth outcomes tool.

2. **d.** *Explanation:* This infant has concerns for vein of Galen malformation, which is a malformation with arteriovenous shunting resulting in high output heart failure, pulmonary congestion, pulmonary hypertension, and multisystem organ failure. Presentation at the time of birth carries a high rate of mortality.

3. **c.** *Explanation:* Pulmonary hyper-expansion causes decreased venous return and cardiac compression, leading to abdominal ascites, impaired cardiac output, and nonimmune hydrops.

4. **b.** Balloon atrial septostomy is the best corrective measure when there are parallel circuits with restrictive mixing at the level of the atrium with an intact ventricular septum. Maintaining patency of the ductus arteriosus is a corrective measure, although, with severe restrictive atrium, hypoxemia will continue to occur with two parallel circuits, continued hypoxemia, and acidosis, leading to a failure in drop of pulmonary pressures and resulting in sustained pulmonary hypertension with right to left shunting across the PDA and failure of saturations of >80%, which can be expected for TGA with mixing capabilities. Performing an arterial switch is the corrective operation, but it is not done in the first hours of life due to high pulmonary pressures and higher risk of mortality following surgery.

Chapter 72

1. **a.** *Explanation:* Knowing the elimination half-life would allow you to determine how long it would take to reach steady state. Because the drug is constantly infused and has constant first-order clearance, after each half-life, the drug concentration would increase closer to steady state—first to 50% after one half-life, then 75% in two half-lives, and 90% of steady state in 3.3 half-lives. The half-life time itself is affected by the clearance rate and the volume of distribution. The dosage rate (infusion rate) will affect the final drug level (i.e., a higher dosage rate would have a higher steady state), but the time to reach that steady-state level would not be different. The bioavailability of the drug would also not affect the time to reach steady state, especially considering the drug is given IV. As mentioned, the volume of distribution does impact the half-life of the drug, which affects the kinetics of the drug, but knowing this value would not allow you to calculate the time to reach steady state. Finally, saturation kinetics, which describe zero order elimination, do not apply to this drug, which you know is cleared by first-order elimination.

2. **e.** *Explanation:* The best answer choice is the bioavailability of the drug, which refers to the fraction of administered drug that reaches systemic circulation in its active form. When considering placental transfer of drugs from maternal to fetal circulation, the drug has already reached systemic circulation, and, as such, its bioavailability does not play a role in its transplacental passage. Most drugs with MW <500 Da cross the placenta, and most drugs with MW >1000 Da do not cross the placenta. Drugs with molecular weights greater than 500 Da have an incomplete transfer across the human placenta. The pKa of the drug refers to the pH at which 50% of the drug is ionized. The degree of ionization of a drug plays a role in the transplacental passage of the drug in the same fashion as it may dictate the initial absorption of the drug. In this manner, the pH of the maternal plasma and infant's plasma will also play a role in the transplacental passage of the drug. The extent of drug binding to plasma proteins will also affect the transplacental passage of the drug; increasingly protein-bound drugs will pass at a lesser extent than those drugs that are increasingly free in the maternal plasma. Although there are several methods of transplacental movement of drugs, including simple diffusion, facilitated diffusion using a carrier, active transport using ATP, and pinocytosis, the former two methods specifically depend on a concentration gradient of the drug, which will affect the extent of drug movement, as well.

3. **d.** *Explanation:* The correct answer choice is that phase II reactions involve sulfation, acetylation, glucuronidation, and methylation. These are all examples of conjugation to an endogenous molecule that ultimately facilitates excretion of the drug. This conjugation occurs after phase I reactions. Phase I reactions are also referred to as "nonsynthetic reactions" (vs. phase II reactions, which are referred to as "synthetic reactions"). Phase I reactions include oxidation, reduction, hydrolysis, and hydroxylation and also include dehydrogenases, esterases, and monoxygenases, which may also be involved in the cytochrome P450 system. Notably, cytochrome P450 enzymes can be inhibited or induced by drugs, which can result in clinically significant drug–drug interactions that may lead to unanticipated adverse reactions or therapeutic failures.

Chapter 73

1. **b.** Phenytoin is contraindicated in pregnancy for the risk of developing fetal hydantoin syndrome. The mnemonic PHEN can help you remember the resulting characteristics: cleft *p*alate/cleft lip; small *h*ead, *h*eart defects, *h*irsutism, midface *h*ypoplasia, and *h*ypoplastic nails and digits; *e*mbryopathy; and *n*eurologic defects (mental deficits).

2. **a.** *Explanation:* Enalapril. Angiotensin-converting enzyme inhibitors (ACEIs) harm the fetus and present a risk for congenital heart disease, CNS malformations, growth restriction, skull ossification defects, and, most notably, renal tubular dysplasia that is a result of absent or low numbers of differentiated proximal tubules. This leads to severe renal dysfunction with anuria and oligohydramnios and subsequently can manifest as Potter's syndrome. ACEIs are contraindicated in pregnancy.

3. **b.** *Explanation:* Requires description of adverse outcomes that includes all of the following: structural abnormalities; embryo, fetal, and infant mortality; functional impairment; and alterations to growth.

4. **d.** *Explanation:* Amiodarone is an iodine-containing compound. Its active metabolite can have unpredictable levels when a neonate is breastfed, and it affects thyroid function in infants in addition to having cardiac effects.

Chapter 74

1. **a.** *Explanation:* Milrinone is an effective phosphodiesterase III inhibitor that decreases cAMP breakdown and improves cardiac contractility (inotropy) and cardiac relaxation (lusitropy) with minimal effects on chronotropy.

2. **c.** Cefazolin (first-generation cephalosporin) does not penetrate the CSF well compared to third- and fourth-generation cephalosporins.

3. **d.** Amphotericin B can result in hypokalemia, hyponatremia, hypomagnesemia, and hypocalcemia, thus warranting close serum monitoring throughout the duration of coverage.

4. **c.** Sildenafil is a selective phosphodiesterase type-5 (PDE5) inhibitor. PDE5 hydrolyzes the pulmonary vasodilator cyclic guanosine monophosphate (cGMP) to its inactive form GMP. Preventing the breakdown of cGMP to GMP prolongs the pulmonary vasodilatory effects of cGMP. Additionally, this enhances the effect of endogenous nitric oxide on pulmonary vascular smooth muscle.

Chapter 75

1. **d.**
2. **c.**
3. **a.**
4. **e.**
5. **c.**

Chapter 76

1. **d.**
2. **c.**

Chapter 77

1. **b.** *Explanation:* Traditional statistics test the null hypothesis of no difference between groups. A p value describes the likelihood of being able to accept the null hypothesis, given the observed value, specifically that a distribution based on no difference would produce a result as or more extreme as the observed difference. In this particular example, it is very possible that both methods are effective in preventing IVH (although we do not have an untreated group to compare), but the new method is more effective than the old one.

2. **c.** *Explanation:* Parametric tests are most appropriate for comparing groups of continuous data, with normal distribution, of reasonably large size. Although the t test is reasonably *robust* (resistant to error) even if these parameters are violated, nonparametric tests may be more appropriate.

3. **a.** *Explanation:* ANOVA tests the null hypothesis that, among mean values derived from multiple groups, no group differs from any other group. A statistically significant result suggests that there is a difference among the groups but does not suggest which or how many groups differ. Further testing of individual comparisons with appropriate correction for multiple comparisons is needed.

4. **b.** *Explanation:* Type II error is the error of concluding, based on a sample, that no difference between groups exists when a difference actually does exist in the population. The likelihood of making a type II error decreases as sample size increases. A more stringent p value would reduce the chance of type I error (concluding a difference exists when it does not). Fisher's exact test would also be an appropriate statistical test, but it would not address a type II error. One could argue that neither of the surgical dressings is any good, and the investigators should move on.

5. **b.** *Explanation:* Correlation can range from 0 (no correlation) to 1 (complete correlation). Correlation coefficients above about 0.70 to 0.75 describe strong correlations. The coefficient of determination (r^2) describes the variance in one measure that can be attributed to another (and is, in this case, 0.81, or 81%). In the absence of a gold standard measure, it is not possible to determine whether one measure is superior to another in this example.

6. **a.** *Explanation:* Sensitivity is the ability of a test to detect those with disease = true positive tests (in this case, test positive in the presence of NEC) divided by all cases of disease (in this example, all NEC) = 15/(15 + 5) = 15/20 = 75%.

7. **c.** *Explanation:* Specificity is the ability of a test to detect those without disease = true negative tests/all without disease = 40/(10 + 40) = 40/50 = 80%.

8. **b.** *Explanation:* Positive predictive value is the ability of a test, when positive, to predict disease = true positive tests/all positive tests = 15/(15 + 10) = 15/25 = 60%.

9. **d.** *Explanation:* Negative predictive value is the ability of a test, when negative, to predict absence of disease = true negative tests/all negative tests = 40/(5 + 40) = 40/45 = 89%. (Note that the relatively high prevalence of NEC in this population [20/70 = 29%] pushes the test's PPV up and NPV down compared to a lower prevalence.)

10. **c.** *Explanation:* An ideal test (sensitivity and specificity of 100% each) has an AUC of 1.0. A test that performs no better than chance (sensitivity marches straight to 0 as specificity marches straight to 100% and vice versa) has an AUC of 0.50. This test is unlikely to have a good combination of sensitivity and specificity. By comparison, the AUC of Fig. 77.12 is about 0.80. Although ROC curves describe the relationship between sensitivity and specificity, the AUC itself does not directly describe a particular relationship (e.g., what sensitivity will be at a particular specificity or vice versa). The AUC also does not directly describe positive predictive value (a).

Chapter 78

1. **c.** *Explanation:* Case–control studies, by virtue of selecting currently existing cases (outcomes), can accrue a large number of cases without needing to follow large numbers of patients waiting for an outcome to occur. Neither case–control studies nor cohort studies are the gold standard for assessing causation. Because exposure data must be collected retrospectively in case–control studies, such data are sometimes incomplete or biased. Relative risk cannot be assessed from case–control studies. (Odds ratios can be calculated; see Chapter 77.)

2. **a.** *Explanation:* Because they are experimental studies in which only the intervention differs between groups, randomized controlled trials are more likely than observation trials to allow investigators to conclude that an exposure causes an outcome. Randomized controlled trials are resource intensive and time consuming, and, unlike observational studies, they involve the investigators exposing participants to interventions that could carry risk. (There may be the same risks in an observational study, but they are accrued in the course of treatment, not imposed by the study.)

3. **b.** *Explanation:* Double blinding of studies is a method of decreasing bias in reporting of events, particularly if the events are subjective. Avoiding the use of a placebo would likely increase rather than decrease bias. A priori definition of event severity is likely to avoid misclassification of events that are reported (and could avoid investigator bias) but would not be likely to change reports from participants. More frequent ascertainment of side effects is likely to improve the reliability of reports but may not decrease bias in reporting.

4. **b.** *Explanation:* Multivariate analysis is one method of detecting and controlling for confounding factors. Other methods include matching and experimental (rather than observational) study designs. Because confounding factors are, by definition, related to both the exposure of interest and the outcome, targeting data collection toward suspected confounding factors would increase the likelihood confounding would be detected.

5. **c.** *Explanation:* Dose response, biological plausibility, and consistency with other studies all support a causal effect of A on B. If A always preceded B, then the temporal sequence would also support causation. However, experimental studies remain the best method for testing causal hypotheses.

6. **d.** *Explanation:* Incidence is a rate, implying that the time over which risk accrues must be included in reporting it. An alternative way of expressing this incidence would be five cases per 10,000 child-years. A prevalence (e.g., of survivors of childhood sepsis) could be expressed as a percentage or a number per 10,000. A rate without a denominator does not fully express incidence.

7. **b.** *Explanation:* Presence of a presymptomatic period during which an effective treatment could minimize later harm, combined with a high-sensitivity, high-specificity test and a relatively high prevalence of disease, all improve the suitability of a screening test. Other factors that make a screening test more suitable include high severity of the disease, low invasiveness of the test, and reasonable cost.

8. **c.** *Explanation:* To review, decision analysis attempts to quantify both the frequencies of outcomes of a given decision and the value (expected utility [EU]) of those outcomes for patients, with a goal to combine these to predict the best decision for the average patient in that situation. A decision that clear data suggest leads to a high likelihood of an outcome for which there is high agreement on the value of that outcome (e.g., return to former state of good health vs. death) would be supported. Because decision analysis depends on applying only a few factors derived from population data to an individual case, it can serve only as a general guide for patient care.

9. **c.** *Explanation:* In expanding from one rater to two, it would be most reasonable to assess the interrater reliability of reads. Another measure of reliability (and a close second for a correct answer) would be internal consistency (Do the various components of the scoring system correlate with one another?). Validity (Does the test work?) is separate from reliability (reproducibility: Can the test be applied?). Face validity (the subjective impression that brain injury might be associated with neurodevelopmental impairment) and predictive validity (previously shown to have high sensitivity and specificity for predicting outcome) have already been assessed for this test.

10. **d.** *Explanation:* Answer (a) is both accurate (estimates the true pressure correctly) and precise (little scatter). Answer (b) is precise but inaccurate. Answer (c) is both inaccurate and imprecise. Answer (d), although imprecise, estimates the pulmonary pressure accurately on average.

Chapter 79

1. **b.** *Explanation:* Brainstem auditory evoked response at 6 months of age is correlated with and predicts behavioral audiometry results. A measure before therapy begins would not test the effect of the therapy (and is temporally more distant from the definitive outcome). Death is a competing outcome rather than a surrogate. Although cholestatic jaundice might be affected by therapy, it is less clear that it would predict hearing outcomes.

2. **a.** *Explanation:* Larger expected difference between groups, larger α error, smaller variability (e.g., standard deviation), or a larger β (= lower power $[1 - \beta]$) allows a smaller sample size for a study. See Table 79.2 for an illustration.

3. **c.** *Explanation:* Surrogate endpoints are typically used in clinical trials when a definitive clinical endpoint may only occur long after an intervention occurs, when the clinical endpoint is prohibitively expensive to assess, or when the clinical outcome is not possible to measure (for example, due to safety concerns). It is important to choose an appropriate surrogate outcome considering cost, safety, and length of time until it can be measured.

The association needs to be stronger than a correlation but cannot be guaranteed.

4. **b.** *Explanation:* The relative risk reduction is the change in risk compared to the original risk—in this case, $0.20/0.70 = 0.29$ or 29%. The absolute risk reduction is the absolute change in risk— in this case, 20%. Relative risk or risk ratio (RR) is the ratio of risks, shown in these examples as both (risk untreated):(risk treated) $= 0.70/0.50 = 1.4$ and (risk treated):(risk untreated) $= 0.50/0.70 = 0.71$. The odds ratio (OR) of treated to untreated is $(0.5/0.5)/(0.7/0.3) = 0.43$, compared to RR 0.71, showing how ORs can exaggerate effects.

5. **a.** *Explanation:* The number needed to treat (i.e., number who would need to receive an intervention in order for one patient to have an improvement) is 1/(absolute risk difference)—in this case, $1/0.07 \approx 14$. Note that the number needed to treat (NNT) does not depend on the initial risk, so changes from 97% to 90%, 40% to 33%, and 8% to 1% all have the same NNT.

6. **d.** *Explanation:* Although an absolute definition of statistical significance is open to debate, $p < 0.05$ is usually accepted as statistically significant. A difference of 2 hours of cough, with wide overlap of groups, is not likely to be clinically important. The statistical significance is due to the large sample size (this result is for 500 subjects per group), which can show statistical significance for even small differences.

7. **c.** *Explanation:* The sensitivity and specificity of a diagnostic test are best measured by comparison to a gold standard in a group of subjects all receiving both the new test and the gold standard evaluation.

8. **a.** *Explanation:* Case–control studies provide the opportunity to oversample for rare conditions and are particularly useful for the study of the antecedents of rare diseases.

9. **d.** *Explanation:* Longitudinal evaluations allow assessment of disease prognosis. Full ascertainment of outcomes is important for full understanding of prognosis. A comparison group allows more certainty about whether a particular outcome is related to the disease itself but is not always necessary. For example, assessment of death from a primary cancer might not require a comparison group, but assessment of death from second cancers following cancer therapy might benefit from a comparison to incidence of the same cancers in the general population. Other possible, but less appropriate, answers would be (a) and (b). Cohort studies can also assess the association of disease with earlier exposure, but the sample often must be quite large and the earlier exposure must be predefined (in order to be able to establish the cohort). Cohort studies, particularly if they are large, can also assess the harm of a therapy that might not be detected in a clinical trial. Phase IV registry studies are, in fact, cohort studies.

10. **b.** *Explanation:* Experimental studies such as randomized controlled trials allow the investigator to isolate the effect of a therapy by assigning groups of otherwise similar subjects (with variation minimized by randomization) to receive the therapy (intervention group) or not (control group).

Chapter 80

1. **b.**
2. **c.**
3. **b.**
4. **a.**

Chapter 81

1. **b.** *Explanation:* The characteristics of effective feedback include the following:
   - Timely
   - Nonjudgmental
   - Focused on changeable behaviors or attainable goals
   - Specific and based on observed behaviors
   - Focused on positive consequences of change

   The main purpose of formative feedback is to help individuals learn new knowledge or skills, improve upon existing knowledge or skills, and reinforce behaviors that are desirable. Formative feedback should provide examples of observed behaviors (e.g., "When the mother asked how long her daughter needed to stay in the hospital, you estimated 1 to 2 days."), followed by a suggestion to improve upon the behavior (e.g., "I also suggest letting her know what her baby should accomplish before going home ...") and why that suggestion is important (e.g., "... so that she understands the discharge criteria, just in case her baby does not respond to phototherapy as anticipated"). In this vignette, telling the medical student that he did a "great job talking to the mother about jaundice" does not help him understand what was great about his communication skills. Specific information is needed to reinforce desirable behaviors (e.g., "You did a great job talking to the mother about jaundice by helping her understand why jaundice is important to follow"). Although helping the learner practice how he may discuss the need for phototherapy with parents, (c) is not a form of providing feedback.

2. **d.** *Explanation:* Well-formulated learning objectives are specific (a), measurable (c), and outcome based (d), stating what the learner should be able to do after a learning activity. These learning objectives set clear expectations and can serve as an educational guide for both learners and educators. Choice (c) is the incorrect response because goals are different from learning objectives; goals provide aspiration toward a long-term outcome, whereas learning objectives provide more focused short-term steps toward achieving the long-term goal. In addition, the verb used in (c), "understand," is nonspecific and not measurable. Neither learners nor educators would be able to define how understanding would be measured. The statements in choices (a) and (b) would serve as learning objectives that define how understanding is measured.

3. **b.** *Explanation:* Key concepts in creating an effective learning environment include making the learning relevant and based on clear learning objectives, respecting the experiences that adult learners bring to the environment, ensuring a safe space where all learners' opinions

are valued, and creating an interactive environment. Interactive teaching styles engage the learner and allow them to bring their experiences, insights, and opinions to the group, reinforcing the relevance to the learner and their individual needs. The physical environment should have appropriate lighting, rather than very bright lighting, to ensure that the learner is not distracted by physical discomfort. Although educational sessions may follow learning objectives outlined in a textbook, they should also allow for some flexibility to tailor education to individual learning needs. Similarly, sessions that utilize a large number of slides to deliver educational content may not allow time for questions or in-depth group discussion of specific teaching points. In addition, teaching that focuses strictly on board content specifications may not necessarily align with knowledge needed to provide day-to-day patient care.

4. **a.** *Explanation:* Bedside teaching enables the facilitator to explore the application of learner knowledge, as the facilitator can explore the learner's critical thinking skills and rationales for decision-making. Lectures enable the delivery of large amounts of material to a larger group of learners but lack the ability to deliver content in an individualized manner. Simulation-based training enables standardization of learning exposure because learners can be exposed to the same clinical conditions, presentations, and changes in patient status. In small group discussions, facilitators should create a more interactive environment to help learners feel more comfortable in sharing ideas and opinions. Virtual learning can be delivered to large or small groups of learners; as such, the facilitator-to-learner ratio may be variable.

5. **Correct D.** Direct observation and formative feedback in the clinical environment provide an opportunity to identify individual learning needs and set longitudinal learning goals. The other responses are incorrect. Multiple-choice exams, although an efficient means to assess a breadth of knowledge, do not accurately assess the depth of conceptual understanding or the ability to apply that knowledge. Short-answer questions are better suited to the assessment of knowledge and the application of knowledge (e.g., questions assessing the ability to diagnose a problem, integrate information, and formulate management plans). Although the OSCE exam can also assess domain-specific knowledge, it is a good tool to assess other important skills such as communication, team leadership, and collaboration. Finally, formative assessments are not used to make high-stakes decisions; such forms of assessment are known as *summative assessments.* Formative assessments are used to provide constructive feedback and identify learning needs and goals (e.g., direct assessments, review of portfolios, in-training examinations)

Chapter 82

1. **c.** *Explanation:* Respect for persons is applied as informed consent. Beneficence is applied as assessment of risks and benefits. Justice is applied as subject selection. Data analysis is extremely important but not mentioned as a primary application in *The Belmont Report.*

2. **a.** *Explanation:* The investigator has only two realistic choices: completely remove his/her financial interest or

completely remove himself/herself from any aspect of performing the trial. Performing the trial after divesting all financial and patent interests in the system is also a possibility, but, given the investigator's nonfinancial conflicts (this is his/her invention), this might not be as optimal a solution. Unfortunately, this is based on a real case, where option (d) was chosen, resulting in poor choices and the death of the first subject.

3. **b.** *Explanation:* Some things are just too good to be true. The figures are identical. The *right-hand bars* are exactly half the *left-hand bars*, each time! The drug effect is consistently astounding. The standard errors (if that is what the whiskers depict) are nice, small, and equal. These figures are fabricated. If Figs. 1 and 4 differed from one another, but they were still too pretty, you might believe that the investigator was falsifying the data by cleaning it up to make his/her point. If the introduction of the author's paper looked exactly like the discussion of your last paper, the author would be plagiarizing. This is extremely unlikely to be an honest difference of opinion.

4. **a.** *Explanation:* You have made substantial contributions to the conception, design, analysis, and interpretation of the work. You helped draft and revise the manuscript critically. You would, presumably, before this, have agreed to be accountable for the work. You were not, however, allowed to give the manuscript final approval. If you and your coauthors can work out your differences and you approve the version to be published, you will be eligible for authorship. Authors do not need to have performed or reviewed primary data from all of the assays or have drafted the entire manuscript.

5. **a.** *Explanation:* The American College of Obstetricians and Gynecologists recommends low-dose aspirin for the reduction of preeclampsia. Screening without revealing risk to the mothers and using placebo rather than an active control (aspirin) withholds potential benefits without clear scientific rationale. Studying a drug with an incomplete side-effect profile in a large number of women poses an avoidable risk. There is no clear justification for including the low-risk group. (An observational study of known low-risk women without using a placebo could establish baseline rates, should the investigators truly need to do so.) A more appropriate strategy would be a smaller study with better to define risks and potential efficacy, followed by an active control study in only women at high risk.

6. **b.** *Explanation:* Clinical equipoise describes overall uncertainty in the medical community about the risk/benefit balance of a proposed therapy. The data suggest that equipoise exists: there are promising signs of efficacy but no definitive studies. Although individuals may have strong opinions that drive their treatment decisions, these do not in themselves signal a lack of equipoise in the community. If there were strong evidence of efficacy, equipoise would be lost, and the trial might be inappropriate.

7. **d.** *Explanation:* The mistaking of an experimental intervention in a research setting for treatment in a clinical setting is termed *therapeutic misconception* (or fallacy). Although it can happen with any study, it is a particular risk in early-phase studies of drugs for life-threatening

conditions, where patients or parents feel as if they have no other therapeutic option. Note that, although it is unclear whether the drug will be effective, there is a possibility for direct benefit for the infant, making the study both ethical and approvable. The problem, rather, is that the parents, presumably despite explanation, have not been able to articulate their understanding of the experimental nature of the biologic. Appropriate informed consent would entail further explanation of the nature of the study—the opposite of deception. (Emotional expressions of hope can coexist with an intellectual understanding of the risks and benefits. The goal is not to stamp out hope but rather to ensure understanding.) The infant is too young to assent.

8. **d.** *Explanation:* Children cannot provide informed consent, so parental permission is appropriate. In general, a child with some capacity to understand a research study (*e.g.,* school-age children) should provide assent for the study after having it explained at a level appropriate to his/her development. Although assent may be waived in the setting of a study that might have direct benefit, this study is not testing a therapy. It is correct to be concerned about risks, but this study likely represents a minor increase over minimal risk and would thus potentially be approvable with two parents providing permission (see Table 82.2).

9. **c.** *Explanation:* Despite legal precedents that give women control over their bodies, even while pregnant, federal research regulations specifically consider risks and potential benefits to the fetus. Although research with the prospect of direct benefit for mother, fetus, or both is approvable, research without benefit to either is not approvable if it entails greater than minimal risk to the fetus. Interestingly, if the prospect of direct benefit is only to the fetus, both the mother's and the father's consent is needed. (In the example of an experimental fetal surgery, a woman could agree to take anesthesia and hysterotomy risks on herself, but both parents would need to consent to experimentation on the fetus.)

10. **d.** *Explanation:* This research represents more than a minor increase over minimal risk (risks experienced in daily living), and, although it offers the prospect of societal benefit, it does not offer the prospect of direct benefit to the participants. It falls into the "not otherwise approvable" category and would require special permission. If it were approved, the parents would also need to give permission and the children assent (see Table 82.2).

Chapter 83

1. **b.**
2. **d.** *Explanation:* Venous infarcts may be caused from compression of deep terminal veins, and cerebral palsy is associated with grade III and IV hemorrhages.
3. **d.** *Explanation:* Ischemic change is high signal in the basal ganglia on T1 MRI and increased echogenicity on ultrasound.
4. **c.** Dandy-Walker is characterized by absent cerebellar vermis.

Chapter 84

1. **c.**
2. **c.** *Explanation:* BPD has increased markings with rounded areas of lucency and hyperexpansion.
3. **a.** *Explanation:* Meconium aspirations demonstrate hyperexpansion, asymmetric pulmonary opacities, and increased markings and may have pneumothorax or pleural effusion.
4. **a3, b1, c2**

Chapter 85

1. **b.** *Explanation:* An esophageal pouch will be seen with or without fistula.
2. **a.** *Explanation:* Malrotation is not associated with microcolon.
3. **c.** *Explanation:* Portal venous air but not biliary air is associated with NEC.
4. **e.**

Chapter 86

1. **d.** *Explanation:* Posterior urethral valves are a congenital obstruction of the urethra and cause of uropathy where there is hydronephrosis, bladder hypertrophy with trabecula and diverticula, and a dilated posterior urethra (keyhole sign) seen on an ultrasound secondary to obstruction. The condition frequently has vesicoureteral reflux.
2. **b.** *Explanation:* Umbilical arterial catheters travel through the umbilicus and extend inferiorly toward the groin in the umbilical artery, followed by traveling through the anterior division of the internal iliac artery, then traveling through the common iliac artery and aorta with optimal position of tip between T7 and T9. In the absence of vascular anomalies or isomerism, catheters typically traverse to the left of the spine.
3. **c.** *Explanation:* Umbilical venous catheters travel through the umbilicus and extend superiorly toward the chest in the umbilical vein, passing posteriorly through the ductus venous and into the inferior vena cava. The optimal positioning of the tip is above the diaphragm to avoid hepatic hematomas and around T7 and T8 to avoid the catheter sitting in the atrial chamber, which can result in tachyarrhythmias or pericardial hematoma from perforation.
4. **d.** *Explanation:* Achondroplasia is a nonlethal congenital skeletal dysplasia that exhibits radiographic findings of short femora and humeri lengths, metaphyseal flaring, small trident pelvis, anterior flaring of the ribs, large cranium with small base of skull, and widening of the intervertebral discs. Platyspondyly is widening of the vertebral bodies and is associated with thanatophoric deformity, which is a lethal form of skeletal dysplasia.

Index

Note: Page numbers followed by "*f*" indicate figures, "*t*" indicate tables, and "*b*" indicate boxes.